The Health Consequences of Involuntary Exposure to Tobacco Smoke

A Report of the Surgeon General

D1473478

2006

U.S. DEPARTMENT OF HEALTH AND HUMAN SERVICES
Public Health Service
Office of the Surgeon General
Rockville, MD

National Library of Medicine Cataloging in Publication

The health consequences of involuntary exposure to tobacco smoke : a report of the
   Surgeon General. – [Atlanta, Ga.] : U.S. Dept. of Health and Human Services, Centers
   for Disease Control and Prevention, Coordinating Center for Health Promotion,
   National Center for Chronic Disease Prevention and Health Promotion, Office on
   Smoking and Health, [2006]

   Includes bibliographical references.

   1.   Tobacco Smoke Pollution -- adverse effects. I. United States. Public Health
        Service. Office of the Surgeon General. II. United States. Office on Smoking
        and Health.

O2NLM: WA 754 H4325 2006

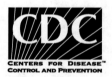

Centers for Disease Control and Prevention
Coordinating Center for Health Promotion
National Center for Chronic Disease Prevention and Health Promotion
Office on Smoking and Health

This publication is available on the World Wide Web at
http://www.surgeongeneral.gov/library

Suggested Citation
U.S. Department of Health and Human Services. *The Health Consequences of Involuntary
Exposure to Tobacco Smoke: A Report of the Surgeon General.* Atlanta, GA: U.S. Department
of Health and Human Services, Centers for Disease Control and Prevention, Coordinating
Center for Health Promotion, National Center for Chronic Disease Prevention and Health
Promotion, Office on Smoking and Health, 2006.

For sale by the Superintendent of Documents, U.S. Government Printing Office,
Washington, DC 20402. ISBN 0-16-076152-2

Use of trade names is for identification only and does not constitute endorsement by the
U.S. Department of Health and Human Services.

For sale by the Superintendent of Documents, U.S. Government Printing Office
Internet: bookstore.gpo.gov Phone: toll free (866) 512-1800; DC area (202) 512-1800
Fax: (202) 512-2250 Mail: Stop IDCC, Washington, DC 20402-0001

ISBN 0-16-076152-2

Message from Michael O. Leavitt
Secretary of Health and Human Services

This Surgeon General's report returns to the topic of the health effects of involuntary exposure to tobacco smoke. The last comprehensive review of this evidence by the Department of Health and Human Services (DHHS) was in the 1986 Surgeon General's report, *The Health Consequences of Involuntary Smoking*, published 20 years ago this year. This new report updates the evidence of the harmful effects of involuntary exposure to tobacco smoke. This large body of research findings is captured in an accompanying dynamic database that profiles key epidemiologic findings, and allows the evidence on health effects of exposure to tobacco smoke to be synthesized and updated (following the format of the 2004 report, *The Health Consequences of Smoking*). The database enables users to explore the data and studies supporting the conclusions in the report. The database is available on the Web site of the Centers for Disease Control and Prevention (CDC) at http://www.cdc.gov/tobacco. I am grateful to the leadership of the Surgeon General, CDC's Office on Smoking and Health, and all of the contributors for preparing this important report and bringing this topic to the forefront once again.

Secondhand smoke, also known as environmental tobacco smoke, is a mixture of the smoke given off by the burning end of tobacco products (sidestream smoke) and the mainstream smoke exhaled by smokers. People are exposed to secondhand smoke at home, in the workplace, and in other public places such as bars, restaurants, and recreation venues. It is harmful and hazardous to the health of the general public and particularly dangerous to children. It increases the risk of serious respiratory problems in children, such as a greater number and severity of asthma attacks and lower respiratory tract infections, and increases the risk for middle ear infections. It is also a known human carcinogen (cancer-causing agent). Inhaling secondhand smoke causes lung cancer and coronary heart disease in nonsmoking adults.

We have made great progress since the late 1980s in reducing the involuntary exposure of nonsmokers in this country to secondhand smoke. The proportion of nonsmokers aged 4 and older with a blood cotinine level (a metabolite of nicotine) indicating exposure has declined from 88 percent in 1988–1991 down to 43 percent in 2001–2002, a decline that exceeds the *Healthy People 2010* objective for this measure. Despite the great progress that has been made, involuntary exposure to secondhand smoke remains a serious public health hazard that can be prevented by making homes, workplaces, and public places completely smoke-free. As of the year 2000, more than 126 million residents of the United States aged 3 or older still are estimated to be exposed to secondhand smoke. Smoke-free environments are the most effective method for reducing exposures. *Healthy People 2010* objectives address this issue and seek optimal protection of nonsmokers through policies, regulations, and laws requiring smoke-free environments in all schools, workplaces, and public places.

Foreword

This twenty-ninth report of the Surgeon General documents the serious and deadly health effects of involuntary exposure to tobacco smoke. Secondhand smoke is a major cause of disease, including lung cancer and coronary heart disease, in healthy nonsmokers.

In 2005, it was estimated that exposure to secondhand smoke kills more than 3,000 adult nonsmokers from lung cancer, approximately 46,000 from coronary heart disease, and an estimated 430 newborns from sudden infant death syndrome. In addition, secondhand smoke causes other respiratory problems in nonsmokers such as coughing, phlegm, and reduced lung function. According to the CDC's National Health Interview Survey in 2000, more than 80 percent of the respondents aged 18 years or older believe that secondhand smoke is harmful and nonsmokers should be protected in their workplaces.

Components of chemical compounds in secondhand smoke, including nicotine, carbon monoxide, and tobacco-specific carcinogens, can be detected in body fluids of exposed nonsmokers. These exposures can be controlled. In 2005, CDC released the *Third National Report on Human Exposure to Environmental Chemicals,* which found that the median cotinine level (a metabolite of nicotine) in nonsmokers had decreased across the life stages: by 68 percent in children, 69 percent in adolescents, and 75 percent in adults, when samples collected between 1999 and 2002 were compared with samples collected a decade earlier. These dramatic declines are further evidence that smoking restrictions in public places and workplaces are helping to ensure a healthier life for all people in the United States.

However, too many people continue to be exposed, especially children. The recent data indicate that median cotinine levels in children are more than twice those of adults, and non-Hispanic blacks have levels that are more than twice as high as those of Mexican Americans and non-Hispanic whites. These disparities need to be better understood and addressed.

Research reviewed in this report indicates that smoke-free policies are the most economic and effective approach for providing protection from exposure to secondhand smoke. But do they provide the greatest health impact. Separating smokers and nonsmokers in the same airspace is not effective, nor is air cleaning or a greater exchange of indoor with outdoor air. Additionally, having separately ventilated areas for smoking may not offer a satisfactory solution to reducing workplace exposures. Policies prohibiting smoking in the workplace have multiple benefits. Besides reducing exposure of nonsmokers to secondhand smoke, these policies reduce tobacco use by smokers and change public attitudes about tobacco use from acceptable to unacceptable.

Research indicates that the progressive restriction of smoking in the United States to protect nonsmokers has had the additional health impact of reducing active smoking. In November 2005, CDC's Tobacco-Free Campus policy took full effect in all facilities owned by CDC in the Atlanta area. As the Director of the nation's leading health promotion and disease prevention agency, I am proud to support this effort. With this commitment, CDC continues to protect the health and safety of all of its employees and serves as a role model for workplaces everywhere.

Julie Louise Gerberding, M.D., M.P.H.
Director
Centers for Disease Control and Prevention
and
Administrator
Agency for Toxic Substances and Disease Registry

Preface

from the Surgeon General,
U.S. Department of Health and Human Services

Twenty years ago when Dr. C. Everett Koop released the Surgeon General's report, *The Health Consequences of Involuntary Smoking*, it was the first Surgeon General's report to conclude that involuntary exposure of nonsmokers to tobacco smoke causes disease. The topic of involuntary exposure of nonsmokers to secondhand smoke was first considered in Surgeon General Jesse Steinfeld's 1972 report, and by 1986, the causal linkage between inhaling secondhand smoke and the risk for lung cancer was clear. By then, there was also abundant evidence of adverse effects of smoking by parents on their children.

Today, massive and conclusive scientific evidence documents adverse effects of involuntary smoking on children and adults, including cancer and cardiovascular diseases in adults, and adverse respiratory effects in both children and adults. This 2006 report of the Surgeon General updates the 1986 report, *The Health Consequences of Involuntary Smoking*, and provides a detailed review of the epidemiologic evidence on the health effects of involuntary exposure to tobacco smoke. This new report also uses the revised standard language of causality that was applied in the 2004 Surgeon General's report, *The Health Consequences of Smoking*.

Secondhand smoke is similar to the mainstream smoke inhaled by the smoker in that it is a complex mixture containing many chemicals (including formaldehyde, cyanide, carbon monoxide, ammonia, and nicotine), many of which are known carcinogens. Exposure to secondhand smoke causes excess deaths in the U.S. population from lung cancer and cardiac related illnesses. Fortunately, exposures of adults are declining as smoking becomes increasingly restricted in workplaces and public places. Unfortunately, children continue to be exposed in their homes by the smoking of their parents and other adults. This exposure leads to unnecessary cases of bronchitis, pneumonia and worsened asthma. Among children younger than 18 years of age, an estimated 22 percent are exposed to secondhand smoke in their homes, with estimates ranging from 11.7 percent in Utah to 34.2 percent in Kentucky.

As this report documents, exposure to secondhand smoke remains an alarming public health hazard. Approximately 60 percent of nonsmokers in the United States have biologic evidence of exposure to secondhand smoke. Yet compared with data reviewed in the 1986 report, I am encouraged by the progress that has been made in reducing involuntary exposure in many workplaces, restaurants, and other public places. These changes are most likely the major contributing factors to the more than 75 percent reduction in serum cotinine levels that researchers have observed from 1988 to 1991. However, more than 126 million nonsmokers are still exposed. We now have substantial evidence on the efficacy of different approaches to control exposure to secondhand smoke. Restrictions on smoking can control exposures effectively, but technical approaches involving air cleaning or a greater exchange of indoor with outdoor air cannot. Consequently, nonsmokers need protection through the restriction of smoking in public places and workplaces and by a voluntary adherence to policies at home, particularly to eliminate exposures of children. Since the release of the 1986 Surgeon General's report, the public's attitude and social norms toward secondhand smoke exposure have changed significantly—a direct result of the growing body of scientific evidence on the health effects of exposure to secondhand smoke that is summarized in this report.

Finally, clinicians should routinely ask about secondhand smoke exposure, particularly in susceptible groups or when a child has had an illness caused by secondhand smoke, such as pneumonia. Because of the high levels of exposure among young children, their exposure should be considered a significant pediatric issue. Additionally, exposure to secondhand smoke poses significant risks for people with lung and heart disease. The large body of evidence documenting that secondhand smoke exposures produce substantial and immediate effects on the cardiovascular system indicates that even brief exposures could pose significant acute risks to older adults or to others at high risk for cardiovascular disease. Those caring for relatives with heart disease should be advised not to smoke in the presence of the sick relative.

An environment free of involuntary exposure to secondhand smoke should remain an important national priority in order to reach the *Healthy People 2010* objectives.

Richard Carmona, M.D., M.P.H., F.A.C.S.
Surgeon General

Acknowledgments

This report was prepared by the U.S. Department of Health and Human Services under the general direction of the Centers for Disease Control and Prevention, Coordinating Center for Health Promotion, National Center for Chronic Disease Prevention and Health Promotion, Office on Smoking and Health.

Richard H. Carmona, M.D., M.P.H., F.A.C.S., Surgeon General, United States Public Health Service, Office of the Surgeon General, Office of the Secretary, Washington, D.C.

Kenneth P. Moritsugu, M.D., M.P.H., Deputy Surgeon General, Office of the Surgeon General, United States Public Health Service, Office of the Secretary, Washington, D.C.

Robert C. Williams, P.E., DEE, Chief of Staff, Office of the Surgeon General, United States Public Health Service, Office of the Secretary, Washington, D.C.

Karen A. Near, M.D., M.S., Senior Science Advisor, Office of the Surgeon General, United States Public Health Service, Office of the Secretary, Washington, D.C.

Ron Schoenfeld, Ph.D., Senior Science Advisor, Office of the Surgeon General, United States Public Health Service, Office of the Secretary, Washington, D.C.

Julie Louise Gerberding, M.D., M.P.H., Director, Centers for Disease Control and Prevention, Atlanta, Georgia.

Janet Collins, Ph.D., Director, National Center for Chronic Disease Prevention and Health Promotion, Coordinating Center for Health Promotion, Centers for Disease Control and Prevention, Atlanta, Georgia.

Barbara Bowman, Ph.D., Associate Director for Science (acting), National Center for Chronic Disease Prevention and Health Promotion, Coordinating Center for Health Promotion, Centers for Disease Control and Prevention, Atlanta, Georgia.

Corinne G. Husten, M.D., M.P.H., Director (acting), Office on Smoking and Health, National Center for Chronic Disease Prevention and Health Promotion, Coordinating Center for Health Promotion, Centers for Disease Control and Prevention, Atlanta, Georgia.

Terry F. Pechacek, Ph.D., Associate Director for Science, Office on Smoking and Health, National Center for Chronic Disease Prevention and Health Promotion, Coordinating Center for Health Promotion, Centers for Disease Control and Prevention, Atlanta, Georgia.

The editors of the report were

Jonathan M. Samet, M.D., M.S., Senior Scientific Editor, Professor and Chairman, Department of Epidemiology, Bloomberg School of Public Health, The Johns Hopkins University, Baltimore, Maryland.

Leslie A. Norman, Managing Editor, Office on Smoking and Health, National Center for Chronic Disease Prevention and Health Promotion, Coordinating Center for Health Promotion, Centers for Disease Control and Prevention, Atlanta, Georgia.

Caran Wilbanks, Technical Editor, Office on Smoking and Health, National Center for Chronic Disease Prevention and Health Promotion, Coordinating Center for Health Promotion, Centers for Disease Control and Prevention, Atlanta, Georgia.

Audrey Pinto, Technical Editor, Barrington, Rhode Island.

Contributing authors were

Stephen Babb, M.P.H., Health Education Specialist, Office on Smoking and Health, National Center for Chronic Disease Prevention and Health Promotion, Coordinating Center for Health Promotion, Centers for Disease Control and Prevention, Atlanta, Georgia.

John T. Bernert, Ph.D., Supervisory Research Chemist, Emergency Response and Air Toxicants Branch, Division of Laboratory Sciences, National Center for Environmental Health, Coordinating Center for Environmental Health and Injury Prevention, Centers for Disease Control and Prevention, Atlanta, Georgia.

Derek G. Cook, Ph.D., Professor of Epidemiology, Division of Community Health Sciences, St. George's, University of London, London, England.

David B. Coultas, M.D., Professor and Chairman, Department of Internal Medicine, University of Texas Health Center at Tyler, Tyler, Texas.

Dawn DeMeo, M.D., Associate Physician, Brigham and Women's Hospital, Channing Laboratory, Instructor in Medicine, Harvard Medical School, Harvard University, Boston, Massachusetts.

Karen Emmons, Ph.D., Professor, Harvard School of Public Health, Deputy Director of Community-Based Research, Department of Medical Oncology, Dana-Farber Cancer Institute, Boston, Massachusetts.

Stanton Glantz, Ph.D., Professor of Medicine, Division of Cardiology, University of California, San Francisco, California.

Steven N. Goodman, M.D., M.H.S., Ph.D., Associate Professor of Oncology, Pediatrics, Epidemiology, and Biostatistics, Department of Oncology, School of Medicine, The Johns Hopkins University, Baltimore, Maryland.

S. Katharine Hammond, Ph.D., C.I.H., Professor of Environmental Health Sciences, School of Public Health, University of California, Berkeley, California.

Stephen S. Hecht, Ph.D., Professor, University of Minnesota Cancer Center, Minneapolis, Minnesota.

John R. Hoidal, M.D., The Clarence M. and Ruth N. Birrer Presidential Professor and Chairman of Medicine, School of Medicine, University of Utah Health Sciences Center, Salt Lake City, Utah.

Jerelyn H. Jordan, Program Consultant, Office on Smoking and Health, National Center for Chronic Disease Prevention and Health Promotion, Coordinating Center for Health Promotion, Centers for Disease Control and Prevention, Atlanta, Georgia.

Ichiro Kawachi, M.D., Ph.D., Professor of Social Epidemiology, Harvard School of Public Health, Harvard University, and Associate Professor of Medicine, Channing Laboratory, Harvard Medical School, Harvard University, Boston, Massachusetts.

Nora L. Lee, Research Program Coordinator, Center for Autism and Developmental Disabilities Epidemiology, Department of Epidemiology, Bloomberg School of Public Health, The Johns Hopkins University, Baltimore, Maryland.

David M. Mannino, M.D., Associate Professor of Medicine, Pulmonary Epidemiology Research Laboratory, Division of Pulmonary, Critical Care and Sleep Medicine, University of Kentucky, Lexington, Kentucky.

John F. McCarthy, Sc.D., C.I.H., President, Environmental Health and Engineering, Inc., Newton, Massachusetts.

Murray A. Mittleman, M.D., Dr.P.H., Associate Professor of Medicine and Epidemiology, Harvard University at Beth Israel Deaconess Medical Center, Boston, Massachusetts.

Patricia J. O'Campo, Ph.D., Alma and Baxter Ricard Chair in Inner City Health, Director, Centre for Research on Inner City Health, St. Michael's Hospital, Toronto, Ontario.

William Parmley, M.D., The Seventy, Salt Lake City, Utah.

Terry F. Pechacek, Ph.D., Associate Director for Science, Office on Smoking and Health, National Center for Chronic Disease Prevention and Health Promotion, Coordinating Center for Health Promotion, Centers for Disease Control and Prevention, Atlanta, Georgia.

Jonathan M. Samet, M.D., M.S., Professor and Chairman, Department of Epidemiology, Bloomberg School of Public Health, The Johns Hopkins University, Baltimore, Maryland.

Donald R. Shopland Sr., U.S. Public Health Service (retired), Ringgold, Georgia.

John D. Spengler, Ph.D., Akira Yamaguchi Professor of Environmental Health and Human Habitation, Director, Environmental Health Department, School of Public Health, Harvard University, Boston, Massachusetts.

David P. Strachan, M.D., Professor of Epidemiology, Division of Community Health Sciences, St. George's, University of London, London, England.

Scott T. Weiss, M.D., M.S., Professor of Medicine, Harvard Medical School, and Director, Respiratory, Environmental, and Genetic Epidemiology, Channing Laboratory, Brigham and Women's Hospital, Harvard Medical School, Boston, Massachusetts.

Anna H. Wu, Ph.D., Professor, Department of Preventive Medicine, Keck School of Medicine, University of Southern California, Los Angeles, California.

Reviewers were

Duane Alexander, M.D., Director, National Institute of Child Health and Human Development, National Institutes of Health, Bethesda, Maryland.

David L. Ashley, Ph.D., Chief, Emergency Response and Air Toxicants Branch, Division of Laboratory Sciences, National Center for Environmental Health, Coordinating Center for Environmental Health and Injury Prevention, Centers for Disease Control and Prevention, Atlanta, Georgia.

Edward L. Avol, M.S., Professor, Department of Preventive Medicine, Keck School of Medicine, University of Southern California, Los Angeles, California.

Cathy L. Backinger, Ph.D., M.P.H., Acting Chief, Tobacco Control Research Branch, Behavioral Research Program, Division of Cancer Control and Population Sciences, National Cancer Institute, National Institutes of Health, Rockville, Maryland.

Stephen W. Banspach, Ph.D., Associate Director for Science, Division of Adolescent and School Health, National Center for Chronic Disease Prevention and Health Promotion, Coordinating Center for Health Promotion, Centers for Disease Control and Prevention, Atlanta, Georgia.

John Baron, M.D., Professor, Departments of Medicine and Community and Family Medicine, Dartmouth Medical School, Hanover, New Hampshire.

Rebecca Bascom, M.D., M.P.H., Professor of Medicine, Division of Pulmonary, Allergy and Critical Care Medicine, Department of Medicine, Pennsylvania State University College of Medicine, Milton S. Hershey Medical Center, Hershey, Pennsylvania.

Glen C. Bennett, M.P.H., Coordinator, Advanced Technologies Applications in Health Education, Office of Prevention, Education, and Control, National Heart, Lung, and Blood Institute, National Institutes of Health, Bethesda, Maryland.

Neal Benowitz, M.D., Professor of Medicine, Psychiatry, and Biopharmaceutical Sciences, and Chief, Division of Clinical Pharmacology and Experimental Therapeutics, University of California, San Francisco, California.

Valerie Beral, F.R.C.P., Professor of Epidemiology, Nuffield Department of Clinical Medicine, University of Oxford, United Kingdom.

Michele Bloch, M.D., Ph.D., Medical Officer, Tobacco Control Research Branch, Behavioral Research Program, Division of Cancer Control and Population Sciences, National Cancer Institute, National Institutes of Health, Bethesda, Maryland.

William Blot, Ph.D., Chief Executive Officer, International Epidemiology Institute, Ltd., Rockville, Maryland, and Professor, Vanderbilt-Ingram Cancer Center, Vanderbilt University Medical Center, Nashville, Tennessee.

Paolo Boffetta, M.D., M.P.H., Coordinator, Genetics and Epidemiology Cluster, International Agency for Research on Cancer, Lyon, France.

Michael B. Bracken, Ph.D., M.P.H., Susan Dwight Bliss Professor of Epidemiology, Center for Perinatal, Pediatric, and Environmental Epidemiology, Yale University, New Haven, Connecticut.

Patrick Breysse, Ph.D., Professor, Division of Environmental Health Sciences, and Director, Division of Environmental Health Engineering, Bloomberg School of Public Health, The Johns Hopkins University, Baltimore, Maryland.

John R. Britton, Professor of Epidemiology, Division of Epidemiology and Public Health, University of Nottingham, Nottingham, England.

Arnold R. Brody, Ph.D., Professor and Vice Chairman, Department of Pathology and Laboratory Medicine, Tulane University Health Sciences Center, New Orleans, Louisiana.

David M. Burns, M.D., Professor of Family and Preventive Medicine, School of Medicine, University of California, San Diego, California.

Carl J. Caspersen, Ph.D., M.P.H., Associate Director for Science, Division of Diabetes Translation, National Center for Chronic Disease Prevention and Health Promotion, Coordinating Center for Health Promotion, Centers for Disease Control and Prevention, Atlanta, Georgia.

Terence L. Chorba, M.D., Associate Director for Science, National Center for HIV, STD, and TB Prevention, Coordinating Center for Infectious Diseases, Centers for Disease Control and Prevention, Atlanta, Georgia.

Ralph J. Coates, Ph.D., Associate Director for Science, Division of Cancer Prevention and Control, National Center for Chronic Disease Prevention and Health Promotion, Coordinating Center for Health Promotion, Centers for Disease Control and Prevention, Atlanta, Georgia.

Graham Colditz, M.D., Dr.P.H., Professor of Medicine, Channing Laboratory, Department of Medicine, Brigham and Women's Hospital, Harvard Medical School, Harvard University, Boston, Massachusetts.

Adolfo Correa, M.D., Ph.D., M.P.H., Medical Epidemiologist, Division of Birth Defects and Developmental Disabilities, National Center for Birth Defects and Developmental Disabilities, Coordinating Center for Health Promotion, Centers for Disease Control and Prevention, Atlanta, Georgia.

Daniel L. Costa, Sc.D., DABT, National Program Director for Air Research, Office of Research and Development, U.S. Environmental Protection Agency, Research Triangle Park, North Carolina.

David B. Coultas, M.D., Professor and Chairman, Department of Internal Medicine, University of Texas Health Center at Tyler, Tyler, Texas.

Linda S. Crossett, R.D.H., Health Scientist, Research Application Branch, Division of Adolescent and School Health, National Center for Chronic Disease Prevention and Health Promotion, Coordinating Center for Health Promotion, Centers for Disease Control and Prevention, Atlanta, Georgia.

Ronald M. Davis, M.D., Director, Center for Health Promotion and Disease Prevention, Henry Ford Health System, Detroit, Michigan.

Mirjana V. Djordevic, Ph.D., Bio-analytical Chemist, Tobacco Control Research Branch, Behavioral Research Program, Division of Cancer Control and Population Sciences, National Cancer Institute, National Institutes of Health, Rockville, Maryland.

Lucinda England, M.D., M.S.P.H., Medical Epidemiologist, Maternal and Infant Health Branch, Division of Reproductive Health, National Center for Chronic Disease Prevention and Health Promotion, Coordinating Center for Health Promotion, Centers for Disease Control and Prevention, Atlanta, Georgia.

Michael P. Eriksen, Sc.D., Professor and Director, Institute of Public Health, Georgia State University, Atlanta, Georgia.

Brenda Eskenazi, Ph.D., Professor of Maternal and Child Health and Epidemiology, and Director, Center for Children's Environmental Health Research, School of Public Health, University of California, Berkeley, California.

Jing Fang, M.D., M.S., Epidemiologist, Epidemiology and Surveillance Team, Division of Heart Disease and Stroke Prevention, National Center for Chronic Disease Prevention and Health Promotion, Coordinating Center for Health Promotion, Centers for Disease Control and Prevention, Atlanta, Georgia.

Elizabeth T.H. Fontham, Dr.P.H., Dean, School of Public Health, Louisiana State University Health Sciences Center, New Orleans, Louisiana.

Alison Freeman, ETS Policy Specialist, Indoor Environments Division, U.S. Environmental Protection Agency, Washington, D.C.

Deborah Galuska, Ph.D., M.P.H., Associate Director for Science, Division of Nutrition and Physical Activity, National Center for Chronic Disease Prevention and Health Promotion, Coordinating Center for Health Promotion, Centers for Disease Control and Prevention, Atlanta, Georgia.

Samuel S. Gidding, M.D., Professor of Pediatrics, Thomas Jefferson University, Nemours Cardiac Center, A.I. duPont Hospital for Children, Wilmington, Delaware.

Frank D. Gilliland, M.D., Ph.D., Professor, University of Southern California, Los Angeles, California.

Gary A. Giovino, Ph.D., M.S., Director, Tobacco Control Research Program, Roswell Park Cancer Institute, Buffalo, New York.

John Girman, Senior Science Advisor, Indoor Environments Division, U.S. Environmental Protection Agency, Washington, D.C.

Thomas J. Glynn, Ph.D., Director, Cancer Science and Trends, American Cancer Society, Washington, D.C.

Keith L. Goddard, D.Sc., P.E., Director, Directorate of Evaluation and Analysis, Occupational Safety and Health Administration, U.S. Department of Labor, Washington, D.C.

Diane R. Gold, M.D., M.P.H., Channing Laboratory, Brigham and Women's Hospital, Associate Professor of Medicine, Harvard Medical School, and Associate Professor of Environmental Health, Harvard School of Public Health, Harvard University, Boston, Massachusetts.

Allan Hackshaw, Deputy Director, Cancer Research UK and UCL Cancer Trials Centre, University College London, London, England.

Thomas P. Houston, M.D., Professor, Public Health and Family Medicine, Louisiana State University Health Sciences Center, New Orleans, Louisiana.

George Howard, Dr.P.H., Chairman, Department of Biostatistics, School of Public Health, University of Alabama at Birmingham, Birmingham, Alabama.

Gary W. Hunninghake, M.D., Professor, Department of Internal Medicine, and Director, Pulmonary Program in Internal Medicine, Department of Internal Medicine, Carver College of Medicine, University of Iowa, Iowa City, Iowa.

Jouni Jaakkola, M.D, Ph.D., D.Sc., Professor and Director, Institute of Occupational and Environmental Medicine, The University of Birmingham, Edgbaston, Birmingham, England.

David R. Jacobs Jr., Ph.D., Professor of Epidemiology, University of Minnesota, Minneapolis, Minnesota.

Martin Jarvis, Professor, Cancer Research UK Health Behaviour Unit, Department of Epidemiology and Public Health, University College London, London, England.

Jennifer Jinot, ETS Risk Assessment Scientist, Mathematical Statistician, Office of Research and Development, U.S. Environmental Protection Agency, Washington, D.C.

Joel Kaufman, M.D., M.P.H., Associate Professor, Department of Environmental and Occupational Health Sciences, University of Washington, Seattle, Washington.

Juliette Kendrick, M.D., Medical Officer, Division of Reproductive Health, National Center for Chronic Disease Prevention and Health Promotion, Coordinating Center for Health Promotion, Centers for Disease Control and Prevention, Atlanta, Georgia.

Neil E. Klepeis, Ph.D., Post-Doctoral Researcher, Stanford University, and Exposure Science Consulting, Watsonville, California.

William Kohn, D.D.S., CAPT, Deputy Associate Director for Science (acting), National Center for Chronic Disease Prevention and Health Promotion, Coordinating Center for Health Promotion, Centers for Disease Control and Prevention, Atlanta, Georgia.

Petros Koutrakis, Ph.D., Professor of Environmental Sciences, Department of Environmental Health, School of Public Health, Harvard University, Boston, Massachusetts.

Darwin Labarthe, M.D., Ph.D., M.P.H., Director (acting), Division of Heart Disease and Stroke Prevention, National Center for Chronic Disease Prevention and Health Promotion, Coordinating Center for Health Promotion, Centers for Disease Control and Prevention, Atlanta, Georgia.

John Lehnherr, Director (acting), Division of Reproductive Health, National Center for Chronic Disease Prevention and Health Promotion, Coordinating Center for Health Promotion, Centers for Disease Control and Prevention, Atlanta, Georgia.

Youlian Liao, M.D., Epidemiologist, Deputy Associate Director for Science (acting), Division of Adult and Community Health, National Center for Chronic Disease Prevention and Health Promotion, Coordinating Center for Health Promotion, Centers for Disease Control and Prevention, Atlanta, Georgia.

Catherine Lorraine, Director, Policy Development and Coordination Staff, Food and Drug Administration, Rockville, Maryland.

William R. Maas, D.D.S., M.P.H., Director, Division of Oral Health, National Center for Chronic Disease Prevention and Health Promotion, Coordinating Center for Health Promotion, Centers for Disease Control and Prevention, Atlanta, Georgia.

Jennifer H. Madans Ph.D., Associate Director for Science, National Center for Health Statistics, Coordinating Center for Health Information and Services, Centers for Disease Control and Prevention, Hyattsville, Maryland.

Fernando D. Martinez, M.D., Director, Arizona Respiratory Center, and Swift-McNear Professor of Pediatrics, University of Arizona, Tucson, Arizona.

Kenneth P. Moritsugu, M.D., M.P.H., Deputy Surgeon General, Office of the Surgeon General, United States Public Health Service, Office of the Secretary, Washington, D.C.

Matthew L. Myers, President, Campaign for Tobacco-Free Kids, Washington, D.C.

Elizabeth G. Nabel, M.D., Director, National Heart, Lung, and Blood Institute, National Institutes of Health, Bethesda, Maryland.

David Nelson, M.D., M.P.H., Senior Scientific Advisor, Office on Smoking and Health, National Center for Chronic Disease Prevention and Health Promotion, Coordinating Center for Health Promotion, Centers for Disease Control and Prevention, Atlanta, Georgia.

F. Javier Nieto, M.D., Ph.D., Professor and Chair, Department of Population Health Sciences, University of Wisconsin Medical School, Madison, Wisconsin.

Thomas E. Novotny, M.D., M.P.H., Education Coordinator, UCSF Global Health Sciences, and Professor, Department of Epidemiology and Biostatistics, University of California, San Francisco, San Francisco, California.

Mark Parascandola, Ph.D., M.P.H., Epidemiologist, Tobacco Control Research Branch, Behavioral Research Program, Division of Cancer Control and Population Sciences, National Cancer Institute, National Institutes of Health, Rockville, Maryland.

Samuel F. Posner, Ph.D., Associate Director for Science, Division of Reproductive Health, National Center for Chronic Disease Prevention and Health Promotion, Coordinating Center for Health Promotion, Centers for Disease Control and Prevention, Atlanta, Georgia.

Bogdan Prokopczyk, Ph.D., Associate Professor of Pharmacology, Department of Pharmacology, Pennsylvania State University College of Medicine, Milton S. Hershey Medical Center, Hershey, Pennsylvania.

Scott Rogers, M.P.H., Epidemiology and Genetics Research Program, Division of Cancer Control and Population Sciences, National Cancer Institute, Rockville, Maryland.

Dale P. Sandler, Ph.D., Chief, Epidemiology Branch, National Institute of Environmental Health Sciences, National Institutes of Health, Research Triangle Park, North Carolina.

Laura A. Schieve, Ph.D., Epidemiologist, National Center on Birth Defects and Developmental Disabilities, Coordinating Center for Health Promotion, Centers for Disease Control and Prevention, Atlanta, Georgia.

Susan Schober, Ph.D., Senior Epidemiologist, National Health and Nutrition Examination Survey (NHANES) Program, National Center for Health Statistics, Centers for Disease Control and Prevention, Hyattsville, Maryland.

Lawrence Schoen, M.S., President and Principal Engineer, Schoen Engineering, Inc., Columbia, Maryland.

Ron Schoenfeld, Ph.D., Senior Science Advisor, Office of the Surgeon General, United States Public Health Service, Office of the Secretary, Washington, D.C.

David Schwartz, M.D., M.P.H., Director, National Institute of Environmental Health Sciences; Director, National Toxicology Program; and Professor of Medicine, Duke University Medical Center, Durham, North Carolina.

Harold E. Seifried, Ph.D., DABT, Chemist, Toxicologist, Industrial Hygenist, Nutritional Science Research Group, Division of Cancer Prevention, National Cancer Institute, National Institutes of Health, Rockville, Maryland.

Frank E. Speizer, M.D., Channing Laboratory, Brigham and Women's Hospital; Edward H. Kass Professor of Medicine, Harvard Medical School; and Professor of Environmental Health, Harvard School of Public Health, Harvard University, Boston, Massachusetts.

Margaret R. Spitz, M.D., M.P.H., Professor and Chair, Department of Epidemiology, M.D. Anderson Cancer Center, University of Texas, Houston, Texas.

Meir J. Stampfer, M.D., Dr.P.H., Department Chair of Epidemiology; Professor of Epidemiology and Nutrition, School of Public Health; and Professor of Medicine, Harvard Medical School, Harvard University, Boston, Massachusetts.

James W. Stephens, Ph.D., Associate Director for Science, National Institute for Occupational Safety and Health, Centers for Disease Control and Prevention, Washington, D.C.

Gary D. Stoner, Ph.D., Professor, Division of Hematology and Oncology, College of Medicine and Public Health, The Ohio State University, Columbus, Ohio.

Esther Sumartojo, Ph.D., M.Sc., Acting Associate Director for Science and Public Health, National Center on Birth Defects and Developmental Disabilities, Coordinating Center for Health Promotion, Centers for Disease Control and Prevention, Atlanta, Georgia.

Ira Tager, M.D., M.P.H., Professor of Epidemiology, Division of Epidemiology, School of Public Health, University of California, Berkeley, California.

Michael J. Thun, M.D., Vice President, Epidemiology and Surveillance Research, American Cancer Society, Atlanta, Georgia.

Edward Trapido, Sc.D., Associate Director, Epidemiology and Genetics Research Program, Division of Cancer Control and Population Sciences, National Cancer Institute, National Institutes of Health, Rockville, Maryland.

Noel S. Weiss, M.D., Dr.P.H., Professor, Department of Epidemiology, School of Public Health and Community Medicine, University of Washington, Seattle, Washington.

Scott T. Weiss, M.D., M.S., Professor of Medicine, Harvard Medical School, and Director, Respiratory, Environmental, and Genetic Epidemiology, Channing Laboratory, Brigham and Women's Hospital, Harvard Medical School, Harvard University, Boston, Massachusetts.

Elizabeth M. Whelan, Sc.D., M.P.H., M.S., President, American Council on Science and Health, New York, New York.

Allen J. Wilcox, M.D., Ph.D., Senior Investigator, National Institute of Environmental Health Sciences, National Institutes of Health, Durham, North Carolina.

Walter C. Willett, M.D., Dr.P.H., Professor of Epidemiology and Nutrition, and Chair, Department of Nutrition, Harvard School of Public Health, Boston, Massachusetts.

Gayle Windham, Ph.D., Research Scientist (Epidemiology), Division of Environmental and Occupational Disease Control, California Department of Health Services, Richmond, California.

Deborah M. Winn, Ph.D., Chief, Clinical and Genetic Epidemiology Research Branch, Epidemiology and Genetics Research Program, Division of Cancer Control and Population Sciences, National Cancer Institute, National Institutes of Health, Rockville, Maryland.

Alistair Woodward, Ph.D., Head, School of Population Health, Faculty of Medical and Health Sciences, The University of Auckland, Auckland, New Zealand.

Other contributors were

Nicole C. Ammerman, Sc.M., Ph.D. Candidate, Research Assistant, Institute for Global Tobacco Control, Department of Epidemiology, Bloomberg School of Public Health, The Johns Hopkins University, Baltimore, Maryland.

Mary Bedford, Proofreader, Cygnus Corporation, Rockville, Maryland.

Caroline M. Fichtenberg, M.S., Ph.D. Candidate, Department of Epidemiology, Bloomberg School of Public Health, The Johns Hopkins University, Baltimore, Maryland.

Charlotte Gerczak, M.L.A., Research Writer and Special Projects Coordinator, Department of Epidemiology, Bloomberg School of Public Health, The Johns Hopkins University, Baltimore, Maryland.

Roberta B. Gray, Senior Administrative Assistant to Dr. Jonathan M. Samet, Department of Epidemiology, Bloomberg School of Public Health, The Johns Hopkins University, Baltimore, Maryland.

Kat Jackson, Statistician, RTI International, Atlanta, Georgia.

Mooim Kang, Graphics Specialist, Cygnus Corporation, Rockville, Maryland.

Teresa Kelly, M.S., Project Director, Cygnus Corporation, Rockville, Maryland.

Elizabeth Khaykin, M.H.S., Sc.M., Ph.D. Candidate, Department of Epidemiology, Bloomberg School of Public Health, The Johns Hopkins University, Baltimore, Maryland.

Nancy Leonard, Administrative Assistant II to Dr. Jonathan M. Samet, Department of Epidemiology, Bloomberg School of Public Health, The Johns Hopkins University, Baltimore, Maryland.

Allison MacNeil, M.P.H., Health Scientist, Office on Smoking and Health, National Center for Chronic Disease Prevention and Health Promotion, Coordinating Center for Health Promotion, Centers for Disease Control and Prevention, Atlanta, Georgia.

William T. Marx, M.L.I.S., Health Communications Specialist, Office on Smoking and Health, National Center for Chronic Disease Prevention and Health Promotion, Coordinating Center for Health Promotion, Centers for Disease Control and Prevention, Atlanta, Georgia.

Linda McLaughlin, Word Processing Specialist, Cygnus Corporation, Rockville, Maryland.

Laura Nelson, M.A., Senior Writer, Cygnus Corporation, Rockville, Maryland.

Alyce Ortuzar, Copy Editor, Cygnus Corporation, Rockville, Maryland.

Margot Raphael, Senior Editor, American Institutes for Research, Silver Spring, Maryland.

Susan Schober, Ph.D., Senior Epidemiologist, National Health and Nutrition Examination Survey (NHANES) Program, National Center for Health Statistics, Centers for Disease Control and Prevention, Hyattsville, Maryland.

Angela Trosclair, M.S., Statistician, Office on Smoking and Health, National Center for Chronic Disease Prevention and Health Promotion, Coordinating Center for Health Promotion, Centers for Disease Control and Prevention, Atlanta, Georgia.

Glenda Vaughn, Public Health Analyst, Office on Smoking and Health, National Center for Chronic Disease Prevention and Health Promotion, Coordinating Center for Health Promotion, Centers for Disease Control and Prevention, Atlanta, Georgia.

Deborah Williams, Desktop Publishing Specialist to Dr. Jonathan M. Samet, Department of Epidemiology, Bloomberg School of Public Health, The Johns Hopkins University, Baltimore, Maryland.

Peggy E. Williams, M.S., Writer-Editor, Quantell, Inc., Marietta, Georgia.

Database contributors were

Mahshid Amini, Health Education Specialist, Office on Smoking and Health, National Center for Chronic Disease Prevention and Health Promotion, Coordinating Center for Health Promotion, Centers for Disease Control and Prevention, Atlanta, Georgia.

Nicole C. Ammerman, Sc.M., Ph.D. Candidate, Research Assistant, Institute for Global Tobacco Control, Department of Epidemiology, Bloomberg School of Public Health, The Johns Hopkins University, Baltimore, Maryland.

Erika Avila-Tang, Ph.D., M.H.S., Project Coordinator, Institute for Global Tobacco Control, Department of Epidemiology, Bloomberg School of Public Health, The Johns Hopkins University, Baltimore, Maryland.

Jeffrey H. Chrismon, P.M.P., Project Manager, Northrup Grumman Mission Systems, Atlanta, Georgia.

Oyelola 'Yomi Faparusi, M.D., Ph.D., Department of Mental Hygiene, Bloomberg School of Public Health, The Johns Hopkins University, Baltimore, Maryland.

Caroline M. Fichtenberg, M.S., Ph.D. Candidate, Department of Epidemiology, Bloomberg School of Public Health, The Johns Hopkins University, Baltimore, Maryland.

Ola Gibson, Software Engineer, Northrup Grumman Mission Systems, Atlanta, Georgia.

Hope L. Johnson, M.P.H., Ph.D. Candidate, Department of International Health, Bloomberg School of Public Health, The Johns Hopkins University, Baltimore, Maryland.

Bindu Kalesan, M.Sc., M.P.H., Biostatistician, Asthma and Allergy Center, The Johns Hopkins University, Baltimore, Maryland.

Elizabeth Khaykin, M.H.S., Sc.M., Ph.D. Candidate, Department of Epidemiology, Bloomberg School of Public Health, The Johns Hopkins University, Baltimore, Maryland.

Georgette Lavetsky, M.H.S., Epidemiologist, Office of Substance Abuse Services, Howard County Health Department, Columbia, Maryland.

Maria Jose Lopez, B.Sc., Ph.D. Candidate, Evaluation and Intervention Methods Service, Public Health Agency, Barcelona, Spain.

Sharon Mc Aleer, Web Designer, Northrop Grumman Mission Systems, Atlanta, Georgia.

Georgiana Onicescu, B.Sc., Master's Candidate in Biostatistics, Bloomberg School of Public Health, The Johns Hopkins University, Baltimore, Maryland.

Patti R. Seikus, M.P.H., Health Communications Specialist, Office on Smoking and Health, National Center for Chronic Disease Prevention and Health Promotion, Coordinating Center for Health Promotion, Centers for Disease Control and Prevention, Atlanta, Georgia.

Stephen Strathdee, User Support Specialist, Department of Epidemiology, Bloomberg School of Public Health, The Johns Hopkins University, Baltimore, Maryland.

The Health Consequences of Involuntary Exposure to Tobacco Smoke

Chapter 1
Introduction, Summary, and Conclusions

Introduction

The topic of passive or involuntary smoking was first addressed in the 1972 U.S. Surgeon General's report (*The Health Consequences of Smoking*, U.S. Department of Health, Education, and Welfare [USDHEW] 1972), only eight years after the first Surgeon General's report on the health consequences of active smoking (USDHEW 1964). Surgeon General Dr. Jesse Steinfeld had raised concerns about this topic, leading to its inclusion in that report. According to the 1972 report, nonsmokers inhale the mixture of sidestream smoke given off by a smoldering cigarette and mainstream smoke exhaled by a smoker, a mixture now referred to as "secondhand smoke" or "environmental tobacco smoke." Cited experimental studies showed that smoking in enclosed spaces could lead to high levels of cigarette smoke components in the air. For carbon monoxide (CO) specifically, levels in enclosed spaces could exceed levels then permitted in outdoor air. The studies supported a conclusion that "an atmosphere contaminated with tobacco smoke can contribute to the discomfort of many individuals" (USDHEW 1972, p. 7). The possibility that CO emitted from cigarettes could harm persons with chronic heart or lung disease was also mentioned.

Secondhand tobacco smoke was then addressed in greater depth in Chapter 4 (Involuntary Smoking) of the 1975 Surgeon General's report, *The Health Consequences of Smoking* (USDHEW 1975). The chapter noted that involuntary smoking takes place when nonsmokers inhale both sidestream and exhaled mainstream smoke and that this "smoking" is "involuntary" when "the exposure occurs as an unavoidable consequence of breathing in a smoke-filled environment" (p. 87). The report covered exposures and potential health consequences of involuntary smoking, and the researchers concluded that smoking on buses and airplanes was annoying to nonsmokers and that involuntary smoking had potentially adverse consequences for persons with heart and lung diseases. Two studies on nicotine concentrations in nonsmokers raised concerns about nicotine as a contributing factor to atherosclerotic cardiovascular disease in nonsmokers.

The 1979 Surgeon General's report, *Smoking and Health: A Report of the Surgeon General* (USDHEW 1979), also contained a chapter entitled "Involuntary Smoking." The chapter stressed that "attention to involuntary smoking is of recent vintage, and only

limited information regarding the health effects of such exposure upon the nonsmoker is available" (p. 11–35). The chapter concluded with recommendations for research including epidemiologic and clinical studies. The 1982 Surgeon General's report specifically addressed smoking and cancer (U.S. Department of Health and Human Services [USDHHS] 1982). By 1982, there were three published epidemiologic studies on involuntary smoking and lung cancer, and the 1982 Surgeon General's report included a brief chapter on this topic. That chapter commented on the methodologic difficulties inherent in such studies, including exposure assessment, the lengthy interval during which exposures are likely to be relevant, and accounting for exposures to other carcinogens. Nonetheless, the report concluded that "Although the currently available evidence is not sufficient to conclude that passive or involuntary smoking causes lung cancer in nonsmokers, the evidence does raise concern about a possible serious public health problem" (p. 251).

Involuntary smoking was also reviewed in the 1984 report, which focused on chronic obstructive pulmonary disease and smoking (USDHHS 1984). Chapter 7 (Passive Smoking) of that report included a comprehensive review of the mounting information on smoking by parents and the effects on respiratory health of their children, data on irritation of the eye, and the more limited evidence on pulmonary effects of involuntary smoking on adults. The chapter began with a compilation of measurements of tobacco smoke components in various indoor environments. The extent of the data had increased substantially since 1972. By 1984, the data included measurements of more specific indicators such as acrolein and nicotine, and less specific indicators such as particulate matter (PM), nitrogen oxides, and CO. The report reviewed new evidence on exposures of nonsmokers using biomarkers, with substantial information on levels of cotinine, a major nicotine metabolite. The report anticipated future conclusions with regard to respiratory effects of parental smoking on child respiratory health (Table 1.1).

Involuntary smoking was the topic for the entire 1986 Surgeon General's report, *The Health Consequences of Involuntary Smoking* (USDHHS 1986). In its 359 pages, the report covered the full breadth of the

Table 1.1   **Conclusions from previous Surgeon General's reports on the health effects of secondhand smoke exposure**

Disease and statement	Surgeon General's report
Coronary heart disease: "The presence of such levels" as found in cigarettes "indicates that the effect of exposure to carbon monoxide may on occasion, depending upon the length of exposure, be sufficient to be harmful to the health of an exposed person. This would be particularly significant for people who are already suffering from. . .coronary heart disease." (p. 7)	1972
Chronic respiratory symptoms (adults): "The presence of such levels" as found in cigarettes "indicates that the effect of exposure to carbon monoxide may on occasion, depending upon the length of exposure, be sufficient to be harmful to the health of an exposed person. This would be particularly significant for people who are already suffering from chronic bronchopulmonary disease. . . ." (p. 7)	1972
Pulmonary function: "Other components of tobacco smoke, such as particulate matter and the oxides of nitrogen, have been shown in various concentrations to affect adversely animal pulmonary. . .function. The extent of the contributions of these substances to illness in humans exposed to the concentrations present in an atmosphere contaminated with tobacco smoke is not presently known." (pp. 7–8)	1972
Asthma: "The limited existing data yield conflicting results concerning the relationship between passive smoke exposure and pulmonary function changes in patients with asthma." (p. 13)	1984
Bronchitis and pneumonia: "The children of smoking parents have an increased prevalence of reported respiratory symptoms, and have an increased frequency of bronchitis and pneumonia early in life." (p. 13)	1984
Pulmonary function (children): "The children of smoking parents appear to have measurable but small differences in tests of pulmonary function when compared with children of nonsmoking parents. The significance of this finding to the future development of lung disease is unknown." (p. 13)	1984
Pulmonary function (adults): ". . .some studies suggest that high levels of involuntary [tobacco] smoke exposure might produce small changes in pulmonary function in normal subjects. . . . Two studies have reported differences in measures of lung function in older populations between subjects chronically exposed to involuntary smoking and those who were not. This difference was not found in a younger and possibly less exposed population." (p. 13)	1984
Acute respiratory infections: "The children of parents who smoke have an increased frequency of a variety of acute respiratory illnesses and infections, including chest illnesses before 2 years of age and physician-diagnosed bronchitis, tracheitis, and laryngitis, when compared with the children of nonsmokers." (p. 13)	1986
Bronchitis and pneumonia: "The children of parents who smoke have an increased frequency of hospitalization for bronchitis and pneumonia during the first year of life when compared with the children of nonsmokers." (p. 13)	1986
Cancers other than lung: "The associations between cancers, other than cancer of the lung, and involuntary smoking require further investigation before a determination can be made about the relationship of involuntary smoking to these cancers." (p. 14)	1986
Cardiovascular disease: "Further studies on the relationship between involuntary smoking and cardiovascular disease are needed in order to determine whether involuntary smoking increases the risk of cardiovascular disease." (p. 14)	1986

Table 1.1   Continued

Disease and statement	Surgeon General's report
Chronic cough and phlegm (children): "Chronic cough and phlegm are more frequent in children whose parents smoke compared with children of nonsmokers." (p. 13)	1986
Chronic obstructive pulmonary disease (COPD): "Healthy adults exposed to environmental tobacco smoke may have small changes on pulmonary function testing, but are unlikely to experience clinically significant deficits in pulmonary function as a result of exposure to environmental tobacco smoke alone." (pp. 13–14) "The implications of chronic respiratory symptoms for respiratory health as an adult are unknown and deserve further study." (p. 13)	1986
Lung cancer: "Involuntary smoking can cause lung cancer in nonsmokers." (p. 13)	1986
Middle ear effusions: "A number of studies report that chronic middle ear effusions are more common in young children whose parents smoke than in children of nonsmoking parents." (p. 14)	1986
Pulmonary function (children): "The children of parents who smoke have small differences in tests of pulmonary function when compared with the children of nonsmokers. Although this decrement is insufficient to cause symptoms, the possibility that it may increase susceptibility to chronic obstructive pulmonary disease with exposure to other agents in adult life, e.g., [*sic*] active smoking or occupational exposures, needs investigation." (p. 13)	1986
Other: "An atmosphere contaminated with tobacco smoke can contribute to the discomfort of many individuals." (p. 7)	1972
"Cigarette smoke can make a significant, measurable contribution to the level of indoor air pollution at levels of smoking and ventilation that are common in the indoor environment." (p. 13)	1984
"Cigarette smoke in the air can produce an increase in both subjective and objective measures of eye irritation." (p. 13)	1984
"Nonsmokers who report exposure to environmental tobacco smoke have higher levels of urinary cotinine, a metabolite of nicotine, than those who do not report such exposure." (p. 13)	1984
"The simple separation of smokers and nonsmokers within the same air space may reduce, but does not eliminate, the exposure of nonsmokers to environmental tobacco smoke." (p. 13)	1986
"Validated questionnaires are needed for the assessment of recent and remote exposure to environmental tobacco smoke in the home, workplace, and other environments." (p. 14)	1986

Sources: U.S. Department of Health, Education, and Welfare 1972; U.S. Department of Health and Human Services 1984, 1986.

topic, addressing toxicology and dosimetry of tobacco smoke; the relevant evidence on active smoking; patterns of exposure of nonsmokers to tobacco smoke; the epidemiologic evidence on involuntary smoking and disease risks for infants, children, and adults; and policies to control involuntary exposure to tobacco smoke. That report concluded that involuntary smoking caused lung cancer in lifetime nonsmoking adults and was associated with adverse effects on respiratory health in children. The report also stated that simply separating smokers and nonsmokers within the same airspace reduced but did not eliminate exposure to secondhand smoke. All of these findings are relevant to public health and public policy (Table 1.1). The lung cancer conclusion was based on extensive information already available on the carcinogenicity of active smoking, the qualitative similarities between secondhand and mainstream smoke, the uptake of tobacco smoke components by nonsmokers, and the epidemiologic data on involuntary smoking. The three major conclusions of the report (Table 1.2), led Dr. C. Everett Koop, Surgeon General at the time, to comment in his preface that "the right of smokers to smoke ends where their behavior affects the health and well-being of others; furthermore, it is the smokers' responsibility to ensure that they do not expose nonsmokers to the potential [*sic*] harmful effects of tobacco smoke" (USDHHS 1986, p. xii).

Two other reports published in 1986 also reached the conclusion that involuntary smoking increased the risk for lung cancer. The International Agency for Research on Cancer (IARC) of the World Health Organization concluded that "passive smoking gives rise to some risk of cancer" (IARC 1986, p. 314). In its monograph on tobacco smoking, the agency supported this conclusion on the basis of the characteristics of sidestream and mainstream smoke, the

absorption of tobacco smoke materials during an involuntary exposure, and the nature of dose-response relationships for carcinogenesis. In the same year, the National Research Council (NRC) also concluded that involuntary smoking increases the incidence of lung cancer in nonsmokers (NRC 1986). In reaching this conclusion, the NRC report cited the biologic plausibility of the association between exposure to secondhand smoke and lung cancer and the supporting epidemiologic evidence. On the basis of a pooled analysis of the epidemiologic data adjusted for bias, the report concluded that the best estimate for the excess risk of lung cancer in nonsmokers married to smokers was 25 percent, compared with nonsmokers married to nonsmokers. With regard to the effects of involuntary smoking on children, the NRC report commented on the literature linking secondhand smoke exposures from parental smoking to increased risks for respiratory symptoms and infections and to a slightly diminished rate of lung growth.

Since 1986, the conclusions with regard to both the carcinogenicity of secondhand smoke and the adverse effects of parental smoking on the health of children have been echoed and expanded (Table 1.3). In 1992, the U.S. Environmental Protection Agency (EPA) published its risk assessment of secondhand smoke as a carcinogen (USEPA 1992). The agency's evaluation drew on toxicologic information on secondhand smoke and the extensive literature on active smoking. A comprehensive meta-analysis of the 31 epidemiologic studies of secondhand smoke and lung cancer published up to that time was central to the decision to classify secondhand smoke as a group A carcinogen—namely, a known human carcinogen. Estimates of approximately 3,000 U.S. lung cancer deaths per year in nonsmokers were attributed to secondhand smoke. The report also covered other respiratory health effects in

Table 1.2   Major conclusions of the 1986 Surgeon General's report, *The Health Consequences of Involuntary Smoking*

1. Involuntary smoking is a cause of disease, including lung cancer, in healthy nonsmokers.

2. The children of parents who smoke compared with the children of nonsmoking parents have an increased frequency of respiratory infections, increased respiratory symptoms, and slightly smaller rates of increase in lung function as the lung matures.

3. The simple separation of smokers and nonsmokers within the same air space may reduce, but does not eliminate, the exposure of nonsmokers to environmental tobacco smoke.

Source: U.S. Department of Health and Human Services 1986, p. 7.

Table 1.3   Selected major reports, other than those of the U.S. Surgeon General, addressing adverse effects from exposure to tobacco smoke

Agency	Publication	Place and date of publication
National Research Council	*Environmental Tobacco Smoke: Measuring Exposures and Assessing Health Effects*	Washington, D.C. United States 1986
International Agency for Research on Cancer (IARC)	*Monographs on the Evaluation of the Carcinogenic Risk of Chemicals to Humans: Tobacco Smoking* (IARC Monograph 38)	Lyon, France 1986
U.S. Environmental Protection Agency (EPA)	*Respiratory Health Effects of Passive Smoking: Lung Cancer and Other Disorders*	Washington, D.C. United States 1992
National Health and Medical Research Council	*The Health Effects of Passive Smoking*	Canberra, Australia 1997
California EPA (Cal/EPA), Office of Environmental Health Hazard Assessment	*Health Effects of Exposure to Environmental Tobacco Smoke*	Sacramento, California United States 1997
Scientific Committee on Tobacco and Health	*Report of the Scientific Committee on Tobacco and Health*	London, United Kingdom 1998
World Health Organization	*International Consultation on Environmental Tobacco Smoke (ETS) and Child Health. Consultation Report*	Geneva, Switzerland 1999
IARC	*Tobacco Smoke and Involuntary Smoking* (IARC Monograph 83)	Lyon, France 2004
Cal/EPA, Office of Environmental Health Hazard Assessment	*Proposed Identification of Environmental Tobacco Smoke as a Toxic Air Contaminant*	Sacramento, California United States 2005

children and adults and concluded that involuntary smoking is causally associated with several adverse respiratory effects in children. There was also a quantitative risk assessment for the impact of involuntary smoking on childhood asthma and lower respiratory tract infections in young children.

In the decade since the 1992 EPA report, scientific panels continued to evaluate the mounting evidence linking involuntary smoking to adverse health effects (Table 1.3). The most recent was the 2005 report of the California EPA (Cal/EPA 2005). Over time, research has repeatedly affirmed the conclusions of the 1986 Surgeon General's reports and studies have further identified causal associations of involuntary smoking with diseases and other health disorders. The epidemiologic evidence on involuntary smoking has

markedly expanded since 1986, as have the data on exposure to tobacco smoke in the many environments where people spend time. An understanding of the mechanisms by which involuntary smoking causes disease has also deepened.

As part of the environmental health hazard assessment, Cal/EPA identified specific health effects causally associated with exposure to secondhand smoke. The agency estimated the annual excess deaths in the United States that are attributable to secondhand smoke exposure for specific disorders: sudden infant death syndrome (SIDS), cardiac-related illnesses (ischemic heart disease), and lung cancer (Cal/EPA 2005). For the excess incidence of other health outcomes, either new estimates were provided or estimates from the 1997 health hazard assessment were used without any revisions (Cal/EPA 1997). Overall, Cal/EPA estimated that about 50,000 excess deaths result annually from exposure to secondhand smoke (Cal/EPA 2005). Estimated annual excess deaths for the total U.S. population are about 3,400 (a range of 3,423 to 8,866) from lung cancer, 46,000 (a range of 22,700 to 69,600) from cardiac-related illnesses, and 430 from SIDS. The agency also estimated that between 24,300 and 71,900 low birth weight or preterm deliveries, about 202,300 episodes of childhood asthma (new cases and exacerbations), between 150,000 and 300,000 cases of lower respiratory illness in children, and about 789,700 cases of middle ear infections in children occur each year in the United States as a result of exposure to secondhand smoke.

This new 2006 Surgeon General's report returns to the topic of involuntary smoking. The health effects of involuntary smoking have not received comprehensive coverage in this series of reports since 1986. Reports since then have touched on selected aspects of the topic: the 1994 report on tobacco use among young people (USDHHS 1994), the 1998 report on tobacco use among U.S. racial and ethnic minorities (USDHHS 1998), and the 2001 report on women and smoking (USDHHS 2001). As involuntary smoking remains widespread in the United States and elsewhere, the preparation of this report was motivated by the persistence of involuntary smoking as a public health problem and the need to evaluate the substantial new evidence reported since 1986. This report substantially expands the list of topics that were included in the 1986 report. Additional topics include SIDS, developmental effects, and other reproductive effects; heart disease in adults; and cancer sites beyond the lung. For some associations of involuntary smoking with adverse health effects, only a few studies were reviewed in 1986 (e.g., ear disease in children); now, the relevant literature is substantial. Consequently, this report uses meta-analysis to quantitatively summarize evidence as appropriate. Following the approach used in the 2004 report (*The Health Consequences of Smoking*, USDHHS 2004), this 2006 report also systematically evaluates the evidence for causality, judging the extent of the evidence available and then making an inference as to the nature of the association.

Organization of the Report

This twenty-ninth report of the Surgeon General examines the topics of toxicology of secondhand smoke, assessment and prevalence of exposure to secondhand smoke, reproductive and developmental health effects, respiratory effects of exposure to secondhand smoke in children and adults, cancer among adults, cardiovascular diseases, and the control of secondhand smoke exposure.

This introductory chapter (Chapter 1) includes a discussion of the concept of causation and introduces concepts of causality that are used throughout this report; this chapter also summarizes the major conclusions of the report. Chapter 2 (Toxicology of Secondhand Smoke) sets out a foundation for interpreting the observational evidence that is the focus of most of the following chapters. The discussion details the mechanisms that enable tobacco smoke components to injure the respiratory tract and cause nonmalignant and malignant diseases and other adverse effects. Chapter 3 (Assessment of Exposure to Secondhand Smoke) provides a perspective on key factors that determine exposures of people to secondhand smoke in indoor environments, including building designs and operations, atmospheric markers of secondhand smoke, exposure models, and biomarkers of exposure to secondhand smoke. Chapter 4 (Prevalence of Exposure to Secondhand Smoke) summarizes findings that focus on nicotine measurements in the air and cotinine measurements in biologic materials. The chapter includes exposures in the home, workplace, public places, and special populations. Chapter 5 (Reproductive and Developmental Effects from Exposure to Secondhand Smoke) reviews the health effects on reproduction, on infants, and on child development. Chapter 6 (Respiratory Effects in Children from Exposure to Secondhand Smoke) examines the effects of parental smoking on the respiratory health of children. Chapter 7 (Cancer Among Adults from Exposure to Secondhand Smoke) summarizes the evidence on cancer of the lung, breast, nasal sinuses, and the cervix. Chapter 8 (Cardiovascular Diseases from Exposure to Secondhand Smoke) discusses coronary heart disease (CHD), stroke, and subclinical vascular disease. Chapter 9 (Respiratory Effects in Adults from Exposure to Secondhand Smoke) examines odor and irritation, respiratory symptoms, lung function, and respiratory diseases such as asthma and chronic obstructive pulmonary disease. Chapter 10 (Control of Secondhand Smoke Exposure) considers measures used to control exposure to secondhand smoke in public places, including legislation, education, and approaches based on building designs and operations. The report concludes with "A Vision for the Future." Major conclusions of the report were distilled from the chapter conclusions and appear later in this chapter.

Preparation of the Report

This report of the Surgeon General was prepared by the Office on Smoking and Health, National Center for Chronic Disease Prevention and Health Promotion, Coordinating Center for Health Promotion, Centers for Disease Control and Prevention (CDC), and U.S. DHHS. Initial chapters were written by 22 experts who were selected because of their knowledge of a particular topic. The contributions of the initial experts were consolidated into 10 major chapters that were then reviewed by more than 40 peer reviewers. The entire manuscript was then sent to more than 30 scientists and experts who reviewed it for its scientific integrity. After each review cycle, the drafts were revised by the scientific editors on the basis of the experts' comments. Subsequently, the report was reviewed by various institutes and agencies within U.S. DHHS. Publication lags, even short ones, prevent an up-to-the-minute inclusion of all recently published articles and data. Therefore, by the time the public reads this report, there may be additional published studies or data. To provide published information as current as possible, this report includes an Appendix of more recent studies that represent major additions to the literature.

This report is also accompanied by a companion database of key evidence that is accessible through the Internet (http://www.cdc.gov/tobacco). The database includes a uniform description of the studies and results on the health effects of exposure to secondhand smoke that were presented in a format compatible with abstraction into standardized tables. Readers of the report may access these data for additional analyses, tables, or figures.

Definitions and Terminology

The inhalation of tobacco smoke by nonsmokers has been variably referred to as "passive smoking" or "involuntary smoking." Smokers, of course, also inhale secondhand smoke. Cigarette smoke contains both particles and gases generated by the combustion at high temperatures of tobacco, paper, and additives. The smoke inhaled by nonsmokers that contaminates indoor spaces and outdoor environments has often been referred to as "secondhand smoke" or "environmental tobacco smoke." This inhaled smoke is the mixture of sidestream smoke released by the smoldering cigarette and the mainstream smoke that is exhaled by a smoker. Sidestream smoke, generated at lower temperatures and under somewhat different combustion conditions than mainstream smoke, tends to have higher concentrations of many of the toxins found in cigarette smoke (USDHHS 1986). However, it is rapidly diluted as it travels away from the burning cigarette.

Secondhand smoke is an inherently dynamic mixture that changes in characteristics and concentration with the time since it was formed and the distance it has traveled. The smoke particles change in size and composition as gaseous components are volatilized and moisture content changes; gaseous elements of secondhand smoke may be adsorbed onto materials, and particle concentrations drop with both dilution in the air or environment and impaction on surfaces, including the lungs or on the body. Because of its dynamic nature, a specific quantitative definition of secondhand smoke cannot be offered.

This report uses the term secondhand smoke in preference to environmental tobacco smoke, even though the latter may have been used more frequently in previous reports. The descriptor "secondhand" captures the involuntary nature of the exposure, while "environmental" does not. This report also refers to the inhalation of secondhand smoke as involuntary smoking, acknowledging that most nonsmokers do not want to inhale tobacco smoke. The exposure of the fetus to tobacco smoke, whether from active smoking by the mother or from her exposure to secondhand smoke, also constitutes involuntary smoking.

Evidence Evaluation

Following the model of the 1964 report, the Surgeon General's reports on smoking have included comprehensive compilations of the evidence on the health effects of smoking. The evidence is analyzed to identify causal associations between smoking and disease according to enunciated principles, sometimes referred to as the "Surgeon General's criteria" or the "Hill" criteria (after Sir Austin Bradford Hill) for causality (USDHEW 1964; USDHHS 2004). Application of these criteria involves covering all relevant observational and experimental evidence. The criteria, offered in a brief chapter of the 1964 report entitled "Criteria for Judgment," included (1) the consistency of the association, (2) the strength of the association, (3) the specificity of the association, (4) the temporal relationship of the association, and (5) the coherence of the association. Although these criteria have been criticized (e.g., Rothman and Greenland 1998), they have proved useful as a framework for interpreting evidence on smoking and other postulated causes of disease, and for judging whether causality can be inferred.

In the 2004 report of the Surgeon General, *The Health Consequences of Smoking*, the framework for interpreting evidence on smoking and health was revisited in depth for the first time since the 1964 report (USDHHS 2004). The 2004 report provided a four-level hierarchy for interpreting evidence (Table 1.4). The categories acknowledge that evidence can be "suggestive" but not adequate to infer a causal relationship, and also allows for evidence that is "suggestive of no causal relationship." Since the 2004 report, the individual chapter conclusions have consistently used this four-level hierarchy (Table 1.4), but

evidence syntheses and other summary statements may use either the term "increased risk" or "cause" to describe instances in which there is sufficient evidence to conclude that active or involuntary smoking causes a disease or condition. This four-level framework also sharply and completely separates conclusions regarding causality from the implications of such conclusions.

That same framework was used in this report on involuntary smoking and health. The criteria dating back to the 1964 Surgeon General's report remain useful as guidelines for evaluating evidence (USDHEW 1964), but they were not intended to be applied strictly or as a "checklist" that needed to be met before the designation of "causal" could be applied to an association. In fact, for involuntary smoking and health, several of the criteria will not be met for some associations. Specificity, referring to a unique exposure-disease relationship (e.g., the association between thalidomide use during pregnancy and unusual birth defects), can be set aside as not relevant, as all of the health effects considered in this report have causes other than involuntary smoking. Associations are considered more likely to be causal as the strength of an association increases because competing explanations become less plausible alternatives. However, based on knowledge of dosimetry and mechanisms of injury and disease causation, the risk is anticipated to be only slightly or modestly increased for some associations of involuntary smoking with disease, such as lung cancer, particularly when the very strong relative risks found for active smokers are compared with those for lifetime nonsmokers. The finding of only a small elevation in risk, as in the

Table 1.4   Four-level hierarchy for classifying the strength of causal inferences based on available evidence

Level 1	Evidence is **sufficient** to infer a causal relationship.
Level 2	Evidence is **suggestive but not sufficient** to infer a causal relationship.
Level 3	Evidence is **inadequate** to infer the presence or absence of a causal relationship (which encompasses evidence that is sparse, of poor quality, or conflicting).
Level 4	Evidence is **suggestive of no causal relationship**.

Source: U.S. Department of Health and Human Services 2004.

example of spousal smoking and lung cancer risk in lifetime nonsmokers, does not weigh against a causal association; however, alternative explanations for a risk of a small magnitude need full exploration and cannot be so easily set aside as alternative explanations for a stronger association. Consistency, coherence, and the temporal relationship of involuntary smoking with disease are central to the interpretations in this report. To address coherence, the report draws not only on the evidence for involuntary smoking, but on the even more extensive literature on active smoking and disease.

Although the evidence reviewed in this report comes largely from investigations of secondhand smoke specifically, the larger body of evidence on active smoking is also relevant to many of the associations that were evaluated. The 1986 report found secondhand smoke to be qualitatively similar to mainstream smoke inhaled by the smoker and concluded that secondhand smoke would be expected to have "a toxic and carcinogenic potential that would

not be expected to be qualitatively different from that of MS [mainstream smoke]" (USDHHS 1986, p. 23). The 2004 report of the Surgeon General revisited the health consequences of active smoking (USDHHS 2004), and the conclusions substantially expanded the list of diseases and conditions caused by smoking. Chapters in the present report consider the evidence on active smoking that is relevant to biologic plausibility for causal associations between involuntary smoking and disease. The reviews included in this report cover evidence identified through search strategies set out in each chapter. Of necessity, the evidence on mechanisms was selectively reviewed. However, an attempt was made to cover all health studies through specified target dates. Because of the substantial amount of time involved in preparing this report, lists of new key references published after these cut-off dates are included in an Appendix. Literature reviews were extended when new evidence was sufficient to possibly change the level of a causal conclusion.

Major Conclusions

This report returns to involuntary smoking, the topic of the 1986 Surgeon General's report. Since then, there have been many advances in the research on secondhand smoke, and substantial evidence has been reported over the ensuing 20 years. This report uses the revised language for causal conclusions that was implemented in the 2004 Surgeon General's report (USDHHS 2004). Each chapter provides a comprehensive review of the evidence, a quantitative synthesis of the evidence if appropriate, and a rigorous assessment of sources of bias that may affect interpretations of the findings. The reviews in this report reaffirm and strengthen the findings of the 1986 report. With regard to the involuntary exposure of nonsmokers to tobacco smoke, the scientific evidence now supports the following major conclusions:

1. Secondhand smoke causes premature death and disease in children and in adults who do not smoke.

2. Children exposed to secondhand smoke are at an increased risk for sudden infant death syndrome (SIDS), acute respiratory infections, ear problems,

and more severe asthma. Smoking by parents causes respiratory symptoms and slows lung growth in their children.

3. Exposure of adults to secondhand smoke has immediate adverse effects on the cardiovascular system and causes coronary heart disease and lung cancer.

4. The scientific evidence indicates that there is no risk-free level of exposure to secondhand smoke.

5. Many millions of Americans, both children and adults, are still exposed to secondhand smoke in their homes and workplaces despite substantial progress in tobacco control.

6. Eliminating smoking in indoor spaces fully protects nonsmokers from exposure to secondhand smoke. Separating smokers from nonsmokers, cleaning the air, and ventilating buildings cannot eliminate exposures of nonsmokers to secondhand smoke.

Chapter Conclusions

Chapter 2. Toxicology of Secondhand Smoke

*Evidence of Carcinogenic Effects
from Secondhand Smoke Exposure*

1. More than 50 carcinogens have been identified in sidestream and secondhand smoke.

2. The evidence is sufficient to infer a causal relationship between exposure to secondhand smoke and its condensates and tumors in laboratory animals.

3. The evidence is sufficient to infer that exposure of nonsmokers to secondhand smoke causes a significant increase in urinary levels of metabolites of the tobacco-specific lung carcinogen 4-(methylnitrosamino)-1-(3-pyridyl)-1-butanone (NNK). The presence of these metabolites links exposure to secondhand smoke with an increased risk for lung cancer.

4. The mechanisms by which secondhand smoke causes lung cancer are probably similar to those observed in smokers. The overall risk of secondhand smoke exposure, compared with active smoking, is diminished by a substantially lower carcinogenic dose.

*Mechanisms of Respiratory Tract Injury and Disease
Caused by Secondhand Smoke Exposure*

5. The evidence indicates multiple mechanisms by which secondhand smoke exposure causes injury to the respiratory tract.

6. The evidence indicates mechanisms by which secondhand smoke exposure could increase the risk for sudden infant death syndrome.

*Mechanisms of Secondhand Smoke Exposure
and Heart Disease*

7. The evidence is sufficient to infer that exposure to secondhand smoke has a prothrombotic effect.

8. The evidence is sufficient to infer that exposure to secondhand smoke causes endothelial cell dysfunctions.

9. The evidence is sufficient to infer that exposure to secondhand smoke causes atherosclerosis in animal models.

Chapter 3. Assessment of Exposure to Secondhand Smoke

Building Designs and Operations

1. Current heating, ventilating, and air conditioning systems alone cannot control exposure to secondhand smoke.

2. The operation of a heating, ventilating, and air conditioning system can distribute secondhand smoke throughout a building.

Exposure Models

3. Atmospheric concentration of nicotine is a sensitive and specific indicator for secondhand smoke.

4. Smoking increases indoor particle concentrations.

5. Models can be used to estimate concentrations of secondhand smoke.

Biomarkers of Exposure to Secondhand Smoke

6. Biomarkers suitable for assessing recent exposures to secondhand smoke are available.

7. At this time, cotinine, the primary proximate metabolite of nicotine, remains the biomarker of choice for assessing secondhand smoke exposure.

8. Individual biomarkers of exposure to secondhand smoke represent only one component of a complex mixture, and measurements of one marker may not wholly reflect an exposure to other components of concern as a result of involuntary smoking.

Chapter 4. Prevalence of Exposure to Secondhand Smoke

1. The evidence is sufficient to infer that large numbers of nonsmokers are still exposed to secondhand smoke.

2. Exposure of nonsmokers to secondhand smoke has declined in the United States since the 1986 Surgeon General's report, *The Health Consequences of Involuntary Smoking*.

3. The evidence indicates that the extent of secondhand smoke exposure varies across the country.

4. Homes and workplaces are the predominant locations for exposure to secondhand smoke.

5. Exposure to secondhand smoke tends to be greater for persons with lower incomes.

6. Exposure to secondhand smoke continues in restaurants, bars, casinos, gaming halls, and vehicles.

Chapter 5. Reproductive and Developmental Effects from Exposure to Secondhand Smoke

Fertility

1. The evidence is inadequate to infer the presence or absence of a causal relationship between maternal exposure to secondhand smoke and female fertility or fecundability. No data were found on paternal exposure to secondhand smoke and male fertility or fecundability.

Pregnancy (Spontaneous Abortion and Perinatal Death)

2. The evidence is inadequate to infer the presence or absence of a causal relationship between maternal exposure to secondhand smoke during pregnancy and spontaneous abortion.

Infant Deaths

3. The evidence is inadequate to infer the presence or absence of a causal relationship between exposure to secondhand smoke and neonatal mortality.

Sudden Infant Death Syndrome

4. The evidence is sufficient to infer a causal relationship between exposure to secondhand smoke and sudden infant death syndrome.

Preterm Delivery

5. The evidence is suggestive but not sufficient to infer a causal relationship between maternal exposure to secondhand smoke during pregnancy and preterm delivery.

Low Birth Weight

6. The evidence is sufficient to infer a causal relationship between maternal exposure to secondhand smoke during pregnancy and a small reduction in birth weight.

Congenital Malformations

7. The evidence is inadequate to infer the presence or absence of a causal relationship between exposure to secondhand smoke and congenital malformations.

Cognitive Development

8. The evidence is inadequate to infer the presence or absence of a causal relationship between exposure to secondhand smoke and cognitive functioning among children.

Behavioral Development

9. The evidence is inadequate to infer the presence or absence of a causal relationship between exposure to secondhand smoke and behavioral problems among children.

Height/Growth

10. The evidence is inadequate to infer the presence or absence of a causal relationship between exposure to secondhand smoke and children's height/growth.

Childhood Cancer

11. The evidence is suggestive but not sufficient to infer a causal relationship between prenatal and postnatal exposure to secondhand smoke and childhood cancer.

12. The evidence is inadequate to infer the presence or absence of a causal relationship between maternal exposure to secondhand smoke during pregnancy and childhood cancer.

13. The evidence is inadequate to infer the presence or absence of a causal relationship between exposure to secondhand smoke during infancy and childhood cancer.

14. The evidence is suggestive but not sufficient to infer a causal relationship between prenatal and postnatal exposure to secondhand smoke and childhood leukemias.

15. The evidence is suggestive but not sufficient to infer a causal relationship between prenatal and postnatal exposure to secondhand smoke and childhood lymphomas.

16. The evidence is suggestive but not sufficient to infer a causal relationship between prenatal and postnatal exposure to secondhand smoke and childhood brain tumors.

17. The evidence is inadequate to infer the presence or absence of a causal relationship between prenatal and postnatal exposure to secondhand smoke and other childhood cancer types.

Chapter 6. Respiratory Effects in Children from Exposure to Secondhand Smoke

Lower Respiratory Illnesses in Infancy and Early Childhood

1. The evidence is sufficient to infer a causal relationship between secondhand smoke exposure from parental smoking and lower respiratory illnesses in infants and children.

2. The increased risk for lower respiratory illnesses is greatest from smoking by the mother.

Middle Ear Disease and Adenotonsillectomy

3. The evidence is sufficient to infer a causal relationship between parental smoking and middle ear disease in children, including acute and recurrent otitis media and chronic middle ear effusion.

4. The evidence is suggestive but not sufficient to infer a causal relationship between parental smoking and the natural history of middle ear effusion.

5. The evidence is inadequate to infer the presence or absence of a causal relationship between parental smoking and an increase in the risk of adenoidectomy or tonsillectomy among children.

Respiratory Symptoms and Prevalent Asthma in School-Age Children

6. The evidence is sufficient to infer a causal relationship between parental smoking and cough, phlegm, wheeze, and breathlessness among children of school age.

7. The evidence is sufficient to infer a causal relationship between parental smoking and ever having asthma among children of school age.

Childhood Asthma Onset

8. The evidence is sufficient to infer a causal relationship between secondhand smoke exposure from parental smoking and the onset of wheeze illnesses in early childhood.

9. The evidence is suggestive but not sufficient to infer a causal relationship between secondhand smoke exposure from parental smoking and the onset of childhood asthma.

Atopy

10. The evidence is inadequate to infer the presence or absence of a causal relationship between parental smoking and the risk of immunoglobulin E-mediated allergy in their children.

Lung Growth and Pulmonary Function

11. The evidence is sufficient to infer a causal relationship between maternal smoking during pregnancy and persistent adverse effects on lung function across childhood.

12. The evidence is sufficient to infer a causal relationship between exposure to secondhand smoke after birth and a lower level of lung function during childhood.

Chapter 7. Cancer Among Adults from Exposure to Secondhand Smoke

Lung Cancer

1. The evidence is sufficient to infer a causal relationship between secondhand smoke exposure and lung cancer among lifetime nonsmokers. This conclusion extends to all secondhand smoke exposure, regardless of location.

2. The pooled evidence indicates a 20 to 30 percent increase in the risk of lung cancer from secondhand smoke exposure associated with living with a smoker.

Breast Cancer

3. The evidence is suggestive but not sufficient to infer a causal relationship between secondhand smoke and breast cancer.

Nasal Sinus Cavity and Nasopharyngeal Carcinoma

4. The evidence is suggestive but not sufficient to infer a causal relationship between secondhand smoke exposure and a risk of nasal sinus cancer among nonsmokers.

5. The evidence is inadequate to infer the presence or absence of a causal relationship between secondhand smoke exposure and a risk of nasopharyngeal carcinoma among nonsmokers.

Cervical Cancer

6. The evidence is inadequate to infer the presence or absence of a causal relationship between secondhand smoke exposure and the risk of cervical cancer among lifetime nonsmokers.

Chapter 8. Cardiovascular Diseases from Exposure to Secondhand Smoke

1. The evidence is sufficient to infer a causal relationship between exposure to secondhand smoke and increased risks of coronary heart disease morbidity and mortality among both men and women.

2. Pooled relative risks from meta-analyses indicate a 25 to 30 percent increase in the risk of coronary heart disease from exposure to secondhand smoke.

3. The evidence is suggestive but not sufficient to infer a causal relationship between exposure to secondhand smoke and an increased risk of stroke.

4. Studies of secondhand smoke and subclinical vascular disease, particularly carotid arterial wall thickening, are suggestive but not sufficient to infer a causal relationship between exposure to secondhand smoke and atherosclerosis.

Chapter 9. Respiratory Effects in Adults from Exposure to Secondhand Smoke

Odor and Irritation

1. The evidence is sufficient to infer a causal relationship between secondhand smoke exposure and odor annoyance.

2. The evidence is sufficient to infer a causal relationship between secondhand smoke exposure and nasal irritation.

3. The evidence is suggestive but not sufficient to conclude that persons with nasal allergies or a history of respiratory illnesses are more susceptible to developing nasal irritation from secondhand smoke exposure.

Respiratory Symptoms

4. The evidence is suggestive but not sufficient to infer a causal relationship between secondhand smoke exposure and acute respiratory symptoms including cough, wheeze, chest tightness, and difficulty breathing among persons with asthma.

5. The evidence is suggestive but not sufficient to infer a causal relationship between secondhand smoke exposure and acute respiratory symptoms including cough, wheeze, chest tightness, and difficulty breathing among healthy persons.

6. The evidence is suggestive but not sufficient to infer a causal relationship between secondhand smoke exposure and chronic respiratory symptoms.

Lung Function

7. The evidence is suggestive but not sufficient to infer a causal relationship between short-term secondhand smoke exposure and an acute decline in lung function in persons with asthma.

8. The evidence is inadequate to infer the presence or absence of a causal relationship between short-term secondhand smoke exposure and an acute decline in lung function in healthy persons.

9. The evidence is suggestive but not sufficient to infer a causal relationship between chronic secondhand smoke exposure and a small decrement in lung function in the general population.

10. The evidence is inadequate to infer the presence or absence of a causal relationship between chronic secondhand smoke exposure and an accelerated decline in lung function.

Asthma

11. The evidence is suggestive but not sufficient to infer a causal relationship between secondhand smoke exposure and adult-onset asthma.

12. The evidence is suggestive but not sufficient to infer a causal relationship between secondhand smoke exposure and a worsening of asthma control.

Chronic Obstructive Pulmonary Disease

13. The evidence is suggestive but not sufficient to infer a causal relationship between secondhand smoke exposure and risk for chronic obstructive pulmonary disease.

14. The evidence is inadequate to infer the presence or absence of a causal relationship between secondhand smoke exposure and morbidity in persons with chronic obstructive pulmonary disease.

Chapter 10. Control of Secondhand Smoke Exposure

1. Workplace smoking restrictions are effective in reducing secondhand smoke exposure.

2. Workplace smoking restrictions lead to less smoking among covered workers.

3. Establishing smoke-free workplaces is the only effective way to ensure that secondhand smoke exposure does not occur in the workplace.

4. The majority of workers in the United States are now covered by smoke-free policies.

5. The extent to which workplaces are covered by smoke-free policies varies among worker groups, across states, and by sociodemographic factors. Workplaces related to the entertainment and hospitality industries have notably high potential for secondhand smoke exposure.

6. Evidence from peer-reviewed studies shows that smoke-free policies and regulations do not have an adverse economic impact on the hospitality industry.

7. Evidence suggests that exposure to secondhand smoke varies by ethnicity and gender.

8. In the United States, the home is now becoming the predominant location for exposure of children and adults to secondhand smoke.

9. Total bans on indoor smoking in hospitals, restaurants, bars, and offices substantially reduce secondhand smoke exposure, up to several orders of magnitude with incomplete compliance, and with full compliance, exposures are eliminated.

10. Exposures of nonsmokers to secondhand smoke cannot be controlled by air cleaning or mechanical air exchange.

Methodologic Issues

Much of the evidence on the health effects of involuntary smoking comes from observational epidemiologic studies that were carried out to test hypotheses related to secondhand smoke and risk for diseases and other adverse health effects. The challenges faced in carrying out these studies reflect those of observational research generally: assessment of the relevant exposures and outcomes with sufficient validity and precision, selection of an appropriate study design, identification of an appropriate and sufficiently large study population, and collection of information on other relevant factors that may confound or modify the association being studied. The challenge of accurately classifying secondhand smoke exposures confronts all studies of such exposures, and consequently the literature on approaches to and limitations of exposure classification is substantial. Sources of bias that can affect the findings of epidemiologic studies have been widely discussed (Rothman and Greenland 1998), both in general and in relation to studies of involuntary smoking. Concerns about bias apply to any study of an environmental agent and disease risk: misclassification of exposures or outcomes, confounding effect modification, and proper selection of study participants. In addition, the generalizability of findings from one population to another (external validity) further determines the value of evidence from a study. Another methodologic concern affecting secondhand smoke literature comes from the use of meta-analysis to combine the findings of epidemiologic studies; general concerns related to the use of meta-analysis for observational data and more specific concerns related to involuntary smoking have also been raised. This chapter considers these methodologic issues in anticipation of more specific treatment in the following chapters.

Classification of Secondhand Smoke Exposure

For secondhand smoke, as for any environmental factor that may be a cause of disease, the exposure assessment might encompass the time and place of the exposure, cumulative exposures, exposure during a particular time, or a recent exposure (Jaakkola and Jaakkola 1997; Jaakkola and Samet 1999). For example, exposures to secondhand smoke across the full life span may be of interest for lung cancer, while only more recent exposures may be relevant to the exacerbation of asthma. For CHD, both temporally remote and current exposures may affect risk. Assessments of exposures are further complicated by the multiplicity of environments where exposures take place and the difficulty of characterizing the exposure in some locations, such as public places or workplaces. Additionally, exposures probably vary qualitatively and quantitatively over time and across locations because of temporal changes and geographic differences in smoking patterns.

Nonetheless, researchers have used a variety of approaches for exposure assessments in epidemiologic studies of adverse health effects from involuntary smoking. Several core concepts that are fundamental to these approaches are illustrated in Figure 1.1 (Samet and Jaakkola 1999). Cigarette smoking is, of course, the source of most secondhand smoke in the United States, followed by pipes, cigars, and other products. Epidemiologic studies generally focus on assessing the exposure, which is the contact with secondhand smoke. The concentrations of secondhand smoke components in a space depend on the number of smokers and the rate at which they are smoking, the volume into which the smoke is distributed, the rate at which the air in the space exchanges with uncontaminated air, and the rate at which the secondhand smoke is removed from the air. Concentration, exposure, and dose differ in their definitions, although the terms are sometimes used without sharp distinctions. However, surrogate indicators that generally describe a source of exposure may also be used to assess the exposure, such as marriage to a smoker or the number of cigarettes smoked in the home. Biomarkers can provide an indication of an exposure or possibly the dose, but for secondhand smoke they are used for recent exposure only.

People are exposed to secondhand smoke in a number of different places, often referred to as "microenvironments" (NRC 1991). A microenvironment is a definable location that has a constant concentration of the contaminant of interest, such as secondhand smoke, during the time that a person is there. Some key microenvironments for secondhand smoke include the home, the workplace, public places, and transportation environments (Klepeis 1999). Based

Figure 1.1   The determinants of exposure, dose, and biologically effective dose that underlie the development of health effects from smoking

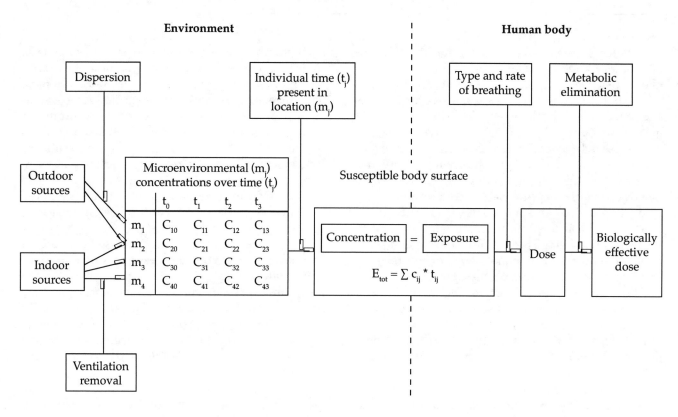

Source: Samet and Jaakkola 1999. Reprinted with permission.

on the microenvironmental model, total exposure can be estimated as the weighted average of the concentrations of secondhand smoke or indicator compounds, such as nicotine, in the microenvironments where time is spent; the weights are the time spent in each microenvironment. Klepeis (1999) illustrates the application of the microenvironmental model with national data from the National Human Activity Pattern Survey conducted by the EPA. His calculations yield an overall estimate of exposure to airborne particles from smoking and of the contributions to this exposure from various microenvironments.

Much of the epidemiologic evidence addresses the consequences of an exposure in a particular microenvironment, such as the home (spousal smoking and lung cancer risk or maternal smoking and risk for asthma exacerbation), or the workplace (exacerbation of asthma by the presence of smokers). Some studies have attempted to cover multiple microenvironments

and to characterize exposures over time. For example, in the multicenter study of secondhand smoke exposure and lung cancer carried out in the United States, Fontham and colleagues (1994) assessed exposures during childhood, in workplaces, and at home during adulthood. Questionnaires that assess exposures have been the primary tool used in epidemiologic studies of secondhand smoke and disease. Measurement of biomarkers has been added in some studies, either as an additional and complementary exposure assessment approach or for validating questionnaire responses. Some studies have also measured components of secondhand smoke in the air.

Questionnaires generally address sources of exposure in microenvironments and can be tailored to address the time period of interest. Questionnaires represent the only approach that can be used to assess exposures retrospectively over a life span, because available biomarkers only reflect exposures over recent days or, at most, weeks. Questionnaires on secondhand smoke exposure have been assessed for their reliability and validity, generally based on comparisons with either biomarker or air monitoring data as the "gold" standard (Jaakkola and Jaakkola 1997). Two studies evaluated the reliability of questionnaires on lifetime exposures (Pron et al. 1988; Coultas et al. 1989). Both showed a high degree of repeatability for questions concerning whether a spouse had smoked, but a lower reliability for responses concerning the quantitative aspects of an exposure. Emerson and colleagues (1995) evaluated the repeatability of information from parents of children with asthma. They found a high reliability for parent-reported tobacco use and for the number of cigarettes to which the child was exposed in the home during the past week.

To assess validity, questionnaire reports of current or recent exposures have been compared with levels of cotinine and other biomarkers. These studies tend to show a moderate correlation between levels of cotinine and questionnaire indicators of exposures (Kawachi and Colditz 1996; Cal/EPA 1997; Jaakkola and Jaakkola 1997). However, cotinine levels reflect not only exposure but metabolism and excretion (Benowitz 1999). Consequently, exposure is only one determinant of variation in cotinine levels among persons; there also are individual variations in metabolism and excretion rates. In spite of these sources of variability, mean levels of cotinine vary as anticipated across categories of self-reported exposures (Cal/EPA 1997; Jaakkola and Jaakkola 1997), and self-reported exposures are moderately associated with measured levels of markers (Cal/EPA 1997; Jaakkola and Jaakkola 1997).

Biomarkers are also used for assessing exposures to secondhand smoke. A number of biomarkers are available, but they vary in their specificity and in the dynamics of the temporal relationship between the exposure and the marker level (Cal/EPA 1997; Benowitz 1999). These markers include specific tobacco smoke components (nicotine) or metabolites (cotinine and tobacco-specific nitrosamines), nonspecific biomarkers (thiocyanate and CO), adducts with tobacco smoke components or metabolites (4-aminobiphenyl–hemoglobin adducts, benzo[a]pyrene–DNA adducts, and polycyclic aromatic hydrocarbon–albumin adducts), and nonspecific assays (urinary mutagenicity). Cotinine has been the most widely used biomarker, primarily because of its specificity, half-life, and ease of measurement in body fluids (e.g., urine, blood, and saliva). Biomarkers are discussed

in detail in Chapter 3 (Assessment of Exposure to Secondhand Smoke).

Some epidemiologic studies have also incorporated air monitoring, either direct personal sampling or the indirect approach based on the microenvironmental model. Nicotine, present in the gas phase of secondhand smoke, can be monitored passively with a special filter or actively using a pump and a sorbent. Hammond and Leaderer (1987) first described a diffusion monitor for the passive sampling of nicotine in 1987; this device has now been widely used to assess concentrations in different environments and to study health effects. Airborne particles have also been measured using active monitoring devices.

Each of these approaches for assessing exposures has strengths and limitations, and preference for one over another will depend on the research question and its context (Jaakkola and Jaakkola 1997; Jaakkola and Samet 1999). Questionnaires can be used to characterize sources of exposures, such as smoking by parents. With air concentrations of markers and time-activity information, estimates of secondhand smoke exposures can be made with the microenvironmental model. Biomarkers provide exposure measures that reflect the patterns of exposure and the kinetics of the marker; the cotinine level in body fluids, for example, reflects an exposure during several days. Air monitoring may be useful for validating measurements of exposure. Exposure assessment strategies are matched to the research question and often employ a mixture of approaches determined by feasibility and cost constraints.

Misclassification of Secondhand Smoke Exposure

Misclassification may occur when classifying exposures, outcomes, confounding factors, or modifying factors. Misclassification may be differential on either exposure or outcome, or it may be random (Armstrong et al. 1992). Differential or nonrandom misclassification may either increase or decrease estimates of effect, while random misclassification tends to reduce the apparent effect and weaken the relationship of exposure with disease risk. In studies of secondhand smoke and disease risk, exposure misclassification has been a major consideration in the interpretation of the evidence, although misclassification of health outcome measures has not been a substantial issue in this research. The consequences for epidemiologic studies of misclassification in general are well established (Rothman and Greenland 1998).

An extensive body of literature on the classification of exposures to secondhand smoke is reviewed in this and other chapters, as well as in some publications on the consequences of misclassification (Wu 1999). Two general patterns of exposure misclassification are of concern to secondhand smoke: (1) random misclassification that is not differential by the presence or absence of the health outcome and (2) systematic misclassification that is differential by the health outcome. In studying the health effects of secondhand smoke in adults, there is a further concern as to the classification of the active smoking status (never, current, or former smoking); in studies of children, the accuracy of secondhand smoke exposure classification is the primary methodologic issue around exposure assessment, but unreported active smoking by adolescents is also a concern.

With regard to random misclassification of secondhand smoke exposures, there is an inherent degree of unavoidable measurement error in the exposure measures used in epidemiologic studies. Questionnaires generally assess contact with sources of an exposure (e.g., smoking in the home or workplace) and cannot capture all exposures nor the intensity of exposures; biomarkers provide an exposure index for a particular time window and have intrinsic variability. Some building-related factors that determine an exposure cannot be assessed accurately by a questionnaire, such as the rate of air exchange and the size of the microenvironment where time is spent, nor can concentrations be assessed accurately by subjective reports of the perceived level of tobacco smoke. In general, random misclassification of exposures tends to reduce the likelihood that studies of secondhand smoke exposure will find an effect. This type of misclassification lessens the contrast between exposure groups, because some truly exposed persons are placed in the unexposed group and some truly unexposed persons are placed in the exposed group. Differential misclassification, also a concern, may increase or decrease associations, depending on the pattern of misreporting.

One particular form of misclassification has been raised with regard to secondhand smoke exposure and lung cancer: the classification of some current or former smokers as lifetime nonsmokers (USEPA 1992; Lee and Forey 1995; Hackshaw et al. 1997; Wu 1999). The resulting bias would tend to increase the apparent association of secondhand smoke with lung cancer, if the misclassified active smokers are also more likely to be classified as involuntary smokers. Most studies of lung cancer and secondhand smoke have used spousal smoking as a main exposure variable. As

smoking tends to aggregate between spouses (smokers are more likely to marry smokers), misclassification of active smoking would tend to be differential on the basis of spousal smoking (the exposure under investigation). Because active smoking is strongly associated with increased disease risk, greater misclassification of an actively smoking spouse as a nonsmoker among spouses of smokers compared with spouses of nonsmokers would lead to risk estimates for spousal smoking that are biased upward by the effect of active smoking. This type of misclassification is also relevant to studies of spousal exposure and CHD risk or other diseases also caused by active smoking, although the potential for bias is less because the association of active smoking with CHD is not as strong as with lung cancer.

There have been a number of publications on this form of misclassification. Wu (1999) provides a review, and Lee and colleagues (2001) offer an assessment of potential consequences. A number of models have been developed to assess the extent of bias resulting from the misclassification of active smokers as lifetime nonsmokers (USEPA 1992; Hackshaw et al. 1997). These models incorporate estimates of the rate of misclassification, the degree of aggregation of smokers by marriage, the prevalence of smoking in the population, and the risk of lung cancer in misclassified smokers (Wu 1999). Although debate about this issue continues, analyses show that estimates of upward bias from misclassifying active smokers as lifetime nonsmokers cannot fully explain the observed increase in risk for lung cancer among lifetime nonsmokers married to smokers (Hackshaw et al. 1997; Wu 1999).

There is one additional issue related to exposure misclassification. During the time the epidemiologic studies of secondhand smoke have been carried out, exposure has been widespread and almost unavoidable. Therefore, the risk estimates may be biased downward because there are no truly unexposed persons. The 1986 Surgeon General's report recognized this methodologic issue and noted the need for further data on population exposures to secondhand smoke (USDHHS 1986). This bias was also recognized in the 1986 report of the NRC, and an adjustment for this misclassification was made to the lung cancer estimate (NRC 1986). Similarly, the 1992 report of the EPA commented on background exposure and made an adjustment (USEPA 1992). Some later studies have attempted to address this issue; for example, in a case-control study of active and involuntary smoking and breast cancer in Switzerland, Morabia and colleagues (2000) used a questionnaire to assess exposure and identified a small group of lifetime nonsmokers who also reported no exposure to secondhand smoke. With this subgroup of controls as the reference population, the risks of secondhand smoke exposure were substantially greater for active smoking than when the full control population was used.

This Surgeon General's report further addresses specific issues of exposure misclassification when they are relevant to the health outcome under consideration.

Use of Meta-Analysis

Meta-analysis refers to the process of evaluating and combining a body of research literature that addresses a common question. Meta-analysis is composed of qualitative and quantitative components. The qualitative component involves the systematic identification of all relevant investigations, a systematic assessment of their characteristics and quality, and the decision to include or exclude studies based on predetermined criteria. Consideration can be directed toward sources of bias that might affect the findings. The quantitative component involves the calculation and display of study results on common scales and, if appropriate, the statistical combination of these results across studies and an exploration of the reasons for any heterogeneity of findings. Viewing the findings of all studies as a single plot provides insights into the consistency of results and the precision of the studies considered. Most meta-analyses are based on published summary results, although they are most powerful when applied to data at the level of individual participants. Meta-analysis is most widely used to synthesize evidence from randomized clinical trials, sometimes yielding findings that were not evident from the results of individual studies. Meta-analysis also has been used extensively to examine bodies of observational evidence.

Beginning with the 1986 NRC report, meta-analysis has been used to summarize the evidence on involuntary smoking and health. Meta-analysis was central to the 1992 EPA risk assessment of secondhand smoke, and a series of meta-analyses supported the conclusions of the 1998 report of the Scientific Committee on Tobacco and Health in the United Kingdom. The central role of meta-analysis in interpreting and applying the evidence related to involuntary smoking and disease has led to focused criticisms of the use of meta-analysis in this context. Several papers that acknowledged support from the tobacco industry have addressed the epidemiologic findings for lung cancer, including the selection and quality of the

studies, the methods for meta-analysis, and dose-response associations (Fleiss and Gross 1991; Tweedie and Mengersen 1995; Lee 1998, 1999). In a lawsuit brought by the tobacco industry against the EPA, the 1998 decision handed down by Judge William L. Osteen, Sr., in the North Carolina Federal District Court criticized the approach EPA had used to select studies for its meta-analysis and criticized the use of 90 percent rather than 95 percent confidence intervals for the summary estimates (*Flue-Cured Tobacco Cooperative Stabilization Corp. v. United States Environmental Protection Agency*, 857 F. Supp. 1137 [M.D.N.C. 1993]). In December 2002, the 4th U.S. Circuit Court of Appeals threw out the lawsuit on the basis that tobacco companies cannot sue the EPA over its secondhand smoke report because the report was not a final agency action and therefore not subject to court review (*Flue-Cured Tobacco Cooperative Stabilization Corp. v. The United States Environmental Protection Agency*, No. 98-2407 [4th Cir., December 11, 2002], *cited in* 17.7 TPLR 2.472 [2003]).

Recognizing that there is still an active discussion around the use of meta-analysis to pool data from observational studies (versus clinical trials), the authors of this Surgeon General's report used this methodology to summarize the available data when deemed appropriate and useful, even while recognizing that the uncertainty around the meta-analytic estimates may exceed the uncertainty indicated by conventional statistical indices, because of biases either within the observational studies or produced by the manner of their selection. However, a decision to not combine estimates might have produced conclusions that are far more uncertain than the data warrant because the review would have focused on individual study results without considering their overall pattern, and without allowing for a full accounting of different sample sizes and effect estimates.

The possibility of publication bias has been raised as a potential limitation to the interpretation of evidence on involuntary smoking and disease in general, and on lung cancer and secondhand smoke exposure specifically. A 1988 paper by Vandenbroucke used a descriptive approach, called a "funnel plot," to assess the possibility that publication bias affected the 13 studies considered in a review by Wald and colleagues (1986). This type of plot characterizes the relationship between the magnitude of estimates and their precision. Vandenbroucke suggested the possibility of publication bias only in reference to the studies of men. Bero and colleagues (1994) concluded that there had not been a publication bias against studies with statistically significant findings, nor against the publication of studies with nonsignificant or mixed findings in the research literature. The researchers were able to identify only five unpublished "negative" studies, of which two were dissertations that tend to be delayed in publication. A subsequent study by Misakian and Bero (1998) did find a delay in the publication of studies with nonsignificant results in comparison with studies having significant results; whether this pattern has varied over the several decades of research on secondhand smoke was not addressed. More recently, Copas and Shi (2000) assessed the 37 studies considered in the meta-analysis by Hackshaw and colleagues (1997) for publication bias. Copas and Shi (2000) found a significant correlation between the estimated risk of exposure and sample size, such that smaller studies tended to have higher values. This pattern suggests the possibility of publication bias. However, using a funnel plot of the same studies, Lubin (1999) found little evidence for publication bias.

On this issue of publication bias, it is critical to distinguish between indirect statistical arguments and arguments based on actual identification of previously unidentified research. The strongest case against substantive publication bias has been made by researchers who mounted intensive efforts to find the possibly missing studies; these efforts have yielded little—nothing that would alter published conclusions (Bero et al. 1994; Glantz 2000). Presumably because this exposure is a great public health concern, the findings of studies that do not have statistically significant outcomes continue to be published (Kawachi and Colditz 1996).

The quantitative results of the meta-analyses, however, were not determinate in making causal inferences in this Surgeon General's report. In particular, the level of statistical significance of estimates from the meta-analyses was not a predominant factor in making a causal conclusion. For that purpose, this report relied on the approach and criteria set out in the 1964 and 2004 reports of the Surgeon General, which involved judgments based on an array of quantitative and qualitative considerations that included the degree of heterogeneity in the designs of the studies that were examined. Sometimes this heterogeneity limits the inference from meta-analysis by weakening the rationale for pooling the study results. However, the availability of consistent evidence from heterogenous designs can strengthen the meta-analytic findings by making it unlikely that a common bias could persist across different study designs and populations.

Confounding

Confounding, which refers in this context to the mixing of the effect of another factor with that of secondhand smoke, has been proposed as an explanation for associations of secondhand smoke with adverse health consequences. Confounding occurs when the factor of interest (secondhand smoke) is associated in the data under consideration with another factor (the confounder) that, by itself, increases the risk for the disease (Rothman and Greenland 1998). Correlates of secondhand smoke exposures are not confounding factors unless an exposure to them increases the risk of disease. A factor proposed as a potential confounder is not necessarily an actual confounder unless it fulfills the two elements of the definition. Although lengthy lists of potential confounding factors have been offered as alternatives to direct associations of secondhand smoke exposures with the risk for disease, the factors on these lists generally have not been shown to be confounding in the particular data of interest.

The term confounding also conveys an implicit conceptualization as to the causal pathways that link secondhand smoke and the confounding factor to

Figure 1.2   Model for socioeconomic status (SES) and secondhand smoke (SHS) exposure

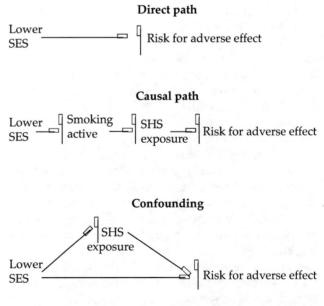

Arrows indicate directionality of association.

disease risk. Confounding implies that the confounding factor has an effect on risk that is independent of secondhand smoke exposure. Some factors considered as potential confounders may, however, be in the same causal pathway as a secondhand smoke exposure. Although socioeconomic status (SES) is often cited as a potential confounding factor, it may not have an independent effect but can affect disease risk through its association with secondhand smoke exposure (Figure 1.2). This figure shows general alternative relationships among SES, secondhand smoke exposure, and risk for an adverse effect. SES may have a direct effect, or it may indirectly exert its effect through an association with secondhand smoke exposure, or it may confound the relationship between secondhand smoke exposure and disease risk. To control for SES as a potential confounding factor without considering underlying relationships may lead to incorrect risk estimates. For example, controlling for SES would not be appropriate if it is a determinant of secondhand smoke exposure but has no direct effect.

Nonetheless, because the health effects of involuntary smoking have other causes, the possibility of confounding needs careful exploration when assessing associations of secondhand smoke exposure with adverse health effects. In addition, survey data from the last several decades show that secondhand smoke exposure is associated with correlates of lifestyle that may influence the risk for some health effects, thus increasing concerns for the possibility of confounding (Kawachi and Colditz 1996). Survey data from the United States (Matanoski et al. 1995) and the United Kingdom (Thornton et al. 1994) show that adults with secondhand smoke exposures generally tend to have less healthful lifestyles. However, the extent to which these patterns of association can be generalized, either to other countries or to the past, is uncertain.

The potential bias from confounding varies with the association of the confounder to secondhand smoke exposures in a particular study and to the strength of the confounder as a risk factor. The importance of confounding to the interpretation of evidence depends further on the magnitude of the effect of secondhand smoke on disease. As the strength of an association lessens, confounding as an alternative explanation for an association becomes an increasing concern. In prior reviews, confounding has been addressed either quantitatively (Hackshaw et al. 1997) or qualitatively (Cal/EPA 1997; Thun et al. 1999). In the chapters in this report that focus on specific diseases, confounding is specifically addressed in the context of potential confounding factors for the particular diseases.

Tobacco Industry Activities

The evidence on secondhand smoke and disease risk, given the public health and public policy implications, has been reviewed extensively in the published peer-reviewed literature and in evaluations by a number of expert panels. In addition, the evidence has been criticized repeatedly by the tobacco industry and its consultants in venues that have included the peer-reviewed literature, public meetings and hearings, and scientific symposia that included symposia sponsored by the industry. Open criticism in the peer-reviewed literature can strengthen the credibility of scientific evidence by challenging researchers to consider the arguments proposed by critics and to rebut them.

Industry documents indicate that the tobacco industry has engaged in widespread activities, however, that have gone beyond the bounds of accepted scientific practice (Glantz 1996; Ong and Glantz 2000, 2001; Rampton and Stauber 2000; Yach and Bialous 2001; Hong and Bero 2002; Diethelm et al. 2004). Through a variety of organized tactics, the industry has attempted to undermine the credibility of the scientific evidence on secondhand smoke. The industry has funded or carried out research that has been judged to be biased, supported scientists to generate letters to editors that criticized research publications, attempted to undermine the findings of key studies, assisted in establishing a scientific society with a journal, and attempted to sustain controversy even as the scientific community reached consensus (Garne et al. 2005). These tactics are not a topic of this report, but to the extent that the scientific literature has been distorted, they are addressed as the evidence is reviewed. This report does not specifically identify tobacco industry sponsorship of publications unless that information is relevant to the interpretation of the findings and conclusions.

References

Armstrong BK, White E, Saracci R, editors. *Principles of Exposure Measurement in Epidemiology*. Monographs in Epidemiology and Biostatistics. Vol. 21. New York: Oxford University Press, 1992.

Benowitz NL. Biomarkers of environmental tobacco smoke. *Environmental Health Perspectives* 1999;107(Suppl 2):349–55.

Bero LA, Glantz SA, Rennie D. Publication bias and public health policy on environmental tobacco smoke. *Journal of the American Medical Association* 1994;272(2):133–6.

California Environmental Protection Agency. *Health Effects of Exposure to Environmental Tobacco Smoke*. Sacramento (CA): California Environmental Protection Agency, Office of Environmental Health Hazard Assessment, Reproductive and Cancer Hazard Assessment Section and Air Toxicology and Epidemiology Section, 1997.

California Environmental Protection Agency. *Proposed Identification of Environmental Tobacco Smoke as a Toxic Air Contaminant. Part B: Health Effects*. Sacramento (CA): California Environmental Protection Agency, Office of Environmental Health Hazard Assessment, 2005.

Copas JB, Shi JQ. Reanalysis of epidemiological evidence on lung cancer and passive smoking. *British Medical Journal* 2000;320(7232):417–8.

Coultas DB, Peake GT, Samet JM. Questionnaire assessment of lifetime and recent exposure to environmental tobacco smoke. *American Journal of Epidemiology* 1989;130(2):338–47.

Diethelm PA, Rielle JC, McKee M. The whole truth and nothing but the truth? The research that Phillip Morris did not want you to see, November 11, 2004; <http://image.thelancet.com/extras/03art7306web.pdf>; accessed: January 6, 2005.

Emerson JA, Hovell MF, Meltzer SB, Zakarian JM, Hofstetter CR, Wahlgren DR, Leaderer BP, Meltzer EO. The accuracy of environmental tobacco smoke exposure measures among asthmatic children. *Journal of Clinical Epidemiology* 1995;48(10):1251–9.

Fleiss JL, Gross AJ. Meta-analysis in epidemiology, with special reference to studies of the association between exposure to environmental tobacco smoke and lung cancer: a critique. *Journal of Clinical Epidemiology* 1991;44(2):127–39.

Flue-Cured Tobacco Cooperative Stabilization Corp. v. United States Environmental Protection Agency (M.D.N.C. June 22, 1993), *cited in* 8.2 TPLR 3.97 (1993).

Flue-Cured Tobacco Cooperative Stabilization Corp. v. The United States Environmental Protection Agency, No. 98-2407 (4th Cir., December 11, 2002), *cited in* 17.7 TPLR 2.472 (2003) (Overturning lower court's decision invalidating EPA's findings that secondhand smoke is a "known human carcinogen").

Fontham ET, Correa P, Reynolds P, Wu-Williams A, Buffler PA, Greenberg RS, Chen VW, Alterman T, Boyd P, Austin DF, Liff J. Environmental tobacco smoke and lung cancer in nonsmoking women: a multicenter study. *Journal of the American Medical Association* 1994;271(22):1752–9.

Garne D, Watson M, Chapman S, Byrne F. Environmental tobacco smoke research published in the journal *Indoor and Built Environment* and associations with the tobacco industry. *Lancet* 2005; 365(9461):804–9.

Glantz SA. The ledger of tobacco control. *Journal of the American Medical Association* 1996;276(11):871–2.

Glantz SA. Lung cancer and passive smoking: nothing new was said. *British Medical Journal* 2000;321(7270):1222–3.

Hackshaw AK, Law MR, Wald NJ. The accumulated evidence on lung cancer and environmental tobacco smoke. *British Medical Journal* 1997;315(7114): 980–8.

Hammond SK, Leaderer BP. A diffusion monitor to measure exposure to passive smoking. *Environmental Science & Technology* 1987;21(5):494–7.

Hong MK, Bero LA. How the tobacco industry responded to an influential study of the health effects of secondhand smoke. *British Medical Journal* 2002;325(7377):1413–6.

International Agency for Research on Cancer. *IARC Monographs on the Evaluation of the Carcinogenic Risk of Chemicals to Humans: Tobacco Smoking*. Vol. 38. Lyon (France): International Agency for Research on Cancer, 1986.

International Agency for Research on Cancer. *IARC Monographs on the Evaluation of Carcinogenic Risks to Humans: Tobacco Smoke and Involuntary Smoking*. Vol. 83. Lyon (France): International Agency for Research on Cancer, 2004.

Jaakkola MS, Jaakkola JJ. Assessment of exposure to environmental tobacco smoke. *European Respiratory Journal* 1997;10(10):2384–97.

Jaakkola MS, Samet JM. Environmental tobacco smoke: risk assessment. *Environmental Health Perspectives* 1999;107(Suppl 6):823–904.

Kawachi I, Colditz GA. Invited commentary: confounding, measurement error, and publication bias in studies of passive smoking. *American Journal of Epidemiology* 1996;144(10):909–15.

Klepeis NE. An introduction to the indirect exposure assessment approach: modeling human exposure using microenvironmental measurements and the recent National Human Activity Pattern Survey. *Environmental Health Perspectives* 1999;107(Suppl 2):365–74.

Lee PN. Difficulties in assessing the relationship between passive smoking and lung cancer. *Statistical Methods in Medical Research* 1998;7(2):137–63.

Lee PN. Simple methods for checking for possible errors in reported odds ratios, relative risks and confidence intervals. *Statistics in Medicine* 1999;18(15):1973–81.

Lee PN, Forey BA. Misclassification of smoking habits as determined by cotinine or by repeated self-report—summary of evidence from 42 studies. *Journal of Smoking-Related Diseases* 1995;6:109–29.

Lee PN, Forey B, Fry JS. Revisiting the association between environmental tobacco smoke exposure and lung cancer risk. III: Adjusting for the biasing effect of misclassification of smoking habits. *Indoor and Built Environment* 2001;10(6):384–98.

Lubin JH. Estimating lung cancer risk with exposure to environmental tobacco smoke. *Environmental Health Perspectives* 1999;107(Suppl 6):879–83.

Matanoski G, Kanchanaraksa S, Lantry D, Chang Y. Characteristics of nonsmoking women in NHANES I and NHANES I Epidemiologic Follow-up Study with exposure to spouses who smoke. *American Journal of Epidemiology* 1995;142(2):149–57.

Misakian AL, Bero LA. Publication bias and research on passive smoking: comparison of published and unpublished studies. *Journal of the American Medical Association* 1998;280(3):250–3.

Morabia A, Bernstein MS, Bouchardy I, Kurtz J, Morris MA. Breast cancer and active and passive smoking: the role of the N-acetyltransferase 2 genotype. *American Journal of Epidemiology* 2000;152(3):226–32.

National Health and Medical Research Council. *The Health Effects of Passive Smoking*. A scientific information paper. Canberra (Commonwealth of Australia): Canberra ACT, 1997.

National Research Council. *Environmental Tobacco Smoke: Measuring Exposures and Assessing Health Effects*. Washington: National Academy Press, 1986.

National Research Council. *Human Exposure Assessment for Airborne Pollutants: Advances and Opportunities*. Washington: National Academy Press, 1991.

Ong EK, Glantz SA. Tobacco industry efforts subverting International Agency for Research on Cancer's second-hand smoke study. *Lancet* 2000;355(9211):1253–9.

Ong EK, Glantz SA. Constructing "sound science" and "good epidemiology": tobacco, lawyers, and public relations firms. *American Journal of Public Health* 2001;91(11):1749–57.

Pron GE, Burch JD, Howe GR, Miller AB. The reliability of passive smoking histories reported in a case-control study of lung cancer. *American Journal of Epidemiology* 1988;127(2):267–73.

Rampton S, Stauber J. *Trust Us, We're Experts: How Industry Manipulates Science and Gambles with Your Future*. Los Angeles: J.P. Tarcher, 2000.

Rothman KJ, Greenland S. *Modern Epidemiology*, 2nd ed. Philadelphia: Lippincott-Raven, 1998.

Samet JM, Jaakkola JJK. The epidemiologic approach to investigating outdoor air pollution. In: Holgate ST, Samet JM, Koren HS, Maynard RL, editors. *Air Pollution and Health*. San Diego: Academic Press, 1999:431–60.

Scientific Committee on Tobacco and Health. *Report of the Scientific Committee on Tobacco and Health*. London: The Stationery Office, 1998.

Thornton A, Lee P, Fry J. Differences between smokers, ex-smokers, passive smokers and non-smokers. *Journal of Clinical Epidemiology* 1994;47(10):1143–62.

Thun M, Henley J, Apicella L. Epidemiologic studies of fatal and nonfatal cardiovascular disease and ETS exposure from spousal smoking. *Environmental Health Perspectives* 1999;107(Suppl 6):841–6.

Tweedie RL, Mengersen KL. Meta-analytic approaches to dose-response relationships, with application in studies of lung cancer and exposure to environmental tobacco smoke. *Statistics in Medicine* 1995;14(5–7):545–69.

U.S. Department of Health and Human Services. *The Health Consequences of Smoking: Cancer. A Report of the Surgeon General*. Rockville (MD): U.S. Department of Health and Human Services, Public Health Service, Office on Smoking and Health. 1982. DHHS Publication No. (PHS) 82-50179.

U.S. Department of Health and Human Services. *The Health Consequences of Smoking: Chronic Obstructive Lung Disease. A Report of the Surgeon General*. Rockville (MD): U.S. Department of Health and Human

Services, Public Health Service, Office on Smoking and Health, 1984. DHHS Publication No. (PHS) 84-50205.

U.S. Department of Health and Human Services. *The Health Consequences of Involuntary Smoking. A Report of the Surgeon General*. Rockville (MD): U.S. Department of Health and Human Services, Public Health Service, Centers for Disease Control, Center for Health Promotion and Education, Office on Smoking and Health, 1986. DHHS Publication No. (CDC) 87-8398.

U.S. Department of Health and Human Services. *Preventing Tobacco Use Among Young People. A Report of the Surgeon General*. Atlanta: U.S. Department of Health and Human Services, Public Health Service, Centers for Disease Control and Prevention, National Center for Chronic Disease Prevention and Health Promotion, Office on Smoking and Health, 1994.

U.S. Department of Health and Human Services. *Tobacco Use Among U.S. Racial/Ethnic Minority Groups—African Americans, American Indians and Alaska Natives, Asian Americans and Pacific Islanders, and Hispanics. A Report of the Surgeon General*. Atlanta: U.S. Department of Health and Human Services, Centers for Disease Control and Prevention, National Center for Chronic Disease Prevention and Health Promotion, Office on Smoking and Health, 1998.

U.S. Department of Health and Human Services. *Women and Smoking. A Report of the Surgeon General*. Rockville (MD): U.S. Department of Health and Human Services, Public Health Service, Office of the Surgeon General, 2001.

U.S. Department of Health and Human Services. *The Health Consequences of Smoking: A Report of the Surgeon General*. Atlanta: U.S. Department of Health and Human Services, Centers for Disease Control and Prevention, National Center for Chronic Disease Prevention and Health Promotion, Office on Smoking and Health, 2004.

U.S. Department of Health, Education, and Welfare. *Smoking and Health: Report of the Advisory Committee to the Surgeon General of the Public Health Service*. Washington: U.S. Department of Health, Education, and Welfare, Public Health Service, Center for Disease Control, 1964. PHS Publication No. 1103.

U.S. Department of Health, Education, and Welfare. *The Health Consequences of Smoking. A Report of the Surgeon General: 1972*. Washington: U.S. Department of Health, Education, and Welfare, Public Health Service, Health Services and Mental Health Administration, 1972. DHEW Publication No. (HSM) 72-7516.

U.S. Department of Health, Education, and Welfare. *The Health Consequences of Smoking. A Report of the Surgeon General, 1975*. Washington: U.S. Department of Health, Education, and Welfare, Public Health Service, Center for Disease Control, 1975. DHEW Publication No. (CDC) 77-8704.

U.S. Department of Health, Education, and Welfare. *Smoking and Health. A Report of the Surgeon General*. Washington: U.S. Department of Health, Education, and Welfare, Public Health Service, Office of the Assistant Secretary for Health, Office of Smoking and Health, 1979. DHEW Publication No. (PHS) 79-50066.

U.S. Environmental Protection Agency. *Respiratory Health Effects of Passive Smoking: Lung Cancer and Other Disorders*. Washington: U.S. Environmental Protection Agency, Office of Research and Development, Office of Air Radiation, 1992. Report No. EPA/600/6-90/0006F.

Vandenbroucke JP. Passive smoking and lung cancer: a publication bias? *British Medical Journal (Clinical Research Edition)* 1988;296(6619):391–2.

Wald NJ, Nanchahal K, Thompson SG, Cuckle HS. Does breathing other people's tobacco smoke cause lung cancer? *British Medical Journal (Clinical Research Edition)* 1986;293(6556):1217–22.

World Health Organization. *International Consultation on Environmental Tobacco Smoke (ETS) and Child Health. Consultation Report*. Geneva: World Health Organization, 1999.

Wu AH. Exposure misclassification bias in studies of environmental tobacco smoke and lung cancer. *Environmental Health Perspectives* 1999;107(Suppl 6):873–7.

Yach D, Bialous SA. Junking science to promote tobacco. *American Journal of Public Health* 2001;91(11):1745–8.

Chapter 2
Toxicology of Secondhand Smoke

Introduction

A full range of scientific evidence, extending from the molecular level to whole populations, supports the conclusion that secondhand smoke causes disease. The scope of this evidence is enormous, and encompasses not only the literature on secondhand smoke but also relevant findings on active smoking and on the toxicity of individual tobacco smoke components. The 2004 report of the Surgeon General provides reviews on biologic considerations in relation to active smoking (U.S. Department of Health and Human Services [USDHHS] 2004). The guidelines for causal inference include coherence, which is defined as the extent to which all lines of scientific evidence converge in support of a causal conclusion. Beginning with the 1964 Surgeon General's report on smoking and health (U.S. Department of Health, Education, and Welfare [USDHEW] 1964), reports in this series have comprehensively evaluated the full scope of evidence supporting causal inference with regard to particular associations of smoking with disease. This chapter reviews the evidence relevant to coherence, and includes the mechanisms relevant to the pathogenesis of diseases caused by secondhand smoke.

Studies reviewed for this chapter were selected from Medline and SciFinder literature searches. Search terms included "carcinogens," "environmental tobacco smoke," "DNA adducts," "protein adducts," "urinary metabolites," "tobacco smoke," and the names of specific carcinogens and their metabolites. Recent reviews and cited references in recent papers provided additional sources for this chapter.

This chapter sets out a foundation for interpreting the observational evidence that is the focus of most of the following chapters. The discussion that follows details the mechanisms that enable tobacco smoke components to injure the respiratory tract and cardiovascular system and to cause nonmalignant and malignant diseases and other adverse effects.

Composition of Tobacco Smoke

The chemical and physical properties of tobacco smoke from mainstream (drawn through the cigarette) and sidestream (released by the smoldering cigarette) smoke have been reviewed in a number of publications (Jenkins et al. 2000; Hoffmann et al. 2001; International Agency for Research on Cancer [IARC] 2004; California Environmental Protection Agency [Cal/EPA] 2005). The IARC (2004) review indicates that some 4,000 mainstream tobacco smoke compounds have been identified (Roberts 1988), and the qualitative composition of the components is nearly identical in mainstream smoke, sidestream smoke, and secondhand smoke. An assessment by the National Research Council (1986) of differences in the composition of mainstream and sidestream smoke indicates that some compounds are emitted at levels up to more than 10 times greater in sidestream smoke compared with mainstream smoke (see also Table III-1 in Cal/EPA 2005). The Cal/EPA (2005) report identified 19 gas-phase and 21 particulate matter compounds in sidestream smoke with known carcinogenic and noncarcinogenic health effects (e.g., pulmonary edema, immune alterations, cardiac arrthythmias, and hepatotoxic and neurologic effects). The National Toxicology Program (USDHHS 2000) estimates that at least 250 chemicals in secondhand smoke are known to be toxic or carcinogenic. Other published reports have additional listings of specific chemical compounds in mainstream and secondhand smoke (Fowles and Dybing 2003; Cal/EPA 2005).

Evidence of Carcinogenic Effects from Secondhand Smoke Exposure

Carcinogens in Sidestream Smoke and Secondhand Smoke

As a result of advances in chemical analytical techniques and an expanded understanding of the mechanisms by which environmental agents are genotoxic, the number of known carcinogens in tobacco smoke increased to 69 in the year 2000 (IARC 2004). Table 2.1 summarizes representative levels of carcinogens found in sidestream and secondhand cigarette smoke, but includes only 30 compounds that have been evaluated by IARC and that have fulfilled certain other criteria: sufficient evidence of carcinogenicity in either laboratory animals or humans and published data on levels found in sidestream or secondhand smoke. Field studies on the carcinogenic composition of secondhand smoke cannot comprehensively evaluate all of the potential carcinogens in secondhand smoke. Some tobacco smoke carcinogens that IARC evaluated were not included in Table 2.1 because there were no published data on their levels in sidestream or secondhand cigarette smoke (Hoffmann et al. 2001). It is likely, however, that these carcinogens (which include some polycyclic aromatic hydrocarbons [PAHs], heterocycles, heterocyclic aromatic amines, nitro compounds, and other miscellaneous organic compounds) are also present in sidestream and secondhand smoke. In addition, there may be carcinogens present that IARC has not yet fully characterized or evaluated.

PAHs are a diverse group of compounds formed in the incomplete combustion of organic material, and are potent, locally acting carcinogens in laboratory animals. PAHs induce tumors of the upper respiratory tract and lung when inhaled, instilled in the trachea, implanted in the lung, or administered by other routes (Shimkin and Stoner 1975), and are found in tobacco smoke, broiled foods, and polluted environments of various types. The best known member of this class of compounds is benzo[*a*]pyrene (B[*a*]P), which induces tumors of the upper respiratory tract and lung when inhaled, instilled in the trachea, implanted in the lung, or administered intraperitoneally, intravenously, subcutaneously, or by other routes (Shimkin and Stoner 1975). When administered systemically, B[*a*]P causes lung tumors in mice but not in rats (IARC 1973, 1983; Culp et al. 1998). Workers in iron and steel foundries and aluminum and coke production plants are exposed to PAHs. These exposures are considered to be a cause of excess cancers among workers in these settings (IARC 1983, 1984).

N-Nitrosamines are a large group of carcinogens that induce cancer in a wide variety of species and tissues and are presumed to cause cancer in humans (Preussmann and Stewart 1984). These carcinogens can be formed endogenously from amines and nitrogen oxides and are found at low levels in foods (Bartsch and Spiegelhalder 1996). Tobacco smoke contains volatile *N*-nitrosamines such as *N*-nitrosodimethylamine and *N*-nitrosopyrrolidine, as well as tobacco-specific *N*-nitrosamines such as *N'*-nitrosonornicotine (NNN) and 4-(methylnitrosamino)-1-(3-pyridyl)-1-butanone (NNK) (Hoffmann and Hecht 1990). Tobacco-specific *N*-nitrosamines are chemically related to nicotine and other tobacco alkaloids and are therefore found only in tobacco products or related materials (Hecht and Hoffmann 1988). In laboratory animals, many *N*-nitrosamines are powerful carcinogens that display a striking organospecificity and affect particular tissues often independently of the route of administration (Preussmann and Stewart 1984). For example, NNN causes tumors of the esophagus and nasal cavity in rats, while the principal target of NNK in rodents is the lung; NNK is the only tobacco smoke carcinogen that induces lung tumors by systemic administration in all three commonly used rodent models—rat, mouse, and hamster (Hecht 1998).

Among the aromatic amines first identified as carcinogens in dye industrial exposures, 2-naphthylamine and 4-aminobiphenyl are well-established human bladder carcinogens (IARC 1973, 1974). These carcinogens are also found in tobacco smoke. Aromatic amines cause tumors at a variety of sites in laboratory animals. Some members of this class, such as 2-toluidine, are only weakly carcinogenic (Garner et al. 1984).

Formaldehyde and acetaldehyde, weaker carcinogens than PAHs, *N*-nitrosamines, and aromatic amines, have been measured in sidestream and secondhand smoke. When inhaled, formaldehyde and acetaldehyde induce respiratory tract tumors in rodents (Kerns et al. 1983; IARC 1999). Butadiene and benzene are volatile hydrocarbons that also occur in considerable quantities in sidestream and secondhand smoke. Butadiene is a multiorgan carcinogen that is particularly potent in mice; benzene causes leukemia

Table 2.1   Levels of carcinogens in sidestream and secondhand cigarette smoke

| Carcinogen | Representative amounts | | Study |
	Sidestream (per cigarette)	Secondhand (per cubic meter [m³])	
Polycyclic aromatic hydrocarbons			
Benz[a]anthracene	201 nanograms (ng)	0.32–1.7 ng	Grimmer et al. 1987; Chuang et al. 1991
Benzo[a]pyrene	45–103 ng	0.37–1.7 ng	Adams et al. 1987; Grimmer et al. 1987; Chuang et al. 1991
Benzo[b]fluoranthene Benzo[j]fluoranthene Benzo[k]fluoranthene	196 ng	0.79–2.0 ng	Grimmer et al. 1987; Chuang et al. 1991
Dibenz[a,h]anthracene	NR*	1 ng	Vu-Duc and Huynh 1989
Indeno[1,2,3-cd]pyrene	51 ng	0.35–1.1 ng	Grimmer et al. 1987; Chuang et al. 1991
5-Methylchrysene	NR	35.5 ng	Vu-Duc and Huynh 1989
N-Nitrosamines			
N-Nitrosodiethanolamine	43 ng	NR	Brunnemann and Hoffmann 1981
N-Nitrosodiethylamine	8.2–73 ng	0–20 ng	Brunnemann et al. 1977; Hoffmann et al. 1987
N-Nitrosodimethylamine	143–1,040 ng	4–240 ng	Brunnemann et al. 1977; Hoffmann et al. 1987; Klus et al. 1992
N-Nitrosoethylmethylamine	3–35 ng	NR	Brunnemann et al. 1977; Hoffmann et al. 1987
N'-Nitrosonornicotine	110–857 ng	0.7–23 ng	Brunnemann et al. 1983, 1992; Adams et al. 1987; Klus et al. 1992
N-Nitrosopiperidine	4.8–19.8 ng	NR	Adams et al. 1987
N-Nitrosopyrrolidine	7–700 ng	3.5–27.0 ng	Brunnemann et al. 1977; Hoffmann et al. 1987; Klus et al. 1992; Mahanama and Daisey 1996
4-(Methylnitrosamino)-1-(3-pyridyl)-1-butanone	201–1,440 ng	0.2–29.3 ng	Brunnemann et al. 1983, 1992; Adams et al. 1987; Klus et al. 1992
Aromatic amines			
2-Naphthylamine	63.1–128 ng	NR	Government of British Columbia Ministry of Health Services 2001
2-Toluidine	3,030 ng	NR	Patrianakos and Hoffmann 1979
4-Aminobiphenyl	11.4–18.8 ng	NR	Government of British Columbia Ministry of Health Services 2001
Aldehydes			
Acetaldehyde	961–1,820 micrograms (µg)	268 µg	Martin et al. 1997; Government of British Columbia Ministry of Health Services 2001
Formaldehyde	233–485 µg	143 µg	Martin et al. 1997; Government of British Columbia Ministry of Health Services 2001

Table 2.1   Continued

Carcinogen	Representative amounts		Study
	Sidestream (per cigarette)	Secondhand (per cubic meter [m³])	
Miscellaneous organics			
Acrylonitrile	42–109 μg	NR	Government of British Columbia Ministry of Health Services 2001
Benzene	163–353 μg	4.2–63.7 μg	Scherer et al. 1995; Heavner et al. 1996; Martin et al. 1997; Government of British Columbia Ministry of Health Services 2001; Kim et al. 2001
Catechol	98–292 μg	1.24 μg	Sakuma et al. 1983; Martin et al. 1997; Government of British Columbia Ministry of Health Services 2001
Isoprene	668–1,260 μg	657 μg	Martin et al. 1997; Government of British Columbia Ministry of Health Services 2001
1,3-Butadiene	98–205 μg	0.3–40 μg	Heavner et al. 1996; Martin et al. 1997; Government of British Columbia Ministry of Health Services 2001; Kim et al. 2001
Inorganic compounds			
Cadmium	330–689 ng	4–38 ng	Wu et al. 1995; Government of British Columbia Ministry of Health Services 2001
Chromium	57–79 ng	NR	Government of British Columbia Ministry of Health Services 2001
Hydrazine	94 ng	NR	Liu et al. 1974
Lead	28.9–46.6 ng	NR	Government of British Columbia Ministry of Health Services 2001
Nickel	51 ng	NR	Government of British Columbia Ministry of Health Services 2001
Polonium-210	0.091–0.139 picocurie	NR	Ferri and Baratta 1966

*NR = Data were not reported.
Source: Adapted from Hoffmann et al. 2001.

in humans (IARC 1982, 1992, 1999). Metals such as nickel, chromium, and cadmium are human carcinogens that are also present in sidestream smoke (IARC 1990, 1994).

Mainstream cigarette smoke consists of a gas phase and a particulate phase specifically composed of several million semiliquid particles per cubic centimeter (cm³) within a mixture of combustion gases (Ingebrethsen 1986; Guerin et al. 1992). Sidestream smoke contains free radicals in about the same concentrations as does mainstream smoke (Pryor et al. 1983). Pryor and colleagues (1998) detected reactive yet long-lived radicals in the gas phase; in the particulate phase, these investigators found a free radical system that is a mixture of semiquinones, hydroquinones, and quinones (Pryor et al. 1998). Whether such agents can induce tumors in laboratory animals is not known.

Carcinogenicity of Sidestream Smoke and Secondhand Smoke

Numerous studies have demonstrated that mainstream cigarette smoke condensate, the solid materials in the smoke, induces tumors on mouse skin and, by implantation, in rat lungs (IARC 1986, 2004). Inhalation experiments with mainstream smoke have demonstrated that cigarette smoke and its particulate phase induce preneoplastic lesions and benign and malignant tumors of the larynx in Syrian golden hamsters (IARC 1986). Studies with rats and mice documented less consistent results (IARC 1986, 2004; Hecht 1999).

The carcinogenicity of sidestream smoke has been less extensively investigated. Sidestream smoke condensate was significantly more carcinogenic than mainstream smoke condensate when tested on mouse skin: mice treated with sidestream smoke developed two to six times more skin tumors than mice treated

with mainstream smoke (Mohtashamipur et al. 1990). In a rat model using implanted sidestream smoke particles, a fraction containing PAHs with four or more rings produced tumors, while a fraction with semivolatiles and a PAH fraction with fewer rings had little effect (Grimmer et al. 1988). Limited histopathologic changes were observed in rats exposed to cigarette sidestream smoke aged in the chamber for 12 months (Haussmann et al. 1998). Researchers have carried out a series of investigations on the effects of secondhand smoke inhalation in A/J mice (Witschi et al. 1995, 1997a,b,c, 1998, 1999, 2000; Witschi 1998, 2000). Table 2.2 summarizes the data from these studies. Lung tumor multiplicity, the most sensitive indicator of response in this model, increased significantly in all experiments, and lung tumor incidence increased in several experiments. The protocol involved exposing mice to secondhand smoke (89 percent sidestream smoke and 11 percent mainstream smoke) for five months followed by a four-month recovery period in air. Other experiments have demonstrated that to observe an increase in lung tumor multiplicity, there must be a recovery period. These same experiments also showed that the response is due to a gas-phase component of secondhand smoke.

Table 2.2   Inhalation studies of secondhand smoke (89% sidestream smoke and 11% mainstream smoke) in A/J mice

Study	Exposure (mg/m³* of total suspended particulates)	Lung tumor multiplicity[†]		Lung tumor incidence[‡]	
		Filtered air control	Smoke	Filtered air control (%)	Smoke (%)
Witschi et al. 1997a	79	0.5 ± 0.1 (24)	1.3 ± 0.3 (26)[§]	42	58
Witschi et al. 1997b	87	0.5 ± 0.2 (24)	1.4 ± 0.2 (24)[§]	38	83[§]
Witschi et al. 1998	83	0.9 ± 0.2 (29)	1.3 ± 0.2 (33)[§]	69	73
Witschi et al. 1999	132	0.6 ± 0.1 (30)	2.1 ± 0.3 (38)[§]	50	86[Δ]
Witschi et al. 2000	137	0.9 ± 0.2 (30)	2.8 ± 0.2 (38)[§]	60	100[Δ]
	137	1.0 ± 0.1 (54)	2.4 ± 0.3 (28)[§]	65	89[Δ]
Witschi et al., unpublished data	134	1.2 ± 0.2 (25)	2.3 ± 0.3 (26)[§]	60	88[Δ]

*mg/m³ = Milligrams per cubic meter.
[†]Mean ± standard error (number of animals is in parentheses).
[‡]Percentage of all animals at risk that had tumors.
[§]Significantly different (p <0.05) compared with air controls by Welsh's alternate test.
[Δ]Significantly different (p <0.05) compared with air controls by Fisher's exact test.
Source: Adapted from Witschi 2000.

Although these results are of interest, there are some poorly understood features of the model. The animals lose weight during exposure and never weigh as much as the air-treated controls even after the recovery period. The consequences of the weight loss are unknown. The reason for the recovery period requirement also is not clear. In addition, the apparent tumor-inducing effect of the gas phase is inconsistent with most of the earlier work on mainstream smoke inhalation and with the tumor-inducing properties of sidestream smoke condensate described above. Finally, recent data from De Flora and colleagues (2003) somewhat contradict the observations of Witschi and colleagues (1995, 1997a,b,c, 1998, 1999, 2000). De Flora and colleagues (2003) exposed Swiss strain mice to environmental tobacco smoke continuously for a period of nine months without a recovery period and observed a significant increase in the lung tumor response.

Collectively, these studies suggest the potential involvement of multiple carcinogens from sidestream and secondhand cigarette smoke in tumor induction. The results of the implanted mouse skin and rat lung carcinogenicity assays demonstrate the importance of PAHs and other nonvolatile carcinogens. Moreover, sidestream and secondhand smoke contain potent lung carcinogens such as NNK. The results of the mouse inhalation studies indicate that gas-phase constituents of secondhand smoke contribute to tumorigenesis. Prominent among these constituents could be formaldehyde, acetaldehyde, butadiene, and benzene because of their tumorigenic activities and relatively high concentrations in secondhand smoke.

Human Carcinogen Uptake from Secondhand Smoke

Tables 2.3 and 2.4 summarize data from biomarker studies on human uptake of specific secondhand smoke carcinogens. These studies demonstrate that human exposures to secondhand smoke lead to the uptake of carcinogens, a topic that Scherer and Richter (1997) have reviewed.

trans,trans-Muconic acid is a urinary metabolite of benzene, a known cause of leukemia, that has been widely used to estimate benzene uptake (Scherer et al. 1998). Studies on the relationship of this metabolite to secondhand smoke exposure have documented mixed results, with some studies showing somewhat higher levels in persons exposed to secondhand smoke while others found no effect (Scherer et al. 1995, 1999; Weaver et al. 1996; Yu and Weisel 1996; Ruppert et al. 1997; Carrer et al. 2000). The interpretation of these findings is complicated by differences in excretion rates among participants and by contributions from sources other than benzene, such as sorbate in food, to levels of this metabolite in urine (Yu and Weisel 1996; Ruppert et al. 1997; Scherer and Richter 1997). Benzene itself can be quantified in exhaled breath. Breath measurements of nonsmokers who reported secondhand smoke exposures at work from smokers showed elevated benzene levels, but nonsmokers living with smokers did not have increased levels (Wallace et al. 1987). A second study detected higher levels of exhaled benzene in nonsmokers living with smokers compared with nonsmokers living with nonsmokers (Scherer et al. 1995). Another study documented no difference in levels of exhaled benzene among children living with smokers compared with children living with nonsmokers (Scherer et al. 1999). Collectively, the biomarker data discussed here indicate that benzene uptake in humans is not consistently found to be associated with secondhand smoke exposure, but there are other sources of benzene exposure that complicate efforts to estimate the contribution of secondhand smoke to biomarker levels.

Several methods have been used to estimate PAH uptake by persons exposed to secondhand smoke. 1-Hydroxypyrene and hydroxyphenanthrene are urinary metabolites of pyrene and phenanthrene, respectively. These metabolites are widely used as biomarkers of PAH uptake although the parent compounds, pyrene and phenanthrene, are noncarcinogenic. Exposure to secondhand smoke does not increase 1-hydroxypyrene and hydroxyphenanthrene levels in urine (Hoepfner et al. 1987; Scherer et al. 1992, 2000; Van Rooij et al. 1994; Siwińska et al. 1999). Other factors such as smoking, occupational exposures, and diet are significant contributors to urinary levels of these compounds. Metabolites of B[*a*]P and other PAHs form covalent binding products (adducts) with hemoglobin and serum albumin and have been measured using a variety of methods, including immunoassay and gas chromatography–mass spectrometry (GC–MS). Studies of adduct formation with hemoglobin and albumin have given mixed results. Using an enzyme-linked immunosorbent technique, one group found increased levels of PAH-albumin adducts in children exposed to secondhand smoke (Crawford et al. 1994; Tang et al. 1999), but two other studies did not find increments in these levels (Autrup et al. 1995; Nielsen et al. 1996). Using GC–MS as the detection method, researchers found no effect of secondhand smoke exposure on B[*a*]P albumin and hemoglobin adducts (Scherer et al. 2000). Thus, the evidence that

Table 2.3   Representative biomarker studies of carcinogens in persons exposed to secondhand smoke

Carcinogen	Exposure data (if reported)	Biomarker levels	Exposed vs. unexposed: significant difference?	Study
Benzene	11.5 μg/m³*, personal exposure (nonsmokers, nonsmoking homes, n = 39)	tt-MA[†] 92 μg/g creatinine	No	Scherer et al. 1995
	13.6 μg/m³ (nonsmokers, smoking homes, n = 43)	126 μg/g creatinine		
Benzene	NR[‡]	tt-MA 3.84 ± 1.6 ng/μL[§] in 53 secondhand smoke-exposed children 4.02 ± 1.1 ng/μL in 26 unexposed children	No	Weaver et al. 1996
		3.5 ± 1.4 ng/μL when urinary cotinine ≤44 ng/mL[Δ] (n = 39) 4.32 ± 1.4 ng/μL when urinary cotinine >44 ng/mL (n = 39)	Yes	
Benzene	<0.19–22 μg/m³, personal exposure, 5 females exposed to secondhand smoke	tt-MA 34–74 μg excreted on nonexposure days	Yes	Yu and Weisel 1996
		42–95 μg excreted on exposure days		
Benzene	2–100 μg/m³, personal exposure (n = 69 nonsmokers from smoking and nonsmoking households)	tt-MA was not correlated with benzene; marginal difference in tt-MA of nonsmokers from smoking homes vs. those from nonsmoking homes	No	Ruppert et al. 1997
Benzene	11.5 μg/m³, personal exposure (children, smoking homes, n = 24)	tt-MA 130 μg/g creatinine	No	Scherer et al. 1999
	19.7 μg/m³ (children, nonsmoking homes, n = 15)	112 μg/g creatinine		
Benzene (geometric means)	16.5 ± 2.3 μg/m³, personal exposure (nonsmokers, no secondhand smoke, n = 42)	tt-MA 38.9 ± 2.4 μg/L	Yes	Carrer et al. 2000
	25.4 ± 2.9 μg/m³ (nonsmokers, secondhand smoke, n = 27)	54.7 ± 2.9 μg/L		

Table 2.3   Continued

Carcinogen	Exposure data (if reported)	Biomarker levels	Exposed vs. unexposed: significant difference?	Study
NNK[¶]	75–263 ng/m³ in a 16 m³ room	Significantly increased levels of NNAL[**] plus NNAL-Gluc[††] in urine of 5 men after secondhand smoke exposure	Yes	Hecht et al. 1993
NNK	NR	Significantly increased levels of NNAL-Gluc in hospital workers (n = 9) exposed to secondhand smoke compared with controls	Yes	Parsons et al. 1998
NNK	2.4–50 ng/m³ in 19 rooms where smoking took place	NNAL plus NNAL-Gluc levels correlated with nicotine on personal sampler in secondhand smoke-exposed persons	Yes	Meger et al. 2000
NNK	NR	NNAL plus NNAL-Gluc levels were significantly higher in women (n = 23) who lived with male smokers compared with women (n = 22) who lived with male nonsmokers	Yes	Anderson et al. 2001
NNK	NR	34% of 204 children with cotinine >5 ng/mL urine; 52/54 of these samples had detectable NNAL plus NNAL-Gluc; NNAL plus NNAL-Gluc levels were significantly higher in secondhand smoke-exposed vs. unexposed children	Yes	Hecht et al. 2001
Polycyclic aromatic hydrocarbons (PAHs)	NR	5 nonsmokers exposed to secondhand smoke from 100 cigarettes (100–180 μg/m³ cotinine in the room) over an 8-hour period; no effect on urinary hydroxyphenanthrenes	No	Hoepfner et al. 1987
PAHs	Benzo[*a*]pyrene (B[*a*]P), 21.5 ng/m³; phenanthrene, 6.8 ng/m³; pyrene, 17.6 ng/m³ in an experimental room with 5 smokers and 5 nonsmokers	No effects on urinary hydroxyphenanthrenes (2.0 vs. 2.2 μg/24 hours before and after secondhand smoke exposure); no effects on urinary 1-HOP[‡‡] (0.24 μg/24 hours before and after secondhand smoke exposure); no effects on ^{32}P-postlabeling of DNA adducts	No	Scherer et al. 1992
PAHs	NR	No differences in PAH-albumin levels in umbilical cord blood from women exposed to secondhand smoke (n = 49) vs. unexposed women (n = 54)	No	Autrup et al. 1995
PAHs	NR	No effect of secondhand smoke on PAH-albumin adduct levels in 73 persons from Aarhus, Denmark	No	Nielsen et al. 1996

Table 2.3   Continued

Carcinogen	Exposure data (if reported)	Biomarker levels	Exposed vs. unexposed: significant difference?	Study
PAHs	NR	No difference in urinary 1-HOP levels of children exposed to secondhand smoke from their parents' smoking (n = 286) vs. unexposed children (n = 126)	No	Siwińska et al. 1999
PAHs	NR	1-HOP: 0.140 μg/24 hours in 19 secondhand smoke-exposed persons (urinary cotinine 12.3 μg/24 hours) vs. 0.171 μg/24 hours in 23 unexposed persons (urinary cotinine 2.3 μg/24 hours)	NR	Scherer et al. 2000
		B[a]P-hemoglobin (Hb) adducts: 0.049 fmol/mg[§§] Hb in secondhand smoke-exposed persons vs. 0.083 fmol/mg Hb in unexposed persons (same persons as above)	No	
		B[a]P-albumin adducts: 0.021 fmol/mg albumin in secondhand smoke-exposed persons vs. 0.019 fmol/mg albumin in unexposed persons (same persons as above)	NR	
PAH and 4-aminobiphenyl	NR	Significantly higher levels of 4-aminobiphenyl–Hb adducts and PAH-albumin adducts in children whose mothers smoked (n = 23 for 4-aminobiphenyl Hb, n = 44 for PAH albumin) compared with unexposed children (n = 10 for 4-aminobiphenyl Hb, n = 24 for PAH albumin)	Yes	Tang et al. 1999
4-Aminobiphenyl	Estimated weekly average nicotine concentration ranged from <0.5 to ≥2.0 μg/m³	Higher 4-aminobiphenyl–Hb adducts (27.8 pg/g[ΔΔ] Hb) in 9 pregnant women with >2.0 μg/m³ nicotine (personal exposure) than in pregnant women with 0.5–1.9 μg/m³ (n = 20, 20.8 pg/g Hb) or in pregnant women with <0.5 μg/m³ (n = 7, 17.6 pg/g Hb)	Yes	Hammond et al. 1993
4-Aminobiphenyl and other aromatic amines	NR	No relationship of aromatic amine-Hb adducts to reported secondhand smoke exposure or cotinine/creatinine ratios in 73 pregnant women	No	Branner et al. 1998

Table 2.3   Continued

Carcinogen	Exposure data (if reported)	Biomarker levels	Exposed vs. unexposed: significant difference?	Study
4-Aminobiphenyl and other aromatic amines	NR	No increase in aromatic amine-Hb adducts among 224 children with increased exposures to secondhand smoke; exposures were confirmed by cotinine testing	No	Richter et al. 2001
Unknown	NR	No effects of secondhand smoke exposure on ^{32}P-postlabeled DNA adducts in monocytes of 5 nonsmokers exposed for 8 hours	No	Holz et al. 1990
Unknown	5 nonsmokers exposed to secondhand smoke in an unventilated room, 4,091 $\mu g/m^3$ respirable suspended particles	A marginal, nonsignificant increase in urinary thioethers was observed	No	Scherer et al. 1992
Unknown	NR	No effect of secondhand smoke exposure on ^{32}P-postlabeled DNA adducts in women (n = 31 exposed, 11 unexposed)	No	Binková et al. 1995
Unknown	NR	No difference in urinary thioethers between persons exposed to low (n = 23) and high (n = 23) levels of secondhand smoke based on plasma cotinine; no difference in urinary thioethers between persons exposed to low (n = 20) and high (n = 19) levels of secondhand smoke exposures in the home	No	Scherer et al. 1996
Unknown	NR	No difference in placental levels of 8-OH-dG[¶¶] in 10 nonsmokers vs. 9 nonsmokers exposed to secondhand smoke, validated by plasma and urine cotinine; no effects of secondhand smoke on adducts were detected by ^{32}P-postlabeling	No	Daube et al. 1997
Unknown	NR	Significantly higher (63%) levels of 8-OH-dG in blood DNA of persons exposed to secondhand smoke in the workplace (n = 38) than in unexposed persons, verified by plasma cotinine (n = 36)	Yes	Howard et al. 1998b

Table 2.3   Continued

Carcinogen	Exposure data (if reported)	Biomarker levels	Exposed vs. unexposed: significant difference?	Study
Unknown	NR	No difference in 8-OH-dG levels in leukocytes of unexposed adults (n = 36), adults exposed 1–4 hours/day to secondhand smoke (n = 35), and adults exposed >4 hours/day (n = 21)	No	van Zeeland et al. 1999
Unknown	NR	Among 194 students in Athens and 77 persons in Halkida, Greece, ^{32}P-postlabeled DNA adducts in lymphocytes showed no relationship to secondhand smoke exposure in the entire group, but did correlate with secondhand smoke exposure measurements in winter in a subgroup living in the Halkida campus area	No/yes	Geordiadis et al. 2001

*μg/m^3 = Micrograms per cubic meter.
†tt-MA = *trans,trans*-Muconic acid.
‡NR = Data were not reported.
§ng/μL = Nanograms per microliter.
ᐃmL = Milliliter.
¶NNK = 4-(Methylnitrosamino)-1-(3-pyridyl)-1-butanone, a tobacco-specific *N*-nitrosamine.
**NNAL = 4-(Methylnitrosamino)-1-(3-pyridyl)-1-butanol.
††NNAL-Gluc = A mixture of 4-(methylnitrosamino)-1-(3-pyridyl)-1-(*O*-β-D-glucopyranuronosyl) butane and 4-(methylnitrosamino)-1-(3-pyridyl-*N*-β-D-glucopyranuronosyl)-1-butanolonium inner salt.
‡‡1-HOP = 1-Hydroxypyrene.
§§fmol/mg = Femtomoles per milligram.
ᐃᐃpg/g = Picograms per gram.
¶¶8-OH-dG = 8-Hydroxydeoxyguanosine.

secondhand smoke exposure significantly increases human uptake of PAHs is inconsistent.

Aromatic amines such as 4-aminobiphenyl form adducts with hemoglobin that GC–MS can quantify, but studies of the effects of secondhand smoke on 4-aminobiphenyl–hemoglobin adducts have provided mixed results. Hammond and colleagues (1993) demonstrated that adduct levels were elevated in pregnant women exposed to secondhand smoke. Maclure and colleagues (1989) observed slightly higher levels of 4-aminobiphenyl– and 3-aminobiphenyl– hemoglobin adducts in persons with confirmed secondhand smoke exposures compared with unexposed persons. 4-Aminobiphenyl–hemoglobin adducts were also elevated in children exposed to secondhand smoke (Tang et al. 1999). However, two other studies, including one of pregnant women,

showed no consistent relationship between adduct levels and secondhand smoke exposures (Bartsch et al. 1990; Branner et al. 1998). A recent study of German children also showed no significant increase in aromatic amine–hemoglobin adduct levels with increased secondhand smoke exposures; in fact, there was a significant decrease in ortho- and meta-toluidine adducts (Richter et al. 2001). There is a background level of aromatic amine–hemoglobin adducts in apparently unexposed humans. The origin of this background is unknown, but it could be due in part to the uptake of corresponding nitro compounds from sources such as diesel emissions. Levels of aromatic amines in urine were unaffected by exposures to secondhand smoke in a study of nonsmokers (Grimmer et al. 2000).

Because tobacco-specific nitrosamines are found only in tobacco products or in related

Table 2.4   Relationship of specific biomarkers of carcinogen uptake to secondhand smoke exposure

Carcinogens in secondhand smoke	Biomarker	Association with secondhand smoke exposure	Study
Aromatic amines	Hemoglobin adducts	Mixed results	Maclure et al. 1989; Bartsch et al. 1990; Hammond et al. 1993; Branner et al. 1998; Tang et al. 1999; Richter et al. 2001
Benzene	*trans,trans*-Muconic acid in urine	Mixed results	Scherer et al. 1995, 1999; Weaver et al. 1996; Yu and Weisel 1996; Ruppert et al. 1997; Carrer et al. 2000
NNK*	NNAL† and NNAL-Gluc‡ in urine	Consistently increased	Hecht et al. 1993, 2001; Parsons et al. 1998; Meger et al. 2000; Anderson et al. 2001
NNK/NNN§	Hemoglobin adducts	None	Branner et al. 1998
PAHs△	1-Hydroxypyrene in urine Hydroxyphenanthrenes in urine Albumin adducts Hemoglobin adducts	None in most studies	Scherer et al. 1992, 2000; Crawford et al. 1994; Van Rooij et al. 1994; Autrup et al. 1995; Nielsen et al. 1996; Siwińska et al. 1999; Tang et al. 1999

*NNK = 4-(Methylnitrosamino)-1-(3-pyridyl)-1-butanone, a tobacco-specific *N*-nitrosamine.
†NNAL = 4-(Methylnitrosamino)-1-(3-pyridyl)-1-butanol.
‡NNAL-Gluc = A mixture of 4-(methylnitrosamino)-1-(3-pyridyl)-1-(*O*-β-D-glucopyranuronosyl) butane and
4-(methylnitrosamino)-1-(3-pyridyl-*N*-β-D-glucopyranuronosyl)-1-butanolonium inner salt.
§NNN = *N*′-Nitrosonornicotine.
△PAHs = Polycyclic aromatic hydrocarbons.
Source: Adapted from Scherer and Richter 1997.

nicotine-containing materials, their adducts or metabolites should be specific biomarkers of tobacco exposure. NNK- and NNN-hemoglobin adducts can be hydrolyzed to release 4-hydroxy-1-(3-pyridyl)-1-butanone (HPB), which GC–MS can then quantify. In smokers, levels of HPB-releasing hemoglobin adducts of NNK and NNN are low compared with hemoglobin adducts of several other carcinogens, possibly attributable to the high reactivity of the alkylating intermediate (Carmella et al. 1990; Hecht et al. 1994). Considering the relatively low levels of these adducts in smokers, nonsmokers exposed to secondhand smoke should not have significantly elevated amounts (Branner et al. 1998). However, urinary metabolites of NNK are readily measured in the urine of persons exposed to secondhand smoke. The metabolite 4-(methylnitrosamino)-1-(3-pyridyl)-1-butanol (NNAL) and its glucuronide conjugate (NNAL-Gluc) can be quantified using GC with thermal energy analyzer (TEA) nitrosamine-selective detection (GC-TEA) (Hecht et al. 1993, 2001; Parsons et al. 1998; Meger et al. 2000; Anderson et al. 2001). All studies reported to date show significantly higher amounts of NNAL plus NNAL-Gluc, or NNAL-Gluc alone, in the urine of secondhand smoke-exposed participants than in the urine of unexposed controls (Tables 2.3–2.5). In one study, the uptake of NNK was more than six times higher in women who lived with smokers compared with women who lived with nonsmokers (Anderson et al. 2001). The amount of NNAL plus NNAL-Gluc in these secondhand smoke-exposed women was about 5 percent as great as in their male partners who smoked. Another study found an uptake of NNK in a group of economically disadvantaged schoolchildren, and the range of levels varied approximately 90-fold (Hecht et al. 2001). Most of the studies demonstrate a correlation between levels of cotinine and NNAL plus NNAL-Gluc in urine (Figure 2.1). Cotinine is a valid biomarker for nicotine uptake in nonsmokers exposed to secondhand smoke. Therefore, NNAL plus NNAL-Gluc is a biomarker for the uptake of the tobacco-specific lung carcinogen NNK in nonsmokers exposed to secondhand smoke. The NNAL plus NNAL-Gluc biomarker is more directly related to cancer risk than cotinine is because NNK (but not nicotine) is carcinogenic. The uptake of NNK by nonsmokers exposed to secondhand smoke thus provides a biochemical link between secondhand smoke exposure and lung cancer risk.

Studies of secondhand smoke exposure have also explored several other less specific markers. 8-Hydroxydeoxyguanosine (8-OH-dG) is a widely used biomarker of oxidative damage to DNA. Two studies observed no increase in 8-OH-dG levels in placentas and leukocytes of persons exposed to secondhand smoke compared with unexposed persons (Daube et al. 1997; van Zeeland et al. 1999). However, in a study of occupational exposure in Reno, Nevada, the average 8-OH-dG level in whole blood DNA of secondhand smoke-exposed workers was 63 percent higher than in unexposed persons; this finding represents a significant difference (Howard et al. 1998b). Urinary 3-ethyladenine is a biomarker of ethylating agents. In one study, exposure to secondhand smoke did not increase urinary concentrations of 3-ethyladenine (Kopplin et al. 1995). ^{32}P-postlabeling is a technique that can estimate levels of hydrophobic DNA adducts. Four investigations did not find effects of secondhand smoke exposure on levels of ^{32}P-postlabeled DNA (Holz et al. 1990; Scherer et al. 1992; Binková et al. 1995; Daube et al. 1997). However, a recent study conducted in Greece did find a relationship between secondhand smoke exposure and ^{32}P-postlabeled DNA adducts in lymphocytes from a subgroup (Georgiadis et al. 2001). Urinary thioethers are conjugates of carbonyl-containing mutagens. Thioethers did not significantly increase as a result of secondhand smoke exposure (Scherer et al. 1992, 1996). 3-Hydroxypropyl mercapturic acid, possibly from acrolein exposure, was identified as a possible secondhand smoke-related product in urine (Scherer et al. 1992). Studies investigating the effects

Table 2.5   4-(Methylnitrosamino)-1-(3-pyridyl)-1-butanol (NNAL) and NNAL-glucuronide (NNAL-Gluc*) in the urine of nonsmokers exposed to secondhand smoke

Study	Population	Analyte	Correlation with cotinine	Mean ± standard deviation pmol/mL[†] (number of samples analyzed)	Range[‡] (fold)
Hecht et al. 1993	Men exposed to secondhand smoke in a chamber	NNAL plus NNAL-Gluc	Yes	0.16 ± 0.10[§] (n = 7)	0.084–0.296 (4)
Parsons et al. 1998	Hospital workers	NNAL-Gluc	Yes	0.059 ± 0.028 (n = 27)	0.005–0.11 (22)
Meger et al. 2000	Nonsmokers exposed to secondhand smoke	NNAL plus NNAL-Gluc	Yes	0.043 ± 0.044[‡] (n = 16)	0.0038–0.148 (39)
Anderson et al. 2001	Women married to smokers	NNAL plus NNAL-Gluc	No	0.050 ± 0.068 (n = 23)	0.009–0.28 (31)
Hecht et al. 2001	Elementary school-age children	NNAL plus NNAL-Gluc	Yes	0.056 ± 0.076 (n = 74)	0.004–0.373 (93)

*NNAL-Gluc = A mixture of 4-(methylnitrosamino)-1-(3-pyridyl)-1-(*O-β*-D-glucopyranuronosyl) butane and 4-(methylnitrosamino)-1-(3-pyridyl-*N-β*-D-glucopyranuronosyl)-1-butanolonium inner salt.
[†]pmol/mL = Picomoles per milliliter.
[‡]Detected values only.
[§]Approximate, based on the assumption of 1,200 mL of urine excreted per day.
Source: Meger et al. 2000.

Figure 2.1 The correlation between levels of cotinine plus cotinine 4-(methylnitrosamino)-1-(3-pyridyl)-1-butanol (NNAL) plus NNAL-glucuronide (NNAL-Gluc) conjugates in the urine of 74 school-age children exposed to secondhand smoke*

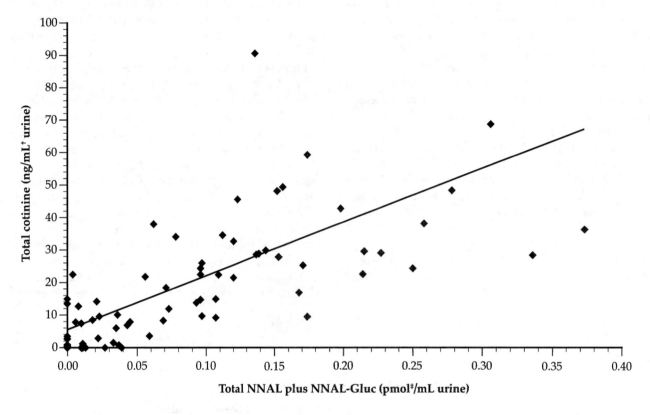

*r = 0.71; p <0.001.
†ng/mL = Nanograms per milliliter.
‡pmol = Picomoles.
Source: Hecht et al. 2001. Reprinted with permission.

of secondhand smoke on urinary mutagenicity have demonstrated conflicting results (Scherer et al. 1992; Scherer and Richter 1997). In general, there seem to be small and sometimes significant effects of secondhand smoke exposure on urinary mutagenicity when diet is controlled (Scherer et al. 1996; Smith et al. 2000a). In a recent study of 1,249 Italian women whose husbands smoked, there was an inverse dose-response relationship between the intensity of the secondhand smoke and concentrations of plasma beta-carotene and L-ascorbic acid found in the women. There also was a significant inverse association between urinary cotinine and plasma beta-carotene (Farchi et al. 2001).

Mechanisms of Carcinogenesis of Secondhand Smoke

Figure 2.2 presents a framework for considering mechanisms of secondhand smoke carcinogenesis. An analogous scheme proposes how cigarette smoke generally can induce lung cancer (Hecht 1999). The broad mechanisms of cancer induction from exposures to secondhand and mainstream cigarette smoke are probably similar because the same carcinogens are present in both, although in different concentrations. The major difference is the significantly lower carcinogenic dose from inhaling secondhand smoke compared with active smoking.

Exposure to secondhand smoke leads to a small but measurable uptake of NNK and perhaps other carcinogens, as discussed in the previous section. Carcinogens are enzymatically transformed into a series of metabolites as the exposed organism attempts to convert them into compounds that are easily excreted from the body (Miller 1994), a process called metabolic detoxification. An unintended consequence of this detoxification process is that the carcinogen sometimes converts to a form that is reactive with DNA and other cellular macromolecules. These reactive forms usually have an electron-deficient (or electrophilic) center that is reactive with the electron-rich (or nucleophilic) centers in DNA. This process, called metabolic activation, forms adducts in DNA, RNA, and protein.

Because most of the carcinogens in Table 2.1 require metabolic activation to induce cancer, the metabolism of a carcinogen is in most cases a key component of the mechanism of cancer induction. The balance between metabolic activation and detoxification will be important in determining individual risks for cancer upon exposure to carcinogens in secondhand smoke. The initial enzymatic steps are frequently catalyzed by cytochrome P-450 enzymes, which are encoded by the *CYP* family of genes (Guengerich 1997). These enzymes generally oxygenate the carcinogen. Other enzymes, such as cyclooxygenases, myeloperoxidases, lipoxygenases, and monoamine oxidases, may also be involved. The oxygenated intermediates formed in the initial reactions may undergo further transformations by glutathione *S*-transferases, uridine-5'-diphosphate-glucuronosyl-transferases, sulfatases, hydratases, and other enzymes (Armstrong 1997; Burchell et al. 1997; Duffel 1997). All of these enzymes occur in multiple forms with different substrate specificity. Some of the forms are polymorphic in humans (i.e., they occur in variants with different types of metabolic activation). For example,

the glutathione *S*-transferase form M1 (GSTM1) is null in 50 percent of the population.

The complexity of carcinogen metabolism is illustrated for B[*a*]P and NNK in Figure 2.3 (Hecht 1999). The major metabolic activation pathway of B[*a*]P is its conversion to 7,8-diol-9,10-epoxide metabolites. One of the four enantiomers produced is highly carcinogenic and reacts with DNA to form an adduct with deoxyguanosine, BPDE-*N*2-dG. GSTM1 is one of the enzymes competing for the metabolically activated intermediates in this pathway. The major metabolic activation pathways of NNK and NNAL occur by hydroxylating the carbons adjacent to the *N*-nitroso group (α-hydroxylation), resulting in the formation of a variety of DNA adducts including 7-methylguanine, O^6-methylguanine, and pyridyloxobutyl adducts (Hecht 1998). No specific carcinogen–DNA adducts have been detected in nonsmokers exposed to secondhand smoke, probably because of the low carcinogenic dose. The characterization of such adducts in human tissues is difficult even in smokers, but has been accomplished for a number of different tobacco smoke carcinogens (Hecht 1999). The same adducts probably are present in nonsmokers exposed to secondhand smoke, but at considerably lower levels.

Two studies examined the role of GSTM1 and glutathione *S*-transferase form T1 (GSTT1) variants as modifiers of risk for lung cancer in nonsmokers exposed to secondhand smoke (Bennett et al. 1999; Malats et al. 2000). Neither study found an effect of GSTT1 variants, although opposing results were obtained for GSTM1 null. One study documented an increased risk for lung cancer in secondhand smoke-exposed nonsmoking women (Bennett et al. 1999); the other found no significant effect in secondhand smoke-exposed nonsmokers (Malats et al. 2000).

Figure 2.2 **Scheme showing the steps linking secondhand smoke exposure and cancer via tobacco smoke carcinogens**

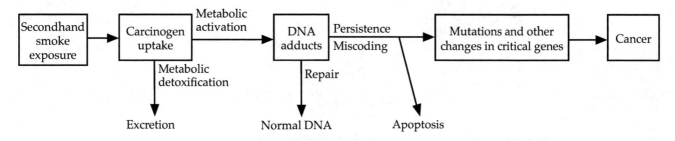

Figure 2.3 Metabolic pathways of benzo[*a*]pyrene (B[*a*]P) and 4-(methylnitrosamino)-1-(3-pyridyl)-1-butanone (NNK)

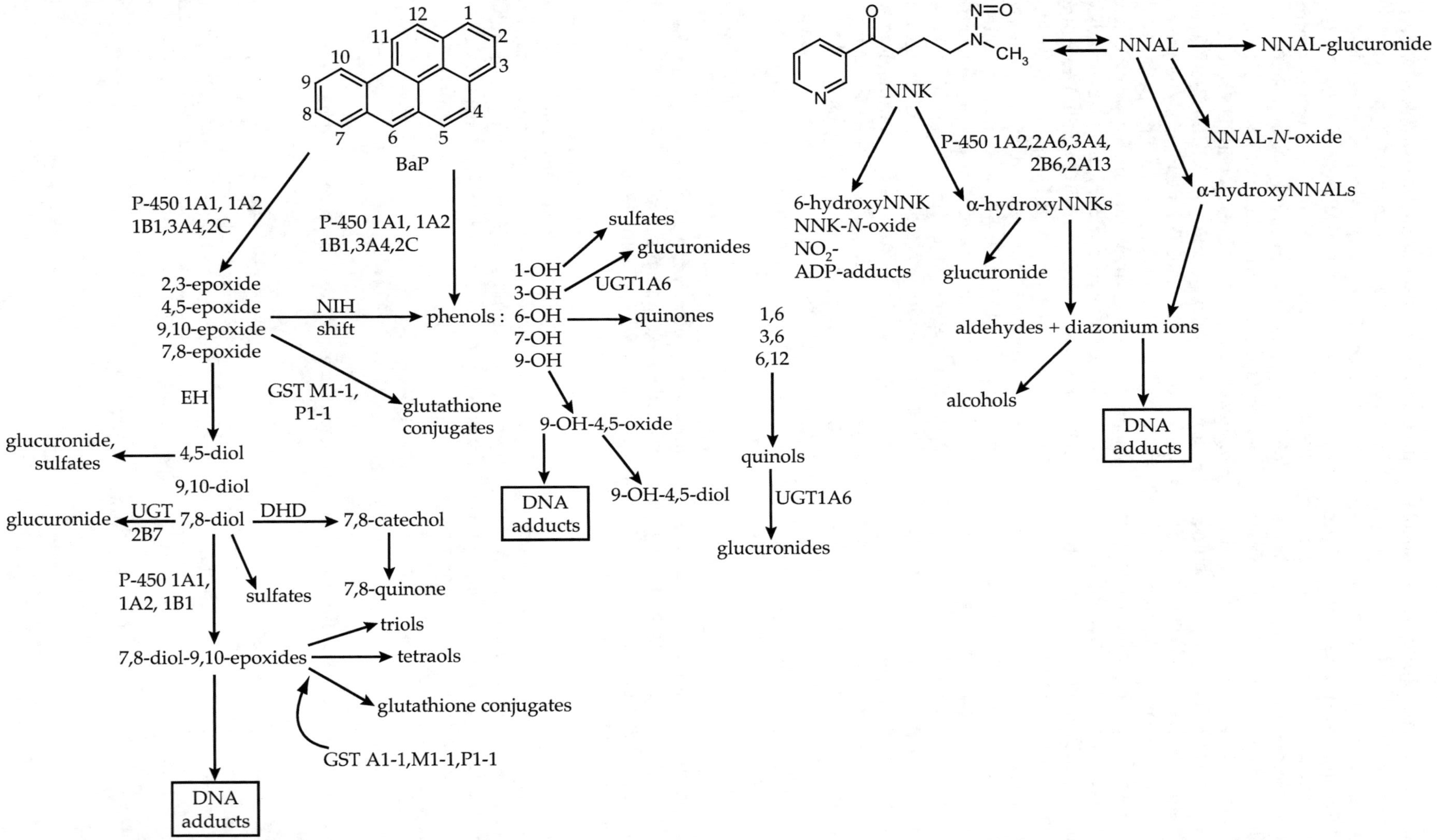

Note: Metabolic pathways of B[*a*]P and NNK were modified from Cooper et al. 1983 and Hecht 1996, 1998. Some human enzymes involved in the various reactions are indicated (Gelboin 1980; Pelkonen and Nebert 1982; Cooper et al. 1983; Ketterer et al. 1992; Smith et al. 1992; Yamazaki et al. 1992; Yun et al. 1992; Tiano et al. 1993; Conney et al. 1994; Friedberg et al. 1994; Shou et al. 1994; Bauer et al. 1995; Smith et al. 1995; Hecht 1996; Jernström et al. 1996; Patten et al. 1996; Shimada et al. 1996; Baird and Ralston 1997; Staretz et al. 1997; Sundberg et al. 1997; Kim et al. 1998; Penning et al. 1999). ADP = adenosine diphosphate; DHD = 4 dihydrodiol dehydrogenase; EH = 4 epoxide hydrolase; GST = 4 glutathione *S*-transferase; NNAL = 4-(methylnitrosamino)-1-(3-pyridyl)-1-butanol; NO_2 = nitrogen dioxide; P-450 = 4 cytochrome P-450; UGT = 4 UDP(uridine 5'-diphosphate)-glucuronosyl transferase; 1-OH, 3-OH: 4 1-hydroxy B[*a*]P, 3-hydroxy B[*a*]P; National Institutes of Health shift (where the shift [a biochemical process] was first identified) = intramolecular hydrogen migration, which can be observed in enzymatic and chemical hydroxylations of aromatic rings.
Source: Hecht 1999. Adapted with permission.

DNA adducts are critical for the induction of tumors by carcinogens. A great deal of mechanistic information is now available about the structures of DNA adducts and their potential to produce mutations (Hemminki et al. 1994; Geacintov et al. 1997). Cellular repair mechanisms exist to protect the DNA from persistent adduction. There are five main mechanisms of DNA repair: direct repair, base excision repair, nucleotide excision repair, mismatch repair, and double-strand break repair (Pegg et al. 1995; Sancar 1996; Singer and Hang 1997). If the adducts are not repaired, cells with damaged DNA may be removed by apoptosis (programmed cell death). When DNA adducts persist they may cause miscoding, resulting in a permanent mutation. Depending on the DNA polymerase involved, the sequence context, and other factors, DNA adducts will typically cause specific mutations. For example, O^6-methylguanine causes mainly G to A mutations, while BPDE-$N2$-dG frequently results in G to T mutations (Loechler et al. 1984; Shukla et al. 1997). If a permanent mutation occurs in a critical region of a growth control gene, it can lead to the loss of normal growth control mechanisms and ultimately to cancer. There are six proposed hallmarks of cancer: self-sufficiency in growth signals, evasion of apoptosis, insensitivity to anti-growth signals, sustained angiogenesis, tissue invasion and metastasis, and limitless replicative potential (Hanahan and Weinberg 2000). Virtually all of these processes are controlled by specific genes that can lose their normal function when miscoding occurs. The intricate circuitry of the cell, which involves multiple pathways of signal transduction, can be subverted by inappropriate carcinogen–DNA adduction and miscoding. Multiple events of this type lead to aberrant cells with the loss of normal growth control. For example, lung carcinogenesis involves changes that include the loss of heterozygosity at 3p, 5q, 8p, 9p, 9q, 11p, 11q, 13q, 17p, and 17q loci, which are known or possible sites of tumor suppressor genes such as *p53*, *p16*, and others (Sekido et al. 1998; Vähäkangas et al. 2001).

Although numerous studies describe mutations in the *p53* tumor suppressor gene and *K-ras* oncogene in lung tumors from smokers (Hecht 1999), few investigations include lung tumors from nonsmokers with documented exposures to secondhand smoke, mainly because lung cancer in nonsmokers is relatively uncommon. Two studies have addressed *p53* mutations in nonsmokers. In one study, the risk of mutation in the *p53* gene doubled (odds ratio = 2.0 [95 percent confidence interval (CI), 0.5–8.7]) with exposure to spousal secondhand smoke only compared with unexposed spouses (Husgafvel-Pursiainen et al. 2000). The risk was 1.5 (95 percent CI, 0.2–8.8) for those ever exposed to spousal or workplace secondhand smoke compared with those who were never exposed. These estimates are statistically unstable because of the small numbers of cases. The findings that G:C to A:T transversions were the most common among lifetime nonsmokers are in agreement with other studies. The second investigation reported a variety of mutations in the *p53* gene from tumors of lifetime nonsmokers exposed to secondhand smoke (Vähäkangas et al. 2001). Mutations in codons 12 and 13 of the *K-ras* gene were also observed. The observed *p53* and *K-ras* gene mutations are plausibly related to DNA adduct formation from carcinogens in secondhand smoke. It is difficult to specify which carcinogen may be responsible for a particular mutation, but the predominance of G mutations observed in these studies is consistent with the generally higher reactivity of G in DNA with metabolically activated carcinogens.

Summary

The evidence indicates that sidestream smoke, the principal component of secondhand smoke, contains carcinogens. Exposure to secondhand smoke results in the uptake by nonsmokers of many of these carcinogens. Although data are sparse on the specific elements in Figure 2.2 linking secondhand smoke exposure and tumor induction in humans via exposure to tobacco smoke carcinogens, substantial data from active smokers support this framework of biologic steps toward cancer. The most plausible mechanisms involved in lung cancer reflect the continuing exposure of the lungs to DNA-damaging material, which leads to multiple genetic changes that culminate in lung cancer. Available evidence points to these same mechanisms as the cause of lung cancer in persons exposed to carcinogens in secondhand smoke.

Conclusions

1. More than 50 carcinogens have been identified in sidestream and secondhand smoke.

2. The evidence is sufficient to infer a causal relationship between exposure to secondhand smoke and its condensates and tumors in laboratory animals.

3. The evidence is sufficient to infer that exposure of nonsmokers to secondhand smoke causes a significant increase in urinary levels of metabolites of the tobacco-specific lung carcinogen 4-(methylnitrosamino)-1-(3-pyridyl)-1-butanone (NNK). The presence of these metabolites links exposure to secondhand smoke with an increased risk for lung cancer.

4. The mechanisms by which secondhand smoke causes lung cancer are probably similar to those observed in smokers. The overall risk of secondhand smoke exposure, compared with active smoking, is diminished by a substantially lower carcinogenic dose.

Mechanisms of Respiratory Tract Injury and Disease Caused by Secondhand Smoke Exposure

Although attention has centered primarily on secondhand smoke and the risk for lung cancer and coronary heart disease (CHD), extensive epidemiologic data support a broader range of adverse effects, particularly related to respiratory health. Information on the underlying mechanisms of these effects is central to the interpretation of the epidemiologic data and in the understanding of the pathogenesis of the non-malignant related disorders associated with secondhand smoke exposure. This review focuses primarily on pathogenetic mechanisms that likely contribute to secondhand smoke-induced respiratory diseases other than lung cancer. Respiratory effects of secondhand smoke exposure include a higher rate, an earlier onset, and an exacerbation of asthma (Wahlgren et al. 2000); spirometric indicators of lung impairment (Cook and Strachan 1999); an increased risk of lower respiratory tract illnesses in children (Strachan and Cook 1997); sudden infant death syndrome (SIDS) (Cook and Strachan 1999); and possibly chronic obstructive pulmonary disease (COPD) (Jaakkola 2002). This review also briefly discusses mechanisms of nonrespiratory disorders affected by secondhand smoke.

The respiratory system is the portal of entry for secondhand smoke and one of the key systems at risk for damage by secondhand smoke. Its structure and function are relevant to understanding the adverse effects of secondhand smoke. The respiratory tract includes the upper (nose, pharynx, and larynx) and lower (trachea, bronchi, and bronchioles) airways and the alveoli of the lung. Odor and irritant receptors are found primarily in the nose, but there are irritant receptors in the upper and lower airways as well. The airways conduct air to the alveoli where gas exchange occurs across the alveolar–capillary membrane, with

oxygen taken up by red blood cells and carbon dioxide removed from the bloodstream. In addition, the upper and lower airways have defense mechanisms against inhaled particles and gases that impact or are adsorbed onto the airway walls. The upper airways, which clean and condition the inhaled air, prevent most large particles and water-soluble vapors from reaching the airways of the lower respiratory tract. The removal of small particles that reach the lower airways and alveoli is accomplished by mechanisms that include the mucociliary apparatus, macrophages, and epithelial cells. This anatomical framework of the respiratory tract provides a large area for deposition and adsorption of secondhand smoke components.

Secondhand Smoke and Asthma

Extensive data describe an association that connects secondhand smoke exposure, particularly from maternal smoking, with asthma in children (Strachan and Cook 1998) (Chapter 6, Respiratory Effects in Children from Exposure to Secondhand Smoke). Studies also link secondhand smoke exposure with asthma in adults (Dayal et al. 1994; Flodin et al. 1995; Hu et al. 1997; Larsson et al. 2001) (Chapter 9, Respiratory Effects in Adults from Exposure to Secondhand Smoke). This section considers biologic mechanisms that could underlie these associations as they reflect exposures during different points of the life span.

The biologic basis by which maternal smoking during pregnancy increases the risk of asthma is not fully understood, but a number of possible mechanisms have been identified. One mechanism is the impairment of fetal airway development. A number of studies have reported that infants of mothers who had smoked during pregnancy had abnormal results on lung function tests, including decreased expiratory flow rates (Hanrahan et al. 1992; Cunningham et al. 1994; Tager et al. 1995) and increased airway resistance (Dezateux et al. 1999; Milner et al. 1999). These changes in lung mechanics that result from in utero tobacco smoke exposures persist through late childhood (Cunningham et al. 1994) and perhaps into adulthood (Upton et al. 1998). Also, diminished respiratory function in neonates precedes and is predictive of wheeze in early childhood (Martinez et al. 1988b; Dezateux et al. 1999; Young et al. 2000). Alterations in airway wall structure, particularly increased airway wall thickness, were found in infants exposed to maternal smoking (Elliot et al. 1998). This increased wall thickness could explain a major effect of maternal smoking on expiratory flow rates because it results in a smaller airway lumen, thereby increasing airway resistance. Supporting evidence comes from studies in rats that also indicated that exposure to smoking during pregnancy impaired fetal airway development and function (Collins et al. 1985).

A possible explanation for the impaired airway development, supported by recent data obtained in monkeys, is that the changes in airway structure are attributable to in utero effects of nicotine on extracellular matrix synthesis (Sekhon et al. 1999, 2002). Nicotine readily crosses the feto-placental barrier and attains concentrations in amniotic fluid that are equivalent to or higher than maternal serum nicotine levels (Luck and Nau 1984; Luck et al. 1985). At these concentrations, nicotine can exert profound biologic effects by targeting specific ionotropic channel receptors termed nicotinic acetylcholine receptors (nAChRs). These receptors are a family of ligand-gated, pentameric ion channels. In humans, 16 different subunits have been identified that form a large number of homopentameric and heteropentameric receptors with distinct structural and pharmacologic properties (Leonard and Bertrand 2001). Although the main focus on this receptor family has been to elucidate its role in transmitting signals for the neurotransmitter acetylcholine at neuromuscular junctions, recent interest has included its role in signaling events in nonneuronal cells. In the developing lung, $\alpha 7$ nAChRs are the most abundant form of nAChRs. Prenatal nicotine exposure strikingly increases $\alpha 7$ nAChR expression and binding. Acting through $\alpha 7$ nAChRs, nicotine markedly affects lung development. For example, prenatal exposure of primates to nicotine significantly alters lung structure (Sekhon et al. 1999). Specifically,

paralleling the increase in $\alpha 7$ expression is a substantial increase in collagen expression surrounding large airways and vessels (Sekhon et al. 1999). Nicotine also increases collagen type I and type III mRNA expressions (i.e., copies of information carried by a gene on the DNA) in airways and alveolar walls (Sekhon et al. 2002). Collectively, these studies suggest that nicotine may be an important component of cigarette smoke responsible for increasing the airway wall thickness in infants of mothers who smoke during pregnancy.

A second mechanism that may cause a predisposition to asthma as a result of secondhand smoke exposure is the induction of bronchial hyperreactivity (BHR). Secondhand smoke exposure reportedly increases BHR in both children and adults. Martinez and colleagues (1988a) reported an increase in BHR following exposure to secondhand smoke in 70 percent of nine-year-old children whose mothers had smoked regularly during pregnancy. Young and colleagues (1991) reported a modest increase in BHR from inhaled histamine in infants (mean age four and one-half weeks) of parents who smoked compared with unexposed infants. That study was unable to separate the effects of prenatal and postnatal exposure to cigarette smoke. Recent results from the multicenter European Community Respiratory Health Survey demonstrated that secondhand smoke was also significantly associated with BHR in adults (Janson et al. 2001). This analysis included data from more than 7,800 adults who had never smoked. There were also significant dose-related trends between secondhand smoke and BHR. The increase in BHR caused by secondhand smoke may be attributable, in part, to cigarette smoke-induced increases of neuroendocrine cells in the lung. Located in the airway epithelium, neuroendocrine cells synthesize and release bronchoconstrictors, including serotonin, endothelin, and bombesin. Airways of persons with asthma also contained a higher number of neuroendocrine cells (Schuller at al. 2003). In rats, in utero and postnatal secondhand smoke exposure caused BHR and increased the number of neuroendocrine cells in the lungs (Joad et al. 1995). That study exposed pregnant rats to filtered air or to secondhand smoke under controlled conditions from day three of gestation until birth. The female rat pups were then exposed postnatally to either filtered air or secondhand smoke for 7 to 10 weeks. Exposure to prenatal and postnatal secondhand smoke resulted in lungs that were less compliant and more reactive to methacholine, with a 22-fold increase in the number of pulmonary neuroendocrine cells.

Nicotine may also be responsible for this increase in neuroendocrine cells. Sekhon and colleagues (1999) demonstrated that in utero nicotine exposure substantially increased neuroendocrine cells in the lungs of monkeys. Studies also suggest that nicotine may cause the release of bronchoconstrictors. Schuller and colleagues (2003) recently demonstrated that nicotine and its nitrosated carcinogenic derivative NNK bind to α7 nAChRs on pulmonary neuroendocrine cells. This results in the influx of calcium, the release of bronchoconstrictors, and the activation of (1) a mitogenic pathway mediated by protein kinase C, (2) the serine/threonine protein kinase Raf-1, (3) the mitogen-activated protein kinase, and (4) the proto-oncogene *c-myc*. These findings thus identify a possible effector cell for the increased BHR resulting from secondhand smoke exposure and indicate plausible mechanisms.

Researchers have also determined that secondhand smoke exposure affects the neural control of airways. In particular, there are extensive studies on the role of secondhand smoke exposure on the lung C-fiber central nervous system (CNS) reflex. The stimulation of sensory nonmyelinated bronchopulmonary C-fibers can trigger intense respiratory responses through local and CNS reflexes. Responses include bronchoconstriction, mucous secretion, and increased microvascular leakage, which are all hallmarks of asthma (Coleridge and Coleridge 1994). C-fibers are stimulated by components of secondhand smoke including nicotine (Saria et al. 1988), acrolein (Lee et al. 1992), and oxidants (Coleridge et al. 1993). In studies examining the role of secondhand smoke in neural control, Bonham and colleagues (2001) exposed one-week-old guinea pigs to filtered air or secondhand smoke for five weeks. Secondhand smoke exposure increased the excitability of afferent lung C-fibers and neurons in the CNS reflex pathway. This pathway could underline the increased risk for respiratory symptoms attributable to secondhand smoke exposure.

Altered immune responses may also play a role in the increased incidence of asthma in secondhand smoke-exposed children. Active smoking is associated with higher concentrations of total serum immunoglobulin E (IgE) (Sapigni et al. 1998; Oryszczyn et al. 2000). Magnusson (1986) extended these studies and demonstrated that cord blood IgE concentration was elevated significantly in infants whose mothers had smoked during pregnancy and that maternal smoking during pregnancy might predispose infants to subsequent sensitization and allergy. Studies have also associated high serum IgE levels with secondhand smoke exposure in children (Wjst

et al. 1994) and in adults (Sapigni et al. 1998; Oryszczyn et al. 2000), although not all studies observed this association (Janson et al. 2001). Such enhanced IgE values might predict a later development of allergies (Marini et al. 1996).

Cigarette smoke exposure may also modify the balance of immune cells in airways. Studies on immune cells in airways have primarily addressed active smoking, and the effects of secondhand smoke exposure on airway immune cells remain unknown. Hagiwara and colleagues (2001) examined whether cigarette smoking could affect the distribution in the human airway of cells secreting T-helper 1 (Th1) or Th2 cytokines by identifying and quantifying the frequencies of cells spontaneously secreting cytokines in bronchoalveolar lavage fluid (BALF). The researchers collected BALF from nonsmokers or heavy cigarette smokers and performed cytokine assays to quantify cells secreting interleukin-2 (IL-2), IL-4, and interferon gamma (IFN-γ) with or without phorbol 12-myristate 13-acetate stimulation. No cells spontaneously secreting IL-2 were detected in BALF from smokers, whereas the BALF from most nonsmokers had detectable cells secreting IL-2. The number of cells secreting IFN-γ also decreased substantially in smokers compared with nonsmokers. Cells secreting IL-4 were not detected in samples from either group. There were also significant decreases in mitogen-stimulated Th1 cytokine-secreting cells in the airways of smokers. The frequency of cells secreting IL-2 and the lymphocyte CD4/CD8 ratio in BALF had a weak positive correlation. These results indicate that cigarette smoking depletes Th1 cytokine-secreting cells in the human airway and may explain the susceptibility of smokers to certain airway disorders, including allergic diseases.

Nicotine can impair antigen receptor-mediated signal transduction in lymphocytes, possibly contributing further to the asthma phenotype among the huge number of other sensitizing chemicals in tobacco smoke (Geng et al. 1995). Nicotine can inhibit both T cell-dependent and T cell-independent antibody forming cell responses and thus contribute to the immunosuppression that leads to an increased risk of respiratory infections, which are common triggers of BHR.

Nitric oxide (NO) plays an important role in the physiologic regulation of human airways. Changes in its production are implicated in the pathophysiology of airway diseases associated with cigarette smoking (Barnes and Belvisi 1993). Studies show that NO is a mild bronchodilator in persons with asthma when administered exogenously (Hogman et al. 1993). The inhibition of endogenous NO synthesis by nitro-L-arginine methyl ester, a NO synthase (NOS) inhibitor, increases BHR in response to histamine in persons with asthma (Taylor et al. 1998). This reaction suggests that there are protective effects against bronchoconstriction by the NO that is released within the airways. Of note, inhalation of NG-monomethyl-L-arginine, another NOS inhibitor, increases BHR to bradykinin in patients with mild asthma (Ricciardolo et al. 1996), but not in those with more severe asthma (Ricciardolo et al. 1997), indicating a possible relationship between disease severity and the bronchodilatory role of endogenous NO. Several studies have demonstrated that exhaled NO levels, indicators of endogenous production, were lower in smokers than in nonsmokers (Persson et al. 1994; Schilling et al. 1994; Kharitonov et al. 1995). Those studies were more recently extended to secondhand smoke exposure. Yates and colleagues (2001) demonstrated a rapid (within 15 minutes) fall in exhaled NO levels during secondhand smoke exposure. The decreases in exhaled NO were observed at levels of secondhand smoke exposure frequently experienced in community settings (Yates et al. 1996). The inhibitory effect of cigarette smoke on exhaled NO has also been demonstrated in vitro, where cigarette smoke decreased NO production (Edwards et al. 1999). Thus, the decreased generation of NO in airways provides an additional mechanism for the increased BHR in persons exposed to secondhand smoke.

A number of plausible mechanisms could account for the decrease in exhaled NO associated with secondhand smoke exposure. Cigarette smoke contains high concentrations of oxides of nitrogen, and the reduction in exhaled NO may be attributable to the decreased production of NOS by a negative feedback mechanism (Kharitonov et al. 1995). Other possible mechanisms include an accelerated uptake of NO following tobacco smoke exposure, or an increased breakdown or modification of NO by oxidants in cigarette smoke. NO reacts rapidly with superoxide anion, yielding the harmful oxidant peroxynitrite. This mechanism would be similar to that observed in cystic fibrosis where nitrite levels, indicators of NO oxidative metabolism, are elevated in breath condensate of afflicted persons but exhaled NO is not (Ho et al. 1998).

The induction of BHR following exposure to secondhand smoke might also result from smoke-induced inflammation. Lee and colleagues (2002) demonstrated that airway inflammation markedly increased BHR. Saetta (1999) demonstrated that cigarette smoking caused a profound inflammatory response in airways and lung parenchyma. Cigarette

smokers had increases in total inflammatory cell counts and polymorphonuclear leukocyte (PMN) counts (tested by BAL), and nonsmokers exposed to secondhand smoke for as little as three hours experienced an increase in circulating PMNs, enhanced PMN chemotaxis, and the augmented release of oxidants upon stimulation (Anderson et al. 1991). Airway epithelial cells are likely involved in producing this inflammatory reaction because they line the respiratory tract and interact directly with inhaled cigarette smoke to elaborate proinflammatory cytokines (Yu et al. 2002). Human bronchial epithelial cell cultures exposed to cigarette smoke extract exhibited significantly greater PMN chemotactic activity compared with the control cell cultures (Mio et al. 1997).

Secondhand Smoke and Infection

The topic of active smoking and host defenses against infectious agents has been covered in previous reports of the Surgeon General (USDHHS 1990, 2004). Epidemiologic studies show that secondhand smoke exposure enhances susceptibility to respiratory infections and/or worsens infections in both adults and children (Porro et al. 1992; Strachan and Cook 1997; Jaakkola 2002). Although mechanisms underlying the increased risk of infection associated with secondhand smoke exposure have not been fully evaluated, several studies have identified mechanisms that are likely to be involved. As reviewed earlier (Geng et al. 1995), secondhand smoke can inhibit antibody responses that are either T cell-dependent or T cell-independent, thus contributing to impaired immune responses. Secondhand smoke hinders macrophage responsiveness, further impairing the proper functioning of the immune system (Edwards et al. 1999). It also impairs mucociliary clearance (Wanner et al. 1996), enhances bacterial adherence, and disrupts the respiratory epithelium (Fainstein and Musher 1979; Dye and Adler 1994), a critical host defense barrier. Secondhand smoke exposure may also alter bacterial flora in pharyngeal mucosa of infants, thus providing an additional mechanism for enhanced susceptibility to infection (Kilian et al. 1995).

Secondhand Smoke and Chronic Obstructive Pulmonary Disease

As a slowly progressive condition, COPD is characterized by airflow limitation that is largely irreversible. Characteristic pathologic changes are the accumulation of inflammatory cells in airways and lung parenchyma and the extensive derangement of the extracellular matrix, resulting in small distinct airspaces that coalesce into much larger abnormal ones (Niewoehner et al. 1974; Cosio et al. 1980; Jeffery 2001). The inflammatory cells are regarded as the source of enzymes (e.g., elastases) that cause the matrix destruction. Oxidative stress is also thought to play an important role in the development of COPD. A number of studies have shown an increased oxidant burden and consequently increased markers of oxidative stress in the airspaces, breath, blood, and urine of smokers and of patients with COPD (MacNee 2001). Sources of the increased oxidative burden in COPD patients include cigarette smoke, which contains abundant amounts of oxygen-based free radicals, peroxides, peroxynitrites, and phagocytes (Pryor 1992). Alveolar macrophages and PMN from smokers release increased amounts of reactive oxygen species under certain conditions when compared with the same cell types from nonsmokers (Hoidal et al. 1981; Ludwig and Hoidal 1982). The consequences of oxidative stress may include oxidative inactivation of antiproteinases, airspace epithelial injury, and expression of proinflammatory mediators (MacNee 2001), which are all elements of the inflammatory process underlying the development of COPD.

Although secondhand smoke clearly causes an increased oxidant burden in the lungs, only a few publications address secondhand smoke and COPD, and the magnitudes of the associations observed are modest. A few studies have suggested an increased risk of COPD with a high level of exposure (Coultas 1998). One approach investigators have taken to determine the potential risk of COPD from secondhand smoke exposure is to examine the relationship between lung function level and secondhand smoke. Although longitudinal data on the effects of active or involuntary smoking and the development of COPD are not available from childhood through adulthood, evidence suggests that COPD in adults may result from impaired lung development and growth, the premature onset of a decline in lung function, and/or an accelerated decline in lung function (Samet and Lange 1996; Kerstjens et al. 1997). As discussed earlier in this chapter (see "Secondhand Smoke and Asthma"), exposure to secondhand smoke in infancy and childhood and active smoking during childhood and adolescence contribute to impaired lung growth (Collins et al. 1985). In general, however, although studies have identified plausible mechanisms, there is a need for additional evidence on the relationship between secondhand smoke and COPD.

Secondhand Smoke and Sudden Infant Death Syndrome

Many epidemiologic studies document that maternal smoking during pregnancy and after birth is a major risk factor for SIDS (Haglund and Cnattingius 1990; Klonoff-Cohen et al. 1995; Taylor and Sanderson 1995). Earlier reports have concluded that maternal smoking during pregnancy causes SIDS (USDHHS 2001, 2004). Research has identified mechanisms in SIDS infants related to arousal failure, inadequate cardiorespiratory compensatory motor responses, and sleep apnea that are attributable to developmental abnormalities in the brainstem and autonomic nervous system (Avery and Frantz 1983; Harper 2000; Slotkin 2004; Spitzer 2005; Adgent 2006). Researchers have studied the potential mechanisms by which prenatal, perinatal, and postnatal exposures to secondhand smoke are related to neurodevelopmental abnormalities. The data suggest that the potent neurotoxic effects of nicotine are important (Slotkin et al. 1997; Önal et al. 2004; Slotkin 2004; Adgent 2006). Children who die from SIDS have higher concentrations of nicotine in their lungs compared with children who die of other causes (Milerad et al. 1998; McMartin et al. 2002). This association holds even when the parents report a nonsmoking environment. The specific role of nicotine and other tobacco smoke constituents in the pathogenesis of SIDS is not known. Research, however, particularly animal exposure models, suggests that many cardiorespiratory control deficiencies are associated with nicotinic receptors within the peripheral and central nervous systems (Neff et al. 1998; Adgent 2006). Animal studies have documented effects that can be related to several potential mechanisms that could cause SIDS, including the effects of perinatal exposure to secondhand smoke on increased nAChR production in brains of monkeys (Slotkin et al. 2002); the disruptions in brain development through cholinergic mechanisms (Slotkin 2004); and adverse effects on brain cell development, synaptic development and function, and neurobehavioral activity. Perinatal exposure to secondhand smoke also has adverse effects on neurobehavioral development (Makin et al. 1991), and recent studies indicate that perinatal exposure to secondhand smoke induces adenylyl cyclase (AC) activity and alters receptor-mediated cell signaling in brains of neonatal rats (Slotkin et al. 2001). In those studies, rats were exposed to secondhand smoke during gestation or during the early neonatal period or both. Brains were examined for alterations in AC activity and for changes in beta-adrenergic and

M2 muscarinic cholinergic receptors and their linkage to AC. Secondhand smoke exposure induced an increase in total AC activity, which was monitored with forskolin, the direct enzymatic stimulant. In the brain, the specific coupling of beta-adrenergic receptors to AC was inhibited in the groups exposed to secondhand smoke despite a normal complement of receptor-binding sites. Because alterations in AC signaling are known to affect cardiorespiratory function, the results provide a possible mechanistic link to the action of secondhand smoke, including postnatal secondhand smoke exposure, in disturbances culminating in SIDS. Secondhand smoke exposure causes the same changes in AC signaling seen previously with prenatal nicotine exposure: increases in AC production and the loss of specific receptor coupling to AC. In a recent independent analysis of perinatal and postnatal exposure to secondhand smoke in rhesus monkeys, researchers observed significant neural cellular effects from postnatal exposures alone, including specific damage in the occipital cortex, in the midbrain, and in temporal cortex cell development. These effects are similar to those previously observed in other animal models for either prenatal nicotine or perinatal secondhand smoke exposure, or for continuous prenatal and postnatal exposures (Slotkin et al. 2006).

A second possible mechanism for the increased incidence of SIDS following secondhand smoke exposure relates to earlier cited evidence from a guinea pig model of postnatal secondhand smoke exposure. That model demonstrated an increase in the production or release of lung C-fiber CNS reflex responses to secondhand smoke (Bonham et al. 2001). The responses invoked by the increased excitability of afferent lung C-fibers and nucleus tractus solitarius (NTS) neurons in the CNS reflex pathway include changes in breathing patterns, such as prolonged expiratory apnea. The findings suggest that an increase in secondhand smoke-induced excitability of NTS neurons augmenting C-fiber reflex output may contribute to SIDS.

Findings of a study that used a piglet model suggest that nicotine interferes with normal autoresuscitation (Frøen et al. 2000). The effect of nicotine was augmented by the additional administration of IL-1B, which is released during infections. Studies with a piglet model also suggest that early involuntary, postnatal nicotine exposure may be responsible for some neuropathologic changes in apoptotic markers that researchers have observed in SIDS infants (Machaalani et al. 2005).

Although investigators have not established a specific role for apnea as a potential cause of SIDS,

one study of human newborns evaluated this theoretical potential of apnea in relation to SIDS (Chang et al. 2003). A controlled sleeping experiment included 10 infants either prenatally or postnatally exposed to tobacco smoke and 10 unexposed control infants. The researchers found that five of the exposed infants did not have a behavioral arousal response to a standard sequence of audiology stimuli, whereas all of the unexposed infants were aroused.

Secondhand Smoke and Nasal or Sinus Disease

Some studies indicate an association, particularly in children, between secondhand smoke exposure and acute or chronic nasal and sinus symptoms (Barr et al. 1992; Moyes et al. 1995; Benninger 1999). In children aged 4 through 11 years, frequent colds and general sinus symptoms were significantly associated with maternal smoking (Barr et al. 1992). Normal healthy persons have also developed nasal congestion, irritation, and increased rhinitis from exposure to moderate levels of secondhand smoke (Willes et al. 1998). Researchers have examined a number of potential mechanisms (Samet 2004). Tobacco smokers have abnormal nasal mucociliary clearance, and a study by Bascom and colleagues (1995) demonstrated differential nasal responsiveness to secondhand smoke. Using the clearance of ^{99m}Tc-sulfur colloid as an indicator of mucociliary function, decreased clearance occurred in 3 out of 12 persons following exposure. Persons with delayed clearances all had a history of secondhand smoke rhinitis (Bascom et al. 1995). In a follow-up study comparing persons who were not sensitive with persons who were sensitive to secondhand smoke, those who were sensitive had more rhinorrhea following the intranasal administration of capsaicin, thus suggesting a role for C-fiber stimulation (Bascom et al. 1991). The researchers observed no changes in nasal vascular permeability or inflammation following secondhand smoke exposure. Studies have also shown secondhand smoke-induced increases in epithelial permeability to environmental allergens, thus enhancing allergic reactions to inhaled allergens (Kjellman 1981; Zetterstrom et al. 1981).

Summary

Cellular, animal, and human studies indicate a number of mechanisms by which secondhand smoke injures the respiratory tract. There is extensive information on the harm from active smoking as well.

There are limitations to many of the cited studies. Most clinical studies base secondhand smoke exposure on self-reports and have not included objective measurements of exposure, such as salivary, serum, or urine cotinine concentrations. An additional limitation is that studies of secondhand smoke exposure frequently use a cross-sectional design and provide little data on the duration of the exposure. In addition, mechanistic studies frequently rely on animal models or in vitro studies. Both have limitations, particularly in relation to the level and duration of the exposures and difficulties in simulating human exposures. There is very little information about the concentrations of specific tobacco smoke constituents following secondhand smoke exposure in the alveolar milieu and limited information about the interactions among the various constituents.

Obviously, the closer a model mimics human exposure the more relevant this information will be. In addition to more closely simulating conditions of human exposure, future studies should focus on individual susceptibilities. This approach will lead to the recognition of genetic profiles that influence susceptibility to adverse effects of secondhand smoke and will provide insights into the underlying mechanisms of the health consequences.

Animal and human studies indicate several potential mechanisms by which exposure to secondhand smoke may affect the neuroregulation of breathing, apneic spells, and sudden infant death. The role of nicotine and other tobacco smoke constituents in the pathogenesis of SIDS is not known. However, the neurotoxicity of prenatal and neonatal exposures to nicotine and secondhand smoke in animal models can be related to several potential causal mechanisms, including adverse effects on brain cell development, synaptic development and function, and neurobehavioral activity.

Conclusions

1. The evidence indicates multiple mechanisms by which secondhand smoke exposure causes injury to the respiratory tract.

2. The evidence indicates mechanisms by which secondhand smoke exposure could increase the risk for sudden infant death syndrome.

Mechanisms of Secondhand Smoke Exposure and Heart Disease

When the association of CHD with secondhand smoke was first reported, its plausibility and the magnitude of the observed risk were questioned. The observed risk for involuntary smoking was thought to be relatively strong compared with the well-documented risk of active smoking. In addition, it was uncertain whether the mechanisms underlying the association of active smoking with CHD risk were relevant, considering the lower doses of smoke components associated with typical secondhand smoke exposures. Subsequently, an understanding of the potential mechanisms associating CHD with involuntary smoking has deepened, largely as a result of findings from human and animal experiments involving secondhand smoke exposure.

Clinical and experimental evidence continues to accumulate regarding the mechanisms by which active smoking causes CHD (USDHHS 1990,

1994, 1998, 2001, 2004). Active smoking promotes atherogenesis by unfavorably affecting many elements in the interface of the blood with the arterial wall and the cellular elements of the artery itself. Atherosclerosis is, in part, considered an inflammatory process (Ross 1993, 1999), and smoking results in a potent, systemic inflammatory stimulus (USDHHS 2004). Active smoking is associated with dysfunctional endothelial cells, the cells lining the inner arterial wall that are in contact with the circulating blood. This dysfunction leads to the secretion of inflammatory cytokines, the adhesion of monocytes and lymphocytes and their migration to the endothelium, the proliferation of smooth muscle cells, and the reduction of the normal antithrombotic properties of the endothelium. Compared with nonsmoking controls, smokers also have less endothelium-dependent vasodilatation (Celermajer et al. 1993).

The balance of the tightly regulated coagulation–fibrinolytic system is critical to the prevention of atherothrombotic events such as acute coronary syndromes, which include unstable angina and myocardial infarction (MI) (Corti et al. 2003). Smoking has a prothrombotic effect, tipping this system toward clot formation, which comes from a variety of actions of smoking including impaired endothelial cell functioning, increased platelet aggregation, and reduced fibrinolysis (USDHHS 2004).

Smoking is also associated with an adverse lipid profile (USDHHS 1990, 2004). Smokers tend to have higher concentrations of total low-density lipoprotein (LDL) and very low-density lipoprotein and decreased levels of high-density lipoprotein (HDL). Smoking also increases oxygen demand while reducing oxygen-delivering capacity.

This section reviews mechanisms that are considered to be the basis of the association between exposure to secondhand smoke and CHD. The following section reviews the relevant body of research and covers each of the systems affected unfavorably by active smoking for which there is also research on secondhand smoke exposure. The discussion also provides a foundation for considering the observational evidence in Chapter 8, Cardiovascular Diseases from Exposure to Secondhand Smoke.

Platelets

Exposure to secondhand smoke activates blood platelets (i.e., makes them sticky), and thereby increases the likelihood of a thrombus. These activated platelets can damage the lining of the coronary arteries and may facilitate the development and progression of atherosclerotic lesions (Pittilo et al. 1982; Sinzinger and Kefalides 1982; Burghuber et al. 1986; Davis et al. 1989; Sinzinger and Virgolini 1989; Steinberg et al. 1989). Increased platelet activation is associated with an increased risk for ischemic heart disease (Elwood et al. 1991). Thus, increases in platelet activation observed in persons exposed to secondhand smoke would be expected to have acute adverse effects.

In one experiment, two groups each smoked two cigarettes: individuals who by history were nonsmokers and individuals who were reported smokers (Burghuber et al. 1986). At the beginning of the experiment, the platelets of the chronic smokers were less sensitive to stimulation by exogenous prostacyclin than those of the nonsmokers; platelet sensitivity did not significantly change in the smokers in response to smoking the two cigarettes (Figure 2.4). In contrast to these findings, nonsmokers who smoked just two cigarettes had a significantly ($p < 0.01$) decreased level of response to the same stimulus, reaching a level close

Figure 2.4   Effect of active and involuntary smoking on platelet aggregation in smokers and nonsmokers

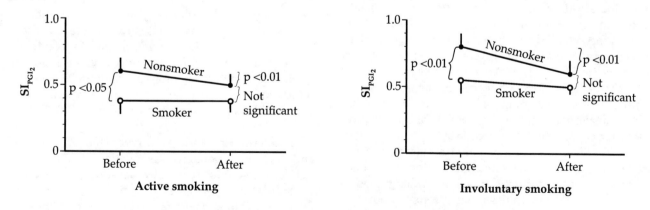

Note: The sensitivity index, SI_{PGI_2}, is defined as the inverse of the concentration of prostaglandin I_2, which is necessary to inhibit adenosine disphosphate-induced platelet aggregation by 50 percent. Lower values of SI_{PGI_2} indicate greater platelet aggregation.
Source: Burghuber et al. 1986. Adapted with permission.

to that of the smokers. The findings indicate differing acute responses of platelets of nonsmokers and smokers to the toxins in cigarette smoke.

In an experiment more relevant to involuntary smoking, the same investigators used the same platelet assay in another group of smokers and nonsmokers before and after they sat in a room for 20 minutes where cigarettes had just been smoked (Figure 2.4) (Burghuber et al. 1986). The researchers again found no significant change among smokers, but a significant increase in platelet sensitivity to prostacyclin among nonsmokers brought them to a level similar to that of the smokers. These data, together with findings from other human experiments (Davis et al. 1989), indicate that nonsmokers are sensitive to secondhand smoke, and even very low levels of secondhand smoke exposure can have a major impact on platelet function in nonsmokers. Animal data also show an effect of secondhand smoke exposure. Bleeding time, another measure of platelet function, is significantly shortened by secondhand smoke exposure (meaning more activated platelet activity) in both rabbits (Zhu et al. 1993b; Sun et al. 1994) and rats (Zhu et al. 1994).

With regard to the mechanisms, studies of cigarette smoke extract on platelet function suggest that the toxins in cigarette smoke increase platelet function by interfering with and degrading platelet-activating factor acetylhydrolase (PAF-AH) (Miyaura et al. 1992). Exposure of serum to cigarette smoke extract reduces the effectiveness of PAF-AH and may thus increase the concentration of platelet-activating factor. The reduced efficacy of PAF-AH may explain the increased serum concentration of platelet-activating factor in smokers. Nicotine appears to be one of the active agents in tobacco smoke, but other specific compounds may also contribute to the effects of exposure on platelets (Davis et al. 1985; Miyaura et al. 1992). This in vitro finding complements results of clinical studies that compared the effects of smoking and transdermal nicotine on platelets and on hemostatic function. Benowitz and colleagues (1993) carried out a crossover trial that compared the effects of cigarette smoking and transdermal nicotine on eicosanoid formation and hemostatic function. Although both active smoking and transdermal nicotine produced similar nicotine levels, there was an increase in the urinary excretion of several markers of platelet function while smoking cigarettes that was not seen with transdermal therapy (Benowitz et al. 1993).

Some investigators have reported conflicting findings and have questioned whether platelet aggregation is an underlying mechanism of the

association between CHD and secondhand smoke exposure (Smith et al. 2000b, 2001). Smith and colleagues (2001) conducted an observational study that compared secondhand smoke-exposed and unexposed adult nonsmokers and did not find differences in urinary metabolites of thromboxane and prostacyclin.

Endothelial Function and Vasodilation

Arteries are lined by a cell layer known as the vascular endothelium. The endothelium plays a critical role in controlling the ability of arteries to dilate and constrict as they regulate blood flow. In addition, damage to the vascular endothelium facilitates the development of atherosclerosis. Evidence in both animals (Hutchison et al. 1995, 1996, 1997a,b, 1998, 1999; Jorge et al. 1995; Zhu and Parmley 1995; Schwarzacher et al. 1998; Török et al. 2000) and humans (Celermajer et al. 1996; Sumida et al. 1998; Otsuka et al. 2001) shows that secondhand smoke interferes with endothelium-dependent vasodilation. Moreover, these effects can be attenuated by increasing the amount of L-arginine, an amino acid that is a precursor of NO, the mediator of endothelium-dependent vasodilation (Hutchison et al. 1996, 1997a, 1998, 1999; Schwarzacher et al. 1998). Studies in rats have also demonstrated that involuntary smoking reduces NOS in the penis (Xie et al. 1997), indicating that secondhand smoke specifically interferes with the production of NO.

Consistent with other results from animal studies, most human studies indicate that endothelium-dependent vasodilation in nonsmokers is sensitive to secondhand smoke following both chronic (Celermajer et al. 1996; Sumida et al. 1998) and acute (Otsuka et al. 2001) exposures. Indeed, the effects of secondhand smoke on endothelium-dependent vasodilation in human coronary circulation are comparable in magnitude to the effects observed in smokers when compared with nonsmokers (Sumida et al. 1998; Otsuka et al. 2001).

Celermajer and colleagues (1996) studied endothelium-dependent vasodilation in 78 healthy persons aged 15 to 30 years by measuring the extent of reactive hyperemia in the brachial artery after occluding it with a blood pressure cuff (with the flow increase determined by endothelium-dependent vasodilation) before and after administering nitroglycerine (an endothelium-independent vasodilator). Involuntary smokers were classified by self-reported levels of chronic exposure to secondhand smoke. Investigators found similar impairments in flow-mediated dilation in both involuntary and active smokers when compared with unexposed nonsmoking controls (Figure 2.5). Among those exposed to secondhand smoke, there was an inverse relationship between the intensity of the exposure and flow-mediated dilation ($r = -0.67$, $p < 0.001$). Using similar methods, Woo and colleagues (1997) studied 72 rural Chinese persons and 72 White persons in Australia and England. These researchers did not find a smoking effect among adults living in rural China, but the analysis grouped active with involuntary smokers. An effect of exposure was observed in White participants, but results were also reported with active and involuntary smokers combined.

The adverse effects of chronic secondhand smoke exposure may be partially reversible. In a cross-sectional study of young adults, there was less evidence for arterial endothelial dysfunction in former involuntary smokers compared with current involuntary smokers (Raitakari et al. 1999). Kato and colleagues (1999) experimentally tested whether the reduction in endothelium-dependent vasodilation from secondhand smoke is an acute phenomenon in nonsmokers. The experiment included a brief, acute exposure to secondhand smoke (15 minutes). There were similar responses before and after exposure in the brachial artery flow to acetylcholine, which stimulates endothelium-dependent vasodilation, and to nitroprusside, which stimulates endothelium-independent vasodilation. The investigators concluded that the consequences of exposure to secondhand smoke were attributable to chronic rather than acute effects on the brachial artery.

Two studies document the effects of secondhand smoke on human coronary arteries (Sumida et al. 1998; Otsuka et al. 2001). Sumida and colleagues (1998) studied 38 women aged 40 to 60 years with no known risk factors for CHD other than age and exposure to tobacco smoke. The participants included three groups: nonsmokers who had never smoked and had never been regularly exposed to secondhand smoke, nonsmokers with a self-reported history of exposure for at least an hour a day for at least 10 years, and active smokers. The study examined the changes in the diameter of the epicardial coronary artery (proximal and distal segments of the left anterior descending and left circumflex coronary arteries) in response to an intracoronary injection of acetylcholine. Acetylcholine constricted most coronary arteries in both exposed nonsmokers and active smokers to a similar extent and dilated the coronary arteries in unexposed nonsmokers. This result suggests possibly similar levels of coronary endothelial dysfunction among involuntary and active smokers.

Otsuka and colleagues (2001) used ultrasound in healthy young adult nonsmokers and smokers to measure coronary flow velocity changes in response to acetylcholine as a measure of endothelium-dependent vasodilation (quantified as coronary flow velocity reserve). The measurements were made before and 30 minutes after breathing secondhand smoke for 30 minutes in a hospital smoking room in Japan. Before the exposure, nonsmokers had a significantly higher coronary flow velocity reserve compared with smokers (Figure 2.6). The 30 minutes of exposure had no effect on the coronary flow velocity reserve among smokers, but significantly reduced the reserve in nonsmokers to a level that almost equaled the level found in smokers (Figure 2.6). This substantial acute response is similar in magnitude to the effect observed with chronic exposures on brachial (Celermajer et al. 1996) and coronary (Sumida et al. 1998) arteries. However, the finding differs from the lack of effect seen for short-term (15 minutes) acute exposures on the brachial artery (Kato et al. 1999). The different findings in these two studies (Sumida et al. 1998; Otsuka et al. 2001) may be attributable to the duration of the exposure (30 versus 15 minutes) or to differences in the responses of the coronary arteries and the brachial arteries to secondhand smoke exposure.

An experiment in humans also showed that an acute exposure to secondhand smoke reduces the distensibility of the aorta (Stefanadis et al. 1998). In this study, the nonsmokers were exposed to secondhand smoke for five minutes at a mean carbon monoxide (CO) level of 30 parts per million; the smokers smoked one cigarette. The distensibility of the aorta in nonsmokers exposed to secondhand smoke for just five minutes was reduced significantly by 21 percent compared with a 27 percent reduction in the active smokers. There was no change in the sham-exposed patients.

Human experiments have indicated that even short-term exposures to active smoking (Přerovský and Hladovec 1979) or to other tobacco product constituents significantly increase the number of nuclear endothelial cell carcasses in the blood (Davis et al. 1989). The presence of these cell carcasses suggests damage to the endothelium. The number of endothelial cell carcasses (i.e., remains of dead cells) in nonsmokers after they were exposed to secondhand smoke was almost as great as the number of carcasses observed in active smokers.

Figure 2.5   Flow-mediated (endothelium-dependent) and nitroglycerin-induced (endothelium-independent) vasodilation in human brachial arteries

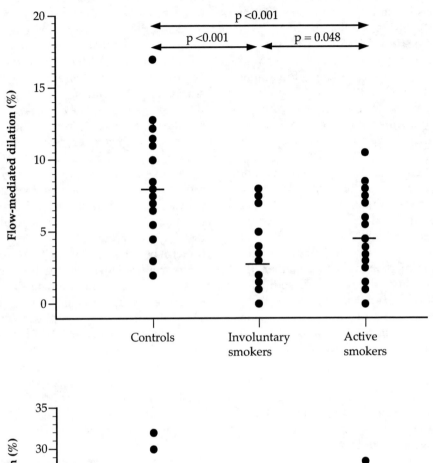

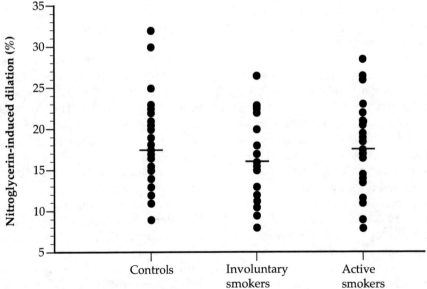

Note: Flow-mediated (endothelium-dependent) vasodilation in human brachial arteries was significantly impaired in chronically exposed involuntary smokers and in active smokers to a similar degree, compared with the controls, whereas nitroglycerine-induced (endothelium-independent) vasodilation was similar in all three groups.
Source: Celermajer et al. 1996. Adapted with permission.

Figure 2.6   Coronary flow velocity changes before and after secondhand smoke exposure

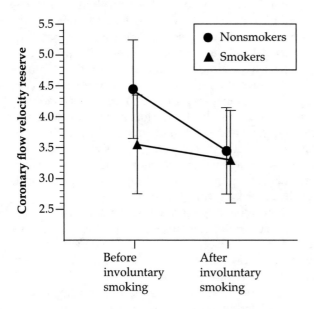

Note: Data are mean (standard deviation). Coronary flow velocity reserve (CFVR) before involuntary smoking was significantly higher in nonsmokers than in smokers. However, CFVR after involuntary smoking was reduced significantly in nonsmokers, but only slightly among smokers. Source: Otsuka et al. 2001. Adapted with permission.

Atherosclerosis

Endothelial dysfunction may also contribute to the development of atherosclerosis. Normal endothelial cells promote vasodilation and inhibit atherosclerosis and thrombosis, in part through the release of NO (Harrison 1997). Dysfunctional cells, on the other hand, contribute to vasoconstriction, atherogenesis, and thrombosis. Risk factors contribute collectively to endothelial dysfunction. For example, active smoking interacts with LDL in a way that damages the endothelium (Heitzer et al. 1996). One unifying hypothesis for the effects of cardiovascular risk factors is a combined action to increase damaging oxidative stress (Oskarsson and Heistad 1997). Thus, reducing exposure to risk factors may improve endothelial function and lessen the risk for clinical coronary events. For example, lipid reduction improves endothelial function in patients with hyperlipidemia both acutely (Tamai et al. 1997) and chronically (Treasure et al. 1995).

Platelets are also relevant to the development of atherosclerosis (Ross 1986; Steinberg et al. 1989). Following damage to the arterial endothelium, platelets interact with or adhere to the subendothelial connective tissue and initiate a sequence that leads to the formation of atherosclerotic plaque. When platelets interact with or adhere to subendothelial connective tissue, they are stimulated to release their granule contents.

Endothelial cells normally prevent platelet adherence because of the nonthrombogenic character of their surface and their capacity to form antithrombotic substances such as prostacyclin (Corti et al. 2003). However, platelets can stick to damaged endothelial cells and release mitogens such as platelet-derived growth factor and chemoattractants, which encourage the migration and proliferation of smooth muscle cells in the region of the endothelial injury (Ross 1993). When platelet aggregation increases as a result of exposure to secondhand smoke, platelet accumulation at the injured site is also expected to increase. Tobacco smoke exposure has also been associated with the accumulation of glycosaminoglycans and glycoproteins in vascular tissues of rats, another early event in atherogenesis (Latha et al. 1991).

Effects on Children

Adverse cardiovascular effects of secondhand smoke exposure may begin in childhood. Adolescents and children whose parents smoked exhibited lower HDL levels than children who were not exposed to secondhand smoke (Moskowitz et al. 1990; Feldman et al. 1991). White and Froeb (1991) reported similar results among adults exposed at work. These findings indicate a less favorable lipid profile in persons exposed to secondhand smoke.

Cross-cultural comparisons suggest that genetic differences may influence how children are affected by secondhand smoke. There was a small exposure effect on HDL cholesterol in Japanese children (Misawa et al. 1989) and no effect in Turkish children (İşcan et al. 1996), but the LDL cholesterol level and the ratio of LDL to HDL cholesterol were adversely affected in Turkish children (İşcan et al. 1996). These effects were similar to those found in smokers and may be mediated by inhibiting the activity of the enzyme plasma lecithin: cholesterol acyltransferase in plasma and altered clearance of chylomicron remnants by the liver (Bielicki et al. 1995; Pan et al. 1997). In children with severe hypercholesterolemia, a lower HDL cholesterol level was associated with parental smoking (Neufeld et al. 1997).

Chemical Interactions with Low-Density Lipoprotein Cholesterol

Several animal studies (Albert et al. 1977; Penn et al. 1981, 1996; Majesky et al. 1983; Revis et al. 1984; Penn and Snyder 1993, 1996a,b) demonstrated that PAHs, in particular 7,12-dimethylbenz[*a,h*] anthracene and B[*a*]P, as well as 1,3 butadiene (Penn and Snyder 1996a,b), accelerate the development of atherosclerosis. PAHs, including B[*a*]P and 1,3 butadiene, are constituents of secondhand smoke. PAHs appear to bind preferentially to both LDL and HDL subfragments of cholesterol and may facilitate the incorporation of toxic compounds into the cells lining the coronary arteries. Thus, exposure to PAHs may contribute to both cell injury and hyperplasia in the atherosclerotic process. Adults who inhaled secondhand smoke for only five and one-half hours exhibited compromised antibiochemical defenses and an increased accumulation of LDL cholesterol in macrophages (Valkonen and Kuusi 1998).

Experimental Atherosclerosis

In addition to the studies of single tobacco smoke components, animal experiments have demonstrated that exposure to secondhand smoke for only a few weeks significantly speeds the atherosclerotic process (Table 2.6). These animal models provide an indication of the effect of exposure to more than one component of tobacco smoke.

Zhu and colleagues (1993b) exposed three groups of rabbits to a high-cholesterol diet. Two of the groups were also exposed to 10 weeks of secondhand smoke from Marlboro cigarettes for six hours a day, five days a week. One group was exposed to levels comparable to a smoky bar and the other group was exposed to much higher levels, with a nicotine level 30 times higher. The high-dose group experienced levels comparable to those observed in a car with the windows rolled up while four cigarettes per hour were smoked (Ott et al. 1992). With just 10 weeks of exposure (a total of 300 hours), the fraction of pulmonary artery and aorta covered with lipid deposits was nearly twice as high in the high-exposure group compared with the control animals. There was a smaller increase in the low-exposure group (Figure 2.7) (Zhu et al. 1993b).

This effect appears to be directly attributable to components in the cigarette smoke itself, rather than to an increase in adrenergic tone resulting from the discomfort associated with the forced breathing of secondhand smoke. Sun and colleagues (1994) exposed rabbits to secondhand smoke in an experiment similar to that of Zhu and colleagues (1993b) and gave half of the rabbits the beta-blocking drug metoprolol. As expected, the animals receiving metoprolol developed fewer lipid deposits than those receiving a placebo (saline), but this effect was independent of whether the rabbits were breathing secondhand smoke. Therefore, increased levels of catacholamines did not mediate the effect of secondhand smoke on the development of atherosclerotic-type lesions in the arteries.

Experiments exposing rabbits to secondhand smoke from standard (Marlboro) and nicotine-free cigarettes produced similar levels of lipid deposits. This finding suggests that nicotine is not the primary atherogenic agent, and there are other combustion products in cigarette smoke that may be responsible for the atherosclerosis (Sun et al. 2001).

Critics have questioned the findings of this rabbit model of atherosclerosis because the animals are fed a high-cholesterol diet in order to develop lesions within a reasonable time (Wu 1993). This experimental model of atherosclerosis has been used since 1908 (Zhu et al. 1993a). Supporting findings come from a different model of plaque development that used young cockerels between the ages of 6 and 22 weeks that were exposed to secondhand smoke for six hours a day, five days a week, for 12 weeks (Penn and Snyder 1993; Penn et al. 1994). The cockerels ate a normal, low-cholesterol diet and were exposed to lower secondhand smoke levels than the rabbits were. The incidence of plaque development was the same in the cockerels breathing secondhand smoke and those breathing clean air. However, the growth rate of the plaques was greater in the exposed animals.

Some specific components have been evaluated in that same model with effects that are not likely to be attributable to the CO in the smoke because exposure of cockerels to high doses of CO (Penn et al. 1992), to tobacco-specific nitrosamines (Penn and Snyder 1996b), or to the tar fraction of the smoke (Penn et al. 1996) did not produce similar effects. Thus, agents in the vapor phase of the smoke appear to be the atherogenic agents; 1,3 butadiene (Penn and Snyder 1996a,b) and 7,12-dimethylybenz[*a*]anthracene (Penn et al. 1981) did increase the amount of atherosclerotic plaque in this experimental model.

Gairola and colleagues (2001) studied the effects of secondhand smoke on apolipoprotein E -/- mice that were on a high-cholesterol diet, which is another model for human atherosclerosis. After exposure to secondhand smoke from University of Kentucky 1R4F research cigarettes for six hours a day, five days a week, for up to 14 weeks, there was a dose-dependent increase in the fraction of the aorta that was covered with atherosclerotic lesions. The exposed mice had significant increases compared with control animals on the same diet who had breathed clean air for just seven days, with the effect increasing over time. The exposed mice had lesions that were about twice the size of those found in the clean-air controls; there were similar increases in the cholesterol content of the aortas in the exposed mice.

Elements in the smoke rapidly affect the process of incorporating LDL cholesterol into the linings of arteries. Roberts and colleagues (1996) used isolated perfused carotid arteries from rats exposed to secondhand smoke for two or four hours. The researchers demonstrated a synergistic effect between secondhand smoke and LDL that facilitated the binding of oxidized LDL to the vessel wall (Roberts et al. 1996). Rats exposed to secondhand smoke for just two hours had higher rates of incorporation of LDL cholesterol into their carotid arteries.

Secondhand smoke exposure induces atherosclerotic-like changes in four different species of experimental animals after only a few weeks of exposure to secondhand smoke at levels similar to those experienced by people in normal day-to-day life. These findings provide strong support for the epidemiologic evidence that exposure to secondhand smoke causes heart disease. The experimental studies on rabbits, cockerels, mice, and rats were not affected by potential confounding and support a causal conclusion by showing that atherosclerosis can be induced in experimental animals exposed to secondhand smoke.

Oxygen Delivery, Processing, and Exercise

Secondhand smoke reduces the ability of the blood to deliver oxygen to the myocardium. The CO in secondhand smoke competes with oxygen for binding sites on hemoglobin and thus displaces oxygen (USDHHS 1983, 1986; Leone et al. 1991; U.S. Environmental Protection Agency 1991). Children of smoking parents have elevated levels of 2,3-diphosphoglycerate, a compound that increases in red blood cells to compensate for reduced oxygen availability (Moskowitz et al. 1990, 1993) and is associated with serum thiocyanate levels, a measure of secondhand smoke exposure (Moskowitz et al. 1990).

Evidence from animal studies shows that in addition to reducing the ability of the blood to deliver oxygen to the heart, secondhand smoke may reduce the ability of the heart muscle to convert oxygen into the "energy molecule" adenosine triphosphate (ATP). In a rabbit model, there was an approximate 25 percent reduction in cytochrome oxidase activity after a

single 30-minute exposure to secondhand smoke, and the activity continued to drop with a prolonged exposure; after eight weeks of exposure for 30 minutes per day, its activity was 50 percent of the level found in controls (Gvozdják et al. 1987). Thus, not only does secondhand smoke exposure reduce the ability of the blood to deliver oxygen to the myocardium, it may also reduce the ability of the myocardium to effectively use the oxygen it receives (Gvozdjáková et al. 1984, 1985, 1992; Gvozdják et al. 1987).

Secondhand smoke also significantly increases the amount of lactate in venous blood with an exercise challenge (McMurray et al. 1985). Eight women with and without exposure to tobacco smoke through a mouthpiece (concentration not given) engaged in exercises. Compared with the unexposed group, the exposed group documented a lower maximum oxygen uptake and a higher blood lactate. People with CHD cannot exercise as long or reach a level of exercise as high after breathing secondhand smoke, even relatively briefly, compared with breathing clean air (Aronow 1978; Khalfen and Klochkov 1987; Leone et al. 1991). Another study showed that 10 persons with a past MI were more likely to develop increased arrhythmias from exercise following secondhand smoke exposure (Leone et al. 1992).

Free Radicals and Ischemic Damage

Free radicals are highly reactive oxygen products (Church and Pryor 1985; Ferrari et al. 1991) that are destructive to the heart muscle cell membrane as well as to other processes within the cell. Tobacco smoke contains high levels of activated oxygen species, and the inflammatory consequences of tobacco smoke components in various organs are thought to be a critical path of injury. Antioxidants provide protection against the free radicals, but levels of antioxidants, such as beta-carotene and vitamin C, tend to be lower in active smokers (USDHHS 2004) and possibly in involuntary smokers (Farchi et al. 2001).

Experiments have demonstrated that exposure to secondhand smoke worsens the outcome of an ischemic event in the heart through the activity of free radicals during reperfusion injury. Animal studies indicate that low exposures to nicotine or to other cigarette smoke constituents significantly worsen reperfusion injury. Intravenous administration of the amount of nicotine delivered by just one cigarette doubled the reperfusion injury in a dog model of MI (Przyklenk 1994). This dose was low and had no effect on heart rate, blood pressure, regional myocardial shortening,

Table 2.6   Studies of experimental atherosclerosis in animals exposed to secondhand smoke

Study	Species	Secondhand smoke exposure		
		Source	Duration	Measure
Penn and Snyder 1993	Cockerel	1R4F research cigarettes	6 hours/day, 5 days/ week for 16 weeks	Nicotine: 365–414 $\mu g/m^{3}$* CO[†]: 35 ppm[‡] Particulates: 8 mg[§]/m^3
Zhu et al. 1993a	Rabbit	Marlboro	6 hours/day, 5 days/ week for 10 weeks	<u>Low exposure</u> Air nicotine: 30 $\mu g/m^3$ CO: 19 ppm Particulates: 4 mg/m^3 <u>High exposure</u> Air nicotine: 1,000 $\mu g/m^3$ CO: 60 ppm Particulates: 33 mg/m^3
Penn et al. 1994	Cockerel	1R4F research cigarettes	1 cigarette/day, 5 days/week for 16 weeks	Nicotine: 90–130 $\mu g/m^3$ CO: 4 ppm Particulates: 2.5 mg/m^3
Sun et al. 1994	Rabbit	Marlboro	6 hours/day, 5 days/ week for 10 weeks	Air nicotine: 1,100 $\mu g/m^3$ CO: 60–70 ppm Particulates: 38 mg/m^3
Roberts et al. 1996	Rat	Data were not reported	2 or 4 hours	Nicotine: 615 $\mu g/m^3$ CO: 18 ± 2 ppm Particulates: 3 $\mu g/m^3$
Gairola et al. 2001	Mouse	1R4F research cigarettes	6 hours/day, 5 days/ week for 7, 10, and 14 weeks	Blood CO hemoglobin: 10% in secondhand smoke-exposed mice Particulates: 25 mg/m^3
Sun et al. 2001	Rabbit	Standard or nicotine-free research cigarettes	6 hours/day, 5 days/ week for 10 weeks	CO: 45–54 ppm Particulates: 24–35 mg/m^3

*$\mu g/m^3$ = Micrograms per cubic meter.
[†]CO = Carbon monoxide.
[‡]ppm = Parts per million.
[§]mg = Milligram.
[Δ]LDL = Low-density lipoprotein.

End point	Findings
Number and size of plaques in aortic segments	• Exposure had no effect on the number of plaques • Plaques in exposed animals were significantly larger (median size about 1.5 times larger in each aortic segment) than in unexposed animals
Area of atherosclerotic lesions by planimetry in aorta and pulmonary artery; bleeding time (to measure platelet activity)	• High-exposure secondhand smoke group had dose-dependent lipid deposits with lesion size about 1.7 times larger than those in the low-exposure group • Low-exposure group was between the high-exposure and control groups • Bleeding times were shorter in rabbits that breathed secondhand smoke • No differences between high-dose and low-dose exposures for serum triglycerides, cholesterol, and high-lipoprotein cholesterol
Number and size of plaques in aortic segments	• Exposure had no effect on the number of plaques • Plaques in exposed animals were significantly larger (median size about 1.5 times larger in each aortic segment) than those in unexposed animals
Area of atherosclerotic lesions by planimetry in aorta and pulmonary artery; bleeding time (to measure platelet activity)	• Secondhand smoke exposure was associated with greater lipid deposits and shorter bleeding times • Metoprolol did not block these effects, indicating that they are not mediated by increased circulating catecholamines
Uptake of LDL[a] cholesterol in isolated perfused carotid artery	• Rate of LDL uptake more than quadrupled
Area of atherosclerotic lesions at several places in aorta measured by planimetry; cholesterol content of aortic segments	• Increasing lesion size and cholesterol content over time in both groups • Secondhand smoke-exposed mice had approximately twice the level of atherosclerosis as controls at any given time
Area of atherosclerotic lesions by planimetry in aorta and pulmonary artery	• Secondhand smoke increased the area of arteries with lipid deposits by about 50% • There was no significant difference between nicotine and nicotine-free cigarette smoke

Figure 2.7   Secondhand smoke exposure and lipid deposits in rabbits

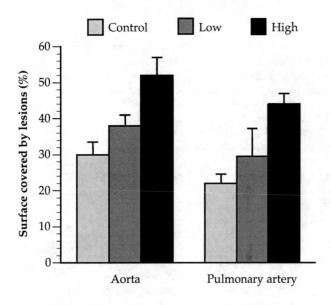

Note: Exposure to secondhand smoke increased lipid deposits in arteries of rabbits in a dose-dependent manner. Bars are for controls (clear air), and low doses and high doses of secondhand smoke exposures. Error bars represent standard error of the mean.
Source: Zhu et al. 1993b. Reprinted with permission.

or on other hemodynamic measures of cardiac function that are commonly affected by nicotine in active and involuntary smokers (Benowitz 1991). After an ischemic episode from ligation of the left anterior descending coronary artery for 15 minutes, the regional shortening during reperfusion was reduced by 50 percent of the pre-ischemic values. When the dog was exposed to nicotine from just a single cigarette, the regional shortening during reperfusion was reduced by 25 percent of control values. When the dog was given a free radical scavenger along with the nicotine, this effect was obliterated. Thus, exposure to a very low dose of nicotine doubled the impact of the reperfusion injury on the myocardium.

The effects of free radicals induced by secondhand smoke have been explored at the cellular level (van Jaarsveld et al. 1992a,b). Rats exposed to secondhand smoke from two cigarettes a day for two months exhibited severely damaged mitochondrial function during reperfusion injury. Thus, the ability of cardiac mitochondrial cells to convert oxygen into ATP

was more compromised during reperfusion injury among rats exposed to these low doses than among control rats.

Secondhand smoke exposure is associated with lower levels of antioxidant vitamins in nonsmoking women (Farchi et al. 2001). Despite a similar dietary intake of beta-carotene, retinol, L-ascorbic acid, and alpha-tocopherol, women whose husbands smoked exhibited a dose-dependent relationship between the extent of exposure and plasma concentrations of beta-carotene and L-ascorbic acid. These associations persisted even after controlling for daily beta-carotene and vitamin C intake and for other potential confounders (vitamin supplementation, alcohol consumption, and body mass index). A similar dose-response relationship was observed when urinary cotinine was used as the measure of exposure.

In a mouse model, a 30-minute exposure to secondhand smoke also produced evidence of oxidative DNA damage in the myocardium assessed by increased levels of 8-OH-dG (Howard et al. 1998a). There are also parallel human data. In a cross-sectional study, persons exposed to secondhand smoke at work exhibited increased levels of 8-OH-dG (Howard et al. 1998b). The plasma cotinine levels were 65 percent higher in the exposed group compared with controls, and increases in 8-OH-dG levels were similar. In workers exposed to secondhand smoke, 8-OH-dG levels fell after 60 days of antioxidant supplementation (Howard et al. 1998c).

There is also evidence that smokers are less sensitive to free radical damage from cigarette smoke than nonsmokers are because of changes in the levels of enzymes that control free radicals (McCusker and Hoidal 1990). When hamsters were exposed to secondhand smoke from six cigarettes a day for eight weeks, the activity of antioxidant enzymes in their lungs nearly doubled. Similar changes found in the lungs of smokers compared with nonsmokers provide further evidence that secondhand cigarette smoke may affect smokers and nonsmokers differently. Chronic exposures to cigarette smoke appear to increase the capacity of free radical scavenging systems in smokers.

In addition, human exposures to secondhand smoke sensitize lung neutrophils (Anderson et al. 1991). As with platelets, neutrophils are an important element of the body's defenses against infection and damage. Inappropriately activated neutrophils, however, release oxidants that can play a role in tissue damage. In a group of nonsmokers exposed to three hours of sidestream smoke at relatively high levels (respirable particles >2,000 micrograms/m³), there were significant increases in circulating leukocyte counts, in stimulated neutrophil migration, and in the release of reactive oxidents by neutrophils.

Myocardial Infarction

Several of the effects discussed above would lead to the expectation that exposure to secondhand smoke would increase the severity of MIs. Direct animal data show that secondhand smoke increases tissue damage following a MI. Dogs exposed to secondhand smoke for one hour daily for 10 days and then subjected to a coronary artery blockage developed MIs that were twice as large as those found in controls breathing clean air (Prentice et al. 1989). This effect was not due to elevated circulating levels of nicotine or carboxy-hemoglobin, because the infarcts were created the day after the last day of secondhand smoke exposure. Zhu and colleagues (1994) conducted an experiment in rats to investigate the effects of secondhand smoke exposure on infarct size. Rats were exposed to secondhand smoke six hours a day for three days, three weeks, or six weeks, and then subjected to a left coronary artery occlusion for 35 minutes followed by reperfusion. There was a dose-dependent increase in infarct size, with the longest exposure of 180 hours yielding infarcts nearly twice as large as in the control group that breathed clean air (Figure 2.8). This effect could be countered by feeding the animals L-arginine (Zhu et al. 1996). This finding suggests that the effect of secondhand smoke in producing an MI comes from interference with the vascular endothelium. There is no evidence indicating a threshold level of exposure that is needed to produce this effect.

Heart Rate Variability

Alterations in heart rates are caused by the opposing effects of the sympathetic and para-sympathetic nervous systems on the sino-atrial node (the pacemaker of the heart) through the elevation of catecholamines. The sympathetic nervous system tends to oppose the rate-slowing effects of the para-sympathetic (vagus) nervous system, and sympathetic activation reduces heart rate variability. If sympathetic tone is reduced and vagal activity enhanced, heart rate variability increases. Clinically, decreased heart rate variability predicts a higher risk of cardiac death or arrhythmic events after an acute MI, presumably reflecting the adverse effects of increased sympathetic tone (Kleiger et al. 1987; Singh et al. 1996).

Figure 2.8 Secondhand smoke exposure and infarct size in rats

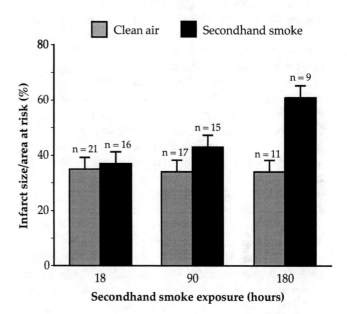

Note: Exposure to secondhand smoke increased infarct size in rats subjected to a 35-minute occlusion of the left coronary artery in a dose-dependent manner. There is no evidence of a threshold effect.
Source: Zhu et al. 1994. Adapted with permission.

Activation of the sympathetic nervous system would tend to reduce heart rate variability. One experimental study has tested this hypothesis. Pope and colleagues (2001) measured heart rate variability in healthy young adults for two hours in the smoke-free areas of a U.S. airport, followed by two hours in the smoking area, and then repeated this protocol. When the experimental participants were in the smoking area, heart rate variability was 12 percent lower. The levels of secondhand smoke were not high enough to affect mean heart rate or blood pressure, but the secondhand smoke exposure was associated with altered cardiac autonomic function in a direction consistent with an increased risk of a cardiac event.

Summary

A source of uncertainty in interpreting evidence on secondhand smoke exposure and heart disease has been the apparently large size of the effect compared with active smoking. Active smoking delivers doses of the toxins in secondhand smoke that are markedly greater than the doses received by a nonsmoker, and active smoking approximately doubles, depending on the amount smoked, the risk of heart disease (USDHHS 1983). Thus, the effect of secondhand smoke may appear large for the associated doses of cigarette smoke components, particularly since secondhand smoke exposure generally does not produce changes in systemic physiologic measures such as heart rate or blood pressure (Celermajer et al. 1996; Hausberg et al. 1997; Sumida et al. 1998; Otsuka et al. 2001). However, findings of a wide variety of clinical and experimental studies of various designs demonstrate that the effects of secondhand smoke on the cardiovascular system occur at low doses in nonsmokers, with some of the effects (on platelets and vascular function) similar to those in active smokers. For this reason, it is not appropriate to scale from the effects of active smoking in a linear, dose-dependent approach to estimate the effects of exposure to secondhand smoke based on comparative doses of smoke components (Howard and Thun 1999).

Secondhand smoke interferes with the normal functioning of the heart, blood, and vascular systems in ways that increase the risk of a cardiac event. For some of these effects (changes in platelet and vascular function), the immediate effects of even short exposures to secondhand smoke appear to be as large as those seen in association with active smoking of one pack of cigarettes a day. Some evidence indicates lower levels of circulating antioxidants associated with secondhand smoke exposure. The experimental and observational evidence reviewed in this chapter supports the plausibility of the findings of the epidemiologic studies reviewed in Chapter 8 (Cardiovascular Diseases from Exposure to Secondhand Smoke). The large body of evidence documenting that secondhand smoke produces substantial and rapid effects on the cardiovascular system demonstrates that even a brief exposure to secondhand smoke has adverse consequences for the heart, blood, and blood vessels (Glantz and Parmley 2001; Barnoya and Glantz 2005).

Conclusions

1. The evidence is sufficient to infer that exposure to secondhand smoke has a prothrombotic effect.

2. The evidence is sufficient to infer that exposure to secondhand smoke causes endothelial cell dysfunctions.

3. The evidence is sufficient to infer that exposure to secondhand smoke causes atherosclerosis in animal models.

Evidence Synthesis

This chapter reviews the substantial amount of data from cellular, animal, and human studies supporting the overall conclusion that exposure to secondhand smoke causes a broad range of adverse effects in both children and adult nonsmokers. These data provide a strong foundation for the biologic plausibility of causal conclusions related to specific diseases and other adverse health effects that are reviewed in Chapters 5 through 9. This chapter provides substantial additional evidence on the underlying pathogenic mechanisms for major adverse health outcomes associated with exposure to secondhand smoke.

Secondhand smoke is a complex mixture of thousands of chemicals emitted from burning tobacco. The toxicologic profiles of a large number of these specific chemicals and compounds are well established (http://www.atsdr.cdc.gov/toxpro2.html). This chemical mixture includes more than 50 carcinogens, and both IARC (2004) and the National Toxicology Program (USDHHS 2000) have classified this mixture as a known human carcinogen. Researchers have thus concluded that exposure to secondhand smoke can cause DNA damage and genetic mutations. For DNA-damaging carcinogens, the occurrence of permanent mutations implies that there is no level of exposure that does not pose a risk.

The complex mixture of chemicals in secondhand smoke also contains a large number of toxicants harmful to the respiratory and cardiovascular systems. Evidence from both animal and human studies indicates that exposures to secondhand smoke can produce substantial and rapid adverse effects on the functioning of the heart, blood, and vascular systems in ways that increase the risk of a cardiac event. Furthermore, many of these acute and chronic changes in blood and vascular function appear to be as large as those seen in active smokers. The immediate effects in some measures of blood and vascular functioning among nonsmokers from even brief exposures (i.e., 30 minutes or less) to secondhand smoke are comparable in magnitude to the effects observed in active smokers. Thus, the evidence reviewed in this chapter supports the biologic plausibility of adverse cardiovascular health outcomes that are associated with exposure to secondhand smoke, which are reviewed in Chapter 8.

As the portal of entry for secondhand smoke, the respiratory system is the initial site of deposition for the particulate and gaseous compounds found in secondhand smoke. This chapter identifies the multiple mechanisms by which secondhand smoke exposure can induce both acute and chronic adverse health effects within the respiratory tract that affect infants, children, and adults. The evidence for underlying mechanisms of respiratory injury from exposure to secondhand smoke suggests that a safe level of exposure may not exist, thus implying that any exposure carries some risk. For infants, children, and adults with asthma or with more sensitive respiratory systems, even very brief exposures to secondhand smoke can trigger intense bronchopulmonary responses that could be life threatening in the most susceptible individuals.

Animal and human studies indicate that prenatal and postnatal exposure to nicotine and other toxicants in tobacco smoke may affect the neuroregulation of breathing, apneic spells, and sudden infant death. Experimental data on the neurotoxicity of prenatal and neonatal exposure to nicotine and secondhand smoke in animal models can be related to several potential causal mechanisms for SIDS, including adverse effects on brain cell development, synaptic development and function, and neurobehavioral activity. Finally, studies have documented that exposure to tobacco smoke from active smoking has a broad effect on immune function and host defenses against infectious agents. Evidence indicates that exposure to secondhand smoke appears to also impair immune function in both children and adult nonsmokers, which increases susceptibility to infection.

Conclusions

Evidence of Carcinogenic Effects from Secondhand Smoke Exposure

1. More than 50 carcinogens have been identified in sidestream and secondhand smoke.

2. The evidence is sufficient to infer a causal relationship between exposure to secondhand smoke and its condensates and tumors in laboratory animals.

3. The evidence is sufficient to infer that exposure of nonsmokers to secondhand smoke causes a significant increase in urinary levels of metabolites of the tobacco-specific lung carcinogen 4-(methylnitrosamino)-1-(3-pyridyl)-1-butanone (NNK). The presence of these metabolites links exposure to secondhand smoke with an increased risk for lung cancer.

4. The mechanisms by which secondhand smoke causes lung cancer are probably similar to those observed in smokers. The overall risk of secondhand smoke exposure, compared with active smoking, is diminished by a substantially lower carcinogenic dose.

Mechanisms of Respiratory Tract Injury and Disease Caused by Secondhand Smoke Exposure

5. The evidence indicates multiple mechanisms by which secondhand smoke exposure causes injury to the respiratory tract.

6. The evidence indicates mechanisms by which secondhand smoke exposure could increase the risk for sudden infant death syndrome.

Mechanisms of Secondhand Smoke Exposure and Heart Disease

7. The evidence is sufficient to infer that exposure to secondhand smoke has a prothrombotic effect.

8. The evidence is sufficient to infer that exposure to secondhand smoke causes endothelial cell dysfunctions.

9. The evidence is sufficient to infer that exposure to secondhand smoke causes atherosclerosis in animal models.

Overall Implications

The biologic mechanisms reviewed in this chapter underlie a wide range of acute and chronic adverse health effects in infants, children, and adults examined in Chapters 5 through 9. This broadly reaching body of evidence on the toxicology of secondhand smoke and on these biologic mechanisms indicates that any exposure to secondhand smoke will increase risk for adverse health outcomes.

References

Adams JD, O'Mara-Adams KJ, Hoffmann D. Toxic and carcinogenic agents in undiluted mainstream smoke and sidestream smoke of different types of cigarettes. *Carcinogenesis* 1987;8(5):729–31.

Adgent MA. Environmental tobacco smoke and sudden infant death syndrome: a review. *Birth Defects Research (Part B)* 2006;77(1):69–85.

Albert RE, Vanderlaan M, Burns FJ, Nishizumi M. Effect of carcinogens on chicken atherosclerosis. *Cancer Research* 1977;37(7 Pt 1):2232–5.

Anderson KE, Carmella SG, Ye M, Bliss RL, Le C, Murphy L, Hecht SS. Metabolites of a tobacco-specific lung carcinogen in nonsmoking women exposed to environmental tobacco smoke. *Journal of the National Cancer Institute* 2001;93(5):378–81.

Anderson R, Theron AJ, Richards GA, Myer MS, van Rensburg AJ. Passive smoking by humans sensitizes circulating neutrophils. *American Review of Respiratory Diseases* 1991;144(3 Pt 1):570–4.

Armstrong RN. Glutathione-*S*-transferases. In: Guengerich FP, editor. *Comprehensive Toxicology: Biotransformation*. Vol. 3. New York: Elsevier Science, 1997:307–27.

Aronow WS. Effect of passive smoking on angina pectoris. *New England Journal of Medicine* 1978;299(1):21–4.

Autrup H, Vestergaard AB, Okkels H. Transplacental transfer of environmental genotoxins: polycyclic aromatic hydrocarbon–albumin in non-smoking women, and the effect of maternal GSTM1 genotype. *Carcinogenesis* 1995;16(6):1305–9.

Avery ME, Frantz ID 3rd. To breathe or not to breathe—what have we learned about apneic spells and sudden infant death [editorial]? *New England Journal of Medicine* 1983;309(2):107–8.

Baird WM, Ralston SL. Carcinogenic polycyclic aromatic hydrocarbons. In: Bowden GT, Fischer SM, editors. *Comprehensive Toxicology: Chemical Carcinogens and Anticarcinogens*. Vol. 12. New York: Elsevier Science, 1997:171–200.

Barnes PJ, Belvisi MG. Nitric oxide and lung disease. *Thorax* 1993;48(10):1034–43.

Barnoya J, Glantz SA. Cardiovascular effects of secondhand smoke: nearly as large as smoking. *Circulation* 2005;111(20):2684–98.

Barr MB, Weiss ST, Segal MR, Tager IB, Speizer FE. The relationship of nasal disorders to lower respiratory tract symptoms and illness in a random sample of children. *Pediatric Pulmonology* 1992;14(2):91–4.

Bartsch H, Caporaso N, Coda M, Kadlubar F, Malaveille C, Skipper P, Talaska G, Tannenbaum SR, Vineis P. Carcinogen hemoglobin adducts, urinary mutagenicity, and metabolic phenotype in active and passive cigarette smokers. *Journal of the National Cancer Institute* 1990;82(23):1826–31.

Bartsch H, Spiegelhalder B. Environmental exposure to *N*-nitroso compounds (NNOC) and precursors: an overview. *European Journal of Cancer Prevention* 1996;5(Suppl 1):11–7.

Bascom R, Kagey-Sobotka A, Proud D. Effect of intranasal capsaicin on symptoms and mediator release. *Journal of Pharmacology and Experimental Therapeutics* 1991;259(3):1323–7.

Bascom R, Kesavanathan J, Fitzgerald TK, Cheng KH, Swift DL. Sidestream tobacco smoke exposure acutely alters human nasal mucociliary clearance. *Environmental Health Perspectives* 1995;103(11):1026–30.

Bauer E, Guo Z, Ueng Y-F, Bell LC, Zeldin D, Guengerich FP. Oxidation of benzo[*a*]pyrene by recombinant human cytochrome P450 enzymes. *Chemical Research in Toxicology* 1995;8(1):136–42.

Bennett WP, Alavanja MCR, Blomeke B, Vähäkangas KH, Castrén K, Welsh JA, Bowman ED, Khan MA, Flieder DB, Harris CC. Environmental tobacco smoke, genetic susceptibility, and risk of lung cancer in never-smoking women. *Journal of the National Cancer Institute* 1999;91(23):2009–14.

Benninger MS. The impact of cigarette smoking and environmental tobacco smoke on nasal and sinus disease: a review of the literature. *American Journal of Rhinology* 1999;13(6):435–8.

Benowitz NL. Nicotine and coronary heart disease. *Trends in Cardiovascular Medicine* 1991;1(8):315–21.

Benowitz NL, Fitzgerald GA, Wilson M, Zhang Q. Nicotine effects on eicosanoid formation and hemostatic function: comparison of transdermal nicotine and cigarette smoking. *Journal of the American College of Cardiology* 1993;22(4):1159–67.

Bielicki JK, McCall MR, van den Berg JJM, Kuypers FA, Forte TM. Copper and gas-phase cigarette smoke inhibit plasma lecithin: cholesterol acyltransferase activity by different mechanisms. *Journal of Lipid Research* 1995;36(2):322–31.

Binková B, Lewtas J, Misková I, Leníček J, Šrám R. DNA adducts and personal air monitoring of carcinogenic polycyclic aromatic hydrocarbons in an environmentally exposed population. *Carcinogenesis* 1995;16(5):1037–46.

Bonham AC, Chen CY, Mutoh T, Joad JP. Lung C-fiber CNS reflex: role in the respiratory consequences of extended environmental tobacco smoke exposure in young guinea pigs. *Environmental Health Perspectives* 2001;109(Suppl 4):573–8.

Branner B, Kutzer C, Zwickenpflug W, Scherer G, Heller W-D, Richter E. Haemoglobin adducts from aromatic amines and tobacco-specific nitrosamines in pregnant smoking and non-smoking women. *Biomarkers* 1998;3(1):35–47.

Brunnemann KD, Cox JE, Hoffmann D. Analysis of tobacco-specific *N*-nitrosamines in indoor air. *Carcinogenesis* 1992;13(12):2415–8.

Brunnemann KD, Hoffmann D. Assessment of the carcinogenic N-nitrosodiethanolamine in tobacco products and tobacco smoke. *Carcinogenesis* 1981; 2(11):1123–7.

Brunnemann KD, Masaryk J, Hoffmann D. Role of tobacco stems in the formation of *N*-nitrosamines in tobacco and cigarette mainstream and sidestream smoke. *Journal of Agricultural and Food Chemistry* 1983;31(6):1221–4.

Brunnemann KD, Yu L, Hoffmann D. Assessment of carcinogenic volatile *N*-nitrosamines in tobacco and in mainstream and sidestream smoke from cigarettes. *Cancer Research* 1977;37(9):3218–22.

Burchell B, McGurk K, Brierley CH, Clarke DJ. UDP-glucuronosyltransferases. In: Guengerich FP, editor. *Comprehensive Toxicology: Biotransformation*. Vol. 3. New York: Elsevier Science, 1997:401–36.

Burghuber OC, Punzengruber C, Sinzinger H, Haber P, Silberbauer K. Platelet sensitivity to prostacyclin in smokers and non-smokers. *Chest* 1986;90(1): 34–8.

California Environmental Protection Agency. *Proposed Identification of Environmental Tobacco Smoke as a Toxic Air Contaminant. Part B: Health Effects*. Sacramento (CA): California Environmental Protection Agency, Office of Environmental Health Hazard Assessment, 2005.

Carmella SG, Kagan SS, Kagan M, Foiles PG, Palladino G, Quart AM, Quart E, Hecht SS. Mass spectrometric analysis of tobacco-specific nitrosamine hemoglobin adducts in snuff dippers, smokers, and nonsmokers. *Cancer Research* 1990;50(17):5438–45.

Carrer P, Maroni M, Alcini D, Cavallo D, Fustinoni S, Lovato L, Visigalli F. Assessment through environmental and biological measurements of total daily exposure to volatile organic compounds of office workers in Milan, Italy. *Indoor Air* 2000;10(4): 258–68.

Celermajer DS, Adams MR, Clarkson P, Robinson J, McCredie R, Donald A, Deanfield JE. Passive smoking and impaired endothelium-dependent arterial dilation in healthy young adults. *New England Journal of Medicine* 1996;334(3):150–4.

Celermajer DS, Sorensen KE, Georgakopoulos D, Bull C, Thomas O, Robinson J, Deanfield JE. Cigarette smoking is associated with dose-related and potentially reversible impairment of endothelium-dependent dilation in healthy young adults. *Circulation* 1993;88(5 Pt 1):2149–55.

Chang AB, Wilson SJ, Masters IB, Yuill M, Williams J, Williams G, Hubbard M. Altered arousal response in infants exposed to cigarette smoke. *Archives of Disease in Childhood* 2003;88(1):30–3.

Chuang JC, Mack GA, Kuhlman MR, Wilson NK. Polycyclic aromatic hydrocarbons and their derivatives in indoor and outdoor air in an eight-home study. *Atmospheric Environment* 1991;25B(3):369–80.

Church DF, Pryor WA. Free-radical chemistry of cigarette smoke and its toxicological implications. *Environmental Health Perspectives* 1985;64:111–26.

Coleridge HM, Coleridge JC. Pulmonary reflexes: neural mechanisms of pulmonary defense. *Annual Review of Physiology* 1994;56:69–91.

Coleridge JC, Coleridge HM, Schelegle ES, Green JF. Acute inhalation of ozone stimulates bronchial C-fibers and rapidly adapting receptors in dogs. *Journal of Applied Physiology* 1993;74(5):2345–52.

Collins MH, Moessinger AC, Kleinerman J, Bassi J, Rosso P, Collins AM, James LS, Blanc WA. Fetal lung hypoplasia associated with maternal smoking: a morphometric analysis. *Pediatric Research* 1985;19(4):408–12.

Conney AH, Chang RL, Jerina DM, Wei S-JC. Studies on the metabolism of benzo[a]pyrene and dose-dependent differences in the mutagenic profile of its ultimate carcinogenic metabolite. *Drug Metabolism Reviews* 1994;26(1-2):125–63.

Cook DG, Strachan DP. Health effects of passive smoking. 10: summary of effects of parental smoking on the respiratory health of children and implications for research. *Thorax* 1999;54(4):357–66.

Cooper CS, Grover PL, Sims P. The metabolism and activation of benzo[a]pyrene. In: Bridges JW, Chasseaud LF, editors. *Progress in Drug Metabolism*. Vol. 7. New York: John Wiley & Sons, 1983: 295–396.

Corti R, Fuster V, Badimon JJ. Pathogenetic concepts of acute coronary syndromes. *Journal of the American College of Cardiology* 2003;41(4):7S–14S.

Cosio MG, Hale KA, Niewoehner DE. Morphologic and morphometric effects of prolonged cigarette smoking on the small airways. *American Review of Respiratory Diseases* 1980;122(2):265–71.

Coultas DB. Health effects of passive smoking. 8: passive smoking and risk of adult asthma and COPD: an update. *Thorax* 1998;53(5):381–7.

Crawford FG, Mayer J, Santella RM, Cooper TB, Ottman R, Tsai W-Y, Simon-Cereijido G, Wang M, Tang D, Perera FP. Biomarkers of environmental tobacco smoke in preschool children and their mothers. *Journal of the National Cancer Institute* 1994;86(18):1398–402.

Culp SJ, Gaylor DW, Sheldon WG, Goldstein LS, Beland FA. A comparison of the tumors induced by coal tar and benzo[*a*]pyrene in a 2-year bioassay. *Carcinogenesis* 1998;19(1):117–24.

Cunningham J, Dockery DW, Speizer FE. Maternal smoking during pregnancy as a predictor of lung function in children. *American Journal of Epidemiology* 1994;139(12):1139–52.

Daube H, Scherer G, Riedel K, Ruppert T, Tricker AR, Rosenbaum P, Adlkofer F. DNA adducts in human placenta in relation to tobacco smoke exposure and plasma antioxidant status. *Journal of Cancer Research and Clinical Oncology* 1997;123(3):141–51.

Davis JW, Shelton L, Eigenberg DA, Hignite CE, Watanabe IS. Effects of tobacco and non-tobacco cigarette smoking on endothelium and platelets. *Clinical Pharmacology and Therapeutics* 1985;37(5):529–33.

Davis JW, Shelton L, Watanabe IS, Arnold J. Passive smoking affects endothelium and platelets. *Archives of Internal Medicine* 1989;149(2):386–9.

Dayal HH, Khuder S, Sharrar R, Trieff N. Passive smoking in obstructive respiratory disease in an industrialized urban population. *Environmental Research* 1994;65(2):161–71.

De Flora S, D'Agostini F, Balansky R, Camoirano A, Bennicelli C, Bagnasco M, Cartiglia C, Tampa E, Grazia Longobardi M, Lubet RA, Izotti A. Modulation of cigarette smoke-related end-points in mutagenesis and carcinogenesis. *Mutation Research* 2003;523-524:237–52.

Dezateux C, Stocks J, Dundas I, Fletcher ME. Impaired airway function and wheezing in infancy: the influence of maternal smoking and a genetic predisposition to asthma. *American Journal of Respiratory and Critical Care Medicine* 1999;159(2):403–10.

Duffel MW. Sulfotransferases. In: Guengerich FP, editor. *Comprehensive Toxicology: Biotransformation*. Vol. 3. New York: Elsevier Science, 1997:365–83.

Dye JA, Adler KB. Effects of cigarette smoke on epithelial cells of the respiratory tract. *Thorax* 1994;49(8):825–34.

Edwards K, Braun KM, Evans G, Sureka AO, Fan S. Mainstream and sidestream cigarette smoke condensates suppress macrophage responsiveness to interferon gamma. *Human & Experimental Toxicology* 1999;18(4):233–40.

Elliot J, Vullermin P, Robinson P. Maternal cigarette smoking is associated with increased inner airway wall thickness in children who die from sudden infant death syndrome. *American Journal of Respiratory and Critical Care Medicine* 1998;158(3):802–6.

Elwood PC, Renaud S, Sharp DS, Beswick AD, O'Brien JR, Yarnell JWG. Ischemic heart disease and platelet aggregation: the Caerphilly Collaborative Heart Disease Study. *Circulation* 1991;83(1):38–44.

Fainstein V, Musher DM. Bacterial adherence to pharyngeal cells in smokers, nonsmokers, and chronic bronchitics. *Infection and Immunity* 1979;26(1):178–82.

Farchi S, Forastiere F, Pistelli R, Baldacci S, Simoni M, Perucci CA, Viegi G, SEASD Group. Exposure to environmental tobacco smoke is associated with lower plasma β-carotene levels among nonsmoking women married to a smoker. *Cancer Epidemiology, Biomarkers & Prevention* 2001;10(8):907–9.

Feldman J, Shenker IR, Etzel RA, Spierto FW, Lilienfeld DE, Nussbaum M, Jacobson MS. Passive smoking alters lipid profiles in adolescents. *Pediatrics* 1991;88(2):259–64.

Ferrari R, Ceconi C, Curello S, Cargnoni A, Alfieri O, Pardini A, Marzollo P, Visioli O. Oxygen free radicals and myocardial damage: protective role of thiol-containing agents. *American Journal of Medicine* 1991;91(Suppl 3C):95S–105S.

Ferri ES, Baratta EJ. Polonium 210 in tobacco, cigarette smoke, and selected human organs. *Public Health Reports* 1966;81(2):121–7.

Flodin U, Jonsson P, Ziegler J, Axelson O. An epidemiologic study of bronchial asthma and smoking. *Epidemiology* 1995;6(5):503–5.

Fowles J, Dybing E. Application of toxicological risk assessment principles to the chemical constituents of cigarette smoke. *Tobacco Control* 2003;12:424–30.

Friedberg T, Becker R, Oesch F, Glatt H. Studies on the importance of microsomal epoxide hydrolase in the detoxification of arene oxides using the heterologous expression of the enzyme in mammalian cells. *Carcinogenesis* 1994;15(2):171–5.

Frøen JF, Akre H, Stray-Pedersen B, Saugstad OD. Adverse effects of nicotine and interleukin-1β on autoresuscitation after apnea in piglets: implications for sudden infant death syndrome. *Pediatrics* 2000;105(4):e52.

Gairola CG, Drawdy ML, Block AE, Daugherty A. Sidestream cigarette smoke accelerates atherogenesis in apolipoprotein E-/- mice. *Atherosclerosis* 2001; 156(1):49–55.

Garner RC, Martin CN, Clayson DB. Carcinogenic aromatic amines and related compounds. In: Searle CE, editor. *Chemical Carcinogens, Second Edition, Revised and Expanded*. ACS Monograph 182. Vol. 1. Washington: American Chemical Society, 1984:175–276.

Geacintov NE, Cosman M, Hingerty BE, Amin S, Broyde S, Patel DJ. NMR solution structures of stereoisomeric covalent polycyclic aromatic carcinogen–DNA adducts: principles, patterns, and diversity. *Chemical Research in Toxicology* 1997; 10(2):111–46.

Gelboin HV. Benzo[a]pyrene metabolism, activation, and carcinogenesis: role and regulation of mixed-function oxides and related enzymes. *Physiological Reviews* 1980;60(4):1107–66.

Geng Y, Savage SM, Johnson LJ, Seagrave J, Sopori ML. Effects of nicotine on the immune response. I: chronic exposure to nicotine impairs antigen receptor-mediated signal transduction in lymphocytes. *Toxicology and Applied Pharmacology* 1995;135(2): 268–78.

Georgiadis P, Topinka J, Stoikidou M, Kaila S, Gioka M, Katsouyanni K, Sram R, Autrup H, Kyrtopoulos SA. Biomarkers of genotoxicity of air pollution (the AULIS project): bulky DNA adducts in subjects with moderate to low exposures to airborne polycyclic aromatic hydrocarbons and their relationship to environmental tobacco smoke and other parameters. *Carcinogenesis* 2001;22(9):1447–57.

Glantz SA, Parmley WW. Even a little secondhand smoke is dangerous [letter]. *Journal of the American Medical Association* 2001;286(4):462–3.

Government of British Columbia Ministry of Health Services. What is in cigarettes?; <http://www.healthservices.gov.bc.ca/ttdr/>; accessed: February 3, 2006.

Grimmer G, Brune H, Dettbarn G, Naujack K-W, Mohr U, Wenzel-Hartung R. Contribution of polycyclic aromatic compounds to the carcinogenicity of sidestream smoke of cigarettes evaluated by implantation into the lungs of rats. *Cancer Letters* 1988;43(3):173–7.

Grimmer G, Dettbarn G, Seidel A, Jacob J. Detection of carcinogenic aromatic amines in the urine of non-smokers. *Science of the Total Environment* 2000;247(1):81–90.

Grimmer G, Naujack K-W, Dettbarn G. Gaschromatographic determination of polycyclic aromatic hydrocarbons, aza-arenes, aromatic amines in the particle and vapor phase of mainstream and sidestream smoke of cigarettes. *Toxicology Letters* 1987;35(1):117–24.

Guengerich FP. Cytochrome P450 enzymes. In: Guengerich FP, editor. *Comprehensive Toxicology: Biotransformation*. Vol. 3. New York: Elsevier Science, 1997:37–68.

Guerin MR, Jenkins RA, Tomkins BA. Mainstream and sidestream cigarette smoke. In: Eisenberg M, editor. *The Chemistry of Environmental Tobacco Smoke: Composition and Measurement*. Chelsea (MI): Lewis Publishers, 1992:43–62.

Gvozdják J, Gvozdjáková A, Kucharska J, Bada V. The effect of smoking on myocardial metabolism. *Czechoslovak Medicine* 1987;10(1):47–53.

Gvozdjáková A, Bada V, Sány L, Kucharská J, Krutý F, Božek P, Trštanský L, Gvozdják J. Smoke cardiomyopathy: disturbance of oxidative process in myocardial mitochondria. *Cardiovascular Research* 1984;18(4):229–32.

Gvozdjáková A, Kucharská J, Gvozdják J. Effect of smoking on the oxidative processes of cardiomyocytes. *Cardiology* 1992;81(2–3):81–4.

Gvozdjáková A, Kucharská J, Sány L, Bada V, Božek, Gvozdják J. (The effect of smoking on the cytochrome and oxidase system of the myocardium) [Slovak]. *Bratislavske Lekarske Listy* 1985;83(1):10–5.

Hagiwara E, Takahashi KI, Okubo T, Ohno S, Ueda A, Aoki A, Odagiri S, Ishigatsubo Y. Cigarette smoking depletes cells spontaneously secreting Th(1) cytokines in the human airway. *Cytokine* 2001;14(2):121–6.

Haglund B, Cnattingius S. Cigarette smoking as a risk factor for sudden infant death syndrome: a population-based study. *American Journal of Public Health* 1990;80(1):29–32. [See also erratum in *American Journal of Public Health* 1992;82(11):1489.]

Hammond SK, Coghlin J, Gann PH, Paul M, Taghizadeh K, Skipper PL, Tannenbaum SR. Relationship between environmental tobacco smoke exposure and carcinogen–hemoglobin adduct levels in non-smokers. *Journal of the National Cancer Institute* 1993;85(6):474–8.

Hanahan D, Weinberg RA. The hallmarks of cancer. *Cell* 2000;100(1):57–70.

Hanrahan JP, Tager IB, Segal MR, Tosteson TD, Castile RG, Van Vunakis H, Weiss ST, Speitzer FE. The effect of maternal smoking during pregnancy on early infant lung function. *American Review of Respiratory Diseases* 1992;145(5):1129–35.

Harper RM. Sudden infant death syndrome: a failure of compensatory cerebellar mechanisms? *Pediatric Research* 2000;48(2):140–2.

Harrison DG. Cellular and molecular mechanisms of endothelial dysfunction. *Journal of Clinical Investigation* 1997;100(9):2153–7.

Hausberg M, Mark AL, Winniford MD, Brown RE, Somers VK. Sympathetic and vascular effects of short-term passive smoke exposure in healthy non-smokers. *Circulation* 1997;96(1):282–7.

Haussmann H-J, Gerstenberg B, Göcke W, Kuhl P, Schepers G, Stabbert R, Stinn W, Teredesai A, Tewes F, Anskeit E, Terpstra P. 12-Month inhalation study on room-aged cigarette sidestream smoke in rats. *Inhalation Toxicology* 1998;10(7):663–97.

Heavner DL, Morgan WT, Ogden MW. Determination of volatile organic compounds and respirable suspended particulate matter in New Jersey and Pennsylvania homes and workplaces. *Environment International* 1996;22(2):159–83.

Hecht SS. Carcinogenesis due to tobacco: molecular mechanisms. In: Bertino JR, editor. *Encyclopedia of Cancer*. Vol. 1. San Diego (CA): Academic Press, 1996:220–32.

Hecht SS. Biochemistry, biology, and carcinogenicity of tobacco-specific N-nitrosamines. *Chemical Research in Toxicology* 1998;11(6):559–603.

Hecht SS. Tobacco smoke carcinogens and lung cancer. *Journal of the National Cancer Institute* 1999; 91(14):1194–210.

Hecht SS, Carmella SG, Murphy SE. Tobacco-specific nitrosamine–hemoglobin adducts. *Methods in Enzymology* 1994;231:657–67.

Hecht SS, Carmella SG, Murphy SE, Akerkar S, Brunnemann KD, Hoffmann D. A tobacco-specific lung carcinogen in the urine of men exposed to cigarette smoke. *New England Journal of Medicine* 1993;329(21):1543–6.

Hecht SS, Hoffmann D. Tobacco-specific nitrosamines, an important group of carcinogens in tobacco and tobacco smoke. *Carcinogenesis* 1988;9(6):875–84.

Hecht SS, Ye M, Carmella SG, Fredrickson A, Adgate

JL, Greaves IA, Church TR. Metabolites of a tobacco-specific lung carcinogen in the urine of elementary school-aged children. *Cancer Epidemiology, Biomarkers & Prevention* 2001;10(11):1109–16.

Heitzer T, Yla-Herttuala S, Luoma J, Kurz S, Munzel T, Just H, Olschewski M, Drexler H. Cigarette smoking potentiates endothelial dysfunction of forearm resistance vessels in patients with hypercholesterolemia: role of oxidized LDL. *Circulation* 1996;93(7):1346–53.

Hemminki K, Dipple A, Shuker DEG, Kadlubar FF, Segerbäck D, Bartsch H, editors. *IARC Monographs on the Evaluation of Carcinogenic Risks to Humans: DNA Adducts: Identification and Biological Significance*. No. 125. Lyon (France): International Agency for Research on Cancer, 1994.

Ho LP, Innes JA, Greening AP. Nitrite levels in breath condensate of patients with cystic fibrosis is elevated in contrast to exhaled nitric oxide. *Thorax* 1998;53(8):680–4.

Hoepfner I, Dettbarn G, Scherer G, Grimmer G, Adlkofer F. Hydroxy-phenanthrenes in the urine of non-smokers and smokers. *Toxicology Letters* 1987;35(1):67–71.

Hoffmann D, Adams JD, Brunnemann KD. A critical look at N-nitrosamines in environmental tobacco smoke. *Toxicology Letters* 1987;35(1):1–8.

Hoffmann D, Hecht SS. Advances in tobacco carcinogenesis. In: Cooper CS, Grover PL, editors. *Handbook of Experimental Pharmacology*. Vol. 94/I. Heidelberg (Germany): Springer-Verlag, 1990:63–102.

Hoffmann D, Hoffmann I, El-Bayoumy K. The less harmful cigarette: a controversial issue. A tribute to Ernst L. Wynder. *Chemical Research in Toxicology* 2001;14(7):767–90.

Hogman M, Frostell CG, Hedenstrom H, Hedenstierna G. Inhalation of nitric oxide modulates adult human bronchial tone. *American Review of Respiratory Diseases* 1993;148(6 Pt 1):1474–8.

Hoidal JR, Fox RB, LeMarbe PA, Perri R, Repine JE. Altered oxidative metabolic responses in vitro of alveolar macrophages from asymptomatic cigarette smokers. *American Review of Respiratory Diseases* 1981;123(1):85–9.

Holz O, Krause T, Scherer G, Schmidt-Preuss U, Rüdiger HW. ^{32}P-postlabelling analysis of DNA adducts in monocytes of smokers and passive smokers. *International Archives of Occupational and Environmental Health* 1990;62(4):299–303.

Howard DJ, Briggs LA, Pritsos CA. Oxidative DNA damage in mouse heart, liver, and lung tissue due to acute side-stream tobacco smoke exposure. *Archives of Biochemistry and Biophysics* 1998a;352(2):293–7.

Howard DJ, Ota RB, Briggs LA, Hampton M, Pritsos CA. Environmental tobacco smoke in the workplace induces oxidative stress in employees, including increased production of 8-hydroxy-2'-deoxyguanosine. *Cancer Epidemiology, Biomarkers & Prevention* 1998b;7(2):141–6.

Howard DJ, Ota RB, Briggs LA, Hampton M, Pritsos CA. Oxidative stress induced by environmental tobacco smoke in the workplace is mitigated by antioxidant supplementation. *Cancer Epidemiology, Biomarkers & Prevention* 1998c;7(11):981–8.

Howard G, Thun MJ. Why is environmental tobacco smoke more strongly associated with coronary heart disease than expected: a review of potential biases and experimental data. *Environmental Health Perspectives* 1999;107(Suppl 6):853–8.

Hu FB, Persky V, Flay BR, Richardson J. An epidemiological study of asthma prevalence and related factors among young adults. *Journal of Asthma* 1997;34(1):67–76.

Husgafvel-Pursiainen K, Boffetta P, Kannio A, Nyberg F, Pershagen G, Mukeria A, Constantinescu V, Fortes C, Benhamou S. p53 Mutations and exposure to environmental tobacco smoke in a multicenter study on lung cancer. *Cancer Research* 2000;60(11):2906–11.

Hutchison SJ, Glantz SA, Zhu B-Q, Sun Y-P, Chou TM, Chatterjee K, Deedwania PC, Parmley WW, Sudhir K. In-utero and neonatal exposure to secondhand smoke causes vascular dysfunction in newborn rats. *Journal of the American College of Cardiology* 1998;32(5):1463–7.

Hutchison SJ, Ibarra M, Chou TM, Sievers RE, Chatterjee K, Glantz SA, Deedwania PC, Parmley WW. L-arginine restores normal endothelium-mediated relaxation in hypercholesterolemic rabbits exposed to tobacco smoke [abstract]. *Journal of the American College of Cardiology* 1996;27(2 Suppl):39A.

Hutchison SJ, Reitz MS, Sudhir K, Sievers RE, Zhu B-Q, Sun Y-P, Chou TM, Deedwania PC, Chatterjee K, Glantz SA, Parmley WW. Chronic dietary L-arginine prevents endothelial dysfunction secondary to environmental tobacco smoke in normocholesterolemic rabbits. *Hypertension* 1997a;29(5):1186–91.

Hutchison SJ, Sievers RE, Zhu B-Q, Sun Y-P, Sudhir K, Deedwania PC, Parmley WW, Chatterjee K. Physiological concentrations of testosterone impair endothelium-dependent vasorelaxation in hypercholesterolemic rabbits exposed to tobacco smoke [abstract]. *Circulation* 1995;92(8 Suppl 1):I-68.

Hutchison SJ, Sudhir K, Chou TM, Sievers RE, Zhu B-Q, Sun Y-P, Deedwania PC, Glantz SA, Parmley WW, Chatterjee K. Testosterone worsens endothelial dysfunction associated with hypercholesterolemia and environmental tobacco smoke exposure in male rabbit aorta. *Journal of the American College of Cardiology* 1997b;29(4):800–7.

Hutchison SJ, Sudhir K, Sievers RE, Zhu B-Q, Sun Y-P, Chou TM, Chatterjee K, Deedwania PC, Cooke JP, Glantz SA, Parmley WW. Effects of L-arginine on atherogenesis and endothelial dysfunction due to secondhand smoke. *Hypertension* 1999;34(1):44–50.

Ingebrethsen BJ. Aerosol studies of cigarette smoke. In: Norman V, chairman. *Recent advances in tobacco science: advances in the analytical methodology of leaf and smoke*. Vol. 12. Symposium of the 40th Tobacco Chemists' Research Conference; October 13–16, 1986; Knoxville (TN): The Conference, 1986: 54–142.

International Agency for Research on Cancer. *IARC Monographs on the Evaluation of Carcinogenic Risk of the Chemicals to Man: Certain Polycyclic Aromatic Hydrocarbons and Heterocyclic Compounds*. Vol. 3. Lyon (France): International Agency for Research on Cancer, 1973.

International Agency for Research on Cancer. *IARC Monographs on the Evaluation of Carcinogenic Risk of Chemicals to Man: Some Aromatic Amines, Hydrazine and Related Substances, N-Nitroso Compounds and Miscellaneous Alkylating Agents*. Vol. 4. Lyon (France): International Agency for Research on Cancer, 1974.

International Agency for Research on Cancer. *IARC Monographs on the Evaluation of the Carcinogenic Risk of Chemicals to Humans: Some Industrial Chemicals and Dyestuffs*. Vol. 29. Lyon (France): International Agency for Research on Cancer, 1982.

International Agency for Research on Cancer. *IARC Monographs on the Evaluation of the Carcinogenic Risk of Chemicals to Humans: Polynuclear Aromatic Compounds, Part 1, Chemical, Environmental and Experimental Data*. Vol. 32. Lyon (France): International Agency for Research on Cancer, 1983.

International Agency for Research on Cancer. *IARC Monographs on the Evaluation of the Carcinogenic Risk of Chemicals to Humans: Polynuclear Aromatic Compounds, Part 3, Industrial Exposures in Aluminum Production, Coal Gasification, Coke Production, and Iron and Steel Founding*. Vol. 34. Lyon (France): International Agency for Research on Cancer, 1984.

International Agency for Research on Cancer. *IARC Monographs on the Evaluation of the Carcinogenic Risk of Chemicals to Humans: Tobacco Smoking.* Vol. 38. Lyon (France): International Agency for Research on Cancer, 1986.

International Agency for Research on Cancer. *IARC Monographs on the Evaluation of Carcinogenic Risks to Humans: Chromium, Nickel and Welding.* Vol. 49. Lyon (France): International Agency for Research on Cancer, 1990.

International Agency for Research on Cancer. *IARC Monographs on the Evaluation of Carcinogenic Risks to Humans: Occupational Exposures to Mists and Vapours from Strong Inorganic Acids; and Other Industrial Chemicals.* Vol. 54. Lyon (France): International Agency for Research on Cancer, 1992.

International Agency for Research on Cancer. *IARC Monographs on the Evaluation of Carcinogenic Risks to Humans: Beryllium, Cadmium, Mercury, and Exposures in the Glass Manufacturing Industry.* Vol. 58. Lyon (France): International Agency for Research on Cancer, 1994.

International Agency for Research on Cancer. *IARC Monographs on the Evaluation of Carcinogenic Risks to Humans: Re-evaluation of Some Organic Chemicals, Hydrazine and Hydrogen Peroxide.* Vol. 71. Lyon (France): International Agency for Research on Cancer, 1999.

International Agency for Research on Cancer. *IARC Monographs on the Evaluation of Carcinogenic Risks to Humans: Tobacco Smoke and Involuntary Smoking.* Vol. 83. Lyon (France): International Agency for Research on Cancer, 2004.

Işcan A, Uyanik BS, Vurgun N, Ece A, Yiğitoğlu MR. Effects of passive exposure to tobacco, socioeconomic status and a family history of essential hypertension on lipid profiles in children. *Japanese Heart Journal* 1996;37(6):917–23.

Jaakkola MS. Environmental tobacco smoke and health in the elderly. *European Respiratory Journal* 2002;19(1):172–81.

Janson C, Chinn S, Jarvis D, Zock JP, Toren K, Burney P, European Community Respiratory Health Survey. Effect of passive smoking on respiratory symptoms, bronchial responsiveness, lung function, and total serum IgE in the European Community Respiratory Health Survey: a cross-sectional study. *Lancet* 2001;358(9299):2103–9. [See also erratum in *Lancet* 2002;359(9303):360.]

Jeffery PK. Remodeling in asthma and chronic obstructive lung disease. *American Journal of Respiratory and Critical Care Medicine* 2001;164(10 Pt 2):S28–S38.

Jenkins RA, Guerin MR, Tomkins BA. Mainstream and sidestream cigarette smoke. In: *Chemistry of Environmental Tobacco Smoke: Composition and Measurement.* 2nd ed. Boca Raton (FL): CRC Press LLC, 2000:49–75.

Jernström B, Funk M, Frank H, Mannervik B, Seidel A. Glutathione S-transferase A1-1-catalysed conjugation of bay and fjord region diol epoxides of polycyclic hydrocarbons with glutathione. *Carcinogenesis* 1996;17(7):1491–8.

Joad JP, Bric JM, Pinkerton KE. Sidestream smoke effects on lung morphology and C-fibers in young guinea pigs. *Toxicology and Applied Pharmacology* 1995;131(2):289–96.

Jorge PA, Ozaki MR, Almeida EA. Endothelial dysfunction in coronary vessels and thoracic aorta of rats exposed to cigarette smoke. *Clinical and Experimental Pharmacology & Physiology* 1995;22(6–7): 410–3.

Kalyoncu AF, Selcuk ZT, Enunlu T, Demir AU, Coplu L, Sahin AA, Artvinli M. Prevalence of asthma and allergic diseases in primary school children in Ankara, Turkey: two cross-sectional studies, five years apart. *Pediatric Allergy and Immunology* 1999;10(4):261–5.

Kato M, Roberts-Thomson P, Phillips BG, Narkiewicz K, Haynes WG, Pesek CA, Somers VK. The effects of short-term passive smoke exposure on endothelium-dependent and independent vasodilation. *Journal of Hypertension* 1999;17(10): 1395–1401.

Kerns WD, Pavkov KL, Donofrio DJ, Gralla EJ, Swenberg JA. Carcinogenicity of formaldehyde in rats and mice after long-term inhalation exposure. *Cancer Research* 1983;43(9):4382–92.

Kerstjens HAM, Rijcken B, Schouten JP, Postma DS. Decline of FEV_1 by age and smoking status: facts, figures, and fallacies. *Thorax* 1997;52(9):820–7.

Ketterer B, Harris JM, Talaska G, Meyer DJ, Pemble SE, Taylor JB, Lang NP, Kadlubar FF. The human glutathione S-transferase supergene family, its polymorphism, and its effects on susceptibility to lung cancer. *Environmental Health Perspectives* 1992;98:87–94.

Khalfen ESH, Klochkov VA. Vliianie "passivnogo kureniia" kureniia na tolerantnost'k fizicheskoî nagruzke u bol'nykh ischemicheskoî bolezn'iu serdtsa (Effect of passive smoking on physical tolerance of ischemic heart disease patients) [Russian]. *Terapevticheskii Arkhiv* 1987;59(5):112–5.

Kharitonov SA, Robbins RA, Yates D, Keatings V, Barnes PJ. Acute and chronic effects of cigarette smoking on exhaled nitric oxide. *American Journal of Respiratory and Critical Care Medicine* 1995;152(2):609–12.

Kilian M, Husby S, Host A, Halken S. Increased proportions of bacteria capable of cleaving IgA1 in the pharynx of infants with atopic disease. *Pediatric Research* 1995;38(2):182–6.

Kim JH, Stansbury KH, Walker NJ, Trush MA, Strickland PT, Sutter TR. Metabolism of benzo[a]pyrene and benzo[a]pyrene-7,8-diol by human cytochrome P450 1B1. *Carcinogenesis* 1998;19(10):1847–53.

Kim YM, Harrad S, Harrison RM. Concentrations and sources of VOCs in urban domestic and public microenvironments. *Environmental Science & Technology* 2001;35(6):997–1004.

Kjellman NI. Effect of parental smoking on IgE levels in children [letter]. *Lancet* 1981;1(8227):993–4.

Kleiger RE, Miller JP, Bigger JT Jr, Moss AJ, Multicenter Post-Infarction Research Group. Decreased heart rate variability and its association with increased mortality after acute myocardial infarction. *American Journal of Cardiology* 1987;59(4):256–62.

Klonoff-Cohen HS, Edelstein SL, Lefkowitz ES, Srinivasan IP, Kaegi D, Chang JC, Wiley KJ. The effect of passive smoking and tobacco exposure through breast milk on sudden infant death syndrome. *Journal of the American Medical Association* 1995;273(10):795–8.

Klus H, Begutter H, Scherer G, Tricker AR, Adlkofer F. Tobacco-specific and volatile N-nitrosamines in environmental tobacco smoke of offices. *Indoor Environment* 1992;1:348–50.

Kopplin A, Eberle-Adamkiewicz G, Glüsenkamp K-H, Nehls P, Kirstein U. Urinary excretion of 3-methyladenine and 3-ethyladenine after controlled exposure to tobacco smoke. *Carcinogenesis* 1995;16(11):2637–41.

Larsson ML, Frisk M, Hallstrom J, Kiviloog J, Lundback B. Environmental tobacco smoke exposure during childhood is associated with increased prevalence of asthma in adults. *Chest* 2001;120(3):711–7.

Latha MS, Vijayammal PL, Kurup PA. Changes in the glycosaminoglycans and glycoproteins in the tissues in rats exposed to cigarette smoke. *Atherosclerosis* 1991;86(1):49–54.

Lee BP, Morton RF, Lee LY. Acute effects of acrolein on breathing: role of vagal bronchopulmonary afferents. *Journal of Applied Physiology* 1992;72(3):1050–6.

Lee LY, Kwong K, Lin YS, Gu Q. Hypersensitivity of bronchopulmonary C-fibers induced by airway mucosal inflammation: cellular mechanisms. *Pulmonary Pharmacology & Therapeutics* 2002;15(3):199–204.

Leonard S, Bertrand D. Neuronal nicotinic receptors: from structure to function. *Nicotine & Tobacco Research* 2001;3(3):203–23.

Leone A, Bertanelli F, Mori L, Fabiato P, Bertoncini G. Ventricular arrhythmias by passive smoke in patients with pre-existing myocardial infarction [abstract]. *American Journal of Cardiology* 1992;19(3 Suppl A):256A.

Leone A, Mori L, Bertanelli F, Fabiano P, Filippelli M. Indoor passive smoking: its effect on cardiac performance. *International Journal of Cardiology* 1991;33(2):247–51.

Liu Y-Y, Schmeltz I, Hoffmann D. Chemical studies on tobacco smoke: quantitative analyses of hydrazine in tobacco and cigarette smoke. *Analytical Chemistry* 1974;46(7):885–9.

Loechler EL, Green CL, Essigmann JM. *In vivo* mutagenesis by O^6-methylguanine built into a unique site in a viral genome. *Proceedings of the National Academy of Sciences of the United States of America* 1984;81(20):6271–5.

Luck W, Nau H. Exposure of the fetus, neonate, and nursed infant to nicotine and cotinine from maternal smoking [letter]. *New England Journal of Medicine* 1984;311(10):672.

Luck W, Nau H, Hansen R, Steldinger R. Extent of nicotine and cotinine transfer to the human fetus, placenta and amniotic fluid of smoking mothers. *Developmental Pharmacology and Therapeutics* 1985;8(6):384–95.

Ludwig PW, Hoidal JR. Alterations in leukocyte oxidative metabolism in cigarette smokers. *American Review of Respiratory Diseases* 1982;126(6):977–80.

Machaalani R, Waters KA, Tinworth KD. Effects of postnatal nicotine exposure on apoptotic markers in the developing piglet brain. *Neuroscience* 2005;132(2):325–33.

Maclure M, Katz RB-A, Bryant MS, Skipper PL, Tannenbaum SR. Elevated blood levels of carcinogens in passive smokers. *American Journal of Public Health* 1989;79(10):1381–4.

MacNee W. Oxidative stress and lung inflammation in airways disease. *European Journal of Pharmacology* 2001;429(1–3):195–207.

Magnusson CG. Maternal smoking influences cord serum IgE and IgD levels and increases the risk for subsequent infant allergy. *Journal of Allergy and Clinical Immunology* 1986;78(5 Pt 1):898–904.

Mahanama KRR, Daisey JM. Volatile *N*-nitrosamines in environmental tobacco smoke: sampling, analysis, emission factors, and indoor air exposures. *Environmental Science & Technology* 1996;30(5):1477–84.

Majesky MW, Yang H-Y, Benditt EP, Juchau MR. Carcinogenesis and atherogenesis: differences in monooxygenase inducibility and bioactivation of benzo[*a*]pyrene in aortic and hepatic tissues of atherosclerosis-susceptible versus resistant pigeons. *Carcinogenesis* 1983;4(6):647–52.

Makin J, Fried PA, Watkinson B. A comparison of active and passive smoking during pregnancy: long-term effects. *Neurotoxicology and Teratology* 1991;13(1):5–12.

Malats N, Camus-Radon A-M, Nyberg F, Ahrens W, Constantinescu V, Mukeria A, Benhamou S, Batura-Gabryel H, Bruske-Hohlfeld I, Simonato L, Menezes A, Lea S, Lang M, Boffetta P. Lung cancer risk in nonsmokers and *GSTM1* and *GSTT1* genetic polymorphism. *Cancer Epidemiology, Biomarkers & Prevention* 2000;9(8):827–33.

Marini A, Agosti M, Motta G, Mosca F. Effects of a dietary and environmental prevention programme on the incidence of allergic symptoms in high atopic risk infants: three years' follow-up. *Acta Paediatrica Supplement* 1996;414:1–21.

Martin P, Heavner DL, Nelson PR, Maiolo KC, Risner CH, Simmons PS, Morgan WT, Ogden MW. Environmental tobacco smoke (ETS): a market cigarette study. *Environment International* 1997;23(1):75–90.

Martinez FD, Antognoni G, Macri F, Bonci E, Midulla F, De Castro G, Ronchetti R. Parental smoking enhances bronchial responsiveness in nine-year-old children. *American Review of Respiratory Diseases* 1988a;138(3):518–23.

Martinez FD, Morgan WJ, Wright AL, Holberg CJ, Taussig LM. Diminished lung function as a predisposing factor for wheezing respiratory illness in infants. *New England Journal of Medicine* 1988b;319(17):1112–7.

McCusker K, Hoidal J. Selective increase of antioxidant enzyme activity in the alveolar macrophages from cigarette smokers and smoke-exposed hamsters. *American Review of Respiratory Disease* 1990;141(3):678–82.

McMartin KI, Platt MS, Hackman R, Klein J, Smialek JE, Vigorito R, Koren G. Lung tissue concentrations of nicotine in sudden infant death syndrome (SIDS). *Journal of Pediatrics* 2002;140(2):205–9.

McMurray RG, Hicks LL, Thompson DL. The effects of passive inhalation of cigarette smoke on exercise performance. *European Journal of Applied Physiology and Occupational Physiology* 1985;54(2):196–200.

Meger M, Meger-Kossien I, Riedel K, Scherer G. Biomonitoring of environmental tobacco smoke (ETS)-related exposure to 4-(methylnitrosamino)-1-(3-pyridyl)-1-butanone (NNK). *Biomarkers* 2000;5(1):33–45.

Milerad J, Vege A, Opdal SH, Rognum TO. Objective measurements of nicotine exposure in victims of sudden infant death syndrome and in other unexpected child deaths. *Journal of Pediatrics* 1998;133(2):232–6.

Miller JA. Research in chemical carcinogenesis with Elizabeth Miller—a trail of discovery with our associates. *Drug Metabolism Reviews* 1994;26(1&2):1–36.

Milner AD, Marsh MJ, Ingram DM, Fox GF, Susiva C. Effects of smoking in pregnancy on neonatal lung function. *Archives of Disease in Childhood Fetal and Neonatal Edition* 1999;80(1):F8–F14.

Mio T, Romberger DJ, Thompson AB, Robbins RA, Heires A, Rennard SI. Cigarette smoke induces interleukin-8 release from human bronchial epithelial cells. *American Journal of Respiratory and Critical Care Medicine* 1997;155(5):1770–6.

Misawa K, Matsuki H, Kasuga H, Yokoyama H, Hinohara S. (An epidemiological study on the relationships among HDL-cholesterol, smoking and obesity) [Japanese]. *Nippon Eiseigaku Zasshi* 1989;44(3):725–32.

Miyaura S, Eguchi H, Johnson JM. Effect of a cigarette smoke extract on the metabolism of the proinflammatory autacoid, platelet-activating factor. *Circulation Research* 1992;70(2):341–7.

Mohtashamipur E, Mohtashamipur A, Germann P-G, Ernst H, Norpoth K, Mohr U. Comparative carcinogenicity of cigarette mainstream and sidestream smoke condensates on the mouse skin. *Journal of Cancer Research and Clinical Oncology* 1990;116(6):604–8.

Moskowitz WB, Mosteller M, Hewitt JK, Eaves LJ, Nance WE, Schieken RM. Univariate genetic analysis of oxygen transport regulation in children: the Medical College of Virginia Twin Study. *Pediatric Research* 1993;33(6):645–8.

Moskowitz WB, Mosteller M, Schieken RM, Bossano R, Hewitt JK, Bodurtha JN, Segrest JP. Lipoprotein and oxygen transport alterations in passive smoking preadolescent children: the MCV Twin Study. *Circulation* 1990;81(2):586–92.

Moyes CD, Waldon J, Ramadas D, Crane J, Pearce N. Respiratory symptoms and environmental factors in schoolchildren in the Bay of Plenty. *New Zealand Medical Journal* 1995;108(1007):358–61.

National Research Council. *Environmental Tobacco Smoke: Measuring Exposures and Assessing Health Effects.* Washington: National Academy Press, 1986.

Neff RA, Humphrey J, Mihalevich M, Mendelowitz D. Nicotine enhances presynaptic and postsynaptic glutamatergic neurotransmission to activate cardiac parasympathetic neurons. *Circulation Research* 1998;83(12):1241–7.

Neufeld EJ, Mietus-Snyder M, Beiser AS, Baker AL, Newburger J. Passive cigarette smoking and reduced HDL cholesterol levels in children with high-risk lipid profiles. *Circulation* 1997;96(5):1403–7.

Nielsen PS, Okkels H, Sigsgaard T, Kyrtopoulos S, Autrup H. Exposure to urban and rural air pollution: DNA and protein adducts and effect of glutathione-S-transferase genotype on adduct levels. *International Archives of Occupational and Environmental Health* 1996;68(3):170–6.

Niewoehner DE, Kleinerman J, Rice DB. Pathologic changes in the peripheral airways of young cigarette smokers. *New England Journal of Medicine* 1974;291(15):755–8.

Önal A, Uysal A, Ülker S, Delen Y, Yurtseven ME, Evinç A. Alterations of brain tissue in fetal rats exposed to nicotine in utero: possible involvement of nitric oxide and catecholamines. *Neurotoxicology and Teratology* 2004;26(1):103–12.

Oryszczyn MP, Annesi-Maesano I, Charpin D, Paty E, Maccario J, Kauffmann F. Relationships of active and passive smoking to total IgE in adults of the Epidemiological Study of the Genetics and Environment of Asthma, Bronchial Hyperresponsiveness, and Atopy (EGEA). *American Journal of Respiratory and Critical Care Medicine* 2000;161(4 Pt 1):1241–6.

Oskarsson HJ, Heistad DD. Oxidative stress produced by angiotensin too: implications for hypertension and vascular injury. *Circulation* 1997;95(3):557–9.

Otsuka R, Watanabe H, Hirata K, Tokai K, Muro T, Yoshiyama M, Takeuchi K, Yoshikawa J. Acute effects of passive smoking on the coronary circulation in healthy young adults. *Journal of the American Medical Association* 2001;286(4):436–41.

Ott W, Langan L, Switzer P. A time series model for cigarette smoking activity patterns: model validation for carbon monoxide and respirable particles in a chamber and an automobile. *Journal of Exposure Analysis and Environmental Epidemiology* 1992;2(Suppl 2):175–200.

Pan X-M, Staprans I, Hardman DA, Rapp JH. Exposure to cigarette smoke delays the plasma clearance of chylomicrons and chylomicron remnants in rats. *American Journal of Physiology* 1997;273(1 Pt 1):G158–G163.

Parsons WD, Carmella SG, Akerkar S, Bonilla LE, Hecht SS. A metabolite of the tobacco-specific lung carcinogen 4-(methylnitrosamino)-1-(3-pyridyl)-1-butanone in the urine of hospital workers exposed to environmental tobacco smoke. *Cancer Epidemiology, Biomarkers & Prevention* 1998;7(3):257–60.

Patrianakos C, Hoffmann D. Chemical studies on tobacco smoke LXIV: on the analysis of aromatic amines in cigarette smoke. *Journal of Analytical Toxicology* 1979;3:150–4.

Patten CJ, Smith TJ, Murphy SE, Wang M-H, Lee J, Tynes RE, Koch P, Yang CS. Kinetic analysis of the activation of 4-(methylnitrosamino)-1-(3-pyridyl)-1-butanone by heterologously expressed human P450 enzymes and the effect of P450-specific chemical inhibitors on this activation in human liver microsomes. *Archives of Biochemistry and Biophysics* 1996;333(1):127–8.

Pegg AE, Dolan ME, Moschel RC. Structure, function, and inhibition of O^6-alkylguanine-DNA alkyltransferase. *Progress in Nucleic Acid Research and Molecular Biology* 1995;51:167–223.

Pelkonen O, Nebert DW. Metabolism of polycyclic hydrocarbons: etiologic role in carcinogenesis. *Pharmacological Reviews* 1982;34(2):189–222.

Penn A, Batastini G, Soloman J, Burns F, Albert R. Dose-dependent size increases of aortic lesions following chronic exposure to 7,12-dimethybenz(*a*)anthracene. *Cancer Research* 1981;41(2):588–92.

Penn A, Chen LC, Snyder CA. Inhalation of steady-state sidestream smoke from one cigarette promotes atherosclerotic plaque development. *Circulation* 1994;90(3):1363–7.

Penn A, Currie J, Snyder C. Inhalation of carbon monoxide does not accelerate arteriosclerosis in cockerels. *European Journal of Pharmacology* 1992;228(2-3):155–64.

Penn A, Keller K, Snyder C, Nadas A, Chen LC. The tar fraction of cigarette smoke does not promote arteriosclerotic plaque development. *Environmental Health Perspectives* 1996;104(10):1108–13.

Penn A, Snyder CA. Inhalation of sidestream cigarette smoke accelerates development of arteriosclerotic plaques. *Circulation* 1993;88(4 Pt):1820–5.

Penn A, Snyder CA. Butadiene inhalation accelerates arteriosclerotic plaque development in cockerels. *Toxicology* 1996a;113(1-3):351–4.

Penn A, Snyder CA. 1,3 butadiene, a vapor phase component of environmental tobacco smoke, accelerates arteriosclerotic plaque development. *Circulation* 1996b;93(3):552–7.

Penning TM, Burczynski ME, Hung C-F, McCoull KD, Palackal NT, Tsuruda LS. Dihydrodiol dehydrogenases and polycyclic aromatic hydrocarbon activation: generation of reactive and redox active *o*-quinones. *Chemical Research in Toxicology* 1999;12(1):1–18.

Persson MG, Zetterstrom O, Agrenius V, Ihre E, Gustafsson LE. Single-breath nitric oxide measurements in asthmatic patients and smokers. *Lancet* 1994;343(8890):146–7.

Pittilo RM, Mackie IJ, Rowles PM, Machine SJ, Woolf N. Effects of cigarette smoking on the ultrastructure of rat thoracic aorta and its ability to produce prostacyclin. *Thrombosis and Haemostasis* 1982;48(2):173–6.

Pope CA III, Eatough DJ, Gold DR, Pang Y, Nielsen KR, Nath P, Verrier RL, Kanner RE. Acute exposure to environmental tobacco smoke and heart rate variability. *Environmental Health Perspectives* 2001;109(7):711–6.

Porro E, Calamita P, Rana I, Montini L, Criscione S. Atopy and environmental factors in upper respiratory infections: an epidemiological survey on 2304 school children. *International Journal of Pediatric Otorhinolaryngology* 1992;24(2):111–20.

Prentice RC, Carroll R, Scanlon PJ, Thomas JX Jr. Recent exposure to cigarette smoke increases myocardial infarct size [abstract]. *Journal of the American College of Cardiology* 1989;13(1):124A.

Přerovský I, Hladovec J. Suppression of the desquamating effect of smoking on the human endothelium by hydroxyethylrutosides. *Blood Vessels* 1979;16:239–40.

Preussmann R, Stewart BW. *N*-Nitroso carcinogens. In: Searle CE, editor. *Chemical Carcinogens, Second Edition*. ACS Monograph 182. Vol. 2. Washington: American Chemical Society, 1984:643–828.

Pryor WA. Biological effects of cigarette smoke, wood smoke, and the smoke from plastics: the use of electron spin resonance. *Free Radical Biology & Medicine* 1992;13(6):659–76.

Pryor WA, Prier DG, Church DF. Electron-spin resonance study of mainstream and sidestream cigarette smoke: nature of the free radicals in gas-phase smoke and in cigarette tar. *Environmental Health Perspectives* 1983;47:345–55.

Pryor WA, Stone K, Zang L-Y, Bermúdez E. Fractionation of aqueous cigarette tar extracts: fractions that contain the tar radical cause DNA damage. *Chemical Research in Toxicology* 1998;11(5):441–8.

Przyklenk K. Nicotine exacerbates postischemic contractile dysfunction of stunned myocardium in the canine model: possible role of free radicals. *Circulation* 1994;89(3):1272–81.

Raitakari OT, Adams MR, McCredies RJ, Celermajer DS. Arterial endothelial dysfunction related to passive smoking is potentially reversible in healthy young adults. *Annals of Internal Medicine* 1999;130(7):578–81.

Revis NW, Bull R, Laurie D, Schiller CA. The effectiveness of chemical carcinogens to induce atherosclerosis in the white carneau pigeon. *Toxicology* 1984;32:215–27.

Ricciardolo FL, Di Maria GU, Mistretta A, Sapienza MA, Geppetti P. Impairment of bronchoprotection by nitric oxide in severe asthma. *Lancet* 1997;350(9087):1297–8.

Ricciardolo FL, Geppetti P, Mistretta A, Nadel JA, Sapienza MA, Bellofiore S, Di Maria GU. Randomised double-blind placebo-controlled study of the effect of inhibition of nitric oxide synthesis in bradykinin-induced asthma. *Lancet* 1996;348(9024):374–7.

Richter E, Rosler S, Scherer G, Gostomzyk JG, Grubl A, Kramer U, Behrendt H. Haemoglobin adducts from aromatic amines in children in relation to area of residence and exposure to environmental tobacco smoke. *International Archives of Occupational and Environmental Health* 2001;74(6):421–8.

Roberts DL. Natural tobacco flavor. *Recent Advances in Tobacco Science: Chemical and Sensory Aspects of Tobacco Flavor* 1988;14:49–81.

Roberts KA, Rezai AA, Pinkerton KE, Rutledge JC. Effect of environmental tobacco smoke on LDL accumulation in the artery wall. *Circulation* 1996;94(9):2248–53.

Ross R. The pathology of atherosclerosis—an update. *New England Journal of Medicine* 1986;314(8):488–500.

Ross R. The pathogenesis of atherosclerosis: a perspective for the 1990s. *Nature* 1993;362(6423):801–9.

Ross R. Atherosclerosis—an inflammatory disease. *New England Journal of Medicine* 1999;340(2):115–26.

Ruppert T, Scherer G, Tricker AR, Adlkofer F. *trans,trans*-Muconic acid as a biomarker of non-occupational environmental exposure to benzene. *International Archives of Occupational and Environmental Health* 1997;69(4):247–51.

Saetta M. Airway inflammation in chronic obstructive pulmonary disease. *American Journal of Respiratory and Critical Care Medicine* 1999;160(5 Pt 2):S17–S20.

Sakuma H, Kusama M, Munakata S, Ohsumi T, Sugawara S. The distribution of cigarette smoke components between mainstream and sidestream smoke. I: acidic components. *Beiträge Zur Tabakforschung International* 1983;12(2):63–71.

Samet JM. Adverse effects of smoke exposure on the upper airway. *Tobacco Control* 2004;13(Suppl 1): i57–i60.

Samet JM, Lange P. Longitudinal studies of active and passive smoking. *American Journal of Respiratory and Critical Care Medicine* 1996;154(6 Pt 2):S257–S265.

Sancar A. DNA excision repair. *Annual Review of Biochemistry* 1996;65:43–81.

Sapigni T, Biavati P, Simoni M, Viegi G, Baldacci S, Carrozzi L, Modena P, Pedreschi M, Vellutini M, Paoletti P. The Po River Delta Respiratory Epidemiological Survey: an analysis of factors related to level of total serum IgE. *European Respiratory Journal* 1998;11(2):278–83.

Saria A, Martling CR, Yan Z, Theodorsson-Norheim E, Gamse R, Lundberg JM. Release of multiple tachykinins from capsaicin-sensitive sensory nerves in the lung by bradykinin, histamine, dimethylphenyl piperazinium, and vagal nerve stimulation. *American Review of Respiratory Diseases* 1988;137(6): 1330–5.

Scherer G, Conze C, Tricker AR, Adlkofer F. Uptake of tobacco smoke constituents on exposure to environmental tobacco smoke (ETS). *Clinical Investigator* 1992;70(3–4):352–67.

Scherer G, Doolittle DJ, Ruppert T, Meger-Kossien I, Riedel K, Tricker AR, Adlkofer F. Urinary mutagenicity and thioethers in nonsmokers: role of environmental tobacco smoke (ETS) and diet. *Mutation Research* 1996;368(3–4):195–204.

Scherer G, Frank S, Riedel K, Meger-Kossien I, Renner T. Biomonitoring of exposure to polycyclic aromatic hydrocarbons of nonoccupationally exposed persons. *Cancer Epidemiology, Biomarkers & Prevention* 2000;9(4):373–80.

Scherer G, Meger-Kossien I, Riedel K, Renner T, Meger M. Assessment of the exposure of children to environmental tobacco smoke (ETS) by different methods. *Human & Experimental Toxicology* 1999;18(4):297–301.

Scherer G, Renner T, Meger M. Analysis and evaluation of *trans,trans*-muconic acid as a biomarker for benzene exposure. *Journal of Chromatography B: Biomedical Sciences and Applications* 1998;717(1–2): 179–99.

Scherer G, Richter E. Biomonitoring exposure to environmental tobacco smoke (ETS): a critical reappraisal. *Human & Experimental Toxicology* 1997; 16(8):449–59.

Scherer G, Ruppert T, Daube H, Kossien I, Riedel K, Tricker AR, Adlkofer F. Contribution of tobacco smoke to environmental benzene exposure in Germany. *Environment International* 1995;21(6): 779–89.

Schilling J, Holzer P, Guggenbach M, Gyurech D, Marathia K, Geroulanos S. Reduced endogenous nitric oxide in the exhaled air of smokers and hypertensives. *European Respiratory Journal* 1994;7(3): 467–71.

Schuller HM, Plummer HK 3rd, Jull BA. Receptor-mediated effects of nicotine and its nitrosated derivative NNK on pulmonary neuroendocrine cells. *Anatomical Record* 2003;270A(1):51–8.

Schwarzacher SP, Hutchison S, Chou TM, Sun Y-P, Zhu B-Q, Chatterjee K, Glantz SA, Deedwania PC, Parmley WW, Sudhir K. Antioxidant diet preserves endothelium-dependent vasodilatation in resistance arteries of hypercholesterolemic rabbits exposed to environmental tobacco smoke. *Journal of Cardiovascular Pharmacology* 1998;31(5):649–53.

Sekhon HS, Jia Y, Raab R, Kuryatov A, Pankow JF, Whisett JA, Lindstrom J, Spindel ER. Prenatal nicotine increases pulmonary α7 nicotinic receptor expression and alters fetal lung development in monkeys. *Journal of Clinical Investigation* 1999; 103(5):637–47.

Sekhon HS, Keller JA, Proskocil BJ, Martin EL, Spindel ER. Maternal nicotine exposure upregulates collagen gene expression in fetal monkey lung: association with α7 nicotinic acetylcholine receptors. *American Journal of Respiratory Cell and Molecular Biology* 2002;26(1):31–41.

Sekido Y, Fong KM, Minna JD. Progress in understanding the molecular pathogenesis of human lung cancer. *Biochimica et Biophysica Acta* 1998;1378(1): F21–F59.

Shimada T, Hayes CL, Yamazaki H, Amin S, Hecht SS, Guengerich FP, Sutter TR. Activation of chemically diverse procarcinogens by human cytochrome P-450 1B1. *Cancer Research* 1996;56(13):2979–84.

Shimkin MB, Stoner GD. Lung tumors in mice: application to carcinogenesis bioassay. *Advances in Cancer Research* 1975;21:1–58.

Shou M, Korzekwa KR, Crespi CL, Gonzalez FJ, Gelboin HV. The role of 12 cDNA-expressed human, rodent, and rabbit cytochromes P450 in the metabolism of benzo[a]pyrene and benzo[a]pyrene *trans*-7,8-dihydrodiol. *Molecular Carcinogenesis* 1994; 10(1):159–68.

Shukla R, Liu T, Geacintov NE, Loechler EL. The major, N²-dG adduct of (+)-*anti*-B[a]PDE shows a dramatically different mutagenic specificity (predominantly, G → A) in a 5'-CGT-3' sequence context. *Biochemistry* 1997;36(33):10256–61.

Singer B, Hang B. What structural features determine repair enzyme specificity and mechanism in chemically modified DNA? *Chemical Research in Toxicology* 1997;10(7):713–32.

Singh N, Mironov D, Armstrong PW, Ross AM, Langer A, GUSTO ECG Substudy Investigators. Heart rate variability assessment early after acute myocardial infarction: pathophysiological and prognostic correlates. *Circulation* 1996;93(7):1388–95.

Sinzinger H, Kefalides A. Passive smoking severely decreases platelet sensitivity to antiaggregatory prostaglandines [letter]. *Lancet* 1982;2(8294):392–3.

Sinzinger H, Virgolini I. Besitzen passiv raucher ein erhöhtes thromboserisiko? [Are passive smokers at greater risk of thrombosis?] [German; English abstract] *Wien Klin Wochenschr* 1989;101(20):694–8.

Siwińska E, Mielżyńska D, Bubak A, Smolik E. The effect of coal stoves and environmental tobacco smoke on the level of urinary 1-hydroxypyrene. *Mutation Research* 1999;445(2):147–53.

Slotkin TA. Cholinergic systems in brain development and disruption by neurotoxicants: nicotine, environmental tobacco smoke, organophosphates. *Toxicology and Applied Pharmacology* 2004;198(2):132–51.

Slotkin TA, Pinkerton KE, Auman JT, Qiao D, Seidler FJ. Perinatal exposure to environmental tobacco smoke upregulates nicotinic cholinergic receptors in monkey brain. *Brain Research Developmental Brain Research* 2002;133(2):175–9.

Slotkin TA, Pinkerton KE, Garofolo MC, Auman JT, McCook EC, Seidler FJ. Perinatal exposure to environmental tobacco smoke induces adenylyl cyclase and alters receptor-mediated cell signaling in brain and heart of neonatal rats. *Brain Research* 2001;898(1):73–81.

Slotkin TA, Pinkerton KE, Seidler FJ. Perinatal environmental tobacco smoke exposure in rhesus monkeys: critical periods and regional selectivity for effects on brain cell development and lipid peroxidation. *Environmental Health Perspectives* 2006;114(1):34–9.

Slotkin TA, Saleh JL, McCook EC, Seidler FJ. Impaired cardiac function during postnatal hypoxia in rats exposed to nicotine prenatally: implications for perinatal morbidity and mortality, and for sudden infant death syndrome. *Teratology* 1997;55(3):177–84.

Smith CJ, Bombick DW, Ryan BA, Morgan WT, Doolittle DJ. Urinary mutagenicity in nonsmokers following exposure to fresh diluted sidestream cigarette smoke. *Mutation Research* 2000a;470(1):53–70.

Smith CJ, Fischer TH, Heavner DL, Rumple MA, Bowman DL, Brown BG, Morton MJ, Doolittle DJ. Urinary thromboxane, prostacyclin, cortisol, and 8-hydroxy-2′-deoxyguanosine in nonsmokers exposed and not exposed to environmental tobacco smoke. *Toxicological Sciences* 2001;59(2):316–23.

Smith CJ, Fisher TH, Sears S. Environmental tobacco smoke, cardiovascular disease, and the nonlinear-dose-response hypothesis. *Toxicological Sciences* 2000b;54(2):462–72.

Smith TJ, Guo Z, Gonzalez FJ, Guengerich FP, Stoner GD, Yang CS. Metabolism of 4-(methylnitrosamino)-1-(3-pyridyl)-1-butanone in human lung and liver microsomes and cytochromes P-450 expressed in hepatoma cells. *Cancer Research* 1992;52(7):1757–63.

Smith TJ, Stoner GD, Yang CS. Activation of 4-(methylnitrosamino)-1-(3-pyridyl)-1-butanone (NNK) in human lung microsomes by cytochromes P450, lipoxygenase, and hydroperoxides. *Cancer Research* 1995;55(23):5566–73.

Spitzer AR. Current controversies in the pathophysiology and prevention of sudden infant death syndrome. *Current Opinion in Pediatrics* 2005;17(2):181–5.

Staretz ME, Murphy SE, Patten CJ, Nunes MG, Koehl W, Amin S, Koenig LA, Guengerich FP, Hecht SS. Comparative metabolism of the tobacco-related carcinogens benzo[*a*]pyrene, 4-(methylnitrosamino)-1-(3-pyridyl)-1-butanone, 4-(methylnitrosamino)-1-(3-pyridyl)-1-butanol, and *N*′-nitrosonornicotine in human hepatic microsomes. *Drug Metabolism and Disposition* 1997;25(2):154–62.

Stefanadis C, Vlachopoulos C, Tsiamis E, Diamantopoulos L, Toutouzas K, Giatrakos N, Vaina S, Tsekoura D, Toutouzas P. Unfavorable effects of passive smoking on aortic function in men. *Annals of Internal Medicine* 1998;128(6):426–34.

Steinberg D, Parthasarathy S, Carew TE, Khoo JC, Witztum JL. Beyond cholesterol: modifications of low-density lipoprotein that increase its atherogenicity. *New England Journal of Medicine* 1989;320(14):915–24.

Strachan DP, Cook DG. Health effects of passive smoking. 1: parental smoking and lower respiratory illness in infancy and early childhood. *Thorax* 1997;52(10):905–14.

Strachan DP, Cook DG. Health effects of passive smoking. 6: parental smoking and childhood asthma: longitudinal and case-control studies. *Thorax* 1998;53(3):204–12.

Sumida H, Watanabe H, Kugiyama K, Ohgushi M, Matsumura T, Yasue H. Does passive smoking impair endothelium-dependent coronary artery dilation in women? *Journal of the American College of Cardiology* 1998;31(4):811–5.

Sun Y-P, Zhu B-Q, Browne AE, Sievers RE, Bekker JM, Chatterjee K, Parmley WW, Glantz SA. Nicotine does not influence arterial lipid deposits in rabbits exposed to second-hand smoke. *Circulation* 2001;104(7):810–4.

Sun Y-P, Zhu B-Q, Sievers RE, Glantz SA, Parmley WW. Metoprolol does not attenuate atherosclerosis in lipid-fed rabbits exposed to environmental tobacco smoke. *Circulation* 1994;89(5):2260–5.

Sundberg K, Widersten M, Seidel A, Mannervik B, Jernström B. Glutathione conjugation of bay- and fjord-region diol epoxides of polycyclic aromatic hydrocarbons by glutathione transferase M1-1 and P1-1. *Chemical Research in Toxicology* 1997;10(11):1221–7.

Tager IB, Ngo L, Hanrahan JP. Maternal smoking during pregnancy: effects on lung function during the first 18 months of life. *American Journal of Respiratory and Critical Care Medicine* 1995;152(3):977–83.

Tamai O, Matsuoka H, Itabe H, Wada Y, Kohno K, Imaizumi T. Single LDL apheresis improves endothelium-dependent vasodilatation in hypercholesterolemic humans. *Circulation* 1997;95(1):76–82.

Tang D, Warburton D, Tannenbaum SR, Skipper P, Santella RM, Cereijido GS, Crawford FG, Perera FP. Molecular and genetic damage from environmental tobacco smoke in young children. *Cancer Epidemiology, Biomarkers & Prevention* 1999;8(5):427–31.

Taylor DA, McGrath JL, Orr LM, Barnes PJ, O'Connor BJ. Effect of endogenous nitric oxide inhibition on airway responsiveness to histamine and adenosine-5'-monophosphate in asthma. *Thorax* 1998;53(6):483–9.

Taylor JA, Sanderson M. A reexamination of the risk factors for the sudden infant death syndrome. *Journal of Pediatrics* 1995;126(6):887–91.

Tiano HF, Hosokawa M, Chulada PC, Smith PB, Wang R-L, Gonzalez FJ, Crespi CL, Langenbach R. Retroviral mediated expression of human cytochrome P450 2A6 in C3H/10T1/2 cells confers transformability by 4-(methylnitrosamino)-1-(3-pyridyl)-1-butanone (NNK). *Carcinogenesis* 1993;14(7):1421–7.

Török J, Gvozdjáková A, Kucharská J, Balažovjech I, Kyselá S, Šimko F, Gvozdják J. Passive smoking impairs endothelium-dependent relaxation of isolated rabbit arteries. *Physiological Research* 2000;49(1):135–41.

Treasure CB, Klein JL, Weintraub WS, Talley JD, Stillabower ME, Kosinski AS, Zhang J, Boccuzzi SJ, Cedarholm JC, Alexander RW. Beneficial effects of cholesterol-lowering therapy on the coronary endothelium in patients with coronary artery disease. *New England Journal of Medicine* 1995;332(8):481–7.

Upton MN, Watt GC, Davey Smith G, McConnachie A, Hart CL. Permanent effects of maternal smoking on offsprings' lung function [letter]. *Lancet* 1998;352(9126):453.

U.S. Department of Health and Human Services. *The Health Consequences of Smoking: Cardiovascular Disease. A Report of the Surgeon General.* Rockville (MD): U.S. Department of Health and Human Services, Public Health Service, Office on Smoking and Health, 1983. DHHS Publication No. (PHS) 84-50204.

U.S. Department of Health and Human Services. *The Health Consequences of Involuntary Smoking. A Report of the Surgeon General.* Rockville (MD): U.S. Department of Health and Human Services, Public Health Service, Centers for Disease Control, Center for Health Promotion and Education, Office on Smoking and Health, 1986. DHHS Publication No. (CDC) 87-8398.

U.S. Department of Health and Human Services. *The Health Benefits of Smoking Cessation. A Report of the Surgeon General.* Atlanta: U.S. Department of Health and Human Services, Public Health Service, Centers for Disease Control, National Center for Chronic Disease Prevention and Health Promotion, Office on Smoking and Health, 1990. DHHS Publication No. (CDC) 90-8416.

U.S. Department of Health and Human Services. *Preventing Tobacco Use Among Young People. A Report of the Surgeon General.* Atlanta: U.S. Department of Health and Human Services, Public Health Service, Centers for Disease Control and Prevention, National Center for Chronic Disease Prevention and Health Promotion, Office on Smoking and Health, 1994.

U.S. Department of Health and Human Services. *Tobacco Use Among U.S. Racial/Ethnic Minority Groups—African Americans, American Indians and Alaska Natives, Asian Americans and Pacific Islanders, and Hispanics. A Report of the Surgeon General.* Atlanta: U.S. Department of Health and Human Services, Centers for Disease Control and Prevention, National Center for Chronic Disease Prevention and Health Promotion, Office on Smoking and Health, 1998.

U.S. Department of Health and Human Services. *9th Report on Carcinogens.* Research Triangle Park (NC): U.S. Department of Health and Human Services, Public Health Service, National Institutes of Health, National Institute of Environmental

Health Sciences, National Toxicology Program, 2000.

U.S. Department of Health and Human Services. *Women and Smoking. A Report of the Surgeon General.* Rockville (MD): U.S. Department of Health and Human Services, Public Health Service, Office of the Surgeon General, 2001.

U.S. Department of Health and Human Services. *The Health Consequences of Smoking: A Report of the Surgeon General.* Atlanta: U.S. Department of Health and Human Services, Centers for Disease Control and Prevention, National Center for Chronic Disease Prevention and Health Promotion, Office on Smoking and Health, 2004.

U.S. Department of Health, Education, and Welfare. *Smoking and Health: Report of the Advisory Committee to the Surgeon General of the Public Health Service.* Washington: U.S. Department of Health, Education, and Welfare, Public Health Service, Center for Disease Control, 1964. PHS Publication No. 1103.

U.S. Environmental Protection Agency. *Air Quality Criteria for Carbon Monoxide.* Research Triangle Park (NC): U.S. Environmental Protection Agency, 1991. Publication No. EPA 800/8-90/045F.

Vähäkangas KH, Bennett WP, Castrén K, Welsh JA, Khan MA, Blömeke B, Alavanja MCR, Harris CC. *p53* and *K-ras* mutations in lung cancers from former and never-smoking women. *Cancer Research* 2001;61(11):4350–6.

Valkonen M, Kuusi T. Passive smoking induces atherogenic changes in low-density lipoprotein. *Circulation* 1998;97(20):2012–6.

van Jaarsveld H, Kuyl JM, Alberts DW. Antioxidant vitamin supplementation of smoke-exposed rats partially protects against myocardial ischaemic/reperfusion injury. *Free Radical Research Communications* 1992a;17(4):263–9.

van Jaarsveld H, Kuyl JM, Alberts DW. Exposure of rats to low concentration of cigarette smoke increases myocardial sensitivity to ischaemia/reperfusion. *Basic Research in Cardiology* 1992b;87(1):393–9.

Van Rooij JGM, Veeger MMS, Bodelier-Bade MM, Scheepers PTJ, Jongeneelen FJ. Smoking and dietary intake of polycyclic aromatic hydrocarbons as sources of interindividual variability in the baseline excretion of 1-hydroxypyrene in urine. *International Archives of Occupational and Environmental Health* 1994;66(1):55–65.

van Zeeland AA, de Groot AJL, Hall J, Donato F. 8-Hydroxydeoxyguanosine in DNA from leukocytes of healthy adults: relationship with cigarette smoking, environmental tobacco smoke, alcohol and coffee consumption. *Mutation Research* 1999;439(2):249–57.

Vu-Duc T, Huynh C-K. Sidestream tobacco smoke constituents in indoor air modelled in an experimental chamber—polycyclic aromatic hydrocarbons. *Environment International* 1989;15:57–64.

Wahlgren DR, Hovell MF, Meltzer EO, Meltzer SB. Involuntary smoking and asthma. *Current Opinion in Pulmonary Medicine* 2000;6(1):31–6.

Wallace L, Pellizzari E, Hartwell TD, Perritt R, Ziegenfus R. Exposures to benzene and other volatile compounds from active and passive smoking. *Archives of Environmental Health* 1987;42(5):272–9.

Wanner A, Salathe M, O'Riordan TG. Mucociliary clearance in the airways. *American Journal of Respiratory and Critical Care Medicine* 1996;154 (6 Pt 1):1868–902.

Weaver VM, Davoli CT, Heller PJ, Fitzwilliam A, Peters HL, Sunyer J, Murphy SE, Goldstein GW, Groopman JD. Benzene exposure, assessed by urinary *trans,trans*-muconic acid, in urban children with elevated blood lead levels. *Environmental Health Perspectives* 1996;104(3):318–23.

White JR, Froeb HF. Serum Lipoproteins in non-smokers chronically exposed to tobacco smoke in the workplace [abstract]. *8th World Conference on Tobacco or Health* (March 30–April 3, 1992). Buenos Aires (Argentina), 1991:118.

Willes SR, Fitzgerald TK, Permutt T, Proud D, Haley NJ, Bascom R. Acute respiratory response to prolonged, moderate levels of sidestream tobacco smoke. *Journal of Toxicology and Environmental Health Part A* 1998;53(3):193–209.

Witschi H. Tobacco smoke as a mouse lung carcinogen. *Experimental Lung Research* 1998;24(4):385–94.

Witschi H. Successful and not so successful chemoprevention of tobacco smoke-induced lung tumors. *Experimental Lung Research* 2000;26(8):743–55.

Witschi H, Espiritu I, Maronpot RR, Pinkerton KE, Jones AD. The carcinogenic potential of the gas phase of environmental tobacco smoke. *Carcinogenesis* 1997a;18(11):2035–42.

Witschi H, Espiritu I, Peake JL, Wu K, Maronpot RR, Pinkerton KE. The carcinogenicity of environmental tobacco smoke. *Carcinogenesis* 1997b;18(3):575–86.

Witschi H, Espiritu I, Uyeminami D. Chemoprevention of tobacco smoke-induced lung tumors in A/J strain mice with dietary *myo*-inositol and dexamethasone. *Carcinogenesis* 1999;20(7):1375–8.

Witschi H, Espiritu I, Yu M, Willits NH. The effects of phenethyl isothiocyanate, *N*-acetylcysteine and green tea on tobacco smoke-induced lung tumors in strain A/J mice. *Carcinogenesis* 1998;19(10): 1789–94.

Witschi H, Joad JP, Pinkerton KE. The toxicology of environmental tobacco smoke. *Annual Review of Pharmacology and Toxicology* 1997c;37:29–52.

Witschi H, Pinkerton KE, Coggins CRE, Penn A, Gori GB. Environmental tobacco smoke: experimental facts and societal issues. *Fundamental and Applied Toxicology* 1995;24(1):3–12.

Witschi H, Uyeminami D, Moran D, Espiritu I. Chemoprevention of tobacco-smoke lung carcinogenesis in mice after cessation of smoke exposure. *Carcinogenesis* 2000;21(5):977-82.

Wjst M, Heinrich J, Liu P, Dold S, Wassmer G, Merkel G, Huelsse C, Wichmann HE. Indoor factors and IgE levels in children. *Allergy* 1994;49(9):766–71.

Woo KS, Robinson JTC, Chook P, Adams MR, Yip G, Mai ZJ, Lam CWK, Sorenson KE, Deanfield JE, Celermajer DS. Differences in the effect of cigarette smoking on endothelial function in Chinese and white adults. *Annals of Internal Medicine* 1997;127(5):372–5.

Wu JM. Increased experimental atherosclerosis in cholesterol-fed rabbits exposed to passive smoke: taking issue with study design and methods of analysis [letter]. *Journal of the American College of Cardiology* 1993;22(6):1751–3.

Wu D, Landsberger S, Larson WM. Evaluation of elemental cadmium as a marker for environmental tobacco smoke. *Environmental Science & Technology* 1995;29(9):2311–6.

Xie Y, Garban H, Ng C, Rajfer J, Gonzalez-Cadavid NF. Effect of long-term passive smoking on erectile function and penile nitric oxide synthase in the rat. *Journal of Urology* 1997;157(3):1121–6.

Yamazaki H, Inui Y, Yun C-H, Guengerich FP, Shimada T. Cytochrome P450 2E1 and 2A6 enzymes as major catalysts for metabolic activation of *N*-nitrosodialkylamines and tobacco-related nitrosamines in human liver microsomes. *Carcinogenesis* 1992;13(10):1789–94.

Yates DH, Breen H, Thomas PS. Passive smoke inhalation decreases exhaled nitric oxide in normal subjects. *American Journal of Respiratory and Critical Care Medicine* 2001;164(6):1043–6. [See also comments in *American Journal of Respiratory and Critical Care Medicine* 2002;165(8):1188.]

Yates DH, Havill K, Thompson MM, Rittano AB, Chu J, Glanville AR. Sidestream smoke inhalation decreases respiratory clearance of 99mTc-DTPA acutely. *Australian and New Zealand Journal of Medicine* 1996;26(4):513–8.

Young S, Arnott J, O'Keeffe PT, Le Souef PN, Landau LI. The association between early life lung function and wheezing during the first 2 yrs of life. *European Respiratory Journal* 2000;15(1):151–7.

Young S, Le Souef PN, Geelhoed GC, Stick SM, Turner KJ, Landau LI. The influence of a family history of asthma and parental smoking on airway responsiveness in early infancy. *New England Journal of Medicine* 1991;324(17):1168–73. [See also erratum in *New England Journal of Medicine* 1991;325(10):747.]

Yu M, Pinkerton KE, Witschi H. Short-term exposure to aged and diluted sidestream cigarette smoke enhances ozone-induced lung injury in B6C3F1 mice. *Toxicological Sciences* 2002;65(1):99–106. [See also comments in *Toxicological Sciences* 2002;65(1): 1–3.]

Yu R, Weisel CP. Measurement of the urinary benzene metabolite *trans,trans*-muconic acid from benzene exposure in humans. *Journal of Toxicology and Environmental Health* 1996;48(5):453–77.

Yun CH, Shimada T, Guengerich FP. Roles of human liver cytochrome P4502C and 3A enzymes in the 3-hydroxylation of benzo[*a*]pyrene. *Cancer Research* 1992;52(7):1868–74.

Zetterstrom O, Osterman K, Machado L, Johansson SG. Another smoking hazard: raised serum IgE concentration and increased risk of occupational allergy. *British Medical Journal (Clinical Research Edition)* 1981;283(6301):1215–7.

Zhu B, Sun Y, Sievers RE, Shuman JL, Glantz SA, Chatterjee K, Parmley WW, Wolfe CL. L-arginine decreases infarct size in rats exposed to environmental tobacco smoke. *American Heart Journal* 1996;132(1 Pt 1):91–100.

Zhu BQ, Parmley WW. Hemodynamic and vascular effects of active and passive smoking. *American Heart Journal* 1995;130(6):1270–5.

Zhu B-Q, Sun Y-P, Sievers RE, Glantz SA, Parmley WW, Wolfe CL. Exposure to environmental tobacco smoke increases myocardial infarct size in rats. *Circulation* 1994;89(3):1282–90.

Zhu B-Q, Sun Y-P, Sievers RE, Isenberg WM, Glantz SA, Parmley WW. Increased experimental atherosclerosis in cholesterol-fed rabbits exposed to passive smoke: taking issue with study design and methods of analysis [reply to letter]. *Journal of the American College of Cardiology* 1993a;22(6):1752–3.

Zhu BQ, Sun YP, Sievers RE, Isenberg WM, Glantz SA, Parlmey WW. Passive smoking increases experimental atherosclerosis in cholesterol-fed rabbits. *Journal of the American College of Cardiology* 1993b;21(1):225–32.

Chapter 3
Assessment of Exposure to Secondhand Smoke

Introduction

This chapter provides a review of key factors that determine exposures of people to secondhand smoke in indoor environments. The discussion describes (1) the dynamic movement of secondhand smoke throughout indoor environments, (2) the factors that determine secondhand smoke concentrations in these environments, (3) the atmospheric markers of secondhand smoke that are measured to assess concentrations, (4) the biomarkers that are measured to assess doses of tobacco smoke components, and (5) the models that can be used to describe patterns of human exposures. Chapter 4 (Prevalence of Exposure to Secondhand Smoke) reports on findings of studies on exposures to secondhand smoke that applied these methods with a focus on measurements of nicotine in the air and cotinine in biologic materials. The validity of nicotine as a marker for secondhand smoke concentrations supports the use of cotinine, a principal metabolite of nicotine, as an exposure biomarker.

As described earlier, the term secondhand smoke refers to a complex mixture of particulate (or solid) and gaseous components. The characteristics of secondhand smoke change over time, particularly the components of sidestream smoke that the smoldering cigarette releases. Sidestream smoke dilutes quickly and changes as the particles release volatile compounds and change in size and composition as they age. Although few studies have made measurements, available data indicate that the estimated median aerodynamic diameter of secondhand smoke particles is 0.4 micrometers (μm), a size range where particles tend to remain suspended in the air unless removed by diffusion to or impaction with a surface, or by air cleaning (Hiller et al. 1982; Jenkins et al. 2000).

The composition of secondhand smoke was addressed in the 1986 report of the Surgeon General, *The Health Consequences of Involuntary Smoking* (U.S. Department of Health and Human Services [USDHHS] 1986), and was the focus of a comprehensive monograph first published in 1992 and updated in 2000 (Guerin et al. 1992; Jenkins et al. 2000). The 1986 report commented on the richness of secondhand smoke as a mixture and its inherent variability over time and space as it moves through the air (USDHHS 1986). Nonetheless, the report concluded that secondhand smoke and mainstream smoke were qualitatively similar, a conclusion that subsequent research supports (U.S. Environmental Protection Agency [USEPA] 1992; Scientific Committee on Tobacco and

Health 1998; International Agency for Research on Cancer [IARC] 2004).

People are exposed to secondhand smoke in multiple places where they spend varying amounts of time. The term "microenvironment" refers to places that have a fairly uniform concentration of a mixture of pollutants across the time that is spent there (National Research Council [NRC] 1991; Klepeis 1999a). In the microenvironmental model, total human exposure to an atmospheric contaminant, such as secondhand smoke, represents the time-integrated sum of the exposures in the multiple microenvironments where time is spent. The source of secondhand smoke—the burning cigarette—produces the resulting concentrations of secondhand smoke in the air of places where people spend time. The concentration depends on the intensity of smoking, dilution by ventilation, and other processes that remove smoke from the air. The consequent exposures lead ultimately to doses of secondhand smoke components that reach and harm target organs and manifest as adverse health effects. This conceptual framework, which is central to this chapter, makes clear distinctions between cigarette smoking as the source, secondhand smoke concentrations in the air (the amount of material present per unit volume), exposures to secondhand smoke (the time spent in contact with secondhand smoke at various concentrations), and the doses from secondhand smoke exposure (the amount of material entering the body). The strength of the source—cigarette smoking—depends on the number of smokers and the rate at which they are smoking. Total human exposure can be estimated by measuring secondhand smoke concentrations in key microenvironments and assessing the time spent in those environments. Concentrations are also determined by aspects of the design and operation of a building (NRC 1986, 1991).

The mass balance model is a conceptual approach that provides a framework for how the design and operation of a building may affect secondhand smoke concentrations within the building (Ott 1999). In this model, which is considered in more detail later in this chapter (see "Exposure Models"), the concentration of indoor air contaminants (such as secondhand smoke) is a function of the strength of the source(s) generating the contaminant, the dilution of the contaminant by the exchange of outdoor with indoor air, and the rate of removal of the contaminant by air cleaning and other processes.

Building Designs and Operations

Determinants of Secondhand Smoke Concentrations

When people are exposed to secondhand smoke in indoor environments, the concentrations to which they are exposed depend not only on the number of cigarettes smoked, which determines the strength of the source, but on how air moves through buildings and at what rate indoor air is exchanged with outdoor air. The exchange of indoor with outdoor air is referred to as ventilation (American Society of Heating, Refrigerating and Air-Conditioning Engineers [ASHRAE] 1989). In general, the concentration of an indoor contaminant in a building or in a space within a building depends on the volume of the space and the rate at which the contaminant is generated and then removed. The removal may be by ventilation, air cleaning, or other processes such as chemical reactions or adsorption onto surfaces. This set of relationships is referred to as the mass balance model. It implies that concentrations of secondhand smoke components in a space (1) increase as the number of cigarettes smoked increases, (2) decrease with an increase in ventilation, and (3) decrease in proportion to the rate of cleaning or removal of secondhand smoke components from the air (Ott 1999). The cleaning or removal processes might include active air cleaning with a device, the naturally occurring passive deposition of particles onto surfaces, and the adsorption of gases onto materials.

The factors in the mass balance model vary across different kinds of buildings. Buildings can be ventilated using natural or mechanical methods. Air can be supplied naturally through windows, louvers, and leakages through building envelopes; air is supplied mechanically through a heating, ventilating, and air conditioning (HVAC) system that usually includes fans, duct work, and a system for delivering air in a controlled manner throughout a building (Figure 3.1). In most homes, ventilation occurs by a naturally occurring exchange of indoor with outdoor air. Commercial and public buildings generally have HVAC systems that move air through buildings to accomplish the exchange of indoor with outdoor air. Important considerations are variations in the range of surfaces and their characteristics across different kinds of buildings and microenvironments. For example, most HVAC systems incorporate a component

for air cleaning that typically removes large particles but not the smaller particles or the gases found in secondhand smoke. The central air cleaning systems in homes and in many commercial buildings generally are not designed to remove smaller particles or gases (Spengler 1999).

Heating, Ventilating, and Air Conditioning Systems

For modern public and commercial buildings, often with sealed windows, air ventilation is required to provide a safe, functional, and comfortable environment for the occupants, and is defined as "outside air" delivered to or brought indoors. For many types of indoor environments, mechanical ventilation systems are used to control contaminant concentrations and to meet the comfort needs of occupants. Such systems are almost always used in hospitals, large office buildings, theaters, hospitality venues, schools, and many other larger buildings. This discussion addresses how these systems affect secondhand smoke concentrations in indoor environments and focuses on public and commercial buildings where HVAC units are generally in place. Mechanical systems are intended to provide thermally conditioned air, dissipate thermal loads, and dilute contaminants (Bearg 2001). These systems can also be used to maintain pressure differentials between areas when air is extracted and exhausted from specific spaces, or to clean and recirculate the air using filters, catalytic converters, and various sorbent beds. The efficiencies and costs for an entire ventilation system vary depending on specific requirements and settings (Liddament 2001). Although mechanical systems are widely used for general ventilation, their potential use as a control strategy for secondhand smoke requires a detailed understanding of the constituents to be controlled, the air distribution patterns within structures, the air cleaning or extraction techniques, and the requirements for ongoing operation and maintenance (Ludwig 2001). If not properly designed and maintained, mechanical systems can increase the risk of exposures by distributing pollutants (including secondhand smoke) throughout the building, by direct recirculation, or by poor pressure control.

Figure 3.1   Schematic of a typical air handling unit

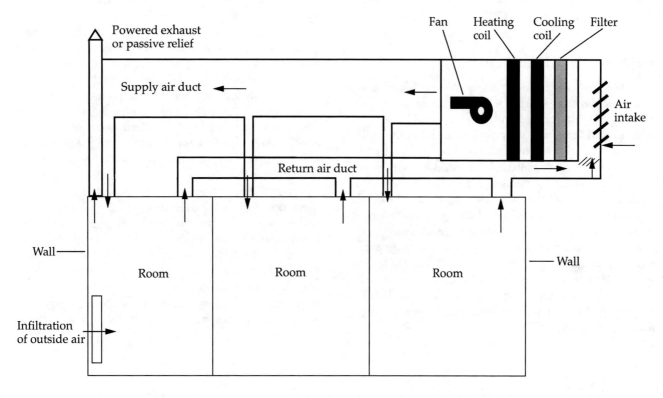

Source: U.S. Environmental Protection Agency 1994, with modifications.

Complex and dynamic processes affect the characteristics and concentrations of secondhand smoke. As a foundation for considering ventilation systems commonly found in buildings, here is a description of the transport and fate of particles and gases released from a burning cigarette. In still air, the smoke plume from a cigarette is often observed rising intact as high as several meters above the burning tip. If plume gases remain concentrated, they are buoyant and have a temperature several degrees higher than the surrounding room air temperature. If the room air is not still, as in buildings with mechanical air handling systems, or if people move within the space, there will be some mixing that breaks up the plume and disperses "pockets" of smoke throughout the air space (Klepeis 1999b). Concentrations of secondhand smoke components are then reduced and, as the smoke spreads and ages, its components change as a result of condensation, evaporation, coagulation, and deposition to surfaces. The characteristics of secondhand smoke within a particular building thus depend, to an extent, on chemical and physical characteristics of spaces that vary among buildings. Volatile components such as nicotine are adsorbed and degassed by materials. As a consequence, the smell of cigarettes emanates from clothing, carpets, air conditioners, and other surfaces without the presence of active smoking, as previously deposited or adsorbed material is re-emitted by air currents (Klepeis 1999b).

Although interactions in the air and at surfaces modify the secondhand smoke mixture, under most circumstances concentrations within the original space will depend strongly on an exchange of air in the space with less contaminated air (Spengler 1999). Mechanically delivered air disperses secondhand smoke constituents through mixing (turbulence) and dilutes secondhand smoke by supplying less contaminated air. Generally, mechanical mixing is significantly more effective in reducing concentrations from a "point source" of pollution in a room, such as a burning cigarette, than is diffusion alone in still air. Air exchange and surface removal processes act together to lower secondhand smoke concentrations. Surface removal is enhanced if air is forced through an air cleaning device and delivered back to the room with a reduced secondhand smoke concentration (McDonald and Ouyang 2001).

Building Ventilation Control

Mechanical HVAC systems that heat, ventilate, and air-condition indoor spaces achieve controlled building ventilation (Spengler 1999). The HVAC systems in buildings are composed of air handling units (AHUs) of various sizes and complexities that filter and condition air supplied to the building with varying degrees of effectiveness, depending upon need, design, and maintenance. Components of AHUs typically include fans, filters, cooling coils, and heat exchangers. Air ventilated by air conditioning (i.e., mechanical cooling) can be ducted to separate areas within a building and removed with an air return system that recirculates and/or exhausts the air. In Figure 3.1, a schematic demonstrates a typical AHU configured for general ventilation and pressure relationship control (USEPA 1994).

Three major categories are used for airborne contaminant control: general or dilution ventilation, displacement ventilation, and local exhaust ventilation. General or dilution ventilation requires mixing large volumes of outdoor air with room air. Although this ventilation system is the most commonly used method in buildings today for thermal comfort, it is not very efficient for controlling contaminant emissions from human activities such as smoking. Its effectiveness is highly dependent upon the number and location of emission sources (the smokers), the volume of air supply to the room, the capacity of materials and surfaces to remove various constituents of secondhand smoke, and the mixing efficiency of the room. Figure 3.2 demonstrates that the term "air exchange rate," when applied to dilution ventilation, is a misnomer. Mixing the supply air within the zone served by the AHU is often not uniform or complete. Even for a well-mixed space, one air change per hour (ACH) means that only 63.2 percent of the original air, including the corresponding airborne contaminants, is removed in one hour. So even though an amount

Figure 3.2   Anticipated changes in concentrations of airborne materials for various air exchange rates

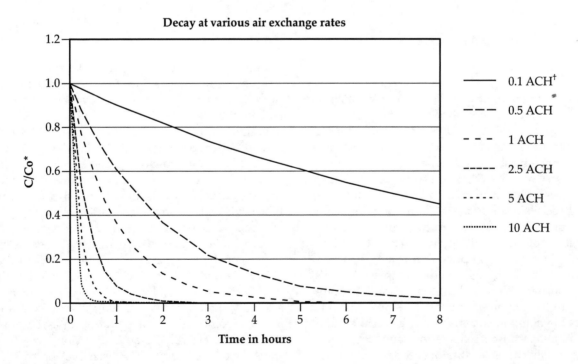

*C/Co = Fraction of original concentration of contaminant at time t.
†ACH = Air changes per hour.

of air equivalent to the volume of the room is introduced during one hour, it does not completely replace all of the air occupying the space previously. Short-circuiting or moving air directly from inlets to the exhaust without mixing, obstructions to supply and exhaust air, and thermal gradients can reduce the mixing efficiency to much less than the theoretical limit. Thus, an air exchange rate greater than that made with simple calculations based on the volume of the space may be required to effect a meaningful reduction in airborne concentrations of various contaminants (Liddament 2001). Simple mass balance and volumetric calculations assume perfect mixing, no sink effects (the adsorption and possible re-emission of pollutants by materials acting as "sinks" [Sparks 2001]), and constant emission sources; these conditions generally are not met in real-world indoor environments. Any occupant of a space, particularly a space near a pollution source, may be exposed to much higher concentrations than estimated for the overall area.

Displacement ventilation, which is also referred to as piston or plug flow, conditions the space and removes contaminants by admitting air at one location and "sweeping" it across the space before exhausting it at the opposite "face." This design often uses low-velocity grills at or near floor level to admit cool supply air into the space that is then exhausted at ceiling level. For maximum effectiveness, displacement ventilation requires a more or less uniform and unidirectional flow. This flow structure might easily be disrupted by large numbers of people moving about a space, or through the use of ceiling fans or supplementary ventilation systems. Displacement ventilation often uses specific characteristics of the contaminant to aid in its capture. For example, a heated plume from a computer, copier, or cigarette develops convective (vertical) flows. If the displacement air is also moving vertically from floor to ceiling, pollutants and excess heat can be captured, treated, or exhausted from the ceiling. With this strategy, however, contaminants on their way to the exhaust stage can still pass through the breathing zones of both smokers and nonsmokers. Furthermore, vertical flows may be disrupted by furniture that is in the space, thus limiting the effectiveness of displacement ventilation.

Local exhaust ventilation extracts the air around a specific point source. It has been used for many decades to effectively control a variety of contaminants from specific activities or processes, often in industrial settings. Its effectiveness relies upon strict compliance with control measures that can include source enclosure, high air exhaust rates, and direct ducting to the outdoors that minimizes entrainment into outdoor air intakes. Restrictive compliance requirements limit its application to secondhand smoke in general indoor environments, except in separately exhausted smoking enclosures.

Operation of Ventilation Systems

Ventilation requirements for spaces such as office buildings, classrooms, and various hospitality venues are expressed as the volume of outside air per unit of time (e.g., liters per second, cubic feet per minute) per person, and/or volume flow rates of outdoor air per square foot of the area of the building. ASHRAE (1999) included the latter criterion in the revised Standard 62-1999 as a result of the recognition that air pollutants are also released by building sources—building materials, furnishings, and the HVAC equipment itself—and that to protect the occupants, ventilation standards should also apply to these sources as well as to the occupants. ASHRAE develops standards to guide building designs and operations that often become part of municipal codes (Chapter 10, Control of Secondhand Smoke Exposure). Consequently, ASHRAE standards are considered relevant to the control of secondhand smoke in the United States (Table 3.1). Building ventilation codes generally specify the total amount of air as well as a minimum percentage of outdoor air that should be supplied to occupied spaces. Minimum amounts between 10 and 20 percent are often specified, but in practice, outdoor air delivery into a building may vary from 0 to 100 percent over time. The variation depends on the design requirements of the space and operational characteristics of the ventilation system.

Ventilation systems are often quite complex and have multiple components. Controls are in place to modulate the air intake louvers, airflow, air temperature, and sometimes the humidity to meet specified thermal conditions (ASHRAE 1999). These control systems often consist of combinations of sensors, signal processors, computerized controllers, switches, dampers, valves, relays, and motors. The operating strategies for ventilation systems can have a major impact on the control of secondhand smoke within buildings. For example, many systems operate on economizer cycles that use the cooling or heating capacity of the outside air. During the economizer phase, the outside louvers open. Often, depending on the climate and season, a temperature range (generally between 50° and 65° F) will completely open the outside dampers (Spengler 1999; Bearg 2001). If ambient conditions become too warm and humid, the outside air vents

Table 3.1   Outdoor air requirements for ventilation*

| Application | Estimated maximum[†] occupancy per 1,000 ft²[‡] or 100 m²[§] | Outdoor air requirements | | Comments |
		cf/m/ person[Δ]	cf/m/ft²	
Food and beverage services				
Dining rooms	70	20	NR[¶]	
Cafeteria, fast food	100	20	NR	
Bars, cocktail lounges	100	30	NR	Supplementary smoke-removal equipment may be required
Kitchen (cooking)	20	15	NR	Make-up air for hood exhaust may require more ventilating air; the sum of the outdoor air and transfer air of acceptable quality from adjacent spaces shall be sufficient to provide an exhaust rate of not less than 1.5 cf/m/ft² (7.5 liters/second/m²)
Hotels, motels, resorts, dormitories			cf/m/room	
Bedrooms	NR	NR	30	
Lobbies	30	15	NR	
Conference rooms	50	20	NR	
Casinos	120	30	NR	Supplementary smoke-removal equipment may be required
Offices				Some office equipment may require local exhaust
Office space	NR	20	NR	
Public spaces				Normally supplied by transfer air; local mechanical exhaust with no recirculation is recommended
Smoking lounge	70	60	NR	

*This table prescribes supply rates of acceptable outdoor air required for acceptable indoor air quality. These values have been chosen to dilute human bioeffluents and other contaminants with adequate margins of safety and to account for health variations and varied activity levels among people.
[†]Net occupiable space.
[‡]ft² = Square feet.
[§]m² = Square meters.
[Δ]cf/m/person = Cubic feet per minute per person.
[¶]NR = Data were not reported.
Source: American Society of Heating, Refrigerating and Air-Conditioning Engineers Standard 62-1999, Table 2.1 (1999).

will return to minimum or closed settings. To protect coils from freezing or to minimize heating, outside air vents might be closed or set at minimum openings during colder temperatures. Thus, contaminants such as secondhand smoke that are generated within a building are often subject to varying amounts of dilution air, and building occupants may face indoor air quality that varies during a day or over longer periods of time (Spengler 1999).

Most large, modern buildings use a building automation system (BAS) to provide direct digital control of ventilation through a central computer. Planned into the BAS is a sequence of operations for the HVAC system (USEPA 1998). Knowledge of routine activities related to building occupancy allow engineers to program HVAC systems through the central BAS to improve comfort and optimize energy efficiency.

However, a BAS is generally not programmed to control indoor air pollutants such as secondhand smoke.

Mechanical air handling systems exchange indoor air with outside air by pressure-driven flows through windows, doors, and cracks. Some buildings are not designed or constructed to be airtight; an estimated 40 percent of commercial buildings have operable windows, and natural ventilation is more common in older and smaller buildings (Liddament 2001). Pressure differentials across the building envelope are caused by wind and by indoor and outdoor temperature differences. The wind that flows around a building creates static positive pressures as well as negative pressures in the wake flow that is downstream of objects. Pressure differences across openings can force air into or out of a building. The HVAC system of pressurized ducts and building exhaust fans also creates an air exchange. Plumbing and electrical chases, elevator shafts, leaky air ducts, and cracks and openings between floors can become unplanned pathways for pressure-driven internal flows. Thus, contaminants such as secondhand smoke are not always controlled by HVAC airflows alone, and the HVAC ducts may transport and distribute secondhand smoke-contaminated air. Entrainment from doors, window cracks, or loading docks can bring tobacco smoke back into a building even when smokers are restricted to smoking outdoors. Even within buildings, secondhand smoke can move along unplanned or uncontrolled pathways to annoy and irritate occupants in other rooms or even on other floors far removed from the smoking areas.

Residential Ventilation

There are more than 100 million residential units in the United States. The most common types are single family (73 percent) followed by multi-family structures that include both low-rise and high-rise apartments (21 percent) and mobile homes (6 percent). The United States has a high rate of owner-occupied households (67 percent); 33 percent of households live in rental units (Diamond 2001).

The age and size of housing vary around the country. In general, older homes are smaller (<2,000 square feet of conditioned space) and are more common in the Northeast and Midwest. The average apartment unit is about half that size (approximately 1,000 square feet). Three million Americans live in public housing, most of which are two-bedroom units built in the 1950s and 1960s; the total size is typically 500 to 600 square feet (Diamond 2001). The south and

southwestern regions of the United States continue to be the fastest growing areas and lead in new housing construction (Joint Center for Housing Studies of Harvard University 2002). Despite a decrease in the size of households, the size of single-family homes has increased with more square feet per person. Homes built in 1995 were 17 percent larger than those built just a decade earlier. During a 15-year period, new apartment units increased in average floor space by almost 10 percent (Diamond 2001).

Most houses and apartments have heating systems. Besides the size of the unit (i.e., volume), the type of heating, cooling, and exhaust system is an important factor in the dispersion, dilution, and removal of indoor-generated secondhand smoke across a room or throughout a residence. More than 50 percent of U.S. residences have central warm air furnaces. These systems include fan-forced directed air distributed to rooms with a gravity or ducted return back to the heat exchange unit of the furnace. Gravitational settling is not intended to remove the smaller particles found in secondhand smoke, nor is it efficient at removing them. Filters upstream of the blower serve to protect the mechanical parts from objects and large particles, but these filters also fail to remove the smaller secondhand smoke particles and gases.

Air conditioning can affect the distribution and concentration of secondhand smoke. Air conditioning systems are common in U.S. residences, including apartments. According to the Residential Energy Conservation Survey (U.S. Department of Energy 1999), 48 percent of residences were equipped with central air conditioning and 27 percent had window units. Forty-seven percent of the respondents with central systems versus only 18 percent with window units reported using their air conditioning "quite a bit" or "just about all summer." Similar to forced warm air mechanical systems, central air-cooling systems can rapidly mix secondhand smoke throughout the conditioned space. Doors and windows are generally closed when the air conditioner is in use and the system is usually set to recirculate the indoor air. These closed conditions tend to reduce the dilution of secondhand smoke.

Wallace (1996) comprehensively reviewed indoor air particle concentrations and sources and quantified the effect of air conditioning on the concentration of secondhand smoke. His review included studies that measured indoor and outdoor particulate matter 2.5 ($PM_{2.5}$) concentrations across six U.S. communities (Dockery and Spengler 1981; Spengler et al. 1981; Spengler and Thurston 1983; Letz et al. 1984; Neas et al. 1994). Estimated concentrations of fine particles were 30 micrograms per cubic meter ($\mu g/m^3$) higher in homes with smokers than in homes without smokers. According to Wallace (1996), "A mass balance model was used to estimate the impact of cigarette smoking on indoor particles. Long-term mean infiltration of outdoor $PM_{2.5}$ was estimated to be 70% for homes without air conditioners, but only 30% for homes with air conditioners. An estimate of 0.88 $\mu g/m^3$ per cigarette (24-h average) was made for homes without air conditioning, while in homes with air conditioning the estimate increased to 1.23 $\mu g/m^3$ per cigarette" (p. 100). The greater estimate for air conditioning is consistent with lowered air exchange rates while the air conditioning is operating, and is supported by a 1994 study (Suh et al. 1994).

Air exchange rates in homes are usually determined by one of two methods: blower door pressurization or tracer gases. Blower door pressurization tests identify air leakage areas that are then used to estimate air exchange rates. Sherman and Matson (1997), who modeled the results of blower door tests, found that a typical single-family house constructed before 1990 has an estimated air exchange rate of 1.0 ACH. Homes built to meet more energy efficient building codes have estimated rates of 0.5 ACH.

Tracer gases are emitted into a home and measured over time to calculate short-term (decay rate) or long-term (mass balance method) air exchange rates. Murray and Burmaster (1995) examined the Brookhaven National Laboratory tracer gas data that included almost 3,000 households. The analysis derived best-fit, log-normal distributions from data classified by four regions or by heating degree days (a measurement used to relate a day's temperature to the demand for fuel to heat buildings: a 65° average daily temperature = the number of heating degree days), and by the four seasons. In general, air exchange rates are higher for homes that are in warmer climates. Air exchange rates across all regions are higher during the summer months followed by spring, fall, and winter. The summer mean air exchange rate is 1.5 h^{-1} (air changes per hour) versus 0.41 h^{-1} for the fall.

Other characteristics of air exchange rates derived from blower door and tracer gas methods indicate that apartment units and multifamily structures with shared interior walls have less external surface area, less unplanned air leakage, and typically lower air exchange rates compared with single-family detached houses.

Conclusions

1. Current heating, ventilating, and air conditioning systems alone cannot control exposure to secondhand smoke.

2. The operation of a heating, ventilating, and air conditioning system can distribute secondhand smoke throughout a building.

Implications

These conclusions suggest that control strategies for indoor exposure to secondhand smoke cannot use approaches based on HVAC system design and operation. The benefits from HVAC systems include a number of critical functions that help to maintain a healthful and comfortable indoor environment. This review of their functioning shows, however, that current HVAC systems cannot fully control exposures to secondhand smoke unless a complete smoking ban is enforced. Furthermore, unless carefully controlled, HVAC operations can distribute air that has been contaminated with secondhand smoke throughout a building. Simple predictions cannot be made about the consequences of these operations because they vary with the building and with the HVAC characteristics. However, to develop models that assess the effects of indoor secondhand tobacco smoke exposures, it is necessary to first develop an understanding of HVAC systems and their effectiveness in a particular structure. However, this review indicates that a complete ban on indoor smoking is the most efficient and effective approach to control exposures to secondhand smoke. Additional implications of these findings are considered in Chapter 10, Control of Secondhand Smoke Exposure.

Atmospheric Markers of Secondhand Smoke

Concepts and Interpretations of Exposure Markers

Secondhand smoke is a dynamic mixture that contains thousands of compounds in its vapor and particle phases. Some of these components are specific to secondhand smoke, such as nicotine, but others have additional sources and are not specific to secondhand smoke, as in the case of carbon monoxide (CO). Some of the more specific markers can be useful indicators of secondhand smoke concentrations, but no particular marker will be predictive of the full range of risks from exposures to secondhand smoke. Additionally, some components of particular interest for disease risk, such as the tobacco-specific nitrosamines, are not easily measured at typical indoor air concentrations (Hecht 1999). Nonetheless, some components of secondhand smoke can be quantified in indoor air. This quantification enables researchers to estimate exposures to secondhand smoke for research purposes and for tracking population exposures. In 1986, the NRC report on involuntary smoking proposed useful atmospheric markers that are believed to be unique to tobacco smoke or that are believed to have cigarette smoking as their primary source in most environments; the mass that is emitted is believed to be similar across cigarette brands (NRC 1986). Subsequent studies have evaluated some of the markers used to detect secondhand smoke in indoor environments (Guerin et al. 1992; Daisey 1999; Jenkins et al. 2000).

Researchers need sensitive and specific markers of secondhand smoke for exposure surveillance and potentially for enforcement of regulations. For research and for population risk assessments, measurements of marker compounds can be used with microenvironmental models to estimate exposures to secondhand smoke (Jaakkola and Samet 1999). Researchers can also estimate the relative contributions of different environments to these exposures and the potential consequences of exposure levels. Furthermore, the concentration of one marker may be used to predict concentrations of other constituents if the concentration ratios between the marker and the other constituents of interest are known.

Evaluation of Specific Markers

Concentrations of secondhand smoke components in indoor air have multiple determinants: the rate of smoking, the volume of the room or space, the air exchange rate, the exchange of volatile components between vapor and particle phases, deposition rates on surfaces, rates of re-emission from the surfaces, and chemical transformations (Daisey 1999). Although studies have measured concentrations of some of these chemicals in laboratory conditions, the behaviors of only a few of these compounds as tracers have been characterized in field settings. Studies document that each component under consideration has potential limitations as a marker. These limitations may be the result of photodegradation, variable partitioning between the particle and vapor phases, or adsorption/re-emission rates that differ from those of other compounds of concern. No single compound or component has been identified as a completely valid marker for every constituent found in secondhand smoke. On the other hand, several useful markers have a sufficient specificity for secondhand smoke and they can be used to characterize exposures of the public in general or of particular groups. Of these markers, nicotine is highly specific and is considered a valid marker of the PM component of secondhand smoke across a wide range of concentrations in indoor environments (Daisey 1999).

Researchers have studied secondhand smoke characteristics in chambers, with different cigarette brands as the source. In these studies, many different brands generated similar steady-state concentrations of both vapor phase nicotine and respirable particles, and the relationship between these two markers was similar among brands (Leaderer and Hammond 1991; Daisey et al. 1998). Sources other than smoking also contribute to background concentrations of particles found indoors, such as cooking and particles that have infiltrated from the outdoors (Leaderer and Hammond 1991). Thus, the models for estimating the relationship between nicotine and respirable particle concentrations involve regression approaches that estimate increases in nicotine concentrations with increases in particle concentrations. In such linear regression models, the intercept estimates the background concentration of particles and the slope describes the relationship between concentrations of nicotine and secondhand smoke particles. In most environments where people spend time, secondhand smoke concentrations are usually much lower than in laboratory chambers, so background particles represent a significant fraction of the particle concentration. The relationship between concentrations of nicotine and respirable particles in indoor air has been consistent across field studies in 47 homes (Leaderer and Hammond 1991), in 44 office samples (Schenker et al. 1990), and in 14 other workplaces (Miesner et al. 1989). The range of slopes for the increase of respirable particulate matter (RPM) concentration with nicotine concentration is narrow: 8.6 to 9.8 μg of RPM per μg of nicotine. Daisey (1999) calculated a slope of 10.9 μg of RPM per μg of nicotine using personal sampling data that Jenkins and colleagues (1996) had compiled from more than 1,500 people in the United States. Thus, for each microgram of atmospheric nicotine in the various environments where people spend time, there is an estimated increase of about 10 μg in secondhand smoke particle concentrations.

Until recently, most studies incorporated either respirable particles or nicotine as markers for secondhand smoke, and they remain the most commonly used markers. The literature on the concentrations of these markers is now substantial. In an early study carried out in the late 1970s, Repace and Lowrey (1980) evaluated secondhand smoke levels by contrasting the concentration of particles measured during a bingo game in a church with the concentration measured during a church service with a similar number of people present who were not smoking. The particle levels were much higher during the bingo game (279 μg/m^3) compared with during the service (30 μg/m^3). Similarly, studies in the early 1980s of respirable particles in homes found that concentrations in the homes of smokers were substantially higher than concentrations in the homes of nonsmokers (approximately 74 μg/m^3 versus 28 μg/m^3, respectively)

(Spengler et al. 1985). However, the high levels of respirable particles from other sources and the variability in the concentrations of these particles make it difficult to use the respirable particle concentration as an indicator of secondhand smoke, particularly if secondhand smoke concentrations are low.

In most environments where the public spends time, nicotine in the air comes only from tobacco smoke, so there is no background concentration to be considered. This very high specificity, in combination with the development of inexpensive, sensitive, and passive methods to measure nicotine concentrations in real-world environments, has led to the widespread use of nicotine as a marker for secondhand smoke (Jenkins et al. 2000). A 1999 review concluded that nicotine was a suitable marker for secondhand smoke (Daisey 1999).

Findings from initial secondhand smoke chamber studies that used nicotine as a marker provide evidence supporting its use (Hammond et al. 1987; Leaderer and Hammond 1991). The ambient concentrations of both nicotine and respirable particles were similar when human volunteers smoked 12 brands of cigarettes in separate tests. Nicotine and tar yields varied in mainstream smoke over an order of magnitude (0.1 milligram [mg] of nicotine per cigarette for ultra-low nicotine cigarettes to 1.3 mg per cigarette for regular cigarettes). Subsequent studies showed that nicotine decay in chambers did not follow first-order kinetics (where the speed of a chemical reaction is proportional to the concentrations of the reactants), and short-term measurements in chambers indicated varying ratios of nicotine when compared with other secondhand smoke constituents (Eatough et al. 1989a; Nelson et al. 1992; Van Loy et al. 1998). However, further investigations showed that these findings were artifacts of the chambers themselves. In real-world settings with longer sampling times, nicotine concentrations closely tracked levels of other secondhand smoke constituents (Van Loy et al. 1998; Daisey 1999; LaKind et al. 1999a).

Concentrations of eight possible tracers for secondhand smoke (nicotine, 3-ethenyl pyridine, myosmine, solanesol, scopoletin, RPM, ultraviolet-absorbing particulate matter [UVPM], and fluorescing particulate matter [FPM]) were measured in 469 personal samples collected in workplaces where smoking was allowed (LaKind et al. 1999a). The first three chemicals were in the gas phase, while the latter five were in the particle phase. Concentrations of the three gas phase markers (nicotine, 3-ethenyl pyridine, and myosmine) were highly correlated ($r^2 > 0.8$, where r^2 = the coefficient of determination describing the strength of the model), as were those for three of the particle phase markers (UVPM, FPM, and solanesol) (Table 3.2). Scopoletin was also correlated with UVPM, but only at higher concentrations. Respirable particle concentrations were not strongly correlated with concentrations of UVPM or of nicotine, probably because respirable particles were present in the workplaces from sources other than smoking. Nicotine concentrations in the gas phase correlated with concentrations of the particle phase marker UVPM and with the other particle phase markers that were correlated with UVPM: FPM, solanesol, and scopoletin.

Several studies examined concentrations of some of the toxic compounds that cigarette smoking emits into the air. Two studies found that different brands of cigarettes released very similar amounts of two nitrosamines, *N*-nitrosodimethylamine and *N*-nitrosopyrrolidine (Mahanama and Daisey 1996). Other toxic volatile organic compounds in secondhand smoke, including benzene, formaldehyde, 1,3-butadiene, and styrene, also exhibited little variation among brands (Daisey et al. 1998). This consistency in emissions among several different brands indicates that changes in the concentration of a particular marker imply proportional changes in the concentrations of other airborne toxic chemicals that are in secondhand smoke.

The level of sensitivity is another key characteristic of a potential marker for secondhand smoke. High sensitivity enables markers to detect low levels of secondhand smoke, which is a necessary quality

Table 3.2 Correlations between various secondhand smoke constituents as selective markers of exposures

Secondhand smoke constituent	Secondhand smoke exposure marker	R^2*
Nicotine	3-EP[†]	.83
	Myosmine	.88
	UVPM[‡]	.63
UVPM	FPM[§]	.96
	Solanesol	.84
	Scopoletin >1	.73
	Scopoletin <1	.10

Note: 469 personal samples collected from workplaces that permitted smoking.
*R^2 = The coefficient of determination describing the strength of the model.
[†]EP = Ethenyl pyridine.
[‡]UVPM = Ultraviolet-absorbing particulate matter.
[§]FPM = Fluorescing particulate matter.
Source: LaKind et al. 1999b (from the 16 Cities Study).

for evaluating control programs and for surveillance. Some markers have this necessary degree of sensitivity. In the 16 Cities Study conducted by Jenkins and colleagues (1996), researchers collected 469 samples of these eight markers during one workday at worksites where smoking was allowed. Three markers were quite sensitive: nicotine, FPM, and UVPM; less than 2 percent of the samples had concentrations below the limit of detection. More than 10 percent of the samples fell below the limit of detection for myosmine, scopoletin, and solanesol (Figure 3.3). In fact, less than half of the samples collected in workplaces where smoking was allowed had detectable levels of solanesol.

Figure 3.3   Sensitivity of markers for secondhand smoke exposure

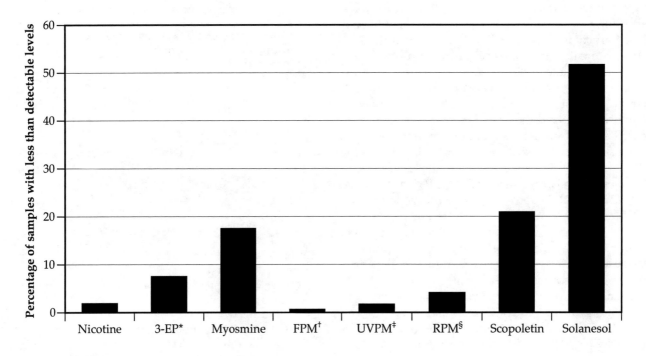

Note: 469 personal samples from workplaces that permitted smoking.
*EP = Ethenyl pyridine.
†FPM = Fluorescing particulate matter.
‡UVPM = Ultraviolet-absorbing particulate matter.
§RPM = Respirable particulate matter.
Source: Calculated from data in LaKind et al. 1999a.

Exposure Models

Models and mathematical representations can also be used to estimate human exposures to secondhand smoke (Ott 1999) because they are useful for predicting secondhand smoke concentrations with different patterns of cigarette smoking and for comparing control measures. The microenvironmental model is a tool that can estimate population exposures to secondhand smoke when there is information on the places where people spend time and whether people are smoking. Secondhand smoke concentrations can be inferred from models that characterize contamination of indoor spaces from smoking or from measurements made in the various microenvironments.

Standard techniques that are used to model concentrations of air contaminants indoors, based on the mass balance model, typically include terms that account for the volume of the room, the generation rate, and the removal rate. For secondhand smoke, the generation rate is the number of cigarettes smoked, and the removal rate may include terms such as the air exchange rate, the rate of deposition on surfaces, and terms for chemical transformations. In some cases, the rate of re-emission from surfaces may also be important. Van Loy and colleagues (1998) have written one such equation:

$$\frac{dC_i}{dt} = \frac{E_i(t)}{V} - ACH * C_i - \frac{1}{V}\sum_{j=1}^{g} S_j \frac{dM_{ij}}{dt}$$

where C_i is the concentration of airborne chemical i, $E_i(t)$ is the emission rate of i, V is the volume of the room, ACH is the air exchange rate, S_j is the area of surface j, and M_{ij} is the mass of i deposited on surface j. The term

$$\frac{dC_i}{dt}$$

gives the rate of change of the concentration. The first term on the right is the emissions rate per volume, the second is the loss of concentration due to air exchange, and the third is the loss to surfaces.

Adapted to secondhand smoke, the model implies that secondhand smoke concentrations depend on the number of smokers and their rate of smoking corresponding to $E_i(t)$ and the space, air exchange rate, and surface deposition—the factors that determine the net removal of secondhand smoke. Ott (1999) has more specifically formulated this model for secondhand smoke, as have others (Daisey et al. 1998; Klepeis 1999a).

$$\frac{}{C(t)} = \frac{n_{ave}g_{cig}}{Q} - \frac{\Delta C}{(ACH)t}$$

The average secondhand smoke concentration at some time ($\overline{C}(t)$) depends on two terms. The first term

$$\frac{n_{ave}g_{cig}}{Q}$$

has the source strength as its numerator: n_{ave} is the number of smokers, and g_{cig} is the emission rate from the cigarette as mass multiplied by time. The denominator is the air flow rate, with higher air flows leading to lower concentrations. The second term

$$\frac{\Delta C}{(ACH)t}$$

captures changes in concentrations over the time of observation (ΔC), the air exchange rate (ACH), and the time of observation t. Thus, the average concentration is determined by source strength (the first term) and

loss rate (the second term). If conditions are stable, then $\Delta C = 0$, and the secondhand smoke concentration depends only on source strength ($n_{ave}g_{cig}$) and dilution rate (Q). This model assumes a uniform mixing of the smoke throughout the space.

Klepeis and colleagues (1996) applied this multismoker model to data collected from observations of respirable particle and CO measurements in smoking lounges in two airports. During 10 visits, the authors carefully tracked the number of cigarettes smoked and measured continuous particle and CO concentrations. A test with a cigar (several cigars at a time) generated substantial concentrations of CO and RPM that were then tracked as they decayed exponentially. Because CO does not react with surfaces, its decay rate was used to determine the mechanical air exchange rate. Calculating the difference between the CO and RPM decay rates provided estimates of the effective decay rate, which takes into account physical and chemical reactions that affect particle concentrations in addition to removal (dilution) by the mechanical ventilation system. The report documented that the removal of RPM by surface deposition and chemical reaction in both lounges was about 19 to 20 percent of the ventilatory removal. Air exchange rates for these airport smoking lounges were high, approximately 11 and 13 ACH. Mechanically induced turbulence will increase particle removal by surface deposition, but if the number of air changes is similar to that found in office buildings (1 to 3 ACH) and homes (0.3 to 3 ACH), the removal of RPM by deposition, evaporation, and agglomeration would be a more substantial fraction of the overall effective ventilation rate.

Surface adsorption also removes gaseous constituents of secondhand smoke. Because different physical and chemical processes are involved, different decay rates are expected for different components. Sorption, or the uptake and release of gaseous components of secondhand smoke, is a complex phenomenon involving physical and chemical processes on surfaces. Coverage of this topic is beyond the scope of this chapter. The model developed by Ott and colleagues (1992) and validated by Klepeis and colleagues (1996) provided realistic estimates of time-varying concentrations of respirable suspended particles associated with secondhand smoke (Figure 3.4) (Klepeis 1999a). The estimated RPM from cigarettes (11.4 mg per cigarette) was similar to the value derived independently by Özkaynak and colleagues (1996), who used a mass balance regression

Figure 3.4   Estimates of time-varying respirable suspended particle (RSP) concentrations associated with secondhand smoke

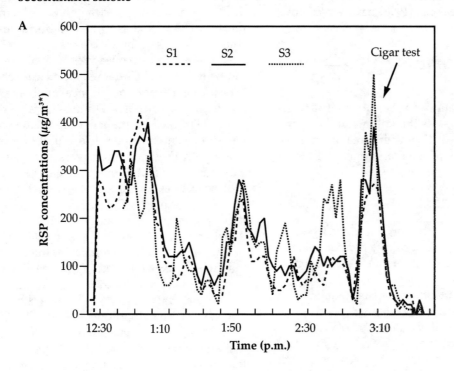

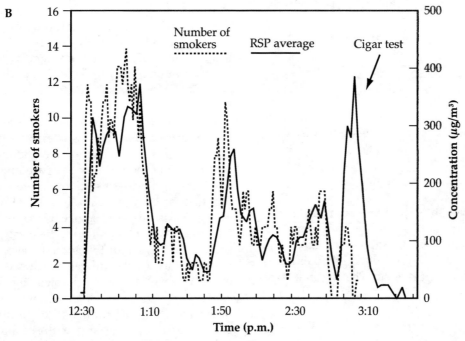

Note: Figure A shows RSP concentration time series measured by piezobalances (labeled S1, S2, and S3) at three widely spaced locations in the smoking lounge taken at the San Jose International Airport (SJC5) fifth study visit. The large decay curve at the end of the trace is for the cigar test conducted to determine the air exchange rate after all persons had departed. Figure B shows the cigarette count time series and the mean RSP concentration time series from the three piezobalances taken at the SJC5 study visit.

*μg/m³ = Micrograms per cubic meter.

Source: Klepeis et al. 1996. Reprinted with permission.

model and indoor $PM_{2.5}$ data from the Particle Total Exposure Assessment Study. The model predicted CO emissions per cigarette similar to the values presented by Owens and Rosanno (1969).

The model for RPM exposures from secondhand smoke that Ott and colleagues (1992) developed is a useful tool for estimating short-term concentrations in settings where the smoking rates and ventilation rates are known. The model could also be used to advance exposure assessment studies and as a design aid for designated smoking areas within buildings. Mass-based models also successfully predict the concentration of nicotine. Repace and colleagues (1998) used a similar model to predict nicotine from secondhand smoke in office air and in salivary cotinine among office workers exposed only in the office; the agreement between the predicted concentrations and the levels observed in field studies was excellent: the mean-predicted concentration was 13.8 $\mu g/m^3$ and the observed mean of 61 samples in nine offices was 15.8 $\mu g/m^3$; the median-predicted salivary cotinine was 0.49 nanograms (ng)/m compared with an observed median of 0.5 ng/milliliter (mL) in 89 nonsmoking office workers who had not been exposed at home.

Both chamber and field studies have validated these models. Experimental chambers differ from many real-world environments such as homes, restaurants, and workplaces in several important aspects. For example, chambers typically have much greater surface to volume ratios, which increase the opportunity for adsorption onto those surfaces, and the air exchange rates are carefully controlled and often kept low to maintain high concentrations. Thus, adsorption onto and desorption from surfaces may have a greater impact in chamber studies than in the field. In fact, the adsorption and desorption of secondhand smoke chemicals onto surfaces have been studied in chambers, and concerns have been raised about the different rates of adsorption and desorption with different markers. However, this phenomenon was less important in field studies than in chamber studies. Thus, the concentrations of secondhand smoke marker chemicals measured in the workplace are well correlated with one another (Table 3.2).

Summary of Atmospheric Markers and Exposure Models

Researchers have suggested several markers for measuring the concentration of secondhand smoke (USDHHS 1986). Of the gas phase markers that researchers have most often used (nicotine, 3-ethenyl pyridine, and myosmine), concentrations were highly correlated in various real-world environments and were correlated with particle phase markers when these markers were detectable (Jenkins et al. 1996). Nicotine, FPM, and UVPM were the most sensitive of these gas and particle phase markers, detecting low levels of secondhand smoke when levels of other markers were below the limit of detection (LaKind et al. 1999b).

Conclusions

1. Atmospheric concentration of nicotine is a sensitive and specific indicator for secondhand smoke.

2. Smoking increases indoor particle concentrations.

3. Models can be used to estimate concentrations of secondhand smoke.

Implications

A set of approaches is available for documenting the exposures of people to secondhand smoke in indoor environments. The atmospheric concentration of nicotine can be readily measured, offering a valid quantitative indicator of the presence of secondhand smoke in the indoor air. Smoking increases levels of other contaminants, including particles. Measurements of nicotine can be used for both research and surveillance purposes. Models have also been developed to estimate concentrations of secondhand smoke in indoor spaces. These models can be used to assess the consequences of various scenarios of controlling for secondhand smoke.

Biomarkers of Exposure to Secondhand Smoke

A biomarker of exposure has been defined by the NRC (1989) as "...an exogenous substance or its metabolite or the product of an interaction between a xenobiotic agent (an external, biologically active agent) and some target molecule or cell that is measured in a compartment within an organism" (p. 12). Thus, measuring specific biomarkers in people can provide evidence that exposure of the individual to secondhand smoke has actually occurred. For some agents, measurements of biomarkers that have interacted with a target site in the body may indicate the biologically effective dose (Sampson et al. 1994; Perera 2000). However, biomarkers do not provide direct information on exposure microenvironments and are therefore complementary to environmental and personal monitoring (NRC 1991). In 1992, the EPA listed several criteria that a biomarker of exposure for a specific air contaminant should meet (USEPA 1992). Based on those criteria, the ideal biomarker of exposure to secondhand smoke should (1) be specific for involuntary smoking, (2) have an appropriate half-life in the body, (3) be measurable with high sensitivity and precision, (4) be measurable in samples collected by noninvasive techniques, (5) be inexpensive to assay, (6) be either an agent associated with health effects or strongly and consistently associated with such an agent, and (7) be related quantitatively to a prior exposure to secondhand smoke. Several biomarkers have been used to assess involuntary smoking, but each has had limitations when matched against these criteria. Nevertheless, these biomarkers have provided information for tracking population exposures to secondhand smoke. There are several published reviews of biomarkers of secondhand smoke exposure (Benowitz 1996, 1999; Jaakkola and Jaakkola 1997; Scherer and Richter 1997; National Cancer Institute 1999; Woodward and Al-Delaimy 1999).

Compounds that have been used as biomarkers for involuntary smoking include CO in exhaled air, carboxyhemoglobin (the complex form of CO found in the blood), thiocyanate, nicotine and its primary metabolite cotinine, polycyclic aromatic hydrocarbon (PAH) adducts in leukocyte DNA or plasma albumin, and hemoglobin (Hb) adducts of tobacco-related aromatic amines such as 3-aminobiphenyl (3AB) and 4AB. A relationship between urinary concentrations of hydroxyproline, an indicator of collagen degradation (a marker of effect), and exposure to secondhand smoke has been proposed (Yanagisawa et al. 1986) but has not been confirmed by other investigators (Adlkofer et al. 1984; Verplanke et al. 1987; Scherer and Richter 1997), and hydroxyproline analyses have not been used in more recent studies. The tobacco-specific nitrosamine 4-(methylnitrosamino)-1-(3-pyridyl)-1-butanol (NNAL) may prove to be quite useful as an exposure marker in the future (Hecht et al. 1993b), although relatively few studies have been conducted of NNAL levels in nonsmokers (Hecht et al. 1993b, 2001; Parsons et al. 1998; Meger et al. 2000; Anderson et al. 2001). Levels of other compounds present in tobacco smoke such as benzene, 2,5-dimethylfuran, and benzo[*a*]pyrene (B[*a*]P) may be significantly higher among smokers compared with nonsmokers, but such compounds are of limited value as biomarkers of involuntary smoking because they are not specific to tobacco smoke. Thus, although some of these compounds may be of value in classifying active smokers and nonsmokers, only those compounds with the highest specificity and sensitivity are potentially useful for assessing variations in exposure to secondhand smoke. Feasibility and cost are additional considerations. The biomarkers most commonly proposed for this purpose have been CO, thiocyanate, and nicotine or its metabolites.

Carbon Monoxide and Thiocyanate

The compound CO is present in both mainstream and sidestream smoke and can be measured in people as either expired breath CO or as carboxyhemoglobin. Such measurements may be useful in confirming the absence of active smoking, but they are of limited value as markers of exposure to secondhand smoke because of a relatively short half-life and because of the nonspecificity of CO as a marker for exposure to tobacco smoke. In addition to tobacco combustion, CO has both indoor and outdoor sources, including vehicle exhaust and incomplete combustion in furnaces, space heaters, and other similar devices. The human body's own metabolic processes also produce CO, and nonsmokers have a typical carboxyhemoglobin concentration of about 1 percent. The half-life of CO in the body is about two to four hours (Castleden and Cole 1974). Therefore, although this time period varies with individual activity levels,

CO is only useful as an indicator of recent exposures. Both expired breath CO and blood level carboxyhemoglobin measurements have been used in studies of exposure to secondhand smoke. In general, however, a definite increase in these markers has only been noted immediately following substantial exposures (Table 3.3). Thus, levels of CO in exhaled breath or in carboxyhemoglobin in blood are of limited value as routine markers of involuntary smoking.

Cigarette smoke also contains significant amounts of hydrogen cyanide, which is detoxified in the body by conversion to thiocyanate. As a marker, thiocyanate is easily measured in serum, urine, or saliva by manual or automated colorimetric methods. Thiocyanate has an estimated half-life of about one week—a period of time that is a fairly long interval for the integration of an exposure (Junge 1985). However, thiocyanate lacks specificity as a marker of involuntary smoking primarily because of dietary contributions from cyanide-containing foods, such as almonds, or from the presence of thiocyanate itself in certain cruciferous vegetables such as cabbage, broccoli, and cauliflower. This lack of specificity restricts the usefulness of thiocyanate in assessing exposure to tobacco smoke. Although some studies have reported significantly increased levels of thiocyanate among nonsmokers exposed to secondhand smoke (Table 3.3), two rather large studies with more than 1,000 persons apiece found no significant difference in serum thiocyanate levels between nonsmokers with and those without reported exposure to secondhand smoke (Table 3.3) (Foss and Lund-Larsen 1986; Woodward et al. 1991). Both expired breath CO and serum thiocyanate levels may be useful as confirmatory markers in smoking cessation studies because no interference from nicotine replacement therapy occurs, but the lack of specificity of these markers limits their application in studies of involuntary smoking.

Nicotine and Cotinine

Nicotine is a highly tobacco-specific component of cigarette smoke that is present in abundant amounts (approximately 7 to 8 mg per cigarette) (IARC 2004). Nicotine can be readily measured in both active and involuntary smokers in a number of biologic materials including serum, urine, and saliva. Most of the nicotine emitted from a cigarette is found in sidestream smoke (NRC 1986), which is the major contributor to secondhand smoke. Nonsmokers inhale nicotine, which is present as a gas, during involuntary smoking. Some of the absorbed nicotine is excreted in urine, but on average, about 90 percent of the nicotine is further metabolized (Benowitz and Jacob 1994). Of this nicotine, about 70 to 80 percent is metabolized to cotinine (range: 60 to 90 percent). Cotinine is the major proximate metabolite of nicotine and the predominant nicotine metabolite present in the blood; cotinine is further metabolized to other chemicals, such as hydroxycotinine and cotinine glucuronide. Nicotine can be measured in physiologic fluids as an exposure biomarker, but its short half-life in the body of approximately one to three hours limits its utility as a marker of chronic exposure (Scherer et al. 1988; Benowitz et al. 1991). Consequently, cotinine, the primary metabolite of nicotine with a substantially longer half-life, is regarded as the biomarker of choice for exposure to secondhand smoke (Jarvis et al. 1987; Watts et al. 1990; Benowitz 1999). Participants in a workshop convened to discuss analytical approaches suitable for assessing involuntary smoking among people concluded with a general consensus "...that the nicotine metabolite, cotinine, has the prerequisites of specificity, retention time in the body, and detectable concentration levels that make it the analyte of choice for quantifying exposures" (Watts et al. 1990, p. 173).

The estimated half-life of cotinine in serum, urine, or saliva averages about 16 to 18 hours (Table 3.4) (Jarvis et al. 1988). Some investigators have reported that the cotinine half-life in nonsmokers may be significantly longer than in smokers, whereas other studies have found a similar half-life in both groups (Table 3.4). Kyerematen and colleagues (1982) used a relatively low dose of nicotine (less than 0.2 mg based on an assumed mean body weight of 70 kilograms) and found a statistical, but small, difference in the half-life of labeled cotinine between smokers and nonsmokers. However, Sepkovic and colleagues (1986) and Haley and colleagues (1989) reported a much longer half-life of cotinine in nonsmokers than in smokers. Both studies used a radioimmunoassay (RIA) for their analyses, and the cross-reactivity or limited sensitivity of their assays during the terminal elimination phase when cotinine concentrations would be low may have contributed to their results. Benowitz (1996) pointed out that more recent data indicate similar cotinine clearance rates for both smokers and nonsmokers. Benowitz (1996) suggested that any increase in the apparent half-life for nonsmokers at low nicotine concentrations may represent residual tissue storage of nicotine with continued release over time. This notion would be consistent with the finding that the mean half-life for the elimination of cotinine derived from labeled nicotine among nonsmokers was slightly

Table 3.3   Expired air carbon monoxide (CO), carboxyhemoglobin, and thiocyanate levels following exposure to secondhand smoke

Study	Analysis	Method	Findings Unexposed	Findings Exposed	Difference
Russell et al. 1973	Carboxy-hemoglobin	CO oximeter	1.6% ± 0.6	2.6% ± 0.7	p <0.001
Jarvis et al. 1983	Expired air CO	Data were not reported	4.7 ppm	10.6 ppm	p <0.001
Poulton et al. 1984	Serum thiocyanate	Colorimetric	54.2 ± 11.3 μmol/L[†] n = 10	97.3 ± 45.3 μmol/L n = 14	p <0.002
Foss and Lund-Larsen 1986	Serum thiocyanate	Colorimetric	Men 29.7 ± 14.2 μmol/L n = 248 Women 30.2 ± 13.6 μmol/L n = 366	30.9 ± 13.5 μmol/L n = 328 31.9 ± 15.8 μmol/L n = 229	NS[‡] NS
Husgafvel-Pursiainen et al. 1987	Carboxy-hemoglobin	CO oximeter	0.6% ± 0.2 n = 20	0.7% ± 0.3 n = 27	NS
	Plasma thiocyanate	Colorimetric	46 ± 16 μmol/L n = 20	58 ± 18 μmol/L n = 27	p <0.01
Robertson et al. 1987	Serum thiocyanate	Colorimetric	44.8 ± 21.2 μmol/L n = 57	Group A 44.1 ± 18.5 μmol/L n = 69 Group B 49.6 ± 27.3 μmol/L n = 21	NS NS
Chen et al. 1990	Serum thiocyanate	Colorimetric	26.9 (9.3–40.9) μmol/L n = 20	35.8 (14.8–78.2) μmol/L n = 26	p <0.05
Woodward et al. 1991	Expired air CO	Ecolyser	Men 2 ppm n = 519 Women 2 ppm n = 817	3 ppm n = 259 2 ppm n = 461	NS NS
	Serum thiocyanate	Colorimetric	Men 37 μmol/L n = 455 Women 40 μmol/L n = 702	35 μmol/L n = 244 39 μmol/L n = 401	NS NS
Otsuka et al. 2001	Carboxy-hemoglobin	Spectrophotometry	0.24% ± 0.18	1.57% ± 0.32	p <0.001

*ppm = Parts per million.
[†]μmol/L = Micromoles per liter.
[‡]NS = Not significant.

Comments

12 nonsmoking volunteers assayed before (unexposed) and immediately after remaining in a smoke-filled room for an average of 79 minutes; mean CO in the room was about 38 ppm*

7 nonsmokers assayed before (unexposed) and after 2 hours of exposure to secondhand smoke in a bar; peak ambient CO in the bar was 13 ppm

24 children or adolescents (mean age 7.6 years), with 14 living in homes with ≥1 smoker in the immediate family (exposed)

Nonsmokers in Norway with self-reported exposures to secondhand smoke at home or at work

Office workers with no reported exposure (unexposed) and restaurant employees exposed an average of 40 hours per week

Nonsmoking office workers who reported no exposure to secondhand smoke; exposure to secondhand smoke only at work (Group A); or exposure to secondhand smoke both at home and at work (Group B)

Median and range of serum levels among infants in the Chang-Ning Epidemiological Study who lived in nonsmoking homes (unexposed) or in homes where ≥20 cigarettes/day were smoked

Nonsmokers in the Scottish Heart Health Study self-reported either "none" or "a lot" of exposure to secondhand smoke

15 healthy nonsmokers assayed before (unexposed) and immediately after remaining in a room for 30 minutes with people who were smoking; the mean CO level in the room was approximately 6 ppm

longer (21 ± 4.6 hours) (Benowitz and Jacob 1993) than the mean half-life measured in nonsmokers (17 ± 3.9 hours) in a separate study that used labeled cotinine (Benowitz and Jacob 1994). Zevin and colleagues (1997) compared labeled nicotine with labeled cotinine and reported similar results. However, a small increase in the effective half-life resulting from tissue distribution effects would not be expected to influence estimates of secondhand smoke exposure based on cotinine measurements made under steady-state conditions. Collier and colleagues (1990) reported a significantly longer cotinine half-life in neonates and children, but a more recent evaluation found a similar half-life in both newborns and adults (Dempsey et al. 2000).

Besides possible differences in the effective half-life of cotinine among smokers and nonsmokers, research suggests that differences based on gender, race, and ethnicity may exist. Two studies found higher levels of serum cotinine per cigarette smoked in Black smokers than in White smokers—a finding that may reflect differences in nicotine metabolism or in the way that cigarettes are smoked (Wagenknecht et al. 1990; Caraballo et al. 1998). Total and nonrenal clearance of cotinine were significantly lower among Black smokers, and the metabolism of nicotine, cotinine, and N-glucuronidation activities were slower among Black smokers than among White smokers (Pérez-Stable et al. 1998; Benowitz et al. 1999). The mean half-life of cotinine among Black smokers (18 hours) was 12.5 percent longer than that found among White smokers (16 hours). One report also suggests that in comparisons with either Latinos or Whites, Chinese Americans metabolized nicotine more slowly; the mean increase in the cotinine half-life among Chinese American smokers was about 14 percent (Benowitz et al. 2002). Although Lynch (1984) found no gender differences in the cotinine half-life, Benowitz and colleagues (1999) found a significantly shorter cotinine half-life in women (14.5 hours) than in men (18.5 hours), a difference that the researchers attributed to a smaller volume of cotinine distribution in women. The same group reported higher metabolic clearance rates and a substantially shorter half-life (about nine hours) for cotinine in pregnant women (Dempsey et al. 2002), a finding that may require a slight revision of classification cutoff levels when assessing active smokers and women exposed to secondhand smoke during pregnancy.

Table 3.4   Half-life of cotinine in smokers and nonsmokers from several studies

Study	Exposure	Assay	Cotinine half-life in hours (mean ± SD*)	Comments
Kyerematen et al. 1982	Intravenous dose of ^{14}C-labeled nicotine at 2.7 µg/kg[†]	LC[‡] separation; then measured radiolabeled metabolite	10.3 ± 2.3 n = 6	6 male smokers; overnight abstention before dosing and throughout the study; plasma assays
		Same	13.3 ± 2.2 n = 6	6 male nonsmokers
Benowitz et al. 1983	Intravenous cotinine infusion	GLC/NPD[§]	15.8 ± 4 n = 8	5 male and 3 female smokers; plasma assays
	Cotinine washout during 3 days of smoking abstention	GLC/NPD	19.7 ± 6.5 n = 12	8 male and 4 female smokers
Lynch 1984	Cotinine washout during 24 hours of smoking abstention	GLC/NPD	14.6 (men) 15.1 (women)	Averages from 47 male and 41 female smokers; cotinine half-life was calculated from 2-point data only; plasma assays
	Cotinine washout during 3 days of smoking abstention	GLC/NPD	15.4 (men) 15.7 (women)	8 male and 11 female smokers in a smoking cessation program; assayed once/day for 3 days
Sepkovic et al. 1986	Smokers abstained for 7 days	RIA[∆]	18.5 (plasma) 21.9 (urine)	10 smokers were followed during 7 days of smoking abstention
	Nonsmokers exposed to secondhand smoke in a chamber	RIA	49.7 (plasma) 32.7 (urine)	4 nonsmokers were exposed to secondhand smoke for 80 minutes/day for 4 days, then followed for an additional 7 days
De Schepper et al. 1987	Oral dose of cotinine at 10 and 20 mg[¶] concentrations	GC–MS**	12.3 ± 2.6 n = 4	4 male nonsmokers; cotinine half-life was independent of dose, so both doses were averaged per person; the same results were obtained with infused cotinine; plasma assays
Jarvis et al. 1988	Oral dose of nicotine at 28 mg/day for 5 days before analysis	GLC/NPD 2 labs performed each assay	16.6 ± 3.4 n = 5	3 male and 2 female nonsmokers; plasma cotinine assays
			15.9 ± 3.1 n = 5	Salivary cotinine assays
			18.0 ± 4.0 n = 9	Urine cotinine assays

Table 3.4   Continued

Study	Exposure	Assay	Cotinine half-life in hours (mean ± SD*)	Comments
Scherer et al. 1988	Cotinine intravenous infusion	GLC/NPD	17.1 ± 4.4 n = 6	6 smokers; 5 days of smoking abstention before infusion; serum assays
Haley et al. 1989	Cotinine washout during 5 days of smoking abstention	RIA	16.6 ± 3.4 n = 9	9 smokers were followed for 5 days beginning with smoking cessation; urine assays
	Nonsmokers exposed to secondhand smoke in a chamber	RIA	27.3 ± 5.9 n = 10	10 nonsmokers were exposed to secondhand smoke for 8 minutes/day for 2 days, then followed for 4 additional days; urine assays
Curvall et al. 1990b	Oral dose of cotinine at indicated amount Followed for 4 days	GLC/NPD	14.9 ± 4.1 n = 3	7 male and 2 female nonsmokers; plasma cotinine assays following 5 mg dose
			15.6 ± 3.7 n = 9	Plasma cotinine assays following 10 mg dose
			14.9 ± 4.3 n = 9	Plasma cotinine assays following 20 mg dose
			16.3 ± 1.9 n = 3	Salivary cotinine assays following 5 mg dose
			15.7 ± 2.9 n = 9	Salivary cotinine assays following 10 mg dose
			14.9 ± 3.7 n = 9	Salivary cotinine assays following 20 mg dose
Benowitz and Jacob 1994	Native and isotopically labeled intravenous cotinine infusion	GC–MS	16.3 ± 4.4 n = 6	3 male and 3 female nonsmokers dosed with an average of 4.4 mg cotinine over 30 minutes (2 μg/minute/kg body weight); plasma half-life was measured for native cotinine
			16.9 ± 4.3 n = 6	Plasma half-life was measured for dideuterated cotinine
			17.2 ± 3.9 n = 6	Plasma half-life was measured for tetradeuterated cotinine

*SD = Standard deviation.
†μg/kg = Micrograms per kilogram.
‡LC = Liquid chromatography.
§GLC/NPD = Gas-liquid chromatography with nitrogen-phosphorus–specific detectors.
ΔRIA = Radioimmunoassay.
¶mg = Milligram.
**GC–MS = Gas chromatography with mass spectrometry.

Cotinine Analytical Procedures

Cotinine can be measured by a variety of techniques, but for application to studies of involuntary exposure, methods of high specificity and sensitivity are needed. The most commonly used methods have included RIAs and enzyme-linked immunoassays, gas-liquid chromatography (GLC) with nitrogen-phosphorus–specific detectors (NPD) or coupled to a mass spectrometer, and high-performance liquid chromatography (HPLC) using either ultraviolet (UV) or mass spectrometric detection. With the development of suitable antibodies (Langone et al. 1973; Knight et al. 1985), RIAs were made available for relatively sensitive and rapid analyses of nicotine and cotinine in biologic matrices. Enzyme-linked immunosorbent assays that use monoclonal antibodies have also been developed (Bjercke et al. 1986) that obviate radioactive reagents and provide a consistent antibody source. Immunoassays are well suited for screening large numbers of samples in epidemiologic investigations, but may be subject to cross-reactivity from other compounds that can limit the specificity. Even the more sensitive immunoassays for serum cotinine provide reliable results only for more heavily exposed nonsmokers who have serum cotinine concentrations of approximately 0.3 to 1 ng/mL or greater (Coultas et al. 1988; Emmons et al. 1996).

Chromatographic procedures for nicotine and cotinine measurements have commonly involved either HPLC with UV detection (Machacek and Jiang 1986; Hariharan et al. 1988; Oddoze et al. 1998), or capillary GLC/NPD (Jacob et al. 1981; Davis 1986; Teeuwen et al. 1989; Feyerabend and Russell 1990). The sensitive GLC/NPD methods of Feyerabend and Russell (1990) and of Jacob and colleagues (1981), with reported detection limits of about 0.1 ng/mL, have been used in support of several studies of exposure to secondhand smoke. There has been a more recent increase in the use of mass spectrometry for these analyses (Daenens et al. 1985; Norbury 1987; Jacob et al. 1991; McAdams and Cordeiro 1993; James et al. 1998). Gas chromatography (GC) with mass spectrometric detection provides a sensitive analytical method with inherently high specificity and enables the optimal use of stable isotopically labeled forms of the analyte as internal standards. This type of analysis is particularly well suited for sensitive cotinine measurements in complex biologic matrices. The recent availability of instrumentation combining HPLC with atmospheric pressure ionization tandem mass spectrometry has enabled the development of methods that provide high sensitivity and analytical specificity. These methods are also well suited for application to epidemiologic studies that analyze large numbers of samples (Bernert et al. 1997; Bentley et al. 1999; Tuomi et al. 1999). Benowitz (1996) has compared the relative sensitivity, specificity, and costs of these analytic procedures (Table 3.5).

Table 3.5   Analytical methods for measuring cotinine in nonsmokers

Study	Method	Sensitivity	Specificity	Cost
Langone et al. 1973; Haley et al. 1983; Knight et al. 1985	Radioimmunoassay	1–2 nanograms/ milliliter (ng/mL)	Variable (poorest in urine)	Low
Jacob et al. 1981; Feyerabend et al. 1986	Gas chromatography	0.1–0.2 ng/mL	Good	Moderate
Hariharan and VanNoord 1991	High-performance liquid chromatography	±1 ng/mL	Good	Moderate
Jacob et al. 1991	Gas chromatography–mass spectrometry	0.1–0.2 ng/mL	Excellent	High
Bernert et al. 1997	Liquid chromatography/atmospheric pressure ionization tandem mass spectrometry	<0.05 ng/mL	Excellent	Extremely high

Source: Benowitz 1996.

Analytical Matrices for Cotinine Measurements

Nicotine and cotinine have been measured in a wide variety of physiologic matrices, including amniotic fluid (Lähdetie et al. 1993; Jauniaux et al. 1999), meconium (Ostrea et al. 1994; Dempsey et al. 1999; Nuesslein et al. 1999), cervical lavage (Jones et al. 1991), seminal plasma (Shen et al. 1997), breast milk (Luck and Nau 1984; Becker et al. 1999), sweat (Balabanova et al. 1992), and pericardial fluid (Milerad et al. 1994). However, most investigations of exposure to secondhand smoke have involved assays of cotinine in blood, urine, or saliva, or of nicotine or cotinine in hair. Nicotine is metabolized to cotinine mainly in the liver, but also in the lungs and kidneys; cotinine then enters the bloodstream. When an individual is subjected to involuntary smoking on a regular basis, a steady-state condition may be achieved in which blood cotinine levels remain fairly constant during the day (Benowitz 1996). Because of this stability in concentration levels, in conjunction with the reliable and well-defined composition of blood samples, blood serum or plasma has been considered the matrix of choice for quantitative cotinine assays (Watts et al. 1990; Benowitz 1996). Thus, in the past few years, plasma or serum cotinine measurements have been used in several large epidemiologic investigations of secondhand smoke exposure (Tunstall-Pedoe et al. 1991; Wagenknecht et al. 1993; Pirkle et al. 1996).

Despite a preference for blood plasma or serum as the matrix for cotinine assays, obtaining a blood sample is invasive, and collecting samples from younger children may be difficult. Consequently, saliva cotinine has been suggested as a useful alternative in many cases (Jarvis et al. 1987; Curvall et al. 1990a; Etzel 1990). Saliva is secreted into the oral cavity primarily by the parotid, sublingual, and submandibular glands. These glands typically produce between 18 and 30 mL of unstimulated saliva per hour (Sreebny and Broich 1987); the flow of stimulated saliva is three to six times greater. Oral fluids are a mixture derived from the individual salivary glandular secretions and oral mucosal transudates (gingival crevicular fluid), which are filtrates of plasma. Specific secretions may be recovered, but mixed or "whole" saliva is most commonly collected for cotinine analysis either by direct collection in an appropriate vessel or by adsorption onto commercially available collection pads (Sreebny and Broich 1987).

Many lipophilic drugs may pass from blood into saliva by simple diffusion through the lipid membranes of acinar cells. Because cotinine is a small, relatively lipophilic molecule with little protein binding (Benowitz et al. 1983), its concentration in saliva tends to closely parallel its concentration in blood. Several investigators have found a linear relationship between blood and saliva cotinine concentrations, with saliva levels typically about 1.1 to 1.5 times higher than the corresponding serum concentrations (Jarvis et al. 1988; Curvall et al. 1990a; Rose et al. 1993; Bernert et al. 2000). Schneider and colleagues (1997) compared cotinine levels in saliva samples that were obtained by using either sugar or paraffin wax to stimulate flow—unstimulated saliva samples were collected from the same persons. The researchers concluded that the significantly lower levels found in stimulated samples resulted from higher salivary flow rates. Other investigators, however, concluded that salivary flow rates did not influence cotinine concentrations in their samples (Van Vunakis et al. 1989; Curvall et al. 1990a), and the use of stimulated saliva with a somewhat higher and more uniform pH may reduce both the interindividual and intraindividual variability in the saliva-plasma ratio of a weak base such as cotinine (Knott 1989). Saliva cotinine assays have proven to be a quite useful noninvasive approach for assessing exposures to secondhand smoke, although a greater consistency in salivary collection methods among studies may facilitate subsequent comparisons of the results (Schneider et al. 1997).

Urine can also be readily obtained. Urine cotinine assays have several additional advantages over blood or saliva assays, such as the availability of the large volumes that can usually be collected, and typical cotinine concentration levels that average about five to six times higher than serum levels for unconjugated cotinine (Jarvis et al. 1984; Benowitz 1996). Besides nicotine and cotinine, urine samples may also contain significant amounts of the cotinine metabolite *trans*-3'-hydroxycotinine (Dagne and Castagnoli 1972; Neurath and Pein 1987) as well as several additional minor metabolites including nicotine-1'-*N*-oxide, cotinine-*N*-oxide, nornicotine, and norcotinine (Beckett et al. 1971; Jacob et al. 1986; Zhang et al. 1990; Benowitz et al. 1994). Two additional metabolites that were described more recently are 4-oxo-4-(3-pyridyl)butanoic acid and 4-hydroxy-4-(3-pyridyl)butanoic acid, which possibly arise from 2'-hydroxylation of nicotine and represent up to 14 percent of the nicotine dose (Hecht et al. 1999b, 2000). Nicotine, cotinine, and hydroxycotinine predominate in urine and are present in both an unconjugated form and as their glucuronides (Byrd et al. 1992), with nicotine and cotinine forming *N*-glucuronides and hydroxycotinine forming an *O*-glucuronide (Byrd et al. 1994; Benowitz et al. 1999).

Hydroxycotinine is often the most abundant nicotine metabolite present in urine, with a half-life of approximately six hours in adults when given alone, which is much shorter than that of cotinine (Scherer et al. 1988; Benowitz and Jacob 2001). In the presence of cotinine, however, the elimination half-life of 3'-hydroxycotinine is similar to that of continine (Dempsey et al. 2004). Consequently, cotinine is the most commonly used biomarker in urine samples. However, this half-life differential may not be present in newborns in whom the half-life is about the same for cotinine and 3'-hydroxycotinine (Dempsey et al. 2000). As with saliva, urine cotinine concentrations are also highly correlated (r ± 0.8) with blood concentrations (Jarvis et al. 1984; Thompson et al. 1990; Benowitz 1996). Measuring a range of nicotine metabolites rather than cotinine alone may also be useful in some circumstances, and for such analyses, urine would often be the matrix of choice.

Higher cotinine concentrations present in urine can enhance sensitivity in an analysis of secondhand smoke exposure. However, urine assays have the disadvantage of being subject to variability that results from hydration differences among participants at the time of collection, because 24-hour urine samples are rarely available and random samples are most often used. Many investigators have attempted to circumvent this limitation by measuring both cotinine and creatinine in the sample and expressing the results as simple cotinine-creatinine ratios (NRC 1986), or by normalizing to a standardized creatinine concentration based on a regression between cotinine and creatinine in urine (Thompson et al. 1990). However, although daily urinary creatinine excretion is rather uniform within individuals, creatinine production is also directly related to muscle mass and varies by age and gender. Despite these potential limitations, creatinine adjustments of cotinine measurements are often used to provide an index of exposure to secondhand smoke from spot urine samples (NRC 1986).

Nicotine and Cotinine in Hair

One of the primary limitations of blood, urine, or saliva cotinine as a biomarker of exposure is the short exposure period that is represented. Assuming that substances such as nicotine are incorporated into the growing hair shaft over time, the use of hair as an analytical matrix has been suggested as an enhanced index of exposure to secondhand smoke covering a period of several months rather than just a few days. Ishiyama and colleagues (1983) first proposed using

hair as a matrix for nicotine analyses, and several investigators have subsequently evaluated both nicotine and cotinine in hair. Unlike other matrices, the concentration of nicotine in hair is greater than that of cotinine (Haley and Hoffmann 1985; Kintz 1992; Koren et al. 1992). Because both concentrations are assumed to be stable once they have been deposited into the hair shaft, many hair analyses have included nicotine measurements or assays of both nicotine and cotinine. Studies of adult nonsmokers have reported a significant increase in hair nicotine concentrations with an increase in self-reported exposures to secondhand smoke (Eliopoulos et al. 1994; Dimich-Ward et al. 1997; Al-Delaimy et al. 2001; Jaakkola et al. 2001). Studies of infants and children have documented similar findings (Nafstad et al. 1995; Pichini et al. 1997; Al-Delaimy et al. 2000). Nafstad and colleagues (1998), however, found no significant differences in hair nicotine levels in a study of 68 nonsmoking women with no known exposure to secondhand smoke and 54 nonsmoking women with reported exposures. Some studies also found that hair nicotine levels for those most heavily exposed to secondhand smoke tended to overlap substantially with levels found in active smokers (Dimich-Ward et al. 1997; Al-Delaimy et al. 2001).

At this point, significant uncertainties remain concerning the use of hair analyses for either nicotine or cotinine to assess exposure to secondhand smoke, including the influence of variations in hair growth rates and in hair treatments such as bleaching or permanents. The mechanism of deposition and the influence of pigmentation are questions that also need to be addressed. The rate of hair growth, which varies among individuals, normally averages about one centimeter per month (Wennig 2000). Selecting nonrepresentative telogen stage (resting phase) hairs is a risk when only a few strands are selected for analysis (Uematsu 1993). Researchers believe that the systemic incorporation of nicotine or cotinine involves the passive diffusion of the substance from the blood into the hair follicle, and then into the growing hair shaft. Findings from studies that administered nicotine to animals are consistent with the systemic incorporation of both nicotine and cotinine into hair in this manner (Gerstenberg et al. 1995; Stout and Ruth 1999). In addition, Gwent and colleagues (1995) administered a single dose of nicotine (Nicorette Plus chewing gum) to six nonsmoking volunteers and demonstrated the incorporation of cotinine (but not nicotine) into beard hair. Cotinine levels peaked on the third day following the exposure. However, drugs may also be deposited in the hair from contact with apocrine and sebaceous gland secretions, as well as directly into the hair shaft from the environment (Henderson 1993). Nicotine is present in apocrine and eccrine sweat (Balabanova et al. 1992), and studies have clearly demonstrated the adsorption of nicotine into hair from the environment (Nilsen et al. 1994; Zahlsen et al. 1996). Thus, multiple sources may contribute to the presence and levels of nicotine found in hair. Although each of these routes still reflects exposure of the nonsmoker to second-hand smoke, the proper interpretation of the results requires a better understanding of the relative contributions of these various factors. Direct environmental adsorption represents a form of personal air monitoring rather than a biomarker assessment. Because the adsorption of cotinine directly from the environment is expected to be quite low (Eatough et al. 1989b), the analysis of cotinine in hair would seem to provide an advantage in minimizing contributions directly from the environment. However, studies have found cotinine hair measurements to be generally less useful than nicotine hair measurements in assessing differences in exposure to secondhand smoke (Kintz 1992; Dimich-Ward et al. 1997; Al-Delaimy et al. 2000).

An additional concern with hair analyses is the influence of hair pigmentation on nicotine incorporation. Studies have documented a significantly greater systemic accumulation of nicotine in pigmented versus unpigmented hair in rodents (Gerstenberg et al. 1995; Stout and Ruth 1999), and in black hairs compared with white hairs from the same persons (Mizuno et al. 1993; Uematsu et al. 1995). This difference presumably reflects the strong binding of nicotine to melanin (Stout and Ruth 1999; Dehn et al. 2001), which is a relevant issue because differences in deposition as a function of either pigmentation or hair structure could lead to a differential sensitivity of detection or exposure classification among participants, including persons of differing ethnicity. This concern may be specific to nicotine deposition, however, because a similar differential response was not seen in a study of hair cotinine levels among children with either light or dark hair (Knight et al. 1996). Although the analysis of nicotine or cotinine in hair is potentially useful in assessing a longer-term exposure to secondhand smoke, this approach needs additional work.

Dietary Sources of Nicotine

Researchers consider the presence of nicotine or its metabolites in the body to be a specific indicator of prior exposures to tobacco smoke. This consideration thus provides an important rationale for the use of nicotine or its metabolites as biomarkers for secondhand smoke exposure. However, researchers have suggested that nicotine could be detected in some samples of tea and in certain vegetables, including potatoes and tomatoes, that belong to the same family (*Solanaceae*) as tobacco (Castro and Monji 1986; Sheen 1988). Idle (1990) subsequently referenced Sheen's (1988) results and suggested that cotinine measurements might be influenced by the ingestion of significant amounts of nicotine from these or other foodstuffs. Idle (1990) hypothesized that the uptake of dietary nicotine would be similar to the nicotine that is absorbed from the vapor phase in the lungs. However, Svensson (1987) proposed that at the acid pH of the stomach, nicotine would be protonated and not readily absorbed. Using direct measurements, Ivey and Triggs (1978) found essentially no absorption of nicotine from the human stomach at pH 1 and an approximate 8 percent absorption at pH 7.4. Even under moderately alkaline conditions (pH 9.8), the mean absorption was less than 20 percent. However, extensive intestinal absorption of nicotine does occur. Benowitz and colleagues (1991) found that the oral bioavailability of encapsulated nicotine administered to 10 smokers averaged about 44 percent. Bioavailability is low because of first-pass metabolism, which is when nicotine is converted to cotinine and other metabolites.

On the basis of their measurements and projections of dietary intake, Davis and colleagues (1991) proposed that from 9 µg to nearly 100 µg of nicotine per day might be ingested from food. However, this projection was based on maximum intakes of each of the foods of interest including large quantities of tea; actual intakes at that level would be unlikely (Benowitz 1999). In contrast, Repace (1994) used the food-nicotine concentrations reported by Domino and colleagues (1993) as well as a more realistic average consumption quantity of potatoes and tomatoes in the diet. The estimated daily nicotine intake from these foods was approximately 0.7 µg/day. Furthermore, more recent analyses of nicotine content in foodstuffs by specific mass spectrometric procedures found values that were somewhat lower than the earlier estimates. Siegmund and colleagues (1999a) developed a validated method for the extraction and recovery of nicotine from foods using capillary GC–mass spectrometry analysis. This method was subsequently applied to an analysis of a variety of foodstuffs including solanaceous vegetables and tea (Siegmund et al. 1999b). The estimated daily intake of nicotine from all dietary sources for 14 countries, including the United States, was about 1.4 μg/day, with an estimated 2.25 μg/day at the 95th percentile. These values, which were derived from a Monte Carlo simulation that used mean daily consumption and measured nicotine contents of the foods, are well below the earlier estimates made by Davis and colleagues (1991) but are closer to those reported by Repace (1994).

Calculations of dietary nicotine contributions are necessarily imprecise. Direct evaluations of dietary intake should be more meaningful, and these measurements tended to produce lower results. For example, the dietary intake of nicotine estimated by Davis and colleagues (1991) included an important contribution from tea. Researchers assessed the contribution from tea in more than 1,800 nonsmokers, including many customary tea drinkers, in the Scottish Heart Health Study; no consistent relationship was found between serum cotinine levels and a daily tea intake of up to 10 cups (Tunstall-Pedoe et al. 1991). Those who consumed 10 or more cups per day had a slight increase in serum cotinine, but the effect of tea was noted to be inconsistent. In a large, national epidemiologic survey conducted in the United States, Pirkle and colleagues (1996) used a 24-hour food recall diary, which was completed by each study participant, to compare the dietary intake of potatoes, tomatoes, eggplants, cauliflowers, green peppers, and both instant and brewed tea with serum cotinine levels. Using regression models, these food items explained less than 2 percent of the variance in serum cotinine levels.

Benowitz and Jacob (1994) proposed a conversion factor between nicotine and serum cotinine and suggested that it can be used to estimate nicotine exposure under steady-state conditions. For example, using the most recent estimate from Siegmund and colleagues (1999b) of 1.4 μg of nicotine per day in the average diet, and assuming that 71.3 percent of the dietary nicotine is absorbed in the same manner as vapor phase nicotine from secondhand smoke (Iwase et al. 1991), applying this conversion factor would result in a predicted mean serum cotinine concentration of no more than 0.013 ng/mL; at the 95th percentile of dietary nicotine intake, the estimate would be 0.020 ng/mL. These estimates are consistent with the results of Pirkle and colleagues (1996) and indicate a minimal dietary contribution to serum cotinine measurements. Thus, trace amounts of nicotine may be consumed in the diet, but any contribution from this source is likely to be quite small for most people compared with the amount of nicotine absorbed from secondhand smoke exposure. Additionally, comparisons of cotinine within individuals over time,

such as before and after an intervention, would probably be unaffected by diet.

Cotinine Measurements as an Index of Nicotine Exposure

Although the potential for overlap of levels always exists between nonsmokers with an extensive exposure to secondhand smoke and occasional or currently abstinent smokers, the use of cotinine measurements to separate smokers from nonsmokers provides a generally valid approach. Benowitz and colleagues (1983) originally proposed 10 ng/mL as a reasonable cutoff level for cotinine in serum to distinguish between smokers and nonsmokers. Consistent with that proposal, Repace and Lowrey (1993) estimated median serum cotinine levels to be about 1 ng/mL for U.S. adult nonsmokers and about 10 ng/mL for the most heavily exposed nonsmokers. In a study of 211 people in London, England, a plasma cutoff of 13.7 ng/mL provided an optimal classification with 94 percent sensitivity and 81 percent specificity based on self-reported exposure levels (Jarvis et al. 1987). The authors attributed the relatively poor specificity to "deception" in the self-reports of some participants with high serum cotinine levels. When the investigators reclassified those believed to be deceptive as smokers, sensitivities were 96 to 97 percent and specificities were 99 to 100 percent using plasma, saliva, or urine cotinine as the biomarker for comparison. The optimal cutoff values in this study were 14.2 ng/mL in saliva and 49.7 ng/mL in urine (Jarvis et al. 1987).

Pirkle and colleagues (1996) used a serum cotinine cutoff level of 15 ng/mL in a large U.S. epidemiologic study. They found a strong agreement with the self-reported nonsmoking status of the participants: those with serum cotinine levels above 15 ng/mL who claimed no tobacco use comprised only about 1.3 percent of the adult participants and 2.6 percent of the adolescents. Caraballo and colleagues (2001) examined the participants in this study aged 17 years and older in detail and used the same nominal cutoff of 15 ng/mL. There was a 92.5 percent agreement between serum cotinine concentrations and self-reported active smoking status and a 98.5 percent agreement among self-reported nonsmokers. The researchers regarded the infrequent or low rate of cigarette use as an explanation for the disagreement with serum cotinine levels among self-reported smokers in most cases. However, there may have been some deception in the 1.5 percent with discrepant results between their serum cotinine levels and self-reported status as nonsmokers, particularly among those with relatively high concentrations of serum cotinine. Wagenknecht and colleagues (1992) found similar results in the Coronary Artery Risk Development in (Young) Adults Study, which had a serum cotinine cutoff value of 15 ng/mL that produced a sensitivity of 94.5 percent and a specificity of 96 percent. In general, self-reports of smoking status validated with biomarker assays were accurate in most studies (Patrick et al. 1994), although small adjustments to customary cutoff values between smokers and nonsmokers may be needed based on gender and race for both males and females and for pregnant women. The accuracy of questionnaire reports in determining the extent of exposure may be higher in population contexts than in clinical studies, particularly in investigations of smoking cessation.

The objective in many studies is not only to identify nonsmokers exposed to secondhand smoke, but also to estimate the relative extent of their exposure. If a quantitative relationship exists between exposure to nicotine in secondhand smoke and cotinine biomarker concentrations, then investigators should be able to estimate the average nicotine exposure of groups of individuals from their biomarker levels. Repace and Lowrey (1993) developed a model that related nicotine exposure to cotinine levels measured in both the plasma and urine of nonsmokers. Subsequent comparisons of the model predictions with data from 10 epidemiologic studies were consistent within 10 to 15 percent for median and peak levels of cotinine. Using the fractional conversion of nicotine to cotinine and estimated cotinine clearances in active smokers, Benowitz and Jacob (1994) proposed a factor (K = 0.08 with a coefficient of variation ±22 percent) that could be used to estimate daily nicotine intake (in milligrams of nicotine) from the steady-state plasma cotinine concentration in ng/mL. The validity of this factor is supported by the data from Galeazzi and colleagues (1985). They administered measured doses of nicotine intravenously to six volunteers on four consecutive days and assessed serum cotinine levels on the fourth day, when steady-state conditions had been reached. The results indicate that plasma cotinine concentrations could be directly and linearly related to daily nicotine intake. Predicted nicotine intake calculations, based on the factor proposed by Benowitz and Jacob (1994), demonstrated a close agreement in all cases with the actual exposures (Table 3.6).

Although Benowitz and Jacob (1994) had derived their factor from smokers, the clearance of cotinine was similar for smokers and nonsmokers (Zevin et al.

Table 3.6   Calculation of nicotine dosage from plasma cotinine concentrations

Nicotine administered* (milligrams [mg]/day)	Mean plasma cotinine[†] (nanograms/ milliliter)	Calculated dose[†] (mg/day)
7.3	92	7.4
14.6	185	14.8
22.0	278	22.2
29.3	381	30.5

*From the dosage and plasma cotinine concentrations given in Galeazzi et al. 1985 (Table 1). Doses were adjusted to mg/day based on the reported mean weight of the participants (61 kilograms, n = 6).
[†]Calculated from plasma cotinine multiplied by 0.08.
Sources: Galeazzi et al. 1985; Benowitz and Jacob 1994.

1997), and Benowitz (1996) noted that the factor for nicotine exposure among nonsmokers should also be similar. The results obtained by Curvall and colleagues (1990b) with short-term exposures and nonsteady-state correlations are in general agreement with that expectation. After administering various low doses of nicotine intravenously to nonsmokers, the researchers concluded that the average intake of nicotine among their participants could be estimated from the following relationship:

$$\text{Cotinine concentration (ng/mL)} \sim 0.5 * [\text{nicotine infusion rate in } \mu g/min] * [\text{absorption time in hours}]$$

where 0.5 represents the somewhat lower fraction of nicotine metabolized to cotinine among nonsmokers as Curvall and colleagues (1990b) had reported. A comparison of this expression with that of Benowitz and Jacob (1994) suggests that both should generate similar results, with the main difference between them reflecting the lower fractional conversion of nicotine to cotinine among nonsmokers as Curvall and colleagues (1990b) had estimated. Curvall and colleagues (1990b) noted that this conversion may represent a true difference, or may have resulted from differences in the experimental setups between the two studies. Zevin and colleagues (1997) reported that the mean conversion of nicotine to cotinine is approximately the same for nonsmokers as for smokers. If that conclusion is correct, then the factor derived by Benowitz and Jacob (1994) should be applicable to both groups.

These estimates are based on studies in which nicotine was infused into people, often at greater concentrations than would result from involuntary smoking. However, the estimates are consistent with a linear relationship between nicotine exposure and mean serum cotinine concentrations when measured under steady-state conditions. These findings suggest that at least an approximate quantitative estimate of nicotine exposures within population groups might be derived from their plasma cotinine concentrations. Because cotinine levels in an individual reflect not only exposure variations but also individual differences in metabolism and excretion, the value of a single measurement within an individual may be limited. However, the application of cotinine measurements in epidemiologic studies that involve large numbers of individuals may provide reliable estimates of average group exposures to nicotine in secondhand smoke (Benowitz 1999).

Protein and DNA Adducts

Measurements of DNA or protein adducts of carcinogens in secondhand smoke may indicate both the exposure (internal dose) and the interaction of the carcinogen or its metabolite with the host tissue, thus reflecting the biologically effective dose. Furthermore, if the adduct is stable, this approach can determine time-integrated exposures over the lifetime of the modified biopolymer. In the case of protein adducts, this exposure interval corresponds to the lifetime of the red cell (approximately 127 days) for Hb adducts and to the 21-day half-life of serum albumin adducts. Based on continuing daily exposures, this integration over time can lead to an approximate 60-fold amplification in Hb adduct levels and to a 30-fold amplification for serum albumin adduct levels (Skipper and Tannenbaum 1990). DNA adducts in human target tissue, such as the lung, are of particular interest because they may be directly relevant to carcinogenesis, but such tissue is available only by surgery or biopsy. Thus, many analyses have used white blood cell DNA adducts as surrogate markers. Many investigators prefer to analyze adducts in lymphocytes because of their significantly longer lifetimes (up to several years) than the lifetime of less than one day that monocytes and granulocytes have (Kriek et al. 1998). However, these assays are limited by the small amount of DNA that is available in peripheral blood, by the low rates of base

modification typically observed, and by the removal of adducts through DNA repair mechanisms. Consequently, studies of adducts in response to the exposure of humans to secondhand smoke have largely focused on the use of protein adducts as surrogate markers because they are more abundant and are not subject to repair mechanisms.

Maclure and colleagues (1989) found that concentrations of both 4AB–Hb and 3AB–Hb adducts were significantly higher in nonsmokers with confirmed exposures to secondhand smoke (based on plasma cotinine concentrations) than in unexposed nonsmokers. The same investigators had previously demonstrated that concentrations of 4AB–Hb were significantly higher in smokers than in nonsmokers, and that the concentrations declined during smoking cessation to levels found in nonsmokers (Bryant et al. 1987; Skipper and Tannenbaum 1990). Hammond and colleagues (1993) found a dose-response relationship for 4AB–Hb concentrations in nonsmokers who were categorized into three levels of exposure to secondhand smoke based on their personal monitoring of nicotine exposure. These authors found that 4AB–Hb concentrations in nonsmokers exposed to secondhand smoke were about 14 percent of those found in smokers, whereas cotinine levels in nonsmokers were about 1 percent of those in smokers. These relative biomarker concentrations are consistent with the higher concentrations of 4AB–Hb and nicotine in sidestream versus mainstream smoke of about 31-fold and 2-fold, respectively (NRC 1986). These results implicate secondhand smoke exposure as a contributing factor to the amount of 4AB adducted to Hb. However, detectable background levels of 4AB–Hb adducts are commonly observed among nonsmokers with no known sources of exposure to secondhand smoke, although they were possibly exposed to other combustion emissions (Bryant et al. 1987; Maclure et al. 1990). As a consequence, the distributions of adduct levels in nonsmokers exposed to secondhand smoke and in those who have no known exposure may not be sharply separated. Additionally, at the time of these studies, secondhand smoke exposure may have been so ubiquitous that few persons were truly unexposed.

In a study of 109 children, 4AB–Hb and PAH–albumin adducts were higher in children whose mothers smoked and in children from households with a smoker other than the mother, compared with children unexposed to secondhand smoke (Crawford et al. 1994; Tang et al. 1999). Cotinine levels also increased with exposure and there were significant differences among the groups for both biomarkers. After adjusting for the exposure group, the researchers found that these markers were higher among African American children than among Hispanic children. Conversely, in a study of 107 nonsmoking women, Autrup and colleagues (1995) found no significant difference in PAH–albumin levels of those exposed and those unexposed to secondhand smoke. Although serum cotinine measurements confirmed the status of the nonsmokers, the researchers did not compare cotinine and PAH–albumin levels of the participating smokers and nonsmokers. Scherer and colleagues (2000) also found no difference in B[*a*]P adducts of either Hb or albumin in a study of 19 nonsmokers exposed to secondhand smoke and 23 unexposed nonsmokers. This study measured nicotine from personal samplers on individual participants and cotinine levels in both plasma and urine. Cotinine levels were significantly higher among those exposed to secondhand smoke; this finding confirmed the differences in exposure. Additional work may be needed to resolve these findings for the PAH adducts.

Tobacco-Specific Nitrosamines

Tobacco-specific nitrosamines (TSNAs) are of considerable interest as biomarkers of exposure to secondhand smoke because they combine both high specificity for tobacco exposure and additional relevancy as presumed carcinogens. The formation, metabolism, and role of these nitrosamines as significant carcinogens in tobacco smoke were discussed in detail in Chapter 2 (Toxicology of Secondhand Smoke). Several recent studies demonstrated that NNAL and its glucuronide can be measured in the urine of nonsmokers exposed to secondhand smoke (Hecht et al. 1993b; Parsons et al. 1998; Meger et al. 2000; Anderson et al. 2001). There were significant correlations with urine cotinine levels (Hecht et al. 1993b; Parsons et al. 1998) and with nicotine exposures measured with personal samplers (Meger et al. 2000). An additional advantage of NNAL and NNAL-glucuronide as biomarkers is that they are reportedly eliminated more slowly than either nicotine or cotinine in smokers following smoking cessation (Hecht et al. 1999a). Hecht and colleagues (1999a) estimated that the elimination half-life of NNAL was 45 days compared with 40 days for NNAL-glucuronide. If a similar extended half-life can be confirmed in nonsmokers, then these markers may offer the promise of monitoring a longer period of exposure than is possible with either nicotine or cotinine. The main limitation of NNAL measurements

is that the concentrations are quite low, even among active smokers, and relatively large urine sample volumes combined with extensive cleanup and sensitive analytical procedures are needed for assays of nonsmokers.

Besides forming urinary metabolites, both 4-(methylnitrosamino)-1-(3-pyridyl)-1-butanone (NNK) and another TSNA, *N*′-nitrosonornicotine, may also form adducts with Hb and DNA that release 4-hydroxy-1-(3-pyridyl)-1-butanone (HPB) on hydrolysis (Hecht et al. 1994). However, the HPB yield has been surprisingly low and was significantly elevated in only a minority of active smokers and in very few nonsmokers. There was also a substantial overlap in values from the samples of both groups. The reason for this finding is unclear; it may reflect individual metabolic differences in Hb alkylation (Hecht et al. 1993a) or limitations in the analytical procedures. If such limitations could be identified and resolved, the analysis of TSNA adducts might offer considerable promise. However, measurements of NNAL and NNAL-glucuronide in urine appear to be the best approach for monitoring exposures to NNK among people exposed to secondhand smoke.

Evidence Synthesis

Biomarkers are valuable for providing an objective index of the internal dose of a component or its metabolite from secondhand smoke following exposure. Biomarkers can be particularly useful in verifying self-reports of exposure to secondhand smoke because individuals may differ in their awareness of the extent and duration of such exposures. Thus, the use of sensitive biomarker measurements may permit the identification of previously unrecognized exposures within nominal control or unexposed groups, and thereby improve the reliability of classifications. However, biomarkers are also limited by interindividual and intraindividual variability, analytical constraints, and limitations on the exposure timeframe that can be monitored.

For example, as tobacco smoke ages and decays, the physical and chemical composition of secondhand smoke changes (NRC 1986), and the ratio of a marker compound such as nicotine to other components of interest may also change. Temporal variations in the ratio of a biomarker to other hazardous compounds in tobacco smoke could thus complicate the interpretation of exposure based on the measurement of that marker. However, as Benowitz (1999) noted, when ratios of nicotine to other constituents such as respirable suspended particulates are averaged over exposure-time intervals of hours or days, as is typical of a human exposure, the ratios remain consistent. This consistency suggests that biomarkers such as nicotine or its cotinine metabolite should provide a valid assessment of exposure to other toxic constituents in secondhand smoke. Nevertheless, the continual changes in composition during aging will complicate the assessment of tobacco smoke exposure based on one specific marker such as nicotine.

Cotinine measurements in blood or other matrices provide the most useful biomarker for assessing exposure to secondhand smoke because these measurements combine high levels of specificity and sensitivity for exposure. However, as noted above, cotinine measurements reflect an exposure only to nicotine; they are limited to monitoring an exposure over the previous few days unless hair cotinine is measured, and are susceptible to short-term fluctuations that reflect metabolic variations. Even regular smokers may display diurnal variations in plasma cotinine that average 30 percent from peak to trough, with higher concentrations occurring later in the day (Benowitz and Jacob 1994); similar fluctuations may be expected in nonsmokers regularly exposed to secondhand smoke. Cotinine may also reflect an exposure to nicotine previously adsorbed onto dust or emitted from room surfaces rather than a direct exposure to secondhand smoke (Hein et al. 1991), although the extent of this indirect mode of exposure is believed to be trivial (Hein et al. 1991; Benowitz 1999). The interpretation of a result from a single cotinine measurement for an individual is difficult, but multiple measurements over time and mean values from groups within a population may provide useful indices of typical exposure levels. As Benowitz (1999) noted, current evidence "...indicates that cotinine levels provide valid and quantitative measures of average ongoing human ETS [environmental tobacco smoke] exposure over time" (p. 353).

Besides cotinine, other promising biomarkers of involuntary smoking include the tobacco-specific nitrosamine NNAL, the 4AB–Hb adduct, and perhaps hair analysis for nicotine. Each of these markers has the potential to provide an index of exposure over a period of at least several weeks rather than the few days afforded by cotinine, and both NNAL and Hb adducts of aromatic amines are directly relevant as indicators of potential adverse health risks.

Conclusions

1. Biomarkers suitable for assessing recent exposures to secondhand smoke are available.

2. At this time, cotinine, the primary proximate metabolite of nicotine, remains the biomarker of choice for assessing secondhand smoke exposure.

3. Individual biomarkers of exposure to secondhand smoke represent only one component of a complex mixture, and measurements of one marker may not wholly reflect an exposure to other components of concern as a result of involuntary smoking.

Implications

There is a need to refine the methodology used to measure biomarkers to increase their sensitivity and for research into their validity as predictors of population risk. There remains a need for a biomarker capable of reliably indicating past exposures over an extended time period. Until such a marker can be identified, long-term exposures to secondhand smoke can only be assessed through the use of questionnaires and similar approaches.

Conclusions

Building Designs and Operations

1. Current heating, ventilating, and air conditioning systems alone cannot control exposure to secondhand smoke.

2. The operation of a heating, ventilating, and air conditioning system can distribute secondhand smoke throughout a building.

Exposure Models

3. Atmospheric concentration of nicotine is a sensitive and specific indicator for secondhand smoke.

4. Smoking increases indoor particle concentrations.

5. Models can be used to estimate concentrations of secondhand smoke.

Biomarkers of Exposure to Secondhand Smoke

6. Biomarkers suitable for assessing recent exposures to secondhand smoke are available.

7. At this time, cotinine, the primary proximate metabolite of nicotine, remains the biomarker of choice for assessing secondhand smoke exposure.

8. Individual biomarkers of exposure to secondhand smoke represent only one component of a complex mixture, and measurements of one marker may not wholly reflect an exposure to other components of concern as a result of involuntary smoking.

References

Adlkofer F, Scherer G, Heller WD. Hydroxyproline excretion in urine of smokers and passive smokers. *Preventive Medicine* 1984;13(6):670–9.

Al-Delaimy W, Fraser T, Woodward A. Nicotine in hair of bar and restaurant workers. *New Zealand Medical Journal* 2001;114(1127):80–3.

Al-Delaimy WK, Crane J, Woodward A. Questionnaire and hair measurement of exposure to tobacco smoke. *Journal of Exposure Analysis and Environmental Epidemiology* 2000;10(4):378–84.

American Society of Heating, Refrigerating and Air-Conditioning Engineers. *ASHRAE Standard 62-1989: Ventilation for Acceptable Indoor Air Quality*. Atlanta: American Society of Heating, Refrigerating and Air-Conditioning Engineers, 1989.

American Society of Heating, Refrigerating and Air-Conditioning Engineers. *ANSI/ASHRAE Standard 62-1999, Ventilation for Acceptable Indoor Air Quality*. Atlanta: American Society of Heating, Refrigerating and Air-Conditioning Engineers, 1999.

Anderson KE, Carmella SG, Ye M, Bliss RL, Le C, Murphy L, Hecht SS. Metabolites of a tobacco-specific lung carcinogen in nonsmoking women exposed to environmental tobacco smoke. *Journal of the National Cancer Institute* 2001;93(5):378–81.

Autrup H, Vestergaard AB, Okkels H. Transplacental transfer of environmental genotoxins: polycyclic aromatic hydrocarbon–albumin in non-smoking women, and the effect of maternal GSTM1 genotype. *Carcinogenesis* 1995;16(6):1305–9.

Balabanova S, Buhler G, Schneider E, Boschek HJ, Schneitler H. Über die Ausscheidung von nikotin mit dem apokrinen und ekkrinen schweiß bei rauchern und passiv-rauchern (Nicotine excretion by the apocrine and eccrine sweat in smokers and passive smokers) [German; English abstract]. *Hautarzt* 1992;43(2):73–6.

Bearg DW. HVAC systems. In: Spengler JD, Samet JM, McCarthy JF, editors. *Indoor Air Quality Handbook*. New York: McGraw-Hill, 2001:7.1–7.18.

Becker AB, Manfreda J, Ferguson AC, Dimich-Ward H, Watson WT, Chan-Yeung M. Breast-feeding and environmental tobacco smoke exposure. *Archives of Pediatrics & Adolescent Medicine* 1999;153(7):689–91.

Beckett AH, Gorrod JW, Jenner P. The analysis of nicotine-1'-N-oxide in urine, in the presence of nicotine and cotinine, and its application to the study of *in vivo* nicotine metabolism in man. *Journal of Pharmacy and Pharmacology* 1971;23:55S–61S.

Benowitz NL. Cotinine as a biomarker of environmental tobacco smoke exposure. *Epidemiologic Reviews* 1996;18(2):188–204.

Benowitz NL. Biomarkers of environmental tobacco smoke exposure. *Environmental Health Perspectives* 1999;107(Suppl 2):349–55.

Benowitz NL, Jacob PJ III. Nicotine and cotinine elimination pharmacokinetics in smokers and nonsmokers. *Clinical Pharmacology and Therapeutics* 1993;53(3):316–23.

Benowitz NL, Jacob P III. Metabolism of nicotine to cotinine studied by a dual stable isotope method. *Clinical Pharmacology and Therapeutics* 1994;56(5):483–93.

Benowitz NL, Jacob P III. *Trans*-3'-hydroxycotinine: disposition kinetics, effects and plasma levels during cigarette smoking. *British Journal of Clinical Pharmacology* 2001;51(1):53–9.

Benowitz NL, Jacob P III, Denaro C, Jenkins R. Stable isotope studies of nicotine kinetics and bioavailability. *Clinical Pharmacology and Therapeutics* 1991;49(3):270–7.

Benowitz NL, Jacob P III, Fong I, Gupta S. Nicotine metabolic profile in man: comparison of cigarette smoking and transdermal nicotine. *Journal of Pharmacology and Experimental Therapeutics* 1994;268(1):296–303.

Benowitz NL, Kuyt F, Jacob P III, Jones RT, Osman A-L. Cotinine disposition and effects. *Clinical Pharmacology and Therapeutics* 1983;34(5):604–11.

Benowitz NL, Pérez-Stable EJ, Fong I, Modin G, Herrera B, Jacob P III. Ethnic differences in N-glucuronidation of nicotine and cotinine. *Journal of Pharmacology and Experimental Therapeutics* 1999;291(3):1196–203.

Benowitz NL, Pérez-Stable EJ, Herrera B, Jacob P III. Slower metabolism and reduced intake of nicotine from cigarette smoking in Chinese-Americans. *Journal of the National Cancer Institute* 2002;94(2):108–15.

Bentley MC, Abrar M, Kelk M, Cook J, Phillips K. Validation of an assay for the determination of cotinine and 3-hydroxycotinine in human saliva using automated solid-phase extraction and liquid chromatography with tandem mass spectrometric detection. *Journal of Chromatography B: Biomedical Sciences and Applications* 1999;723(1–2):185–94.

Bernert JT Jr, McGuffey JE, Morrison MA, Pirkle JL. Comparison of serum and salivary cotinine measurements by a sensitive high-performance liquid chromatography-tandem mass spectrometry method as an indicator of exposure to tobacco smoke among smokers and nonsmokers. *Journal of Analytical Toxicology* 2000;24(5):333–9.

Bernert JT Jr, Turner WE, Pirkle JL, Sosnoff CS, Akins JR, Waldrep MK, Ann Q, Covey TR, Whitfield WE, Gunter EW, et al. Development and validation of sensitive method for determination of serum cotinine in smokers by liquid chromatography/atmospheric pressure ionization tandem mass spectrometry. *Clinical Chemistry* 1997;43(12):2281–91.

Bjercke RJ, Cook G, Rychlik N, Gjika HB, Van Vunakis H, Langone JJ. Stereospecific monoclonal antibodies to nicotine and cotinine and their use in enzyme-linked immunosorbent assays. *Journal of Immunological Methods* 1986;90(2):203–13.

Bryant MS, Skipper PL, Tannenbaum SR, Maclure M. Hemoglobin adducts of 4-aminobiphenyl in smokers and nonsmokers. *Cancer Research* 1987;47(2):602–8.

Byrd GD, Chang K-M, Greene JM, deBethizy JD. Evidence for urinary excretion of glucuronide conjugates of nicotine, cotinine, and *trans*-3′-hydroxycotinine in smokers. *Drug Metabolism and Disposition* 1992;20(2):192–7.

Byrd GD, Uhrig MS, deBethizy JD, Caldwell WS, Crooks PA, Ravard A, Riggs RM. Direct determination of cotinine-*N*-glucuronide in urine using thermospray liquid chromatography/mass spectrometry. *Biological Mass Spectrometry* 1994;23(2):103–7.

Caraballo RS, Giovino GA, Pechacek TF, Mowery PD. Factors associated with discrepancies between self-reports on cigarette smoking and measured serum cotinine levels among persons aged 17 years or older: Third National Health and Nutrition Examination Survey, 1988–1994. *American Journal of Epidemiology* 2001;153(8):807–14.

Caraballo RS, Giovino GA, Pechacek TF, Mowery PD, Richter PA, Strauss WJ, Sharp DJ, Eriksen MP, Pirkle JL, Maurer KR. Racial and ethnic differences in serum cotinine levels of cigarette smokers: Third National Health and Nutrition Examination Survey, 1988–1991. *Journal of the American Medical Association* 1998;280(2):135–9.

Castleden CM, Cole PV. Variations in carboxyhaemoglobin levels in smokers. *British Medical Journal* 1974;4(5947):736–8.

Castro A, Monji N. Dietary nicotine and its significance in studies of tobacco smoking. *Biochemical Archives* 1986;2:91–7.

Chen Y, Pederson LL, Lefcoe NM. Exposure to environmental tobacco smoke (ETS) and serum thiocyanate level in infants. *Archives of Environmental Health* 1990;45(3):163–7.

Collier AM, Goldstein GM, Shrewsbury RP, Zhang CA, Williams RW. International Conference on Indoor Air Quality and Climate. *Indoor Air '90: the Fifth International Conference on Indoor Air Quality and Climate, Toronto, Canada, July 29–August 3, 1990.* Ottawa (Canada): The Conference, 1990:195–200.

Coultas DB, Howard CA, Peake GT, Skipper BJ, Samet JM. Discrepancies between self-reported and validated cigarette smoking in a community survey of New Mexico Hispanics. *American Review of Respiratory Disease* 1988;137(4):810–4.

Crawford FG, Mayer J, Santella RM, Cooper TB, Ottman R, Tsai W-Y, Simon-Cereijido G, Wang M, Tang D, Perera FP. Biomarkers of environmental tobacco smoke in preschool children and their mothers. *Journal of the National Cancer Institute* 1994;86(18):1398–402.

Curvall M, Elwin C-E, Kazemi-Vala E, Warholm C, Enzell CR. The pharmacokinetics of cotinine in plasma and saliva from non-smoking healthy volunteers. *European Journal of Clinical Pharmacology* 1990a;38(3):281–7.

Curvall M, Vala EK, Enzell CR, Wahren J. Simulation and evaluation of nicotine intake during passive smoking: cotinine measurements in body fluids of nonsmokers given intravenous infusions of nicotine. *Clinical Pharmacology and Therapeutics* 1990b;47(1):42–9.

Daenens P, Laruelle L, Callewaert K, De Schepper P, Galeazzi R, Van Rossum J. Determination of cotinine in biological fluids by capillary gas chromatography–mass spectrometry–selected-ion monitoring. *Journal of Chromatography* 1985;342(1):79–87.

Dagne E, Castagnoli N Jr. Structure of hydroxycotinine, a nicotine metabolite. *Journal of Medicinal Chemistry* 1972;15(4):356–60.

Daisey JM. Tracers for assessing exposure to environmental tobacco smoke: what are they tracing? *Environmental Health Perspectives* 1999;107(Suppl 2):319–27.

Daisey JM, Mahanama KR, Hodgson AT. Toxic volatile organic compounds in simulated environmental tobacco smoke: emission factors for exposure assessment. *Journal of Exposure Analysis and Environmental Epidemiology* 1998;8(3):313–34.

Davis RA. The determination of nicotine and cotinine in plasma. *Journal of Chromatographic Science* 1986;24(4):134–41.

Davis RA, Stiles MF, deBethizy JD, Reynolds JH. Dietary nicotine: a source of urinary cotinine. *Food and Chemical Toxicology* 1991;29(12):821–7.

De Schepper PJ, Van Hecken A, Daenens P, Van Rossum JM. Kinetics of cotinine after oral and intravenous administration to man. *European Journal of Clinical Pharmacology* 1987;31(5):583–8.

Dehn DL, Claffey DJ, Duncan MW, Ruth JA. Nicotine and cotinine adducts of a melanin intermediate demonstrated by matrix-assisted laser desorption/ionization time-of-flight mass spectrometry. *Chemical Research in Toxicology* 2001;14(3):275–9.

Dempsey D, Jacob P III, Benowitz NL. Nicotine metabolism and elimination kinetics in newborns. *Clinical Pharmacology and Therapeutics* 2000;67(5):458–65.

Dempsey D, Jacob P III, Benowitz NL. Accelerated metabolism of nicotine and cotinine in pregnant smokers. *Journal of Pharmacology and Experimental Therapeutics* 2002;301(2):594–8.

Dempsey D, Moore C, Deitermann D, Lewis D, Feeley B, Niedbala RS. The detection of cotinine in hydrolyzed meconium samples. *Forensic Science International* 1999;102(2–3):167–71.

Dempsey D, Tutka P, Jacob P III, Allen F, Schoedel K, Tyndale RF, Benowitz NL. Nicotine metabolite ratio as an index of cytochrome P45 2A6 metabolic activity. *Clinical Pharmacology and Therapeutics* 2004;76(1):64–72.

Diamond RC. An overview of the U.S. building stock. In: Spengler JD, Samet JM, McCarthy JF, editors. *Indoor Air Quality Handbook*. New York: McGraw-Hill, 2001:6.3–6.18.

Dimich-Ward H, Gee H, Brauer M, Leung V. Analysis of nicotine and cotinine in the hair of hospitality workers exposed to environmental tobacco smoke. *Journal of Occupational and Environmental Medicine* 1997;39(10):946–8.

Dockery DW, Spengler JD. Indoor-outdoor relationships of respirable sulfates and particles. *Atmospheric Environment* 1981;15(3):335–43.

Domino EF, Hornbach E, Demana T. The nicotine content of common vegetables [letter]. *New England Journal of Medicine* 1993;329(6):437.

Eatough DJ, Benner CL, Bayona JM, Galen R, Lamb JD, Lee ML, Lewis EA, Hansen LD. Chemical composition of environmental tobacco smoke: 1. Gas-phase acids and bases. *Environmental Science and Technology* 1989a;23(6):679–87.

Eatough DJ, Benner CL, Tang H, Landon V, Richards G, Caka FM, Crawford J, Lewis EA, Hansen LD, Eatough NL. The chemical composition of environmental tobacco smoke. III: identification of conservative tracers on environmental tobacco smoke. *Environment International* 1989b;15(1–6):19–28.

Eliopoulos C, Klein J, Phan MK, Knie B, Greenwald M, Chitayat D, Koren G. Hair concentrations of nicotine and cotinine in women and their newborn infants. *Journal of the American Medical Association* 1994;271(8):621–3.

Emmons KM, Marcus BH, Abrams DB, Marshall R, Novotny TE, Kane ME, Etzel RA. Use of a 24-hour recall diary to assess exposure to environmental tobacco smoke. *Archives of Environmental Health* 1996;51(2):146–9.

Etzel RA. A review of the use of saliva cotinine as a marker of tobacco smoke exposure. *Preventive Medicine* 1990;19(2):190–7.

Feyerabend C, Bryant AE, Jarvis MJ, Russell MA. Determination of cotinine in biological fluids of non-smokers by packed column gas-liquid chromatography. *Journal of Pharmacology* 1986;38(12):917–9.

Feyerabend C, Russell MAH. A rapid gas-liquid chromatographic method for the determination of cotinine and nicotine in biological fluids. *Journal of Pharmacy and Pharmacology* 1990;42(6):450–2.

Foss OP, Lund-Larsen PG. Serum thiocyanate and smoking: interpretation of serum thiocyanate levels observed in a large health study. *Scandinavian Journal of Clinical and Laboratory Investigation* 1986;46(3):245–51.

Galeazzi RL, Daenens P, Gugger M. Steady-state concentration of cotinine as a measure of nicotine-intake by smokers. *European Journal of Clinical Pharmacology* 1985;28(3):301–4.

Gerstenberg B, Schepers G, Voncken P, Völkel H. Nicotine and cotinine accumulation in pigmented and unpigmented rat hair. *Drug Metabolism and Disposition* 1995;23(1):143–8.

Guerin MR, Jenkins RA, Tomkins BA. *The Chemistry of Environmental Tobacco Smoke: Composition and Measurement*. Boca Raton (FL): Lewis Publishers, 1992.

Gwent SH, Wilson JF, Tsanaclis LM, Wicks JFC. Time course of appearance of cotinine in human beard hair after a single dose of nicotine. *Therapeutic Drug Monitoring* 1995;17(2):195–8.

Haley NJ, Axelrad CM, Tilton KA. Validation of self-reported smoking behavior: biochemical analyses of cotinine and thiocyanate. *American Journal of Public Health* 1983;73(10):1204–7.

Haley NJ, Hoffmann D. Analysis for nicotine and cotinine in hair to determine cigarette smoker status. *Clinical Chemistry* 1985;31(10):1598–600.

Haley NJ, Sepkovic DW, Hoffmann D. Elimination of cotinine from body fluids: disposition in smokers and nonsmokers. *American Journal of Public Health* 1989;79(8):1046–8.

Hammond SK, Coghlin J, Gann PH, Paul M, Taghizadeh K, Skipper PL, Tannenbaum SR. Relationship between environmental tobacco smoke exposure and carcinogen-hemoglobin adduct levels in nonsmokers. *Journal of the National Cancer Institute* 1993;85(6):474–8.

Hammond SK, Leaderer BP, Roche AC, Schenker M. Collection and analysis of nicotine as a marker for environmental tobacco smoke. *Atmospheric Environment* 1987;21(2):457–62.

Hariharan M, VanNoord T. Liquid chromatographic determination of nicotine and cotinine in urine from passive smokers: comparison with gas chromatography with a nitrogen-specific detector. *Clinical Chemistry* 1991;37(7):1276–80.

Hariharan M, VanNoord T, Greden JF. A high-performance liquid-chromatographic method for routine simultaneous determination of nicotine and cotinine in plasma. *Clinical Chemistry* 1988; 34(4):724–9.

Hecht SS. Tobacco smoke carcinogens and lung cancer. *Journal of the National Cancer Institute* 1999;91(14):1194–210.

Hecht SS, Carmella SG, Chen M, Dor Koch KJ, Miller AT, Murphy SE, Jensen JA, Zimmerman CL, Hatsukami DK. Quantitation of urinary metabolites of a tobacco-specific lung carcinogen after smoking cessation. *Cancer Research* 1999a;59(3):590–6.

Hecht SS, Carmella SG, Foiles PG, Murphy SE. Biomarkers for human uptake and metabolic activation of tobacco-specific nitrosamines. *Cancer Research* 1994;54(7 Suppl):1912s–1917s.

Hecht SS, Carmella SG, Foiles PG, Murphy SE, Peterson LA. Tobacco-specific nitrosamine adducts: studies in laboratory animals and humans. *Environmental Health Perspectives* 1993a;99:57–63.

Hecht SS, Carmella SG, Murphy SE, Akerkar S, Brunnemann KD, Hoffmann D. A tobacco-specific lung carcinogen in the urine of men exposed to cigarette smoke. *New England Journal of Medicine* 1993b;329(21):1543–6.

Hecht SS, Hatsukami DK, Bonilla LE, Hochalter JB. Quantitation of 4-oxo-4-(3-pyridyl)butanoic acid and enantiomers of 4-hydroxy-4-(3-pyridyl)butanoic acid in human urine: a substantial pathway of nicotine metabolism. *Chemical Research in Toxicology* 1999b;12(2):172–9.

Hecht SS, Hochalter JB, Villalta PW, Murphy SE. 2'-Hydroxylation of nicotine by cytochrome P450 2A6 and human liver microsomes: formation of a lung carcinogen precursor. *Proceedings of the National Academy of Sciences of the United States of America* 2000;97(23):12493–7.

Hecht SS, Ye M, Carmella SG, Fredrickson A, Adgate JL, Greaves IA, Church TR, Ryan AD, Mongin SJ, Sexton K. Metabolites of a tobacco-specific lung carcinogen in the urine of elementary school-aged children. *Cancer Epidemiology, Biomarkers & Prevention* 2001;10(11):1109–16.

Hein HO, Suadicani P, Skov P, Gyntelberg F. Indoor dust exposure: an unnoticed aspect of involuntary smoking. *Archives of Environmental Health* 1991;46(2):98–101.

Henderson GL. Mechanisms of drug incorporation into hair. *Forensic Science International* 1993; 63(1–3):19–29.

Hiller FC, McCusker KT, Mazumder MK, Wilson JD, Bone RC. Deposition of sidestream cigarette smoke in the human respiratory tract. *American Review of Respiratory Disease* 1982;125(4):406–8.

Husgafvel-Pursiainen K, Sorsa M, Engström K, Einistö P. Passive smoking at work: biochemical and biological measures of exposure to environmental tobacco smoke. *International Archives of Occupational and Environmental Health* 1987;59(4):337–45.

Idle JR. Titrating exposure to tobacco smoke using cotinine—a minefield of misunderstandings. *Journal of Clinical Epidemiology* 1990;43(4):313–7.

International Agency for Research on Cancer. *IARC Monographs on the Evaluation of Carcinogenic Risks to Humans: Tobacco Smoke and Involuntary Smoking.* Vol. 83. Lyon (France): International Agency for Research on Cancer, 2004.

Ishiyama I, Nagai T, Toshida S. Detection of basic drugs (methamphetamine, antidepressants, and nicotine) from human hair. *Journal of Forensic Science* 1983;28(2):380–5.

Ivey KJ, Triggs EJ. Absorption of nicotine by the human stomach and its effect on gastric ion fluxes and potential difference. *American Journal of Digestive Diseases* 1978;23(9):809–14.

Iwase A, Aiba M, Kira S. Respiratory nicotine absorption in non-smoking females during passive smoking. *International Archives of Occupational and Environmental Health* 1991;63(2):139–43.

Jaakkola JJK, Jaakkola N, Zahlsen K. Fetal growth and length of gestation in relation to prenatal exposure to environmental tobacco smoke assessed by hair nicotine concentration. *Environmental Health Perspectives* 2001;109(6):557–61.

Jaakkola MS, Jaakkola JJK. Assessment of exposure to environmental tobacco smoke. *European Respiratory Journal* 1997;10(10):2384–97.

Jaakkola MS, Samet JM. Occupational exposure to environmental tobacco smoke and health risk assessment. *Environmental Health Perspectives* 1999;107(Suppl 6):829–35.

Jacob P III, Benowitz NL, Yu L, Shulgin AT. Determination of nicotine N-oxide by gas chromatography following thermal conversion to 2-methyl-6-(3-pyridyl)tetrahydro-1,2-oxazine. *Analytical Chemistry* 1986;58(11):2218–21.

Jacob P III, Wilson M, Benowitz NL. Improved gas chromatographic method for the determination of nicotine and cotinine in biologic fluids. *Journal of Chromatography B: Biomedical Sciences and Applications* 1981;222(1):61–70.

Jacob P III, Yu L, Wilson M, Benowitz NL. Selected ion monitoring method for determination of nicotine, cotinine and deuterium-labeled analogs: absence of an isotope effect in the clearance of (S)-nicotine-3′,3′-d$_2$ in humans. *Biological Mass Spectrometry* 1991;20(5):247–52.

James H, Tizabi Y, Taylor R. Rapid method for the simultaneous measurement of nicotine and cotinine in urine and serum by gas chromatography–mass spectrometry. *Journal of Chromatography B: Biomedical Sciences and Applications* 1998;708(1–2):87–93.

Jarvis M, Tunstall-Pedoe H, Feyerabend C, Vesey C, Saloojee Y. Biochemical markers of smoke absorption and self reported exposure to passive smoking. *Journal of Epidemiology and Community Health* 1984;38(4):335–9.

Jarvis MJ, Russell MAH, Benowitz NL, Feyerabend C. Elimination of cotinine from body fluids: implications for noninvasive measurement of tobacco smoke exposure. *American Journal of Public Health* 1988;78(6):696–8.

Jarvis MJ, Russell MAH, Feyerabend C. Absorption of nicotine and carbon monoxide from passive smoking under natural conditions of exposure. *Thorax* 1983;38(11):829–33.

Jarvis MJ, Tunstall-Pedoe H, Feyerabend C, Vesey C, Saloojee Y. Comparison of tests used to distinguish smokers from nonsmokers. *American Journal of Public Health* 1987;77(11):1435–8.

Jauniaux E, Gulbis B, Acharya G, Thiry P, Rodeck C. Maternal tobacco exposure and cotinine levels in fetal fluids in the first half of pregnancy. *Obstetrics and Gynecology* 1999;93(1):25–9.

Jenkins RA, Guerin MR, Tomkins BA. *The Chemistry of Environmental Tobacco Smoke: Composition and Measurement.* 2nd ed. Boca Raton (FL): Lewis Publishers, 2000.

Jenkins RA, Palausky A, Counts RW, Bayne CK, Dindal AB, Guerin MR. Exposure to environmental tobacco smoke in sixteen cities in the United States as determined by personal breathing zone air sampling. *Journal of Exposure Analysis and Environmental Epidemiology* 1996;6(4):473–502.

Joint Center for Housing Studies of Harvard University. *The State of the Nation's Housing.* Cambridge (MA): Harvard University, 2002.

Jones CJ, Schiffman MH, Kurman R, Jacob P III, Benowitz NL. Elevated nicotine levels in cervical lavages from passive smokers. *American Journal of Public Health* 1991;81(3):378–9.

Junge B. Changes in serum thiocyanate concentration on stopping smoking. *British Medical Journal (Clinical Research Edition)* 1985;291(6487):22.

Kintz P. Gas chromatographic analysis of nicotine and cotinine in hair. *Journal of Chromatography B: Biomedical Sciences and Applications* 1992;580(1–2):347–53.

Klepeis NE. An introduction to the indirect exposure assessment approach: modeling human exposure using microenvironmental measurements and the recent National Human Activity Pattern Survey. *Environmental Health Perspectives* 1999a;107(Suppl 2):365–74.

Klepeis NE. Validity of the uniform mixing assumption: determining human exposure to environmental tobacco smoke. *Environmental Health Perspectives* 1999b;107(Suppl 2):357–63.

Klepeis NE, Ott WR, Switzer P. A multiple-smoker model for predicting indoor air quality in public lounges. *Environmental Science and Technology* 1996;30(9):2813–20.

Knight GJ, Wylie P, Holman MS, Haddow JE. Improved ^{125}I radioimmunoassay for cotinine by selective removal of bridge antibodies. *Clinical Chemistry* 1985;31(1):118–21.

Knight JM, Eliopoulos C, Klein J, Greenwald M, Koren G. Passive smoking in children: racial differences in systemic exposure to cotinine by hair and urine analysis. *Chest* 1996;109(2):446–50.

Knott C. Excretion of drugs into saliva. In: Tenovuo JO, editor. *Human Saliva: Clinical Chemistry and Microbiology.* Vol. II. Boca Raton (FL): CRC Press, 1989:177–201.

Koren G, Klein J, Forman R, Graham K, Phan M-K. Biological markers of intrauterine exposure to cocaine and cigarette smoking. *Developmental Pharmacology and Therapeutics* 1992;18(3–4):228–36.

Kriek E, Rojas M, Alexandrov K, Bartsch H. Polycyclic aromatic hydrocarbon-DNA adducts in humans: relevance as biomarkers for exposure and cancer risk. *Mutation Research* 1998;400(1–2):215–31.

Kyerematen GA, Damiano MD, Dvorchik BH, Vesell ES. Smoking-induced changes in nicotine disposition: application of a new HPLC assay for nicotine and its metabolites. *Clinical Pharmacology and Therapeutics* 1982;32(6):769–80.

Lähdetie J, Engström K, Husgafvel-Pursiainen K, Nylund L, Vainio H, Sorsa M. Maternal smoking induced cotinine levels and genotoxicity in second trimester amniotic fluid. *Mutation Research* 1993;300(1):37–43.

LaKind JS, Ginevan ME, Naiman DQ, James AC, Jenkins RA, Dourson ML, Felter SP, Graves CG, Tardiff RG. Distribution of exposure concentrations and doses for constituents of environmental tobacco smoke. *Risk Analysis* 1999a;19(3):375–90.

LaKind JS, Jenkins RA, Naiman DQ, Ginevan ME, Graves CG, Tardiff RG. Use of environmental tobacco smoke constituents as markers for exposure. *Risk Analysis* 1999b;19(3):359–73.

Langone JJ, Gjika HB, Van Vunakis H. Nicotine and its metabolites: radioimmunoassays for nicotine and cotinine. *Biochemistry* 1973;12(24):5025–30.

Leaderer BP, Hammond SK. Evaluation of vapor-phase nicotine and respirable suspended particle mass as markers for environmental tobacco smoke. *Environmental Science & Technology* 1991;25(4):770–7.

Letz R, Ryan PB, Spengler JD. Estimated distributions of personal exposure to respirable particles. *Environmental Monitoring and Assessment* 1984;4:351–9.

Liddament MW. Ventilation strategies. In: Spengler JD, Samet JM, McCarthy JF, editors. *Indoor Air Quality Handbook.* New York: McGraw-Hill, 2001: 13.1–13.24.

Luck W, Nau H. Nicotine and cotinine concentrations in serum and milk of nursing smokers. *British Journal of Clinical Pharmacology* 1984;18(1):9–15.

Ludwig JF. HVAC subsystems. In: Spengler JD, Samet JM, McCarthy JF, editors. *Indoor Air Quality Handbook.* New York: McGraw-Hill, 2001:8.1–8.37.

Lynch CJ. Half-lives of selected tobacco smoke exposure markers. *European Journal of Respiratory Diseases Supplement* 1984;133:63–7.

Machacek DA, Jiang N-S. Quantification of cotinine in plasma and saliva by liquid chromatography. *Clinical Chemistry* 1986;32(6):979–82.

Maclure M, Bryant MS, Skipper PL, Tannenbaum SR. Decline of the hemoglobin adduct of 4-aminobiphenyl during withdrawal from smoking. *Cancer Research* 1990;50(1):181–4.

Maclure M, Katz RB-A, Bryant MS, Skipper PL, Tannenbaum SR. Elevated blood levels of carcinogens in passive smokers. *American Journal of Public Health* 1989;79(10):1381–4.

Mahanama KRR, Daisey JM. Volatile N-nitrosamines in environmental tobacco smoke: sampling, analysis, source emission factors, and indoor air exposures. *Environmental Science & Technology* 1996;30(5):1477–84.

McAdams SA, Cordeiro ML. Simple selected ion monitoring capillary gas chromatographic–mass spectrometric method for the determination of cotinine in serum, urine and oral samples. *Journal of Chromatography* 1993;615(1):148–53.

McDonald B, Ouyang M. Air cleaning—particles. In: Spengler JD, Samet JM, McCarthy JF, editors. *Indoor Air Quality Handbook.* New York: McGraw-Hill, 2001.

Meger M, Meger-Kossien I, Riedel K, Scherer G. Biomonitoring of environmental tobacco smoke (ETS)-related exposure to 4-(methylnitrosamino)-1-(3-pyridyl)-1-butanone (NNK). *Biomarkers* 2000; 5(1):33–45.

Miesner EA, Rudnick SN, Hu FC, Spengler JD, Preller L, Ozkaynak H, Nelson W. Particulate and nicotine sampling in public facilities and offices. *Journal of the Air Pollution Control Association* 1989;39(12): 1577–82.

Milerad J, Rajs J, Gidlund E. Nicotine and cotinine levels in pericardial fluid in victims of SIDS. *Acta Paediatrica* 1994;83(1):59–62.

Mizuno A, Uematsu T, Oshima A, Nakamura M, Nakashima M. Analysis of nicotine content of hair for assessing individual cigarette-smoking behavior. *Therapeutic Drug Monitoring* 1993;15(2):99–104.

Murray DM, Burmaster DE. Residential air exchange rates in the United States: empirical and estimated parametric distributions by season and climatic regions. *Risk Analysis* 1995;15(4):459–65.

Nafstad P, Botten G, Hagen JA, Zahlsen K, Nilsen OG, Silsand T, Kongerud J. Comparison of three methods for estimating environmental tobacco smoke exposure among children aged between 12 and 36 months. *International Journal of Epidemiology* 1995;24(1):88–94.

Nafstad P, Fugelseth D, Qvigstad E, Zahlsen K, Magnus P, Lindemann R. Nicotine concentration in the hair of nonsmoking mothers and size of offspring. *American Journal of Public Health* 1998;88(1):120–4.

National Cancer Institute. *Health Effects of Exposure to Environmental Tobacco Smoke: The Report of the California Environmental Protection Agency.* Smoking and Tobacco Control Monograph No. 10. Bethesda (MD): U.S. Department of Health and Human Services, National Institutes of Health, National Cancer Institute, 1999. NIH Publication No. 99-4645.

National Research Council. *Environmental Tobacco Smoke: Measuring Exposures and Assessing Health Effects.* Washington: National Academy Press, 1986.

National Research Council. *Biologic Markers in Pulmonary Toxicology.* Washington: National Academy Press, 1989.

National Research Council. *Human Exposure Assessment for Airborne Pollutants: Advances and Opportunities.* Washington: National Academy Press, 1991.

Neas LM, Dockery DW, Ware JH, Spengler JD, Ferris BG Jr, Speizer FE. Concentration of indoor particulate matter as a determinant of respiratory health in children. *American Journal of Epidemiology* 1994;139(11):1088–99.

Nelson PR, Heavner DL, Collie BB, Maiolo KC, Ogden MW. Effect of ventilation and sampling time on environmental tobacco smoke component ratios. *Environmental Science & Technology* 1992;26(10):1909–15.

Neurath GB, Pein FG. Gas chromatographic determination of *trans*-3'-hydroxycotinine, a major metabolite of nicotine in smokers. *Journal of Chromatography* 1987;415(2):400–6.

Nilsen T, Zahlsen K, Nilsen OG. Uptake of nicotine in hair during controlled environmental air exposure to nicotine vapour: evidence for a major contribution of environmental nicotine to the overall nicotine found in hair from smokers and non-smokers. *Pharmacology and Toxicology* 1994;75(3–4):136–42.

Norbury CG. Simplified method for the determination of plasma cotinine using gas chromatography–mass spectrometry. *Journal of Chromatography* 1987;414(2):449–53.

Nuesslein TG, Beckers D, Rieger CHL. Cotinine in meconium indicates risk for early respiratory tract infections. *Human & Experimental Toxicology* 1999;18(4):283–90.

Oddoze C, Pauli AM, Pastor J. Rapid and sensitive high-performance liquid chromatographic determination of nicotine and cotinine in nonsmoker human and rat urines. *Journal of Chromatography B: Biomedical Sciences and Applications* 1998;708(1–2):95–101.

Ostrea EM Jr, Knapp DK, Romero A, Montes M, Ostrea AR. Meconium analysis to assess fetal exposure to nicotine by active and passive maternal smoking. *Journal of Pediatrics* 1994;124(3):471–6.

Otsuka R, Watanabe H, Hirata K, Tokai K, Muro T, Yoshiyama M, Takeuchi K, Yoshikawa J. Acute effects of passive smoking on the coronary circulation in healthy young adults. *Journal of the American Medical Association* 2001;286(4):436–41.

Ott WR. Mathematical models for predicting indoor air quality from smoking activity. *Environmental Health Perspectives* 1999;107(Suppl 2):375–81.

Ott WR, Langan L, Switzer P. A time series model for cigarette smoking activity patterns: model validation for carbon monoxide and respirable particles in a chamber and an automobile. *Journal of Exposure Analysis and Environmental Epidemiology* 1992;2(Suppl 2):175–200.

Owens DF, Rosanno AJ. Design procedures to control cigarette smoke and other air pollutants. *ASHRAE Transactions* 1969;75:93–102.

Özkaynak H, Xue J, Weker R, Butler D, Koutrakis P, Spengler J. The Particle Team (PTEAM) study: analysis of the data. Final Report, Volume III. Research Triangle Park (NC): U.S. Environmental Protection Agency, 1996. Publication No. EPA/600/R-95/098.

Parsons WD, Carmella SG, Akerkar S, Bonilla LE, Hecht SS. A metabolite of the tobacco-specific lung carcinogen 4-(methylnitrosamino)-1-(3-pyridyl)-1-butanone in the urine of hospital workers exposed to environmental tobacco smoke. *Cancer Epidemiology, Biomarkers & Prevention* 1998;7(3):257–60.

Patrick DL, Cheadle A, Thompson DC, Diehr P, Koepsell T, Kinne S. The validity of self-reported smoking: a review and meta-analysis. *American Journal of Public Health* 1994;84(7):1086–93.

Perera FP. Molecular epidemiology: on the path to prevention? *Journal of the National Cancer Institute* 2000;92(8):602–12.

Pérez-Stable EJ, Herrera B, Jacob P III, Benowitz NL. Nicotine metabolism and intake in black and white smokers. *Journal of the American Medical Association* 1998;280(2):152–6.

Pichini S, Altieri I, Pellegrini M, Pacifici R, Zuccaro P. The analysis of nicotine in infants' hair for measuring exposure to environmental tobacco smoke. *Forensic Science International* 1997;84(1–3):253–8.

Pirkle JL, Flegal KM, Bernert JT, Brody DJ, Etzel RA, Maurer KR. Exposure of the US population to environmental tobacco smoke: the Third National Health and Nutrition Examination Survey, 1988 to 1991. *Journal of the American Medical Association* 1996;275(16):1233–40.

Poulton J, Rylance GW, Taylor AW, Edwards C. Serum thiocyanate levels as indicator of passive smoking in children [letter]. *Lancet* 1984;2(8416):1405–6.

Repace JL. Dietary nicotine: won't mislead on passive smoking...: new insight into myocardial protection. *British Medical Journal* 1994;308(6920):61–2.

Repace JL, Jinot J, Bayard S, Emmons K, Hammond SK. Air nicotine and saliva cotinine as indicators of workplace passive smoking exposure and risk. *Risk Analysis* 1998;18(1):71–83.

Repace JL, Lowrey AH. Indoor air pollution, tobacco smoke, and public health. *Science* 1980;208(4443):464–72.

Repace JL, Lowrey AH. An enforceable indoor air quality standard for environmental tobacco smoke in the workplace. *Risk Analysis* 1993;13(4):463–75.

Robertson AS, Burge PS, Cockrill BL. A study of serum thiocyanate concentrations in office workers as a means of validating smoking histories and assessing passive exposure to cigarette smoke. *British Journal of Industrial Medicine* 1987;44(5):351–4.

Rose JE, Levin ED, Benowitz N. Saliva nicotine as an index of plasma levels in nicotine skin patch users. *Therapeutic Drug Monitoring* 1993;15(5):431–5.

Russell MAH, Cole PV, Brown E. Absorption by non-smokers of carbon monoxide from room air polluted by tobacco smoke. *Lancet* 1973;1(7803):576–9.

Sampson EJ, Needham LL, Pirkle JL, Hannon WH, Miller DT, Patterson DG, Bernert JT, Ashley DL, Hill RH, Gunter EW, Paschal DC, Spierto FW, Rich MJ. Technical and scientific developments in exposure marker methodology. *Clinical Chemistry* 1994;40(7 Pt 2):1376–84.

Schenker MB, Samuels SJ, Kado NY, Hammond SK, Smith TJ, Woskie SR. Markers of exposure to diesel exhaust in railroad workers. *Research Report (Health Effects Institute)* 1990;(33):1–51.

Scherer G, Frank S, Riedel K, Meger-Kossien I, Renner T. Biomonitoring of exposure to polycyclic aromatic hydrocarbons of nonoccupationally exposed persons. *Cancer Epidemiology, Biomarkers & Prevention* 2000;9(4):373–80.

Scherer G, Jarczyk L, Heller W-D, Biber A, Neurath GB, Adlkofer F. Pharmacokinetics of nicotine, cotinine, and 3'-hydroxycotinine in cigarette smokers. *Klinische Wochenschrift* 1988;66(Suppl XI):5–11.

Scherer G, Richter E. Biomonitoring exposure to environmental tobacco smoke (ETS): a critical re-appraisal. *Human & Experimental Toxicology* 1997;16(8):449–59.

Schneider NG, Jacob P III, Nilsson F, Leischow SJ, Benowitz NL, Olmstead RE. Saliva cotinine levels as a function of collection method. *Addiction* 1997;92(3):347–51.

Scientific Committee on Tobacco and Health. *Report of the Scientific Committee on Tobacco and Health.* London: The Stationery Office, 1998.

Sepkovic DW, Haley NJ, Hoffmann D. Elimination from the body of tobacco products by smokers and passive smokers [letter]. *Journal of the American Medical Association* 1986;256(7):863.

Sheen SJ. Detection of nicotine in foods and plant materials. *Journal of Food Science* 1988;53(5):1572–3.

Shen H-M, Chia S-E, Ni Z-Y, New A-L, Lee B-L, Ong C-N. Detection of oxidative DNA damage in human sperm and the association with cigarette smoking. *Reproductive Toxicology* 1997;11(5):675–80.

Sherman M, Matson N. Residential ventilation and energy characteristics. *ASHRAE Transactions* 1997;103(Pt 1):717–30.

Siegmund B, Leitner E, Pfannhauser W. Determination of the nicotine content of various edible nightshades (Solanaceae) and their products and estimation of the associated dietary nicotine intake. *Journal of Agricultural and Food Chemistry* 1999a;47(8):3113–20.

Siegmund B, Leitner E, Pfannhauser W. Development of a simple sample preparation technique for gas chromatographic–mass spectrometric determination of nicotine in edible nightshades (Solanaceae). *Journal of Chromatography A* 1999b;840(2):249–60.

Skipper PL, Tannenbaum SR. Protein adducts in the molecular dosimetry of chemical carcinogens. *Carcinogenesis* 1990;11(4):507–18.

Sparks LE. Indoor air quality modeling. In: Spengler JD, Samet JM, McCarthy JF, editors. *Indoor Air Quality Handbook.* New York: McGraw-Hill, 2001.

Spengler JD. Building operations and ETS exposure. *Environmental Health Perspectives* 1999;107(Suppl 2):313–7.

Spengler JD, Dockery DW, Turner WA, Woolfson JM, Ferris BG Jr. Long-term measurements of respirable sulfates and particles inside and outside homes. *Atmospheric Environment* 1981;15(1):23–30.

Spengler JD, Thurston GD. Mass and elemental composition of fine and coarse particles in 6 U.S. cities. *Journal of the Air Pollution Control Association* 1983;33(12):1162–71.

Spengler JD, Treitman RD, Tosteson T, Mage DT, Soczek ML. Personal exposures to respirable particulates and implications for air pollution epidemiology. *Environmental Science & Technology* 1985;19(8):700–7.

Sreebny LM, Broich G. Xerostomia (dry mouth). In: Sreebny LM, editor. *The Salivary System.* Boca Raton (FL): CRC Press, 1987:179–202.

Stout PR, Ruth JA. Deposition of [$_3$H]cocaine, [$_3$H]nicotine, and [$_3$H]flunitrazepam in mouse hair melanosomes after systemic administration. *Drug Metabolism and Disposition* 1999;27(6):731–5.

Suh HH, Koutrakis P, Spengler JD. The relationship between airborne acidity and ammonia in indoor environments. *Journal of Exposure Analysis and Environmental Epidemiology* 1994;4(1):1–22.

Svensson CK. Clinical pharmacokinetics of nicotine. *Clinical Pharmacokinetics* 1987;12(1):30–40.

Tang D, Warburton D, Tannenbaum SR, Skipper P, Santella RM, Cereijido GS, Crawford FG, Perera FP. Molecular and genetic damage from environmental tobacco smoke in young children. *Cancer Epidemiology, Biomarkers & Prevention* 1999;8(5):427–31.

Teeuwen HWA, Aalders RJ, Van Rossum JM. Simultaneous estimation of nicotine and cotinine levels in biological fluids using high-resolution capillary-column gas chromatography combined with solid phase extraction work-up. *Molecular Biology Reports* 1989;13(3):165–75.

Thompson SG, Barlow RD, Wald NJ, Van Vunakis H. How should urinary cotinine concentrations be adjusted for urinary creatinine concentration? *Clinica Chimica Acta* 1990;187(3):289–95.

Tunstall-Pedoe H, Woodward M, Brown CA. Tea drinking, passive smoking, smoking deception and serum cotinine in the Scottish Heart Health Study. *Journal of Clinical Epidemiology* 1991;44(12):1411–4.

Tuomi T, Johnsson T, Reijula K. Analysis of nicotine, 3-hydroxycotinine, cotinine, and caffeine in urine of passive smokers by HPLC-tandem mass spectrometry. *Clinical Chemistry* 1999;45(12):2164–72.

U.S. Department of Energy. *A Look at Residential Energy Consumption in 1997.* Washington: U.S. Department of Energy, 1999.

U.S. Department of Health and Human Services. *The Health Consequences of Involuntary Smoking. A Report of the Surgeon General.* Rockville (MD): U.S. Department of Health and Human Services, Public Health Service, Centers for Disease Control, Center for Health Promotion and Education, Office on Smoking and Health, 1986. DHHS Publication No. (CDC) 87-8398.

U.S. Environmental Protection Agency. *Respiratory Health Effects of Passive Smoking: Lung Cancer and Other Disorders.* Washington: Environmental Protection Agency, Office of Research and Development, Office of Air and Radiation, 1992. Publication No. EPA/600/6-90/006F.

U.S. Environmental Protection Agency. *Orientation to Indoor Air Quality.* Washington: U.S. Environmental Protection Agency, 1994.

U.S. Environmental Protection Agency. Architecture, engineering, and planning guidelines. *EPA Facilities Manual,* Vol. 1. Washington: U.S. Environmental Protection Agency, 1998.

Uematsu T. Utilization of hair analysis for therapeutic drug monitoring with a special reference to ofloxacin and to nicotine. *Forensic Science International* 1993;63(1–3):261–8.

Uematsu T, Mizuno A, Nagashima S, Oshima A, Nakamura M. The axial distribution of nicotine content along hair shaft as an indicator of changes in smoking behaviour: evaluation in a smoking-cessation programme with or without the aid of nicotine chewing gum. *British Journal of Clinical Pharmacology* 1995;39(6):665–9.

Van Loy MD, Nazaroff WW, Daisey JM. Nicotine as a marker for environmental tobacco smoke: implications of sorption on indoor surface materials. *Journal of the Air & Waste Management Association* 1998;48(10):959–68.

Van Vunakis H, Tashkin DP, Rigas B, Simmons M, Gjika HB, Clark VA. Relative sensitivity and specificity of salivary and serum cotinine in identifying tobacco-smoking status of self-reported nonsmokers and smokers of tobacco and/or marijuana. *Archives of Environmental Health* 1989;44(1):53–8.

Verplanke AJW, Remijn B, Hoek F, Houthuijs D, Brunekreef B, Boleij JSM. Hydroxyproline excretion in schoolchildren and its relationship to measures of indoor air pollution. *International Archives of Occupational and Environmental Health* 1987;59(3):221–31.

Wagenknecht LE, Burke GL, Perkins LL, Haley NJ, Friedman GD. Misclassification of smoking status in the CARDIA study: a comparison of self-report with serum cotinine levels. *American Journal of Public Health* 1992;82(1):33–6.

Wagenknecht LE, Cutter GR, Haley NJ, Sidney S, Manolio TA, Hughes GH, Jacobs DR. Racial differences in serum cotinine levels among smokers in the Coronary Artery Risk Development in (Young) Adults Study. *American Journal of Public Health* 1990;80(9):1053–6.

Wagenknecht LE, Manolio TA, Sidney S, Burke GL, Haley NJ. Environmental tobacco smoke exposure as determined by cotinine in black and white young adults: the CARDIA Study. *Environmental Research* 1993;63(1):39–46.

Wallace L. Indoor particles: a review. *Journal of the Air & Waste Management Association* 1996;46(2):98–126.

Watts RR, Langone JJ, Knight GJ, Lewtas J. Cotinine analytical workshop report: consideration of analytical methods for determining cotinine in human body fluids as a measure of passive exposure to tobacco smoke. *Environmental Health Perspectives* 1990;84:173–82.

Wennig R. Potential problems with the interpretation of hair analysis results. *Forensic Science International* 2000;107(1–3):5–12.

Woodward A, Al-Delaimy W. Measures of exposure to environmental tobacco smoke: validity, precision, and relevance. *Annals of the New York Academy of Sciences* 1999;895:156–72.

Woodward M, Tunstall-Pedoe H, Smith WCS, Tavendale R. Smoking characteristics and inhalation biochemistry in the Scottish population. *Journal of Clinical Epidemiology* 1991;44(12):1405–10.

Yanagisawa Y, Nishimura H, Matsuki H, Osaka F, Kasuga H. Personal exposure and health effect relationship for NO_2 with urinary hydroxyproline to creatinine ratio as indicator. *Archives of Environmental Health* 1986;41(1):41–8.

Zahlsen K, Nilsen T, Nilsen OG. Interindividual differences in hair uptake of air nicotine and significance of cigarette counting for estimation of environmental tobacco smoke exposure. *Pharmacology and Toxicology* 1996;79(4):183–90.

Zevin S, Jacob P III, Benowitz N. Cotinine effects on nicotine metabolism. *Clinical Pharmacology and Therapeutics* 1997;61(6):649–54.

Zhang Y, Jacob P III, Benowitz NL. Determination of nornicotine in smokers' urine by gas chromatography following reductive alkylation to N'-propylnornicotine. *Journal of Chromatography B: Biomedical Sciences and Applications* 1990;525(2):349–57.

Chapter 4
Prevalence of Exposure to Secondhand Smoke

Introduction

The 1986 U.S. Surgeon General's report, *The Health Consequences of Involuntary Smoking*, outlined the need for valid and reliable methods to more accurately determine and assess the health consequences of exposure to secondhand smoke (U.S. Department of Health and Human Services [USDHHS] 1986). The report concluded that reliable methods were necessary to research the health effects and to characterize the public health impact of exposure to secondhand tobacco smoke in the home, at work, and in other environments. The report noted that without valid and reliable evidence, policymakers could not draft and implement effective policies to reduce and eliminate exposures: "Validated questionnaires are needed for the assessment of recent and remote exposure to environmental tobacco smoke in the home, workplace, and other environments" (USDHHS 1986, p. 14).

Since the publication of that report, public health investigators have made significant advances in the development and application of reliable and valid research methods to assess exposure to secondhand smoke (Jaakkola and Samet 1999; Samet and Wang 2000). Several investigators have recently developed new methods to measure tobacco smoke concentrations in indoor environments and have discovered sensitive biologic markers of active and involuntary exposures (Jaakkola and Samet 1999; Samet and Wang 2000). These advances have generated a substantial amount of data on exposure of nonsmokers to secondhand smoke and have improved the capability of researchers to measure a recent exposure. However, many public health investigators agree that more accurate tools are still needed to measure temporally remote exposures, which, by necessity, are still assessed using questionnaires (Jaakkola and Samet 1999).

The main methods researchers rely on to evaluate secondhand smoke exposure are questionnaires, measurements of concentrations of the airborne components of secondhand smoke, and measurements of biomarkers (Chapter 3, Assessment of Exposure to Secondhand Smoke). The discussion that follows on the prevalence of secondhand smoke exposure includes current metrics of exposure, changes in exposure over time, exposure of special populations such as children with asthma and persons in prisons, and international differences in exposure.

Methods

To identify research publications on biomarkers of secondhand smoke, the authors of this chapter reviewed the published literature for studies on population exposures to and concentrations of secondhand smoke in different environments by conducting a Medline search with the following terms: tobacco smoke pollution, environmental tobacco smoke, and secondhand smoke. These terms were then paired with the term population or survey. The authors then reviewed abstracts of articles to specifically identify studies that used representative surveys of the U.S. population for inclusion in this report.

To specifically identify articles on concentrations of secondhand smoke, the authors used Boolean logic to search Medline and Web of Science, pairing the selected terms for secondhand smoke (secondhand smoke, environmental tobacco smoke, passive smoking, and involuntary smoking) with terms indicative of a location that included home, work, workplace, occupation and restaurants, bars, public places, sports, transportation, buses, trains, cars, airplanes, casinos, bingo, nightclubs, prisons, correctional institutions, nursing homes, and mental institutions. The authors searched for these terms with and without other selected terms such as exposure, concentration, and level of exposure. The authors also included data from a review of studies on the composition and measurement of secondhand smoke (Jenkins et al. 2000).

This chapter focuses on measured concentrations of airborne nicotine—nicotine is a specific tracer for secondhand smoke and has therefore been widely used in many studies. This discussion also focuses on biomarker levels of cotinine, the metabolite of nicotine. Thus, the abstracts of articles identified through the literature search were further reviewed for data that contained measured values of nicotine in the air of selected environments.

Metrics of Secondhand Smoke Exposure

This chapter considers how researchers have used the techniques for assessing exposure to secondhand smoke to determine the extent of exposure among populations. The discussion includes the strengths and limitations of these techniques.

Questionnaires

A questionnaire-based assessment of exposure to secondhand smoke is the most widely used method to evaluate an exposure. Questionnaires have important advantages: they are relatively inexpensive; they can be feasibly administered in a variety of ways, including mail surveys, telephone surveys, or in person; and they are able to assess both current and past exposures (Jaakkola and Jaakkola 1997; Jaakkola and Samet 1999). The disadvantages include difficulties in validation, particularly of a past exposure, and the potential for misclassification. Misclassification may result from a respondent's lack of knowledge about a current or past exposure, the difficulty in characterizing an exposure in complex indoor environments, and biased recall, whether intentional or unintentional (USDHHS 1986).

Investigators have developed numerous questionnaires that assess exposures to secondhand smoke. The questionnaires address fundamental factors such as duration, source strength (the number of smokers or number of cigarettes smoked), room size, and distance from smokers, as well as the perception of an exposure such as observations of tobacco smoke, odor, and irritation. For example, the indirect index of being married to a smoker or of being in the presence of smokers has been widely used to examine the long-term effects of secondhand smoke exposure (Hirayama 1984; Sandler et al. 1989). However, a misclassification of total exposure may occur with indirect measures because they do not capture exposures outside of the home, and because some smokers may not smoke in the house. Nevertheless, compared with persons living in smoke-free homes, Hammond (1999) demonstrated that persons who are married to or living with smokers have higher exposures to secondhand smoke.

Several investigators have used questionnaires to quantitatively estimate exposures by ascertaining the number of hours per day of exposure and the number of cigarettes smoked in a specific location, such as in the home, at work, or in public places (Coghlin et al. 1989; Fontham et al. 1994; Pirkle et al. 1996). These estimates may be made either collectively or separately in each location where the respondents spend time. Although it may be necessary to ask many questions to cover all possible microenvironments of exposure, questionnaires that capture objective measures may provide more accurate estimates of an exposure, and measured concentrations of airborne components of secondhand smoke can be used to calculate summary measures across exposure locations.

Studies have assessed secondhand smoke exposure by asking respondents to rate their perceived level of exposure (e.g., none, slight, moderate, heavy) in various environments (Haley et al. 1989). However, this type of assessment cannot be readily standardized and could potentially result in both random and nonrandom misclassification. For example, persons with a respiratory disease such as asthma may be more likely to perceive exposures to secondhand smoke and to classify them toward the higher end of the scale.

Questionnaires are the only means of assessing remote past exposures to secondhand smoke, absent stored samples for biomarker measurements. For example, Sandler and colleagues (1989) used the smoking status of the spouse as a surrogate for determining household exposures to secondhand smoke. These researchers found that 30 percent of nonsmoking men and 64 percent of nonsmoking women in Washington County, Maryland, reported an exposure in 1963. This information was used to assign an exposure in assessing subsequent disease risk. In a community-based study in California, 60 percent of nonsmoking participants reported secondhand smoke exposure during their lifetime, defined as at least one hour per day for at least one year (Berglund et al. 1999). However, biomarker data from other studies indicate higher percentages for secondhand smoke exposure. Data from the Third National Health and Nutrition Examination Survey (NHANES III) showed a detectable level of cotinine in 88 percent of nonsmoking adults (Pirkle et al. 1996).

Many investigators have validated questionnaire assessments of current exposures to secondhand smoke using biomarkers, specifically cotinine (Haley et al. 1989; Jarvis et al. 1991; Hammond et al. 1993; Pirkle et al. 1996; Al-Delaimy et al. 2000; Mannino et al. 2001). These studies have demonstrated that persons who were classified as having high levels of secondhand smoke exposure (often defined as living with a smoker) had higher levels of biomarkers in biologic samples of serum, urine, saliva, or hair when compared with persons who had low levels of exposure (often defined as not living with a smoker). Because there is no known biomarker that assesses long-term or temporally remote exposures, researchers still use questionnaires. For example, Coghlin and colleagues (1989) evaluated the reliability of a questionnaire and a personal diary by measuring the individual exposure of each study participant during a one-week period. The questionnaire and the personal diary were both used to collect information on the number of smokers the participants were exposed to, and the proximity and duration of exposure. The investigators found a high correlation (r^2 [prediction values] = 0.98) between the exposure score derived from data recorded in the personal diaries and the log of nicotine concentrations (r^2 measures the strength of the linear model that was used).

Airborne Concentrations

Measuring airborne concentrations of secondhand smoke constituents provides estimates of the level of an exposure and identifies the environments in which the exposure occurred. These measurements can be made using personal monitors, a form of assessing direct exposures (Hammond et al. 1987, 1988, 1993; Coghlin et al. 1989; Mattson et al. 1989; Kado et al. 1991; Emmons et al. 1994; Jenkins et al. 1996a), or monitors that evaluate the concentrations in various microenvironments, a form of assessing

indirect exposures (Henderson et al. 1989; Leaderer and Hammond 1991; Marbury et al. 1993; Hammond 1999). Measurements of airborne contaminants can also evaluate the efficacy of various control measures (Vaughan and Hammond 1990; Hammond et al. 1995; Emmons et al. 2001; Hammond 2002). Concentrations are typically assessed by measuring specific components of secondhand smoke referred to as tracers.

Studies have used several airborne constituents of tobacco as tracers, and their advantages and disadvantages are reviewed in Chapter 3 (Assessment of Exposure to Secondhand Smoke) of this report. As noted in that chapter, the concentration of secondhand smoke in any given location will depend on the number of cigarettes smoked in that location, the size of the room, the exchange of air in that room with outdoor air (whether windows are open, or how much air is circulated by natural means and by mechanical systems), and the interaction of the tobacco smoke with surfaces in the room. Because each of these factors has a range of values across locations, the concentration of secondhand smoke varies across settings. This variation results in a distribution of secondhand smoke concentrations in each type of setting. For example, Rogge and colleagues (1994) found a wider range of concentrations in locations such as workplaces and restaurants than in the home because a wider range exists in the number of smokers, the size of the rooms, and the exchange rates of indoor with outdoor air.

Biomarkers

Biomarkers provide an indicator of the internal dose of secondhand smoke and reflect exposure (Chapter 3, Assessment of Exposure to Secondhand Smoke). Persons with comparable exposures to secondhand smoke can have different levels of a marker because of individual variations in factors that determine uptake, metabolism, and elimination of the biomarker (Pirkle et al. 1996; Jaakkola and Samet 1999). Cotinine is the biomarker most frequently used to measure tobacco smoke doses, including doses from secondhand smoke (Benowitz 1999). Cotinine has a half-life ranging from 7 to 40 hours in adults and 32 to 38 hours in children (Jaakkola and Jaakkola 1997) and can be measured in serum, urine, saliva, hair, and breast milk. Studies show that cotinine measurements separated current active smokers from current nonsmokers with a high degree of validity and were used to identify people with current and high levels of secondhand smoke exposure (Pirkle et al. 1996; Mannino et al. 2001). Given its half-life, investigators have demonstrated that cotinine levels are generally not influenced by an exposure that occurred more than two to four days before the testing (Benowitz 1996). However, cotinine levels increased in people using nonsmoking-related sources of nicotine, such as nicotine patches or spit tobacco. Other biomarkers of tobacco smoke exposure, such as 4-aminobiphenyl adducts or nitrosamines, have not been widely used in population studies and are not discussed in this chapter (Jaakkola and Samet 1999).

Estimates of Exposure

National Trends in Biomarkers of Exposure

Beginning in 1988, researchers used serum cotinine measurements to assess exposures to secondhand smoke in the United States within the NHANES. The NHANES is conducted by the National Center for Health Statistics (NCHS), Centers for Disease Control and Prevention (CDC), and is designed to examine a nationally representative sample of the U.S. civilian (noninstitutionalized) population based upon a complex, stratified, multistage probability cluster sampling design (see http://www.cdc.gov/nchs/nhanes.htm). The protocols include a home interview followed by a physical examination in a mobile examination center, where blood samples are drawn for serum cotinine analysis. NHANES III, conducted from 1988 to 1994, was the first national survey of secondhand smoke exposure of the entire U.S. population aged 4 through 74 years. There were two phases: Phase I from 1988 to 1991, and Phase II from 1991 to 1994. There were no further studies between 1995 and 1998. In 1999, NCHS resumed NHANES on a continuous basis and completed a new nationally representative sample every two years. This more recent NHANES (1999) also began to draw blood samples for serum cotinine analyses from participants aged three years and older.

Researchers have reported serum cotinine levels in nonsmokers from the NHANES for four distinct intervals within the overall time period of 14 years, from 1988 through 2002: Phase I and Phase II of NHANES III, NHANES 1999–2000, and NHANES 2001–2002 (Pirkle et al. 1996, 2006). Researchers have reported additional data on serum cotinine levels in nonsmokers from NHANES 1999–2002 in the *National Report on Human Exposure to Environmental Chemicals* (CDC 2001a, 2003, 2005). To maintain comparability among survey intervals, trend data are only reported for participants aged four or more years in each study interval (Pirkle et al. 2006). Factors that affect nicotine metabolism, such as age, race, and the level of exposure to secondhand smoke, also influence cotinine levels (Caraballo et al. 1998; Mannino et al. 2001). Because cotinine levels reflect exposures that occurred within two to three days, they represent patterns of usual exposure (Jarvis et al. 1987; Benowitz 1996; Jaakkola and Jaakkola 1997).

Studies document NHANES serum cotinine levels in both children and adult nonsmokers (Pirkle et al. 1996, 2006; CDC 2001a, 2003, 2005). Nonsmoking adults were defined in these studies as persons whose serum cotinine concentrations were 10 nanograms per milliliter (ng/mL) or less, who reported no tobacco or nicotine use in the five days before the mobile examination center visit, and who were self-reported former smokers or lifetime nonsmokers. In NHANES III, the laboratory limit of detection was 0.050 ng/mL. However, the laboratory methods have continued to improve, and the detection limit was recently lowered to 0.015 ng/mL (CDC 2005; Pirkle et al. 2006). Additionally, researchers have categorized serum cotinine concentrations by age, race, and ethnicity. The racial and ethnic categories are non-Hispanic White, non-Hispanic Black, Mexican American, or "Other," and are self-reported. The category of "Other" was included in these reports in mean and percentile estimates for the total population but not in the geometric mean estimates because of small sample sizes (CDC 2005; Pirkle et al. 2006).

Figure 4.1 shows the overall proportion of all nonsmokers aged four or more years with serum cotinine levels of 0.050 ng/mL or greater for the four survey periods. Pirkle and colleagues (1996) reported detectable levels of serum cotinine among nearly all nonsmokers (87.9 percent) during Phase I (1988–1991) of NHANES III. Exposures among nonsmokers have declined significantly since that time

Figure 4.1   Trends in exposure* of nonsmokers[†] to secondhand smoke in the U.S. population, NHANES[‡] 1988–2002

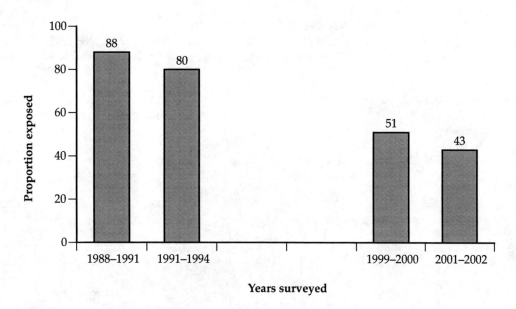

*Serum cotinine ≥0.05 nanograms per milliliter.
[†]Aged ≥4 years.
[‡]NHANES = National Health and Nutrition Examination Survey.
Source: Adapted from Pirkle et al. 2006.

(CDC 2005). The proportion of U.S. nonsmokers with cotinine concentrations of 0.050 ng/mL or greater fell to 43 percent in NHANES 2001–2002 (Pirkle et al. 2006).

Pirkle and colleagues (2006) provided additional data on the levels and distribution of serum cotinine concentrations in U.S. nonsmokers during 1988–2002. Trends in the adjusted geometric mean cotinine concentrations (adjusted for age, race, and gender) are in Table 4.1. Since Phase I of NHANES III, secondhand smoke exposures measured by serum cotinine concentrations in U.S. nonsmokers aged four or more years have declined by about 75 percent (from 0.247 ng/mL to 0.061 ng/mL). While declines among children aged 4 through 11 years and young persons aged 12 through 19 years also have been notable, the declines have been smaller than those among adults aged 20 through 74 years. Trends among racial and ethnic categories were also stratified by age: 4 through 11 years, 12 through 19 years, and 20 through 74 years. Pirkle and colleagues (2006) noted that serum cotinine levels in NHANES differed by race and ethnicity. Overall, in the order of the adjusted mean cotinine

concentrations during each of the four time periods, concentrations among Mexican Americans were less than those of non-Hispanic Whites, which were less than those of non-Hispanic Blacks; the non-Hispanic Black mean cotinine concentrations were significantly higher during each of the four time periods (Pirkle et al. 2006).

Current patterns of secondhand smoke exposure are reflected in the NHANES 1999–2002 serum cotinine concentrations (Table 4.2). As noted in Figure 4.1, the proportion of U.S. nonsmokers with serum cotinine levels of 0.050 ng/mL or greater has declined since NHANES III to less than 45 percent. However, the proportion of children and nonsmoking adults with serum cotinine levels of 0.050 ng/mL or greater in NHANES 1999–2002 differs significantly by age, from 59.6 percent among children aged 3 through 11 years to 35.7 percent among nonsmoking adults aged 60 through 74 years. Additionally, the median cotinine concentration in the serum is significantly higher in children aged 3 through 11 years (0.09 ng/mL) than in older adults (0.035 ng/mL) (CDC 2005). Children aged 3 through 11 years and

Table 4.1 Trends in serum cotinine levels (nanograms per milliliter) of nonsmokers* stratified by age, gender, race, and ethnicity, United States, 1988–2002

Population		NHANES III, Phase I 1988–1991	NHANES III, Phase II 1991–1994	NHANES 1999–2000	NHANES 2001–2002	% decline from 1988–1991 to 2001–2002
Overall						
Aged ≥4 years	Geometric mean[†]	0.247	0.182	0.106	0.061	75.3
	95% CI[‡]	0.219–0.277	0.165–0.202	0.094–0.119	0.049–0.076	
Aged 4–11 years						
Male	Geometric mean	0.283	0.234	0.166	0.098	65.4
	95% CI	0.223–0.360	0.188–0.291	0.105–0.262	0.064–0.151	
Female	Geometric mean	0.328	0.285	0.172	0.115	64.9
	95% CI	0.240–0.449	0.235–0.345	0.113–0.262	0.075–0.177	
Race and ethnicity						
Non-Hispanic White	Geometric mean	0.295	0.255	0.171	0.100	
	95% CI	0.226–0.385	0.214–0.303	0.100–0.293	0.061–0.165	
Non-Hispanic Black	Geometric mean	0.534	0.460	0.284	0.261	
	95% CI	0.387–0.738	0.393–0.538	0.249–0.324	0.188–0.361	
Mexican American	Geometric mean	0.192	0.125	0.080	0.060	
	95% CI	0.148–0.250	0.107–0.145	0.066–0.097	0.042–0.086	
Aged 12–19 years						
Male	Geometric mean	0.346	0.239	0.189	0.090	74.0
	95% CI	0.255–0.470	0.190–0.300	0.138–0.258	0.061–0.132	
Female	Geometric mean	0.280	0.228	0.156	0.078	72.1
	95% CI	0.223–0.353	0.175–0.298	0.124–0.197	0.048–0.126	
Race and ethnicity						
Non-Hispanic White	Geometric mean	0.301	0.219	0.170	0.074	
	95% CI	0.228–0.396	0.174–0.276	0.139–0.210	0.044–0.123	
Non-Hispanic Black	Geometric mean	0.515	0.460	0.263	0.227	
	95% CI	0.392–0.677	0.374–0.567	0.229–0.303	0.191–0.270	
Mexican American	Geometric mean	0.179	0.143	0.095	0.063	
	95% CI	0.139–0.229	0.126–0.162	0.082–0.110	0.045–0.089	

Table 4.1   Continued

Population		NHANES III, Phase I 1988–1991	NHANES III, Phase II 1991–1994	NHANES 1999–2000	NHANES 2001–2002	% decline from 1988–1991 to 2001–2002
Aged ≥20 years						
Male	Geometric mean	0.293	0.199	0.106	0.067	77.1
	95% CI	0.259–0.332	0.178–0.222	0.092–0.122	0.054–0.082	
Female	Geometric mean	0.188	0.138	0.078	0.042	77.7
	95% CI	...215	0.120–0.159	0.072–0.085	0.035–0.050	
			0.151	0.085	0.044	
		...244	0.133–0.172	0.077–0.095	0.036–0.055	
			0.299	0.135	0.129	
		...494	0.271–0.330	0.116–0.157	0.101–0.163	
			0.138	0.078	0.058	
		...251	0.117–0.162	0.066–0.093	0.040–0.083	

Survey (NHANES) study intervals.
...atory limit of detection (LOD) were assigned a value of LOD/square

Environmental Sites of Exposure

The principal places where studies have measured exposures to secondhand smoke represent key microenvironments: homes, worksites, and public places such as restaurants, malls, and bars. The contributions of these different locations to total personal exposures vary across different groups. For example, the dominant site of exposure for children is the home, whereas worksites are typically important exposure locations for nonsmoking adults who may not be exposed at home.

People spend most of their time at home, which is potentially the most important location of secondhand smoke exposure for people who live with regular smokers (Klepeis 1999). Because the workplace is second only to the home as the location where adults spend most of their time, smoking in the workplace has been a major contributor to total secondhand smoke exposure. The National Human Activity Pattern

Table 4.2   Serum cotinine levels among nonsmokers aged 3 years and older, NHANES* 1999–2002

Age group	Median cotinine level (SE†) (95% CI‡)	% with levels ≥0.05 ng/mL§ (SE) (95% CI)	% with at least 1 smoker in the home (SE) (95% CI)	Total population (2000)	Estimated number of persons (in millions) with serum cotinine levels ≥0.05 ng/mL
≥3 years	<LODᐃ (<LOD–0.52)	47.0 (1.9) (43.0–50.9)	11.1 (0.45) (10.2–12.0)	270,005,230	126.9
3–19 years	0.08 (0.01) (0.06–0.11)	57.7 (2.8) (52.0–63.3)	22.6 (1.4) (19.9–25.6)	69,056,589	39.8
3–11 years	0.09 (0.02) (0.06–0.12)	59.6 (2.9) (53.5–65.4)	24.9 (1.8) (21.5–28.7)	36,697,776	21.9
12–19 years	0.07 (0.01) (0.05–0.10)	55.6 (3.1) (49.1–61.9)	19.9 (1.3) (17.4–22.7)	32,358,813	18.0
≥20 years	<LOD (<LOD–<LOD)	42.8 (1.9) (39.0–46.6)	6.56 (0.32) (5.93–7.25)	200,948,641	86.0
20–39 years	<LOD (<LOD–0.066)	49.2 (2.9) (43.3–55.2)	6.85 (0.77) (5.43–8.61)	81,562,389	40.1
40–59 years	<LOD (<LOD–<LOD)	41.6 (2.2) (37.1–46.2)	7.3 (0.86) (5.73–9.26)	73,589,052	30.6
≥60 years	<LOD (<LOD–<LOD)	35.7 (1.7) (32.3–39.4)	5.12 (0.52) (4.15–6.3)	45,797,200	16.3

*NHANES = National Health and Nutrition Examination Survey.
†SE = Standard error.
‡CI = Confidence interval.
§ng/mL = Nanograms per milliliter.
ᐃLOD = Limit of detection (0.05 ng/mL).
Sources: U.S. Bureau of the Census 2005; Centers for Disease Control and Prevention, National Center for Health Statistics, unpublished data.

Survey (NHAPS), conducted from 1992 to 1994, interviewed 9,386 randomly chosen U.S. residents about their activities and exposures to secondhand smoke (Klepeis 1999; Klepeis et al. 2001). For those persons reporting secondhand smoke exposure of at least one minute, the average daily duration of the exposure and the percentage of respondents who reported an exposure in each indoor locale were as follows:

- 305 minutes in the home (58 percent);
- 363 minutes in the office or factory (10 percent);
- 249 minutes in schools or public buildings (6 percent);
- 143 minutes in bars or restaurants (23 percent);
- 198 minutes in malls or stores (7 percent);
- 79 minutes in vehicles (33 percent); and
- 255 minutes in other indoor locations (6 percent) (Klepeis 1999).

Even for adults who live in homes where smoking routinely occurs, the workplace can add significantly to this exposure. Among NHANES III participants who lived in smoke-free homes, a workplace that permitted smoking was typically the major contributor to their total secondhand smoke exposure (Pirkle et al. 1996).

Studies have shown that restaurants can be important sites of exposures to children as well as adults (Maskarinec et al. 2000; McMillen et al. 2003; Skeer and Siegel 2003; Siegel et al. 2004), and other public places may also contribute substantially to exposures of selected segments of the population. Finally, persons who cannot move about freely, such as those who live in nursing homes, mental institutions, or correctional facilities, may find such exposures unavoidable.

Exposure in the Home

Secondhand smoke exposure at home can be substantial for both children and adults (Jenkins et al. 1996a; Pirkle et al. 1996; Klepeis 1999; Klepeis et al. 2001). This section considers children exposed to secondhand smoke at home separately from adults who are exposed at home because the patterns are different for the two groups (Mannino et al. 1996, 1997). The definition of "children" varies across the studies cited in this report. There are also separate data for special populations, including children with asthma, pregnant women, and persons living in the inner city.

Representative Surveys of Children

Researchers have conducted a number of local (Greenberg et al. 1989), state (King et al. 1998), and national (Mannino et al. 1996) surveys of childhood exposure to secondhand smoke. One of the best data sources available on children's secondhand smoke exposure in the home is the National Health Interview Survey (NHIS). This information can be derived from NHIS data by correlating data on smoking in the home with data on households with children. NHIS data shows that the proportion of children aged 6 years and younger who are regularly exposed to secondhand smoke in their homes fell from 27 percent in 1994 to 20 percent in 1998. Most surveys were primarily based on the indirect indicator of one or more smoking adults in a home; estimates of the percentages exposed in the home ranged from 54 to 75 percent of the children (Lebowitz and Burrows 1976; Schilling et al. 1977; Ferris et al. 1985). A 1988 survey using an indirect indicator estimated that 48.9 percent of the children studied had experienced postnatal exposures to secondhand smoke (Overpeck and Moss 1991). Exposure prevalence was higher for children in poverty (63.6 percent) or for those whose mothers had less than 12 years of education (66.7 percent). An analysis of National Health Interview Survey (NHIS) data for 1994 showed that 35 percent of U.S. children lived in homes where they had contact with a smoker at least one day per week (Schuster et al. 2002).

Use of the indirect approach assumes that the presence of a smoking adult in the household results in exposure of children to secondhand smoke. Over time, as more people recognized the health effects from exposure in the home and implemented in-home smoking policies, the presence of smoking adults in the home has become a less valid indicator of exposure. In a 1991 survey of U.S. adults, 11.8 percent of current smokers reported that because no smoking had occurred in their homes in the two weeks before the survey, their children had not been exposed to secondhand smoke in the home (Mannino et al. 1996). Using data from the California Tobacco Survey, Gilpin and colleagues (2001) found that the proportion of households prohibiting smoking increased from 50.9 percent in 1993 to 72.8 percent in 1999 (Gilpin et al. 2001). The increase was greater in homes with smokers, from 20.1 percent in 1993 to 47.2 percent in 1999 (Pierce et al. 1998; Gilpin et al. 2001). The survey did not capture data from nonfamily members who may have smoked in the home, nor would it have addressed the contamination of one dwelling from smokers in another within a multiresidence building.

Other analyses have used questionnaires that ask specifically about the number of cigarettes smoked in the home to determine whether children were exposed to secondhand smoke. A 1991 nationally representative survey estimated that 31.2 percent of U.S. children were exposed daily to secondhand smoke in their homes, with an additional 5.8 percent exposed at home at least one day in the previous two weeks (Mannino et al. 1996). This exposure varied significantly by socioeconomic status (SES) (46.5 percent for a lower SES versus 22.5 percent for a higher SES) and by region of the country, with the lowest exposure (24.3 percent) in the western part of the United States (Mannino et al. 1996). In Phase I of the NHANES III (collected from 1988 to 1991), 43 percent of children aged 2 months through 11 years lived in a home with at least one smoker (Pirkle et al. 1996). In NHANES 1999–2002, the proportion of children aged 3 through 11 years living with one or more smokers in the household was 24.9 percent (Table 4.2). However, 59.6 percent of children aged 3 through 11 years had a serum cotinine concentration of 0.05 ng/mL or higher. State and local surveys have documented higher levels of reported exposure. In a 1985 study from New Mexico, 60 to 70 percent of the children had been exposed to secondhand smoke (Coultas et al. 1987). In a 1986 study of North Carolina infants, 56 percent had been exposed (Margolis et al. 1997). On the basis of self-reported data on smoking among household residents, CDC estimated in 1996 that 21.9 percent of U.S. children had been exposed to secondhand smoke in their homes (CDC 1997). The prevalence of exposure varied by state, from a low of 11.7 percent in Utah to a high of 34.2 percent in Kentucky. However, the data on serum cotinine concentrations suggest that these estimates are low.

As noted above, since 1988 the NHANES has provided nationally representative measurements of serum cotinine levels in both children and adults (Pirkle et al. 1996, 2006; CDC 2001a, 2003, 2005). Figure 4.1 and Table 4.1 show overall U.S. trends in exposure measured by serum cotinine concentrations. Although exposures have declined among both children and adults since Phase I of NHANES III (1988–1991), the percentage of the decline was smaller among children aged 4 through 11 years. In the NHANES 2001–2002, mean cotinine levels were highest among children aged 4 through 11 years (non-Hispanic Black children in particular) (Pirkle et al. 2006). Measured cotinine concentrations were more than twice as high among children aged 4 through 11 years than among nonsmoking adults aged 20 or more years, and the levels of non-Hispanic Black children were two to three times higher than those of non-Hispanic White and Mexican American children. While metabolic factors can also influence cotinine levels (Caraballo et al. 1998; Mannino et al. 2001), the racial and ethnic differences in serum cotinine concentrations overall, and particularly among children, presumably reflect greater exposures to secondhand smoke among non-Hispanic Black populations (Pirkle et al. 2006).

Table 4.2 compares current estimates of national exposure by age. In Phases I and II of NHANES III (1988–1994), 84.7 percent of children aged 4 through 11 years had a serum cotinine concentration of 0.05 ng/mL or greater; 99.1 percent of children with a reported exposure in the home and 75.6 percent of children without any reported exposure had measurable cotinine levels (Mannino et al. 2001). The strongest predictor of cotinine levels in children was the number of cigarettes smoked daily in the home, but other factors were also significant predictors, including race, ethnicity, age of the child, size of the home, and region of the country (Mannino et al. 2001). In the most recent estimates of exposure (Table 4.2), 59.6 percent of children aged 3 through 11 years had a serum cotinine concentration of 0.05 ng/mL or greater, and 24.9 percent reported living with at least one smoker in the household. Based upon this estimate of the proportion of children aged 3 through 11 years living with a smoker in the household, an estimated nine million children or more in this age range may be exposed to secondhand smoke. However, serum cotinine measurements indicate an even greater exposed population of almost 22 million children aged 3 through 11 years in the year 2000.

Trends in exposure of children to secondhand smoke indicate that levels of exposure have declined significantly since Phase I of NHANES III (Pirkle et al. 2006). The multiple factors related to this decline are still being studied. Several researchers have suggested that a major component of this decline is related to the decrease in parental smoking (Shopland et al. 1996) and to the increase in household smoking restrictions (Gilpin et al. 2001). Data from the 1992 and 2000 NHIS (Soliman et al. 2004) indicate that self-reported exposure of nonsmokers to secondhand smoke in homes with children declined significantly in the 1990s from 36 percent in 1992 to 25 percent in 2000. Because researchers have identified parental smoking in the home as a major source for exposure among younger

children (Mannino et al. 2001), this decline in reported home exposures to secondhand smoke suggests that voluntary changes in home policies and smoking practices of adults in homes where children reside are a major contributing factor to the observed declines in serum cotinine concentrations among children since Phase I of NHANES III.

Protecting children from secondhand smoke exposure in homes has been the focus of the U.S. Environmental Protection Agency's parental outreach and educational programs to promote smoke-free home rules for the last decade. The potential for exposing children to secondhand smoke has dropped even further as more local and state governments restrict smoking in public areas (CDC 1999). Jarvis and colleagues (2000) documented similar findings in data from Great Britain. From 1988 to 1996, the proportion of homes without smokers increased from 48 to 55 percent. During this same period, the geometric mean salivary cotinine levels decreased from 0.47 to 0.28 ng/mL among children with nonsmoking parents, and from 3.08 to 2.25 ng/mL among children with two smoking parents (Jarvis et al. 2000).

Additional studies that document exposure of children in the United States to secondhand smoke in the home include three studies that reported the presence of some form of smoking ban at home in many households (Norman et al. 1999; Kegler and Malcoe 2002; McMillen et al. 2003). Norman and colleagues (1999) surveyed a representative sample of 6,985 California adults. Kegler and Malcoe (2002) studied 380 rural, low-income Native American and White parents from northeastern Oklahoma. McMillan and colleagues (2003) conducted a telephone survey of more than 4,500 eligible adults across the United States. Two other studies also focused on prevalence and patterns of childhood household secondhand smoke exposure in the United States: CDC (2001b) reported on the Behavioral Risk Factor Surveillance System (BRFSS) telephone interviews that took place in 20 states, and Schuster and colleagues (2002) reported on personal interviews with 45,335 respondents from around the country in the 1994 NHIS.

Representative Surveys of Adults

Representative surveys of adult household exposures to secondhand smoke in the United States were conducted at the national, state, and local levels to determine the prevalence of exposure in the home (Mannino et al. 1997; King et al. 1998). When analyzing these surveys, researchers need to consider that some current smokers may misclassify themselves as lifetime nonsmokers or as former smokers (Haley et al. 1983; Coultas et al. 1988). Exposures at home were assessed using questionnaires and cotinine levels. In a California study that was conducted from 1979 to 1980, 24 percent of 37,881 adult lifetime nonsmokers and former smokers reported household exposures (Friedman et al. 1983). When data from Phase I of NHANES III (1988–1991) were analyzed, Pirkle and colleagues (1996) showed that 17.4 percent of nonsmokers reported exposures to secondhand smoke in the home. Mannino and colleagues (1997) reported similar findings when they analyzed data from another national survey that was conducted in 1991: 16.4 percent of lifetime nonsmokers and 19.2 percent of former smokers reported exposures in the home. In findings similar to those among children, there is also evidence that certain subgroups of adults are more likely to be exposed to secondhand smoke. For example, in a 1985–1986 study of 4,200 persons in Philadelphia, an industrialized and urban population, 60 percent reported household exposures (Dayal et al. 1994).

Table 4.1 shows trends in exposure among U.S. nonsmoking adults aged 20 or more years measured by serum cotinine levels. Among all adults in this age group, the geometric mean serum cotinine concentration declined more than 77 percent between Phase I of NHANES III (1988–1991) and NHANES 2001–2002: from 0.293 to 0.067 ng/mL among men and from 0.188 to 0.042 ng/mL among women. Analyses indicate that serum cotinine levels of adult nonsmokers were higher among adults who reported exposures at home or in the workplace (Pirkle et al. 1996). Recent data from NHANES 1999–2002 (CDC, NCHS, unpublished data) indicate that among younger nonsmoking adults aged 20 through 39 years, the proportion who reported living with at least one smoker is much lower (6.9 percent) compared with nonsmoking adults aged 20 through 39 years with a current job who reported that they could smell smoke at work (13.2 percent). However, among older nonsmoking adults aged 40 through 59 years, the proportion who reported living with a smoker (7.3 percent) was similar to the proportion of nonsmoking adults aged 40 through 59 years with a current job who reported smelling smoke at work (9.8 percent). Finally, while older nonsmoking adults reported a slightly lower portion of nonsmokers living with at least one smoker (5.1 percent), a significantly lower proportion of that age group with a current job reported smelling smoke at work (2.0 percent). Thus, particularly for adults aged 20 through 59 years, the worksite remains an important environment for exposure to secondhand smoke.

Susceptible Populations

Some populations may be particularly susceptible to secondhand smoke exposure. Examples include persons with asthma or other chronic respiratory diseases, and fetuses exposed to tobacco smoke components in utero either by maternal smoking or maternal exposure to secondhand smoke. In one 1994 community-based study in Seattle, 31 percent of children with asthma reported household exposures to secondhand smoke, but only 17 percent of children without asthma reported an exposure (Maier et al. 1997).

Studies have tracked smoking by pregnant women using several different data collection systems including natality surveys, NHIS, BRFSS, National Survey of Family Growth, and since 1989, birth certificates in nearly all states and the District of Columbia (CDC 2001a). The estimates from these different sources generally agree that the proportion of women who report smoking during pregnancy has decreased in recent years, from between 30 and 40 percent in the early 1980s to between 10 and 15 percent in the late 1990s. By 2003, only an estimated 10.7 percent of mothers of a live-born infant reported smoking during pregnancy. However, the prevalence of reported smoking was not uniform across all population groups or education levels. For example, a CDC report (CDC 2005) documented that 18 percent of American Indian or Alaska Native women reported smoking during pregnancy, but only 3 percent of Hispanic women reported smoking during pregnancy. And women with 9 to 11 years of education were far more likely to report smoking (25.5 percent) compared with women with 16 or more years of education (1.6 percent) (CDC 2005). Ebrahim and colleagues (2000) showed that the declining trend in smoking during pregnancy in recent years is primarily attributable to a decrease in smoking prevalence among women of childbearing age, rather than to an increase in smoking cessation during pregnancy. Of the women who reported smoking during pregnancy, most (68.6 percent) said that they had smoked 10 or fewer cigarettes daily.

Researchers have also found that pregnant women may conceal their smoking from clinicians (Windsor et al. 1993; Ford et al. 1997). Thus, smoking during pregnancy may be underestimated. Estimates of the prevalence of smoking during pregnancy are also sensitive to how smoking was defined in a study, which may range from any smoking at any time during pregnancy to smoking during the final three months of pregnancy.

Complicating the interpretation of findings on health effects of secondhand smoke exposure in very young children is evidence that a large proportion of children are exposed both prenatally and postnatally. Overpeck and Moss (1991) used CDC data to show that 96 percent of children with prenatal exposures also had postnatal exposures. The investigators found that 29 percent of the children had been exposed prenatally to maternal smoking and that an additional 21 percent had been exposed to secondhand smoke postnatally. A second source of involuntary smoking for a developing fetus is the exposure of a pregnant woman to secondhand smoke. The factors that predicted prenatal maternal exposure to secondhand smoke were similar to those associated with secondhand smoke exposure in general, such as low SES, low levels of education, and living in a small home (Overpeck and Moss 1991).

Although national surveys have not specifically asked about secondhand smoke exposure during pregnancy, they have provided estimates of exposure among women of childbearing age. In NHANES III, 18 percent of nonsmoking females aged 17 years and older reported exposures to secondhand smoke. However, the percentages of reported exposures were higher among women of childbearing age: 31 percent for 17- through 19-year-olds, 30 percent for 20- through 29-year-olds, and 26 percent for 30- through 39-year-olds (Pirkle et al. 1996). Of the nontobacco users surveyed in 1988–1991, 88 percent had detectable levels of serum cotinine (>0.050 ng/mL), a finding that suggests an unreported or unknown exposure. These findings are consistent with results from a 1985 study of 1,231 nonsmoking pregnant women in Maine, which found that 70 percent of the participants had cotinine levels above 0.5 ng/mL (Haddow et al. 1987).

Measurements of Airborne Tracers in Homes

Numerous studies have measured secondhand smoke concentrations in homes (Leaderer and Hammond 1991; Hammond et al. 1993; Marbury et al. 1993; Manning et al. 1994; O'Connor et al. 1995; Jenkins et al. 1996a,b; Phillips et al. 1996, 1997a,b, 1998a–h, 1999a,b). Concentrations of secondhand smoke components are higher at the time that the cigarettes are smoked compared with a few hours later. Measurements taken only during periods of smoking document higher concentrations than samples measured during both smoking and nonsmoking periods. For example, Muramatsu and colleagues (1984) measured both nicotine and particulate matter sequentially for 10 hours in an office. They found that the 30-minute

nicotine samples ranged from 2 to 26 micrograms per cubic meter ($\mu g/m^3$) during the workday; most values ranged between 5 and 15 $\mu g/m^3$. The 10-hour averaged concentration was 10 $\mu g/m^3$, which was based on a shorter time period than that used by other studies to obtain stable estimates. Most studies have measured concentrations averaged over longer periods of time, which include periods with and without smoking.

Studies have demonstrated a high correlation (Spearman rho correlation coefficient = 0.74, p <0.001) between nicotine concentrations measured in the family activity rooms and in the kitchens (Emmons et al. 2001), as well as between concentrations in the activity rooms and in the bedrooms (Spearman correlation coefficient = 0.91; 0.90 for homes of smokers only) (Marbury et al. 1993).

The results of several studies that measured nicotine concentrations in the homes of smokers in the United States are presented in Figure 4.2 and Table 4.3. Median nicotine concentrations were generally between 1 and 3 $\mu g/m^3$ (averaged over 14 hours to several weeks), with nicotine concentrations ranging from <0.1 to 8 $\mu g/m^3$ across the span from minimum to the 95th percentile. An exception was a study of 291 low-income homes in New England that found 4 homes with concentrations above 18 $\mu g/m^3$ (Emmons et al. 2001). Homes where smoking was restricted to the basement or the outdoors had lower mean nicotine concentrations of 0.3 $\mu g/m^3$ (Marbury et al. 1993).

Personal sampling of secondhand smoke exposure has yielded similar results with measured home exposure. In a study of exposure away from work (predominantly at home, lasting 16 hours), 306 nonsmokers who reported secondhand smoke exposure had a mean nicotine exposure of 2.7 $\mu g/m^3$ (median 1.2 $\mu g/m^3$), with a 95th percentile value of 7.9 in 1993 and 1994 (Jenkins et al. 1996a). Personal sampling of 100 people in Massachusetts during 1987 and 1988 found the median of a weekly average of nicotine concentrations to be 1.0 $\mu g/m^3$ for nonsmokers married to nonsmokers and 3.5 $\mu g/m^3$ for those married to smokers; the respective maximum values were 9.5 and 14 $\mu g/m^3$. These values included all exposures throughout the week in homes, workplaces, and public places (Coghlin et al. 1989, 1991). To evaluate secondhand smoke exposure among pregnant women, participants in two studies wore passive samplers (small personal monitors that measure secondhand smoke exposure) for one week. Although the two studies had similar designs, the investigators reported quite different results. Among 36 low-income pregnant women in Massachusetts, 80 percent were exposed to

Figure 4.2   Concentrations of nicotine in homes of U.S. smokers

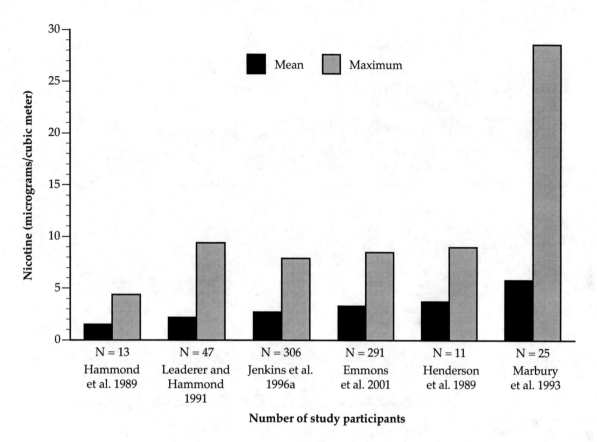

Note: Data are provided in detail in Table 4.3.

nicotine at 0.5 μg/m^3 or greater, and 25 percent were exposed at a concentration above 2.0 μg/m^3 (Hammond et al. 1993). The measured exposure was lower for 131 pregnant upper-middle-class women in Connecticut who reported secondhand smoke exposure, with a median of 0.1 μg/m^3 and a 90th percentile of 0.6 μg/m^3 (O'Connor et al. 1995).

International studies of secondhand smoke exposure sponsored by the tobacco industry (Jenkins et al. 1996a; Phillips et al. 1996, 1997a,b, 1998a–h, 1999a,b) followed a similar protocol where participants wore a sampling device for 16 to 24 hours. Figure 4.3 illustrates the median nicotine concentrations observed "away from work" (predominantly at home) in the United States compared with homes in Australia and in several European and Asian locations. U.S. homes had the second highest reported values after Beijing, which reported a median of 1.3 μg/m^3. Hong Kong homes reported 0.3 μg/m^3, which was consistent with a study of 300 Chinese homes in 18 provinces that

reported a 0.1 μg/m^3 weekly average concentration of nicotine in the homes of smokers (Hammond 1999).

Exposure in the Workplace

This section reviews studies that measured secondhand smoke exposure in the workplace, an important source of secondhand smoke exposure for nonsmoking adults (Klepeis 1999; Klepeis et al. 2001). These studies include surveys, biomarkers (Pirkle et al. 1996), or (more commonly) measurements of airborne nicotine (Vaughan and Hammond 1990; Hammond et al. 1995; Jenkins et al. 1996a; Hammond 1999).

Surveys of Workplaces with Policies Regarding Smoking

Large representative surveys of secondhand smoke workplace exposure have looked at patterns of exposure and the impact of policies to reduce

Table 4.3   Concentrations of nicotine in homes of U.S. smokers

Study	Population Year sampled	Measurement duration	Number of study participants
Hammond et al. 1989	North Carolina 1988	Weekly	13
Henderson et al. 1989	Lower income North Carolina 1987	14 hours	11
Leaderer and Hammond 1991	Randomly chosen New York 1986	1 week (winter)	47
Marbury et al. 1993	Children aged <2 years Living room and bedroom Minnesota 1989	1 week[†]	25
Jenkins et al. 1996a	Adults Personal sampling 16 cities	16 hours	306
Emmons et al. 2001	Lower income Massachusetts 1997–1998	Weekly	291

*NR = Data were not reported.
[†] Following the initial measure of exposure, measures were taken weekly for 8 weeks.

exposure. Although not all workplaces are smoke-free, policies toward smoking in workplace settings have changed dramatically since the publication of the 1986 Surgeon General's report (USDHHS 1986). For example, using data from the California Tobacco Survey, Gilpin and colleagues (2001) showed that the percentage of indoor workers in California who reported smoke-free workplaces had increased from 35 percent in 1990 to 93 percent in 1999. Shopland and colleagues (2001) analyzed data from the national Current Population Survey (CPS), a monthly survey of about 50,000 households conducted by the Bureau of the Census for the Bureau of Labor Statistics, and found that the proportion of workers who reported a smoke-free workplace policy had increased from 46 percent in 1993 to 69 percent in 1999. The 1999 data documented a low of 49 percent in Nevada and a high of 84 percent in Utah (Shopland et al. 2001). In an analysis of the 1993 CPS data, Farrelly and colleagues (1999) noted that the proportion of workers in smoke-free worksites also varied by industry, from a low of

30 percent in wholesale or retail trades to 73 percent in medical services. A similar analysis of the 1996 CPS data showed that the proportion of smoke-free work-sites ranged from a low of 44 percent in agriculture, forestry, fishing, mining, and construction to 82 percent in professional and related services (Sweeney et al. 2000).

However, having a smoke-free policy in the workplace does not assure workers that they will not be exposed to secondhand smoke. In a 1990 study from California, 9.3 percent of nonsmokers who worked in a "smoke-free" worksite reported at least one episode of exposure at work during the two weeks before the survey (Borland et al. 1992). This proportion was higher at 51 percent among nonsmokers working in sites without a smoking policy (Brancker 1990). In data from Phase I of NHANES III (1988–1991), 47.7 percent of adult nontobacco users who currently worked reported exposures at home or at the work-site (Pirkle et al. 1996). Nonsmoking workers who reported workplace exposures had higher geometric

	Concentrations of nicotine (micrograms per cubic meter [µg/m³])							
Geometric mean	Standard deviation	Median	25th percentile	90th percentile	95th percentile	Minimum	Maximum
1.5	1.1	1.4	NR*	NR	NR	1.1	4.4
3.74	0.5	3.6	NR	NR	7.5	0.8	9.0
2.2	2.4	1.0	0.2	8.0	8.5	<0.1	9.4
Living room 5.8	NR	3.0	NR	NR	9.0	0.1	28.6
Bedroom 2.7	NR	2.1	NR	NR	NR	NR	7.2
2.7	NR	1.2	NR	NR	7.9	NR	NR
3.3	5.0	1.6	0.3	8.5	10.4	0.3	45.1

mean levels of cotinine (0.32 ng/mL) compared with workers who did not report workplace or home exposures (0.13 ng/mL) (Pirkle et al. 1996). Recent data suggest that worksite exposures may be declining significantly since Phase I of NHANES III (1988–1991). In NHANES 1999–2002, the proportion of adults aged 20 or more years with a current job who reported smelling smoke at work was 8.94 percent (95 percent CI, 7.84–10.10) (CDC, NCHS, unpublished data).

Workplace Surveys

Hammond (1999) reviewed studies of exposures to secondhand smoke among U.S. workers. The earliest personal sampling of workplace secondhand smoke exposure involved railroad workers studied between 1981 and 1984. Investigators collected more than 625 nicotine samples from participants wearing personal samplers at four railroad locations (Hammond et al. 1988; Schenker et al. 1990). In 1983 and 1984, 275 personal samples were collected and levels were

analyzed by job type; 84 samples were collected from smokers and 191 from nonsmokers (Schenker et al. 1986, 1992; Hammond 1999). Among workers such as clerks and brakers who worked in small spaces, nonsmokers and smokers were exposed to similar levels of nicotine. For workers in other types of jobs (notably the repair shop workers), exposure was lower by more than an order of magnitude, possibly because of the large open space and ventilation of the shop. The range of nicotine exposure at work was notably greater among the nonsmoking railroad workers compared with exposures at home; minimum concentration values for all job categories were less than 0.1 µg/m³ and maximum values ranged up to 38 µg/m³. Half of the nonsmoking workers were exposed to more than 1 µg/m³ on at least one sampling day.

Many investigators have studied offices in the United States. Where smoking was allowed, there was a wide range of nicotine concentrations, from less than

Figure 4.3   Concentrations of nicotine away from work in 12 locations

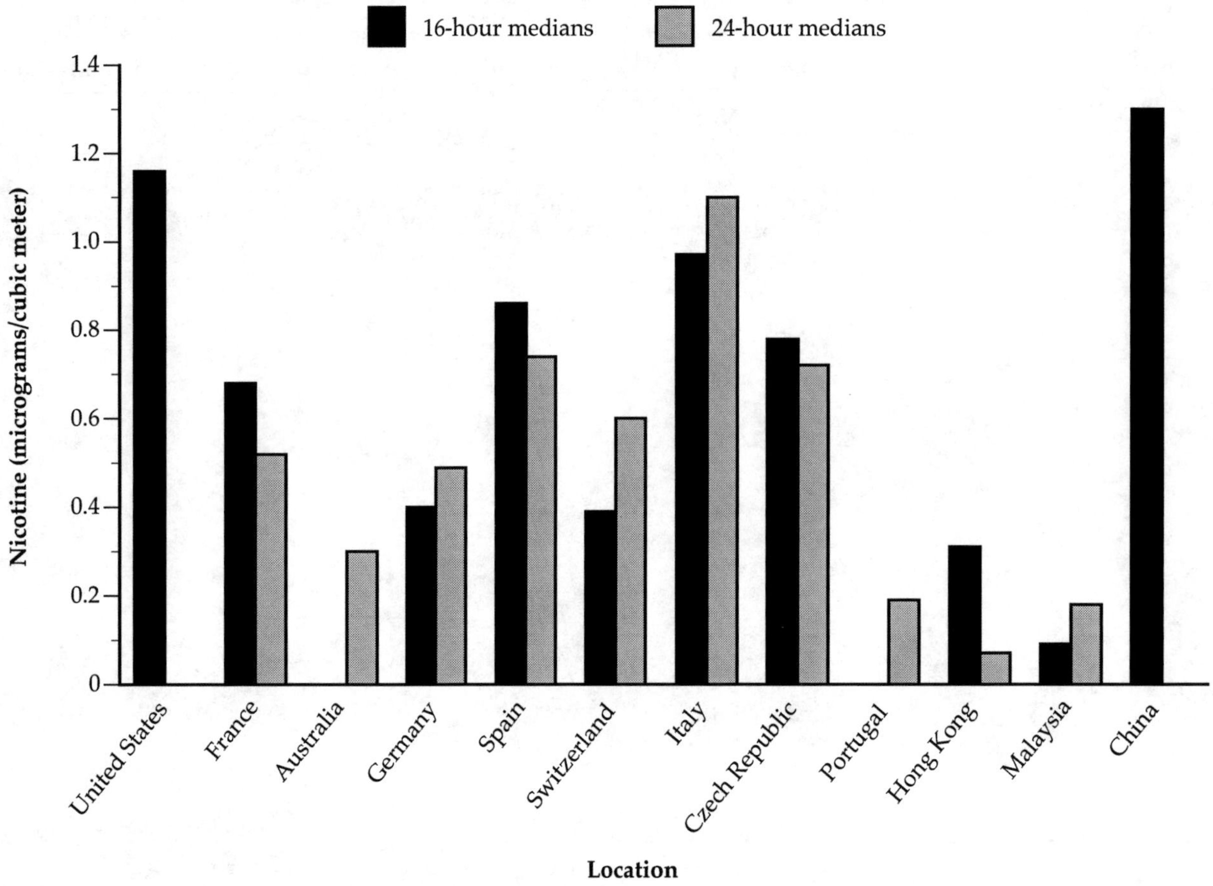

Sources: Jenkins et al. 1996a; Phillips et al. 1996, 1997a,b, 1998a–h, 1999a,b.

0.05 μg/m³ to about 70 μg/m³ (Table 4.4). For nearly half of the offices, the minimum value was more than 1 μg/m³. For offices where five or more samples were collected, median values were between 1 and 17 μg/m³, and average values were between 2 and 24.8 μg/m³. Most worksites had at least one sample above 10 μg/m³, and many studies reported concentrations greater than 40 μg/m³.

Offices at worksites that restricted smoking to designated areas generally had much lower concentrations of nicotine (Table 4.4 and Figure 4.4). Half of these worksites had a median concentration of less than 1 μg/m³, and only one site (Newspaper A) exceeded 2.5 μg/m³. The maximum concentrations in five out of eight workplaces were 1 to 2 μg/m³, but in the other three the maximum concentrations were 6.3, 13.7, and 16.7 μg/m³. Workplaces with smoking bans had much lower concentrations, with the medians and

averages at all worksites less than 1 μg/m³, except for one worksite, the weapons systems worksite that had a mean of 2.8 μg/m³. The maximum concentrations at three of these worksites were less than 1 μg/m³; the maximum concentrations for the other three were 1.9, 2.4, and 8.5 μg/m³. In one workplace, lower secondhand smoke concentrations were observed at the same location comparing measurements taken before and after smoking was restricted. Concentrations had declined by more than 90 percent as a result of restricting smoking (Vaughan and Hammond 1990). Thus, workplace policies decrease nicotine concentrations substantially but do not completely eliminate them. These results are consistent with questionnaire survey results cited above, where 9.3 percent of nonsmoking California workers in "smoke-free worksites" reported some secondhand smoke exposure.

A number of studies have measured the nicotine concentrations in a variety of other workplaces, including fire stations and manufacturing, printing, and medical facilities (Table 4.5). Although concentrations were lower in these settings than in offices, the results of the analyses showed that one-third of the workplaces that allowed smoking still had minimum values above 1 $\mu g/m^3$, and most workplaces had detectable levels of nicotine on all of the collected samples (Table 4.5). Two workplaces had maximum values above 50 $\mu g/m^3$, and most had at least one sample above 10 $\mu g/m^3$. Most of the median values were between 1 and 4 $\mu g/m^3$. Where smoking was restricted, the median dropped from 2.3 to 0.7 $\mu g/m^3$. Where smoking was banned, it dropped to 0.2 $\mu g/m^3$ (Hammond et al. 1995). Thus, smoking policies also effectively reduced secondhand smoke concentrations in these nonoffice settings (Figure 4.5).

Exposure in Public Places

Exposures to secondhand smoke in public places have been particular public health concerns for more than two decades. Although these sites are workplaces for some, they may now be the only source of secondhand smoke exposure for most of the U.S. population with no home or work exposures. Studies using biomarkers confirm that secondhand smoke exposure in public places continues to affect nonsmokers. Using NHANES III data, several investigators have shown that persons with no home or workplace exposures still had detectable levels of cotinine in their serum (Pirkle et al. 1996; Mannino et al. 2001). This finding suggests that many people are exposed to secondhand smoke in other locations.

Restaurants, Cafeterias, and Bars

Restaurants, cafeterias, and bars are worksites as well as public places where smoking is frequently unrestricted or restricted in a manner that does not effectively decrease exposure. Servers and bartenders working in environments where smoking is permitted may be exposed to high levels of secondhand smoke (Jarvis et al. 1992; Jenkins and Counts 1999). In a survey of 1,224 residents from Olmsted County, Minnesota, 57 percent of the respondents reported exposures to secondhand smoke: 44 percent reported exposures in restaurants, 21 percent reported exposures at work, and 19 percent reported exposures in bars (Kottke et al. 2001). A quarter of the respondents in the NHAPS study reported exposures in restaurants or bars on the

previous day for an average of two and one-half hours (Klepeis 1999; Klepeis et al. 2001). Restaurants may be the principal point of secondhand smoke exposure for children from nonsmoking homes, and an exposure of even a short duration may be relevant to acute effects, such as inducing or exacerbating an asthma attack (Chapter 6, Respiratory Effects in Children from Exposure to Secondhand Smoke).

In eating establishments, a wide variability in factors determines the concentration of secondhand smoke, including the size of the room, ventilation rate, number of smokers, and smoking rate. Furthermore, these concentrations vary throughout the day and evening. Concentrations measured for one to two hours during lunch or dinner are likely to be much higher than the average concentrations measured during a full day or week. The nicotine concentrations measured in restaurants have ranged from less than detectable to values of 70 $\mu g/m^3$ (Table 4.6).

Tobacco smoke has long been considered a nuisance that interferes with the enjoyment of food. One approach to reducing exposures of nonsmokers has been to establish smoking and nonsmoking sections in restaurants. Nonsmoking sections generally do have lower concentrations of secondhand smoke (Lambert et al. 1993; Hammond 1999), but they neither eliminate secondhand smoke nor reduce secondhand smoke concentrations to insignificant levels. The concentrations of nicotine in nonsmoking sections of restaurants persist at high levels. For example, a study of seven restaurants in Albuquerque, New Mexico, found that half of them had concentrations above 1 $\mu g/m^3$ in the nonsmoking sections (Lambert et al. 1993). Similar results were noted in more than half of 71 restaurants surveyed in Indiana where nicotine concentrations were above 2 $\mu g/m^3$ in the nonsmoking sections (Hammond and Perrino 2002). In a study of waiters exposed to secondhand smoke, the average nicotine concentration was as high as 5.8 $\mu g/m^3$, with the upper end of the range at 68 $\mu g/m^3$ (Maskarinec et al. 2000).

Hammond (1999) reported that nicotine concentrations in cafeterias were somewhat higher than in restaurants; average values were between 6 and 14 $\mu g/m^3$. Out of the 37 samples from company cafeterias in Massachusetts that allowed or restricted workplace smoking, two-thirds had nicotine concentrations that were above 5 $\mu g/m^3$. Secondhand smoke concentrations measured during lunchtime at a medical center cafeteria revealed large gradients between the smoking and nonsmoking sections. The concentrations were generally 25 to 40 $\mu g/m^3$ in the smoking section, 2 to 5 $\mu g/m^3$ in a nonsmoking section that was

Table 4.4   Occupational exposures to nicotine among nonsmoking office workers stratified by the smoking policy in effect at the time of the measurements

Study	Worksite description	Year sampled	Number of samples
	Smoking permitted		
Schenker et al. 1986, 1990, 1992	Railroad clerks (personal)	1983–1984	31
Carson and Erikson 1988	Multiple worksites	Before 1988	28
Crouse and Carson 1989	Multiple worksites	Before 1989	32
Eatough et al. 1989	Multiple worksites	NR	28
Miesner et al. 1989	Two office buildings	1987–1988	3
Coultas et al. 1990	Social worker office (personal)	1986–1987	1
	Attorney office (personal)	1986–1987	1
	Stockbroker (personal)	1986–1987	1
	Multiple worksites (personal)	1986–1987	5
	Travel agent (personal)	1986–1987	2
Oldaker et al. 1990	Multiple worksites	Before 1990	156
Turner and Binnie 1990	Multiple worksites	Before 1990	33
	Multiple worksites (naturally ventilated)	Before 1990	17
Vaughan and Hammond 1990	Telephone company	1987	13
Guerin et al. 1992	Multiple worksites	Before 1990	194
Hammond et al. 1995; Hammond 1999	Labels and paper products	1991–1992	7
	Tool manufacturing	1991–1992	7
	Die manufacturer	1991–1992	4
	Textile finishing B	1991–1992	2
	Sintering metal	1991–1992	7
	Specialty chemicals	1991–1992	7
	Textile finishing A	1991–1992	3
	Newspaper B	1991–1992	19
	Union headquarters[‡]	1991–1992	15
Jenkins et al. 1996a	Multiple sites (personal)	1993–1994	<136
Sterling et al. 1996	Building 2 (personal)	1994	12
	Building 1 (personal)	1994	13
	Smoking restricted		
Miesner et al. 1989	Two office buildings	1987–1988	2
Vaughan and Hammond 1990	Telephone company	1988	19
Hammond et al. 1995; Hammond 1999	Filtration products	1991–1992	6
	Fiber optics	1991–1992	4
	Work clothing	1991–1992	4
	Film and imaging	1991–1992	7
	Valve manufacturer	1991–1992	8
	Newspaper A	1991–1992	7

Concentrations of nicotine (micrograms per cubic meter [$\mu g/m^3$])					
Mean	Standard deviation	Geometric mean	Minimum	Median	Maximum
Smoking permitted					
6.9	6.7	3.2	<0.1	5.7	25.7
NR*	NR	7.2	LD[†]	NR	70.0
NR	NR	3.8	1.2	NR	24.0
6.0	NR	NR	4.1	NR	7.8
1.7	2.3	0.8	LD	0.6	4.3
2.5	NR	2.5	NR	2.5	NR
5.9	NR	5.9	NR	5.9	NR
7.2	NR	7.2	NR	7.2	NR
24.8	22.8	16.8	2.5	10.0	50.0
48.4	2.3	48.3	1.0	48.4	50.0
NR	NR	4.8	LD	NR	69.7
7.2	NR	NR	NR	LD	41.9
10.0	NR	NR	NR	LD	41.9
2.5	1.7	2.1	0.9	1.9	6.7
3.5	8.3	1.7	<1.6	NR	71.5
2.7	1.9	1.4	<0.05	2.6	6.0
3.5	4.9	3.5	0.8	1.4	14.5
5.0	4.2	3.2	0.7	5.1	9.1
5.1	2.8	4.7	3.1	5.1	7.1
5.8	8.9	1.6	0.3	0.9	20.2
6.2	7.8	2.0	<0.05	3.7	22.4
9.7	0.9	9.6	8.8	9.6	10.6
15.8	14.5	8.0	0.2	10.8	47.7
22.0	12.4	17.2	1.1	17.0	45.1[§]
NR	NR	NR	NR	1.9	>20.0[§]
1.8	NR	NR	1.1	1.7	2.3
2.0	NR	NR	0.3	1.6	4.7
Smoking restricted					
1.0	NR	NR	LD	1.0	2.0
0.3	0.2	0.2	<0.1	0.2	0.7
0.4	0.7	0.1	<0.05	0.1	1.7
0.5	0.4	0.4	0.2	0.4	1.0
0.6	0.5	0.5	0.3	0.4	1.4
2.7	2.2	2.0	0.6	1.8	6.3
4.2	4.5	2.5	0.5	2.5	13.7
7.9	5.9	5.2	0.6	7.6	16.7

Table 4.4   Continued

Study	Worksite description	Year sampled	Number of samples
	Smoking prohibited		
Miesner et al. 1989	Office building	1987–1988	2
Hammond et al. 1995; Hammond 1999	Hospital products	1991–1992	9
	Radar communications	1991–1992	4
	Computer chip equipment	1991–1992	1
	Infrared and imaging systems	1991–1992	8
	Aircraft components	1991–1992	5
	Weapons systems	1991–1992	3

*NR = Data were not reported.
†LD = Less than detectable.
‡Omits one data point, 130 μg/m³.
§95th percentile, as given in paper.
Source: Hammond 1999.

Figure 4.4   Occupational exposures to nicotine among groups of nonsmoking office workers

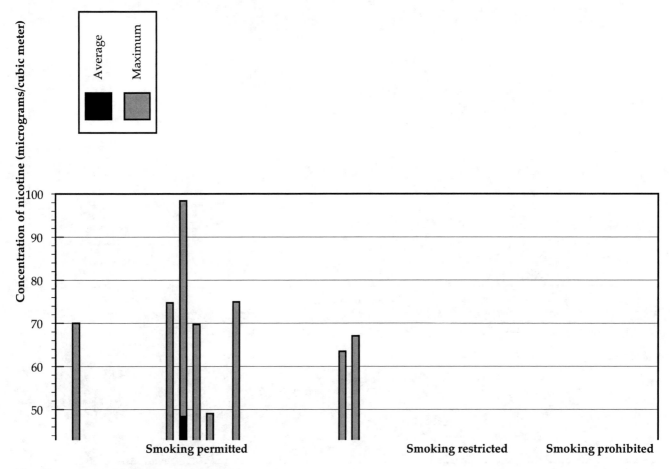

Note: Data are provided in detail in Table 4.4.

	Concentrations of nicotine (micrograms per cubic meter [$\mu g/m^3$])				
Mean	Standard deviation	Geometric mean	Minimum	Median	Maximum
		Smoking prohibited			
0.2	NR	NR	LD	0.2	0.4
0.1	0.2	0.1	<0.05	<0.05	0.4
0.4	0.3	0.2	<0.05	0.3	0.8
0.6	NR	NR	NR	0.6	NR
0.7	0.8	0.3	<0.05	0.4	1.9
0.8	1.0	0.4	<0.05	0.4	2.4
2.8	4.9	0.2	<0.05	<0.05	8.5

Figure 4.5   **Mean concentrations of nicotine in nonoffice workplace settings with different smoking policies**

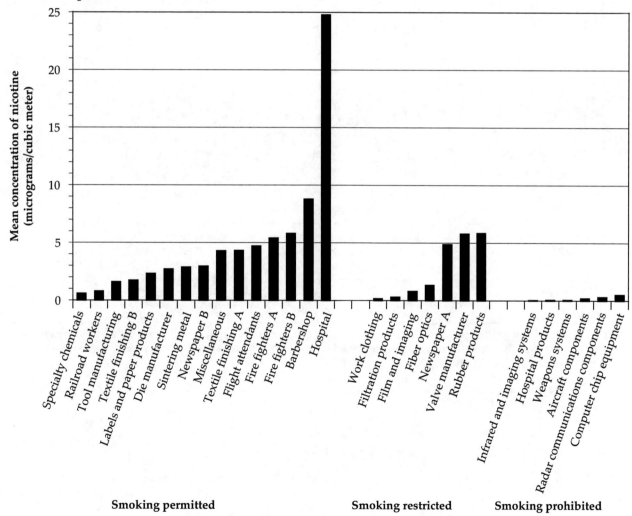

Note: Data are provided in detail in Table 4.5.

Table 4.5   Occupational exposures to nicotine in nonoffice workplace settings among nonsmokers only, stratified by the smoking policy in effect at the time of the measurements

Study	Type of company	Year sampled	Number of samples
Smoking permitted			
Schenker et al. 1986, 1990, 1992	Railroad workers (personal)	1983–1984	152
Mattson et al. 1989	Flight attendants (personal)	1988	16
Coultas et al. 1990	Barbershop (personal)	1986–1987	2
	Hospital (personal)	1986–1987	5
Guerin et al. 1992	Miscellaneous	Before 1990	282
Hammond et al. 1995;	Specialty chemicals	1991–1992	8
Hammond 1999	Tool manufacturing	1991–1992	13
	Textile finishing B	1991–1992	11
	Labels and paper products	1991–1992	1
	Die manufacturer	1991–1992	12
	Sintering metal	1991–1992	12
	Newspaper B	1991–1992	5
	Textile finishing A	1991–1992	11
	Firefighters A[†]	1991–1992	16
	Firefighters B	1991–1992	24
Smoking restricted			
Hammond et al. 1995;	Work clothing	1991–1992	9
Hammond 1999	Filtration products	1991–1992	10
	Film and imaging	1991–1992	6
	Fiber optics	1991–1992	13
	Newspaper A	1991–1992	4
	Valve manufacturer	1991–1992	10
	Rubber products	1991–1992	2
Smoking prohibited			
Hammond et al. 1995;	Infrared and imaging systems	1991–1992	1
Hammond 1999	Hospital products	1991–1992	5
	Weapons systems	1991–1992	12
	Aircraft components	1991–1992	12
	Radar communications components	1991–1992	13
	Computer chip equipment	1991–1992	10

Note: Concentrations were calculated by assuming that all smoking occurred during the workweek, although samplers were in place for 1 full week. Therefore, the nicotine was assumed to have been collected over 45 hours. The exceptions were the fire stations, where 112 hours were assumed.

*NR = Data were not reported.

[†]Omits one data point, 101 $\mu g/m^3$.

Source: Hammond 1999.

Concentrations of nicotine (micrograms per cubic meter [μg/m^3])					
Mean	Standard deviation	Geometric mean	Minimum	Median	Maximum
Smoking permitted					
0.8	3.3	0.2	<0.1	0.1	38.1
4.7	4.0	2.3	0.1	4.2	10.5
8.8	NR*	NR	4.0	NR	13.7
24.8	22.8	16.8	6.3	10.0	53.2
4.3	11.8	1.7	<1.6	<1.6	126.0
0.6	0.9	0.2	<0.05	0.5	2.8
1.6	1.0	1.2	0.2	1.8	3.4
1.7	1.7	1.1	0.3	0.9	5.1
2.3	NR	NR	NR	2.3	NR
2.7	1.3	2.5	1.2	2.4	5.4
2.9	2.6	2.1	0.6	2.2	9.7
3.0	1.4	2.7	1.2	2.8	4.6
4.3	8.8	1.8	0.5	1.4	30.7
5.4	3.8	4.1	1.2	4.8	13.4
5.8	6.8	3.8	0.7	3.6	27.5
Smoking restricted					
0.2	0.3	0.06	<0.05	<0.05	0.9
0.3	0.9	0.08	<0.05	<0.05	2.8
0.8	0.8	0.4	<0.05	0.7	2.2
1.3	2.8	0.6	0.2	0.6	10.6
4.9	6.6	2.6	0.9	1.8	14.8
5.8	7.8	3.6	1.2	3.3	27.3
5.8	5.4	4.2	2.1	5.8	9.6
Smoking prohibited					
<0.05	NR	NR	NR	<0.05	NR
0.08	0.17	<0.05	<0.05	<0.05	0.39
0.08	0.20	<0.05	<0.05	<0.05	0.63
0.20	0.18	0.13	<0.05	0.21	0.61
0.31	0.36	0.14	<0.05	0.26	1.08
0.51	0.33	0.41	0.15	0.39	1.08

Table 4.6   Concentrations of nicotine in restaurants

Study	Year sampled	State	Number of restaurants	Number of days	Number of samples
All sections					
Coghlin et al. 1989	1987	Massachusetts	6	NR*	NR
Crouse and Carson 1989	NR	NR	36	NR	NR
Miesner et al. 1989	1987–1988	NR	2	NR	NR
Thompson et al. 1989	NR	NR	34	NR	NR
Coultas et al. 1990	1986–1987	NR	1	NR	NR
Crouse and Oldaker 1990	NR	NR	21	NR	NR
	NR	NR	21	NR	NR
Oldaker et al. 1990	NR	NR	170	NR	NR
Jenkins et al. 1991	1991	NR	7	NR	NR
Lambert et al. 1993	1989	New Mexico	7	NR	NR
McFarling 1994	1994	Massachusetts	1	NR	NR
Maskarinec et al. 2000	1996–1997	Tennessee	NR	NR	32
	1996–1997 Waiters	Tennessee	NR	NR	83
Nonsmoking sections					
Lambert et al. 1993	1989	New Mexico	7	NR	NR
Moschandreas and Vuilleumier 1999	Before 1998	Illinois	1 theme restaurant	8	NR
	Before 1998	Illinois	1 gourmet restaurant	8	NR
Hammond and Perrino 2002	1998–1999	Indiana	71	NR	NR

*NR = Data were not reported.
†LD = Less than detectable.

Concentrations of nicotine (micrograms per cubic meter [μg/m³])					
Mean	Standard deviation	Geometric mean	Minimum	Median	Maximum
All sections					
NR	NR	NR	18.0	NR	70.0
NR	NR	4.1	1.0	NR	36.0
4.1	NR	NR	2.0	4.1	6.2
5.4	6.4	3.5	0.5	4.1	37.2
NR	NR	NR	NR	45.0	NR
4.3	NR	NR	LD[†]	2.9	24.0
6.3	NR	NR	0.3	4.2	24.8
NR	NR	5.1	LD	NR	23.8
3.4	NR	NR	LD	NR	16.1
NR	NR	NR	1.5	3.2	3.8
13.8	NR	NR	NR	NR	NR
6.0	11.9	NR	<0.24	0.8	49.3
5.8	11.9	NR	<0.24	1.2	67.9
Nonsmoking sections					
NR	NR	NR	0.2	1.0	2.8
0.5	NR	NR	0.1	NR	1.2
1.1	NR	NR	0.1	NR	1.6
3.7	5.1	NR	0.02	2.2	26.7

within 25 feet of the smoking section, and less than 0.5 $\mu g/m^3$ in a nonsmoking section that was 30 feet from the smoking section (although on one day, the average in that section was 1.8 $\mu g/m^3$).

Among the highest concentrations of nicotine measured in public places were those found in bars and lounges, where reported values were generally greater than 50 $\mu g/m^3$ and occasionally were above 100 $\mu g/m^3$ (Table 4.7). Bartenders had higher exposures than waiters, at an average concentration of 14 $\mu g/m^3$ and a maximum exposure of more than 100 $\mu g/m^3$ (Maskarinec et al. 2000).

Other Locations

Casinos and bingo halls are other public locations where both nonsmoking workers and the public are exposed to high concentrations of secondhand smoke (Table 4.7). A 1986 study in California found a median nicotine concentration of 65.5 $\mu g/m^3$ (Kado et al. 1991). A study in Massachusetts the following year reported a median concentration of 56 $\mu g/m^3$ (Coghlin et al. 1989). In 1995, a study of casino workers in Atlantic City, New Jersey, showed increased levels of serum cotinine at baseline (geometric mean cotinine 1.34 ng/mL) that rose following a workshift (geometric mean cotinine 1.85 ng/mL) (Trout et al. 1998); nicotine levels in the personal breathing zone of casino workers ranged from 6 to 12 $\mu g/m^3$.

Reported nicotine concentrations in bowling alleys were between 10 and 23 $\mu g/m^3$ (Coghlin et al. 1989; Jenkins et al. 1996a) (Table 4.7). And although indoor exposures are expected to be higher than outdoor exposures, McFarling (1994) reported one nicotine sample at an outdoor baseball game that was at a concentration of 2.4 $\mu g/m^3$. Researchers have previously reported data for commercial aircraft, an environment now entirely smoke-free in the United States (Holm and Davis 2004).

Special Populations

Prisoners

Some of the highest concentrations of secondhand smoke in living quarters have been measured in correctional facilities (Hammond and Emmons 2005). Although most living and sleeping areas averaged 3 to 10 $\mu g/m^3$, Hammond and Emmons (2005) reported nicotine concentrations that averaged 25 $\mu g/m^3$ in a gym that was used as a bunkroom.

Evidence Synthesis

Since 1986, investigators have reported a substantial amount of new evidence on exposure to secondhand smoke. The more recent data provide insights into typical patterns of exposure, exposure in key microenvironments, and the consequences of various policies intended to reduce exposure. As noted in Figure 4.1 and Table 4.1, exposures of nonsmokers to secondhand smoke have declined significantly between 1988 and 2002. These declines have been observed in both children and nonsmoking adults, in both men and women, and in all racial and ethnic categories. However, significant levels of exposure persist for the U.S. population in general and for susceptible populations. Table 4.2 notes estimates for 2000; approximately 127 million children and nonsmoking adults were exposed to secondhand smoke. This estimated total includes almost 22 million children aged 3 through 11 years, and 18 million nonsmoking youth aged 12 through 19 years.

The findings consistently show the importance of two microenvironments as places for secondhand smoke exposure: the home and the workplace. Although microenvironments such as bars and restaurants may also be important for patrons, the home and the workplace are particularly significant because of the amount of time spent in these two locations. For the workplace, restrictions and smoking bans lead to much lower concentrations of secondhand smoke than in locations where smoking is allowed.

National surveys indicate that progress in reducing secondhand smoke exposure has been variable across the country. Certain states, such as California, Maryland, and Utah, have made significant advances in protecting nonsmokers, but others, such as Kentucky and Nevada, have not (Gilpin et al. 2001; Shopland et al. 2001). Even in locales with smoking restrictions in place, significant pockets of exposure remain, most notably in homes, some worksites such as restaurants and bars, and in automobiles. Exposures in some of these locations can be remedied by changing public policy. Exposures in other locations, particularly homes and automobiles, can perhaps only be addressed through education that alters lifestyle behaviors.

It is likely that geographic differences in secondhand smoke exposure are related to trends in tobacco use and policies that determine where tobacco use is permitted (Giovino et al. 1995; Gilpin et al. 2001). Wide regional differences exist within the United States in secondhand smoke exposure and cotinine levels. In the NHANES III data, children with and without reported exposures had lower cotinine levels if they lived in the western part of the United States (Mannino et al. 2001)—a finding that may reflect lower community exposures to secondhand smoke. Where smoking is allowed, especially at worksites and in public places, concentrations are highly variable, so concentrations in individual locations may be significantly higher than average. Concentrations of secondhand smoke are also typically higher in the workplace and in restaurants than in the home (Figure 4.6). Policies that restrict smoking to particular areas reduce but do not eliminate secondhand smoke exposure. Smoke-free polices reduce secondhand smoke concentrations far more effectively.

Figure 4.6   Average concentrations of nicotine in homes, offices, other workplaces, and restaurants where smoking is permitted

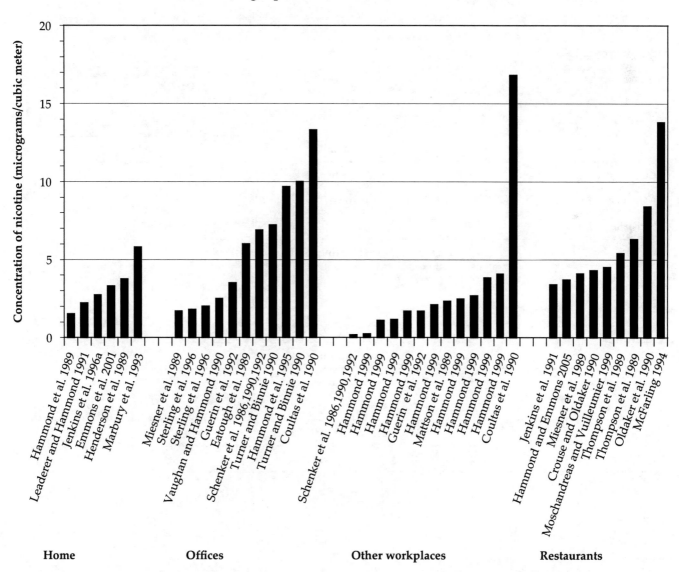

Note: Data are provided in detail in Tables 4.3, 4.4, 4.5, and 4.6.

Table 4.7   Concentrations of nicotine in bars, lounges, and other public venues

Study	Year sampled	State	Number of venues	Number of days	Number of samples
Bars					
Coghlin et al. 1989	1987	Massachusetts	11	NR*	NR
Loefroth et al. 1989	NR	North Carolina	1	2	NR
Miesner et al. 1989	1987–1988	NR	3	NR	5
Oldaker and Conrad 1989	NR	NR	NR	NR	NR
Jenkins et al. 1991	NR	NR	8	NR	NR
Guerin et al. 1992	NR	NR	2	NR	NR
Bergman et al. 1996	NR	NR	3	NR	17
Maskarinec et al. 2000	1996–1997	Tennessee	NR	NR	53
	1996–1997 Bartenders	NR	NR	NR	80
Bingo halls					
Coghlin et al. 1989	1987	Massachusetts	NR	NR	2
Kado et al. 1991	1986	California	NR	NR	6
McFarling 1994	1994	NR	NR	NR	1
Casinos and other betting establishments					
Jenkins et al. 1991	NR	NR	NR	NR	2
Kado et al. 1991	NR	NR	NR	NR	NR
Trout et al. 1998	1996	New Jersey	1	NR	1
Bowling alleys					
Coghlin et al. 1989	1987	Massachusetts	NR	NR	2
Jenkins et al. 1991	NR	NR	NR	NR	4
Professional baseball games					
McFarling 1994	1994	Massachusetts	NR	NR	1

*NR = Data were not reported.

Concentrations of nicotine (micrograms per cubic meter [$\mu g/m^3$])					
Mean	Standard deviation	Geometric mean	Minimum	Median	Maximum
Bars					
NR	NR	NR	6.0	NR	82.0
65.5	NR	NR	60.0	NR	71.0
7.4	4.4	6.0	1.1	7.0	13.0
59.2	NR	NR	6.1	NR	109.0
17.6	NR	NR	1.8	NR	91.0
12.9	NR	NR	4.1	NR	21.6
37.1	6.9	36.0	28.0	34.9	50.0
14.4	16.9	NR	<0.2	5.8	61.1
14.1	20.9	NR	<0.2	4.4	116.0
Bingo halls					
NR	NR	NR	53.0	56.0	60.0
NR	NR	NR	4.4	65.5	85.4
NR	NR	NR	NR	7.8	NR
Casinos and other betting establishments					
10.7	NR	NR	NR	NR	NR
NR	NR	NR	NR	65.5	NR
10.0	NR	8.0	6.0	NR	12.0
Bowling alleys					
18.0	NR	NR	13.0	18.0	23.0
10.7	NR	NR	NR	NR	NR
Professional baseball games					
2.4	NR	NR	NR	NR	NR

Conclusions

1. The evidence is sufficient to infer that large numbers of nonsmokers are still exposed to secondhand smoke.

2. Exposure of nonsmokers to secondhand smoke has declined in the United States since the 1986 Surgeon General's report, *The Health Consequences of Involuntary Smoking*.

3. The evidence indicates that the extent of secondhand smoke exposure varies across the country.

4. Homes and workplaces are the predominant locations for exposure to secondhand smoke.

5. Exposure to secondhand smoke tends to be greater for persons with lower incomes.

6. Exposure to secondhand smoke continues in restaurants, bars, casinos, gaming halls, and vehicles.

Overall Implications

Exposure to secondhand smoke remains a serious public health problem in the United States, with exposure of almost 60 percent of children aged 3 through 11 years and more than 40 percent of nonsmoking adults. Since the publication of the 1986 Surgeon General's report, measured levels of exposure in the United States have declined significantly. However, the proportional decrease has been larger among adults than among children, and the most recent data suggest that children aged 3 through 11 years have serum cotinine concentrations that are more than twice as high as those among nonsmoking adults. Data suggest that the home remains the most important target for reducing exposures to secondhand smoke, particularly for children but also for middle-aged and older adults. Although progress has been made to protect nonsmoking workers, continuing efforts are needed to protect these workers, and particularly younger workers, in all occupational categories.

Research questions remain regarding exposure to secondhand smoke. As noted in the 1986 report, no indicator has been developed that can objectively estimate long-term exposure or early-life exposure. Secondhand smoke exposure from "shared air spaces" within a building is also of concern, as a significant proportion of the population lives in apartment buildings or condominiums where smoking in another part of the building might increase tobacco smoke exposure for households of nonsmokers.

References

Al-Delaimy WK, Crane J, Woodward A. Questionnaire and hair measurement of exposure to tobacco smoke. *Journal of Exposure Analysis and Environmental Epidemiology* 2000;10(4):378–84.

Benowitz NL. Cotinine as a biomarker of environmental tobacco smoke exposure. *Epidemiologic Reviews* 1996;18(2):188–204.

Benowitz NL. Biomarkers of environmental tobacco smoke exposure. *Environmental Health Perspectives* 1999;107(Suppl 2):349–55.

Berglund DJ, Abbey DE, Lebowitz MD, Knutsen SF, McDonnell WF. Respiratory symptoms and pulmonary function in an elderly nonsmoking population. *Chest* 1999;115(1):49–59.

Bergman TA, Johnson DL, Boatright DT, Smallwood KG, Rando RJ. Occupational exposure of nonsmoking nightclub musicians to environmental tobacco smoke. *American Industrial Hygiene Association Journal* 1996;57(8):746–52.

Borland R, Pierce JP, Burns DM, Gilpin E, Johnson M, Bal D. Protection from environmental tobacco smoke in California: the case for a smoke-free workplace. *Journal of the American Medical Association* 1992;268(6):749–52.

Brancker A. Lung cancer and smoking prevalence in Canada. *Health Reports* 1990;2(1):67–83.

Caraballo RS, Giovino GA, Pechacek TF, Mowery PD, Richter PA, Strauss WJ, Sharp DJ, Eriksen MP, Pirkle JL, Maurer KR. Racial and ethnic differences in serum cotinine levels of cigarette smokers: Third National Health and Nutrition Examination Survey, 1988–1991. *Journal of the American Medical Association* 1998;280(2):135–9.

Carson JR, Erikson CA. Results from survey of environmental tobacco smoke in offices in Ottawa, Ontario. *Environmental Technology* 1988;9(6):501–8.

Centers for Disease Control and Prevention. State-specific prevalence of cigarette smoking among adults, and children's and adolescents' exposure to environmental tobacco smoke—United States, 1996. *Morbidity and Mortality Weekly Report* 1997;46(44):1038–43.

Centers for Disease Control and Prevention. State laws on tobacco control—United States, 1998. *Morbidity and Mortality Weekly Report* 1999;48(3):21–40.

Centers for Disease Control and Prevention. *National Report on Human Exposure to Environmental Chemicals.* Atlanta: U.S. Department of Health and Human Services, Centers for Disease Control and Prevention, 2001a.

Centers for Disease Control and Prevention. State-specific prevalence of current cigarette smoking among adults, and policies and attitudes about secondhand smoke—United States, 2000. *Morbidity and Mortality Weekly Report* 2001b;50(49):1101–6.

Centers for Disease Control and Prevention. *Second National Report on Human Exposure to Environmental Chemicals.* Atlanta: U.S. Department of Health and Human Services, Centers for Disease Control and Prevention, National Center for Environmental Health, 2003. NCEH Publication No. 02-0716.

Centers for Disease Control and Prevention. *Third National Report on Human Exposure to Environmental Chemicals.* Atlanta: U.S. Department of Health and Human Services, Centers for Disease Control and Prevention, National Center for Environmental Health, 2005. NCEH Publication No. 05-0570.

Coghlin J, Gann PH, Hammond SK, Skipper PL, Taghizadeh K, Paul M. 4-Aminobiphenyl hemoglobin adducts in fetuses exposed to the tobacco smoke carcinogen in utero. *Journal of the National Cancer Institute* 1991;83(4):274–80.

Coghlin J, Hammond SK, Gann PH. Development of epidemiologic tools for measuring environmental tobacco smoke exposure. *American Journal of Epidemiology* 1989;130(4):696–704.

Coultas DB, Howard CA, Peake GT, Skipper BJ, Samet JM. Salivary cotinine levels and involuntary tobacco smoke exposure in children and adults in New Mexico. *American Review of Respiratory Disease* 1987;136(2):305–9.

Coultas DB, Howard CA, Peake GT, Skipper BJ, Samet JM. Discrepancies between self-reported and validated cigarette smoking in a community survey of New Mexico Hispanics. *American Review of Respiratory Disease* 1988;137(4):810–4.

Coultas DB, Samet JM, McCarthy JF, Spengler JD. A personal monitoring study to assess workplace exposure to environmental tobacco smoke. *American Journal of Public Health* 1990;80(8):988–90.

Crouse WE, Carson J. Surveys of environmental tobacco smoke (ETS) in Washington, D.C., offices and restaurants [abstract]. To be submitted to the 43rd Tobacco Chemists' Research Conference,

October 2–5, 1989. Richmond (VA) 1989. Lorillard. Bates No. 87733746. <http://legacy.library.ucsf.edu/tid/gpr99d00>.

Crouse WE, Oldaker GB. Comparison of area and personal sampling methods for determining nicotine in environmental tobacco smoke. In: *Measurement of Toxic and Related Air Pollutants*. Proceedings of the 1990 EPA/A&WMA International Symposium; May 1990; Raleigh (NC): U.S. Environmental Protection Agency and Air & Waste Management Association, 1990:562–6. Air & Waste Management Association Publication VIP-17; Publication No. EPA 600/9–90/026.

Dayal HH, Khuder S, Sharrar R, Trieff N. Passive smoking in obstructive respiratory disease in an industrialized urban population. *Environmental Research* 1994;65(2):161–71.

Eatough DJ, Benner CL, Tang H, Landon V, Richares G, Caka FM, Crawford J, Lewis EA, Hansen LD, Eatough NL. The chemical composition of environmental tobacco smoke III: identification of conservative tracers of environmental tobacco smoke. *Environment International* 1989;15(1–6):19–28.

Ebrahim SH, Floyd RL, Merritt RK II, Decoufle P, Holtzman D. Trends in pregnancy-related smoking rates in the United States, 1987–1996. *Journal of the American Medical Association* 2000;283(3):361–6.

Emmons KM, Hammond SK, Abrams DB. Smoking at home: the impact of smoking cessation on nonsmokers' exposure to environmental tobacco smoke. *Health Psychology* 1994;13(6):516–20.

Emmons KM, Hammond SK, Fava JL, Velicer WF, Evans JL, Monroe AD. A randomized trial to reduce passive smoke exposure in low-income households with young children. *Pediatrics* 2001;108(1):18–24.

Farrelly MC, Evans WN, Sfekas AE. The impact of workplace smoking bans: results from a national survey. *Tobacco Control* 1999;8(3):272–7.

Ferris BG Jr, Ware JH, Berkey CS, Dockery DW, Spiro A III, Speizer FE. Effects of passive smoking on health of children. *Environmental Health Perspectives* 1985;62:289–95.

Fontham ET, Correa P, Reynolds P, Wu-Williams A, Buffler PA, Greenberg RS, Chen VW, Alterman T, Boyd P, Austin DF, Liff J. Environmental tobacco smoke and lung cancer in nonsmoking women. A multicenter study. *Journal of the American Medical Association* 1994;271(22):1752–9.

Ford RP, Tappin DM, Schluter PJ, Wild CJ. Smoking during pregnancy: how reliable are maternal self reports in New Zealand? *Journal of Epidemiology and Community Health* 1997;51(3):246–51.

Friedman GD, Petitti DB, Bawol RD. Prevalence and correlates of passive smoking. *American Journal of Public Health* 1983;73(4):401–5.

Gilpin EA, Emery SL, Farkas AJ, Distefan JM, White MM, Pierce JP. *The California Tobacco Control Program: A Decade of Progress, Results from the California Tobacco Surveys, 1990–1999*. La Jolla (CA): University of California, San Diego, 2001.

Giovino GA, Henningfield JE, Tomar SL, Escobedo LG, Slade J. Epidemiology of tobacco use and dependence [review]. *Epidemiologic Reviews* 1995;17(1):48–65.

Greenberg RA, Bauman KE, Glover LH, Strecher VJ, Kleinbaum DG, Haley NJ, Stedman HC, Fowler MG, Loda FA. Ecology of passive smoking by young infants. *Journal of Pediatrics* 1989;114(5):774–80.

Guerin MR, Jenkins RA, Tompkins BA. *The Chemistry of Environmental Tobacco Smoke: Composition and Measurement*. Boca Raton (FL): Lewis Publishers, 1992.

Haddow JE, Knight GJ, Palomaki GE, Kloza EM, Wald NJ. Cigarette consumption and serum cotinine in relation to birthweight. *British Journal of Obstetrics and Gynaecology* 1987;94(7):678–81.

Haley NJ, Axelrad CM, Tilton KA. Validation of self-reported smoking behavior: biochemical analyses of cotinine and thiocyanate. *American Journal of Public Health* 1983;73(10):1204–7.

Haley NJ, Colosimo SG, Axelrad CM, Harris R, Sepkovic DW. Biochemical validation of self-reported exposure to environmental tobacco smoke. *Environmental Research* 1989;49(1):127–35.

Hammond SK. Exposure of U.S. workers to environmental tobacco smoke [review]. *Environmental Health Perspectives* 1999;107(Suppl 2):329–40.

Hammond SK. The efficacy of strategies to reduce environmental tobacco smoke concentrations in homes, workplaces, restaurants, and correctional facilities. In: Levin H, editor. *Indoor Air 2000*. Proceedings of the 9th International Conference on Indoor Air Quality and Climate; June 30–July 5, 2002; Monterey (CA). Vol. 2. Santa Cruz (CA): Indoor Air, 2002:115–20.

Hammond SK, Coghlin J, Gann PH, Paul M, Taghizadeh K, Skipper PL, Tannenbaum SR. Relationship between environmental tobacco smoke exposure and carcinogen–hemoglobin adduct levels in nonsmokers. *Journal of the National Cancer Institute* 1993; 85(6):474–8.

Hammond SK, Emmons KM. Inmate exposure to secondhand smoke in correctional facilities and the impact of smoking restrictions. *Journal of*

Exposure Analysis and Environmental Epidemiology 2005;15(3):205–11.

Hammond SK, Leaderer BP, Roche AC, Schenker M. Collection and analysis of nicotine as a marker for environmental tobacco smoke. *Atmospheric Environment* 1987;21(2):457–62.

Hammond SK, Mumford JL, Henderson FW, Lewtas J. Exposures to environmental tobacco smoke in homes. In: *Measurement of Toxic and Related Air Pollutants*. Proceedings of the 1989 EPA/A&WMA International Symposium; May 1989; Raleigh (NC): U.S. Environmental Protection Agency and Air & Waste Management Association, 1989:590–5. Air & Waste Management Association Publication VIP-13; Publication No. EPA 600/9–89/060.

Hammond SK, Perrino C. Passive smoking in nonsmoking sections of 71 Indiana restaurants [abstract]. *Epidemiology* 2002;13(4):S145–S146.

Hammond SK, Smith TJ, Woskie SR, Leaderer BP, Bettinger N. Markers of exposure to diesel exhaust and cigarette smoke in railroad workers. *American Industrial Hygiene Association Journal* 1988;49(10):516–22.

Hammond SK, Sorensen G, Youngstrom R, Ockene JK. Occupational exposure to environmental tobacco smoke. *Journal of the American Medical Association* 1995;274(12):956–60.

Henderson FW, Reid HF, Morris R, Wang OL, Hu PC, Helms RW, Forehand L, Mumford J, Lewtas J, Haley NJ, Hammond SK. Home air nicotine levels and urinary cotinine excretion in preschool children. *American Review of Respiratory Disease* 1989;140(1):197–201.

Hirayama T. Cancer mortality in nonsmoking women with smoking husbands based on a large-scale cohort study in Japan. *Preventive Medicine* 1984;13(6):680–90.

Holm AL, Davis RM. Clearing the airways: advocacy and regulation for smoke-free airlines. *Tobacco Control* 2004;13(Suppl 1):i30–i36.

Jaakkola MS, Jaakkola JJ. Assessment of exposure to environmental tobacco smoke. *European Respiratory Journal* 1997;10(10):2384–97.

Jaakkola MS, Samet JM. Summary: workshop on health risks attributable to ETS exposure in the workplace. *Environmental Health Perspectives* 1999;107(Suppl 6):823–8.

Jarvis MJ, Foulds J, Feyerabend C. Exposure to passive smoking among bar staff. *British Journal of Addiction* 1992;87(1):111–3.

Jarvis MJ, Goddard E, Higgins V, Feyerabend C, Bryant A, Cook DG. Children's exposure to passive smoking in England since the 1980s: cotinine evidence from population surveys. *British Medical Journal* 2000;321(7257):343–5.

Jarvis MJ, McNeill AD, Bryant A, Russell MA. Factors determining exposure to passive smoking in young adults living at home: quantitative analysis using saliva cotinine concentrations. *International Journal of Epidemiology* 1991;20(1):126–31.

Jarvis MJ, Tunstall-Pedoe H, Feyerabend C, Vesey C, Saloojee Y. Comparison of tests used to distinguish smokers from nonsmokers. *American Journal of Public Health* 1987;77(11):1435–8.

Jenkins RA, Counts RW. Personal exposure to environmental tobacco smoke: salivary cotinine, airborne nicotine, and nonsmoker misclassification. *Journal of Exposure Analysis and Environmental Epidemiology* 1999;9(4):352–63.

Jenkins RA, Guerin MR, Tomkins BA. *The Chemistry of Environmental Tobacco Smoke: Composition and Measurement.* 2nd ed. Boca Raton (FL): Lewis, 2000.

Jenkins RA, Moody RL, Higgins CE, Moneyhun JH. Nicotine in environmental tobacco smoke (ETS): comparison of mobile personal and stationary area sampling. Philip Morris Collection. 1991. Bates No. 2021007252/7256. <http://legacy.library.ucsf.edu/tid/noj52d00>; accessed: April 10, 2006.

Jenkins RA, Palausky A, Counts RW, Bayne CK, Dindal AB, Guerin MR. Exposure to environmental tobacco smoke in sixteen cities in the United States as determined by personal breathing zone air sampling. *Journal of Exposure Analysis and Environmental Epidemiology* 1996a;6(4):473–502.

Jenkins RA, Palausky MA, Counts RW, Guerin MR, Dindal AB, Bayne CK. Determination of personal exposure of non-smokers to environmental tobacco smoke in the United States. *Lung Cancer* 1996b;14(Suppl 1):S195–S213.

Kado NY, McCurdy SA, Tesluk SJ, Hammond SK, Hsieh DP, Jones J. Measuring personal exposure to airborne mutagens and nicotine in environmental tobacco smoke. *Mutation Research* 1991;261(1):75–82.

Kegler MC, Malcoe LH. Smoking restrictions in the home and car among rural Native American and white families with young children. *Preventive Medicine* 2002;35(4):334–42.

King G, Strouse R, Hovey DA, Zehe L. Cigarette smoking in Connecticut: home and workplace exposure. *Connecticut Medicine* 1998;62(9):531–9.

Klepeis NE. An introduction to the indirect exposure assessment approach: modeling human exposure using microenvironmental measurements and the recent National Human Activity Pattern Survey.

Environmental Health Perspectives 1999;107(Suppl 2):365–74.

Klepeis NE, Nelson WC, Ott WR, Robinson JP, Tsang AM, Switzer P, Behar JV, Hern SC, Engelmann WH. The National Human Activity Pattern Survey (NHAPS): a resource for assessing exposure to environmental pollutants. *Journal of Exposure Analysis and Environmental Epidemiology* 2001;11(3):231–52.

Kottke TE, Aase LA, Brandel CL, Brekke MJ, Brekke LN, DeBoer SW, Hoffman RS, Menzel PA, Thomas RJ. Attitudes of Olmsted County, Minnesota, residents about tobacco smoke in restaurants and bars. *Mayo Clinic Proceedings* 2001;76(2):134–7.

Lambert WE, Samet JM, Spengler JD. Environmental tobacco smoke concentrations in no-smoking and smoking sections of restaurants. *American Journal of Public Health* 1993;83(9):1339–41.

Leaderer BP, Hammond SK. Evaluation of vapor-phase nicotine and respirable suspended particle mass as markers for environmental tobacco smoke. *Environmental Science & Technology* 1991;25(4):770–7.

Lebowitz MD, Burrows B. Respiratory symptoms related to smoking habits of family adults. *Chest* 1976;69(1):48–50.

Loefroth G, Burton RM, Forehand L, Hammond SK, Seila RL, Zweidinger RB, Lewtas J. Characterization of environmental tobacco smoke. *Environmental Science & Technology* 1989;23(5):610–4.

Maier WC, Arrighi HM, Morray B, Llewellyn C, Redding GJ. Indoor risk factors for asthma and wheezing among Seattle school children. *Environmental Health Perspectives* 1997;105(2):208–14.

Manning SC, Wasserman RL, Silver R, Phillips DL. Results of endoscopic sinus surgery in pediatric patients with chronic sinusitis and asthma. *Archives of Otolaryngology—Head & Neck Surgery* 1994;120(10):1142–5.

Mannino DM, Caraballo R, Benowitz N, Repace J. Predictors of cotinine levels in US children: data from the Third National Health and Nutrition Examination Survey. *Chest* 2001;120(3):718–24.

Mannino DM, Siegel M, Husten C, Rose D, Etzel R. Environmental tobacco smoke exposure and health effects in children: results from the 1991 National Health Interview Survey. *Tobacco Control* 1996;5(1):13–8.

Mannino DM, Siegel M, Rose D, Nkuchia J, Etzel R. Environmental tobacco smoke exposure in the home and worksite and health effects in adults: results from the 1991 National Health Interview Survey. *Tobacco Control* 1997;6(4):296–305.

Marbury MC, Hammond SK, Haley NJ. Measuring exposure to environmental tobacco smoke in studies of acute health effects. *American Journal of Epidemiology* 1993;137(10):1089–97.

Margolis PA, Keyes LL, Greenberg RA, Bauman KE, LaVange LM. Urinary cotinine and parent history (questionnaire) as indicators of passive smoking and predictors of lower respiratory illness in infants. *Pediatric Pulmonology* 1997;23(6):417–23.

Maskarinec MP, Jenkins RA, Counts RW, Dindal AB. Determination of exposure to environmental tobacco smoke in restaurant and tavern workers in one US city. *Journal of Exposure Analysis and Environmental Epidemiology* 2000;10(1):36–49.

Mattson ME, Boyd G, Byar D, Brown C, Callahan JF, Corle D, Cullen DW, Greenblatt J, Haley NJ, Hammond SK, Lewtas J, Reeves W. Passive smoking on commercial airline flights. *Journal of the American Medical Association* 1989;261(6):867–72.

McFarling UL. Air quality survey finds a haze of lingering smoke. *Boston Globe* July 17, 1994;Metro Sect 1.

McMillen RC, Winickoff JP, Klein JD, Weitzman M. US adult attitudes and practices regarding smoking restrictions and child exposure to environmental tobacco smoke: changes in the social climate from 2000–2001. *Pediatrics* 2003;112(1 Pt 1):E55–E60.

Miesner EA, Rudnick SN, Hu FC, Spengler JD, Preller L, Ozkaynak H, Nelson W. Particulate and nicotine sampling in public facilities and offices. *Journal of the Air Pollution Control Association* 1989;39(12):1577–82.

Moschandreas DJ, Vuilleumier KL. ETS levels in hospitality environments satisfying ASHRAE standard 62-1989: "Ventilation for acceptable indoor air quality." *Atmospheric Environment* 1999;33(26):4327–40.

Muramatsu M, Umemura S, Okada T, Tomita H. Estimation of personal exposure to tobacco smoke with a newly developed nicotine personal monitor. *Environmental Research* 1984;35(1):218–27.

Norman GJ, Ribisl KM, Howard-Pitney B, Howard KA. Smoking bans in the home and car: do those who really need them have them? *Preventive Medicine* 1999;29(6 Pt 1):581–9.

O'Connor TZ, Holford TR, Leaderer BP, Hammond SK, Bracken MB. Measurement of exposure to environmental tobacco smoke in pregnant women. *American Journal of Epidemiology* 1995;142(12):1315–21.

Oldaker GB and Conrad FW Jr. Results from measurements of nicotine in a tavern. In: *Measurement of Toxic and Related Air Pollutants*. Proceedings of the 1989 U.S. EPA/A&WMA International

Symposium. Pittsburgh: Air & Waste Management Association, 1989:577–82.

Oldaker GB III, Perfetti PF, Conrad FC Jr, Conner JM, McBride RL. Results from surveys of environmental tobacco smoke in offices and restaurants. In: Kasuga H, editor. *Indoor Air Quality.* New York: Springer-Vergag, 1990:99–104.

Overpeck MD, Moss AJ. Children's exposure to environmental cigarette smoke before and after birth: health of our nation's children, United States, 1988. *Advances in Data* 1991;(202):1–11.

Phillips K, Bentley MC, Abrar M, Howard DA, Cook J. Low level saliva cotinine determination and its application as a biomarker for environmental tobacco smoke exposure. *Human & Experimental Toxicology* 1999a;18(4):291–6.

Phillips K, Bentley MC, Howard DA, Alván G. Assessment of air quality in Stockholm by personal monitoring of nonsmokers for respirable suspended particles and environmental tobacco smoke. *Scandinavian Journal of Work, Environment & Health* 1996;22(Suppl 1):1–24.

Phillips K, Bentley MC, Howard DA, Alván G. Assessment of air quality in Paris by personal monitoring of nonsmokers for respirable suspended particles and environmental tobacco smoke. *Environment International* 1998a;24(4):405–25.

Phillips K, Bentley MC, Howard DA, Alván G. Assessment of environmental tobacco smoke and respirable suspended particle exposures for nonsmokers in Kuala Lumpur using personal monitoring. *Journal of Exposure Analysis and Environmental Epidemiology* 1998b;8(4):519–42.

Phillips K, Bentley MC, Howard DA, Alván G. Assessment of environmental tobacco smoke and respirable suspended particle exposures for nonsmokers in Prague using personal monitoring. *International Archives of Occupational and Environmental Health* 1998c;71(6):379–90.

Phillips K, Bentley MC, Howard DA, Alván G, Huici A. Assessment of air quality in Barcelona by personal monitoring of nonsmokers for respirable suspended particles and environmental tobacco smoke. *Environment International* 1997a;23(2):173–96.

Phillips K, Howard DA, Bentley MC, Alván G. Assessment of air quality in Turin by personal monitoring of nonsmokers for respirable suspended particles and environmental tobacco smoke. *Environment International* 1997b;23(6):851–71.

Phillips K, Howard DA, Bentley MC, Alván G. Assessment by personal monitoring of respirable suspended particles and environmental tobacco smoke

exposure for non-smokers in Sydney, Australia. *Indoor and Built Environment* 1998d;7(4):188–203.

Phillips K, Howard DA, Bentley MC, Alván G. Assessment of environmental tobacco smoke and respirable suspended particle exposures for nonsmokers in Basel by personal monitoring. *Atmospheric Environment* 1999b;33(12):1889–904.

Phillips K, Howard DA, Bentley MC, Alván G. Assessment of environmental tobacco smoke and respirable suspended particle exposures for nonsmokers in Hong Kong using personal monitoring. *Environment International* 1998e;24(8):851–70.

Phillips K, Howard DA, Bentley MC, Alván G. Assessment of environmental tobacco smoke and respirable suspended particle exposures for nonsmokers in Lisbon by personal monitoring. *Environment International* 1998f;24(3):301–24.

Phillips K, Howard DA, Bentley MC, Alván G. Environmental tobacco smoke and respirable suspended particle exposures for non-smokers in Beijing. *Indoor and Built Environment* 1998g;7(5–6):254–69.

Phillips K, Howard DA, Bentley MC, Alván G. Measured exposures by personal monitoring for respirable suspended particles and environmental tobacco smoke of housewives and office workers resident in Bremen, Germany. *International Archives of Occupational and Environmental Health* 1998h;71(3):201–12.

Pierce JP, Gilpin EA, Emery SL, Farkas AJ, Zhu SH, Choi WS, Berry CC, Distefan JM, White MM, Sorato S, Navarro A. *Tobacco Control in California: Who's Winning the War? An Evaluation of the Tobacco Control Program, 1989–1996.* La Jolla (CA): University of California, San Diego, 1998.

Pirkle JL, Bernert JT, Caudill SP, Sosnoff CS, Pechacek TF. Trends in the exposure of nonsmokers in the U.S. population to secondhand smoke: 1988–2002. *Environmental Health Perspectives* 2006;114(6):853–8

Pirkle JL, Flegal KM, Bernert JT, Brody DJ, Etzel RA, Maurer KR. Exposure of the US population to environmental tobacco smoke: the Third National Health and Nutrition Examination Survey, 1988 to 1991. *Journal of the American Medical Association* 1996;275(16):1233–40.

Rogge WF, Hildemann LM, Mazurek MA, Cass GR, Simonneit BRT. Sources of fine organic aerosol: 6. Cigaret smoke in the urban atmosphere. *Environmental Science & Technology* 1994;28(7):1375–88.

Samet JM, Wang SS. Environmental tobacco smoke. In: Lippman M, editor. *Environmental Toxicants: Human Exposures and Their Health Effects.* 2nd ed. New York: John Wiley & Sons, 2000:319–75.

Sandler DP, Helsing KJ, Comstock GW, Shore DL. Factors associated with past household exposure to tobacco smoke. *American Journal of Epidemiology* 1989;129(2):380–7.

Schenker MB, Hammond SK, Woskie S, Samuels S, Kado N, Smith T. Determinants and markers of environmental tobacco smoke (ETS) exposure in an occupational setting [abstract]. *American Review of Respiratory Disease* 1986;133(4 Pt 2):A158.

Schenker MB, Kado NY, Hammond SK, Samuels SJ, Woskie SR, Smith TJ. Urinary mutagenic activity in workers exposed to diesel exhaust. *Environmental Research* 1992;57(2):133–48.

Schenker MB, Samuels SJ, Kado NY, Hammond SK, Smith TJ, Woskie SR. Markers of exposure to diesel exhaust in railroad workers. *Research Report (Health Effects Institute)* 1990;(33):1–51.

Schilling RS, Letai AD, Hui SL, Beck GJ, Schoenberg JB, Bouhuys A. Lung function, respiratory disease, and smoking in families. *American Journal of Epidemiology* 1977;106(4):274–83.

Schuster MA, Franke T, Pham CB. Smoking patterns of household members and visitors in homes with children in the United States. *Archives of Pediatrics & Adolescent Medicine* 2002;156(11):1094–100.

Shopland DR, Gerlach KK, Burns DM, Hartman AM, Gibson JT. State-specific trends in smoke-free workplace policy coverage: the current population survey tobacco use supplement, 1993 to 1999. *Journal of Occupational and Environmental Medicine* 2001;43(8):680–6.

Shopland DR, Hartman AM, Gibson JT, Mueller MD, Kessler LG, Lynn WR. Cigarette smoking among U.S. adults by state and region: estimates from the current population survey. *Journal of the National Cancer Institute* 1996;88(23):1748–58.

Siegel M, Albers AB, Cheng DM, Biener L, Rigotti NA. Effect of local restaurant smoking regulations on environmental tobacco smoke exposure among youths. *American Journal of Public Health* 2004;94(2):321–5.

Skeer M, Siegel M. The descriptive epidemiology of local restaurant smoking regulations in Massachusetts: an analysis of the protection of restaurant customers and workers. *Tobacco Control* 2003;12(2):221–6.

Soliman S, Pollack HA, Warner KE. Decrease in the prevalence of environmental tobacco smoke exposure in the home during the 1990s in families with children. *American Journal of Public Health* 2004;94(2):314–20.

Sterling TD, Glicksman A, Perry H, Sterling DA, Rosenbaum WL, Weinkam JJ. An alternative explanation for the apparent elevated relative mortality and morbidity risks associated with exposure to environmental tobacco smoke. *Journal of Clinical Epidemiology* 1996;49(7):803–8.

Sweeney CT, Shopland DR, Hartman AM, Gibson JT, Anderson CM, Gower KB, Burns DM. Sex differences in workplace smoking policies: results from the current population survey. *Journal of the American Medical Women's Association* 2000;55(5):311–5.

Thompson CV, Jenkins RA, Higgins CE. A thermal desorption method for the determination of nicotine in indoor environments. *Environmental Science & Technology* 1989;23(4):429–35.

Trout D, Decker J, Mueller C, Bernert JT, Pirkle J. Exposure of casino employees to environmental tobacco smoke. *Journal of Occupational and Environmental Medicine* 1998;40(3):270–6.

Turner S, Binnie PWH. An indoor air quality survey of twenty-six Swiss office buildings. In: Walkinshaw DS, editor. *Indoor Air '90.* Proceedings of the 5th International Conference on Indoor Air Quality and Climate, Toronto, 29 July–3 August 1990. Ottawa: International Conference on Indoor Air Quality and Climate, 1990:27–32.

U.S. Bureau of the Census. Summary File 1 (SF 1), 2000; <http://www.census.gov/Press-Release/www/2001/sumfile1.html>; accessed: May 15, 2006.

U.S. Department of Health and Human Services. *The Health Consequences of Involuntary Smoking. A Report of the Surgeon General.* Rockville (MD): U.S. Department of Health and Human Services, Public Health Service, Centers for Disease Control, Center for Health Promotion and Education, Office on Smoking and Health, 1986. DHHS Publication No. (CDC) 87-8398.

Vaughan WM, Hammond SK. Impact of "designated smoking area" policy on nicotine vapor and particle concentrations in a modern office building. *Journal of the Air & Waste Management Association* 1990;40(7):1012–7.

Windsor RA, Lowe JB, Perkins LL, Smith-Yoder D, Artz L, Crawford M, Amburgy K, Boyd NRF Jr. Health education for pregnant smokers: its behavioral impact and cost benefit. *American Journal of Public Health* 1993;83(2):201–6.

Chapter 5
Reproductive and Developmental Effects from Exposure to Secondhand Smoke

Introduction

This chapter concerns adverse effects on reproduction, infants, and child development from exposure to secondhand smoke. Previous Surgeon General's reports have not comprehensively addressed the relationship between secondhand smoke exposure and reproductive outcomes, infant mortality, or child development. The 2001 Surgeon General's report (*Women and Smoking*) did summarize the literature on developmental and reproductive outcomes in relation to secondhand smoke exposure, focusing on the specific outcomes of fertility and fecundity, fetal growth and birth weight, fetal loss and neonatal mortality,

and congenital malformations (U.S. Department of Health and Human Services [USDHHS] 2001). The effects of active smoking by the mother during pregnancy were comprehensively reviewed in the 2004 report (USDHHS 2004). This new report reviews the possible effects of secondhand smoke exposure on reproductive and developmental outcomes, incorporates the substantial amount of evidence that has emerged since the 1986 Surgeon General's report (*The Health Consequences of Involuntary Smoking*, USDHHS 1986), and expands upon the 2001 report.

Conclusions of Previous Surgeon General's Reports and Other Relevant Reports

The early literature on secondhand smoke exposure and child health focused on adverse respiratory effects. Initial relevant reports were first published in the 1960s (Cameron et al. 1969), followed by larger studies in the 1970s (Colley 1974; Colley et al. 1974). The first summary report to comprehensively address reproductive and perinatal effects of secondhand smoke exposure was prepared by the California

Environmental Protection Agency and released in 1997 (National Cancer Institute [NCI] 1999). These topics were also addressed by a number of other agencies and groups, including the United Kingdom Department of Health (1998), the World Health Organization (WHO 1999), and the University of Toronto (2001). Table 5.1 summarizes the conclusions for reproductive and perinatal outcomes from these reports.

Literature Search Methods

The authors identified most of the literature on secondhand smoke exposure and adverse reproductive and perinatal effects through a systematic search of the National Library of Medicine's indexed journals, which date back to 1966. The relevant Medical Subject Headings (MeSH) terms and text terms were used to search PubMed. Text terms were used because many of the relevant MeSH terms were not introduced into the PubMed key wording scheme until some time

after 1966. For example, the MeSH term "Tobacco Smoke Pollution" was not introduced until 1982. The following text terms were also used in the search for articles: environmental, tobacco, smoke, secondhand smoke, paternal smoking, and passive smoking. By combining these text terms and MeSH terms using "or" as the Boolean connector, nearly 4,500 citations were identified. The authors also used this strategy to identify relevant research on outcomes. The results

Table 5.1   Findings on secondhand smoke exposure and reproductive and perinatal effects

Report	Outcome	Conclusion
Report of the Scientific Committee on Tobacco and Health (United Kingdom Department of Health 1998)	Sudden infant death syndrome	"Sudden infant death syndrome. . .is associated with exposure to environmental tobacco smoke. The association is judged to be one of cause and effect." (p. 10)
Health Effects of Exposure to Environmental Tobacco Smoke: The Report of the California Environmental Protection Agency (National Cancer Institute 1999)	Low birth weight/small for gestational age	"Taken together. . .[the studies] support a slight increase in LBW [low birth weight] or IUGR [intrauterine growth retardation] in association with ETS [environmental tobacco smoke, equivalent to secondhand smoke] exposure." (p. 102)
	Preterm delivery	"There was little evidence found for an association with preterm birth." (p. 102)
	Spontaneous abortion	". . .there is some epidemiologic evidence that ETS exposure may play a role in the etiology of spontaneous abortion. . . ." (p. 113)
	Congenital malformations	". . .it is not possible at this time to determine whether there is an association of ETS exposure with birth defects." (p. 119)
	Sudden infant death syndrome (SIDS)	There is "sufficient evidence that postnatal ETS exposure of the child is an independent risk factor for SIDS." (p. 139)
	Childhood cognition and behavior	"The evidence that ETS exposure of a nonsmoking pregnant woman can result in neuropsychologic deficits in the child. . .is inconclusive." (p. 154)
		"No conclusions regarding causality can be made on the basis of these studies, but they do provide suggestive evidence that [postnatal] ETS exposure may pose a neuropsychological developmental hazard." (p. 155)
	Postnatal physical development	". . .there is little to no epidemiological evidence that ETS exposure has a significant effect on height growth of children." (p. 162)
	Female fertility and fecundability	". . .the data are inadequate to determine whether there is an association of ETS exposure with effects on fertility or fecundability." (p. 178)
	Other female reproductive effects	". . .there is a paucity of data on the association of ETS exposure and lowered age at menopause or other measures of menstrual cycle dysfunction, and conclusions regarding causal associations cannot be reached." (p. 179)
	Male reproductive toxicity	". . .due to the paucity of data it is not possible to determine whether there is a causal association between ETS exposure and male reproductive dysfunction." (p. 180)
	Childhood cancers	". . .the evidence for a role of parental smoking and childhood cancers is inconclusive." (p. 282)

Table 5.1   Continued

Report	Outcome	Conclusion
International Consultation on Environmental Tobacco Smoke (ETS) and Child Health: Consultation Report (World Health Organization 1999)	Low birth weight	"ETS exposure among nonsmoking pregnant women can cause a decrease in birth weight…" (p. 4)
	SIDS	"…infant exposure to ETS may contribute to the risk of SIDS." (p. 4)
	Neurodevelopment	"…the effects of prenatal and postnatal ETS exposure on cognition and behaviour remain unclear." (p. 9)
	Childhood cancer	"…there is suggestive evidence linking exposure to tobacco smoke and childhood cancer." (p. 10)
Women and Smoking: A Report of the Surgeon General (U.S. Department of Health and Human Services 2001)	Low birth weight/small for gestational age	"…maternal exposure to ETS appears to be causally associated with detrimental effects on fetal growth." (p. 364)
	Fertility, spontaneous abortion, perinatal mortality	"Studies of ETS exposure and the risks for delay in conception, spontaneous abortion, and perinatal mortality are few, and the results are inconsistent." (p. 372)
Protection from Second-Hand Tobacco Smoke in Ontario: A Review of the Evidence Regarding Best Practices (University of Toronto 2001)	SIDS	"Exposure to second-hand smoke causes the following diseases and conditions… Sudden infant death syndrome…" (p. v)
	Low birth weight/ small for gestational age	"Exposure to second-hand smoke causes the following diseases and conditions… Fetal growth impairment including low birth-weight and small for gestational age…" (pp. v–vi)
	Spontaneous abortion	"Exposure to second-hand smoke has also been linked to other adverse health effects. The relationships may be causal. These include… Miscarriages…" (p. vi)

of each outcome-relevant search were then combined with the secondhand smoke-relevant search using "and" as the Boolean connector. These citations were imported into a database. Using title and abstract information, the authors selected the relevant articles for review. Finally, the references in the articles were reviewed for additional citations that were not identified through the PubMed searches.

Critical Exposure Periods for Reproductive and Developmental Effects

Assessing exposures to secondhand smoke in studies of fertility, fetal development, infant development, and child health and development is complex. For each of the three biologically relevant periods—preconception, pregnancy, and postdelivery—a number of potentially different biologic mechanisms of injury exist from exposure to secondhand smoke. Even within the nine months of pregnancy, vulnerability to the effects of secondhand smoke may change, reflecting differing mechanisms of injury as fetal organs develop and the fetus grows. Moreover, there are multiple environments where the woman or child is exposed to secondhand smoke (e.g., workplace, home, and day care), as well as multiple sources of secondhand smoke exposure for each of these environments (e.g., household members, day care providers, and coworkers). Finally, because of the potential impact of active maternal smoking (USDHHS 2004), active smoking before and during pregnancy needs to be taken into account when assessing the potential independent effects of exposure to secondhand smoke. Maternal smoking has well-characterized adverse effects for several outcomes, such as fertility, sudden infant death syndrome (SIDS), and child growth and development. Thus, the effects of exposure to secondhand smoke may be confounded by those of maternal smoking.

Secondhand smoke exposure may have adverse effects potentially throughout the reproductive and developmental processes (Table 5.2). During the preconception period, maternal exposure to secondhand smoke can potentially affect female fertility by altering the balance of hormones that affect oocyte production, including growth hormone, cortisol, luteinizing hormones, and prolactin (Mattison 1982; Daling et al. 1987; Mattison and Thomford 1987), or by reducing motility in the female reproductive tract (Mattison 1982; Daling et al. 1987). However, separating the potential effect of secondhand smoke exposure on the mother's reproductive process and the effect of active paternal smoking on the father's reproductive process is very difficult. Although the evidence is mixed, active smoking has been shown to affect sperm morphology, motility, and concentration (Rosenberg 1987; USDHHS 2004). Cigarette smoke may also lead to infertility through a combined effect of decreased sperm motility with active paternal smoking and decreased tubal patency with active maternal smoking and secondhand smoke exposure.

During pregnancy, maternal exposure to secondhand smoke could potentially affect the pregnancy by increasing the risk for spontaneous abortion or by interfering with the developing fetus through growth restrictions or congenital malformations (NCI 1999; WHO 1999). During gestation, windows of susceptibility exist when the developing embryo or fetus is vulnerable to various intrauterine conditions or exposures. Organogenesis occurs mainly during the embryonic period (weeks three through eight of gestation), which is also the time when major malformations are most likely to develop. During weeks 9 through 38 of gestation, susceptibility decreases and insults are more likely to lead to minor malformations or functional defects (Sadler 1990).

Finally, secondhand smoke exposure in the postpartum period could affect the developing infant and child, resulting in a number of adverse health outcomes. Given the developmental processes in progress, infants and children are considered to be more vulnerable to the effects of environmental exposures than are adults (Goldman 1995; Dempsey et al. 2000). Mechanisms that could lead to compromised physical and cognitive development as a result of exposure to secondhand smoke may be similar to the processes that affect fetal development, such as hypoxia (USDHHS 1990; Lambers and Clark 1996). One review of the impact of prenatal exposure to nicotine summarized numerous animal studies that demonstrated the effects of nicotine on cognitive processes among exposed rats and guinea pigs, such as impeded learning abilities or increased attention or memory deficits (Ernst et al. 2001). In animal and human studies, prenatal nicotine exposure affected aspects of neural functioning such as the activation of neurotransmitter systems, which may lead to permanent alterations in the developing brain through changes in gene expression. The proposed consequences of altered gene expression included disturbances in neuronal pathfinding and in cell regulation and differentiation (Ernst et al. 2001). Other animal studies have shown that newborn rats exposed to sidestream smoke have reduced DNA and protein concentrations in the brain (Gospe et al. 1996). Ideally, researchers should have information on secondhand smoke exposures for all relevant periods that relate to the outcome under study, because different physiologic processes may be affected across developmental periods (Table 5.2). However, this information is frequently unavailable in a particular study.

Secondhand smoke exposures most commonly occur in the home or workplace, and exposures in public places tend to be more sporadic. Recent exposure assessment and monitoring studies have shown that the home tends to be a greater source of secondhand smoke exposure than the workplace (Emmons et al. 1994; Pirkle et al. 1996; Hammond 1999), particularly since workplace smoking bans have become more restrictive (Marcus et al. 1992) (Chapter 3, Assessment of Exposure to Secondhand Smoke, and Chapter 4, Prevalence of Exposure to Secondhand Smoke). In the home, the major sources of exposures to secondhand smoke have been smoking by the spouse or partner and other household members. Paternal smoking has been the most commonly

Table 5.2   Potentially relevant exposure periods for reproductive and perinatal outcomes

Outcome	Relevant exposure periods		
	Preconception	Prenatal	Postnatal
Fertility (female)	X		
Spontaneous abortion	X	X	
Low birth weight, small for gestational age, intrauterine growth retardation	X	X	
Congenital malformations	X	X	
Infant death (including sudden infant death syndrome)	X	X	X
Cognitive development	X	X	X
Childhood behavior	X	X	X
Height/growth	X	X	X
Childhood cancer	X	X	X

measured source of secondhand smoke in the home (USDHHS 1986), and paternal smoking status tends to be constant across the three developmental periods: preconception, prenatal, and postnatal (USDHHS 1986). Although many studies have not considered smoking in the home by other household members, some studies have documented that such

smoking could be a significant source of secondhand smoke exposure for women (Pattishall et al. 1985; Rebagliato et al. 1995a; Pirkle et al. 1996; Ownby et al. 2000; Kaufman et al. 2002). Studies on workplace exposure have focused on whether or not the person was exposed, but less attention has been paid to quantifying the exposure (Misra and Nguyen 1999).

Fertility

Biologic Basis

Infertility is commonly defined as a failure to conceive after 12 months of unprotected intercourse. Infertility should not be confused with fecundability, which is defined as the probability of conception during one menstrual cycle and measured by time to pregnancy. Thus, low fecundability is delayed conception. The biologic plausibility that secondhand smoke exposure affects human fertility and fecundability is supported by both animal and human studies of active smoking, which include exposure to the same materials as involuntary smoking. In animal

studies, numerous investigators have demonstrated the biologic effects of nicotine in disrupting oviduct function (Neri and Marcus 1972; Ruckebusch 1975) and in delaying blastocyst formation and implantation (Yoshinaga et al. 1979). Investigations of assisted reproduction among humans who actively smoke have also provided information on possible mechanisms of infertility and delayed conception from secondhand smoke exposure. Several studies of assisted reproductive techniques have suggested that active maternal smoking reduces the estradiol level in follicular fluid (Elenbogen et al. 1991; Van Voorhis et al. 1992), impedes ovulation induction (Van Voorhis et al. 1992; Chung et al. 1997), reduces the fertilization rate (Elenbogen et al. 1991; Rosevear et al. 1992), and retards the embryo cleavage rate (dose-dependent) (Hughes et al. 1992). Metabolites of cigarette smoke have been measured in the follicular fluid of active smokers at assisted reproduction clinics (Trapp et al. 1986; Weiss and Eckert 1989; Rosevear et al. 1992) and in the cervical mucus of active smokers in a cervical cancer study (Sasson et al. 1985).

Together, the evidence from studies of biologic mechanisms and the findings of numerous epidemiologic studies have led to the conclusion that active maternal smoking causes reduced fertility. An early review by Stillman and colleagues (1986) of studies of natural reproduction in addition to the two most recent Surgeon General's reports (USDHHS 2001, 2004) support this conclusion of a causal association, and findings of meta-analyses have provided estimates of the magnitude of the effect of maternal smoking on fertility. Hughes and Brennan (1996) combined the results of seven studies on in vitro fertilization with gamete intrafallopian transfer. Comparing smokers and nonsmokers, the researchers obtained a combined odds ratio (OR) for conception of 0.57 (95 percent confidence interval [CI], 0.42–0.78). Similarly, Augood and colleagues (1998) pooled nine studies that compared smokers with nonsmokers and found a combined OR of 0.66 (95 percent CI, 0.49–0.88) for the number of pregnancies per cycle of in vitro fertilization. In their meta-analysis of 12 studies, Augood and colleagues (1998) compared smokers with nonsmokers and found that the overall OR for infertility was 1.60 (95 percent CI, 1.34–1.91). Several investigators found a dose-response trend between the level of active maternal smoking and decreased fertility (Baird and Wilcox 1985; Suonio et al. 1990; Laurent et al. 1992).

Although active paternal smoking could also play a role in infertility by affecting sperm quality, the 2004 Surgeon General's report found conflicting evidence on active smoking and sperm quality (USDHHS 2004). In another review, investigators performed a meta-analysis of 20 study populations (from 18 published papers) on cigarette smoking and sperm density and found a weighted estimated reduction of 13 percent in sperm density (95 percent CI, 8.0–17.1) among smokers compared with nonsmokers (Vine et

al. 1994). The epidemiologic studies that have examined the effect of active paternal smoking on fertility are not as consistent in their findings as the studies that have investigated active maternal smoking and fertility (Underwood et al. 1967; Tokuhata 1968; Baird and Wilcox 1985; de Mouzon et al. 1988; Dunphy et al. 1991; Pattinson et al. 1991; Hughes et al. 1992; Rowlands et al. 1992; Bolumar et al. 1996; Hull et al. 2000). One review concluded that paternal smoking had no effect on fertility (Hughes and Brennan 1996).

Several studies that were conducted in reproductive clinics measured tobacco smoke biomarkers in nonsmoking men and women exposed to secondhand smoke. Cotinine was measurable in follicular fluid, with measurements related to dose (Zenzes et al. 1996), and benzo[*a*]pyrene adducts were found in ovarian cells (Zenzes et al. 1998). Both nicotine and cotinine were measured in semen of nonsmoking, secondhand smoke-exposed men attending a clinic specializing in infertility (Pacifici et al. 1995).

Epidemiologic Evidence

Although active maternal smoking has been causally associated with infertility (USDHHS 2004), less evidence is available on maternal exposure to secondhand smoke and fertility, and no data were found on paternal secondhand smoke exposure and fertility. Two studies specifically addressed maternal exposure to secondhand smoke in relation to infertility, although they examined different outcome measures (Chung et al. 1997; Hull et al. 2000). Chung and colleagues (1997) studied infertile patients undergoing a gamete intrafallopian transfer procedure (Table 5.3). The researchers found that a higher proportion of active smokers had anovulation and required significantly higher amounts of human menopausal gonadotropins (hMG) to stimulate ovulation than did nonsmokers. However, the investigators found no significant differences in these same parameters when they compared unexposed nonsmokers and secondhand smoke-exposed nonsmokers, defined as having at least one household member who smoked. Among the unexposed nonsmokers, 3.0 percent had anovulation and required an average of 26 vials of hMG. Among the exposed nonsmokers, 7.8 percent had anovulation and required an average of 24 vials of hMG. The two groups also did not differ in pregnancy rates (45.5 percent in the unexposed group and 46.2 percent in the exposed group) or birth rates (33.3 percent versus 23.1 percent, respectively). This study included only 98 patients, of whom 13 were secondhand smoke-exposed only. Hull and colleagues (2000) assessed secondhand smoke exposures from the workplace and the home among more than 8,000 women with a planned pregnancy (Table 5.3). Nonsmoking women with any secondhand smoke exposure (n = 1,987) had an increased risk for conception delay of more than six months compared with unexposed nonsmoking women (n = 4,133) (adjusted OR = 1.17 [95 percent CI, 1.02–1.37]). In this study, the investigators also included an analysis of active paternal smoking (adjusted for active maternal smoking); they found that the fathers who smoked more than 20 cigarettes per day had an increased risk for conception delay of more than six months compared with nonsmoking fathers (OR = 1.39 [95 percent CI, 1.14–1.68]).

Two other studies examined maternal exposure to secondhand smoke in addition to active maternal smoking in relation to fertility (Table 5.3) (Baird and Wilcox 1985; Olsen 1991). Using regression analysis, Baird and Wilcox (1985) adjusted for active maternal smoking to examine the impact of active paternal smoking among 678 pregnant women. No effect was found after adjusting for active maternal smoking, although the data were not presented ($\chi^2 = 0.000$, p = 0.953). Olsen (1991) analyzed only nonsmoking women without a history of infertility treatments. Olsen's analysis categorized paternal smoking as 1 to 9, 10 to 19, and 20 or more cigarettes per day, and calculated the ORs for time to pregnancy of more than 6 and more than 12 months. There were increased risks for both time outcomes. The greatest risks were at exposures of 10 to 19 cigarettes per day for more than 6 months (OR = 1.32 [95 percent CI, 1.10–1.58]) and for more than 12 months (OR = 1.39 [95 percent CI, 1.10–1.75]).

The limited epidemiologic evidence on maternal secondhand smoke exposure and fertility does not warrant a meta-analysis of the relevant studies.

Evidence Synthesis

The observational evidence is quite limited. The four studies that directly address maternal secondhand smoke exposure and fertility differ substantially in study design and methods. For example, Chung and colleagues (1997) investigated patients who were attending a clinic for fertility-related problems and examined the success rate of assisted reproduction. Hull and colleagues (2000), on the other hand, included pregnant women and examined delayed natural conception. In the former study, the investigators did not account for potential confounders and obtained retrospective information about exposure to secondhand smoke from telephone interviews (Chung et al. 1997). Hull and colleagues (2000) relied on a self-administered questionnaire to ascertain exposure information during pregnancy, and used potential confounders in the analysis such as parental age, body mass index, and alcohol consumption. The evidence from this larger study on natural conception is consistent with the biologic framework established by the studies on active maternal smoking and fertility (Hull et al. 2000).

Conclusion

1. The evidence is inadequate to infer the presence or absence of a causal relationship between maternal exposure to secondhand smoke and female fertility or fecundability. No data were found on paternal exposure to secondhand smoke and male fertility or fecundability.

Implications

As exposure of women of reproductive age to secondhand smoke continues, this topic needs further rigorous investigation. In particular, the frequency and extent of current exposures should be characterized. Further epidemiologic studies also merit consideration.

Table 5.3   Studies of secondhand smoke exposure and fertility

Study	Design/population	Source of exposure	Outcome	Exposure categories
Baird and Wilcox 1985	678 pregnant women who were not using contraceptives before conception, recruited through early pregnancy classes and obstetric practices	Husband	Time to pregnancy	Yes/no

Olsen 1991	Population-based survey conducted in Denmark between 1984 and 1987, completed by 10,866 women in their third trimester of pregnancy who had no history of infertility treatments	Father
		Father
		Father
		Father
		
		Father
		Father
		Father
		Father
			Time to pregnancy	>6 months:
				  0 cigarettes/day
				  1–9 cigarettes/day
				  10–19 cigarettes/day
				  ≥20 cigarettes/day
				
				>12 months:
				  0 cigarettes/day
				  1–9 cigarettes/day
				  10–19 cigarettes/day
				  ≥20 cigarettes/day

Chung et al. 1997	98 infertile women undergoing a gamete intrafallopian transfer procedure	Home	Anovulation Pregnancy rate Birth rate	Data were not reported
Hull et al. 2000	12,106 pregnant women with due dates between April 1991 and December 1992	Work and home	Time to pregnancy	Yes/no

*OR = Odds ratio.
†CI = Confidence interval.

Findings	Comments
No effect (data were not presented) $\chi^2 = 0.000$, p = 0.953	Adjusted for maternal smoking and potential risk factors; paternal smoking did not affect fertility
>6 months: OR* = 1.16 (95% CI†, 0.95–1.41) OR = 1.32 (95% CI, 1.10–1.58) OR = 1.32 (95% CI, 0.96–1.80) >12 months: OR = 1.34 (95% CI, 1.05–1.72) OR = 1.39 (95% CI, 1.10–1.75) OR = 1.11 (95% CI, 0.72–1.71)	Results are for nonsmoking mothers

Anovulation:
  3.0% in unexposed group
  7.8% in exposed group
 	
Pregnancy rate:
  45.5% in unexposed group
  46.2% in exposed group
 	
Birth rate:
  33.3% in unexposed group
  23.1% in exposed group
	13 were secondhand smoke-exposed only (nonsmokers); this study demonstrated that active, but not involuntary, cigarette smoking has an adverse impact on the pregnancy and live-birth rates in gamete intrafallopian transfer producers

Conceived after >6 months:
  OR = 1.17 (95% CI, 1.02–1.37)
Conceived after >12 months:
  OR = 1.14 (95% CI, 0.92–1.42)
	Findings are based on 4,133 unexposed and 1,987 secondhand smoke-exposed nonsmokers; trends by categories of cigarettes/day smoked by partners of nonsmoking women were not statistically significant; this study provides new evidence of delayed conception if a woman is exposed to secondhand smoke at home or in the workplace

Pregnancy (Spontaneous Abortion and Perinatal Death)

Biologic Basis

Fetal loss or spontaneous abortion is defined as the involuntary termination of an intrauterine pregnancy before 20 weeks of gestation (Anderson et al. 1998). Because most early fetal losses are underreported and unrecognized, spontaneous abortions are extremely difficult to study. Twenty to 40 percent of all pregnancies may terminate too early to be recognized or confirmed (Wilcox et al. 1988; Eskenazi et al. 1995). Furthermore, the etiology of spontaneous abortion is multifactorial and not fully understood. Some early miscarriages result from chromosomal abnormalities in the developing embryo; others are related to factors associated with maternal age, with the pregnancy itself, or to other types of exposures (e.g., occupational exposure, alcohol consumption, or fever). Moreover, relatively few animal studies have been conducted to gain an understanding of how exposure to sidestream smoke may affect the processes of spontaneous abortion (NCI 1999). In one study of sea urchins, investigators noted that exposure to nicotine prevented the cortical granule reaction, which typically prevents the entry of additional sperm into the egg once fertilization has occurred (Longo and

Table 5.4   Studies of secondhand smoke exposure and pregnancy loss

Study	Design/population	Exposure categories	Source of exposure
Koo et al. 1988	Cross-sectional 136 nonsmoking wives Hong Kong 1981–1983	• Unexposed • Secondhand smoke only • Light (1–20 cigarettes/day) • Heavy (>20 cigarettes/day)	• Husband • Some work exposure
Ahlborg and Bodin 1991	Prospective 4,701 pregnancies Sweden (Orebo County) 1980–1983	• Unexposed • Secondhand smoke only • Active smoking (1–9 cigarettes/day, 10–19 cigarettes/day, or ≥20 cigarettes/day)	• Maternal smoking • Secondhand smoke exposure
Windham et al. 1992	Case-control 626 cases and 1,300 controls United States (Santa Clara County, California) 1986–1987	• Exposure ≥1 hour in a room where someone else was smoking • No maternal smoking • Mother smoked 1–10 cigarettes/day • Mother smoked >10 cigarettes/day • Any smoking	• Smoking behavior 1 month before pregnancy • Any smoking changes during pregnancy • Paternal smoking

*RR = Relative risk.
†CI = Confidence interval.
‡OR = Odds ratio.

Anderson 1970). If this same process occurs in the human fertilized ovum as a result of nicotine exposure, this may be a mechanism by which abnormalities in the developing embryo result in spontaneous abortions (Longo and Anderson 1970; Mattison et al. 1989). Several tobacco components and metabolites are potentially toxic to the developing fetus, including lead, nicotine, cotinine, cyanide, cadmium, carbon monoxide (CO), and polycyclic aromatic hydrocarbons (Lambers and Clark 1996; Werler 1997). Finally, with regard to active smoking and spontaneous abortion, many studies have reported a greater increase in risk for smokers than for nonsmokers, and some studies have demonstrated dose-response relationships (USDHHS 2004).

Epidemiologic Evidence

Among five studies that reported on involuntary smoking and miscarriage or spontaneous abortion, three studies found an increased risk among exposed women compared with unexposed women. In a study conducted in Hong Kong, Koo and colleagues (1988) reported that if husbands were heavy smokers (>20 cigarettes per day), their wives were two times more likely to have a miscarriage or spontaneous abortion than were women whose husbands did not smoke. Windham and colleagues (1992) examined active and secondhand smoke exposures among 1,926 pregnant women and measured exposure to secondhand smoke two ways: the amount smoked by the "father of the unborn child," and maternal exposure to secondhand smoke for more than one hour per day (Table 5.4). After adjusting for maternal

Outcome	Findings	Comments
Miscarriage/abortion	Percentage with ≥1 miscarriage/abortion: 　　Nonsmoking husband: 33% 　　Husband was a light smoker: 43% 　　Husband was a heavy smoker: 59% p value = 0.12 for wives with smoking husbands	Participants were interviewed in their homes by trained interviewers 44% of wives with nonsmoking husbands had been exposed to secondhand smoke at home or at work
Spontaneous abortion Preterm birth Low birth weight (LBW)	• Secondhand smoke exposure at work (RR* = 1.53 [95% CI†, 0.98–2.38]) for spontaneous abortion • Adjusted RR for active exposure from smoking 10–19 cigarettes/day = 2.18 (95% CI, 1.51–3.14) for preterm birth and 2.38 (95% CI, 1.22–4.65) for LBW • RR for active exposure from smoking ≥20 cigarettes/day = 2.30 (95% CI, 1.19–4.44) for preterm birth and 2.71 (95% CI, 0.86–8.53) for LBW	Source exposure data were self-reported (questionnaires)
Spontaneous abortion	• OR‡ = 1.31 (95% CI, 0.92–1.88) for mothers who smoked >10 cigarettes/day • OR = 1.5 (95% CI, 1.2–1.9) for mothers exposed to secondhand smoke for ≥1 hour/day • OR = 2.1 (95% CI, 0.8–6.0) for fathers who smoked 1–10 cigarettes/day • 40% of mothers smoked during pregnancy if fathers smoked (highly correlated)	Source exposure data were self-reported; there was no conclusive evidence of an association between active smoking and spontaneous abortion; a moderate association was observed with secondhand smoke exposure; findings were adjusted for maternal factors of age, race, education, marital status, prior fetal loss, tobacco use, alcohol consumption, bottled water intake, employment, insurance, and nausea

factors of age, race, education, marital status, prior fetal loss, tobacco use, alcohol consumption, bottled water intake, employment, insurance, and nausea, women exposed to secondhand smoke for one hour or more per day had an adjusted OR of 1.5 (95 percent CI, 1.2–1.9) for second trimester losses compared with nonsmokers. Windham and colleagues (1992), however, found no association for their second measure of involuntary smoking, which was paternal smoking (examined by dose). Ahlborg and Bodin (1991) examined involuntary smoking and spontaneous abortion among nonsmoking mothers in Sweden. Women who were exposed to secondhand smoke at work were at an increased risk for first trimester losses (relative risk [RR] = 2.16 [95 percent CI, 1.23–3.81]), but exposure to secondhand smoke at home was not associated with spontaneous abortion. In Finland, Lindbohm and colleagues (1991) examined paternal exposures to occupational lead and paternal smoking among 513 pregnancies (213 of which ended in spontaneous abortion). Without adjusting for potential confounding factors, the authors observed that paternal smoking did not increase the risk of spontaneous abortion (OR = 1.3 [95 percent CI, 0.9–1.9]). Windham and colleagues (1999b) conducted another prospective study that involved 5,000 women who resided in California from 1990 to 1991. The investigators examined exposure to secondhand smoke only among nonsmoking women and ascertained the number of hours per day that a woman was near others who smoked (including paternal smoking). There was little evidence for increased risks, and all ORs were an estimated 1.0.

Evidence Synthesis

The few studies that have examined the relationship between involuntary smoking and spontaneous abortion have inconsistent findings (Table 5.4). Although some studies reported an increased risk for spontaneous abortion among women exposed to secondhand smoke at work or at home, many found no association. However, for the studies that showed no associations, the study samples may have lacked adequate statistical power.

Three studies examined secondhand smoke exposures among women who were nonsmokers. Koo and colleagues (1988) examined rates of miscarriage among 136 nonsmoking wives who were part of a larger study on cancer. These 136 women were the controls in this study, which ascertained lifetime smoking histories of the husbands and reproductive histories of the wives. Social and demographic factors differed between families with smoking and nonsmoking husbands. The crude OR for more than two miscarriages among wives with husbands who smoked was 1.81 (95 percent CI, 0.85–3.85) (adjusted ORs were not reported). Ahlborg and Bodin (1991) reported on nonsmoking women who were exposed to secondhand smoke at home. Two estimates were provided, one for first trimester losses (OR = 0.96 [95 percent CI, 0.50–1.86]) and for one second or third trimester losses (OR = 1.06 [95 percent CI, 0.55–2.05]). Windham and colleagues (1999b) reported adjusted ORs for paternal smoking among women who were nonsmokers. When maternal age, prior spontaneous abortion, alcohol and caffeine consumption, and gestational age at initial interviews were taken into account, the investigators obtained an OR of 1.15 (95 percent CI, 0.86–1.55) for secondhand smoke exposure at home. The pooled estimate from these three studies (with the two estimates from Alborg and Bodin [1991] included separately) for secondhand smoke exposure in the home or from fathers who smoked and who were married to nonsmoking women was 1.18 (95 percent CI, 0.92–1.44).

Future studies not only need to ensure an adequate sample size, but they should give particular attention to the difficult issues of confounding and to accurate estimates of secondhand smoke exposures in the workplace and in the home.

Conclusion

1. The evidence is inadequate to infer the presence or absence of a causal relationship between maternal exposure to secondhand smoke during pregnancy and spontaneous abortion.

Implications

As for other outcomes that have very few studies, further research is warranted (see "Overall Implications" later in this chapter).

Infant Deaths

Infant mortality is defined as the death of a live-born infant within 364 days of birth. Many of the major causes of infant deaths, such as low birth weight (LBW), preterm delivery, and SIDS, are also associated with exposure to tobacco smoke during and after pregnancy. The biologic mechanisms by which secondhand smoke exposure leads to these particular outcomes are discussed in other parts of this chapter and will not be discussed here. In 2002, the infant mortality rate for infants of smokers (11.1 percent) was 68 percent higher than the rate for infants of nonsmokers (6.6 percent) (Mathews et al. 2004). For each race and Hispanic-origin group, the infant mortality rate among infants of smokers was higher compared with the rate among infants of nonsmokers.

Epidemiologic Evidence

Numerous studies have demonstrated associations of active maternal smoking with neonatal and perinatal mortality (Comstock and Lundin 1967; Rush and Kass 1972; Cnattingius 1988; Malloy et al. 1988; Schramm 1997). Even with modern neonatal intensive care, children of smokers are at an increased risk for neonatal mortality (death of a live-born infant within 28 days) (Cnattingius 1988; Malloy et al. 1988; Schramm 1997), with reported OR estimates of 1.2 for infants of smokers compared with infants of nonsmokers. Two studies have assessed neonatal mortality among infants exposed to secondhand smoke. Comstock and Lundin (1967) examined neonatal mortality among a sample of 448 live births, 234 stillbirths, and 431 infant deaths that occurred between 1950 and 1964 in Washington County, Maryland. When comparisons were made between families with paternal smokers only and families with two nonsmoking parents, neonatal mortality rates that were adjusted for gender and paternal education were higher: 17.2 (father smoked) versus 11.9 (neither parent smoked) neonatal deaths per 1,000 live births. Yerushalmy (1971) examined active and involuntary smoking and perinatal outcomes among an estimated 13,000 births in California. After examining crude rates for neonatal mortality, Yerushalmy (1971) found (without considering maternal smoking) that rates for both Blacks and Whites were elevated among infants whose fathers smoked compared with infants of nonsmoking fathers; there were no adjustments for any other confounding factors.

Evidence Synthesis

Only two studies examined the relationship of involuntary smoking with neonatal mortality. Both studies reported associations of secondhand smoke exposure from paternal smoking with neonatal mortality. There is significantly more literature on active smoking by the mother during pregnancy and neonatal outcome. Although the strength of the relationship in these two studies was strong, causality cannot be inferred because of the small number of studies and because of inadequate controls for potential confounders.

Conclusion

1. The evidence is inadequate to infer the presence or absence of a causal relationship between exposure to secondhand smoke and neonatal mortality.

Implications

In addition to the consistent relationship demonstrated between exposure to secondhand smoke and neonatal mortality, numerous studies have reported significant associations between active maternal smoking during pregnancy and infant mortality. Thus, the association of secondhand smoke exposure during pregnancy and infant mortality warrants further investigation. Moreover, the data cited were from older studies, and smoking patterns and levels of secondhand smoke exposure may have changed since the time some of the studies were conducted. To clarify the association between maternal smoking and infant mortality, more evidence is needed.

Sudden Infant Death Syndrome

The sudden, unexplained, unexpected death of an infant before one year of age—referred to as SIDS—has been investigated in relation to exposure of the fetus and infant to smoking by mothers and others during the preconception, prenatal, and postpartum periods. The death rate attributable to SIDS has declined by more than half during the past two decades (Ponsonby et al. 2002; American Academy of Pediatrics [AAP] Task Force on SIDS 2005). SIDS has decreased dramatically because of interventions such as the "Back to Sleep" campaign implemented in the 1990s (Gibson et al. 2000; Malloy 2002; Malloy and Freeman 2004). Numerous studies have examined the association between active smoking among mothers during pregnancy and the subsequent risk of SIDS. The evidence for active smoking has demonstrated a causal association between maternal smoking during pregnancy and SIDS (Anderson and Cook 1997; United Kingdom Department of Health 1998; USDHHS 2001). The 2004 Surgeon General's report concluded that the evidence is sufficient to infer a causal relationship between SIDS and maternal smoking during and after pregnancy (USDHHS 2004). This new 2006 Surgeon General's report considers exposure of the infant to secondhand smoke from the mother, father, or others.

Biologic Basis

Although studies have identified social and behavioral risk factors for SIDS, the biologic mechanism or mechanisms underlying sudden, unexplained, unexpected death before one year of age are still unknown (Joad 2000; AAP Task Force on SIDS 2005). Chapter 2 (Toxicology of Secondhand Smoke) reviews the animal and human studies that provide evidence on how prenatal and postnatal exposure to nicotine and to other toxicants in tobacco smoke may affect the neuroregulation of breathing, apneic spells, and risk for sudden infant death. Experimental data from animal models on the neurotoxicity of prenatal and neonatal exposure to nicotine and secondhand smoke can be related to several potential causal mechanisms for SIDS, including adverse effects on brain cell development, synaptic development and

function, and neurobehavioral activity (Slotkin 1998; Slotkin et al. 2001, 2006; Machaalani et al. 2005). Stick and colleagues (1996) observed newborns in the hospital and reported reductions in respiratory function among infants of smokers compared with infants of nonsmokers. Other proposed mechanisms for postpartum reductions in respiratory function have included irritation of the airways by tobacco smoke, susceptibility to respiratory infections that increases the risk of SIDS, and a change in the ventilatory responses to hypoxia attributable to nicotine (Anderson and Cook 1997).

A diagnosis of SIDS requires supporting evidence from an autopsy so as to exclude other causes. Thus, SIDS is a difficult outcome to study. Numerous studies have examined the association between active smoking among mothers during pregnancy and the subsequent risk of SIDS. The evidence for active smoking has demonstrated a causal association between maternal smoking during pregnancy and SIDS (Anderson and Cook 1997; United Kingdom Department of Health 1998; USDHHS 2001, 2004).

Epidemiologic Evidence

Anderson and Cook (1997) and the California Environmental Protection Agency (Cal/EPA 1997, 2005) have provided systematic reviews of the effects of secondhand smoke exposure on SIDS. The 1997 Cal/EPA review identified and selected 10 epidemiologic studies with the best data that examined the relationship between secondhand smoke and SIDS. On the basis of the the results from the quantitative meta-analysis and the qualitative review of results on paternal and other smokers in the household, Anderson and Cook (1997) concluded that the epidemiologic evidence points to a causal relationship between SIDS and postnatal exposure to tobacco smoke.

The discussion that follows includes a review of the epidemiologic studies that examined the association between household secondhand smoke exposure and SIDS among postpartum infants. Consideration was given to the most appropriate study design that controlled for the confounding factors that are critical to delineating the independent risk related to second-hand smoke exposure and SIDS among postpartum infants. Because researchers have established the causal risk of maternal smoking during pregnancy (USDHHS 2001, 2004), there are epidemiologic studies that provide appropriate controls in the study design for the analysis of prenatal maternal smoking and other potentially important confounding factors (e.g., infant's sleeping position and birth weight, parental use of drugs or alcohol, and the potentially synergistic effect of maternal smoking and bed sharing) (Lahr et al. 2005). Although self-reported information on the smoking behaviors of adults living in the household is an indirect measure of the potential for exposing a newborn to secondhand smoke, researchers evaluate analyses of postnatal secondhand smoke exposure from the father or other smokers in the household because these studies have the potential to more fully control for the possible confounding of maternal smoking during pregnancy. Table 5.5 provides a summary of the design, methods, and findings of the Anderson and Cook (1997) meta-analysis and of the nine primary studies identified in that review, which evaluated the risks of postnatal maternal or paternal smoking. Table 5.5 also includes the four epidemiologic studies that were published subsequent to the review by Anderson and Cook (1997). The methodology varied across these studies; many used autopsies to determine that SIDS was the likely cause of death. The "Comments" column of Table 5.5 provides other important methodologic aspects of each study. Only one study evaluated maternal exposure to secondhand smoke during pregnancy (Klonoff-Cohen et al. 1995), and only one study used urinary cotinine levels to biochemically validate secondhand smoke exposures among newborns (Dwyer et al. 1999). Many studies controlled for potential confounders that included sleeping position, parental bed sharing, social class, parental use of drugs or alcohol, birth weight, gestational age, and prenatal maternal smoking.

Of the 13 individual studies in Table 5.5 that examined the association between household second-hand smoke exposure and SIDS among postpartum infants, 10 studies independently examined the effects of postpartum maternal smoking. Each study found a significant association between postnatal maternal smoking and SIDS (Bergman and Wiesner 1976; McGlashan 1989; Schoendorf and Kiely 1992; Mitchell et al. 1993, 1997; Klonoff-Cohen et al. 1995; Ponsonby et al. 1995; Blair et al. 1996; Brooke et al. 1997;

Dwyer et al. 1999). Two of the studies did not consider potential confounders (Bergman and Wiesner 1976; McGlashan 1989), and three studies did not adjust for maternal smoking during pregnancy (Ponsonby et al. 1995; Brooke et al. 1997; Dwyer et al. 1999). Among the four studies (and five samples, including the separate analyses for Whites and Blacks within the Schoendorf and Kiely [1992] study) with more complete adjustments for important confounders such as prenatal maternal smoking, the adjusted ORs for postnatal maternal smoking were all statistically significant. The ORs ranged from 1.65 (95 percent CI, 1.20–2.28) (Mitchell et al. 1993) and 1.75 (95 percent CI, 1.04–2.95) for White infants and 2.33 (95 percent CI, 1.48–3.67) for Black infants (Schoendorf and Kiely 1992), to 2.28 (95 percent CI, 1.04–4.98) (Klonoff-Cohen et al. 1995) and 2.39 (95 percent CI, 1.01–6.00), respectively (Ponsonby et al. 1995). In one study that controlled for prenatal maternal smoking in addition to many other factors in a multivariate model, the effect for postnatal maternal smoking was no longer significant (p = 0.16), possibly because of the strong correlation between maternal smoking during pregnancy and postnatal smoking (Blair et al. 1996). However, this study observed a significant OR for the additive effect of postnatal maternal smoking to the risk of smoking during pregnancy (OR = 2.93 [95 percent CI, 1.56–5.48]). The remaining three studies in Table 5.5 (Mitchell et al. 1991; Nicholl and O'Cathain 1992; Alm et al. 1998) were included because they provide additional data on paternal and other smoking in the household or on dose-response relationships.

Two studies provided data that assessed exposure of the infant to secondhand smoke with greater precision than with classification by the postpartum smoking status of the mother alone (Klonoff-Cohen et al. 1995; Dwyer et al. 1999). Dwyer and colleagues (1999) assessed urinary cotinine levels in 100 infants as part of a prospective study of more than 10,000 births in the Tasmanian Infant Health Survey. Of the 53 mothers who reported postnatal smoking, only 32 reported smoking sometimes or always in the same room as the infant. Maternal smoking in the same room significantly increased infant urinary cotinine levels (p <0.0001) and the OR of the risk of SIDS (1.96 [95 percent CI, 1.01–3.80]). Klonoff-Cohen and colleagues (1995) collected more extensive interview data on sources of infant exposure to tobacco smoke from the mother, father, and other live-in adults, including data on whether the person smoked in the

Table 5.5   Studies of secondhand smoke exposure and sudden infant death syndrome (SIDS)

Study	Design/population	Exposure categories	Source of exposure
Bergman and Wiesner 1976	Case-control (56 cases, 86 controls, matched for gender, race [all Caucasian], and date of birth) United States (King county, Washington state) 1970–1974	• Mother smoked after pregnancy • Father smoked	• Mother and father
McGlashan 1989	Case-control (167 cases, 334 controls, matched for gender, born in same hospital, and proximate date of birth) Australia (Tasmania) 1980–1986	• Smoking status of parents • Cigarettes/day smoked by mother (habitual, during pregnancy, and during the infant's first year)	• Mother and father
Mitchell et al. 1991	Case-control (128 cases, 503 controls randomly selected from all births) New Zealand 1987–1988	• Cigarettes/day smoked by mother during the 2 weeks before the interview	• Mother
Nicholl and O'Cathain 1992	Case-control (303 cases, 277 controls, matched for date and place of birth) United Kingdom 1976–1979	• Prenatal and postnatal smoking status of the mother's partner	• Mother's partner

Schoendorf and Kiely 1992	Case-control (435 cases ≥2,500 grams [g], 6,098 controls ≥2,500 g) All infant deaths were from causes other than SIDS Sample was stratified by race:
	    Black infants (103 cases, 2,423 controls)
	    White infants (89 cases, 1,987 controls)
	Data from the National Maternal and Infant Health Survey United States 1988
		• None (no prenatal or postnatal maternal smoking), mother smoked after pregnancy (secondhand), and mother smoked during and after pregnancy (combined)
		• Secondhand smoke exposure from other household members (none vs. any)
			• Mother (smoked prenatally and postpartum)
			• Other household members (smoking status at time of survey)

Outcome	Findings	Comments

SIDS	Maternal smoking
	  OR* = 2.42 (95% CI[†], 1.22–4.82)
	Paternal smoking
	  OR = 1.53 (95% CI, 0.78–3.01)
	Unadjusted
		Exposure data were self-reported (mailed questionnaire); all cases were autopsied; OR and CI were calculated from prevalence estimates provided in the paper; exposure to secondhand smoke appears to enhance the risk of SIDS; potential confounders were not assessed

SIDS	Father was habitual smoker
	  RR[‡] = 1.73 (p = 0.05)
	Mother smoked during infant's first year
	  RR = 2.20 (p <0.01)
	During infant's first year, mother smoked
	  >10 cigarettes/day: RR = 2.37 (p <0.05)
	  >20 cigarettes/day: RR = 3.11 (p <0.05)
		Exposure data were self-reported (interview); all cases were autopsied; RR was based on statistical analysis of case-2 matched control "triples"; dose-response for level of paternal smoking was noted but RR was not reported; parental smoking carries a high relative risk for SIDS

SIDS	In the past 2 weeks, mother smoked
	  1–9 cigarettes/day: OR = 1.87 (95% CI, 0.98–3.54)
	  10–19 cigarettes/day: OR = 2.64 (95% CI, 1.47–4.74)
	  ≥20 cigarettes/day: OR = 5.06 (95% CI, 2.86–8.95)
	Unadjusted
		Exposure data were self-reported (interview); all cases were autopsied; maternal smoking is an independent risk factor for SIDS

SIDS	Neither mother nor her partner smoked during pregnancy
	  1.0 (reference)
	Mother did not smoke during pregnancy, partner did smoke prenatally and postnatally
	  RR = 1.63 (95% CI, 1.11–2.40)
		Exposure data were self-reported (interview); all cases were autopsied; adjusted for birth weight, maternal age and gravidity, and condition of the family's housing; RR for paternal smoking increased over 4 age-at-death intervals; postnatal secondhand smoke exposure from the father plays a role in the risk of SIDS

SIDS	From mothers
	Black infants
	  Secondhand: OR = 2.33 (95% CI, 1.48–3.67)
	  Combined: OR = 3.06 (95% CI, 2.19–4.29)
	White infants
	  Secondhand: OR = 1.75 (95% CI, 1.04–2.95)
	  Combined: OR = 3.10 (95% CI, 2.27–4.24)
	Adjusted for marital status and maternal age and education
	
	From other household members (none vs. any)
	Black infants (by mother's smoking category)
	  None: OR = 1.00 (95% CI, 0.62–1.58)
	  Secondhand: OR = 1.03 (95% CI, 0.43–2.47)
	  All infants: OR = 0.93 (95% CI, 0.68–1.27)
	White infants
	  None: OR = 1.33 (95% CI, 0.77–2.27)
	  Secondhand: OR = 1.63 (95% CI, 0.58–4.74)
	  All infants: OR = 1.41 (95% CI, 1.04–1.90)
	  Adjusted for marital status and maternal age and education
		Race of infant defined as Black non-Hispanic and White non-Hispanic; control variables were selected from birth certificates; survey questionnaire was completed by the mother; possible bias in self-reported smoking behaviors of case and control mothers; 92% of cases were autopsied; both intrauterine and secondhand smoke exposures are associated with an increased risk of SIDS

Table 5.5   Continued

Study	Design/population	Exposure categories	Source of exposure
Mitchell et al. 1993	Case-control (485 cases, 1,800 controls randomly selected from all births) Data from the New Zealand Cot Death Study 1987–1990	• Mother smoked during pregnancy • Father smoked during the past 2 weeks • Other household members smoked during the past 2 weeks • Cigarettes/day smoked by mother during the past 2 weeks, stratified by father's smoking status	Smoking in the past 2 weeks by • Mother • Father • Other household members
Klonoff-Cohen et al. 1995	Case-control (200 cases, 200 controls) United States (southern California) 1989–1992	• Postpartum secondhand smoking status of household members was assessed using multiple methods including any smoking, quantity smoked, smoking in same rooom as the infant, number of hours spent smoking around the infant	• Mother • Father • Other adult live-in residents • Day care providers

Outcome	Findings	Comments

SIDS	Maternal smoking
	    OR = 1.65 (95% CI, 1.20–2.28)
	Paternal smoking
	    OR = 1.37 (95% CI, 1.02–1.84)
	Smoking by other household members
	    OR = 1.17 (95% CI, 0.84–1.63)
	Adjusted for region, time of day, infant's age, maternal marital status, infant's gender, socioeconomic status, birth weight, infant's race, season, maternal age, sleeping position, bed sharing, breastfeeding, and maternal smoking during pregnancy; also adjusted for either maternal smoking during pregnancy, paternal smoking in the 2 weeks before the interview, or smoking by other household members in the past 2 weeks
	
	Father did not smoke
	In the past 2 weeks, mother smoked
	    0 cigarettes: 1.0 (reference)
	    1–19 cigarettes/day: OR = 2.56 (95% CI, 1.73–3.75)
	    ≥20 cigarettes/day: OR = 3.43 (95% CI, 2.04–5.77)
	
	Father smoked
	In the past 2 weeks, mother smoked
	    0 cigarettes: OR = 1.0 (95% CI, 0.64–1.56)
	    1–19 cigarettes/day: OR = 4.40 (95% CI, 3.26–5.95)
	    ≥20 cigarettes/day: OR = 7.40 (95% CI, 4.92–11.13)
	Unadjusted
		Extended the Mitchell et al. 1991 study using similar methods; exposure data were from obstetric records and self-reports (interview); autopsies were carried out in 474/485 (97.7%) of SIDS cases; infants of smoking mothers who were breastfed had a lower risk than infants of mothers who were not; secondhand smoke exposure is causally related to SIDS

SIDS	Maternal smoking
	    Any: OR = 2.28 (95% CI, 1.04–4.98)
	    In same room as infant: OR = 4.62 (95% CI, 1.82–11.77)
	Paternal smoking
	    Any: OR = 3.46 (95% CI, 1.91–6.28)
	    In same room as infant: OR = 8.49 (95% CI, 3.33–21.63)
	Smoking by other live-in adults
	    Any: OR = 2.18 (95% CI, 1.09–4.38)
	    In same room as infant: OR = 4.99 (95% CI, 1.69–14.75)
	All combined household smoking
	    Any: OR = 3.50 (95% CI, 1.81–6.75)
	    In same room as infant: OR = 4.99 (95% CI, 2.35–10.99)
	
	Exposure to cigarettes from all sources (mother, father, live-in adults, and day care providers
	Total number of household smokers
	    One: OR = 3.00 (95% CI, 1.51–5.97)
	    Two: OR = 5.31 (95% CI, 1.94–14.54)
	    Three–four: OR = 5.13 (95% CI, 0.72–36.61)
	Number smoking in same room as infant
	    One: OR = 3.67 (95% CI, 1.66–8.13)
	    Two–four: OR = 20.91 (95% CI, 4.02–108.7)
	Total daily cigarette exposure
	    1–10: OR = 2.40 (95% CI, 1.06–5.44)
	    11–20: OR = 3.62 (95% CI, 1.50–8.75)
	    ≥20: OR = 22.67 (95% CI, 4.80–107.2)
		Exposure data were self-reported (interview); all reported ORs were adjusted for birth weight (in grams), routine sleep position, medical conditions at birth, prenatal care, breastfeeding, and maternal smoking during pregnancy; breastfeeding was protective in nonsmokers but not in smokers; secondhand smoke exposure in the same room as an infant increases the risk for SIDS; risk of SIDS associated with secondhand smoke exposure was similar among different racial groups

Table 5.5   Continued

Study	Design/population	Exposure categories	Source of exposure
Ponsonby et al. 1995	Case-control (58 cases, 62 age- and region-matched controls, 58 age-, region-, and birth weight-matched controls) Australia (Tasmania) 1988–1991	• Postpartum smoking status of mother	• Mother
Blair et al. 1996	Case-control (195 cases, 780 controls, 4 per case matched for age) United Kingdom (Southwest, Yorkshire, and Trent) 1993–1995	• Smoking status of mother, father, and others in household • Number of smokers in household • Number of cigarettes smoked daily in household	Postpartum exposure from • Mother • Father • Other household members
Anderson and Cook 1997	Meta-analysis Systematic qualitative review of epidemiologic evidence (studies were identified by electronically searching EMBASE§ and Medline) 39 relevant studies were assessed (43 papers)	• Maternal prenatal and postnatal smoking	• Mother

Outcome	Findings	Comments
SIDS	Mother smoked postnatally (full multivariate model) OR = 2.39 (95% CI, 1.01–6.00) Mother smoked postnatally (multivariate model excluding family history of asthma) OR = 3.10 (95% CI, 1.36–7.09)	Exposure data were self-reported (questionnaire); all cases were autopsied; adjusted for maternal age, usual sleeping position, employment status, and family history of asthma; postpartum maternal smoking is a predictor of SIDS
SIDS	<u>Parental smoking status</u> Only father smoked: OR = 3.41 (95% CI, 1.98–5.88) Only mother smoked: OR = 7.01 (95% CI, 3.91–12.56) Both parents smoked: OR = 8.41 (95% CI, 5.08–13.92) Adjusted for maternal smoking during pregnancy <u>Multivariate analysis</u> Postnatal paternal smoking, additive to maternal smoking OR = 2.50 (95% CI, 1.48–4.22) Adjusted for mother's age, mothers without partners, parity, multiple births, short gestation, socioeconomic status, sleeping position, maternal alcohol consumption, parental use of illegal drugs, parental bed sharing, breastfeeding, and birth weight Postnatal paternal smoking, additional adjustment for maternal smoking during pregnancy Nonsignificant (p = 0.1601) <u>Number of smokers at home</u> 1 smoker: OR = 2.44 (95% CI, 1.36–4.37) 2 smokers: OR = 5.15 (95% CI, 3.24–8.21) >2 smokers: OR = 10.43 (95% CI, 3.34–32.54) <u>Cigarettes/day smoked at home</u> 1–19 cigarettes/day: OR = 2.47 (95% CI, 1.29–4.73) 20–39 cigarettes/day: OR = 3.96 (95% CI, 2.40–6.55) >39 cigarettes/day: OR = 7.57 (95% CI, 4.00–14.32) <u>Infant's daily exposure to tobacco smoke (hours)</u> 1–2: OR = 1.99 (95% CI, 1.14–3.46) 3–5 : OR = 3.84 (95% CI, 1.97–7.48) 6–8: OR = 6.78 (95% CI, 3.17–14.49) >8: OR = 8.29 (95% CI, 4.28–16.05)	Exposure data were self-reported (questionnaire); multivariate analysis found nonsignificant effect for other smoking members of household; unclear if postnatal dose-response analyses adjusted for maternal prenatal smoking or other confounding factors; dose-response analyses were limited to households where smoking was allowed in the same room as the infant; exposure to secondhand smoke in the home has an independent effect on the risk of SIDS
SIDS	Prenatal maternal smoking OR = 2.08 (95% CI, 1.96–2.21) Postnatal maternal smoking OR = 1.94 (95% CI, 1.55–2.43)	Pooled adjusted ORs were calculated using a fixed effects model; calculated results are also available using a random effects model; results are also available for pooled unadjusted ORs; the relationship between maternal smoking and SIDS is almost certainly causal—maternal smoking doubled the risk

Table 5.5   Continued

Study	Design/population	Exposure categories	Source of exposure
Brooke et al. 1997	Case-control (147 cases, 276 controls, 2 controls per case from births immediately before and after index case, thus matched for age, season, and maternity unit) Scotland 1992–1995	• Smoking status of mother and father	• Mother and father
Mitchell et al. 1997	Case-control (232 cases, 1,200 population controls) New Zealand 1991–1993	• Maternal cigarettes/day and paternal smoking status when infant was 2 months old	• Mother and father
Alm et al. 1998	Case-control (244 cases, 869 controls, matched for gender, date of birth, and hospital) Denmark, Norway, and Sweden 1992–1995	• Postnatal household secondhand smoke exposure	• Mother • Father • Other household members

Outcome	Findings	Comments

SIDS	Only father smoked
	    OR = 2.12 (95% CI, 0.99–4.55)
	Only mother smoked
	    OR = 5.05 (95% CI, 1.85–13.77)
	Both parents smoked
	    OR = 5.19 (95% CI, 2.26–11.91)
		Exposure data were self-reported (questionnaire); all cases were autopsied; adjusted for sleeping position, old mattress, maternal age, deprivation score, moved under sheets, maternal marital status, social class, use of cot bumper, sleeping with parents, symptoms in previous week, gestational age, was usually swaddled in previous week, history of infant death in family, sweaty upon waking, warmth, maternal education, beastfeeding, parity, and birth weight; parental smoking is confirmed as a modifiable risk factor for SIDS

SIDS	<u>Maternal smoking (at 2 months home visit)</u>
	0 cigarettes/day: 1.0 (reference)
	1–19 cigarettes/day: OR = 4.90 (95% CI, 2.65–9.06)
	≥20 cigarettes/day: OR = 21.42 (95% CI, 6.89–66.52)
	
	<u>Paternal smoking (at 2 months home visit)</u>
	No: 1.0 (reference)
	Yes: OR = 3.21 (95% CI, 1.81–5.71)
	
	<u>Risks from maternal/paternal smoking combinations</u>
	Nonsmoking mother
	    Smoking father: OR = 1.54 (95% CI, 0.67–3.45)
	Smoking mother:
	    Nonsmoking father: OR = 4.15 (95% CI, 2.05–8.38)
	    Smoking father: OR = 10.09 (95% CI, 5.89–17.37)
	
	<u>Adjusted OR (maternal smoking and bed sharing</u>
	Nonsmoking/no bed sharing: 1.0 (reference)
	Nonsmoking/bed sharing: OR = 1.03 (95% CI, 0.21–5.06)
	Smoking/no bed sharing: OR = 1.43 (95% CI, 0.58–3.51)
	Smoking/bed sharing: OR = 5.02 (95% CI, 1.05–24.05)
	
	Adjusted for maternal age, marital status, age mother left school, number of previous pregnancies, infant's gender, ethnicity of infant, birth weight, sleep position, breasfeeding, and the combination of bed sharing and maternal smoking
		Exposure data were self-reported (interviews conducted at postpartum and at 2 months postpartum); maternal smoking and bed sharing increase risk; maternal smoking is a significant risk factor for SIDS

SIDS	Maternal postnatal smoking
	    OR = 3.7 (95% CI, 2.5–5.5)
	Paternal postnatal smoking
	    OR = 1.2 (95% CI, 0.8–1.9)
	Smoking by other household members (after pregnancy)
	    OR = 1.2 (95% CI, 0.6–2.2)
		Exposure data were self-reported (questionnaire); all cases were autopsied; adjusted for age, maternal age, and maternal education; exposure to secondhand smoke is an independent risk factor for SIDS

Table 5.5   Continued

Study	Design/population	Exposure categories	Source of exposure
Dwyer et al. 1999	Nested case-control study with prospective cohort study (35 cases, 9,765 controls); urinary samples for cotinine analysis were collected from 105 infants (August–October 1995) Australia (Tasmania) 1988–1995	• Postnatal household secondhand smoke exposure	• Mother • Other household members

*OR = Odds ratio.
†CI = Confidence interval.
‡RR = Relative risk.
§EMBASE = Excerpta Medica Database.

same room as the infant and the number of hours the adult spent smoking in the presence of the infant. Although the researchers did not report the proportion of smoking mothers who smoked in the same room as the infant, the OR for any maternal postpartum smoking was 2.28 (95 percent CI, 1.04–4.98), adjusted for birth weight, routine sleeping position, medical conditions at birth, prenatal care, breastfeeding, and prenatal maternal smoking. The adjusted OR increased to 4.62 (95 percent CI, 1.82–11.77) when limited to mothers who reported smoking in the same room as the infant.

Of the 10 studies that independently evaluated postnatal maternal smoking, researchers observed a significant dose response in risk with the level of postnatal maternal smoking in the unadjusted ORs from 5 studies (Bergman and Wiesner 1976; McGlashan 1989; Mitchell et al. 1993, 1997; Dwyer et al. 1999), and in other measures of overall household postnatal smoking levels (maternal, paternal, and/or other) from 2 studies (Klonoff-Cohen et al. 1995; Blair et al. 1996). One study examined the risk of SIDS associated with increasing levels of postnatal exposure to cigarettes from all sources in three ways: total number of household smokers, total cigarette exposure per day, and the number of adults smoking in the same room as the infant (Klonoff-Cohen et al. 1995). Using these

three approaches to classify increasing exposures of newborns to secondhand smoke, the investigators estimated unadjusted and adjusted ORs (controlling for birth weight, routine sleeping position, medical conditions at birth, prenatal care, breastfeeding, and maternal smoking during pregnancy). Although the OR was decreased slightly for one measure (total number of household smokers) by adjustment for other factors, the adjusted ORs for the other two measures were somewhat stronger than the unadjusted measures. The adjusted ORs were 3.67 (95 percent CI, 1.66–8.13) if one adult smoked in the same room as the infant, and 20.91 (95 percent CI, 4.02–108.7) if two to four adults smoked in the same room as the infant compared with infants from nonsmoking households. Using the total cigarette exposure per day as the measure of exposure, the OR for 1 to 10 cigarettes in comparison with nonsmoking households was 2.40 (95 percent CI, 1.06–5.44), which increased to 22.67 (95 percent CI, 4.80–107.2) for 21 or more cigarettes per day.

Nine studies examined paternal smoking as a source of exposure to secondhand smoke (Bergman and Wiesner 1976; McGlashan 1989; Nicholl and O'Cathain 1992; Mitchell et al. 1993, 1997; Klonoff-Cohen et al. 1995; Blair et al. 1996; Brooke et al. 1997; Alm et al. 1998). Three of the nine (McGlashan 1989;

Outcome	Findings	Comments
SIDS	<u>Postnatal smoking</u> Maternal postnatal smoking (breastfed infants) OR = 5.29 (95% CI, 1.16–24.11) Maternal postnatal smoking (bottle-fed infants) OR = 2.35 (95% CI, 0.73–7.62) Smoking by other household members OR = 0.69 (95% CI, 0.34–1.40) <u>Dose-response of maternal postnatal smoking</u> None (no maternal postnatal smoking): OR = 1.0 1–10 cigarettes/day: OR = 2.80 (95% CI, 1.08–7.27) 11–20 cigarettes/day: OR = 3.01 (95% CI, 1.22–7.42) ≥21 cigarettes/day: OR = 5.31 (95% CI, 2.04–13.81)	Exposure data are from self-reports (interview) and from urinary cotinine measures (results from n = 100); all cases were autopsied; adjusted for breastfeeding, birth weight, and smoking in same room as infant; analyses of postnatal smoking among 34 cases and 9,464 controls; cotinine data provide estimates of exposure levels by self-reported categories; there is a positive association between maternal smoking and SIDS, but cannot separate risks from prenatal and postnatal smoking

Mitchell et al. 1997; Alm et al. 1998) observed a significant risk for SIDS from paternal smoking without adjustment for several potential confounding factors, including maternal smoking during pregnancy. Four of the remaining six studies reported significantly higher risks of SIDS among infants whose fathers were smokers compared with infants whose fathers were nonsmokers (Nicholl and O'Cathain 1992; Mitchell et al 1993; Klonoff-Cohen et al. 1995; Blair et al. 1996). The fifth and sixth studies reported an association of borderline significance (OR = 1.76, p <0.20) (Bergman and Wiesner 1976) and (OR = 2.12 [95 percent CI, 0.99–4.55]) (Brooke et al. 1997). Across the five studies with controls for maternal smoking, ORs ranged from 1.37 to 3.46, with the higher OR in the study with the stronger assessment of infant exposure to paternal smoking (Klonoff-Cohen et al. 1995). This study also reported an OR of 8.49 (95 percent CI, 3.33–21.63) for infants of fathers who smoked in the same room compared with infants of nonsmoking fathers, after adjustment for birth weight, routine sleeping position, medical conditions at birth, prenatal care, breastfeeding, and maternal smoking during pregnancy (Klonoff-Cohen et al. 1995). Five studies that measured paternal smoking provided the opportunity to examine secondhand smoke among families where

the mothers were nonsmokers. Of the four studies that evaluated households with smoking fathers and nonsmoking mothers compared with nonsmoking households, two studies reported significant ORs and one study reported a borderline significance for the risk of SIDS. Blair and colleagues (1996) reported an OR of 3.41 (95 percent CI, 1.98–5.8); Nicholl and O'Cathain (1992) reported an OR of 1.63 (95 percent CI, 1.11–2.40); and Brooke and colleagues (1997) reported an adjusted OR of 2.12 (95 percent CI, 0.99–4.55). In the study with nonsignificant results for paternal smoking (OR = 1.54 [95 percent CI, 0.67–3.45]), smoking by both parents significantly increased the risk above maternal smoking only (OR = 10.09 [95 percent CI, 5.89–17.37] versus 4.15 [95 percent CI, 2.05–8.38]) (Mitchell et al. 1997). In a case-control study, Alm and colleagues (1998) reported that when the mother did not smoke during pregnancy but the father smoked after pregnancy, the OR was 1.2 (95 percent CI, 0.8–1.9) compared with nonsmoking parents. The results reported by Mitchell and colleagues (1997) and Alm and colleagues (1998) suggest that postnatal paternal exposure has a stronger effect if it augments the effect of prenatal maternal smoking. However, the significant effects for paternal smoking noted by

Mitchell and colleagues (1993), Klonoff-Cohen and colleagues (1995), and Blair and colleagues (1996), adjusting for prenatal maternal smoking and compared with households with nonsmoking mothers, indicate a likely effect from exposure to postnatal paternal smoking that is independent of prenatal maternal smoking. In addition, as noted above for maternal smoking, data from the two studies that provided more complete assessments of the infant's exposure (Klonoff-Cohen et al. 1995; Dwyer et al. 1999) suggest that using the smoking status of the father as an indirect indicator for exposure of the infant to tobacco smoke may result in a misclassification that would bias the estimated risk downward. Specifically, Klonoff-Cohen and colleagues (1995) reported that the adjusted OR for paternal smoking increased from 3.46 (95 percent CI, 1.91–6.28), based on the postpartum smoking status of the father, to 8.49 (95 percent CI, 3.33–21.63) when the father smoked in the same room as the infant.

Assessments of postnatal exposures from "other" smokers in the household are likely subject to more misclassification errors and may thus provide a weaker measure of exposure. In addition, sometimes these "other" exposures were reported for "other than maternal," thus including paternal smoking. Of the six studies that examined such "other" smoker estimates of postnatal exposure, two included smoking fathers in the "other" category and found nonsignificant overall effects (Schoendorf and Kiely 1992; Dwyer et al. 1999). But one of the studies that limited the "other" category to "mother's partner or other adult sometimes or always smokes while in the same room as infant" reported an OR of 1.96 (95 percent CI, 1.01–3.80) (Dwyer et al. 1999, p. 596). Four studies excluded postnatal parental smoking in the assessment of smoking by other adult residents (Klonoff-Cohen et al. 1995; Blair et al. 1996; Mitchell et al. 1997; Alm et al. 1998). Each of these studies observed a statistically significant effect without adjustment for other confounders; three of the studies provided adjusted ORs. The one study without adjustment found a weak dose-response effect for the amount smoked by others, but found an unadjusted OR of 4.12 (95 percent CI, 1.85–9.08) for 20 or more cigarettes per day smoked by other members of the household (excluding the parents) (Blair et al. 1996). Of the three studies with adjusted ORs, two were nonsignificant: 1.17 (95 percent CI, 0.84–1.63) (Mitchell et al. 1997)

and 1.2 (95 percent CI, 0.6–2.2) (Alm et al. 1998); one remained significant: 2.18 (95 percent CI, 1.09–4.38) (Klonoff-Cohen et al. 1995). In this study by Klonoff-Cohen and colleagues (1995), the OR for other live-in adults who smoked in the same room as the infant was 4.99 (95 percent CI, 1.69–14.75), adjusted for birth weight, routine sleeping position, medical conditions at birth, prenatal care, breastfeeding, and maternal smoking during pregnancy.

A recent report by the European Concerted Action on SIDS (ECAS) provides additional supportive evidence (Carpenter et al. 2004). ECAS conducted a multicenter case-control study involving 745 SIDS cases (all with autopsies) and two or more live-birth controls per case (n = 2,411) matched by age and survey area. The multivariate analysis confirmed a significant increase in risk for SIDs after adjusting for sleeping position, older maternal age, more previous live births, and lower birth weight. The multivariate analysis of maternal smoking and household postnatal smoking (controlling for sleeping position, maternal age, number of previous live births, birth weight, and other variables) found no significant increase in risk for SIDs associated with bed sharing among mothers who did not smoke (OR = 1.56 [95 percent CI, 0.91–2.68]), but a highly significant risk associated with bed sharing among mothers who smoked (OR = 17.7 [95 percent CI, 10.3–30.3]). Among mothers who did not bed share, postnatal maternal smoking (unadjusted for prenatal smoking) significantly increased the risk of SIDs (<10 cigarettes per day, OR = 1.52 [95 percent CI, 1.10–2.09]; ≥10 cigarettes per day, OR = 2.43 [95 percent CI, 1.76–3.36]). In the multivariate analysis (adjusting for all of the above factors including maternal smoking but not prenatal smoking directly), researchers observed a risk associated with postnatal smoking by others in the household that increased from an OR of 1.07 (95 percent CI, 0.71–1.61) for 1 to 9 cigarettes per day to 1.54 (95 percent CI, 1.11–2.14) for 10 to 19 cigarettes per day, 1.73 (95 percent CI, 1.21–2.48) for 20 to 29 cigarettes per day, and 3.31 (95 percent CI, 1.84–5.96) for 30 or more cigarettes per day. These data provide additional evidence that postnatal smoking by other adults in the household independently increases the risk of SIDS.

Three studies used a case-control design to evaluate nicotine or cotinine as a biomarker of exposure at postmortem examinations in relation to the risk for SIDS. Rajs and colleagues (1997) measured nicotine and cotinine in pericardial fluid of SIDS and non-SIDS victims, all younger than one year of age at the time of their death. Mean values were similar in the two groups, but the children who died from SIDS included a greater proportion with cotinine values above 30 ng/mL. In a 1998 report based on a study with a similar design, Milerad and colleagues (1998) documented higher cotinine levels in children younger than seven years of age who had died suddenly compared with controls who had died of an infection. Because involuntary smoking increases the risk for childhood respiratory infection, the use of this control group may have underestimated the association of cotinine with a risk for sudden death. In addition, the inclusion of children up to seven years of age extends well beyond the traditional newborn period associated with SIDS. Finally, McMartin and colleagues (2002) compared lung tissue concentrations of nicotine and cotinine in deceased SIDS and non-SIDS infants who were younger than one year of age when they died. Both nicotine and cotinine concentrations were higher in the lungs of the SIDS victims.

Evidence Synthesis

The biologic evidence, especially from animal models, indicates multiple mechanisms by which exposure to secondhand smoke could cause SIDS (Chapter 2, Toxicology of Secondhand Smoke). The evidence for secondhand smoke exposure and the risk of SIDS consistently demonstrates an association between postpartum maternal smoking and SIDS (Table 5.5). The 1997 meta-analysis of 39 relevant studies produced an adjusted OR for postnatal maternal smoking of 1.94 (95 percent CI, 1.55–2.43), a level of risk that the authors concluded was almost certainly causal (Anderson and Cook 1997). Data from the four studies in Table 5.5 published since the 1997 meta-analysis add additional support for this conclusion. Nine of the thirteen studies in Table 5.5 more fully controlled for the major potential confounders (e.g., maternal smoking during pregnancy and routine sleeping position), and many controlled for a broad range of other relevant factors including maternal age, birth weight, and bed sharing. The nine studies all observed significant positive associations between postpartum maternal smoking and SIDS. Moreover, several studies demonstrated a dose-response relationship for secondhand smoke exposure attributable to postpartum maternal smoking, with increasing ORs for higher levels of postpartum maternal smoking. Finally, among the studies of postnatal maternal smoking with better adjustment for confounding, the adjusted ORs are sufficiently large, all greater than 1.5 and three of the five greater than 2.0. These ORs make it unlikely that this association is attributable to any residual confounding from unmeasured factors.

The epidemiologic evidence for secondhand smoke exposure from postpartum maternal smoking associated with the risk of SIDS is consistent and strong, and demonstrates a dose-response relationship. Evidence for secondhand smoke exposures from fathers and "other" smokers (as well as higher concentrations of nicotine and cotinine in children who die from SIDS compared with children who die of other causes) provides additional supporting evidence that secondhand smoke exposure increases the risk of SIDS. Although measures of paternal and "other" smokers in the household are not typically considered to be a comprehensive indicator of the infant's exposure to secondhand smoke, designs that can evaluate paternal smoking have the potential to more fully control for the possible confounding of maternal smoking during pregnancy. However, when considering evidence that supports an association between SIDS and paternal and "other" smokers, researchers also recognize the possible misclassification of actual infant exposures to tobacco smoke from these sources (Klonoff-Cohen et al. 1995; Dwyer et al. 1999). Despite this methodologic challenge, researchers observed an elevated OR in all nine studies of paternal smoking, ranging from 1.4 to 3.5, with many estimates around 2 or higher. Of these nine studies, five observed an elevated OR for households where the fathers smoked compared with households where neither parent smoked, and an OR of 8.5 for infants of fathers who smoked in the same room as the infant, adjusting for maternal smoking during pregnancy, routine sleeping position, and other factors. Also, out of the nine studies that examined paternal smoking, five found a statistically significant association between paternal smoking and SIDS after adjusting for maternal smoking during pregnancy. Despite the potential for misclassification bias linking paternal smoking to an actual exposure of the infant to secondhand smoke, the pooled risk estimate was 1.9 (95 percent CI, 1.01–2.80) from the five studies of paternal smoking with stronger designs that used meta-analytic approaches and random effects modeling. Finally, all of the studies of "other" smokers in the household observed an elevated OR; however, the results that adjusted for maternal smoking during pregnancy and other important confounders were more mixed. The one study with the strongest assessment of infant exposures from "other" smoking residents (i.e., live-in adults smoking in the same room as the infant) reported an OR of 4.99 (95 percent CI, 1.69–14.75), with adjustment for multiple risk factors including maternal smoking during pregnancy and routine sleeping position (Klonoff-Cohen et al. 1995).

Researchers have established prenatal maternal smoking as a major preventable risk for SIDS (USDHHS 2001, 2004; AAP Task Force on SIDS 2005). Evidence indicates that exposure of infants to secondhand smoke from postpartum maternal smoking has a significant additive effect on risk if the mother smoked during pregnancy. In studies that accounted for maternal smoking during pregnancy, evidence indicates that postpartum maternal smoking, particularly in proximity to the infant, significantly increases the risk of SIDS. In addition, epidemiologic evidence indicates that postnatal exposure of infants to secondhand smoke from fathers or other live-in smokers can also increase the risk of SIDS. Thus, the full range of biologic and epidemiologic data are consistent and indicate that exposure of infants to secondhand smoke causes SIDS.

Conclusion

1. The evidence is sufficient to infer a causal relationship between exposure to secondhand smoke and sudden infant death syndrome.

Implications

On the basis of the epidemiologic risk data, researchers have estimated that the population attributable risk of SIDS associated with postnatal exposure to secondhand smoke is about 10 percent (Cal/EPA 2005). Therefore, the evidence indicates that these exposures are one of the major preventable risk factors for SIDS, and all measures should be taken to protect infants from exposure to secondhand smoke.

There is a need for additional research to further characterize the risk of SIDS associated with prenatal and postnatal exposure to secondhand smoke, and to evaluate the relationship between maternal smoking and infant sleeping positions and bed sharing. Future research should also focus on better assessments of actual exposures of infants to secondhand smoke using biochemical assessments and/or more detailed interviews, rather than indirect assessments based on the smoking status of household adults. Because of the continuing and significant racial disparities in infant mortality from SIDS (Malloy and Freeman 2004), there is a need to study the preventable risks factors that could be involved.

Preterm Delivery

Biologic Basis

Pregnancy complications, including premature labor, placenta previa, abruptio placentae, and premature membrane rupture may lead to preterm delivery (<37 completed weeks of gestation). Although the underlying mechanisms are not yet fully characterized, maternal active smoking is associated with

these pregnancy complications (U.S. Department of Health, Education, and Welfare [USDHEW] 1979b; USDHHS 1980, 2001; Andres and Day 2000). Preterm delivery is also associated with active maternal smoking (USDHEW 1979a; USDHHS 1980, 2001; van den Berg and Oechsli 1984; Andres and Day 2000). Smoking cessation during pregnancy appears to reduce the risk for preterm delivery (van den Berg and Oechsli

1984; Li et al. 1993; Mainous and Hueston 1994b; USDHHS 2001), placenta previa (Naeye 1980), abruptio placentae (Naeye 1980), and premature membrane rupture (Harger et al. 1990; Williams et al. 1992); but the risk remains high for those who continue to smoke throughout pregnancy. Tobacco-specific nitrosamines and cotinine have been measured in the cervical mucus of women who were active smokers and women who were nonsmokers (McCann et al. 1992; Prokopczyk et al. 1997). Given that active maternal smoking is associated with preterm delivery, this finding provided further support for the biologic plausibility that secondhand smoke has a role in the injurious processes leading to preterm delivery. Although the biologic pathway from active maternal smoking to preterm delivery is not clear, the evidence for this association is strong enough to infer that maternal secondhand smoke exposure may also lead to preterm delivery.

Epidemiologic Evidence

Few data are available on the effects of maternal secondhand smoke exposure on preterm delivery, and published findings are inconsistent across studies. Four studies did not find a statistically significant association between maternal secondhand smoke exposure and preterm delivery (Table 5.6) (Martin and Bracken 1986; Ahlborg and Bodin 1991; Mathai et al. 1992; Fortier et al. 1994), but several others did report significantly increased risks with exposure to secondhand smoke (Ahluwalia et al. 1997; Hanke et al. 1999; Windham et al. 2000; Jaakkola et al. 2001). Hanke and colleagues (1999) reported an adjusted OR of 1.86 (95 percent CI, 1.05–3.45) for preterm delivery among nonsmoking mothers who were exposed to secondhand smoke for at least seven hours per day compared with unexposed mothers. Using the same secondhand smoke exposure category—exposed for at least seven hours per day—Windham and colleagues (2000) found an adjusted OR of 1.6 (95 percent CI, 0.87–2.9) for exposed, nonsmoking mothers compared with unexposed mothers. The risk increased to 2.8 (95 percent CI, 1.2–6.6) among women aged 30 or more years. Similarly, Ahluwalia and colleagues

(1997) classified secondhand smoke exposure dichotomously as yes/no and also found an increased risk among nonsmoking women aged 30 or more years for preterm delivery when exposed to secondhand smoke (OR = 1.88 [95 percent CI, 1.22–2.88]), but the risk was not observed among nonsmoking women younger than 30 years of age (OR = 0.92 [95 percent CI, 0.76–1.13]). Jaakkola and colleagues (2001) used the hair nicotine level, a biologic measure of exposure to secondhand smoke among nonsmoking women. Those with the highest hair concentrations of nicotine ($\geq$4.0 μg/gram [g]) had an adjusted OR of 6.12 (95 percent CI, 1.31–28.7) for preterm delivery when compared with women with the lowest or undetectable concentrations of hair nicotine. The limited epidemiologic evidence on maternal secondhand smoke exposure and preterm delivery currently does not warrant a meta-analysis of the relevant studies.

Evidence Synthesis

The few studies that have evaluated the association between secondhand smoke exposure and preterm delivery have shown inconsistent findings. Of the four studies that found significant associations, two studies documented that the risk was significant only for women aged 30 years or older. Jaakkola and colleagues (2001) provided the strongest evidence for an association using hair nicotine measurements, which reduce the probability of exposure misclassification. There is a biologic basis for considering this association to be causal.

Conclusion

1. The evidence is suggestive but not sufficient to infer a causal relationship between maternal exposure to secondhand smoke during pregnancy and preterm delivery.

Implications

Further research should be carried out, although studies of substantial size will be needed.

Table 5.6   Studies of secondhand smoke exposure and preterm delivery

Study	Design/population	Source of exposure	Outcome	Exposure categories
Martin and Bracken 1986	3,891 antenatal women seen between 1980 and 1982	Home and work, ≥2 hours/day	Preterm delivery	Yes/no
Ahlborg and Bodin 1991	4,687 prenatal women between October 1980 and June 1983	Home only Work only Both	Preterm delivery	Yes/no
Mathai et al. 1992	994 nonsmoking women receiving obstetric care at a hospital between January and May 1990	Home	Preterm delivery	Yes/no
Fortier et al. 1994	Sample of 4,644 women delivering between January and October 1989	Home only Work only Both	Preterm delivery	Yes/no
Ahluwalia et al. 1997	17,412 low-income women who received services from public maternal and child health clinics	Household members	Preterm delivery	Yes/no
Hanke et al. 1999	1,751 nonsmoking women from a randomly selected group of women who gave birth between June 1996 and May 1997	Home Work Other	Preterm delivery	No exposure 0–1 hour/day 2–3 hours/day 4–6 hours/day ≥7 hours/day
Windham et al. 2000	4,454 pregnant women in their first trimester at their first prenatal appointment through a health plan	Home and work	Preterm delivery Very preterm (<35 weeks)	No exposure: 0 to <0.5 hour/day Moderate exposure: 0.5–6.5 hours/day N = 625 High exposure: ≥7 hours/day N = 134
Jaakkola et al. 2001	389 nonsmoking women who gave birth between May 1996 and April 1997	Home and work	Preterm delivery	Hair nicotine concentrations: <0.75 µg/g[Δ] 0.75 to <4.0 µg/g ≥4.0 µg/g

*RR = Relative risk.
[†]CI = Confidence interval.
[‡]OR = Odds ratio.
[§]AOR = Adjusted odds ratio.
[Δ]µg/g = Micrograms per gram.

Findings	Comments
4.64% in unexposed nonsmokers 4.66% in exposed nonsmokers	No change in crude findings using regression analysis (data were not presented); secondhand smoke exposure showed no effect on preterm delivery
RR* = 0.49 (95% CI†, 0.23–1.06) RR = 1.86 (95% CI, 1.0–3.48) RR = 0.84 (95% CI, 0.53–1.33)	Adjusted; secondhand smoke exposure in the workplace was weakly associated with preterm birth
3.8% in unexposed nonsmokers 5.8% in exposed nonsmokers	Not statistically significant (data were not presented)
OR‡ = 0.93 (95% CI, 0.58–1.51) OR = 0.92 (95% CI, 0.64–1.31) OR = 0.98 (95% CI, 0.56–1.73)	Adjusted; secondhand smoke exposure was not related to preterm birth

Nonsmokers aged <30 years
    OR = 0.92 (95% CI, 0.76–1.13)
Nonsmokers aged ≥30 years
    OR = 1.88 (95% CI, 1.22–2.88)
	The association between secondhand smoke exposure and adverse pregnancy outcomes appears to be modified by maternal age

AOR§ = 0.54 (95% CI, 0.77–4.45) AOR = 1.24 (95% CI, 0.68–2.27) AOR = 1.73 (95% CI, 0.86–3.19) AOR = 1.86 (95% CI, 1.05–3.45)	Urine cotinine was measured in 71 women to verify nonsmoking status; maternal secondhand smoke exposure lasting ≥7 hours was a significant risk factor for preterm delivery; adjusted for maternal age, height, parity, employment, and marital status

Nonsmokers, high secondhand smoke exposure
    Preterm: AOR = 1.6 (95% CI, 0.87–2.9)
    Very preterm: AOR = 2.4 (95% CI, 1.0–5.3)
 	
Aged <30 years, high secondhand smoke exposure
    Preterm: AOR = 1.1 (95% CI, 0.46–2.6)
    Very preterm: AOR = 2.2 (95% CI, 0.75–6.6)
 	
Aged ≥30 years, high secondhand smoke exposure
    Preterm: AOR = 2.8 (95% CI, 1.2–6.6)
    Very preterm: AOR = 2.7 (95% CI, 0.74–9.7)
	High secondhand smoke exposure was moderately associated with preterm birth and most strongly associated with very preterm birth; adjusted by logarithmic regression for prior pregnancy history, race, body mass index, life events, and education

AOR = 1.30 (95% CI, 0.30–5.58) AOR = 6.12 (95% CI, 1.31–28.7)	Adjusted for gender, birth order, maternal age, body mass index before pregnancy, marital status, socioeconomic status, alcohol consumption during pregnancy, and employment during pregnancy; results suggest an increase in the risk of preterm delivery

Low Birth Weight

Biologic Basis

Low birth weight (LBW), defined as less than 2,500 g or less than 5.5 pounds, can result from preterm delivery or intrauterine growth retardation (IUGR), which can occur simultaneously in a pregnancy. Reduced fetal physical growth during gestation, or IUGR, can lead to a small for gestational age (SGA) infant (≤10th percentile of expected birth weight for a given gestational age) that is either preterm or full term (≥37 weeks of gestation), and may or may not be LBW. The established link between active maternal smoking and LBW is known to occur mainly through IUGR rather than through premature birth (Chamberlain 1975; Coleman et al. 1979; Wilcox 1993). Fetal growth is greatest during the third trimester, and studies of active smoking during pregnancy demonstrate no reduction of infant birth weight if smoking ceases before the third trimester (USDHHS 1990, 2004). In 2003, 12.4 percent of births among smokers were LBW (Martin et al. 2005).

A number of researchers have postulated that the limitation of fetal growth from active maternal smoking comes from reduced oxygen to the fetus, which is directly attributable to CO exposure and nicotine-induced vasoconstriction leading to reduced uterine and umbilical blood flow (USDHHS 1990, 2004; Bruner and Forouzan 1991; Rajini et al. 1994; Lambers and Clark 1996; Werler 1997; Andres and Day 2000). Studies have shown elevated nucleated red blood cell counts, a marker of fetal hypoxia, among neonates of women who actively smoked during pregnancy (Yeruchimovich et al. 1999) and among women who were exposed to secondhand smoke (Dollberg et al. 2000). Several investigators have also found elevated erythropoietin, the protein that stimulates red blood cell production and another indicator of hypoxia, in cord blood of newborns whose mothers had smoked during pregnancy (Jazayeri et al. 1998; Gruslin et al. 2000). Because erythropoietin does not cross the placenta, it most likely originated from the fetus. A number of researchers have also reported that the concentration of erythropoietin is positively correlated with the concentration of cotinine measured in cord blood ($r = 0.41$, $p = 0.04$) (Gruslin et al. 2000), the number of cigarettes smoked per day by the mother ($r = 0.26$, $p < 0.0001$) (Jazayeri et al. 1998), and fetal growth retardation (r was not presented, $p < 0.01$) (Maier et al. 1993).

Studies have detected nicotine and its metabolites perinatally in umbilical cord serum in infants born to nonsmoking mothers, and in the cervical mucus of nonsmoking women; consequently, many researchers agree that the information on active maternal smoking is directly relevant to understanding the possible association of maternal secondhand smoke exposure and preterm delivery and LBW (USDHHS 2001). More direct evidence supports the hypothesis that maternal secondhand smoke exposure, specifically to nicotine, may lead to LBW through a pathway of fetal hypoxia (Çolak et al. 2002). One would expect attenuated physiologic effects from exposures to secondhand smoke than from active smoking based on relative dose levels, but the same biologic mechanisms of effect may apply.

Epidemiologic Evidence

A large body of literature is available on secondhand smoke exposure and LBW (Table 5.7). The first studies that reported an association were conducted in the 1960s (MacMahon et al. 1965; Comstock and Lundin 1967; Underwood et al. 1967; Terris and Gold 1969). These early studies found reductions in mean birth weight that ranged from 3 g (Underwood et al. 1967) to 42 g (Comstock and Lundin 1967) (CIs were not calculated) among infants with fathers who smoked compared with infants of nonsmoking fathers. A few relevant studies were published in the 1970s (Yerushalmy 1971; Mau and Netter 1974; Borlee et al. 1978), and one showed a statistically significant association. Borlee and colleagues (1978) found that the mean birth weight of infants of nonsmoking mothers and smoking fathers was 228 g less than the mean birth weight of infants with two nonsmoking parents. This study has been criticized, however, because the study population came from a case-control study of infants with malformations, and some evidence now indicates that both LBW (Xiao 1989; Xu 1992; Lin 1993; Samuelsen et al. 1998) and paternal smoking (Knorr 1979; Davis 1991; Savitz et al. 1991; Zhang et al. 1992; Fraga et al. 1996; Wasserman et al. 1996) are associated with birth defects.

Interest in the topic of LBW and secondhand smoke grew in the 1980s after the association between active maternal smoking during pregnancy and LBW had been established (USDHHS 1980; Stillman et al. 1986). Several investigators have reported RR estimates and adjusted OR estimates from studies published in the last two decades. These estimates have ranged from an OR of less than 1.0 (Sadler et al. 1999; Matsubara et al. 2000) to an OR of 2.31 (Mainous and Hueston 1994a) and, as a whole, have suggested that having a LBW infant is associated with maternal exposure to secondhand smoke. Some investigators have compared mean birth weights of infants whose mothers were exposed to secondhand smoke with infants of unexposed mothers. The results from these studies showed reductions in birth weights among the exposed groups that ranged from 1 g (Sadler et al. 1999; Haug et al. 2000) to 253 g (Luciano et al. 1998). In a 1998 meta-analysis of 11 studies, Peacock and colleagues (1998) found that the mean birth weight for infants of secondhand smoke-exposed mothers was 31 g less (95 percent CI, 19–44) than infants of unexposed mothers. Similarly, in a 1999 meta-analysis of secondhand smoke and LBW literature (19 studies), the summary estimates were an OR of 1.2 for LBW at term or SGA (95 percent CI, 1.1–1.3), and a difference in mean adjusted birth weights of -28 g (95 percent CI, -41 to -16) for infants of nonsmoking mothers exposed to secondhand smoke compared with infants of unexposed mothers (Windham et al. 1999a). The 1999 meta-analysis included most of the studies that were in the earlier 1998 analysis, plus a retrospective study of 992 nonsmoking pregnant women contacted by Windham and colleagues. The estimated reductions for the meta-analysis in mean birth weight were statistically significant in both meta-analyses, but a reduction of 30 g (approximately 1.24 ounces) would not be clinically significant to individual infants at low risk. On a population level, however, a slight shift in the birth weight distribution could put infants already at risk into greater risk for complications associated with LBW.

Some investigators have evaluated dose-response associations using cotinine or nicotine measures (Haddow et al. 1988; Nafstad et al. 1998), self-reported levels of exposure to secondhand smoke (Zhang and Ratcliffe 1993; Mainous and Hueston 1994a), or both (Rebagliato et al. 1995b). Of the five studies that examined these trends, findings in two studies (Haddow et al. 1988; Mainous and Hueston 1994a) suggested that a dose-response relationship

exists between secondhand smoke exposure and birth weight. Haddow and colleagues (1988) measured maternal serum cotinine during the second trimester and found higher levels among nonsmoking mothers whose infants had lower mean birth weights. The adjusted mean birth weights were 3,535 g, 3,531 g, and 3,481 g for low, medium, and high cotinine levels, respectively. These results led Haddow and colleagues (1988) to "suggest that the linear model may not best reflect the true dose-response relationship" (p. 484). The difference in adjusted mean birth weights between the low- and high-exposure groups was statistically significant (p <0.001). Mainous and Hueston (1994a) obtained secondhand smoke exposure information from the 1988 National Health Interview Survey and found statistically significant trends between increasing levels of maternal secondhand smoke exposure and an increase in proportions of LBW infants (p = 0.01) and a decrease in mean birth weights (p = 0.007).

Although the other three studies that evaluated dose-response relationships did not find any trends, two of those studies did find evidence of an association between maternal secondhand smoke exposure and reduced birth weight. Nafstad and colleagues (1998) measured hair nicotine levels and found that nonsmoking mothers whose nicotine levels were within the two middle quartiles were at an increased risk for having a SGA child compared with nonsmoking mothers whose nicotine levels were within the lowest quartile (OR = 3.4 [95 percent CI, 1.3–8.6]). For nonsmoking mothers with hair nicotine levels in the highest quartile, the estimated risk of having a SGA child was 2.1 (95 percent CI, 0.4–10.1). Zhang and Ratcliffe (1993) used paternal smoking as a measure of exposure to secondhand smoke and found that, compared with infants from the unexposed group, the exposed group had a mean birth weight that was 30 g lower. The mean birth weights did not decrease in a linear or monotonic manner with increasing exposure levels. Rebagliato and colleagues (1995b) also examined dose-response associations and did not find any significant trends with exposures at home, at work, from the partner, from all reported sources combined, or with measured cotinine levels. Increases in maternal exposures to secondhand smoke in public places, however, did show a significant dose-response trend with decreases in mean birth weights (p = 0.028).

Another means of looking for an exposure-response trend is by dividing exposure sources into home and work. One would expect that

Table 5.7   Summary of published literature on secondhand smoke and low birth weight (LBW)

Study Location	Design	Population size	Source of secondhand smoke	Cotinine measure	Findings
MacMahon et al. 1965 United States	Cohort	12,192	Husband	NR*	• Mean birth weight difference: -0.7 ounces (oz.) in boys • Mean birth weight difference: -0.8 oz. in girls • No association
Comstock and Lundin 1967 United States	Cohort	448	Husband	NR	• Mean birth weight difference: -42 g[†] • No association
Underwood et al. 1967 United States	Cohort	24,674	Husband	NR	• Mean birth weight difference: -3 g • No association
Terris and Gold 1969 United States	Case-control	197 197	Husband	NR	• No significant difference • No association
Yerushalmy 1971 United States	Cohort	13,000	Husband	NR	• Significant association with LBW among Whites but not among Blacks • Possible association
Mau and Netter 1974 Germany	Cohort	3,696	Husband	NR	• RR = 1.2 for IUGR[‡] • RR = 1.4 for LBW • No significant association
Borlee et al. 1978 Belgium	Cohort	238	Husband	NR	• Mean birth weight difference: -228 g (statistically significant) • Significant association
Hauth et al. 1984 United States	Cohort	163	All (serum thiocyanate)	NR	• No difference in birth weights for infants of involuntary smokers compared with those of nonsmokers • No association
Magnus et al. 1984 Norway	Cohort	3,130	Husband	NR	• Mean birth weight difference: -4.9 (standard deviation = 9.3) per 10 cigarettes/day • No association
Karakostov 1985 Bulgaria	Cohort	NR	NR	NR	• Mean birth weight difference: -84 g • Mean height difference: -0.5 cm[§] • No significant association
Martin and Bracken 1986 United States	Cohort	4,186	Both home and work	NR	• Mean birth weight difference: -23.5 g (95% CI[Δ], -59.9–12.8) • RR[¶] = 2.17 (95% CI, 1.05–4.50)
Rubin et al. 1986 Denmark	Cohort	500	Husband	NR	• Mean birth weight difference: -120 g/pack/day • Mean birth weight difference: -6.1 g/cigarette/day (p <0.03) • RR = 2.17 (95% CI, 1.05–4.50)

Table 5.7   Continued

Study Location	Design	Population size	Source of secondhand smoke	Cotinine measure	Findings
MacArthur and Knox 1987 Britain	Cohort	180	Husband	NR	• Mean birth weight difference: 123 g (p <0.02) • No association
Schwartz-Bickenbach et al. 1987 Germany	Cohort	38	Home	Breast milk and infant's urine	• Mean birth weight difference: -200 g • Association
Campbell et al. 1988 Britain	Cohort	518	Husband	NR	• Mean birth weight difference: -113 g (95% CI, -216 to -8), p = 0.03 • Significant association
Haddow et al. 1988 United States	Cohort	1,231	Both home and work	Serum	• Mean birth weight difference: -108 g (p <0.0001) • 29% had LBW • Sufficient evidence for an association (possible nonlinear dose-response)
Brooke et al. 1989 Britain	Cohort	1,018	Home	NR	• -0.5% in birth weight ratio (p = 0.56) • Mean birth weight difference: -18 g • No association
Chen et al. 1989 China	Cohort	1,058	Home	NR	• Mean birth weight difference: -15 g (p = 0.92) • 0.7% had LBW (p = 0.67) • No association
Ueda et al. 1989 Japan	Cohort	259	Both home and work	Maternal urine, umbilical cord blood	• No specified findings • Significant association
Lazzaroni et al. 1990 Italy	Cohort	1,002	Both home and work	NR	• Mean birth weight difference: -16 g/ hour/day of secondhand smoke exposure (p <0.07); -38.16 g (95% CI, -106.9–30.7) overall birth weight • -0.26 cm (95% CI, -5.6–0.03) overall length • Possible association
Mathai et al. 1990 Britain	Cohort	300	Home	Urine	• Mean birth weight difference: -66 g (questionnaire) • Nonsignificant association
Ahlborg and Bodin 1991 Sweden	Cohort	4,687	Both home and work	NR	• RR = 0.99 (95% CI, 0.45–2.21) for both home and work • RR = 0.69 (95% CI, 0.21–2.27) for home only • RR = 1.09 (95% CI, 0.33–3.62) for work only • RR = 1.83 (95% CI, 0.53–6.28) for work in the third trimester • Nonsignificant association

Table 5.7   Continued

Study Location	Design	Population size	Source of secondhand smoke	Cotinine measure	Findings
Ogawa et al. 1991 Japan	Cohort	5,336	Both home and work	NR	• Mean birth weight difference: -24 g (95% CI, -5 to -54) • RR for IUGR = 1.0 (95% CI, 0.7–1.5) • No association
Saito 1991 Japan	Cohort	3,025	Husband	NR	• RR = 1.21 • Significant association
Mathai et al. 1992 India	Cohort	994	Both home and work	NR	• Mean birth weight difference: -63 g (95% CI, -114 to -12) • Significant association
Pan 1992 China	Cohort	253	Husband	NR	• Higher SGA** rate in the exposed group • No specified association
Zhang and Ratcliffe 1993 China	Cohort	1,785	Husband	NR	• Mean birth weight: -30 g (95% CI, -66–7) • LBW: 0.17% • SGA: 0.20% • Possible association
Fortier et al. 1994 Canada	Cohort	4,644	Both home and work	NR	• OR[††] = 0.94 (95% CI, 0.60–1.49) for both home and work • OR = 0.98 (95% CI, 0.67–1.44) for home only • OR = 1.18 (95% CI, 0.90–1.56) for work only • Nonsignificant association/inconclusive
Mainous and Hueston 1994a United States	Cohort	3,253	Both home and work	NR	• Mean birth weight difference: -84 g • 3.6% had LBW • OR for LBW = 1.59 (95% CI, 0.92–2.73) • OR for LBW in non-Whites = 2.31 (95% CI, 1.06–4.99) • Association with high exposure (threshold effect)
Martinez et al. 1994 United States	Cohort	1,219	Husband	Cord serum	• Mean birth weight difference: -88 g • Significant association
Chen and Petitti 1995 United States	Case-control	111 124	Both home and work	NR	• OR = 0.50 (95% CI, 0.14–1.74) • No association
Eskenazi et al. 1995 United States	Cohort	3,896	NR	Serum	• Mean birth weight difference: -42 g • RR for LBW = 1.35 (95% CI, 0.60–3.03) • Nonsignificant association

Table 5.7   Continued

Study Location	Design	Population size	Source of secondhand smoke	Cotinine measure	Findings
Rebagliato et al. 1995b Spain	Cohort	710	Both home and work	Saliva	• Mean birth weight difference: -88 g (measured by cotinine); -41 g (questionnaire) • Nonsignificant association
Roquer et al. 1995 Spain	Cohort	76	Both home and work	NR	• Mean birth weight difference: -192 g • Association
Jedrychowski and Flak 1996 Poland	Cohort	1,165	NR	Serum	• Mean birth weight difference: -73.1 g • Significant association
Ahluwalia et al. 1997 United States	Cohort	17,412	Home	NR	• Mothers aged <30 years Mean birth weight difference: -8.8 g (95% CI, -43.7–26.1) • Mothers aged ≥30 years Mean birth weight difference: 90.0 g (95% CI, -0.8–180.9) • Inconclusive for SGA • Association for LBW in the group aged ≥30 years
Dejin-Karlsson et al. 1998 Sweden	Cohort	872	Both home and work	NR	• OR for SGA = 2.3 (95% CI, 1.1–4.6) • OR for LBW = 1.3 (95% CI, 0.7–2.5) • SGA crude OR in nonsmokers = 2.4 (95% CI, 1.02–5.8)
Luciano et al. 1998 Italy	Cohort	112	Both home and work	NR	• Mean birth weight difference: -253.5 g
Nafstad et al. 1998 Norway	Case-control	58 105	Both home and work	Hair	• OR in nonsmokers = 1.4 (95% CI, 0.4–4.4)
Hanke et al. 1999 Poland	Cohort	1,751	Both home and work	NR	NR
Sadler et al. 1999 United States	Cohort	2,283	Both home and work	NR	• OR for SGA = 0.82 (95% CI, 0.51–1.33) • Mean birth weight difference: -1.2 g (95% CI, -43.3–41.0)
Windham et al. 1999a United States	Cohort	992	Husband	NR	• OR for LBW = 1.8 (95% CI, 0.64–4.8) • OR for SGA = 1.4 (95% CI, 0.79–2.5)
Haug et al. 2000 Norway	Cohort	34,799	Husband	NR	• Mean birth weight difference: -1 g • No association

Matsubara et al. 2000 Japan	Cohort	7,411	Husband Both home and work	NR	Husband
					    RR for LBW = 0.92 (95% CI, 0.71–1.20)
					    RR for IUGR = 0.95 (95% CI, 0.72–1.26)
					Both home and work
					    RR for LBW = 0.99 (95% CI, 0.77–1.30)
					    RR for IUGR = 0.95 (95% CI, 0.71–1.26)
					No association

Table 5.7   Continued

Study Location	Design	Population size	Source of secondhand smoke	Cotinine measure	Findings
Windham et al. 2000 United States	Cohort	4,454	Both home and work	NR	• Adjusted OR for LBW = 1.8 (95% CI, 0.82–4.1) • Moderate association
Jaakkola et al. 2001 Finland	Cohort	389	Both home and work	Postpartum maternal hair nicotine	• OR for LBW = 1.06 (95% CI, 0.96–1.17) • OR for SGA = 1.04 (95% CI, 0.92–1.19) • Nonsignificant association

*NR = Data were not reported.
†g = Grams.
‡IUGR = Intrauterine growth retardation.
§cm = Centimeters.
ΔCI = Confidence interval.
¶RR = Relative risk.
**SGA = Small for gestational age.
††OR = Odds ratio.

combined exposures from both sources would lead to greater risks of LBW than would exposure from only one of the two sources, but Ahlborg and Bodin (1991) did not find this to be the case. The adjusted RR for LBW among nonsmokers with any secondhand smoke exposure either at home or at work was 0.99 (95 percent CI, 0.45–2.21), but the risks with exposure in the home only and in the workplace only were 0.69 (95 percent CI, 0.21–2.27) and 1.09 (95 percent CI, 0.33–3.62), respectively. Similarly, Fortier and colleagues (1994) did not find any exposure-response trend for SGA when risks were estimated for secondhand smoke exposure in the home only (OR = 0.98 [95 percent CI, 0.67–1.44]), at work only (OR = 1.18 [95 percent CI, 0.90–1.56]), and at both home and work (OR = 0.94 [95 percent CI, 0.60–1.49]). For any exposure either at home or at work, the estimated risk for SGA was 1.09 (95 percent CI, 0.85–1.39).

Evidence Synthesis

The risk estimates for secondhand smoke exposure and LBW have generally been small and have been consistent with the expectation that exposure to secondhand smoke should produce a smaller effect than exposure to active smoking. Most studies show a reduction in the mean birth weight and an increased risk for LBW among infants whose mothers were exposed to secondhand smoke. Across the studies, diverse potential confounding factors have been considered. Despite the lack of statistical significance in many of the studies, the consistencies seen in the literature have been summarized in several published reviews and have provided the strongest argument for an association between secondhand smoke and LBW. There are several plausible mechanisms by which secondhand smoke exposure could influence birth weight. Three comprehensive reviews of the literature on secondhand smoke and LBW that were published in the past decade all found a small increase in risk for LBW or SGA associated with secondhand smoke exposure (Misra and Nguyen 1999; Windham et al. 1999a; Lindbohm et al. 2002). Based on all of the studies that reported on LBW at term or SGA and secondhand smoke exposure, a meta-analysis provided a weighted pooled risk estimate of 1.2 (95 percent CI, 1.1–1.3) for this association (Windham et al. 1999a). Given the published review and meta-analysis by Windham and colleagues (1999a), an updated meta-analysis of the relevant studies on maternal secondhand smoke exposure and birth weight currently is not warranted.

Conclusion

1. The evidence is sufficient to infer a causal relationship between maternal exposure to secondhand smoke during pregnancy and a small reduction in birth weight.

Implications

Secondhand smoke exposure represents an avoidable contribution to birth weight reductions. Women, when pregnant, should not smoke or be exposed to secondhand smoke.

Congenital Malformations

Biologic Basis

Because of the direct fetal effects observed with exposure to tobacco smoke and because of the chemically complex and teratogenic nature of cigarette smoke, researchers have addressed the association between exposure to tobacco smoke and congenital malformations. Most of this literature has focused on active smoking during pregnancy by the mother, but a few studies have examined secondhand smoke exposure. The etiology of most congenital malformations is not fully elaborated (Werler 1997), and no studies have been conducted to identify the mechanisms by which exposure to secondhand smoke may result in congenital malformations in humans. The few studies that have assessed the effects of sidestream smoke in animals have produced little evidence to support an association of secondhand smoke exposure and malformations (NCI 1999). Some recent studies suggest that susceptibility to some malformations may depend in part on the presence of genes that increase susceptibility to tobacco smoke (Wyszynski et al. 1997). Other proposed mechanisms include teratogenic effects of high concentrations of carboxyhemoglobin and nicotine, or malformations that are the result of exposure to some yet unidentified component of the tobacco plant shown to be teratogenic if ingested by animals (Seidman and Mashiach 1991).

The evidence on the relationship between maternal smoking during pregnancy and congenital malformations is inconsistent. Most studies have reported no association between maternal smoking and congenital malformations as a whole. However, for selected malformations, particularly oral clefts, several studies have reported positive associations with active smoking during pregnancy by the mother (Little et al. 2004a,b; Meyer et al. 2004). In fact, recent studies on gene-environment interactions have furthered the etiologic understanding of oral clefts and the role of

smoking (Hwang et al. 1995; Shaw et al. 1996; van Rooij et al. 2001, 2002; Lammer et al. 2004).

Epidemiologic Evidence

Of six studies that collected data on involuntary smoking and congenital malformations, two had very large sample sizes (Table 5.8). Holmberg and Nurminen (1980) examined occupational exposures among parents of infants born with congenital malformations and of control infants matched for date of birth and geographic area in Finland from 1976 to 1978. The researchers found that the distribution of paternal smoking around the time that the woman became pregnant was similar in the cases with CNS defects and their matched controls. Savitz and colleagues (1991) analyzed data collected between 1964 and 1967 on children five years of age from the Child Health and Development Studies (N = 14,685). The researchers examined 33 different malformations in relation to paternal smoking and 4 malformations—cleft lip with or without cleft palate, hydrocephalus, ventricular septal defect, and urethral stenosis—for dose-response relationships. Although prevalence ORs were 2.0 or greater for selected outcomes, the lower 95 percent confidence limits reached below 1.0 once adjustments for potential confounders were made for maternal smoking, maternal age, maternal race, and maternal education. These selected outcomes were hydrocephalus (OR = 2.4 [95 percent CI, 0.06–9.3]), ventricular septal defect (OR = 2.0 [95 percent CI, 0.9–4.3]), and urethral stenosis (OR = 2.0 [95 percent CI, 0.6–6.4]). Strabismus (OR = 0.7 [95 percent CI, 0.5–0.9]) and pyloric stenosis (OR = 0.2 [95 percent CI, 0.2–0.8]), however, occurred in significantly fewer infants with smoking fathers compared with infants of nonsmoking fathers.

Table 5.8   Studies of secondhand smoke exposure and congenital malformations

Study	Design/population	Exposure categories	Source of exposure
Holmberg and Nurminen 1980	Case-control (200) Children who were reported to the national birth defects registry and matched controls Finland	NR*	• Paternal secondhand smoke • Mothers were nonsmokers
Seidman et al. 1990	Retrospective cohort (17,152) Women on first or second postpartum day Israel	0 packs/day <1 pack/day ≥1 pack/day	• Maternal prenatal
Savitz et al. 1991	Prospective longitudinal (14,685) Children enrolled in Child Health and Development Studies between 1964 and 1967 in the San Francisco East Bay area of California United States	<20 cigarettes/day ≥20 cigarettes/day	• Paternal secondhand smoke
Zhang et al. 1992	Case-control (2,024) Birth defects were identified in the Shanghai Municipality during October 1986–September 1987 China	Nonsmokers 1–9 cigarettes/day 10–19 cigarettes/day ≥20 cigarettes/day	• Paternal
Shaw et al. 1996	Population-based case-control study Mothers of infants with orofacial cleft (731) and nonmalformed controls (734)	0 cigarettes/day 1–19 cigarettes/day ≥20 cigarettes/day	• Paternal periconceptional

Outcome	Findings	Comments
Congenital defects of the CNS[†]	• No significant association was found between smoking and CNS defects	All data were self-reported through maternal interviews; smoking was not the primary aim of the study; no adjustments were made except for maternal smoking status
Congenital anomalies	• No correlation was found between smoking behaviors and malformations of the cardiovascular, gastrointestinal, and CNS, or incidence of hypospadias • Slightly higher but not statistically significant incidence of cleft palate, cleft lip, spina bifida, and genitourinary system anomalies • Together with increased age (>35 years), smoking increased the risk of congenital malformations (p <0.002) • Maternal age alone was associated with congenital malformations (p <0.005)	Reproductive histories were self-reported through maternal interviews; maternal smoking may be a preventable risk factor for congenital anomalies among mothers aged ≥35 years
Congenital anomalies	• Urethral stenosis (POR[‡] = 2.4 [95% CI, 0.7–8.5]), cleft lip, and cleft palate (POR = 1.9 [95% CI, 0.5–7.3]) were more commonly seen in children of fathers who were heavy smokers	Source exposure data were reported through maternal intake interviews; assessment of paternal age, smoking, and alcohol consumption on fetal birth outcomes; outcomes were assessed independently by two physicians; this study does not strongly support the hypothesis that paternal smoking behavior is associated with birth defects
Congenital anomalies	• A modest relationship was detected between overall birth defects and paternal smoking behavior (OR[§] = 1.21 [95% CI, 1.01–1.45]) • Higher overall ORs (not broken down by the amount of exposure) for parental smoking and anencephalus (OR = 2.1), spina bifida (OR = 1.9), pigmentary anomalies of the skin (OR = 3.3), and varus/valgus deformities of the feet (OR = 1.8)	Source exposure data were reported through maternal interviews; a paternally mediated effect of smoking on birth defects is suggested and further research is encouraged
Orofacial cleft	• OR = 2.1 (95% CI, 1.3–3.6) for cleft lip with or without cleft palate and OR = 2.2 (95% CI, 1.1–4.5) for isolated cleft palate when mothers smoked ≥20 cigarettes/day • Clefting risks were even greater for infants with the transforming growth factor α (TGFα), ranging from 3-fold to 11-fold across phenotypic groups in White infants • Paternal smoking was not associated with clefting among the offspring of nonsmoking mothers • Secondhand smoke exposures were associated with slightly increased risks	Parental smoking information was obtained from telephone interviews with mothers; DNA was obtained from newborn screening blood spots and genotyped for the allelic variants of TGFα; controlling for the potential influence of other variables did not reveal substantially different results

Table 5.8   Continued

Study	Design/population	Exposure categories	Source of exposure
Wasserman et al. 1996	Case-control Mothers of infants with conotruncal heart defects (207), neural tube defects (264), limb deficiencies (178), and live-born controls (481)	0 cigarettes/day 1–19 cigarettes/day ≥20 cigarettes/day	• Maternal prenatal and postnatal • Paternal prenatal and postnatal • Home environment • Work environment • Any environment

*NR = Data were not reported.
†CNS = Central nervous system.
‡POR = Prevalence odds ratio.
§OR = Odds ratio.

Seidman and colleagues (1990) conducted immediate postpartum interviews with mothers of 17,152 infants from the three largest obstetrics units in Jerusalem; the data yielded crude ORs that showed no significant associations between paternal smoking and major anomalies (e.g., chromosomal anomalies, CNS anomalies, heart defects, cleft lip with or without cleft palate, omphalocele, diaphragmatic hernia, bowel atresias, hermaphroditism, and conjoined twins). Zhang and colleagues (1992) studied 1,012 infants with birth defects and 1,012 infants without birth defects (control group) from 10 urban districts and 29 hospitals in Shanghai. Mothers were interviewed while in the hospital. Although no adjustments were made for potential confounding variables, the investigators noted that the sample had very few families with characteristics pointing to potential confounders and that the two mothers who smoked were eliminated from the sample. In age-adjusted analyses, the investigators found that paternal smoking was associated with a slightly elevated risk among infants with birth defects (OR = 1.2 [95 percent CI, 1.01–1.45]).

The researchers also investigated 25 types of malformations and observed that selected malformations were associated with paternal smoking when dose-response relationships were examined. Infants with pigmentary anomalies of the skin were more likely to have fathers who were moderate smokers (10 to 19 cigarettes per day, OR = 4.1 [95 percent CI, 1.2–14.7]); infants with spina bifida were more likely to have fathers who were heavy smokers (≥20 cigarettes per day, OR = 3.2 [95 percent CI, 1.1–9.2]); and infants with multiple defects were more likely to have fathers who smoked 1 to 9 cigarettes per day (OR = 1.74 [95 percent CI, 1.16–2.61]). Most malformations, however, were not associated with involuntary smoking.

Using maternal interviews, Shaw and colleagues (1996) assessed the association between secondhand smoke exposure during pregnancy and oral clefts. There were conflicting results for nonsmoking mothers exposed to secondhand smoke, with very few significant associations among seemingly small numbers of observations. Wasserman and colleagues (1996) examined associations between secondhand smoke exposure among nonsmoking women and risks for

Outcome	Findings	Comments
Conotruncal heart defects Neural tube defects Limb deficiencies	• OR = 1.9 (95% CI, 1.2–3.1) for conotruncal heart defects when both parents smoked compared with neither • OR = 1.7 (95% CI, 0.96–2.9) for limb deficiencies when both parents smoked compared with neither • No significant increase in risk was associated with maternal smoking in the absence of paternal smoking • An increased risk was associated with heavy paternal smoking in the absence of maternal smoking for limb deficiencies in offspring (OR = 2.1 [95% CI, 1.3–3.6]) • For conotruncal defects, the risks associated with parental smoking differed among racial and ethnic groups • Parental smoking was not associated with increased risks for neural tube defects (Father only, OR = 1.1 [95% CI, 0.76–1.7]; Mother only, OR = 0.56 [95% CI, 0.30–1.0]; Both parents, OR = 1.0 [95% CI, 0.62–1.7])	All data were self-reported through maternal interviews; observed risks did not change substantially when adjusted for maternal vitamin use, alcohol use, and gravidity

heart malformations, neural tube defects, and limb defects. With one exception, secondhand smoke exposure was not associated with these congenital malformations. For tetralogy of Fallot, nonsmoking women exposed at work (but not at home or at "any location") had an OR of 2.9 (95 percent CI, 1.3–6.5) for exposure to secondhand smoke compared with those who were not exposed. However, given the multiple associations examined in this study, and given the inconsistent results for this malformation and the other sources of secondhand smoke, this particular association may have resulted by chance alone.

Evidence Synthesis

The evidence regarding the relationship between involuntary smoking and congenital malformations is inconsistent. The few studies that have been conducted have reported no association between involuntary smoking and specific or all congenital malformations.

Investigating congenital malformations is challenging because of the sample size that is necessary to study specific malformations. To date, few clues are available regarding the hypothesized biologic mechanisms of tobacco smoke and congenital malformations. Although two studies have reported elevated rates of neural tube defects in association with involuntary smoking, this association should be examined further in future studies.

Conclusion

1. The evidence is inadequate to infer the presence or absence of a causal relationship between exposure to secondhand smoke and congenital malformations.

Implications

The topic of tobacco smoke exposure and congenital malformations merits further investigation, particularly in part because of the teratogenic nature of tobacco smoke.

Cognitive, Behavioral, and Physical Development

Biologic Basis

In recent years, studies have suggested that exposure to tobacco smoke during pregnancy and childhood may affect the physical and cognitive development of the growing child. Researchers who examine the effects of these exposures on childhood outcomes need to account for potential confounding factors that reflect the various correlates of secondhand smoke exposure that also affect development. For example, factors that may affect physical and cognitive development include social class, parental education, the home environment as it relates to stimulation and developmentally appropriate exposures, and pregnancy-related factors such as voluntary and involuntary smoking and alcohol and substance use. Birth weight may also be a confounding factor because it is associated with both smoking (voluntary and involuntary) and physical and cognitive development. However, some researchers argue that adjusting for birth weight may overcontrol because it may be in the causal pathway from exposure to tobacco before birth to the time when childhood outcomes are assessed (Baghurst et al. 1992).

Another methodologic challenge lies in differentiating the effects of exposure to tobacco during and after pregnancy. This differentiation is often not possible because of the high correlation of tobacco smoke exposure for these two time periods. Studies with sufficient populations and detailed information on smoking status during both pregnancy and the postpartum period have been able to stratify participants into exposure groups: no prenatal or postpartum exposure, no prenatal but some postpartum exposure, and both prenatal and postpartum exposures. Other studies have examined the effects of secondhand smoke exposure from adults other than the mother among those children whose mothers did not smoke during pregnancy. These categories have served to partially address the timing of the exposures and, in particular, to control for exposures during pregnancy.

The mechanisms by which exposures to secondhand smoke may lead to compromised physical and cognitive development have not been fully explained and may be complex. Some of the mechanisms may be similar to those proposed for maternal smoking during pregnancy, such as hypoxia or the potentially teratogenic effects of tobacco smoke (USDHHS 1990;

Bruner and Forouzan 1991; Lambers and Clark 1996; Werler 1997). Studies document that components of secondhand and mainstream smoke are qualitatively similar to those of sidestream smoke, but quantitative data for doses of tobacco smoke components that reach the fetus across the placenta from active and involuntary maternal smoking have not been available (Slotkin 1998). This consideration is particularly important for outcomes assessed after one year of age because the child's exposure will have occurred for a period of time longer than the exposure of the fetus during the nine months of pregnancy.

For cognitive development, investigators have proposed a number of effects on CNS development from smoking in general and nicotine in particular. First, the fetus may suffer from hypoxia as a result of reduced blood flow or reduced oxygen levels (USDHHS 1990; Lambers and Clark 1996). Alterations in the peripheral autonomic pathways may lead to an increased susceptibility to hypoxia-induced, short-term and long-term brain damage (Slotkin 1998). In one review of prenatal nicotine exposure, Ernst and colleagues (2001) summarized numerous animal studies that document the impact of nicotine on cognitive processes of exposed rats and guinea pigs, such as slowed learning or increased attention or memory deficits. These investigators identified animal as well as human studies that have demonstrated adverse effects of nicotine exposure on neural functioning. Exposure to nicotine alters enzyme activity and thus affects brain development, and alters molecular processes that affect neurotransmitter systems and lead to permanent neural abnormalities (Ernst et al. 2001).

Cognitive Development

Epidemiologic Evidence

Twelve studies have examined the effects of secondhand smoke exposure on cognitive development in children (Table 5.9) (Rantakallio 1983; Bauman et al. 1989, 1991; Makin et al. 1991; Baghurst et al. 1992; Roeleveld et al. 1992; Schulte-Hobein et al. 1992; Byrd and Weitzman 1994; McCartney et al. 1994; Olds et al. 1994; Fried et al. 1997, 1998). The age ranges of the children varied from infants to older adolescents. Hence, the tools used to assess cognitive development also varied and included measures of intelligence, reading and language scores, school grade retention (staying in a grade for an additional year), and various standardized cognitive functioning tests. Four studies found no association between second-hand smoke exposure and cognitive outcomes among infants and children (Baghurst et al. 1992; Schulte-Hobein et al. 1992; McCartney et al. 1994; Fried et al. 1997); four other studies reported findings that varied across outcome measures (Bauman et al. 1991; Makin et al. 1991; Olds et al. 1994; Fried et al. 1998). For example, Makin and colleagues (1991) used standardized assessments to measure skills in the following areas: speech, language, intelligence, and visual and spatial processing. The authors examined involuntary smoking during pregnancy and controlled for potential confounders such as maternal education, maternal age, and family income. Results from 14 specific standardized tests indicated significant differences between exposed and unexposed groups in 11 of the tests. Similarly, Fried and colleagues (1997) examined the effects of pre-natal and postpartum secondhand smoke exposures on 131 children aged 9 through 12 years who were given standardized reading and language assessments. For the prenatal period, the investigators considered only those mothers who were not smokers and found no association between prenatal or postpartum exposures and reading skills. For language skills, however, post-partum secondhand smoke exposures were associated with lower language levels among exposed versus the unexposed children (Fried et al. 1997). Several other investigators also reported associations with cognitive development (Rantakallio 1983; Bauman et al. 1989), mental retardation (Roeleveld et al. 1992), or school performance (Byrd and Weitzman 1994). Roeleveld and colleagues (1992) examined cigarette, pipe, and cigar smoking; only secondhand smoke exposures to pipe and cigar smoke during pregnancy and in the first six months of the infant's life were associated with an increased risk for mental retardation. Bauman and colleagues (1989) studied unexposed adolescents and adolescents who had been exposed to second-hand smoke from family members. The investigators examined overall and domain-specific California Achievement Test scores for math, language, reading, and spelling to identify differences between these two groups of adolescents. After considering several potential confounding factors, including active adolescent smoking, the investigators found that test performance decreased as smoking levels of the family increased.

Evidence Synthesis

The literature cited in this discussion examined the effects of involuntary smoking on children's cognitive development. However, it is difficult to synthesize the results of these studies because the ages of the children, the assessed exposures, and the outcomes vary across and even within studies. Moreover, some of the findings across and within studies are inconsistent. Eight of the 12 studies that examined associations between involuntary smoking and children's cognitive development reported associations between secondhand smoke exposures and reduced levels of cognitive development; these investigators had used a variety of assessments, such as performance on standardized tests, grade retention, or a diagnosis of mental retardation. The use of various cognitive measures across studies precludes an assessment of consistency with specific associations. Yet the finding that secondhand smoke exposure was associated with several different outcomes suggests that exposure may, indeed, impact the cognitive development of children. More studies are clearly needed; of the studies that have been conducted, there is a need for additional efforts to replicate findings.

Conclusion

1. The evidence is inadequate to infer the presence or absence of a causal relationship between exposure to secondhand smoke and cognitive functioning among children.

Implications

Further research is needed but there are complex challenges to carrying out such studies, given the need for longitudinal design and consideration of the many factors affecting cognitive functioning.

Behavioral Development

Epidemiologic Evidence

Three studies examined associations between secondhand smoke exposures and behavioral problems among children (Table 5.10) (Makin et al. 1991; Weitzman et al. 1992; Fergusson et al. 1993). Weitzman and colleagues (1992) studied children aged 4 through 11 years and reported that after adjusting for several potential confounders, heavy maternal smoking after delivery was associated with greater behavioral problems reported by the parents.

Table 5.9   Studies of secondhand smoke exposure and cognitive development

Study	Design/population	Exposure categories	Source of exposure
Rantakallio 1983	Prospective cohort (3,392) Mothers who smoked during pregnancy and controls from two northernmost provinces in Finland	• Light smokers (<10 cigarettes/day) • Heavy smokers (≥10 cigarettes/ day at end of second month of pregnancy) • Father never smoked • Father formerly smoked • Father currently smoked	• Prenatal and involuntary exposure to parental smoking
Bauman et al. 1989	Secondary data analysis (2,008) Eighth-grade students from Guilford County Public Schools in North Carolina United States	• None • 1 cigarette–1 pack/day • 1–2 packs/day • >2 packs/day • Adolescent CO* levels of ≥9 parts per million, an indication of smoking	• Secondhand smoke exposure to family smoking behaviors • Alveolar breath specimens • Adolescent reports of sibling smoking behaviors
Bauman et al. 1991	Longitudinal cohort (year 5 exam, n = 5,342; year 10 exam, n = 3,737; adolescent exam, n = 2,020) Pregnancies from 1960–1967 among women enrolled in the Kaiser Foundation Health Plan in the San Francisco East Bay area Children were all from the Child Health and Development Studies United States 1987	• Mother smoked at time of exam • Father smoked at time of exam • Average number of cigarettes smoked/day by mother and father	• Parental smoking and in utero exposure from maternal smoking during pregnancy
Makin et al. 1991	Cross-sectional (91 children) Aged 6–9 years Canada (Ottawa)	During pregnancy, mother was • Active smoker • Exposed to secondhand smoke • Nonsmoker, not exposed to secondhand smoke	• Mother • Others

Outcome	Findings	Comments
Respiratory disease School performance Retarded growth	• Children of smoking parents had the most frequent incidences of hospital admissions for respiratory illness (p <0.024) • Significant height reduction among children of smokers at 6 months (p <0.001), 12 months (p <0.004), and 14 years of age (p <0.023) • Controlling for height, children of maternal smokers had highly significantly reduced school performance (p <0.001 by F-test) • Maternal and paternal sources of secondhand smoke exposures had similar associations with physiologic and performance outcomes	Source exposure data were from maternal self-reports (mailed questionnaires), school public health nurses, and hospital admission records from 5–10 years ago; these findings are a subset of overall characteristic studies within this birth cohort; school performance was based on school office reports; maternal smoking had an effect on children's physical and mental development, even when these factors were controlled with regression analysis
Test performance	• Stepwise regression identified 8 significant control variables • Pair-wise interactive analysis identified 6 interactive social and psychologic control variables • Controlling for all 14 variables, a statistically significant relationship remained overall between family smoking and CAT[†] scores (p <0.017)	Source exposure data were from maternal self-reports; test performance was based on the CAT; CAT test scores significantly decreased as family smoking increased (p <0.001); other potential variables accounting for an observed association may be active maternal smoking during pregnancy, tobacco smoke ingredients other than CO, and short-term exposures to secondhand tobacco smoke
Cognitive performance in 3 testing periods (aged 5, 9–11, and 15–17 years)	• PPVT[‡] scores and RAVEN[§] scores for children of nonsmoking parents were statistically significant, averaging 5.9% higher than for children of smokers (p <0.05) • Analyses of covariance confirmed that parental smoking had a significant effect on PPVT and RAVEN scores at the 10-year exam • Following adjustments for covariates (e.g., age, low birth weight, race, parental education, and income), a linear dose-response relationship was observed between parental smoking and cognitive performance • No significant interactions were identified between maternal prenatal and current smoking status	Source exposure data were from maternal self-reports; cognitive measurements were made with Goodenough-Harris Drawing test, the Quick Test, PPVT, and RAVEN; husband's smoking status was not measured in one 5-year examination group and in adolescent measurements; child physiologic responses, such as middle-ear effusion and respiratory illness, were related to secondhand tobacco smoke and might influence cognitive performance; family cigarette smoking is associated with selected child cognitive performance skills, and some outcomes exhibited a dose-response relationship with exposure to smoking
Speech and language, intellectual, motor, visual/spatial, academic achievement, and behavior skills	• Children of nonsmoking, unexposed mothers performed better than children of smoking or secondhand smoke-exposed mothers on tests of speech and language skills, intelligence, visual/spatial abilities, and on mother's rating of behavior	Source exposure data were self-reported (interview); children of active and secondhand smoke-exposed mothers are at risk for a pattern of negative developmental outcomes

Table 5.9   Continued

Study	Design/population	Exposure categories	Source of exposure
Baghurst et al. 1992	Prospective cohort (548) Children enrolled in the Port Pine Cohort Study, aged birth to 4 years, whose mothers attended antenatal care between May 1979 and May 1982 Australia	• Nonsmokers (never smoked or smoked ≤5 cigarettes during pregnancy) • Smokers (>5 cigarettes ever)	• Prenatal and involuntary exposures to maternal smoking
Roeleveld et al. 1992	Epidemiologic (628) Cases and referent group were 0–15 years of age, selected from medical files of the Pediatric or Child Neurology Department of Nijmegen University Hospital, or from local rehabilitation centers between 1979 and 1987 Netherlands	• Average number of cigarettes/day reported by parents • Daily amount of paternal pipe or cigar smoking	• Prenatal and secondhand smoke exposures to parental smoking
Schulte-Hobein et al. 1992	Prospective longitudinal matched pair (69 cases, 69 controls) Mothers were selected soon after delivery from 3 maternity hospitals Germany (Berlin)	• Smoked >5 cigarettes/day during pregnancy • Never smoked	• Mother's milk and secondhand smoke exposures during first year of life
Byrd and Weitzman 1994	Cross-sectional data analyses (9,996) Children aged 0–17 years whose parents participated in the National Health Interview Survey, a nationally representative civilian population United States	• Household exposures to cigarette smoke at time of survey	• Maternal prenatal and involuntary exposures

Outcome	Findings	Comments
Neuropsychologic development	• Children with postnatal exposures had significantly lower scores on the MDI$^\Delta$ (p <0.03) and MSCA¶ verbal (p <0.03), perceptual performance (p <0.01), and motor (p <0.01) • A statistically significant inverse association was found between maternal smoking behavior and neuropsychologic development until other determinants of development were controlled (e.g., gender, mother's intelligence, birth weight, and socioeconomic status) • Children of smoking mothers performed significantly lower (2.4–4.1%) in testing sessions (p <0.03) • There was no strong evidence that maternal smoking exerted an independent effect on neuropsychologic development in early childhood	Self-reports and interviews with trained nurse interviewers were used to assess postpartum secondhand smoke exposures; neuropsychologic development was measured by the BSID**, MSCA, and MDI; social and environmental factors are major confounders of the association between maternal smoking and neuropsychologic development in childhood; more precise measures of exposures to secondhand tobacco smoke and a comprehensive assessment of confounders are required for future studies
Mental and psychomotor retardation	• Paternal pipe or cigar smoking was associated with an OR†† of 2.4 (95% CI‡‡, 1.2–5.1) for cases to referents	Source exposure data were from parental reports obtained in a structured interview; paternal smoking before, during, and after pregnancy is a risk factor for mental retardation among offspring
Somatic development Mental development Infant cotinine levels	• 41% of children of smokers and 32% of children of nonsmoking mothers suffered from bronchitis and pneumonia • Cotinine levels present in infants of smokers were 3-fold to 10-fold higher than in infants of nonsmokers • No confirmation of mental/developmental retardation among exposed infants	Physiologic measurements (weight and head circumference) and secondhand smoke exposures were gathered through home interviews with mothers (self-reports) and from medical records (biologic markers); BSID measured development; to prevent health risks to infants, mothers should be encouraged to stop smoking during pregnancy and while nursing, and both parents should avoid smoking when children are present
History of repeating kindergarten or first grade	• OR = 1.4 (95% CI, 1.1–1.7) for children repeating kindergarten or first grade who had a history of exposures to household smoke	Source exposure data were from maternal self-reports (questionnaires); behavior problem assessments were dropped from the analyses because behavior interviews were conducted after the child had repeated kindergarten or first grade, an experience that may account for behavior; the survey was designed to assess a multitude of social and environmental exposures; smoking in the home may contribute to social and individual factors that influence the decision to retain a child in kindergarten or first grade

Table 5.9   Continued

Study	Design/population	Exposure categories	Source of exposure
McCartney et al. 1994	Longitudinal (quasi-experimental) (190) Children aged 6–10 years enrolled in the OPPS[§§] Canada	• Nonsmoking controls • Light (>0 mg[ΔΔ] nicotine/day to 16 mg nicotine/day) • Heavy (>16 mg nicotine/day)	• Prenatal and postnatal secondhand smoke exposures
Olds et al. 1994	Prospective follow-up (400) Children aged 1–4 years from a semirural county in New York state participating in a home nurse visitation program United States	• 0 cigarettes/day • 1–9 cigarettes/day • ≥10 cigarettes/day	• Prenatal exposure
Fried et al. 1997	Longitudinal (131) Children aged 9–12 years enrolled in OPPS Canada	• Nonsmoking controls • Light (>0 mg nicotine/day to 16 mg nicotine/day) • Heavy (>16 mg nicotine/day)	• Maternal prenatal exposure
Fried et al. 1998	Longitudinal (131) Children aged 9–12 years enrolled in OPPS Canada	• Nonsmoking controls • Light (>0 mg nicotine/day to 16 mg nicotine/day) • Heavy (>16 mg nicotine/day)	• Maternal prenatal exposure

*CO = Carbon monoxide.
[†]CAT = California Achievement Test.
[‡]PPVT = Peabody Picture Vocabulary Test.
[§]RAVEN = Raven Colored Progressive Matrices Test.
[Δ]MDI = Mental Development Index.
[¶]MSCA = McCarthy Scales of Children's Abilities.
**BSID = Bayley Scales of Infant Development.
[††]OR = Odds ratio.
[‡‡]CI = Confidence interval.
[§§]OPPS = Ottawa Prenatal Prospective Study.
[ΔΔ]mg = Milligrams.
[¶¶]WISC = Weschler Intelligence Scale for Children.

Outcome	Findings	Comments
Central auditory processing task (SCAN)	• Secondhand smoke exposures both during and after pregnancy were not significantly associated with SCAN results	Source exposure data were from maternal self-reports obtained through interviews with a woman interviewer; maternal smoking rates were averaged over the trimester interview recordings
Intellectual functioning during the first 4 years	• Children whose mothers reported smoking ≥10 cigarettes/day during pregnancy had reduced and adjusted Stanford-Binet scores by 4.35 points (95% CI, 0.02–8.68, p <0.049)	Source exposure data were obtained from maternal self-reports; BSID, MDI, Cattell, and Stanford-Binet were used to measure intellectual functioning outcomes; smoking during pregnancy poses a unique risk of neurodevelopmental impairment for exposed children
Reading scores Language scores	• Maternal prenatal secondhand smoke exposure was not associated with language or reading outcomes • Postnatal exposure to secondhand smoke was associated with lower language scores • An association was observed between prenatal cigarette smoking and altered (reduced) auditory functioning among offspring	Source exposure data were obtained from maternal self-reports through interviews in the home of the participant; multiple measures used to assess reading and language abilities included the WISC^{TM}-III, Wide Range Achievement Test—Revised, PPVT, Fluency Test, Woodcock Reading Mastery Test, Oral Cloze Task, Seashore Rhythm Test, and Regular and Exceptional Pseudoword Task; maternal smoking negatively impacts reading and language capabilities of exposed children
Cognitive performance	• After discriminant functional analysis and key covariate adjustments, a strong linear association persisted with prenatal exposures among the 3 smoking categories (p <0.01) • After discriminant functional analysis and key covariate adjustments, a strong linear association persisted with postnatal secondhand smoke exposure and the 3 smoking categories (p <0.05)	Source exposure data were from maternal self-reports obtained through interviews in the home of the participant; a battery of cognitive performance tests included WISC-III, Fluency Test, Auditory Working Memory, Tactual Performance Task, Category Test, Gordon Delay Task, and the Gordon Vigilance Task; there was a dose-response association between prenatal cigarette exposure and lower global intelligence scores

Table 5.10   Studies of secondhand smoke exposure and behavioral problems among children

Study	Design/population	Exposure categories	Source of exposure
Makin et al. 1991	Prospective longitudinal study (90) Children aged 6–9 years Subsample of Ottawa Prenatal Prospective Study Canada	• Nonsmokers • Involuntary smokers • Active smokers	• Maternal prenatal and postnatal secondhand smoke exposures
Weitzman et al. 1992	Longitudinal (2,256) Children aged 4–11 years participating in the National Longitudinal Survey of Youth United States	• <1 pack/day • ≥1 pack/day • Prenatal (mother smoked during pregnancy only) • Involuntary smoking (mother smoked only after pregnancy) • Prenatal and involuntary smoking (in utero and postnatal exposures to maternal smoking)	• Prenatal and involuntary exposures to parental smoking
Fergusson et al. 1993	Longitudinal (1,265) Children aged 8, 10, and 12 years born in Christchurch, New Zealand, enrolled in the Christchurch Health and Development Study	• Mean number of cigarettes smoked/day during pregnancy (reported during each trimester) • Annual questions regarding daily maternal smoking habits for the first 5 postnatal years and converted to a daily cigarette intake amount	• Maternal smoking during and after pregnancy

Outcome	Findings	Comments
Behavioral, language, and mental development	• The active smoking group demonstrated the poorest performance on the speech, language, intellectual, and behavioral battery of exams • Involuntary smokers had intermediate scores • Nonsmokers had the best scores of the 3 groups • Stepwise discriminant analysis was performed between the involuntary smoking and nonsmoking groups and identified a significant difference ($\chi^2 = 28.15$, $p < 0.001$) • Children in active and involuntary smoking groups rated higher in behavioral problems, with an apparent dose-response relationship	This study was designed to assess a spectrum of long-term consequences of active and involuntary smoking during pregnancy; secondhand smoke exposure was primarily based on the husband's smoking habits; source exposure data were obtained from maternal self-reports through controlled interviews; pregnant mothers, and other persons who may be sources of secondhand smoke, need education and factual information about the deleterious effects smoking can have on the developing fetus
Behavioral problems	• Increased rates of children's behavioral problems were independently associated with all categories of maternal smoking behaviors and with evidence of a dose-response relationship • Among children exposed during and after pregnancy, there were 1.17 additional problems associated with smoking <1 pack/day and 2.04 with ≥1 pack/day ($p < 0.001$) • Odds ratios for extreme behavioral problems = 1.41 for <1 pack/day ($p < 0.01$) and 1.54 for ≥1 pack/day ($p < 0.02$)	Source exposure data were obtained from maternal self-reports through interviews; behavioral problems were measured by the 32-item Child Behavior Problem Index and six subscales; this study suggests that increased behavioral problems among children should be added to the spectrum of adverse health conditions associated with children's prenatal and involuntary exposures to maternal smoking
Behavioral outcomes (disruptive)	• There was a consistent dose-response relationship between the amount smoked during pregnancy and mean problem behavior scores; all behavior assessment measures that compared exposures from 0 to >20 cigarettes/day were statistically significant ($p < 0.001$) • Postnatal exposures identified associations between maternal smoking during preschool years and child behavioral problems ($p < 0.01$) • Assessments of the independent influence of prenatal vs. postnatal exposures indicated that behavioral problems were typically associated with smoking during pregnancy	Source exposure data were from maternal self-reports; outcomes were adjusted for confounding factors potentially associated with maternal smoking and childhood behavioral problems; smoking during pregnancy is associated with a small but detectable increase in the risk of childhood behavioral problems; there was no association between behavioral problems and exposure to maternal postnatal smoking

Makin and colleagues (1991) also noted that compared with children of nonsmokers, children exposed to secondhand smoke had higher levels of maternal-reported behavioral problems even after considering potential confounders. Fergusson and colleagues (1993) studied behavioral problems reported by mothers and teachers of middle school children in New Zealand. After adjusting for confounders, the researchers found small but statistically detectable increases in rates of childhood problem behaviors associated with smoking during pregnancy, but did not observe any associations between exposures to maternal smoking after pregnancy and behavioral outcomes (Fergusson et al. 1993).

Evidence Synthesis

The evidence for an association between exposure to secondhand smoke and behavioral problems in children is inconsistent. Because so few studies have been carried out on this topic, more studies are clearly warranted.

Conclusion

1. The evidence is inadequate to infer the presence or absence of a causal relationship between exposure to secondhand smoke and behavioral problems among children.

Implications

Further research is needed, but the same challenges remain that confront research on other effects such as cognitive functioning.

Height/Growth

Epidemiologic Evidence

Five studies examined the association between children's growth and secondhand smoke exposure (Table 5.11) (Rona et al. 1981, 1985; Rantakallio 1983; Chinn and Rona 1991; Eskenazi and Bergmann 1995). Two of the studies (Chinn and Rona 1991; Eskenazi and Bergmann 1995) reported no association for children aged 5 years and for children aged 5 through

11 years. Eskenazi and Bergmann (1995) used biochemical confirmation of secondhand smoke exposure and proposed that the height differences between exposed and unexposed children were attributable to the effect of tobacco smoke exposure on fetal growth. After adjusting for birth weight, however, any associations between secondhand smoke exposure and height were eliminated. Rona and colleagues (1981) found that differences in height remained among children of smokers even after adjusting for birth weight. Rantakallio (1983) examined secondhand smoke exposures from fathers during pregnancy and found that after adjusting for potential confounding factors, children exposed to paternal smoking during pregnancy were shorter than were children of nonsmoking fathers. Similarly, Rona and colleagues (1985) examined height among children aged 5 through 11 years and found small decreases among children exposed to secondhand smoke. Both of these studies found relatively small differences (1 centimeter or less) even among children exposed to heavy smokers.

Evidence Synthesis

The evidence for an association between secondhand smoke exposure and children's height/growth is mixed (Table 5.11). Those studies that do report associations find relatively consistent deficits associated with secondhand smoke exposure. However, the magnitude of the effect is small and could reflect residual confounding.

Conclusion

1. The evidence is inadequate to infer the presence or absence of a causal relationship between exposure to secondhand smoke and children's height/growth.

Implications

The evidence suggests that any effect of secondhand smoke exposure on height is likely to be small and of little significance. Research on secondhand smoke exposure and height is complicated by the many potential confounding factors.

Childhood Cancer

Biologic Basis

Tobacco smoke contains numerous carcinogens and is a well-established cause of cancer (USDHEW 1964, 1974; USDHHS 1980, 1986; Smith et al. 1997, 2000a,b). Numerous animal studies elucidate evidence for, and mechanisms of, transplacental carcinogenesis (Rice 1979; Schuller 1984; Napalkov et al. 1989). For example, when the oncogenic compound ethylnitrosourea (ENU) was administered intravenously or intraperitoneally to pregnant rabbits, the offspring developed renal and neural cancers (Stavrou et al. 1984). Monkeys are also susceptible to transplacental carcinogenesis, with offspring developing vascular and a variety of other tumors following prenatal administration of ENU to the mother (Rice et al. 1989). The strongest human evidence that transplacental carcinogenesis is biologically plausible may be the occurrence of vaginal clear-cell adenocarcinoma among young women whose mothers were prescribed diethylstilbesterol during pregnancy (Vessey 1989).

Limited biologic evidence suggests that involuntary exposure to cigarette smoke may also lead to transplacental carcinogenesis. Maternal secondhand smoke exposure during pregnancy, as with maternal active smoking during pregnancy, can result in increased measurable metabolites of cigarette smoke in amniotic fluid (Andresen et al. 1982; Smith et al. 1982) and in fetal blood (Bottoms et al. 1982; Coghlin et al. 1991). For example, thiocyanate levels in fetal blood were less than 50 micromoles per liter (μmol/L) when the mother was not exposed to secondhand smoke during pregnancy (Bottoms et al. 1982). Among mothers who were prenatally exposed to secondhand smoke, fetal blood levels of thiocyanate were as high as 90 μmol/L, and among mothers who actively smoked, the measurements were about 170 μmol/L. Notably, however, two studies that measured thiocyanate levels in umbilical cord blood found no differences between secondhand smoke-exposed and unexposed nonsmoking women (Manchester and Jacoby 1981; Hauth et al. 1984). Hauth and colleagues (1984) found thiocyanate levels of 23 μmol/L in umbilical cord blood from unexposed infants of nonsmoking mothers and levels of 26 μmol/L in secondhand smoke-exposed infants of nonsmoking mothers (defined as living

and/or working with someone who smoked at least 10 cigarettes per day). Manchester and Jacoby (1981) also found similar cord blood levels of thiocyanate in unexposed (34 $\pm$ 3 μmol/L) and secondhand smoke-exposed (35 $\pm$ 3 μmol/L) infants of nonsmoking mothers (exposure was defined as living with someone who smoked).

Studies of maternal smoking during pregnancy found enhanced transplacental enzyme activation (Nebert et al. 1969; Manchester and Jacoby 1981) and placental DNA adducts (Everson et al. 1986, 1988; Hansen et al. 1992), and several animal studies suggested that embryonic exposure to tobacco smoke components increased tumor rates (Mohr et al. 1975; Nicolov and Chernozemsky 1979). For example, diethylnitrosamine administered to female hamsters in the last days of pregnancy produced offspring that developed respiratory tract neoplasms in nearly 95 percent of the animals. Cigarette smoke condensate in olive oil that was used in another study of pregnant hamsters was injected intraperitoneally; it produced a variety of tumors in the offspring, including tumors of the pancreas, adrenal glands, liver, uterus, and lung (Nicolov and Chernozemsky 1979). Human studies document an increased frequency of genomic deletions in the *hypoxanthine-guanine phosphoribosyl-transferase* gene found in the cord blood of newborns whose mothers were exposed to secondhand smoke (compared with newborns of unexposed mothers). This finding strongly supports a carcinogenic effect of prenatal secondhand smoke exposure, particularly since these mutations are characteristic of those found in childhood leukemia and lymphoma (Finette et al. 1998). Prenatal exposure to secondhand smoke may also play a role by enhancing any effect of postnatal exposure on the development of childhood cancer (Napalkov 1973), but the potential effects of prenatal and postnatal exposures are difficult to separate given the high correlation between prenatal and postnatal parental smoking. Several studies have assessed postnatal exposures by measuring cotinine and nicotine concentrations in the saliva and urine of infants. The investigators found that those infants with reported secondhand smoke exposures had significantly higher concentrations than those infants with no reported exposure in the 24 hours before measuring the concentrations (Greenberg et al. 1984; Crawford et al. 1994).

Table 5.11   Studies of secondhand smoke exposure and children's growth

Study	Design/population	Exposure categories	Source of exposure
Rona et al. 1981	Longitudinal (1,800) Children aged 5–11 years from England and Scotland who participated in the National Study of Health and Growth United Kingdom	• Children with no smokers in the home • One smoker in the home • Two or more smokers in the home	• Parental secondhand smoke exposure at home
Rantakallio 1983	Longitudinal (12,068) Finnish children (mothers enrolled during pregnancy and children followed until 14 years of age) Finland	• Maternal smoking • Paternal smoking (exposures were not clearly defined)	• Mother • Father
Rona et al. 1985	Editorial prospective (5,000–6,000) Primary school children (aged 5–11 years) from England and Scotland United Kingdom	NR*	• Prenatal and secondhand smoke exposures from parental smoking
Chinn and Rona 1991	Observational study (11,224) English and Scottish inner-city and representative children aged 5–11 years United Kingdom	• Number of cigarettes smoked by parents at home (recorded as a continuous variable) = 0, 1–4, 5–14, 15–24, 25–34, and ≥35	• Secondhand smoke

Eskenazi and Bergmann 1995	Longitudinal cohort (2,622) Children (aged 5 years ± 6 months) enrolled in Child Health and Development Studies between 1964 and 1967 in the San Francisco East Bay area United States	• Nonsmokers exposed to secondhand smoke (cotinine levels 2–10 ng/mL†)
		• Unexposed nonsmokers
		• Serum cotinine levels of smokers:
		  0–79 ng/mL
		  80–163 ng/mL
		  164–569 ng/mL
			• Maternal secondhand smoke exposure during pregnancy and prenatal maternal smoking
			• Serum cotinine sample during pregnancy

*NR = Data were not reported.
†mm = Millimeters.
‡ng/mL = Nanograms per milliliter.

Outcome	Findings	Comments
Height	• There was a strong inverse association between height and the number of household smokers (p <0.001 in England and p <0.01 in Scotland) • After adjusting for confounding variables such as maternal smoking during pregnancy, paternal social class, maternal and paternal heights, and the number of siblings, a significant trend remained only in the English sample (p <0.01)	Source exposure data were obtained from parental self-reports through questionnaires; children's heights were measured across all 28 study areas; persons identified regarding exposures smoked ≥5 cigarettes/day at home; secondhand smoke at home seems to affect the growth of children

Height at 14 years of age	• Children of smokers were shorter at 14 years of age compared with children of nonsmokers
	• Regression coefficient:
	   -0.034 (maternal smoking, p = 0.056)
	   -0.032 (paternal smoking, p = 0.072)
		Source exposure data were self-reported (questionnaire); children of smokers were shorter than children of nonsmokers

Height (in mm⁺)	• Children of mothers who smoked during pregnancy and whose parents smoked at home had significantly reduced (p <0.01) heights by 2 mm for children aged 5–11 years	NR
Height, respiratory illness (wheeze)	• There were no regression coefficients of height standard deviation scores on involuntary smoking; controlling for confounders was significantly different from zero • Significant usual coughs were observed in English inner-city boys and girls (p <0.01 and p <0.05, respectively) • Persistent wheeze was significant for Scottish boys (p <0.05)	Source exposure data were from maternal self-reports (questionnaires); heights were measured by Holtian stadiometer, and respiratory symptoms were gathered from maternal reports; overall risk of respiratory conditions resulting from secondhand smoke is small but not negligible
Height	• Children of smokers and those of nonsmokers in unadjusted analyses were 0.1, 0.2, and 0.5 centimeters shorter for each smoker's cotinine tertile, respectively • Only the adjusted heights of children of mothers who smoked prenatally and postnatally were significantly different from those of nonsmokers (p <0.05), but when birth weight and gestational length were added to the model, the finding was no longer significant	Source exposure data were from maternal self-reports of smoking status; secondhand smoke exposure was measured using cotinine as a biomarker; self-reported smoking status and serum cotinine levels showed good agreement in height measurements collected by trained personnel; children whose mothers were heavy smokers during pregnancy were shorter at 5 years of age compared with children of nonsmokers; this effect appears to be attributable to in utero exposure rather than to postnatal secondhand smoke exposure

Epidemiologic Evidence

In the case of active maternal smoking during pregnancy, investigators who have reviewed the evidence have not found an association between maternal smoking and a transplacental effect on childhood cancer (Pershagen 1989; Tredaniel et al. 1994; Sasco and Vainio 1999). One meta-analysis found a 10 percent increase in risk (RR = 1.10 [95 percent CI, 1.03–1.19]) for all cancers based on 12 studies, but the quality of the available studies and the diversity of the cancer types considered precluded establishing a causal relationship (Boffetta et al. 2000). In a recent monograph on involuntary smoking, the International Agency for Research on Cancer (2004) concluded that the evidence regarding exposure to parental smoking and childhood cancer is inconsistent. Similarly, two other literature reviews of secondhand smoke exposure and childhood cancer also found no strong evidence of an association (Tredaniel et al. 1994; Sasco and Vainio 1999), but a pooled risk estimate that combined studies of specific cancer sites as well as all cancer sites was 1.23 (95 percent CI, 1.14–1.33) for paternal smoking (Sorahan et al. 1997a). Another meta-analysis of paternal smoking and risk of childhood cancer yielded a statistically significant increase in risk for non-Hodgkin's lymphoma based on 4 studies (RR = 2.0 [95 percent CI, 1.08–3.98]) and for brain tumors based on 10 studies (RR = 1.22 [95 percent CI, 1.05–1.40]) (Boffetta et al. 2000). The summary estimate from the meta-analysis for acute lymphocytic leukemia (ALL), the most common type of childhood leukemia, was not statistically significant (RR = 1.17 [95 percent CI, 0.96–1.42]). A separate review of the available studies on childhood brain tumors and tobacco smoke found mixed results for maternal exposure to secondhand smoke during pregnancy (Norman et al. 1996b).

Given the relative rarity of childhood cancer, the epidemiologic evidence on secondhand smoke exposure and childhood cancer comes almost exclusively from case-control studies (Table 5.12). One cohort study that addressed cancer outcomes among offspring (including adults) who had reported at least one parent with lung cancer assumed that these offspring had been exposed to secondhand smoke (Seersholm et al. 1997). Lung cancer patients were identified using the Danish Cancer Registry and their offspring were identified through the Danish Population Registry. Records of the offspring were then linked back to the cancer registry to obtain the overall cancer rate in this cohort, which was lower than the cancer rate for the general Danish population (standardized incidence ratio 0.9, 90 percent CI, 0.6–1.2). The cohort also did not have any statistically significant excesses for any specific cancer sites.

Seven of the case-control studies on secondhand smoke exposure evaluated all cancer types together as well as some specific types of cancers (Stjernfeldt et al. 1986; John et al. 1991; Sorahan et al. 1995, 1997a,b, 2001; Ji et al. 1997). Of another nine studies that examined only CNS tumors (Preston-Martin et al. 1982; Howe et al. 1989; Kuijten et al. 1990; Gold et al. 1993; Bunin et al. 1994; Filippini et al. 1994, 2000; McCredie et al. 1994; Norman et al. 1996a), four focused on leukemias (Magnani et al. 1990; Shu et al. 1996; Brondum et al. 1999; Infante-Rivard et al. 2000)—one included non-Hodgkin's lymphoma (Magnani et al. 1990)—and two other studies analyzed soft-tissue sarcomas (Grufferman et al. 1982; Magnani et al. 1989). Four of the seven studies that examined the overall cancer risk were conducted by the same primary investigator who studied cancer deaths in the United Kingdom during four time periods: 1953–1955 (Sorahan et al. 1997a), 1971–1976 (Sorahan et al. 1997b), 1977–1981 (Sorahan et al. 1995), and 1980–1983 (Sorahan et al. 2001). All four of these studies as well as a study from China (Ji et al. 1997) found positive exposure-response trends that were also statistically significant for the amount of paternal smoking and overall cancers, with ORs ranging from 1.08 (adjusted, 95 percent CI, 1.03–1.13) (Sorahan et al. 1995) to 1.9 (adjusted, 95 percent CI, 1.3–2.7) (Ji et al. 1997).

Because of the heterogeneity in the quality of the epidemiologic evidence on maternal secondhand smoke exposure and childhood cancers, a meta-analysis of the relevant studies is not currently warranted. In addition, the level of epidemiologic evidence on individual types of childhood cancers is limited.

Leukemia

The studies that focused on childhood leukemia (Magnani et al. 1990; Shu et al. 1996; Brondum et al. 1999; Infante-Rivard et al. 2000) did not find statistically significant associations with paternal smoking. Findings from one of these studies, which also investigated the modifying effect of three polymorphisms of the *CYP1A1* gene, showed no effect of paternal smoking on childhood leukemia (nonsignificant OR of 1.0 for all levels of reported paternal smoking), but did suggest a protective effect with postnatal paternal smoking for children with the *CYP1A1*2B* allele but not for children without it (OR = 0.2 [95 percent CI, 0.04–0.9]) (Infante-Rivard et al. 2000). Two of the studies that examined overall and specific cancers did find significantly increased risks for ALL at the highest levels of paternal smoking, with ORs of 3.8 (95 percent CI, 1.3–12.3) for five or more pack-years[1] of smoking before conception (p for trend = 0.01) (Ji et al. 1997) and 5.29 (95 percent CI, 1.31–21.30) for 40 or more cigarettes per day before the pregnancy (p trend = 0.06) (Sorahan et al. 2001).

Lymphoma

Lymphoma was significantly associated with paternal smoking in three of the studies that analyzed multiple cancer sites (Ji et al. 1997; Sorahan et al. 1997b, 2001). The highest risk was associated with 10 or more pack-years of smoking (among nonsmoking mothers) before conception and postnatally (adjusted OR = 5.7 [95 percent CI, 1.3–26.0], p for trend = 0.03) (Ji et al. 1997). One study that was based on 17 cases of non-Hodgkin's lymphoma found large, increased risks with paternal smoking before the birth of the child (overall and by levels of smoking), although these estimates had lower confidence limits of 0.9 and 1.0, respectively (Magnani et al. 1990). Using the broader category of reticuloendothelial system neoplasms, Sorahan and colleagues (2001) also found a large increased risk (RR = 3.69 [95 percent CI, 1.49–9.15]) with paternal cigarette smoking of 20 to 29 cigarettes per day when cases were compared with controls identified from the general practitioners of the cases.

Central Nervous System

Four of the nine studies that analyzed only CNS tumors found statistically significant associations with maternal secondhand smoke exposure during pregnancy ranging from 1.5 (p = 0.03) (Preston-Martin et al. 1982) to 2.2 (95 percent CI, 1.1–4.6, p for trend = 0.02) (Filippini et al. 1994). One study of multiple cancer outcomes found significant associations for neuroblastoma and CNS cancers with paternal smoking after combining three study populations from different time periods (Sorahan et al. 1997b).

Evidence Synthesis

The strongest evidence for any childhood cancer risk from maternal secondhand smoke exposure is specific to leukemias, lymphomas, and brain tumors, although the causal pathway may actually be through DNA damage to the father's sperm from active smoking rather than through maternal secondhand smoke exposure during pregnancy. Some of the epidemiologic studies suggest a slightly increased risk in childhood cancers from prenatal and postnatal secondhand smoke exposures, but most of the studies were small and did not have the power to detect statistically significant associations. In addition, most of the studies lacked exposure assessments for relevant exposure periods (preconception, prenatal, and postnatal), which may also have reduced the risk estimates because of nondifferential misclassification of exposure status. Risk estimates may be inflated by recall bias, especially since interviews to assess exposures took place up to 15 years after birth. Parents of children with cancer may be more likely to think about possible causes for their child's illness, thereby improving their recall of exposure experiences around the time of the pregnancy and birth. Parents of healthy children, however, have no particular reason to think about their exposure experiences and their recall may not be as good. Differential recall is a potential problem common to all case-control studies. If differential positive recall between cases and controls is present, it will inflate the risk estimate for childhood cancer.

Researchers have observed exposure-response trends for overall cancers as well as for leukemia, lymphoma, and brain tumors in a number of studies. Most of the studies adjusted for potentially confounding factors such as the child's date of birth, age at diagnosis, parental education level, parental age at child's birth, socioeconomic status, residence, and race by multivariate adjustment or case-control matching. Only four studies, however, considered other cancer risk factors such as maternal x-rays, drug use, and consumption of foods containing sodium nitrite (Preston-Martin et al. 1982; Howe et al. 1989; Kuijten et al. 1990; Bunin et al. 1994). Although active maternal smoking during pregnancy does not appear to be related to childhood cancer, it was not clear in some studies whether mothers who actively smoked were excluded from the various analyses that estimated risks from

---

[1]Pack-years = The number of years of smoking multiplied by the number of packs of cigarettes smoked per day.

Table 5.12   Case-control studies of childhood cancer by cancer type

Study	Population	Exposure period	Source of exposure
		All cancers combined	
John et al. 1991	Children aged 0–14 years, diagnosed in Denver between 1976 and 1983; controls were selected by random-digit dialing	1 year before birth	Father smoked
		1 year before birth	Father smoked Father smoked 1–10 cigarettes/day Father smoked 11–20 cigarettes/day Father smoked ≥21 cigarettes/day
Sorahan et al. 1995	Cancer deaths among children in England, Wales, and Scotland between 1977 and 1981; included less than 50% of population cancer cases	Prenatal	Father smoked <10 cigarettes/day Father smoked 10–19 cigarettes/day Father smoked 20–29 cigarettes/day Father smoked 30–39 cigarettes/day Father smoked ≥40 cigarettes/day
		Prenatal	Father smoked <10 years Father smoked 10–19 years Father smoked ≥20 years
		Prenatal	Father smoked <10 cigarettes/day Father smoked 10–19 cigarettes/day Father smoked 20–29 cigarettes/day Father smoked 30–39 cigarettes/day Father smoked ≥40 cigarettes/day
		Prenatal	Father smoked

Risk (95% CI*)	Maternal smoking status	Confounding	Comments
All cancers combined			
1.2 (0.8–2.1)	Nonsmokers	Matched for age, gender, and geographic area; adjusted for paternal education	None
1.3 (0.9–2.0) 1.9 (0.9–3.9) 1.3 (0.8–2.1) 1.0 (0.6–1.8)	Smokers and nonsmokers	Matched for age, gender, and geographic area; no adjustments	
1.20 (0.81–1.78) 1.24 (0.98–1.56) 1.26 (1.05–1.50) 1.35 (1.03–1.78) 1.47 (1.07–2.01), p trend <0.001	Smokers and nonsmokers	Matched for gender and date of birth; no adjustments	None
1.41 (1.16–1.72) 1.24 (1.04–1.47) 1.10 (0.81–1.50)	Smokers and nonsmokers	Matched for gender and date of birth; no adjustments	
1.23 (0.82–1.86) 1.17 (0.92–1.49) 1.24 (1.02–1.49) 1.30 (0.98–1.73) 1.39 (1.00–1.92), p trend = 0.003	Smokers and nonsmokers	Matched for gender, date of birth, and paternal alcohol consumption; adjusted for maternal smoking and alcohol consumption	
1.37 (1.12–1.68)	Nonsmokers	Matched for gender and date of birth; adjusted for alcohol consumption, SES†, and maternal age at child's birth	

Table 5.12   Continued

Study	Population	Exposure period	Source of exposure
		All cancers combined	
Ji et al. 1997	Children aged <15 years in Shanghai (China), diagnosed between 1985 and 1991; population-based controls were from household registry	NR[‡]	Father smoked <10 cigarettes/day Father smoked 10–14 cigarettes/day Father smoked ≥15 cigarettes/day
		NR	Father smoked <10 years Father smoke 10–14 years Father smoked ≥15 years

		Preconception	Father smoked <5 years:
			    <10 cigarettes/day
			    10–14 cigarettes/day
			    ≥15 cigarettes/day

		Preconception	Father smoked 5–9 years:
			    <10 cigarettes/day
			    10–14 cigarettes/day
			    ≥15 cigarettes/day

		Preconception	Father smoked ≥10 years:
			    <10 cigarettes/day
			    10–14 cigarettes/day
			    ≥15 cigarettes/day

		Preconception	Father smoked ≤2 pack-years[§] Father smoked >2 to <5 pack-years Father smoked ≥5 pack-years
		Postnatal	Father smoked ≤2 pack-years Father smoked >2 to <5 pack-years Father smoked ≥5 pack-years
		Preconception	Father smoked

Risk (95% CI)	Maternal smoking status	Confounding	Comments
All cancers combined			
1.5 (1.1–2.3) 1.1 (0.8–1.6) 1.5 (1.0–2.3), p trend = 0.07	Nonsmokers	For all analyses: Matched for gender and birth year; adjusted for: birth weight; income; and paternal age, education, and alcohol consumption	Data were not collected on paternal smoking during mother's pregnancy; interviews took place ≥10 years after pregnancy
1.2 (0.7–1.8) 1.1 (0.8–1.7) 1.7 (1.2–2.5), p trend = 0.007	Nonsmokers		
1.2 (0.7–2.1) 0.9 (0.5–1.9) 0.7 (0.2–2.9)	Nonsmokers		
1.2 (0.7–2.0) 1.2 (0.8–1.9) 2.4 (1.3–4.4)	Nonsmokers		
1.5 (0.9–2.5) 1.3 (0.8–2.3) 2.0 (1.2–3.4)	Nonsmokers		
1.2 (0.8–1.8) 1.3 (0.9–2.0) 1.7 (1.2–2.5), p trend = 0.006	Nonsmokers		
1.2 (0.9–1.7) 1.4 (1.0–2.0) 1.1 (0.8–1.7), p trend = 0.57	Nonsmokers		
Diagnosis at 0–4 years of age 1.8 (1.2–2.6) Diagnosis at 5–9 years of age 0.9 (0.5–1.5) Diagnosis at 10–14 years of age 1.9 (0.5–1.8)	Nonsmokers		

Table 5.12   Continued

Study	Population	Exposure period	Source of exposure
All cancers combined			
Sorahan et al. 1997a	Deaths of children in England, Wales, and Scotland between 1953 and 1955; included 79% of population cancer cases	Current	Father smoked 1–9 cigarettes/day Father smoked 10–20 cigarettes/day Father smoked >20 cigarettes/day
		Current	Father smoked
		Current	Father smoked
Sorahan et al. 1997b	Deaths of children in England, Wales, and Scotland between 1971 and 1976; included 51% of population cases	Current	Father smoked 1–9 cigarettes/day Father smoked 10–19 cigarettes/day Father smoked 20–29 cigarettes/day Father smoked 30–39 cigarettes/day Father smoked ≥40 cigarettes/day
		Current	Father smoked
		Current	Father smoked
Sorahan et al. 2001	Children aged <15 years in the United Kingdom, diagnosed between 1980 and 1983; hospital controls were acute surgical and accident patients; general practitioner controls were population based	Preconception	Father smoked <10 cigarettes/day Father smoked 10–19 cigarettes/day Father smoked 20–29 cigarettes/day Father smoked 30–39 cigarettes/day Father smoked ≥40 cigarettes/day
		Preconception	Father smoked (same as above)

Risk (95% CI)	Maternal smoking status	Confounding	Comments
All cancers combined				

Risk (95% CI)	Maternal smoking status	Confounding	Comments
1.03 (0.81–1.29) 1.31 (1.06–1.62) 1.42 (1.08–1.87), p trend <0.001	Smokers and nonsmokers	Matched for gender, date of birth, and residence; adjusted for SES, age of father and mother at child's birth, sibship position, obstetric radiography, and maternal smoking	Exposure assessment for current smoking only; time from birth to interviews was not reported
1.13 (1.05–1.23), p <0.01	Smokers and nonsmokers	Matched for gender, date of birth, and residence; adjusted for maternal smoking	
1.30 (1.10–1.53), p <0.01	Nonsmokers	Matched for gender, date of birth, and residence; adjusted for SES, age of father and mother at child's birth, sibship position, and obstetric radiography	
1.02 (0.78–1.34) 1.37 (1.13–1.65) 1.33 (1.13–1.55) 1.42 (1.09–1.84) 1.63 (1.23–2.15), p trend <0.001	Smokers and nonsmokers	Matched for gender, date of birth, and residence; adjusted for SES, age of father and mother at child's birth, sibship position, obstetric radiography, and maternal smoking	Exposure assessment for current smoking only; median time between birth and interviews for cases was 8.5 years, and 97% of cases were interviewed before the fourth anniversary of the child's death; nonsmokers included former smokers
1.29 (1.10–1.51), p <0.01	Nonsmokers	Matched for gender, date of birth, and residence; adjusted for SES, age of father and mother at child's birth, sibship position, and obstetric radiography	
1.09 (1.05–1.14), p <0.001	Smokers and nonsmokers	Matched for gender, date of birth, and residence; adjusted for maternal smoking	

General practitioner controls
  0.94 (0.53–1.66)
  1.63 (1.10–2.41)
  1.46 (1.05–2.03)
  0.95 (0.52–1.73)
  1.77 (0.94–3.34), p trend = 0.02
	Smokers and nonsmokers	No adjustments (nonsignificant in analysis: paternal age at child's birth, SES, and ethnic origin)	None

General practitioner controls p trend = 0.03 (risks were not reported)	Smokers and nonsmokers	Adjusted for maternal smoking	

Table 5.12   Continued

Study	Population	Exposure period	Source of exposure
		Acute lymphocytic leukemia	
Magnani et al. 1990	Pediatric hospital cases in Italy, diagnosed between 1974 and 1984 and still under observation (prevalent cases)	Preconception and prenatal (up to child's birth)	Father smoked Father smoked 1–15 cigarettes/day Father smoked ≥16 cigarettes/day
John et al. 1991	Children aged 0–14 years in Denver, diagnosed between 1976 and 1983; controls were selected by random-digit dialing	1 year before birth	Father smoked
		1 year before birth	Father smoked Father smoked 1–10 cigarettes/day Father smoked 11–20 cigarettes/day Father smoked ≥21 cigarettes/day
Sorahan et al. 1995	Deaths of children in England, Wales, and Scotland between 1977 and 1981; included less than 50% of population cancer cases	Prenatal	Father smoked
Shu et al. 1996	Cases aged ≤18 months, diagnosed between 1983 and 1988; identified through clinical trial registries in the United States, Canada, and Australia	1 month before conception	Father smoked
		Prenatal	Father smoked
		1 month before conception	Father smoked 1–10 cigarettes/day Father smoked 11–20 cigarettes/day Father smoked >20 cigarettes/day
Ji et al. 1997	Children aged <15 years in Shanghai (China), diagnosed between 1985 and 1991; population-based controls were from household registry	NR	Father smoked <10 cigarettes/day Father smoked 10–14 cigarettes/day Father smoked ≥15 cigarettes/day
		NR	Father smoked <10 years Father smoked 10–14 years Father smoked ≥15 years
		Preconception	Father smoked ≤2 pack-years Father smoked >2 to <5 pack-years Father smoked ≥5 pack-years
		Postnatal	Father smoked ≤2 pack-years Father smoked >2 to <5 pack-years Father smoked ≥5 pack-years
Sorahan et al. 1997a	Deaths among children in England, Wales, and Scotland between 1953 and 1955; included 79% of population cancer cases	Current	Father smoked

Risk (95% CI)	Maternal smoking status	Confounding	Comments
		Acute lymphocytic leukemia	
0.9 (0.6–1.5) 0.9 (0.5–1.6) 0.9 (0.6–1.5)	Smokers and nonsmokers	No adjustments (nonsignificant in analysis: years of smoking, age at smoking initiation, and cumulative cigarette smoking)	Findings did not differ when considering paternal smoking from birth to diagnosis or during the year before birth
1.4 (0.6–3.1)	Nonsmokers	Matched for age, gender, and geographic area; adjusted for father's education	None
1.9 (1.0–3.7) 2.6 (0.9–7.9) 1.6 (0.7–3.7) 1.6 (0.7–4.0)	Smokers and nonsmokers	Matched for age, gender, and geographic area; no adjustments	
1.16 (1.06–1.27)	Smokers and nonsmokers	Matched for gender and date of birth	Risk is for 1 level increase in daily amount of cigarettes smoked (e.g., 6 levels from nonsmokers to ≥40 cigarettes/day)
1.56 (1.03–2.36) 1.45 (0.95–2.19) 2.40 (1.00–5.72) 1.33 (0.79–2.34) 1.51 (0.82–2.77), p trend = 0.12	Smokers and nonsmokers Smokers and nonsmokers Smokers and nonsmokers	Matched for telephone area code and exchange number; adjusted for gender, paternal age and education, and maternal alcohol consumption during pregnancy	None
1.5 (0.7–3.9) 0.9 (0.4–1.5) 1.9 (0.8–4.6), p trend = 0.27 0.9 (0.3–2.3) 1.0 (0.5–2.2) 1.7 (0.8–3.7), p trend = 0.23 0.8 (0.2–2.5) 1.0 (0.4–2.7) 3.8 (1.3–12.3), p trend = 0.01 1.1 (0.4–2.8) 1.8 (0.6–5.2) 1.8 (0.6–5.5), p trend = 0.33	Nonsmokers Nonsmokers Nonsmokers Nonsmokers	For all analyses: Matched for gender and birth year; adjusted for: birth weight; income; and paternal age, education, and alcohol consumption	Data were not collected on paternal smoking during mother's pregnancy; interviews took place ≥10 years after pregnancy
1.08 (0.91–1.27)	Smokers and nonsmokers	Matched for gender, date of birth, and residence; adjusted for maternal smoking	Exposure assessment for current smoking only; time from birth to interviews was not reported; risk is for 1 level increase in daily amount of cigarettes smoked (e.g., 4 levels from <1 cigarette/day to >20 cigarettes/day)

Table 5.12 Continued

Study	Population	Exposure period	Source of exposure
— **Acute lymphocytic leukemia**			
Sorahan et al. 1997b	Deaths among children in England, Wales, and Scotland between 1971 and 1976; included 51% of population cancer cases	Current	Father smoked
Brondum et al. 1999	Children aged <15 years, diagnosed between 1989 and 1993; identified through clinical trial registries in the United States	Ever	Father smoked
		Ever	Father smoked
		1 month before conception and prenatal	Father smoked
		Father's lifetime	Father smoked <10 cigarettes/day Father smoked 10 to <20 cigarettes/day Father smoked ≥20 cigarettes/day
		Father's lifetime	Father smoked <10 years Father smoked 10 to <20 years Father smoked ≥20 years
Infante-Rivard et al. 2000	Children aged 0–9 years in Quebec (Canada), diagnosed between 1980 and 1993; identified from tertiary care centers for childhood cancers	Postnatal up to diagnosis	Father smoked 1–20 cigarettes/day Father smoked >20 cigarettes/day
Sorahan et al. 2001	Children aged <15 years in the United Kingdom, diagnosed between 1980 and 1983; hospital controls were acute surgical and accident patients; general practitioner controls were population based	Preconception	Father smoked <10 cigarettes/day Father smoked 10–19 cigarettes/day Father smoked 20–29 cigarettes/day Father smoked 30–39 cigarettes/day Father smoked ≥40 cigarettes/day
— **Lymphoma**			
Magnani et al. 1990	Non-Hodgkin's lymphoma cases admitted to a pediatric hospital in Italy, diagnosed between 1974 and 1984 and still under observation (prevalent cases)	Preconception and prenatal (up to child's birth)	Father smoked Father smoked 1–15 cigarettes/day Father smoked ≥16 cigarettes/day

Risk (95% CI)	Maternal smoking status	Confounding	Comments
Acute lymphocytic leukemia			
1.07 (0.99–1.16)	Smokers and nonsmokers	Matched for gender, date of birth, and residence; adjusted for maternal smoking	Exposure assessment for current smoking only; median time between birth and interviews for cases was 8.5 years, and 97% of cases were interviewed before the fourth anniversary of the child's death; nonsmokers included former smokers; risk is for 1 level increase in daily amount of cigarettes smoked (e.g., 6 levels from nonsmokers to ≥40 cigarettes/day)
1.04 (0.90–1.20)	Smokers and nonsmokers	Adjusted for income and paternal race and education	None
1.04 (0.86–1.26)	Nonsmokers	Adjusted for income and parental race and education	
1.07 (0.91–1.25)	Smokers and nonsmokers	Adjusted for income and paternal race and education	
1.16 (0.88–1.51) 1.04 (0.83–1.31) 1.06 (0.88–1.26), p trend = 0.56	Smokers and nonsmokers	Adjusted for income and paternal race and education	
1.12 (0.91–1.38) 1.22 (1.00–1.47) 0.91 (0.72–1.14), p trend = 0.79	Smokers and nonsmokers	Adjusted for income and paternal race and education	
1.0 (0.7–1.4) 1.0 (0.7–1.3)	Smokers and nonsmokers	Matched for age and gender; adjusted for maternal age and education	None
General practitioner controls: 0.99 (0.35–2.85) 1.34 (0.62–2.91) 1.32 (0.72–2.45) 2.33 (0.71–7.63) 5.29 (1.31–21.30), p trend = 0.06	Smokers and nonsmokers	No adjustments	None
Lymphoma			
6.7 (1.0–43.4) 6.4 (1.0–45.5) 5.6 (0.9–37.5)	Smokers and nonsmokers	No adjustments	None

Table 5.12   Continued

Study	Population	Exposure period	Source of exposure
		Lymphoma	
Sorahan et al. 1995	Deaths among children in England, Wales, and Scotland between 1977 and 1981; included less than 50% of population cancer cases	Prenatal	Father smoked
Ji et al. 1997	Children aged <15 years in Shanghai (China), diagnosed with lymphoma between 1985 and 1991; population-based controls were from household registry	NR	Father smoked <10 cigarettes/day Father smoked 10–14 cigarettes/day Father smoked ≥15 cigarettes/day
		NR	Father smoked <10 years Father smoke 10–14 years Father smoked ≥15 years
		Preconception	Father smoked ≤2 pack-years Father smoked >2 to <5 pack-years Father smoked ≥5 pack-years
		Postnatal	Father smoked ≤2 pack-years Father smoked >2 to <5 pack-years Father smoked ≥5 pack-years
Sorahan et al. 1997a	Deaths among children in England, Wales, and Scotland between 1953 and 1955; included 79% of population cancer cases	Current	Father smoked
Sorahan et al. 1997b	Deaths among children in England, Wales, and Scotland between 1971 and 1976; included 51% of population cancer cases	Current	Father smoked
Sorahan et al. 2001	Children aged <15 years in the United Kingdom, diagnosed with cancer (other reticuloendothelial system cancers) between 1980 and 1983; hospital controls were acute surgical and accident patients; general practitioner controls were population based	Preconception	Father smoked <10 cigarettes/day Father smoked 10–19 cigarettes/day Father smoked 20–29 cigarettes/day Father smoked 30–39 cigarettes/day Father smoked ≥40 cigarettes/day

Risk (95% CI)	Maternal smoking status	Confounding	Comments
		Lymphoma	
1.14 (0.99–1.31)	Smokers and nonsmokers	Matched for gender and date of birth	Risk is for 1 level increase in daily amount of cigarettes smoked (e.g., 6 levels from nonsmokers to ≥40 cigarettes/day)
3.4 (0.8–14.0) 1.1 (0.3–4.8) 3.8 (0.9–16.5), p trend = 0.09 1.3 (0.2–7.0) 3.4 (0.9–12.7) 3.5 (0.9–13.7), p trend = 0.05 3.1 (0.8–11.4) 1.8 (0.4–7.8) 4.5 (1.2–16.8), p trend = 0.07 3.9 (0.9–16.0) 2.7 (0.8–9.6) 5.0 (1.2–22.4), p trend = 0.08	Nonsmokers Nonsmokers Nonsmokers Nonsmokers	For all analyses: Matched for gender and birth year; adjusted for: birth weight; income; and paternal age, education, and alcohol consumption	Data were not collected on paternal smoking during mother's pregnancy; interviews took place ≥10 years after pregnancy
1.37 (1.02–1.83), p <0.05	Smokers and nonsmokers	Matched for gender, date of birth, and residence; adjusted for maternal smoking	Exposure assessment for current smoking only; time from birth to interviews was not reported; risk is for 1 level increase in daily amount of cigarettes smoked (e.g., 4 levels from <1 cigarette/day to >20 cigarettes/day)
1.07 (0.92–1.23)	Smokers and nonsmokers	Matched for gender, date of birth, and residence; adjusted for maternal smoking	Exposure assessment for current smoking only; median time between birth and interviews for cases was 8.5 years, and 97% of cases were interviewed before the fourth anniversary of the child's death; nonsmokers included former smokers; risk is for a 1 level increase in daily amount of cigarettes smoked (e.g., 6 levels from nonsmokers to ≥40 cigarettes/day)

General practitioner controls:
    1.32 (0.32–5.51)
    2.65 (0.83–8.46)
    3.69 (1.49–9.15)
    0.29 (0.03–2.56)
    1.20 (0.29–5.05), p trend = 0.35
	Smokers and nonsmokers	No adjustments	None

Table 5.12   Continued

Study	Population	Exposure period	Source of exposure
	Central nervous system (CNS) cancers		
Preston-Martin et al. 1982	Brain tumor cases aged <25 years, residents of Los Angeles County, diagnosed between 1972 and 1977; identified through the Los Angeles County Cancer Surveillance Program	Prenatal	Mother lived with a smoker
Howe et al. 1989	Brain tumor cases aged ≤19 years, diagnosed at two hospitals in Toronto between 1977 and 1983	Prenatal	Father smoked
Kuijten et al. 1990	Astrocytoma cases aged <15 years, diagnosed between 1980 and 1986; identified through tumor registries in 8 hospitals in Pennsylvania, New Jersey, and Delaware; controls were selected by random-digit dialing	Prenatal	Maternal exposure to secondhand smoke
Gold et al. 1993	Brain tumor cases aged <18 years, diagnosed between 1977 and 1981; identified through 8 SEER[a] Program registries	During the year of child's birth 2 years before child's birth	Father smoked <1 pack/day Father smoked ≥1 pack/day Father smoked <1 pack/day Father smoked ≥1 pack/day
Bunin et al. 1994	Astrocytoma cases aged <6 years, diagnosed between 1986 and 1989; identified through clinical trial registries in the United States	Prenatal Prenatal	Maternal exposure to secondhand smoke Father smoked
Filippini et al. 1994	Brain tumor cases aged ≤15 years, diagnosed between 1985 and 1988; identified through 8 hospitals in northern Italy	3 months before conception Before mother was aware of pregnancy After mother was aware of pregnancy	Father smoked ≤2 hours/day secondhand smoke exposure >2 hours/day secondhand smoke exposure ≤2 hours/day secondhand smoke exposure >2 hours/day secondhand smoke exposure
McCredie et al. 1994	Brain tumor cases aged <15 years in New South Wales (Australia), diagnosed between 1985 and 1989; identified through the New South Wales Central Cancer Registry	Preconception Prenatal	Father ever smoked Father smoked

Risk (95% CI)	Maternal smoking status	Confounding	Comments
Central nervous system (CNS) cancers			
1.5 (p = 0.03)	Smokers and nonsmokers	Matched for gender, race, and birth year (within 3 years)	None
1.13 (0.615–2.09)	Smokers and nonsmokers	Matched for gender; adjusted for age at diagnosis	None
0.8 (0.5–1.3)	Smokers and nonsmokers	Matched for age, race, and telephone area code and exchange	None
0.68 (0.39–1.19) 1.07 (0.79–1.45) 0.90 (0.53–1.51) 1.15 (0.85–1.56)	Smokers and nonsmokers	Matched for age, gender, and maternal race	None
0.9 (0.6–1.5) 1.0 (0.6–1.7)	Smokers and nonsmokers	Matched for race, birth year, and telephone area code and prefix; adjusted for income	None
1.3 (0.8–2.2) 1.5 (0.7–3.5) 1.7 (0.8–3.7), p trend = 0.08 1.7 (0.8–3.8) 2.2 (1.1–4.6), p trend = 0.02	Smokers and nonsmokers Nonsmokers Nonsmokers	For all analyses: Matched for birth date, gender, and area of residence; adjusted for paternal education	Mean age at diagnosis was 8.5 years, so interviews took place more than 8 years after birth
2.0 (1.0–4.1) 2.2 (1.2–3.8)	Nonsmokers Smokers and nonsmokers	Matched for age and gender; adjusted for paternal education	None

Table 5.12   Continued

Study	Population	Exposure period	Source of exposure
		Central nervous system (CNS) cancers	
Norman et al. 1996a	Brain tumor cases aged ≤19 years, diagnosed between 1984 and 1991; identified through 19 U.S. West Coast SEER Program registries	Prenatal	Father smoked
Sorahan et al. 1997a	CNS cancer deaths among children in England, Wales, and Scotland between 1953 and 1955; included 79% of population cancer cases	Current	Father smoked
Sorahan et al. 1997b	CNS cancer deaths among children in England, Wales, and Scotland between 1971 and 1976; included 51% of population cancer cases	Current	Father smoked
Filippini et al. 2000	CNS tumor cases aged ≤15 years in northern Italy, diagnosed between 1988 and 1993; cases were identified through hospital records	5 years before conception	Father smoked
		Before mother was aware of pregnancy	≤2 hours/day secondhand smoke >2 hours/day secondhand smoke
		After mother was aware of pregnancy	≤2 hours/day secondhand smoke >2 hours/day secondhand smoke
		Before mother was aware of pregnancy	Secondhand smoke
		After mother was aware of pregnancy	Secondhand smoke

*CI = Confidence interval.
†SES = Socioeconomic status.
‡NR = Data were not reported.
§Pack-years = The number of years of smoking multiplied by the number of packs of cigarettes smoked per day.
ΔSEER = Surveillance, Epidemiology, and End Results.

Risk (95% CI)	Maternal smoking status	Confounding	Comments
Central nervous system (CNS) cancers			
1.2 (0.9–1.5)	Nonsmokers	Adjusted for gender, age at diagnosis or selection as control participant, birth year of child, and maternal race	None

CNS cancers
    1.20 (0.96–1.51)
Neuroblastoma
    1.48 (1.09–2.02), p <0.05
	Smokers and nonsmokers	Matched for gender, date of birth, and residence; adjusted for maternal smoking	Exposure assessment for current smoking only; time from birth to interviews was not reported; risk is for 1 level increase in daily amount of cigarettes smoked (e.g., 4 levels from <1 cigarette/day to >20 cigarettes/day)

CNS cancers
    1.02 (0.93–1.11)
Neuroblastoma
    1.13 (0.99–1.29)
	Smokers and nonsmokers	Matched for gender, date of birth, and residence; adjusted for SES, age of father and mother at child's birth, sibship position, obstetric radiography, and maternal smoking	Exposure assessment for current smoking only; median time between birth and interviews for cases was 8.5 years, and 97% of cases were interviewed before the fourth anniversary of the child's death; nonsmokers included former smokers; risk is for 1 level increase in daily amount of cigarettes smoked (e.g., 6 levels from nonsmokers to ≥40 cigarettes/day)

1.2 (0.9–1.7)	Smokers and nonsmokers	Adjusted for age, gender, and residence	Time from birth to interviews was ≤20 years
1.7 (1.1–2.7) 1.8 (1.1–2.9)	Nonsmokers		
1.7 (1.1–2.6) 1.7 (1.1–2.6)	Nonsmokers		
Astroglial: 2.0 (1.2–3.4)	Nonsmokers		
Astroglial: 1.8 (1.1–3.0)	Nonsmokers		

paternal smoking. Thus, some of the elevated risks for cancer in their offspring from paternal smoking may have been compounded by the child's postnatal exposure to active maternal smoking.

Conclusions

1. The evidence is suggestive but not sufficient to infer a causal relationship between prenatal and postnatal exposure to secondhand smoke and childhood cancer.

2. The evidence is inadequate to infer the presence or absence of a causal relationship between maternal exposure to secondhand smoke during pregnancy and childhood cancer.

3. The evidence is inadequate to infer the presence or absence of a causal relationship between exposure to secondhand smoke during infancy and childhood cancer.

4. The evidence is suggestive but not sufficient to infer a causal relationship between prenatal and postnatal exposure to secondhand smoke and childhood leukemias.

5. The evidence is suggestive but not sufficient to infer a causal relationship between prenatal and postnatal exposure to secondhand smoke and childhood lymphomas.

6. The evidence is suggestive but not sufficient to infer a causal relationship between prenatal and postnatal exposure to secondhand smoke and childhood brain tumors.

7. The evidence is inadequate to infer the presence or absence of a causal relationship between prenatal and postnatal exposure to secondhand smoke and other childhood cancer types.

Implications

Childhood cancers are diverse in their characteristics and etiology. Although the evidence is inadequate for some sources and periods of exposure, there is some evidence indicative of associations of childhood cancer risk with secondhand smoke exposure. Further research is needed to provide a better understanding of the potential causal relationships between types of exposures to secondhand smoke and childhood cancer risks.

Conclusions

Fertility

1. The evidence is inadequate to infer the presence or absence of a causal relationship between maternal exposure to secondhand smoke and female fertility or fecundability. No data were found on paternal exposure to secondhand smoke and male fertility or fecundability.

Pregnancy (Spontaneous Abortion and Perinatal Death)

2. The evidence is inadequate to infer the presence or absence of a causal relationship between maternal exposure to secondhand smoke during pregnancy and spontaneous abortion.

Infant Deaths

3. The evidence is inadequate to infer the presence or absence of a causal relationship between exposure to secondhand smoke and neonatal mortality.

Sudden Infant Death Syndrome

4. The evidence is sufficient to infer a causal relationship between exposure to secondhand smoke and sudden infant death syndrome.

Preterm Delivery

5. The evidence is suggestive but not sufficient to infer a causal relationship between maternal exposure to secondhand smoke during pregnancy and preterm delivery.

Low Birth Weight

6. The evidence is sufficient to infer a causal relationship between maternal exposure to secondhand smoke during pregnancy and a small reduction in birth weight.

Congenital Malformations

7. The evidence is inadequate to infer the presence or absence of a causal relationship between exposure to secondhand smoke and congenital malformations.

Cognitive Development

8. The evidence is inadequate to infer the presence or absence of a causal relationship between exposure to secondhand smoke and cognitive functioning among children.

Behavioral Development

9. The evidence is inadequate to infer the presence or absence of a causal relationship between exposure to secondhand smoke and behavioral problems among children.

Height/Growth

10. The evidence is inadequate to infer the presence or absence of a causal relationship between exposure to secondhand smoke and children's height/growth.

Childhood Cancer

11. The evidence is suggestive but not sufficient to infer a causal relationship between prenatal and postnatal exposure to secondhand smoke and childhood cancer.

12. The evidence is inadequate to infer the presence or absence of a causal relationship between maternal exposure to secondhand smoke during pregnancy and childhood cancer.

13. The evidence is inadequate to infer the presence or absence of a causal relationship between exposure to secondhand smoke during infancy and childhood cancer.

14. The evidence is suggestive but not sufficient to infer a causal relationship between prenatal and postnatal exposure to secondhand smoke and childhood leukemias.

15. The evidence is suggestive but not sufficient to infer a causal relationship between prenatal and postnatal exposure to secondhand smoke and childhood lymphomas.

16. The evidence is suggestive but not sufficient to infer a causal relationship between prenatal and postnatal exposure to secondhand smoke and childhood brain tumors.

17. The evidence is inadequate to infer the presence or absence of a causal relationship between prenatal and postnatal exposure to secondhand smoke and other childhood cancer types.

Overall Implications

Because infant mortality for the United States is quite high compared with other industrialized countries, identifying strategies to reduce the number of infant deaths should receive high priority. The epidemiologic evidence for the association of secondhand smoke exposure and an increased risk of SIDS indicates that eliminating secondhand smoke exposures among newborns and young infants should be part of an overall strategy to reduce the high infant mortality rate in the United States.

The available evidence for five reproductive and childhood outcomes—childhood cancer, cognitive development, behaviors, LBW, and spontaneous abortion—calls for further research with improved methodologies. The methodologic challenges and issues that were discussed in relation to exposure assessment and reproductive outcomes might act as a guide for future research on these topics. There is a need for studies that examine exposure to secondhand smoke and childhood cancers to further evaluate the risks for specific cancer types. The evidence reviewed in this chapter points to germ-cell mutations among fathers who smoke as a possible pathway. Additional studies may be warranted that focus on childhood cancer and active paternal smoking, with improved controls for maternal secondhand smoke exposure and active smoking during pregnancy and the exposure of infants to secondhand smoke. For secondhand smoke and spontaneous abortions, studies using samples with adequate statistical power are needed. For all outcomes, investigations should include biochemical measures of exposures, and these measures should be used to determine the presence of dose-response relationships—determining dose-response relationships will greatly facilitate the assessment of causality.

References

Ahlborg G Jr, Bodin L. Tobacco smoke exposure and pregnancy outcome among working women: a prospective study at prenatal care centers in Orebro County, Sweden. *American Journal of Epidemiology* 1991;133(4):338–47.

Ahluwalia IB, Grummer-Strawn L, Scanlon KS. Exposure to environmental tobacco smoke and birth outcome: increased effects on pregnant women aged 30 years or older. *American Journal of Epidemiology* 1997;146(1):42–7.

Alm B, Milerad J, Wennergren G, Skjaerven R, Oyen N, Norvenius G, Daltveit AK, Helweg-Larsen K, Markestad T, Irgens LM. A case-control study of smoking and sudden infant death syndrome in the Scandinavian countries, 1992 to 1995: the Nordic Epidemiological SIDS Study. *Archives of Disease in Childhood* 1998;78(4):329–34.

American Academy of Pediatrics Task Force on Sudden Infant Death Syndrome. The changing concept of sudden infant death syndrome: diagnostic coding shifts, controversies regarding sleeping environment, and new variables to consider reducing risk. *Pediatrics* 2005;116(5):1245–55.

Anderson HR, Cook DG. Passive smoking and sudden infant death syndrome: review of the epidemiological evidence. *Thorax* 1997;52(11):1003–9.

Anderson KN, Anderson LE, Glanze WD, editors. *Mosby's Medical, Nursing, & Allied Health Dictionary.* 5th ed. St. Louis: Mosby-Year Book, 1998.

Andres RL, Day MC. Perinatal complications associated with maternal tobacco use. *Seminars in Neonatology* 2000;5(3):231–41.

Andresen BD, Ng KJ, Iams JD, Bianchine JR. Cotinine in amniotic fluids from passive smokers [letter]. *Lancet* 1982;1(8275):791–2.

Augood C, Duckitt K, Templeton AA. Smoking and female infertility: a systematic review and meta-analysis. *Human Reproduction* 1998;13(6):1532–9.

Baghurst PA, Tong SL, Woodward A, McMichael AJ. Effects of maternal smoking upon neuropsychological development in early childhood: importance of taking account of social and environmental factors. *Paediatric and Perinatal Epidemiology* 1992;6(4):403–15.

Baird DD, Wilcox AJ. Cigarette smoking associated with delayed conception. *Journal of the American Medical Association* 1985;253(20):2979–83.

Bauman KE, Flewelling RL, LaPrelle J. Parental cigarette smoking and cognitive performance of children. *Health Psychology* 1991;10(4):282–8.

Bauman KE, Koch GG, Fisher LA. Family cigarette smoking and test performance by adolescents. *Health Psychology* 1989;8(1):97–105.

Bergman AB, Wiesner LA. Relationship of passive cigarette-smoking to sudden infant death syndrome. *Pediatrics* 1976;58(5):665–8.

Blair PS, Fleming PJ, Bensley D, Smith I, Bacon C, Taylor E, Berry J, Golding J, Tripp J. Smoking and the sudden infant death syndrome: results from 1993–5 case-control study for confidential inquiry into stillbirths and deaths in infancy. *British Medical Journal* 1996;313(7051):195–8.

Boffetta P, Tredaniel J, Greco A. Risk of childhood cancer and adult lung cancer after childhood exposure to passive smoke: a meta-analysis. *Environmental Health Perspectives* 2000;108(1):73–82.

Bolumar F, Olsen J, Boldsen J. Smoking reduces fecundity: a European multicenter study on infertility and subfecundity. *American Journal of Epidemiology* 1996;143(6):578–87.

Borlee I, Bouckaert A, Lechat MF, Misson CB. Smoking patterns during and before pregnancy: weight, length and head circumference of progeny. *European Journal of Obstetrics, Gynecology, and Reproductive Biology* 1978;8(4):171–7.

Bottoms SF, Kuhnert BR, Kuhnert PM, Reese AL. Maternal passive smoking and fetal serum thiocyanate levels. *American Journal of Obstetrics and Gynecology* 1982;144(7):787–91.

Brondum J, Shu XO, Steinbuch M, Severson RK, Potter JD, Robison LL. Parental cigarette smoking and the risk of acute leukemia in children. *Cancer* 1999;85(6):1380–8.

Brooke H, Gibson A, Tappin D, Brown H. Case-control study of sudden infant death syndrome in Scotland, 1992–5. *British Medical Journal* 1997;314(7093):1516–20.

Brooke OG, Anderson HR, Bland JM, Peacock JL, Stewart CM. Effects on birth weight of smoking, alcohol, caffeine, socioeconomic factors, and psychosocial stress. *British Medical Journal* 1989;298(6676):795–801.

Bruner JP, Forouzan I. Smoking and buccally administered nicotine: acute effect on uterine and umbilical artery Doppler flow velocity waveforms. *Journal of Reproductive Medicine* 1991;36(6):435–40.

Bunin GR, Buckley JD, Boesel CP, Rorke LB, Meadows AT. Risk factors for astrocytic glioma and primitive neuroectodermal tumor of the brain in young children: a report from the Children's Cancer Group. *Cancer Epidemiology, Biomarkers & Prevention* 1994;3(3):197–204.

Byrd RS, Weitzman ML. Predictors of early grade retention among children in the United States. *Pediatrics* 1994;93(3):481–7.

California Environmental Protection Agency. *Health Effects of Exposure to Environmental Tobacco Smoke.* Sacramento (CA): California Environmental Protection Agency, Office of Environmental Health Hazard Assessment, Reproductive and Cancer Hazard Assessment Section and Air Toxicology and Epidemiology Section, 1997.

California Environmental Protection Agency. *Proposed Identification of Environmental Tobacco Smoke as a Toxic Air Contaminant. Part B: Health Effects.* Sacramento (CA): California Environmental Protection Agency, Office of Environmental Health Hazard Assessment, 2005.

Cameron P, Kostin JS, Zaks JM, Wolfe JH, Tighe G, Oselett B, Stocker R, Winton J. The health of smokers' and nonsmokers' children. *Journal of Allergy* 1969;43(6):336–41.

Campbell MJ, Lewry J, Wailoo M. Further evidence for the effect of passive smoking on neonates. *Postgraduate Medical Journal* 1988;64(755):663–5.

Carpenter RG, Irgens LM, Blair PS, England PD, Fleming P, Huber J, Jorch G, Schreuder P. Sudden unexplained infant death in 20 regions in Europe: case control study. *Lancet* 2004;363(9409):185–191.

Chamberlain R. Birthweight and length of gestation. In: Chamberlain R, Chamberlain G, Howlett B, Claireaux A, editors. *British Births 1970: A Survey Under the Joint Auspices of the National Birthday Trust Fund and the Royal College of Obstetricians and Gynaecologists, Volume 1: The First Week of Life.* London: William Heinemann Medical Books, 1975:48–88.

Chen LH, Petitti DB. Case-control study of passive smoking and the risk of small-for-gestational-age at term. *American Journal of Epidemiology* 1995;142(2):158–65.

Chen Y, Pederson LL, Lefcoe NM. Passive smoking and low birthweight. *Lancet* 1989;2(8653):54–5.

Chinn S, Rona RJ. Quantifying health aspects of passive smoking in British children aged 5–11 years. *Journal of Epidemiology and Community Health* 1991;45(3):188–94.

Chung PH, Yeko TR, Mayer JC, Clark B, Welden SW, Maroulis GB. Gamete intrafallopian transfer: does smoking play a role? *Journal of Reproductive Medicine* 1997;42(2):65–70.

Cnattingius S. Antenatal screening for small-for-gestational-age, using risk factors and measurements of the symphysis-fundus distance—6 years of experience. *Early Human Development* 1988; 18(2–3):191–7.

Coghlin J, Gann PH, Hammond SK, Skipper PL, Taghizadeh K, Paul M, Tannenbaum SR. 4-Aminobiphenyl hemoglobin adducts in fetuses exposed to the tobacco smoke carcinogen in utero. *Journal of the National Cancer Institute* 1991;83(4):274–80.

Çolak Ö, Alatas Ö, Aydoğdu S, Uslu S. The effect of smoking on bone metabolism: maternal and cord blood bone marker levels. *Clinical Biochemistry* 2002;35(3):247–50.

Coleman S, Piotrow PT, Rinehart W. Tobacco—hazards to health and human reproduction. *Population Reports Series L, Issues in World Health* 1979;(1): L1–L37.

Colley JRT. Respiratory symptoms in children and parental smoking and phlegm production. *British Medical Journal* 1974;2(912):201–4.

Colley JR, Holland WW, Corkhill RT. Influence of passive smoking and parental phlegm on pneumonia and bronchitis in early childhood. *Lancet* 1974;2(7888):1031–4.

Comstock GW, Lundin FE Jr. Parental smoking and perinatal mortality. *American Journal of Obstetrics and Gynecology* 1967;98(5):708–18.

Crawford FG, Mayer J, Santella RM, Cooper TB, Ottman R, Tsai WY, Simon-Cereijido G, Wang M, Tang D, Perera FP. Biomarkers of environmental tobacco smoke in preschool children and their mothers. *Journal of the National Cancer Institute* 1994;86(18):1398–402.

Daling J, Weiss N, Spadoni L, Moore DE, Voigt L. Cigarette smoking and primary tubal infertility. In: Rosenberg MJ, editor. *Smoking and Reproductive Health.* Littleton (MA): PSG Publishing Company, 1987:40–6.

Davis DL. Paternal smoking and fetal health [letter]. *Lancet* 1991;337(8733):123.

de Mouzon J, Spira A, Schwartz D. A prospective study of the relation between smoking and fertility. *International Journal of Epidemiology* 1988;17(2): 378–84.

Dejin-Karlsson E, Hanson BS, Ostergren PO, Sjoberg NO, Marsal K. Does passive smoking in early pregnancy increase the risk of small-for-gestational-age infants? *American Journal of Public Health* 1998;88(10):1523–7.

Dempsey D, Jacob P III, Benowitz NL. Nicotine metabolism and elimination kinetics in newborns. *Clinical Pharmacology and Therapeutics* 2000;67(5):458–65.

Dollberg S, Fainaru O, Mimouni FB, Shenhav M, Lessing JB, Kupferminc M. Effect of passive smoking in pregnancy on neonatal nucleated red blood cells. *Pediatrics* 2000;106(3):E34.

Dunphy BC, Barratt CL, von Tongelen BP, Cooke ID. Male cigarette smoking and fecundity in couples attending an infertility clinic. *Andrologia* 1991;23(3):223–5.

Dwyer T, Ponsonby AL, Couper D. Tobacco smoke exposure at one month of age and subsequent risk of SIDS—a prospective study. *American Journal of Epidemiology* 1999;149(7):593–602.

Elenbogen A, Lipitz S, Mashiach S, Dor J, Levran D, Ben-Rafael Z. The effect of smoking on the outcome of in-vitro fertilization—embryo transfer. *Human Reproduction* 1991;6(2):242–4.

Emmons KM, Abrams DB, Marshall R, Marcus BH, Kane M, Novotny TE, Etzel RA. An evaluation of the relationship between self-report and biochemical measures of environmental tobacco smoke exposure. *Preventive Medicine* 1994;23(1):35–9.

Ernst M, Moolchan ET, Robinson ML. Behavioral and neural consequences of prenatal exposure to nicotine. *Journal of the American Academy of Child and Adolescent Psychiatry* 2001;40(6):630–41.

Eskenazi B, Bergmann JJ. Passive and active maternal smoking during pregnancy, as measured by serum cotinine, and postnatal smoke exposure: I. Effects on physical growth at age 5 years. *American Journal of Epidemiology* 1995;142(9 Suppl):S10–S18.

Eskenazi B, Gold EB, Lasley BL, Samuels SJ, Hammond SK, Wight S, O'Neill Rasor M, Hines CJ, Schenker MB. Prospective monitoring of early fetal loss and clinical spontaneous abortion among female semiconductor workers. *American Journal of Industrial Medicine* 1995;28(6):833–46.

Everson RB, Randerath E, Santella RM, Avitts TA, Weinstein IB, Randerath K. Quantitative associations between DNA damage in human placenta and maternal smoking and birth weight. *Journal of the National Cancer Institute* 1988;80(8):567–76.

Everson RB, Randerath E, Santella RM, Cefalo RC, Avitts TA, Randerath K. Detection of smoking-related covalent DNA adducts in human placenta. *Science* 1986;231(4733):54–7.

Fergusson DM, Horwood LJ, Lynskey MT. Maternal smoking before and after pregnancy: effects on behavioral outcomes in middle childhood. *Pediatrics* 1993;92(6):815–22.

Filippini G, Farinotti M, Ferrarini M. Active and passive smoking during pregnancy and risk of central nervous system tumours in children. *Paediatric and Perinatal Epidemiology* 2000;14(1):78–84.

Filippini G, Farinotti M, Lovicu G, Maisonneuve P, Boyle P. Mothers' active and passive smoking during pregnancy and risk of brain tumours in children. *International Journal of Cancer* 1994;57(6):769–74.

Finette BA, O'Neill JP, Vacek PM, Albertini RJ. Gene mutations with characteristic deletions in cord blood T lymphocytes associated with passive maternal exposure to tobacco smoke. *Nature Medicine* 1998;4(10):1144–51.

Fortier I, Marcoux S, Brisson J. Passive smoking during pregnancy and the risk of delivering a small-for-gestational-age infant. *American Journal of Epidemiology* 1994;139(3):294–301.

Fraga CG, Motchnik PA, Wyrobek AJ, Rempel DM, Ames BN. Smoking and low antioxidant levels increase oxidative damage to sperm DNA. *Mutation Research* 1996;351(2):199–203.

Fried PA, Watkinson B, Gray R. Differential effects on cognitive functioning in 9- to 12-year olds prenatally exposed to cigarettes and marihuana. *Neurotoxicology and Teratology* 1998;20(3):293–306.

Fried PA, Watkinson B, Siegel LS. Reading and language in 9- to 12-year olds prenatally exposed to cigarettes and marijuana. *Neurotoxicology and Teratology* 1997;19(3):171–83.

Gibson E, Dembofsky CA, Rubin S, Greenspan JS. Infant sleep position practices 2 years into the "Back to Sleep" campaign. *Clinical Pediatrics* 2000;39(5):285–9.

Gold EB, Leviton A, Lopez R, Gilles FH, Hedley-Whyte ET, Kolonel LN, Lyon JL, Swanson GM, Weiss NS, West D. Parental smoking and risk of childhood brain tumors. *American Journal of Epidemiology* 1993;137(6):620–8.

Goldman LR. Children—unique and vulnerable: environmental risks facing children and recommendations for response. *Environmental Health Perspectives* 1995;103(Suppl 6):13–8.

Gospe SM Jr, Zhou SS, Pinkerton KE. Effects of environmental tobacco smoke exposure in utero and/or postnatally on brain development. *Pediatric Research* 1996;39(3):494–8.

Greenberg RA, Haley NJ, Etzel RA, Loda FA. Measuring the exposure of infants to tobacco smoke: nicotine and cotinine in urine and saliva. *New England Journal of Medicine* 1984;310(17):1075–8.

Grufferman S, Wang HH, DeLong ER, Kimm SY, Delzell ES, Falletta JM. Environmental factors in the etiology of rhabdomyosarcoma in childhood. *Journal of the National Cancer Institute* 1982;68(1):107–13.

Gruslin A, Perkins SL, Manchanda R, Fleming N, Clinch JJ. Maternal smoking and fetal erythropoietin levels. *Obstetrics and Gynecology* 2000;95(4):561–4.

Haddow JE, Knight GJ, Palomaki GE, McCarthy JE. Second-trimester serum cotinine levels in nonsmokers in relation to birth weight. *American Journal of Obstetrics and Gynecology* 1988;159(2):481–4.

Hammond SK. Exposure of U.S. workers to environmental tobacco smoke. *Environmental Health Perspectives* 1999;107(Suppl 2):329–40.

Hanke W, Kalinka J, Florek E, Sobala W. Passive smoking and pregnancy outcome in central Poland. *Human & Experimental Toxicology* 1999;18(4):265–71.

Hansen C, Sorensen LD, Asmussen I, Autrup H. Transplacental exposure to tobacco smoke in human-adduct formation in placenta and umbilical cord blood vessels. *Teratogenesis, Carcinogenesis, and Mutagenesis* 1992;12(2):51–60.

Harger JH, Hsing AW, Tuomala RE, Gibbs RS, Mead PB, Eschenbach DA, Knox GE, Polk BF. Risk factors for preterm premature rupture of fetal membranes: a multicenter case-control study. *American Journal of Obstetrics and Gynecology* 1990;163(1 Pt 1):130–7.

Haug K, Irgens LM, Skjaerven R, Markestad T, Baste V, Schreuder P. Maternal smoking and birthweight: effect modification of period, maternal age and paternal smoking. *Acta Obstetricia et Gynecologica Scandinavica* 2000;79(6):485–9.

Hauth JC, Hauth J, Drawbaugh RB, Gilstrap LC 3rd, Pierson WP. Passive smoking and thiocyanate concentrations in pregnant women and newborns. *Obstetrics and Gynecology* 1984;63(4):519–22.

Holmberg PC, Nurminen M. Congenital defects of the central nervous system and occupational factors during pregnancy: a case-referent study. *American Journal of Industrial Medicine* 1980;1(2):167–76.

Howe GR, Burch JD, Chiarelli AM, Risch HA, Choi BC. An exploratory case-control study of brain tumors in children. *Cancer Research* 1989;49(15):4349–52.

Hughes EG, Brennan BG. Does cigarette smoking impair natural or assisted fecundity? *Fertility and Sterility* 1996;66(5):679–89.

Hughes EG, YoungLai EV, Ward SM. Cigarette smoking and outcomes of in-vitro fertilization and embryo transfer: a prospective cohort study. *Human Reproduction* 1992;7(3):358–61.

Hull MG, North K, Taylor H, Farrow A, Ford WC. Delayed conception and active and passive smoking. *Fertility and Sterility* 2000;74(4):725–33.

Hwang SJ, Beaty TH, Panny SR, Street NA, Joseph JM, Gordon S, McIntosh I, Francomano CA. Association study of transforming growth factor alpha (TGF alpha) TaqI polymorphism and oral clefts: indication of gene-environment interaction in a population-based sample of infants with birth defects. *American Journal of Epidemiology* 1995;141(7):629–36.

Infante-Rivard C, Krajinovic M, Labuda D, Sinnett D. Parental smoking, CYP1A1 genetic polymorphisms and childhood leukemia (Quebec, Canada). *Cancer Causes and Control* 2000;11(6):547–53.

International Agency for Research on Cancer. *IARC Monographs on the Evaluation of Carcinogenic Risks to Humans: Tobacco Smoke and Involuntary Smoking.* Vol. 83. Lyon (France): International Agency for Research on Cancer, 2004.

Jaakkola JJ, Jaakkola N, Zahlsen K. Fetal growth and length of gestation in relation to prenatal exposure to environmental tobacco smoke assessed by hair nicotine concentration. *Environmental Health Perspectives* 2001;109(6):557–61.

Jazayeri A, Tsibris JC, Spellacy WN. Umbilical cord plasma erythropoietin levels in pregnancies complicated by maternal smoking. *American Journal of Obstetrics and Gynecology* 1998;178(3):433–5.

Jedrychowski W, Flak E. Impact of active and passive smoking during pregnancy on birth weight of the newborn [Polish]. *Polski Merkuriusz Lekarski* 1996;1(6):379–82.

Ji BT, Shu XO, Linet MS, Zheng W, Wacholder S, Gao YT, Ying DM, Jin F. Paternal cigarette smoking and the risk of childhood cancer among offspring of nonsmoking mothers. *Journal of the National Cancer Institute* 1997;89(3):238–44.

Joad JP. Smoking and pediatric respiratory health. *Clinics in Chest Medicine* 2000;21(1):37–46, vii–viii.

John EM, Savitz DA, Sandler DP. Prenatal exposure to parents' smoking and childhood cancer. *American Journal of Epidemiology* 1991;133(2):123–32.

Karakostov P. Passive smoking among pregnant women and its effect on the weight and growth of the newborn infant [Bulgarian]. *Akusherstvo i Ginekologiia* 1985;24(2):28–31.

Kaufman FL, Kharrazi M, Delorenze GN, Eskenazi B, Bernert JT. Estimation of environmental tobacco smoke exposure during pregnancy using a single question on household smokers versus serum cotinine. *Journal of Exposure Analysis and Environmental Epidemiology* 2002;12(4):286–95.

Klonoff-Cohen HS, Edelstein SL, Lefkowitz ES, Srinivasan IP, Kaegi D, Chang JC, Wiley KJ. The effect of passive smoking and tobacco exposure through breast milk on sudden infant death syndrome. *Journal of the American Medical Association* 1995;273(10):795–8.

Knorr K. The effect of tobacco and alcohol on pregnancy course and child development [German]. *Bulletin der Schweizerischen Akademie der Medizinischen Wissenschaften* 1979;35(1–3):137–46.

Koo LC, Ho JH, Rylander R. Life-history correlates of environmental tobacco smoke: a study on nonsmoking Hong Kong Chinese wives with smoking versus nonsmoking husbands. *Social Science and Medicine* 1988;26(7):751–60.

Kuijten RR, Bunin GR, Nass CC, Meadows AT. Gestational and familial risk factors for childhood astrocytoma: results of a case-control study. *Cancer Research* 1990;50(9):2608–12.

Lahr MB, Rosenberg KD, Lapidus JA. Bedsharing and maternal smoking in a population-based survey of new mothers. *Pediatrics* 2005;116(4):e530–e542.

Lambers DS, Clark KE. The maternal and fetal physiologic effects of nicotine. *Seminars in Perinatology* 1996;20(2):115–26.

Lammer EJ, Shaw GM, Iovannisci DM, Van Waes J, Finnell RH. Maternal smoking and the risk of orofacial clefts: susceptibility with *NAT1* and *NAT2* polymorphisms. *Epidemiology* 2004;15(2):150–6.

Laurent SL, Thompson SJ, Addy C, Garrison CZ, Moore EE. An epidemiologic study of smoking and primary infertility in women. *Fertility and Sterility* 1992;57(3):565–72.

Lazzaroni F, Bonassi S, Manniello E, Morcaldi L, Repetto E, Ruocco A, Calvi A, Cotellessa G. Effect of passive smoking during pregnancy on selected perinatal parameters. *International Journal of Epidemiology* 1990;19(4):960–6.

Li CQ, Windsor RA, Perkins L, Goldenberg RL, Lowe JB. The impact on infant birth weight and gestational age of cotinine-validated smoking reduction during pregnancy. *Journal of the American Medical Association* 1993;269(12):1519–24.

Lin RX. Maternal, medical and obstetric complications are major risk factors for low birth weight infant [Chinese]. *Chinese Journal of Obstetrics and Gynecology* 1993;28(1):24–6.

Lindbohm ML, Sallmen M, Anttila A, Taskinen H, Hemminki K. Paternal occupational lead exposure and spontaneous abortion. *Scandinavian Journal of Work, Environment and Health* 1991;17(2):95–103.

Lindbohm ML, Sallmen M, Taskinen H. Effects of exposure to environmental tobacco smoke on reproductive health. *Scandinavian Journal of Work, Environment and Health* 2002;28(Suppl 2):84–96.

Little J, Cardy A, Arslan MT, Gilmour M, Mossey PA. Smoking and orofacial clefts: a United Kingdom-based case-control study. *The Cleft Palate-Craniofacial Journal* 2004a;41(4):381–6.

Little J, Cardy A, Munger RG. Tobacco smoking and oral clefts: a meta-analysis. *Bulletin of the World Health Organization* 2004b;82(3):213–8.

Longo FJ, Anderson E. The effects of nicotine on fertilization in the sea urchin, *Arbacia punctulata*. *Journal of Cell Biology* 1970;46(2):308–25.

Luciano A, Bolognani M, Biondani P, Ghizzi C, Zoppi G, Signori E. The influence of maternal passive and light active smoking on intrauterine growth and body composition of the newborn. *European Journal of Clinical Nutrition* 1998;52(10):760–3.

MacArthur C, Knox EG. Passive smoking and birthweight. *Lancet* 1987;1(8523):37–8.

Machaalani R, Waters KA, Tinworth KD. Effects of postnatal nicotine exposure on apoptotic markers in the developing piglet brain. *Neuroscience* 2005;132(2):325–33.

MacMahon B, Alpert M, Salber EJ. Infant weight and parental smoking habits. *American Journal of Epidemiology* 1965;82(3):247–61.

Magnani C, Pastore G, Luzzatto L, Carli M, Lubrano P, Terracini B. Risk factors for soft tissue sarcomas in childhood: a case-control study. *Tumori* 1989;75(4):396–400.

Magnani C, Pastore G, Luzzatto L, Terracini B. Parental occupation and other environmental factors in the etiology of leukemias and non-Hodgkin's lymphomas in childhood: a case-control study. *Tumori* 1990;76(5):413–9.

Magnus P, Berg K, Bjerkedal T, Nance WE. Parental determinants of birth weight. *Clinical Genetics* 1984;26(5):397–405.

Maier RF, Bohme K, Dudenhausen JW, Obladen M. Cord blood erythropoietin in relation to different markers of fetal hypoxia. *Obstetrics and Gynecology* 1993;81(4):575–80.

Mainous AG 3rd, Hueston WJ. Passive smoke and low birth weight: evidence of a threshold effect. *Archives of Family Medicine* 1994a;3(10):875–8.

Mainous AG 3rd, Hueston WJ. The effect of smoking cessation during pregnancy on preterm delivery and low birthweight. *Journal of Family Practice* 1994b;38(3):262–6.

Makin J, Fried PA, Watkinson B. A comparison of active and passive smoking during pregnancy: long-term effects. *Neurotoxicology and Teratology* 1991;13(1):5–12.

Malloy MH. Trends in postneonatal aspiration deaths and reclassification of sudden infant death syndrome: impact of the "Back to Sleep" program. *Pediatrics* 2002;109(4):661–5.

Malloy MH, Freeman DH. Age at death, season, and day of death as indicators of the effect of the Back to Sleep program on sudden infant death syndrome in the United States, 1992–1999. *Archives of Pediatrics and Adolescent Medicine* 2004;158(4):359–65.

Malloy MH, Kleinman JC, Land GH, Schramm WF. The association of maternal smoking with age and cause of infant death. *American Journal of Epidemiology* 1988;128(1):46–55.

Manchester DK, Jacoby EH. Sensitivity of human placental monooxygenase activity to maternal smoking. *Clinical Pharmacology and Therapeutics* 1981;30(5):687–92.

Marcus BH, Emmons KM, Abrams DB, Marshall RJ, Kane M, Novotny TE, Etzel RA. Restrictive workplace smoking policies: impact on nonsmokers' tobacco exposure. *Journal of Public Health Policy* 1992;13(1):42–51.

Martin JA, Hamilton BE, Sutton PD, Ventura SJ, Menacker F, Munson ML. Births: final data for 2003. *National Vital Statistics Reports* 2005;54(2):1–116.

Martin TR, Bracken MB. Association of low birth weight with passive smoke exposure in pregnancy. *American Journal of Epidemiology* 1986;124(4):633–42.

Martinez FD, Wright AL, Taussig LM. The effect of paternal smoking on the birthweight of newborns whose mothers did not smoke. *American Journal of Public Health* 1994;84(9):1489–91.

Mathai M, Skinner A, Lawton K, Weindling AM. Maternal smoking, urinary cotinine levels and birth-weight. *Australian and New Zealand Journal of Obstetrics and Gynaecology* 1990;30(1):33–6.

Mathai M, Vijayasri R, Babu S, Jeyaseelan L. Passive maternal smoking and birthweight in a south Indian population. *British Journal of Obstetrics and Gynaecology* 1992;99(4):342–3.

Mathews TJ, Menacker F, MacDorman MF. Infant mortality statistics from the 2002 period: linked birth/infant death data set. *National Vital Statistics Reports* 2004;53(10):1–32.

Matsubara F, Kida M, Tamakoshi A, Wakai K, Kawamura T, Ohno Y. Maternal active and passive smoking and fetal growth: a prospective study in Nagoya, Japan. *Journal of Epidemiology* 2000; 10(5):335–43.

Mattison DR. The effects of smoking on fertility from gametogenesis to implantation. *Environmental Research* 1982;28(2):410–33.

Mattison DR, Plowchalk DR, Meadows MJ, Miller MM, Malek A, London S. The effect of smoking on oogenesis, fertilization, and implantation. *Seminars in Reproductive Endocrinology* 1989;7(4):291–304.

Mattison DR, Thomford PJ. The effect of smoking on reproductive ability and reproductive lifespan. In: Rosenberg MJ, editor. *Smoking and Reproductive Health.* Littleton (MA): PSG Publishing Company, 1987:47–54.

Mau G, Netter P. The effects of paternal cigarette smoking on perinatal mortality and the incidence of malformations (author's translation). *Deutsche Medizinische Wochenschrift* 1974;99(21):1113–8.

McCann MF, Irwin DE, Walton LA, Hulka BS, Morton JL, Axelrad CM. Nicotine and cotinine in the cervical mucus of smokers, passive smokers, and nonsmokers. *Cancer Epidemiology, Biomarkers & Prevention* 1992;1(2):125–9.

McCartney JS, Fried PA, Watkinson B. Central auditory processing in school-age children prenatally exposed to cigarette smoke. *Neurotoxicology and Teratology* 1994;16(3):269–76.

McCredie M, Maisonneuve P, Boyle P. Antenatal risk factors for malignant brain tumours in New South Wales children. *International Journal of Cancer* 1994;56(1):6–10.

McGlashan ND. Sudden infant deaths in Tasmania, 1980–1986: a seven year prospective study. *Social Science and Medicine* 1989;29(8):1015–26.

McMartin KI, Platt MS, Hackman R, Klein J, Smialek JE, Vigorito R, Koren G. Lung tissue concentrations of nicotine in sudden infant death syndrome (SIDS). *Journal of Pediatrics* 2002;140(2):205–9.

Meyer KA, Williams P, Hernandez-Diaz S, Cnattingius S. Smoking and the risk of oral clefts: exploring the impact of study designs. *Epidemiology* 2004;15(6):671–8.

Milerad J, Vege A, Opdal SH, Rognum TO. Objective measurements of nicotine exposure in victims of sudden infant death syndrome and in other unexpected child deaths. *Journal of Pediatrics* 1998;133(2):232–6.

Misra DP, Nguyen RH. Environmental tobacco smoke and low birth weight: a hazard in the workplace?

Environmental Health Perspectives 1999;107(Suppl 6): 897–904.

Mitchell EA, Ford RP, Stewart AW, Taylor BJ, Becroft DM, Thompson JM, Scragg R, Hassall IB, Barry DM, Allen EM. Smoking and the sudden infant death syndrome. *Pediatrics* 1993;91(5):893–6.

Mitchell EA, Scragg R, Stewart AW, Becroft DM, Taylor BJ, Ford RP, Hassall IB, Barry DM, Allen EM, Roberts AP. Results from the first year of the New Zealand cot death study. *New Zealand Medical Journal* 1991;104(906):71–6.

Mitchell EA, Tuohy PG, Brunt JM, Thompson JM, Clements MS, Stewart AW, Ford RP, Taylor BJ. Risk factors for sudden infant death syndrome following the prevention campaign in New Zealand: a prospective study. *Pediatrics* 1997;100(5):835–40.

Mohr U, Reznik-Schuller H, Reznik G, Hilfrich J. Transplacental effects of diethylnitrosamine in Syrian hamsters as related to different days of administration during pregnancy. *Journal of the National Cancer Institute* 1975;55(3):681–3.

Naeye RL. Abruptio placentae and placenta previa: frequency, perinatal mortality, and cigarette smoking. *Obstetrics and Gynecology* 1980;55(6):701–4.

Nafstad P, Fugelseth D, Qvigstad E, Zahlen K, Magnus P, Lindemann R. Nicotine concentration in the hair of nonsmoking mothers and size of offspring. *American Journal of Public Health* 1998;88(1):120–4.

Napalkov NP. Some general considerations on the problem of transplacental carcinogenesis. In: Tomatis L, Mohr U, Davis W, editors. *Transplacental Carcinogenesis*. IARC Scientific Publications No. 4. Lyon (France): International Agency for Research on Cancer, 1973:1–13.

Napalkov NP, Rice JM, Tomatis L, Yamasaki H, editors. *Perinatal and Multigeneration Carcinogenesis*. IARC Scientific Publications No. 96. Lyon (France): International Agency for Research on Cancer, 1989.

National Cancer Institute. *Health Effects of Exposure to Environmental Tobacco Smoke: The Report of the California Environmental Protection Agency*. Smoking and Tobacco Control Monograph No. 10. Bethesda (MD): U.S. Department of Health and Human Services, National Institutes of Health, National Cancer Institute, 1999. NIH Pub. No. 99-4645.

Nebert DW, Winker J, Gelboin HV. Aryl hydrocarbon hydroxylase activity in human placenta from cigarette smoking and nonsmoking women. *Cancer Research* 1969;29(10):1763–9.

Neri A, Marcus SL. Effect of nicotine on the motility of the oviducts in the rhesus monkey: a pre-liminary report. *Journal of Reproduction and Fertility* 1972;31(1):91–7.

Nicholl J, O'Cathain A. Antenatal smoking, postnatal passive smoking, and sudden infant death syndrome. In: Poswillo D, Alberman E, editors. *Effects of Smoking on the Fetus, Neonate, and Child*. New York: Oxford University Press, 1992:138–49.

Nicolov IG, Chernozemsky IN. Tumors and hyperplastic lesions in Syrian hamsters following transplacental and neonatal treatment with cigarette smoke condensate. *Journal of Cancer Research and Clinical Oncology* 1979;94(3):249–56.

Norman MA, Holly EA, Ahn DK, Preston-Martin S, Mueller BA, Bracci PM. Prenatal exposure to tobacco smoke and childhood brain tumors: results from the United States West Coast childhood brain tumor study. *Cancer Epidemiology, Biomarkers & Prevention* 1996a;5(2):127–33.

Norman MA, Holly EA, Preston-Martin S. Childhood brain tumors and exposure to tobacco smoke. *Cancer Epidemiology, Biomarkers & Prevention* 1996b; 5(2):85–91.

Ogawa H, Tominaga S, Hori K, Noguchi K, Kanou I, Matsubara M. Passive smoking by pregnant women and fetal growth. *Journal of Epidemiology and Community Health* 1991;45(2):164–8.

Olds DL, Henderson CR Jr, Tatelbaum R. Intellectual impairment in children of women who smoke cigarettes during pregnancy. *Pediatrics* 1994;93(2): 221–7.

Olsen J. Cigarette smoking, tea and coffee drinking, and subfecundity. *American Journal of Epidemiology* 1991;133(7):734–9.

Ownby DR, Johnson CC, Peterson EL. Passive cigarette smoke exposure in infants: importance of nonparental sources. *Archives of Pediatrics and Adolescent Medicine* 2000;154(12):1237–41.

Pacifici R, Altieri I, Gandini L, Lenzi A, Passa AR, Pichini S, Rosa M, Zuccaro P, Dondero F. Environmental tobacco smoke: nicotine and cotinine concentration in semen. *Environmental Research* 1995;68(1):69–72.

Pan MM. Influence of passive smoking on the fetus during pregnancy [Chinese]. *Zhonghua Fu Chan Ke Za Zhi* 1992;27(6):348–50, 380.

Pattinson HA, Taylor PJ, Pattinson MH. The effect of cigarette smoking on ovarian function and early pregnancy outcome of in vitro fertilization treatment. *Fertility and Sterility* 1991;55(4):780–3.

Pattishall EN, Strope GL, Etzel RA, Helms RW, Haley NJ, Denny FW. Serum cotinine as a measure of tobacco smoke exposure in children. *American Journal of Diseases of Children* 1985;139(11):1101–4.

Peacock JL, Cook DG, Carey IM, Jarvis MJ, Bryant AE, Anderson HR, Bland JM. Maternal cotinine level during pregnancy and birthweight for gestational age. *International Journal of Epidemiology* 1998;27(4):647–56.

Pershagen G. Childhood cancer and malignancies other than lung cancer related to passive smoking. *Mutation Research* 1989;222(2):129–35.

Pirkle JL, Flegal KM, Bernert JT, Brody DJ, Etzel RA, Maurer KR. Exposure of the US population to environmental tobacco smoke: the Third National Health and Nutrition Examination Survey, 1988 to 1991. *Journal of the American Medical Association* 1996;275(16):1233–40.

Ponsonby AL, Dwyer T, Cochrane J. Population trends in sudden infant death syndrome. *Seminars in Perinatology* 2002;26(4):296–305.

Ponsonby AL, Dwyer T, Kasl SV, Cochrane JA. The Tasmanian SIDS Case-Control Study: univariable and multivariable risk factor analysis. *Paediatric and Perinatal Epidemiology* 1995;9(3):256–72.

Preston-Martin S, Yu MC, Benton B, Henderson BE. *N*-Nitroso compounds and childhood brain tumors: a case-control study. *Cancer Research* 1982; 42(12):5240–5.

Prokopczyk B, Cox JE, Hoffmann D, Waggoner SE. Identification of tobacco-specific carcinogen in the cervical mucus of smokers and nonsmokers. *Journal of the National Cancer Institute* 1997;89(12):868–73.

Rajini P, Last JA, Pinkerton KE, Hendrickx AG, Witschi H. Decreased fetal weights in rats exposed to sidestream cigarette smoke. *Fundamental and Applied Toxicology* 1994;22(3):400–4.

Rajs J, Råsten-Almqvist P, Falck G, Eksborg S, Andersson BS. Sudden infant death syndrome: postmortem findings of nicotine and cotinine in pericardial fluid of infants in relation to morphological changes and position at death. *Pediatric Pathology and Laboratory Medicine* 1997;17(1):83–97.

Rantakallio P. A follow-up study up to the age of 14 of children whose mothers smoked during pregnancy. *Acta Paediatrica Scandinavica* 1983;72(5):747–53.

Rebagliato M, Bolumar F, Florey C du V. Assessment of exposure to environmental tobacco smoke in nonsmoking pregnant women in different environments of daily living. *American Journal of Epidemiology* 1995a;142(5):525–30.

Rebagliato M, Florey C, Bolumar F. Exposure to environmental tobacco smoke in nonsmoking pregnant women in relation to birth weight. *American Journal of Epidemiology* 1995b;142(5):531–7.

Rice JM. Perinatal period and pregnancy: intervals of high risk for chemical carcinogens. *Environmental Health Perspectives* 1979;29:23–7.

Rice JM, Rehm S, Donovan PJ, Perantoni AO. Comparative transplacental carcinogenesis by directly acting and metabolism-dependent alkylating agents in rodents and nonhuman primates. In: Napalkov NP, Rice JM, Tomatis L, Yamasaki H, editors. *Perinatal and Multigeneration Carcinogenesis.* IARC Scientific Publications No. 96. Lyon (France): International Agency for Research on Cancer, 1989:17–34.

Roeleveld N, Vingerhoets E, Zielhuis GA, Gabreëls F. Mental retardation associated with parental smoking and alcohol consumption before, during, and after pregnancy. *Preventive Medicine* 1992;21(1): 110–9.

Rona RJ, Chinn S, Florey CD. Exposure to cigarette smoking and children's growth. *International Journal of Epidemiology* 1985;14(3):402–9.

Rona RJ, Florey CD, Clarke GC, Chinn S. Parental smoking at home and height of children. *British Medical Journal (Clinical Research Edition)* 1981; 283(6303):1363.

Roquer JM, Figueras J, Botet F, Jimenez R. Influence on fetal growth of exposure to tobacco smoke during pregnancy. *Acta Paediatrica* 1995;84(2):118–21.

Rosenberg MJ. Does smoking affect sperm? In: Rosenberg MJ, editor. *Smoking and Reproductive Health.* Littleton (MA): PSG Publishing Company, 1987: 54–62.

Rosevear SK, Holt DW, Lee TD, Ford WC, Wardle PG, Hull MG. Smoking and decreased fertilisation rates in vitro. *Lancet* 1992;340(8829):1195–6.

Rowlands DJ, McDermott A, Hull MG. Smoking and decreased fertilisation rates in vitro [letter]. *Lancet* 1992;340(8832):1409–10.

Rubin DH, Krasilnikoff PA, Leventhal JM, Weile B, Berget A. Effect of passive smoking on birth-weight. *Lancet* 1986;2(8504):415–7.

Ruckebusch Y. Relationship between the electrical activity of the oviduct and the uterus of the rabbit in vivo. *Journal of Reproduction and Fertility* 1975;45(1):73–82.

Rush D, Kass EH. Maternal smoking: a reassessment of the association with perinatal mortality. *American Journal of Epidemiology* 1972;96(3):183–96.

Sadler TW. *Langman's Medical Embryology.* 6th ed. Baltimore: Williams and Wilkins, 1990.

Sadler L, Belanger K, Saftlas A, Leaderer B, Hellenbrand K, McSharry JE, Bracken MB. Environmental tobacco smoke exposure and small-for-gestational-age birth. *American Journal of Epidemiology* 1999;150(7):695–705.

Saito R. The smoking habits of pregnant women and their husbands, and the effect on their infants [Japanese]. *Japanese Journal of Public Health* 1991;38(2):124–31.

Samuelsen SO, Magnus P, Bakketeig LS. Birth weight and mortality in childhood in Norway. *American Journal of Epidemiology* 1998;148(10):983–91.

Sasco AJ, Vainio H. From in utero and childhood exposure to parental smoking to childhood cancer: a possible link and the need for action. *Human & Experimental Toxicology* 1999;18(4):192–201.

Sasson IM, Haley NJ, Hoffman D, Wynder EL, Hellberg D, Nilsson S. Cigarette smoking and neoplasia of the uterine cervix: smoke constituents in cervical mucus [letter]. *New England Journal of Medicine* 1985;312(5):315–6.

Savitz DA, Schwingl PJ, Keels MA. Influence of paternal age, smoking, and alcohol consumption on congenital anomalies. *Teratology* 1991;44(4):429–40.

Schoendorf KC, Kiely JL. Relationship of sudden infant death syndrome to maternal smoking during and after pregnancy. *Pediatrics* 1992;90(6):905–8.

Schramm WF. Smoking during pregnancy: Missouri longitudinal study. *Paediatric and Perinatal Epidemiology* 1997;11(Suppl 1):73–83.

Schuller HM, editor. *Comparative Perinatal Carcinogenesis*. Boca Raton (FL): CRC Press, 1984.

Schulte-Hobein B, Schwartz-Bickenbach D, Abt S, Plum C, Nau H. Cigarette smoke exposure and development of infants throughout the first year of life: influence of passive smoking and nursing on cotinine levels in breast milk and infant's urine. *Acta Paediatrica* 1992;81(6–7):550–7.

Schwartz-Bickenbach D, Schulte-Hobein B, Abt S, Plum C, Nau H. Smoking and passive smoking during pregnancy and early infancy: effects on birth weight, lactation period, and cotinine concentrations in mother's milk and infant's urine. *Toxicology Letters* 1987;35(1):73–81.

Seersholm N, Hertz H, Olsen JH. Cancer in the offspring of parents with lung cancer. *European Journal of Cancer* 1997;33(14):2376–9.

Seidman DS, Ever-Hadani P, Gale R. Effect of maternal smoking and age on congenital anomalies. *Obstetrics and Gynecology* 1990;76(6):1046–50.

Seidman DS, Mashiach S. Involuntary smoking and pregnancy. *European Journal of Obstetrics, Gynecology, and Reproductive Biology* 1991;41(2):105–16.

Shaw GM, Wasserman CR, Lammer EJ, O'Malley CD, Murray JC, Basart AM, Tolarova MM. Orofacial clefts, parental cigarette smoking, and transforming growth factor-alpha gene variants. *American Journal of Human Genetics* 1996;58(3):551–61.

Shu XO, Ross JA, Pendergrass TW, Reaman GH, Lampkin B, Robison LL. Parental alcohol consumption, cigarette smoking, and risk of infant leukemia: a Childrens Cancer Group study. *Journal of the National Cancer Institute* 1996;88(1):24–31.

Slotkin TA. Fetal nicotine or cocaine exposure: which one is worse? *Journal of Pharmacology and Experimental Therapy* 1998;285(3):931–45.

Slotkin TA, Pinkerton KE, Garofolo MC, Auman JT, McCook EC, Seidler FJ. Perinatal exposure to environmental tobacco smoke induces adenyl cyclase and alters receptor-mediated cell signaling in brain and heart of neonatal rats. *Brain Research* 2001;898(1):73–81.

Slotkin TA, Pinkerton KE, Seidler FJ. Perinatal environmental tobacco smoke exposure in rhesus monkeys: critical periods and regional selectivity for effects on brain cell development and lipid peroxidation. *Environmental Health Perspectives* 2006;114(1):34–9.

Smith CJ, Livingston SD, Doolittle DJ. An international literature survey of "IARC Group I carcinogens" reported in mainstream cigarette smoke. *Food and Chemical Toxicology* 1997;35(10–11):1107–30.

Smith CJ, Perfetti TA, Mullens MA, Rodgman A, Doolittle DJ. "IARC group 2B Carcinogens" reported in cigarette mainstream smoke. *Food and Chemical Toxicology* 2000a;38(9):825–48.

Smith CJ, Perfetti TA, Rumple MA, Rodgman A, Doolittle DJ. "IARC group 2A Carcinogens" reported in cigarette mainstream smoke. *Food and Chemical Toxicology* 2000b;38(4):371–83.

Smith N, Austen J, Rolles CJ. Tertiary smoking by the fetus [letter]. *Lancet* 1982;1(8283):1252–3.

Sorahan T, Lancashire R, Prior P, Peck I, Stewart A. Childhood cancer and parental use of alcohol and tobacco. *Annals of Epidemiology* 1995;5(5):354–9.

Sorahan T, Lancashire RJ, Hulten MA, Peck I, Stewart AM. Childhood cancer and parental use of tobacco: deaths from 1953 to 1955. *British Journal of Cancer* 1997a;75(1):134–8.

Sorahan T, McKinney PA, Mann JR, Lancashire RJ, Stiller CA, Birch JM, Dodd HE, Cartwright RA. Childhood cancer and parental use of tobacco: findings from the Inter-Regional Epidemiological Study of Childhood Cancer (IRESCC). *British Journal of Cancer* 2001;84(1):141–6.

Sorahan T, Prior P, Lancashire RJ, Faux SP, Hulten MA, Peck IM, Stewart AM. Childhood cancer and parental use of tobacco: deaths from 1971 to 1976. *British Journal of Cancer* 1997b;76(11):1525–31.

Stavrou D, Dahme E, Haenichen T. Transplacental carcinogenesis in the rabbit. In: Schuller HM, editor. *Comparative Perinatal Carcinogenesis.* Boca Raton (FL): CRC Press, 1984:23–43.

Stick SM, Burton PR, Gurrin L, Sly PD, LeSouef PH. Effects of maternal smoking during pregnancy and a family history of asthma on respiratory function in newborn infants. *Lancet* 1996;348(9034):1060–4.

Stillman RJ, Rosenberg MJ, Sachs BP. Smoking and reproduction. *Fertility and Sterility* 1986;46(4): 545–66.

Stjernfeldt M, Berglund K, Lindsten J, Ludvigsson J. Maternal smoking during pregnancy and risk of childhood cancer. *Lancet* 1986;1(8494):1350–2.

Suonio S, Saarikoski S, Kauhanen O, Metsapelto A, Terho J, Vohlonen I. Smoking does affect fecundity. *European Journal of Obstetrics, Gynecology, and Reproductive Biology* 1990;34(1–2):89–95.

Terris M, Gold EM. An epidemiologic study of prematurity: I. Relation to smoking, heart volume, employment, and physique. *American Journal of Obstetrics and Gynecology* 1969;103(3):358–70.

Tokuhata GK. Smoking in relation to infertility and fetal loss. *Archives of Environmental Health* 1968;17(3):353–9.

Trapp M, Kemeter P, Feichtinger W. Smoking and in-vitro fertilization. *Human Reproduction* 1986;1(6): 357–8.

Trédaniel J, Boffetta P, Little J, Saracci R, Hirsch A. Exposure to passive smoking during pregnancy and childhood, and cancer risk: the epidemiological evidence. *Paediatric and Perinatal Epidemiology* 1994;8(3):233–55.

Ueda Y, Morikawa H, Funakoshi T, Kobayashi A, Yamasaki A, Takeuchi K, Mochizuki M, Jimbo T, Sato A. Estimation of passive smoking during pregnancy by cotinine measurement and its effect on fetal growth [Japanese]. *Nippon Sanka Fujinka Gakkai Zasshi* 1989;41(4):454–60.

Underwood PB, Kesler KF, O'Lane JJ, Callagan DA. Parental smoking empirically related to pregnancy outcome. *Obstetrics and Gynecology* 1967;29(1):1–8.

United Kingdom Department of Health. *Report of the Scientific Committee on Tobacco and Health.* Norwich (United Kingdom): The Stationery Office, 1998. (See also <http://www.archive.official-documents. co.uk/document/doh/tobacco/contents.htm>; accessed: June 26, 2003.)

U.S. Department of Health and Human Services. *The Health Consequences of Smoking for Women. A Report of the Surgeon General.* Washington: U.S. Department of Health and Human Services, Public Health Service, Office of the Assistant Secretary for Health, Office on Smoking and Health, 1980.

U.S. Department of Health and Human Services. *The Health Consequences of Involuntary Smoking. A Report of the Surgeon General.* Rockville (MD): U.S. Department of Health and Human Services, Public Health Service, Centers for Disease Control, Center for Health Promotion and Education, Office on Smoking and Health, 1986. DHHS Publication No. (CDC) 87-8398.

U.S. Department of Health and Human Services. *The Health Benefits of Smoking Cessation. A Report of the Surgeon General.* Atlanta: U.S. Department of Health and Human Services, Public Health Service, Centers for Disease Control, National Center for Chronic Disease Prevention and Health Promotion, Office on Smoking and Health, 1990. DHHS Publication No. (CDC) 90-8416.

U.S. Department of Health and Human Services. *Women and Smoking. A Report of the Surgeon General.* Rockville (MD): U.S. Department of Health and Human Services, Public Health Service, Office of the Surgeon General, 2001.

U.S. Department of Health and Human Services. *The Health Consequences of Smoking: A Report of the Surgeon General.* Atlanta: U.S. Department of Health and Human Services, Centers for Disease Control and Prevention, National Center for Chronic Disease Prevention and Health Promotion, Office on Smoking and Health, 2004.

U.S. Department of Health, Education, and Welfare. *Smoking and Health: Report of the Advisory Committee to the Surgeon General of the Public Health Service.* Washington: U.S. Department of Health, Education, and Welfare, Public Health Service, Center for Disease Control, 1964. PHS Publication No. 1103.

U.S. Department of Health, Education, and Welfare. *The Health Consequences of Smoking. A Report of the Surgeon General, 1974.* Washington: U.S. Department of Health, Education, and Welfare, Public Health Service, Center for Disease Control, 1974. DHEW Publication No. (CDC) 74-8704.

U.S. Department of Health, Education, and Welfare. *Smoking and Health. A Report of the Surgeon General.* Washington: U.S. Department of Health, Education, and Welfare, Public Health Service, Office of the Assistant Secretary for Health, Office of Smoking and Health, 1979a. DHEW Publication No. (PHS) 79-50066.

U.S. Department of Health, Education, and Welfare. *The Health Consequences of Smoking. A Report of the Surgeon General, 1977–1978.* Rockville (MD): U.S. Department of Health and Human Services, Public Health Service, Office of the Assistant Secretary for Health, Office on Smoking and Health, 1979b. DHEW Publication No. (CDC) 79-50065.

University of Toronto. *Protection From Second-Hand Tobacco Smoke in Ontario: A Review of the Evidence Regarding Best Practices.* Toronto: University of Toronto, Ontario Tobacco Research Unit, 2001.

van den Berg BJ, Oechsli FW. Prematurity. In: Bracken MB, editor. *Perinatal Epidemiology.* New York: Oxford University Press, 1984:69–85.

van Rooij IALM, Groenen PMW, van Drongelen M, te Morsche RHM, Peters WHM, Steegers-Theunissen RPM. Orofacial clefts and spina bifida: *N*-acetyltransferase phenotype, maternal smoking, and medication use. *Teratology* 2002;66(5):260–6.

van Rooij IALM, Wegerif MJM, Roelofs HMJ, Peters WHM, Kuijpers-Jagtman A-M, Zielhuis GA, Merkus HMWM, Steegers-Theunissen RPM. Smoking, genetic polymorphisms in biotransformation enzymes, and nonsyndromic oral clefting: a gene-environment interaction. *Epidemiology* 2001;12(5):502–7.

Van Voorhis BJ, Syrop CH, Hammitt DG, Dunn MS, Snyder GD. Effects of smoking on ovulation induction for assisted reproductive techniques. *Fertility and Sterility* 1992;58(5):981–5.

Vessey MP. Epidemiological studies of the effects of diethylstilbestrol. In: Napalkov NP, Rice JM, Tomatis L, Yamasaki H, editors. *Perinatal and Multigeneration Carcinogenesis.* IARC Scientific Publications No. 96. Lyon (France): International Agency for Research on Cancer, 1989:335–48.

Vine MF, Margolin BH, Morrison HI, Hulka BS. Cigarette smoking and sperm density: a meta-analysis. *Fertility and Sterility* 1994;61(1):35–43.

Wasserman CR, Shaw GM, O'Malley CD, Tolarova MM, Lammer EJ. Parental cigarette smoking and risk for congenital anomalies of the heart, neural tube, or limb. *Teratology* 1996;53(4):261–7.

Weiss T, Eckert A. Cotinine levels in follicular fluid and serum of IVF patients: effect on granulosa-luteal cell function in vitro. *Human Reproduction* 1989;4(5):482–5.

Weitzman M, Gortmaker S, Sobol A. Maternal smoking and behavior problems of children. *Pediatrics* 1992;90(3):342–9.

Werler MM. Teratogen update: smoking and reproductive outcomes. *Teratology* 1997;55(6):382–8.

Wilcox AJ. Birth weight and perinatal mortality: the effect of maternal smoking. *American Journal of Epidemiology* 1993;137(10):1098–104.

Wilcox AJ, Weinberg CR, O'Connor JF, Baird DD, Schlatterer JP, Canfield RE, Armstrong EG, Nisula BC. Incidence of early loss of pregnancy. *New England Journal of Medicine* 1988;319(4):189–94.

Williams MA, Mittendorf R, Stubblefield PG, Lieberman E, Schoenbaum SC, Monson RR. Cigarettes, coffee, and preterm premature rupture of the membranes. *American Journal of Epidemiology* 1992;135(8):895–903.

Windham GC, Eaton A, Hopkins B. Evidence for an association between environmental tobacco smoke exposure and birthweight: a meta-analysis and new data. *Paediatric and Perinatal Epidemiology* 1999a;13(1):35–57.

Windham GC, Hopkins B, Fenster L, Swan SH. Prenatal active or passive tobacco smoke exposure and the risk of preterm delivery or low birth weight. *Epidemiology* 2000;11(4):427–33.

Windham GC, Swan SH, Fenster L. Parental cigarette smoking and the risk of spontaneous abortion. *American Journal of Epidemiology* 1992;135(12):1394–403.

Windham GC, Von Behren J, Waller K, Fenster L. Exposure to environmental and mainstream tobacco smoke and risk of spontaneous abortion. *American Journal of Epidemiology* 1999b;149(3):243–7.

World Health Organization. *International Consultation on Environmental Tobacco Smoke (ETS) and Child Health: Consultation Report.* Geneva: World Health Organization, Tobacco Free Initiative, 1999. Report No. WHO/NCD/TFI/99.10.

Wyszynski DF, Duffy DL, Beaty TH. Maternal cigarette smoking and oral clefts: a meta-analysis. *Cleft Palate-Craniofacial Journal* 1997;34(3):206–10.

Xiao KZ. A survey on the constitutional status of perinates in China [Chinese]. *Chinese Medical Journal* 1989;69(4):185–8, 214.

Xu J. 126 Small gestational age infants: clinical characteristics and long-term observation [Chinese]. *Chinese Medical Journal* 1992;72(8):459–61, 508.

Yeruchimovich M, Dollberg S, Green DW, Mimouni FB. Nucleated red blood cells in infants of smoking mothers. *Obstetrics and Gynecology* 1999;93(3):403–6.

Yerushalmy J. The relationship of parents' cigarette smoking to outcome of pregnancy—implications as to the problem of inferring causation from observed associations. *American Journal of Epidemiology* 1971;93(6):443–56.

Yoshinaga K, Rice C, Krenn J. Effects of nicotine on early pregnancy in the rat. *Biology of Reproduction* 1979;20(2):294–303.

Zenzes MT, Puy LA, Bielecki R. Immunodetection of benzo[*a*]pyrene adducts in ovarian cells of women exposed to cigarette smoke. *Molecular Human Reproduction* 1998;4(2):159–65.

Zenzes MT, Reed TE, Wang P, Klein J. Cotinine, a major metabolite of nicotine, is detectable in follicular fluids of passive smokers in in vitro fertilization therapy. *Fertility and Sterility* 1996;66(4):614–9.

Zhang J, Ratcliffe JM. Paternal smoking and birthweight in Shanghai. *American Journal of Public Health* 1993;83(2):207–10.

Zhang J, Savitz DA, Schwingl PJ, Cai WW. A case-control study of paternal smoking and birth defects. *International Journal of Epidemiology* 1992;21(2):273–8.

Chapter 6
Respiratory Effects in Children from Exposure to Secondhand Smoke

Introduction

Adverse effects of parental smoking on the respiratory health of children have been a clinical and public health concern for decades. As early as 1974, two articles published in the journal *Lancet* alerted readers to a possible link between parental smoking and the risk of a lower respiratory illness (LRI) among infants (Colley et al. 1974; Harlap and Davies 1974). Although adverse effects on children from exposure to secondhand tobacco smoke had already been suggested (Cameron et al. 1969; Norman-Taylor and Dickinson 1972), the association with early episodes of acute chest illnesses was of immediate and continuing interest because of the suspected long-term consequences for lung growth, chronic respiratory morbidity in childhood, and adult chronic obstructive lung disease (Samet et al. 1983).

Subsequently, many epidemiologic studies have associated parental smoking with respiratory diseases and other adverse health effects throughout childhood. The exposures covered include maternal smoking during pregnancy and afterward, paternal smoking, parental smoking generally, and smoking by others. In 1986, the evidence was sufficient for the U.S. Surgeon General to conclude that the children of parents who smoked had an increased frequency of acute respiratory illnesses and related hospital admissions during infancy (U.S. Department of Health and Human Services [USDHHS] 1986). The 1986 Surgeon General's report also noted that in older children, there was an increased frequency of cough and phlegm and some evidence of an association with middle ear disease. The report also commented on an association between slowed lung growth in children and parental smoking. Several authoritative reviews by various agencies followed the 1986 report (U.S. Environmental Protection Agency [EPA] 1992; National Cancer Institute [NCI] 1999). Some researchers have systematically reviewed the literature and, where appropriate, carried out meta-analyses (DiFranza and Lew 1996; Uhari et al. 1996; Li et al. 1999); the most comprehensive systematic review was commissioned by the Department of Health in England (Scientific Committee on Tobacco and Health 1998). Updated versions of these reviews were then published as a series of articles in the journal *Thorax* (Cook and Strachan 1997, 1998, 1999; Strachan and Cook 1997, 1998a,b,c; Cook et al. 1998). These papers later served as a foundation for the 1999 World Health Organization (WHO) consultation report on environmental tobacco smoke and child health (WHO 1999). This chapter of the Surgeon General's report presents a major update of those reviews based on literature searches carried out through March 2001. The methodology for these reviews is described later in this chapter (see "Methods Used to Review the Evidence"). Selected key references published subsequent to these reviews are included in an appendix of significant additions to the literature at the end of this report.

The section that follows focuses on the biologic basis for respiratory health effects; Chapter 2 (Toxicology of Secondhand Smoke) of this report provides further background. Separate sections review the evidence for different adverse effects of secondhand smoke exposure of children: LRIs in infancy and early childhood, middle ear disease and adenotonsillectomy, frequency of respiratory symptoms and prevalent asthma in school-age children, and cohort and case-control studies of the onset of asthma in childhood. There is also a review of the evidence for the effects of parental smoking on several physiologic measures, lung function, bronchial reactivity, and atopic sensitization. Each section concludes with a summary and an interpretation of the evidence.

Mechanisms of Health Effects from Secondhand Tobacco Smoke

This section reviews the biologic impact of secondhand smoke on the respiratory system of the child. Subsequent sections summarize the evidence for adverse health effects on infants and children and describe postulated mechanisms for these effects. Chapter 2 of this report provides additional general data on these mechanisms.

Introduction

Pregnant women who smoke expose the fetus to tobacco smoke components during a critical window of lung development, with consequences that may be persistent. In infancy and early childhood, the contributions of prenatal versus postnatal exposures to secondhand smoke are difficult to separate because women who smoke during pregnancy almost invariably continue to smoke after their children are born. For children, exposure to secondhand smoke may lead to respiratory illnesses as a result of adverse effects on the immune system and on lung growth and development.

Lung Development and Growth

Active smoking by the mother during pregnancy has causal adverse effects on pregnancy outcomes that are well documented (USDHHS 2001, 2004). Exposure of pregnant women to secondhand tobacco smoke has also been associated with prematurity (Hanke et al. 1999), reduced birth weight (Mainous and Hueston 1994; Misra and Nguyen 1999), and small for gestational age outcomes in some studies (Dejin-Karlsson et al. 1998). However, the developmental effects on the respiratory system from maternal smoking during pregnancy extend beyond those that might be expected based on prematurity alone—the airways are particularly affected. Studies have demonstrated that lower measured airflows associated with secondhand smoke exposure are not completely explained by the reduction in somatic growth caused by maternal smoking (Young et al. 2000b). Researchers suspect that fetal growth limitations are mediated in part by the vasoconstrictive effects of nicotine, which may limit uterine blood flow and induce fetal hypoxia (Philipp et al. 1984). Fetal hypoxia, in turn, may lead to slowed fetal growth and may have direct effects on

the lung, possibly affecting lung mechanics by suppressing the fetal respiratory rate. Studies have demonstrated a decrease in fetal movement for at least one hour after maternal smoking, which is consistent with fetal hypoxia (Thaler et al. 1980). Smoking during pregnancy may also negatively affect the control of respiration in the fetus (Lewis and Bosque 1995).

Researchers have proposed several mechanisms that explain the effects of maternal smoking during pregnancy on infant lung function. Animal and human studies suggest that morphologic and metabolic alterations result from in utero exposure to tobacco smoke components that cross the placental barrier (Bassi et al. 1984; Philipp et al. 1984; Collins et al. 1985; Chen et al. 1987). One study with monkeys that involved infusion of nicotine into the mother during pregnancy showed lung hypoplasia and changes in the developing alveoli (Sekhon et al. 1999). The investigators postulated that the effect was mediated by the nicotine cholinergic receptors, which showed an increased expansion and binding with nicotine administration. Further research with this model indicated altered collagen in the developing lung (Sekhon et al. 2002). Studies with this and similar models have shown a variety of effects from nicotine on the neonatal lung (Pierce and Nguyen 2002). The programming of fetal growth genes in utero may have a lifelong effect on lung development and disease susceptibility, areas of ongoing research in other diseases. There is now substantial research in progress on early life events and future disease risk that follows the general hypothesis proposed by Barker and colleagues (1996).

Exposure to secondhand smoke may also lead to structural changes in the developing lung. In a rat model, Collins and colleagues (1985) found that intrauterine exposure of the pregnant rat to secondhand smoke was associated with pulmonary hypoplasia in the baby rats with decreased lung volumes; in this rat model, exposure reduced the number of sacules but increased their size. Brown and colleagues (1995) assessed respiratory mechanics in 53 healthy infants, and interpreted the pattern of findings to suggest that prenatal tobacco smoke exposure from smoking by the mother may lead to a reduction in airway size and changes in lung properties.

Lung maturation in utero is regulated by the endocrine environment, and the timing of secondhand smoke exposures with regard to lung development may have a lifelong impact on respiratory function. Secondhand smoke components may increase in utero stress responses that then speed lung maturation at the expense of lung growth. Several studies have demonstrated an effect on the fetal endocrine milieu secondary to secondhand smoke exposure (Divers et al. 1981; Catlin et al. 1990; Lieberman et al. 1992). Studies have also associated maternal smoking with more advanced lung maturity measured by lectin/sphingomyelin (L/S) ratios that were out of proportion to fetal size in human infants (Mainous and Hueston 1994). Cotinine levels measured in the amniotic fluid were positively correlated with L/S ratios. Studies also noted an increase in free, conjugated, and total cortisol levels, suggesting a potentially direct or indirect role for hormonal effects of secondhand smoke on the fetus (Lieberman et al. 1992). Other researchers have demonstrated higher levels of catecholamines in amniotic fluid in pregnant smokers compared with pregnant nonsmokers, further supporting an endocrine mechanism for the effect of secondhand smoke (Divers et al. 1981).

Multiple studies suggest that the effect of secondhand smoke on the development of the respiratory system begins with in utero exposure (Tager et al. 1995; Stick et al. 1996; Lodrup Carlsen et al. 1997). Stick and colleagues (1996) reported a dose-dependent effect of in utero cigarette smoke exposure in decreasing tidal flow patterns that were measured during the first three days of life (i.e., before any postnatal exposure). This effect was independent of the effect of smoking on birth weight. Hoo and colleagues (1998) evaluated respiratory function in preterm infants of mothers who did and did not smoke during pregnancy, with the goal of investigating whether the effect of prenatal tobacco smoke exposure is limited to an influence during the last weeks of gestation. The researchers observed that respiratory function was impaired in infants born preterm (an average of seven weeks early), suggesting that the adverse effect of prenatal tobacco smoke exposure is not limited to the last weeks of in utero development. The ratio of time to peak tidal expiratory flow to expiratory time (T_{PTEF}:T_E) was lower in infants exposed to secondhand smoke in utero compared with unexposed infants (mean 0.369 standard deviation [SD] 0.109 versus mean 0.426 SD 0.135, $p \leq 0.02$). Because T_{PTEF}:T_E is associated with airway caliber, these data imply that cigarette smoke exposure in utero may affect airway development. Lower maximal forced expiratory flow at functional residual capacity ($Vmax_{FRC}$) (Hanrahan et al. 1992) and diminished expiratory flows (Brown et al. 1995) in infants exposed in utero to secondhand smoke provide further support for the contention that infants of mothers who smoke during pregnancy have smaller airways. Increased airway wall thickness and increased smooth muscle, which can both lead to a decreased airway diameter, were found in infants exposed to tobacco smoke in utero who had died of sudden infant death syndrome (SIDS) (Elliot et al. 1999). In animal models of secondhand smoke exposure, fetuses of rats exposed to mainstream smoke (from active smoking) or to secondhand (sidestream) smoke had reduced lung volume, decreased elastic tissue within the parenchyma, increased density of interstitial tissue, and inadequate development of elastin and collagen (Collins et al. 1985; Vidic 1991). These animal and human data provide clear evidence for an adverse effect of in utero exposure to tobacco smoke on the developing lung. Studies also document structural changes in animal models and in exposed children who have died from SIDS. The physiologic findings suggest altered lung mechanics and reduced airflow consistent with changes in structure.

Immunologic Effects and Inflammation

The development of lung immunophenotype (i.e., the pattern of immunologic response in the lung) is considered to have a key role in determining the risk for asthma, particularly in regard to the T-helper 1 (Th1) pathway (which mediates cellular immunity) and the Th2 pathway (which mediates allergic responses). Secondhand smoke exposure may promote immunologic development along Th2 pathways, thus contributing to the intermediate phenotypes associated with asthma and with a predilection to chronic respiratory disease. Gene-environment interactions that begin in utero and persist during critical periods of development after birth represent the least understood, but potentially the most important, mechanistic route for a lasting influence of secondhand smoke. Although a meta-analysis of epidemiologic evidence suggests that parental smoking before birth (or early childhood secondhand smoke exposure) does not increase the risk for allergic sensitization, other lines of mechanistic investigation do show a variety of influences from secondhand smoke on immune and inflammatory responses (Strachan and Cook 1998b).

Secondhand smoke effects on T cells may influence gene regulation, inflammatory cell function, cytokine production, and immunoglobulin E (IgE) synthesis. These effects are particularly important to consider in regard to immune system ontogeny and for the subsequent development of allergies in childhood. Researchers have demonstrated that mainstream and sidestream smoke condensates selectively suppress the interferon gamma induction of several macrophage functions, including phagocytosis of Ig-opsonized sheep red blood cells, class II major histocompatibility complex expression, and nitric oxide synthesis, which are all representative of effects on immunity (Braun et al. 1998; Edwards et al. 1999). Alterations in antigen presentation may occur not only in the respiratory tract but also in the rest of the body where absorbed toxicants are distributed. Macrophages are potent effector cells for immune responsiveness; suppression of their ability to respond to environmental challenges could have lifelong consequences on immune function.

Immune responses may also be increased as a result of secondhand smoke exposure. Animal studies demonstrate increases in IgE, eosinophils, and Th2 cytokines (especially interleukin [IL]-4 and IL-10) with exposure to secondhand smoke. These increases may augment the potential for allergic sensitization and the development of an atopy phenotype. In mice sensitized to the ovalbumin (OVA) antigen and exposed to secondhand smoke for six hours per day, five days per week, for six weeks, researchers measured increases in total IgE, OVA-specific immunoglobulin G1, and eosinophils in the blood (Seymour et al. 1997). These measures indicate an increase in the allergic response to inhaled antigens. On the basis of the results from this mouse model, the investigators concluded that allergen sensitization with the increase in Th2 responses may contribute to the development of allergies in individuals exposed to secondhand smoke (Seymour et al. 1997). Other studies have demonstrated an increase in IL-5, granulocyte-macrophage colony-stimulating factor, and IL-2 in bronchoalveolar lavage fluid in mice exposed to OVA along with secondhand smoke. In these mouse models, interferon gamma levels decreased. Because mice exposed to OVA alone did not experience these cytokine changes, secondhand smoke appears able to induce a sensitization phenotype to a usually neutral antigen (Rumold et al. 2001). Although the animal data are stronger than the human epidemiologic data, studies in humans are supportive of an effect of tobacco smoke exposure on allergic phenotypes.

Allergies are caused by multiple interacting factors in people with underlying susceptibility. Secondhand smoke exposure both in utero and after birth may promote the development of an allergic phenotype. Antigens presented during the neonatal period in mice skew the immune development and response along a Th2 pathway (i.e., toward an allergic phenotype) (Forsthuber et al. 1996). Human fetuses, under the influence of the maternal system mediated through the placenta, may develop a Th2 preference as a response to an antigen (Michie 1998). Magnusson (1986) studied newborn children of nonallergic parents and found evidence suggesting that tobacco smoke exposure in utero may promote an allergic phenotype. A threefold increase in risk for an elevated IgE level was observed in children whose mothers smoked compared with the IgE levels in children born to nonsmoking mothers. Total cord blood IgE concentrations were substantially higher in infants of mothers who smoked (60.8 international units [IU]) compared with infants of nonsmoking mothers (9.8 IU).

Atopy may be characterized by either a positive IgE-mediated skin test or elevated specific IgE serum levels. Atopy represents a risk factor for asthma, and an increase in bronchial responsiveness has been associated with higher serum IgE levels. Human studies provide mixed evidence as to whether secondhand smoke exposures are associated with an increase in IgE-mediated responses (Weiss et al. 1985; Martinez et al. 1988; Ownby and McCullough 1988; Stankus et al. 1988). Weiss and colleagues (1985) demonstrated that maternal smoking was associated with atopy in children aged five through nine years who were evaluated by skin tests to four common allergens. Ronchetti and colleagues (1990) demonstrated an effect of exposure on IgE levels and on eosinophil counts. Eosinophil counts were at least three times higher in boys exposed to secondhand smoke compared with unexposed boys. There was a dose-response relationship between the number of cigarettes to which each boy had been exposed and the level of eosinophilia (Ronchetti et al. 1990).

Researchers showed decades ago that mainstream cigarette smoke causes airway inflammation (Niewoehner et al. 1974) and an increase in airway permeability to small and large molecules in young smokers (Simani et al. 1974; Jones et al. 1980). Given the qualitative similarities between mainstream smoke and secondhand smoke, these effects may be relevant to involuntary smoking (USDHHS 1986).

There are many specific components of secondhand smoke that may adversely affect a child's lung. For example, a bacterial endotoxin known as lipopolysaccharide (LPS) can be detected in both mainstream and sidestream tobacco smoke. Studies have detected biologically active LPS in mainstream and sidestream smoke from regular and light experimental reference cigarettes used in the studies (mainstream: 120 ± 64 nanograms [ng] per regular cigarette, 45.3 ± 16 ng per light cigarette; sidestream: 18 ± 1.5 ng per regular cigarette, 75 ± 49 ng per light cigarette). The investigators suggested that chronic LPS exposure from cigarette smoke may contribute to the inflammatory effects of secondhand smoke (Hasday et al. 1999). Other studies show that LPS exposure may alter responses to allergen challenge (Tulić et al. 2000).

Researchers need to consider this hypothesized role of endotoxin because of the known pathologic effects of endotoxins on susceptible individuals. As a component of the cell wall of gram-negative bacteria, endotoxins are ubiquitous in the environment and may be found in high concentrations in household dust (Michel et al. 1996) and in ambient air pollution (Bonner et al. 1998). Macrophage activation may result from exposure to low concentrations of an endotoxin, leading to a cascade of inflammatory cytokines (such as IL-1, IL-6, and IL-8) and arachidonic acid metabolites, which are important in the formation of prostaglandin molecules (Bayne et al. 1986; Michie et al. 1988; Ingalls et al. 1999). Studies have documented increased levels of neutrophils in bronchoalveolar lavage fluid after a challenge with dust that contained endotoxins (Hunt et al. 1994). Reversible airflow obstruction has been associated with the inhalation of endotoxins in the air. In a cohort study of infants in Boston, Park and colleagues (2001) used a univariate model and found a significant association of wheeze in the first year of life with elevated dust endotoxin levels (relative risk [RR] = 1.29 [95 percent confidence interval (CI), 1.03–1.62]). In a multivariate model, elevated endotoxin levels in dust were associated with an increased risk for repeated wheeze illness in the first year of life (RR = 1.56 [95 percent CI, 1.03–2.38]) (Park et al. 2001). Exposure to endotoxins from secondhand smoke in utero, during infancy, and in childhood may increase airway inflammation and may interact synergistically with additional secondhand smoke exposures.

Smoking contributes generally to the particulate load in indoor air, and research documents that inhaling particles in the respirable size range contributes to pulmonary inflammation (National Research Council 2004). One consequence of particle-induced inflammation may be an intermediate phenotype with cough and wheeze in early childhood. Investigators used a guinea pig model of secondhand smoke exposure to study sensory nerve pathways for cough and airway narrowing in an effort to explain the development of cough and wheeze symptoms in children of smokers. When guinea pigs were exposed to sidestream smoke for six hours per day, five days per week, from one through six weeks of age, they demonstrated an increase in excitability of pulmonary C fibers (Mutoh et al. 1999) and rapidly adapting receptors (Bonham et al. 1996), which are believed to be primarily responsible for eliciting the reflex responses in defending the lungs against inhaled irritants and toxins (Lee and Widdicombe 2001). These studies have led to the conclusion that cough and wheeze may be produced by neural pathway stimulation and irritation.

Summary

Childhood respiratory disease covers a spectrum of diseases and underlying pathogenetic mechanisms that include infection, prenatal alterations in lung structure, inflammation, and allergic responses. There is a potential for secondhand smoke to contribute over the long term to the development of respiratory disease through altered organ maturation and immune function. Mechanisms underlying the adverse health effects of secondhand smoke vary across the phases of lung growth and development, extending from the in utero period to the completion of lung growth in late adolescence. The long-term effects of secondhand smoke is a field of ongoing research. These effects may vary among individuals because of individual genetic susceptibilities and gene-environment interactions. The discussions that follow summarize the available observational evidence concerning health effects of secondhand tobacco smoke on children, which are presumed to reflect the mechanisms reviewed above. The discussions also interpret the evidence in the context of this mechanistic understanding.

Methods Used to Review the Evidence

The search strategies and statistical methods for pooling that were used for this report were identical to those applied to the earlier reviews of this topic carried out by Strachan and Cook (1997). The authors conducted an electronic search of the EMBASE Excepta Medica and Medline databases using Medical Subject Headings (MeSH) to select published papers, letters, and review articles relating to secondhand tobacco smoke exposure in children. The EMBASE strategy was based on text word searches of titles, keywords, and related abstracts; non-English language articles were not included. The search was carried out through 2001.

Information relating to the odds ratio (OR) for the outcome of interest among children with and without smokers in the family was extracted from each study. Data regarding children exposed and unexposed to maternal smoking prenatally or postnatally were extracted separately. This review also specifically addresses the effects on children of smoking by other household members (usually the father) when the mother was not a smoker. Not every study provided information on all of these indices. The most common measures were smoking by either parent versus neither parent, and the effects of smoking by the mother versus only by the father or by neither parent. Few studies distinguished in any detail between prenatal and postnatal maternal smoking, but those that did were included in the discussion. The ORs for the effects of smoking by both parents compared with neither parent were also extracted from cross-sectional surveys of school-age children.

Because most studies have used self-reported parental smoking behaviors as the principal exposure indicator, and because the major sources of exposure in western countries are overwhelmingly maternal followed by paternal smoking (Cook et al. 1994), the terms parental, maternal, and paternal smoking are used throughout this chapter to refer to major sources of secondhand tobacco smoke exposure for children. The OR was chosen as a measure of association because it can be derived from all types of studies—case-control, cross-sectional, and cohort. In general, ORs and their 95 percent CIs were calculated from data in published tabulations using the actual numbers of participants, or numbers estimated from percentages of published column or row totals. This approach allowed for flexibility in combining categories of household tobacco smoke exposure for comparability across studies. If the number of participants was not provided, the published OR and its 95 percent CI were used. For some studies, it was necessary to derive an approximate standard error (for the log OR) based on the marginal values of the relevant multiplication table (2×2). In situations where ORs were given separately for different genders, a pooled OR and 95 percent CI were calculated by taking a weighted average (on the log scale) using weights inversely proportional to the variances. The papers that quoted an incidence rate ratio rather than an OR are identified in the summary tabulations.

The literature review also identified information on the extent to which the effects of parental smoking were altered by adjustment for potential confounding variables, and whether there was evidence of an exposure-response relationship with, for example, the amount smoked by either parent. Where the presented data could be standardized for age, gender, or occasionally for another confounder, the Mantel-Haenszel method was used to provide an adjusted value. Because there may be multiple published reports for a single study, only one paper from each study (usually the most recently published) was included in the quantitative meta-analyses. In some studies, however, information from other papers contributed to the assessment of potential confounding or a dose-response relationship.

Updated meta-analyses of the health effects from parental smoking were conducted specifically for this chapter. All pooled estimates were calculated using both fixed and random effects models (Egger et al. 2001). All updated analyses were carried out using Stata. For some outcomes, studies were grouped according to the timing of the secondhand smoke exposure (e.g., maternal smoking during pregnancy, parental smoking from infancy to four years of age, and parental smoking at five or more years of age).

The meta-analysis of the cross-sectional evidence relating parental smoking to spirometric indices in children updates the 1998 meta-analysis (Cook et al. 1998). Both the earlier and the more recent meta-analyses used the same effect measure: the average difference in the spirometric index between exposed and unexposed children, expressed as a percentage of the level in the unexposed group. The updated synthesis considered four different spirometric indices: forced vital capacity (FVC), forced expiratory volume in one second (FEV₁), mid-expiratory flow rate (MEFR), and flow rates at end expiration. Pooled estimates of the percentage differences were calculated using both fixed and random effects models (Egger et al. 2001).

To determine whether the exposure classification influenced the relationship between parental smoking and lung function, studies were pooled within the following exposure groups: both parents did versus did not smoke, mother did versus did not smoke, either parent versus neither parent smoked, the highest versus the lowest cotinine category, and high levels of household secondhand smoke versus none. To test for effects on the relationship between parental smoking and lung function from adjustment for variables other than age, gender, and body size, studies were pooled separately depending on adjustment for other variables. Lastly, this meta-analysis also assessed whether adjusting for socioeconomic measures, such as parental education and social class, affected the pooled results.

Lower Respiratory Illnesses in Infancy and Early Childhood

This section summarizes the evidence relating specifically to acute LRIs in the first two or three years of life and updates the previous review by Strachan and Cook (1997). Separate discussions review studies of asthma incidence, prognosis, and severity as well as studies (mostly cross-sectional) of school-age children.

In developed countries, the specific microbial etiology and determinants of some common lower respiratory tract illnesses in infancy remain a subject of uncertainty and research (Silverman 1993; Wilson 1994; Monto 2002; Klig and Chen 2003). Although many LRIs result from viral infections, there is an indication of a prenatally determined susceptibility related to lung function abnormalities that is already detectable at birth (Dezateux and Stocks 1997). As reviewed in the introduction to this chapter, lasting effects of in utero exposure to tobacco smoke from maternal smoking may increase airway resistance and the likelihood of a more severe LRI with infection. This review covers the full spectrum of LRIs, including categories considered to reflect infection and the category of wheeze, which may be a consequence of infection but may also indicate an asthma phenotype.

There is also an emerging consensus that there are several phenotypes of childhood wheeze, each with a different pattern of incidence, prognosis, and risk factors (Wilson 1994; Christie and Helms 1995). However, there is much less certainty about how these different "asthma phenotypes" should be characterized for either research or clinical purposes. Findings from the Tucson (Arizona) birth cohort study suggest physiologic and immunologic differences between the phenotypic syndromes of early childhood wheeze, the onset of asthma symptoms later in childhood, and persistent disease (Martinez et al. 1995; Stein et al. 1997). These findings have yet to be replicated in a comprehensive way in other large population samples, and few large cohort studies are in progress that provide the needed longitudinal data. The classification of phenotype in the epidemiologic studies is relevant to secondhand smoke if the association of secondhand smoke with risk varies across the phenotypes.

Relevant Studies

In the 1997 review, 75 publications were considered in detail as possibly relevant to illnesses in infancy and early childhood. Of those studies, 50 were included in the review, and 38 of those 50 were included in quantitative meta-analyses: 21 cohort studies, 10 case-control studies, 2 controlled trials, and 5 cross-sectional surveys of school-age children (Strachan and Cook 1997). The latter were included because they related parental smoking to a retrospective history of chest illness before two years of age, information that was obtained using the American Thoracic Society's children's questionnaire (Ferris 1978). No additional references were identified by citations in the above papers or in previous overviews.

Of 26 papers published since 1997, 17 contain quantitative information relevant to this review without duplicating the content of the other papers (Margolis et al. 1997; Nafstad et al. 1997; Baker et al. 1998; Gergen et al. 1998; Chen and Millar 1999; Dezateux et al. 1999; Gold et al. 1999; Karaman et al.

1999; Mrazek et al. 1999; Nuesslein et al. 1999; Rusconi et al. 1999; Yau et al. 1999; Diez et al. 2000; Gürkan et al. 2000b; Hjern et al. 2000; Lux et al. 2000; Young et al. 2000a). Most of these papers are community studies of wheeze illnesses: seven cohort studies, two case-control studies, and four surveys that ask about past illnesses. Only a few studies included data on the effects of smoking by only the father. The two most substantial papers analyze data from the Third National Health and Nutrition Examination Survey (NHANES III) (Gergen et al. 1998) and from a large Swedish study of hospital admissions that focused mostly on pneumonia (Hjern et al. 2000). A complement to the Swedish study examined asthma admissions, but only from two years of age and older, and was therefore not included in the quantitative synthesis (Hjern et al. 1999). That study does provide evidence relevant to effect modification by age.

Publications listed in another systematic review (Li et al. 1999) were also considered, but those studies were already included in other reviews for either LRI or asthma. Three studies from this new search were excluded: one Danish study of hospitalizations for any reason that described findings of respiratory problems, but presented no data related to secondhand smoke (Wisborg et al. 1999); a case-control study from The Gambia that considered admissions for acute LRI and implied that neither maternal nor paternal smoking was significantly associated with the outcome at p <0.05, but presented no data (Weber et al. 1999); and a cohort study of acute respiratory infections in children younger than five years of age that reported increased risks of 2.5 for pneumonia and 2.3 for other "severe disease" in children of smoking parents, but included no standard errors (Deb 1998).

Evidence Review

Community Studies of Lower Respiratory Illnesses

Combining studies from the 1997 review with subsequent publications, 34 community studies were related to parental smoking and LRIs in a community or ambulatory clinic setting (Table 6.1). There were 20 prospective cohort studies, 1 panel (short-term cohort) study, 1 cohort study carried out through record linkage, 2 controlled trials, 4 case-control studies, and 6 prevalence surveys of schoolchildren that asked parents about past illnesses. Seven studies combined all lower respiratory diagnoses (Gardner et al. 1984; Ferris et al. 1985; Pedreira et al. 1985;

Wright et al. 1991; Forastiere et al. 1992; Marbury et al. 1996; Richards et al. 1996), six contributed information on bronchitis and pneumonia (Leeder et al. 1976; Fergusson and Horwood 1985; Chen et al. 1988a; Håkansson and Carlsson 1992; Gergen et al. 1998; Nuesslein et al. 1999), and two focused on illnesses diagnosed as bronchiolitis (McConnochie and Roghmann 1986b; Hayes et al. 1989). Twenty-three studies focused specifically on illnesses associated with wheeze (Fergusson and Horwood 1985; Bisgaard et al. 1987; Chen et al. 1988a; Burr et al. 1989; Lucas et al. 1990; Halken et al. 1991; Arshad et al. 1993; Tager et al. 1993; Martinez et al. 1995; Elder et al. 1996; Margolis et al. 1997; Nafstad et al. 1997; Baker et al. 1998; Gergen et al. 1998; Chen and Millar 1999; Dezateaux et al. 1999; Gold et al. 1999; Karaman et al. 1999; Mrazek et al. 1999; Rusconi et al. 1999; Yau et al. 1999; Diez et al. 2000; Lux et al. 2000; Young et al. 2000a). The studies by Baker and colleagues (1998) and Lux and colleagues (2000) both reported on the Avon Longitudinal Study of Pregnancy and Childhood (ALSPAC), and three publications contributed independent data on both bronchitis/pneumonia and wheeze illnesses (Fergusson and Horwood 1985; Chen et al. 1988a; Gergen et al. 1998).

Table 6.2 and Figures 6.1–6.3 summarize the results of these studies. All except one study (Nuesslein et al. 1999) found an elevated risk of LRI associated with parental smoking, including by the father only, among the studies where that exposure variable was included. The one study not finding an increased OR associated with maternal smoking reported a significant association with cotinine levels measured in meconium (Nuesslein et al. 1999). Table 6.3 presents the results of meta-analyses that pooled the results from studies of early wheeze separately from those of an unspecified LRI, bronchitis, bronchiolitis, or pneumonia. Although the effect of smoking by either parent was similar for both wheeze and LRI, maternal smoking appeared to have a somewhat greater effect than paternal smoking in studies that specifically ascertained wheeze illnesses (Table 6.3).

Studies of Hospitalizations for Lower Respiratory Illnesses

The literature search identified 14 studies on hospitalizations for lower respiratory complaints in early life (Harlap and Davies 1974; Sims et al. 1978; Mok and Simpson 1982; Ekwo et al. 1983; Hall et al. 1984; Taylor and Wadsworth 1987; Anderson et al. 1988; Stern et al. 1989b; Reese et al. 1992; Jin and Rossignol 1993; Victora et al. 1994; Rylander et al. 1995;

Table 6.1 **Design, sample size, and recruitment criteria for studies of illness associated with parental smoking included in meta-analyses**

Study	Design/population	Sample size	Case definition	Source of cohort or controls	Outcome
		Community studies of lower respiratory illnesses (LRIs)			
Leeder et al. 1976	Cohort Aged <1 year United Kingdom	2,074	Acute bronchitis (BR)/pneumonia (PN) (reported)	Population-based birth cohort	BR/PN
Gardner et al. 1984	Panel Aged <1 year United States (Texas)	131	LRI (reported)	Virologic surveillance panel	LRI
Fergusson and Horwood 1985	Cohort Aged <2 years New Zealand	1,144	BR/PN consultation	Population-based birth cohort	BR/PN
Ferris et al. 1985	Survey Aged <2 years United States (Six cities)	8,528	Physician-diagnosed respiratory illness before 2 years of age	Population survey (children aged 6–9 years)	LRI
Pedreira et al. 1985	Cohort Aged <1 year United States (District of Columbia)	1,144	LRI consultation	Pediatric practice	LRI
McConnochie and Roghmann 1986b	Case-control Aged <2 years United States (New York)	212	First physician-diagnosed acute bronchiolitis (BL)/ wheeze	Pediatric outpatient lists (no wheeze)	BL/wheeze
Chen et al. 1988a	Cohort Aged <18 months China	2,227	Physician-diagnosed BR/PN	Population-based birth cohort	BR/PN
Hayes et al. 1989	Case-control Aged <1 year Samoa	80	Respiratory syncytial virus (RSV); epidemic LRI	Well-child clinics	BL
Wright et al. 1991	Cohort Aged <1 year United States (Arizona)	797	Physician-diagnosed LRI	Health maintenance organization (HMO)-based cohort	LRI
Forastiere et al. 1992	Survey Aged <2 years Italy	2,797	BR/BL/PN before 2 years of age	Population survey (children aged 7–11 years)	LRI
Hakansson and Carlsson 1992	Cohort Aged <12 months Sweden	192	Antibiotics for BR/PN	Population-based birth cohort	BR/PN
Marbury et al. 1996	Cohort Aged <2 years United States (Minnesota)	1,424	LRI consultation	HMO-based cohort	LRI

Table 6.1   Continued

Study	Design/population	Sample size	Case definition	Source of cohort or controls	Outcome
	**Community studies of LRIs**				
Richards et al. 1996	Survey Aged <2 years South Africa	726	Physician-diagnosed respiratory illness before 2 years of age	Survey of 2 schools (children aged 14–18 years)	LRI
Gergen et al. 1998	Survey Aged 2–36 months United States	7,680	Parental report/ recall of physician-diagnosed asthma (ever)	Representative sample from NHANES III*	Chronic BR
Nuesslein et al. 1999	Cohort Aged <6 months Germany	65	Parental report/ recall of cold with cough	Population-based birth cohort	LRI
	**Community studies of wheeze illnesses**				
Fergusson and Horwood 1985	Cohort Aged <2 years New Zealand	1,144	Wheeze/chest cold	Population-based birth cohort	Wheeze
Bisgaard et al. 1987	Cohort Aged <1 year Denmark	5,953	>1 episode of wheeze	Population-based birth cohort	Wheeze
Chen et al. 1988a	Cohort Aged <18 months China	2,227	Physician-diagnosed asthma	Population-based birth cohort	Wheeze
Burr et al. 1989	Trial Aged <1 year United Kingdom	480	Wheeze by 1 year of age (reported)	Infants from families with allergies	Wheeze
Lucas et al. 1990	Trial Aged <18 months United Kingdom	777	>3 episodes of wheeze or asthma	Infants <37 weeks of gestation	Wheeze
Halken et al. 1991	Cohort Aged <18 months Denmark	276	>2 episodes of wheeze	Random sample of births	Wheeze
Arshad et al. 1993	Cohort Aged <2 years United Kingdom	1,172	>3 episodes of wheeze	Population-based birth cohort	Wheeze
Tager et al. 1993	Cohort Aged <12 months United States (Massachusetts)	97	Wheeze or LRI admission	Special lung function study	Wheeze
Martinez et al. 1995	Cohort Aged <3 years United States (Arizona)	762	LRI with wheeze	HMO-based birth cohort	Wheeze

Table 6.1   Continued

Study	Design/population	Sample size	Case definition	Source of cohort or controls	Outcome
		Community studies of wheeze illnesses			
Elder et al. 1996	Cohort Aged <1 year Australia	525	Bronchodilator therapy	Infants <33 weeks of gestation	Wheeze
Margolis et al. 1997	Cohort Aged ≤12 months United States	325	Parental report/ recall of cough or wheeze	Population-based birth cohort (no high-risk infants)	Wheeze
Nafstad et al. 1997	Cohort Aged ≤24 months Norway	3,038	Bronchial obstruction confirmed by physician diagnosis	Births in 2 clinics (no high-risk infants)	Bronchial obstruction
Baker et al. 1998; Lux et al. 2000	Cohort Aged ≤30 months United Kingdom	8,561	Parental report/ recall of wheeze by 6 months of age	ALSPAC[†] birth cohort	Wheeze
Gergen et al. 1998	Survey Aged 2–36 months United States	7,680	Parental report/ recall of physician diagnosis (ever) of asthma	Representative sample from NHANES III	Asthma
			Parental report/ recall of ≤3 episodes in 12 months		Wheeze
Chen and Millar 1999	Survey Aged ≤36 months Canada	5,888	Parental report/ recall of physician diagnosis of asthma (ever)	Representative sample of Canadian population	Asthma
Dezateux et al. 1999	Cohort Aged <12 months United Kingdom	101	>1 episode of physician-diagnosed wheeze	Population-based birth cohort	Wheeze
Gold et al. 1999	Cohort Aged <12 months United States (Massachusetts)	499	Parental report/ recall of >1 episode of wheeze	Birth cohort of parents with asthma and allergies	Wheeze
Karaman et al. 1999	Case-control Aged 6–24 months Turkey	68	Parental report/ recall of >1 episode of wheeze	A general practice (children with no allergies)	Wheeze
Mrazek et al. 1999	Cohort Aged ≤36 months United States (Colorado)	150	Recurrent asthma in medical records	Birth cohort of mothers with asthma	Wheeze
Rusconi et al. 1999	Survey Aged ≤24 months Italy	16,333	Parental report/ recall of wheeze at 6–7 years of age	Population survey (children aged 6–7 years)	LRI with wheeze

Table 6.1   Continued

Study	Design/population	Sample size	Case definition	Source of cohort or controls	Outcome
Community studies of wheeze illnesses					
Yau et al. 1999	Cohort Aged <24 months Taiwan	71	Parental report/ recall of LRI with wheeze	Healthy full-term infants	Wheeze
Diez et al. 2000	Nested case-control Aged ≤12 months Germany	310	Parental report/ recall of wheeze	Premature infants or others at high risk	Wheeze
Young et al. 2000a	Cohort Aged <24 months Australia	160	Parental report/ recall and/or physician diagnosis of wheeze	Population-based birth cohort	Wheeze
Community studies of upper and lower respiratory illnesses (U/LRIs)					
Ogston et al. 1987	Cohort Aged <12 months United Kingdom	1,542	U/LRIs recorded by a health visitor to the home	Population-based birth cohort	U/LRIs
Woodward et al. 1990	Case-control Aged 1–3 years Australia	489	High U/LRIs "score" based on values assigned to responses to questionnaires	Population survey (children with low scores)	U/LRIs
Hospitalizations for LRIs					
Harlap and Davies 1974	Cohort Aged <1 year Israel	10,672	BR/PN admission	Population-based birth cohort	BR/PN (inpatients)
Sims et al. 1978	Case-control Infants United Kingdom	70	RSV-positive BL admission	Schoolmates at 8 years of age	BL (inpatients)
Mok and Simpson 1982	Case-control Aged <1 year United Kingdom	400	LRI admission	Classmates at 7 years of age	BR/PN (inpatients)
Ekwo et al. 1983	Survey Aged <2 years United States (Iowa)	1,139	LRI admission before 2 years of age	Population survey (children aged 6–12 years)	LRI (inpatients)
Hall et al. 1984	Case-control Aged <2 years United States (New York)	87	RSV and LRI admission	Acute nonrespiratory admission	BL (inpatients)
Taylor and Wadsworth 1987	Cohort Aged <5 years United Kingdom	12,727	LRI admission	Population-based birth cohort	LRI (inpatients)

Table 6.1   Continued

Study	Design/population	Sample size	Case definition	Source of cohort or controls	Outcome
Hospitalizations for LRIs					
Anderson et al. 1988	Case-control Aged <2 years United States (Georgia)	301	PN/BL admission	Outpatient clinics	PN/BL (inpatients)
Stern et al. 1989b	Survey Aged <2 years Canada	4,099	LRI admission before 2 years of age	Population survey (children aged 7–12 years)	LRI (inpatients)
Reese et al. 1992	Case-control Aged 5–15 months Australia	96	BL admission	Nonrespiratory admission	BL (inpatients)
Jin and Rossignol 1993	Cohort Aged <18 months China	1,007	BR/PN admission	Population-based birth cohort	BR/PN (inpatients)
Victora et al. 1994	Case-control Aged <2 years Brazil	1,020	PN (x-ray)	Neighbors	PN (inpatients)
Rylander et al. 1995	Case-control Aged 4–18 months Sweden	308	Wheeze and breathlessness	Population sample (same area)	Wheeze (inpatients)
Gürkan et al. 2000b	Case-control Aged 2–18 months Turkey	58	Symptoms plus RSV antigen	Infants without respiratory distress seen in the emergency room	RSV (outpatients)
Hjern et al. 2000	Record linkage Aged 0–24 months Sweden	350,648 patient-years[‡]	ICD-9[§] 480–487 at discharge	All children in 3 metropolitan areas (1990–1994)	PN (inpatients)
Hospitalizations for URIs or LRIs					
Rantakallio 1978	Cohort Aged <5 years Finland	3,644	URI or LRI admission	Birth cohort drawn from smoking and nonsmoking mothers	URI or LRI (inpatients)
Ogston et al. 1985	Cohort Aged <12 months United Kingdom	1,542	URI or LRI admission	Population-based birth cohort	URI or LRI (inpatients)
Chen 1994	Cohort Aged <18 months China	3,285	Any respiratory admission	2 population birth cohorts	URI or LRI (inpatients)

*NHANES III = Third National Health and Nutrition Examination Survey.
†ALSPAC = Avon Longitudinal Study of Pregnancy and Childhood.
‡Patient-years only were reported in this study.
§ICD-9 = *International Classification of Diseases, 9th Revision* (USDHHS 1989).

Table 6.2   Unadjusted relative risks (odds ratios) of illness associated with parental smoking

Study	Cases/ controls	Dose- response relationship	Outcome	Odds ratio for smoking (95% confidence interval)			
				Either parent	Mother	Father/other*	Both parents
Community studies of lower respiratory illnesses (LRIs)							
Leeder et al. 1976	239/1,835	Yes; number of smokers	Acute bronchitis (BR)/ pneumonia (PN)	1.96 (1.38–2.80)	NR†	NR	2.79 (1.87–4.15)
Gardner et al. 1984	31/‡	NR	LRI	1.25 (0.81–1.93)	NR	NR	NR
Fergusson and Horwood 1985	204/940	Yes; cigarettes/ day by the mother	BR/PN	1.56 (1.15–2.12)	1.83 (1.35–2.49)	1.04 (0.65–1.65)	1.83 (1.22–2.74)
Ferris et al. 1985	820/7,708	Yes; cigarettes/ day by the mother	LRI	1.85 (1.56–2.20)	1.69 (1.47–1.96)	1.51 (1.22–1.86)	1.36 (1.11–1.66)
Pedreira et al. 1985	221/‡	NR	LRI	1.27 (0.97–1.66)	NR	NR	NR
McConnochie and Roghmann 1986b	53/159	NR	Acute bronchiolitis (BL)	3.21 (1.42–7.25)	2.33 (1.19–4.57)	NR	NR
Chen et al. 1988a	925/1,302	Yes; cigarettes/ day in the home	BR/PN	1.25 (1.03–1.52)	None smoked	1.25 (1.03–1.52)	NR
Hayes et al. 1989	20/60	NR	BL	3.86 (0.81–18.4)	NR	NR	NR
Wright et al. 1991	256/541	Yes; cigarettes/ day by the mother	LRI	NR	1.52§ (1.07–2.15)	NR	NR
Forastiere et al. 1992	473/2,324	NR	LRI	1.32 (1.05–1.65)	1.21 (0.99–1.48)	1.25 (0.97–1.62)	1.34 (1.02–1.75)
Hakansson and Carlsson 1992	20/172	NR	BR/PN	3.25 (1.27–8.34)	NR	NR	NR
Marbury et al. 1996	1,107/‡	NR	LRI	NR	1.50§ (1.20–1.80)	NR	NR

Table 6.2   Continued

Study	Cases/ controls	Dose-response relationship	Outcome	Odds ratio for smoking (95% confidence interval)			
				Either parent	Mother	Father/other*	Both parents
Community studies of LRIs							
Richards et al. 1996	100/626	NR	LRI	1.75 (1.07–2.87)	2.18 (1.25–3.78)	NR	NR
Gergen et al. 1998	155/4,264	Yes; cigarettes/ day in the home	Chronic bronchitis	1.97 (1.42–2.61)	2.44△ (1.74–3.40)	NR	NR
Nuesslein et al. 1999	49/16	NR	LRI	1.08¶ (0.17–6.81)	0.87△,¶ (0.17–4.53)	NR	NR
Community studies of wheeze illnesses							
Fergusson and Horwood 1985	733/411	No; cigarettes/ day by the mother	Wheeze	1.32 (1.04–1.69)	1.43 (1.10–1.86)	1.09 (0.77–1.53)	1.50 (1.05–2.12)
Bisgaard et al. 1987	120/5,833	No; cigarettes/ day by the mother	Wheeze	NR	2.85 (1.93–4.19)	NR	NR
Chen et al. 1988a	78/2,149	NR	Wheeze	1.27 (0.71–2.28)	None smoked	1.27 (0.71–2.28)	NR
Burr et al. 1989	166/314	NR	Wheeze	2.04 (1.39–3.01)	2.25 (1.52–3.33)	1.38 (0.81–2.37)	NR
Lucas et al. 1990	175/602	NR	Wheeze	1.70 (1.19–2.42)	NR	NR	NR
Halken et al. 1991	59/217	NR	Wheeze	1.88 (0.97–3.63)	NR	NR	NR
Arshad et al. 1993	127/1,045	NR	Wheeze	NR	2.24 (1.51–3.32)	NR	NR
Tager et al. 1993	59/38	NR	Wheeze	NR	3.16 (1.24–8.04)	NR	NR
Martinez et al. 1995	247/515	NR	Wheeze	NR	2.07 (1.34–3.19)	NR	NR
Elder et al. 1996	76/449	Yes; cigarettes/ day by the mother	Wheeze	NR	1.98 (1.21–3.23)	NR	NR
Margolis et al. 1997	‡	NR	Wheeze	1.62**	NR	NR	NR

Table 6.2   Continued

Study	Cases/ controls	Dose- response relationship	Outcome	Odds ratio for smoking (95% confidence interval)			
				Either parent	Mother	Father/other*	Both parents
Community studies of wheeze illnesses							
Nafstad et al. 1997	271/2,777	Yes; cigarettes/ day by both parents	Bronchial obstruction	1.6¶ (1.3–2.1)	1.6¶ (1.0–2.6)	1.5¶ (1.1–2.2)	1.5¶ (1.0–2.2)
Baker et al. 1998; Lux et al. 2000	1,565/ 6,885	Yes; number of hours/ day of secondhand smoke exposure	Wheeze	1.32 (1.19–1.47)	1.55△ (1.36–1.77)	NR	NR
Gergen et al. 1998	197/4,222	Yes; cigarettes/ day in the home	Asthma	1.33 (0.99–1.77)	1.75△ (1.29–2.39)	NR	NR
	432/3,981	Yes; cigarettes/ day in the home	Wheeze	1.88 (1.54–2.29)	2.15△ (1.74–2.67)	NR	NR
Chen and Millar 1999	326/5,214	NR	Asthma	NR	1.56 (1.24–1.96)	NR	NR
Dezateux et al. 1999	28/73	NR	Wheeze	4.08 (1.12–14.9)	5.10 (1.97–13.3)	NR	NR
Gold et al. 1999	96/403	NR	Wheeze	NR	2.29§,△ (1.44–3.63)	p >0.05	NR
Karaman et al. 1999	38/30	NR	Wheeze	5.6 (1.9–15.9)	4.2△ (1.2–14.6)	NR	NR
Mrazek et al. 1999	14/136	NR	Wheeze	NR	1.5 (0.29–7.16)	NR	NR
Rusconi et al. 1999	1,892/ 14,441	NR	Wheeze	NR	1.55△ (1.37–1.74)	NR	NR
Yau et al. 1999	8/23	NR	Wheeze	1.04 (0.35–3.05)	NR	NR	NR
Diez et al. 2000	64/246	NR	Wheeze	2.0 (1.1–3.5)	NR	NR	NR
Young et al. 2000a	81/79	NR	Wheeze	NR	2.7△ (1.3–5.2)	NR	NR

Table 6.2   Continued

Study	Cases/ controls	Dose-response relationship	Outcome	Odds ratio for smoking (95% confidence interval)			
				Either parent	**Mother**	**Father/other***	**Both parents**
Community studies of upper and lower respiratory illnesses (U/LRIs)							
Ogston et al. 1987	486/1,056	No; number of smokers	U/LRIs	1.68 (1.33–2.11)	1.52 (1.22–1.89)	1.50 (1.12–2.01)	1.74 (1.33–2.27)
Woodward et al. 1990	200/200	NR	U/LRIs	NR	2.43§ (1.63–3.61)	NR	NR
Hospitalizations for LRIs							
Harlap and Davies 1974	1,049/ 9,623	Yes; cigarettes/ day by the mother	BR/PN	NR	1.43 (1.18–1.75)	NR	NR
Sims et al. 1978	35/35	NR	BL	NR	2.65 (0.99–7.11)	NR	NR
Mok and Simpson 1982	200/200	NR	BR/PN	NR	1.26 (0.83–1.92)	NR	NR
Ekwo et al. 1983	53/1,086	Inverse to the number of smokers	LRI	2.09 (1.12–3.89)	1.32 (0.74–2.32)	2.30 (1.13–4.70)	1.59 (0.74–3.44)
Hall et al. 1984	29/58	NR	BL	4.78 (1.76–13.0)	NR	NR	NR
Taylor and Wadsworth 1987	434/ 12,293	Yes; cigarettes/ day by the mother	LRI	1.46 (1.19–1.79)	1.63 (1.34–1.97)	1.05 (0.78–1.41)	1.69 (1.33–2.14)
Anderson et al. 1988	102/199	NR	BL	1.99§ (p <0.05)††	NR	NR	NR
Stern et al. 1989b	NR	NR	LRI	NR	1.85§ (1.53–2.23)	NR	NR
Reese et al. 1992	39/57	Yes; urinary cotinine	BL	2.15 (0.76–6.10)	2.66 (1.15–6.15)	1.27 (0.38–4.22)	3.29 (1.77–6.14)
Jin and Rossignol 1993	164/843	Yes; cigarettes/ day in the home	BR/PN	1.78 (1.18–2.68)	None smoked	1.78 (1.18–2.68)	NR

Table 6.2   Continued

Study	Cases/controls	Dose-response relationship	Outcome	Odds ratio for smoking (95% confidence interval)			
				Either parent	Mother	Father/other*	Both parents
Hospitalizations for LRIs							
Victora et al. 1994	510/510	No; cigarettes/day in the home	PN	0.94 (0.72–1.22)	1.02 (0.79–1.30)	0.89 (0.64–1.24)	0.94 (0.69–1.29)
Rylander et al. 1995	112/196	Yes; urinary cotinine	Wheeze	2.17 (1.38–3.59)	2.04 (1.26–3.28)	1.77 (0.85–3.66)	2.23 (1.23–4.05)
Gürkan et al. 2000b	28/30	NR	Respiratory synctial virus	2.0 (0.6–6.8)	3.6 (0.7–18.3)	1.1 (0.2–4.8)	2.3 (0.5–10.1)
Hjern et al. 2000	‡	NR	LRI	NR	1.3^Δ (1.2–1.4)	NR	NR
Hospitalizations for URIs or LRIs							
Rantakallio 1978	490/3,154	NR	URI or LRI	NR	1.89 (1.55–2.30)	NR	NR
Ogston et al. 1985	41/1,501	Yes; number of smokers	URI or LRI	1.94 (0.94–3.99)	2.68 (1.41–5.10)	0.87 (0.29–2.56)	2.76 (1.28–5.96)
Chen 1994	239/3,046	No; cigarettes/day in the home	URI or LRI	1.49 (1.05–2.10)	None smoked	1.49 (1.05–2.10)	NR

*In households where the mother did not smoke (compared with smoking by neither parent).

†NR = Data were not reported.

‡Results were published as person-time incidence rates; rate ratios, rather than odds ratios, are shown.

§Odds ratio or relative risk was cited in the paper without tabulated numerical data. (Elsewhere, odds ratios were calculated from tabulated numbers or percentages.)

^ΔMaternal smoking during pregnancy. (Elsewhere, maternal postnatal smoking was used.)

¶Adjusted rates only were available (see Table 6.4 for factors adjusted for).

**Based on children exposed to ≤10 cigarettes/day vs. none, as so few were exposed more heavily. Confidence limits for the meta-analysis were assumed to be based on confidence limits for the adjusted analysis (1.20–2.18).

††95% confidence interval was estimated at 1.0–3.96 for purposes of the meta-analysis.

Figure 6.1   Odds ratios for the effect of smoking by either parent on lower respiratory illnesses during infancy

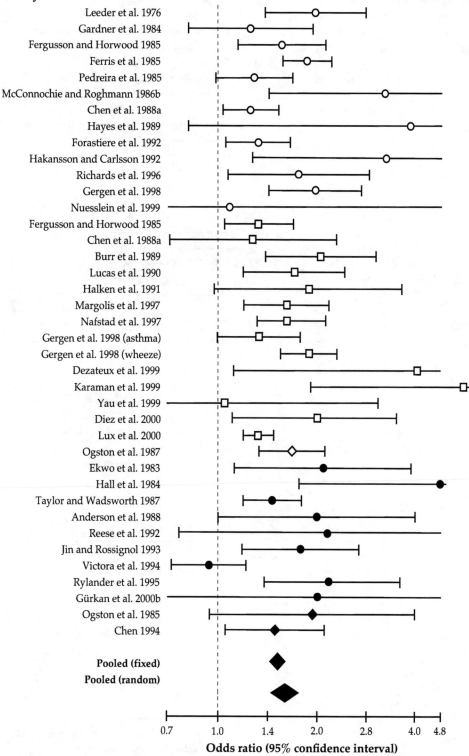

Note: Individual studies are denoted with the following symbols:
 Circles = Studies of lower respiratory illnesses.
 Squares = Studies of wheeze illnesses.
 Diamonds = Studies of upper and lower respiratory illnesses.
 Open symbols = Community studies.
 Closed symbols = Studies of hospitalized illnesses.

Figure 6.2   Odds ratios for the effect of maternal smoking on lower respiratory illnesses during infancy

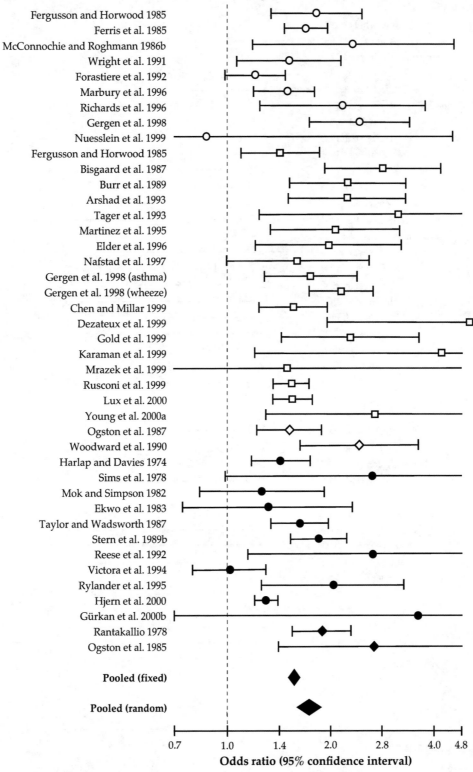

Note: Individual studies are denoted with the following symbols:
  Circles = Studies of lower respiratory illnesses.
  Squares = Studies of wheeze illnesses.
  Diamonds = Studies of upper and lower respiratory illnesses.
  Open symbols = Community studies.
  Closed symbols = Studies of hospitalized illnesses.

Figure 6.3   Odds ratios for the effect of paternal smoking on lower respiratory illnesses during infancy

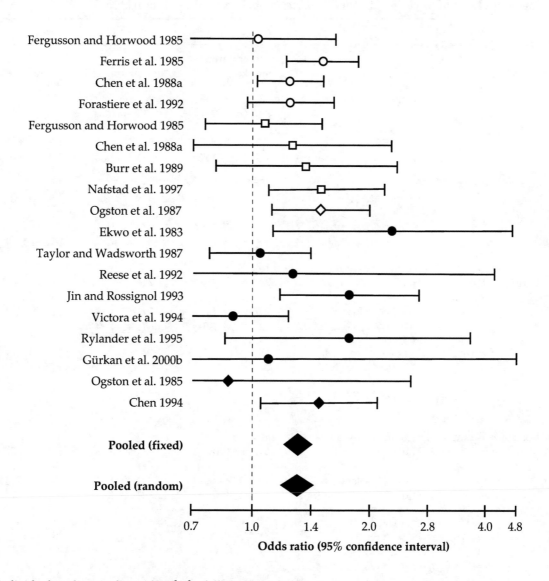

Note: Individual studies are denoted with the following symbols:
 Circles = Studies of lower respiratory illnesses.
 Squares = Studies of wheeze illnesses.
 Diamonds = Studies of upper and lower respiratory illnesses.
 Open symbols = Community studies.
 Closed symbols = Studies of hospitalized illnesses.

Table 6.3   Pooled odds ratios (ORs), 95% confidence intervals (CIs), and heterogeneity tests from meta-analyses of lower respiratory illnesses associated with parental smoking

Study description		Either parent smoked	Mother smoked	Father smoked
		Findings		
All studies	Number of studies	38	41	18
	Heterogeneity χ^2	73.1 (p <0.001)	110.5 (p <0.001)	19.3 (p = 0.311)
	ORs (95% CIs) (fixed)	1.51 (1.44–1.59)	1.56 (1.51–1.62)	1.31 (1.20–1.42)
	ORs (95% CIs) (random)	1.59 (1.47–1.73)	1.72 (1.59–1.86)	1.31 (1.19–1.43)
Excluded studies with upper respiratory illnesses	Number of studies	35	37	15
	Heterogeneity χ^2	71.8 (p <0.001)	99.0 (p <0.001)	17.2 (p = 0.247)
	ORs (95% CIs) (fixed)	1.50 (1.43–1.58)	1.54 (1.48–1.61)	1.28 (1.17–1.40)
	ORs (95% CIs) (random)	1.59 (1.46–1.74)	1.70 (1.56–1.84)	1.28 (1.15–1.42)
Community studies of lower respiratory illnesses (LRIs), bronchitis, and/or pneumonia	Number of studies	13	9	4
	Heterogeneity χ^2	24.7 (p = 0.016)	18.2 (p = 0.020)	3.03 (p = 0.387)
	ORs (95% CIs) (fixed)	1.55 (1.42–1.69)	1.61 (1.47–1.75)	1.31 (1.16–1.48)
	ORs (95% CIs) (random)	1.60 (1.38–1.84)	1.66 (1.42–1.94)	*
Community studies of wheeze illnesses	Number of studies	13	17	4
	Heterogeneity χ^2	23.7 (p = 0.022)	29.9 (p = 0.018)	1.72 (p = 0.633)
	ORs (95% CIs) (fixed)	1.48 (1.38–1.59)	1.71 (1.60–1.83)	1.29 (1.05–1.59)
	ORs (95% CIs) (random)	1.57 (1.39–1.79)	1.85 (1.66–2.06)	*
Studies based on surveys that relied on recall over many years	Number of studies	4	6	3
	Heterogeneity χ^2	6.0 (p = 0.109)	12.08 (p = 0.034)	3.02 (p = 0.221)
	ORs (95% CIs) (fixed)	1.66 (1.46–1.89)	1.58 (1.47–1.71)	1.43 (1.22–1.68)
	ORs (95% CIs) (random)	1.65 (1.33–2.06)	1.58 (1.38–1.81)	*
All studies excluding those that were based on recall over many years	Number of studies	34	35	15
	Heterogeneity χ^2	64.1 (p <0.001)	98.3 (p <0.001)	14.4 (p = 0.419)
	ORs (95% CIs) (fixed)	1.49 (1.41–1.57)	1.56 (1.49–1.63)	1.26 (1.14–1.39)
	ORs (95% CIs) (random)	1.58 (1.45–1.73)	1.77 (1.62–1.94)	1.26 (1.14–1.39)
Hospitalizations for LRIs, bronchitis, bronchiolitis, or pneumonia	Number of studies	9	11	7
	Heterogeneity χ^2	22.5 (p = 0.004)	28.4 (p = 0.002)	11.8 (p = 0.067)
	ORs (95% CIs) (fixed)	1.46 (1.27–1.66)	1.39 (1.31–1.47)	1.20 (1.0–1.44)
	ORs (95% CIs) (random)	1.73 (1.31–2.28)	1.49 (1.29–1.73)	1.31 (0.98–1.76)

*The number of studies was too small for reliable random effects modeling; there was no significant heterogeneity of effects.

Gürkan et al. 2000b; Hjern et al. 2000). Four did not distinguish between different forms of chest illnesses (Ekwo et al. 1983; Taylor and Wadsworth 1987; Stern et al. 1989b; Hjern et al. 2000), four examined bronchitis and/or pneumonia (Harlap and Davies 1974; Mok and Simpson 1982; Jin and Rossignol 1993; Victora et al. 1994), and six focused on hospital admissions for wheeze illnesses (Rylander et al. 1995) or for bronchiolitis with (Sims et al. 1978; Hall et al. 1984; Gürkan et al. 2000b) or without (Anderson et al. 1988; Reese et al. 1992) confirmation of respiratory syncytial virus (RSV) infection.

One cohort study included in the meta-analysis presented detailed findings only for hospital admissions of children from birth to five years of age, and not just for early life (Taylor and Wadsworth 1987). Data presented by age at admission suggest a similar strength of association between maternal smoking and admissions across this age span for bronchitis or pneumonia. The results for all ages were therefore included in the meta-analyses.

Only one of these studies, which was carried out in Brazil, did not find an elevated risk associated with parental smoking (Table 6.2 and Figures 6.1–6.3) (Victora et al. 1994). Table 6.3 summarizes the results of the meta-analyses; the pooled ORs are similar in magnitude to those derived from community studies.

One case-control study from South Africa (Kossove 1982) and one from the United Kingdom (Spencer et al. 1996) were excluded from the quantitative overview because they present only general results for a smoky atmosphere in the home and not specifically for secondhand smoke. In the South African study, the principal source of exposure was wood smoke. In the British study, infants admitted with suspected bronchiolitis were almost three times more likely to have a smoky atmosphere recorded by health visitors after visiting the home when the infant was one month of age (OR = 2.93 [95 percent CI, 1.95–4.41]).

Studies of Upper and Lower Respiratory Illnesses Combined

Five studies related parental smoking to all respiratory illnesses without distinguishing upper from lower respiratory tract diagnoses (Table 6.1) (Rantakallio 1978; Ogston et al. 1985, 1987; Woodward et al. 1990; Chen 1994). Two of these studies were based in the community (Ogston et al. 1987; Woodward et al. 1990), three related to hospitalizations for respiratory illnesses (Rantakallio 1978; Ogston et al. 1985; Chen 1994), and one (Chen 1994) synthesized the results of three earlier papers (Chen et al. 1986, 1988b; Chen 1989).

The findings of these studies are summarized in Table 6.2. Their inclusion in the overall meta-analysis changes the estimates of the effects only slightly (Table 6.3).

Effects of Retrospective Recall

For the six studies based on surveys of school-age children that relied on parental recall of LRIs during early childhood (Ekwo et al. 1983; Ferris et al. 1985; Stern et al. 1989b; Forastiere et al. 1992; Richards et al. 1996; Rusconi et al. 1999), separate meta-analyses were carried out and overall estimates that excluded these studies were calculated (Table 6.3). A separate analysis was carried out because this outcome measure is subject to a greater degree of misclassification than that of a prospective recording of illnesses. There was no clear pattern of differences for the findings of this group of studies compared with the other groups. Excluding the six studies from the overall meta-analysis had only a small effect on the pooled ORs.

Independence of Potential Confounding

About half of the cohort studies, but only a quarter of the case-control or cross-sectional studies, included estimates of the effects of parental smoking both with and without adjustment for potential confounding variables. Although different potential confounding variables were controlled for in each study, the effects of parental smoking changed little or only modestly after adjustment for the potential confounders measured in these studies (Table 6.4).

Exposure-Response Relationships

Of the 22 studies that present evidence of an exposure-response relationship within smoking families, 17 found a statistically significant relationship either with the number of smokers or with the amount smoked in the household, or specifically with the amount of maternal smoking (Table 6.2). However, a formal dose-response meta-analysis could not be carried out because of the nature of the data. In contrast, the risk when both parents smoked compared with smoking by either parent only was not substantially greater. Thirteen studies compared smoking by both parents with smoking by neither parent (Leeder et al. 1976; Ekwo et al. 1983; Fergusson and Horwood 1985; Ferris et al. 1985; Ogston et al. 1985, 1987; Taylor and Wadsworth 1987; Forastiere et al. 1992; Reese et al. 1992; Victora et al. 1994; Rylander et al. 1995; Nafstad et al. 1997; Gürkan et al. 2000b). The pooled OR is 1.67 (95 percent CI, 1.42–1.96).

Table 6.4   **Effects of adjusting for potential confounders of illness associated with parental smoking**

Study	Exposure	Factors adjusted for*	Outcome	Odds ratio Unadjusted	Adjusted
		Community studies of lower respiratory illnesses (LRIs)			
Leeder et al. 1976	Both parents vs. none	Family history of chest symptoms, gender, siblings, sibling illnesses	Acute bronchitis (BR)/pneumonia (PN)	2.95	2.78
Gardner et al. 1984	NR†	None	LRI	NR	NR
Fergusson and Horwood 1985	NR	‡	BR/PN	NR	NR
Ferris et al. 1985	NR	None	LRI	NR	NR
Pedreira et al. 1985	NR	None	LRI	NR	NR
McConnochie and Roghmann 1986b	Mother smoked	(Age), socioeconomic status (SES), breastfeeding, siblings, crowding, family history of asthma	Acute bronchiolitis (BL)	2.33	2.68
Chen et al. 1988a	Mother did not smoke, but others smoked ≥10 cigarettes/day	Gender, birth weight, day care, education, cooking fuel	BR/PN	1.33	1.31
Hayes et al. 1989	NR	(Age)	BL	NR	NR
Wright et al. 1991	Mother smoked ≥10 cigarettes/ day	Family history of chest illness, season of birth, day care, crowding	LRI	1.82	1.74
Forastiere et al. 1992	Either parent smoked	Age, gender, area, SES, siblings, domestic crowding, heating	LRI	1.32	1.3
Hakansson and Carlsson 1992	NR	None	BR/PN	NR	NR
Marbury et al. 1996	Mother smoked	Family history of asthma, breastfeeding, birth order, day care, housing	LRI	§	1.5
Richards et al. 1996	NR	None	LRI	NR	NR
Gergen et al. 1998	Mother smoked prenatally	Age, gender, ethnicity, birth weight, day care, family history of allergy	Chronic bronchitis (CBR)	2.44	2.2
	≥20 cigarettes/ day in the home vs. none	Age, gender, ethnicity, birth weight, day care, family history of allergy	CBR	3.0	2.5
Nuesslein et al. 1999	NR	None	NR	NR	NR

Table 6.4   Continued

Study	Exposure	Factors adjusted for*	Outcome	Odds ratio Unadjusted	Odds ratio Adjusted
community		**Community studies of wheeze illnesses**			
Fergusson and Horwood 1985	NR	‡	Wheeze	NR	NR
Bisgaard et al. 1987	Mother smoked ≥20 cigarettes/day	Gender, SES	Wheeze	2.85	2.7
Chen et al. 1988a	Family members who smoked ≥20 cigarettes/day	None	Wheeze	NR	NR
Burr et al. 1989	NR	None	Wheeze	NR	NR
Lucas et al. 1990	NR	None	Wheeze	NR	NR
Halken et al. 1991	Any smoking	Gender, SES	Wheeze	1.88	2.4
Arshad et al. 1993	Mother smoked	Gender, low birth weight, family history of allergy, season of birth△	Wheeze	2.24	2.2
Tager et al. 1993	NR	None	Wheeze	NR	NR
Martinez et al. 1995	Mother smoked	Gender, ethnicity, past allergy, family history of asthma	Wheeze	2.07	2.25
Elder et al. 1996	Mother smoked	Duration of breastfeeding	Wheeze	1.98	1.77
Margolis et al. 1997	≤10 cigarettes/day in child's presence	Age, season, SES, crowding, family history of respiratory disease, day care	Wheeze	1.6	1.5
Nafstad et al. 1997	Secondhand smoke in the home	Gender, family history of atopy, duration of breastfeeding, day care, having siblings	Wheeze	1.52	1.6
Baker et al. 1998	Mother smoked prenatally at 8 months	(Age), housing tenure, mother's education, persons per room, parity, breastfeeding	Wheeze	NR	1.38

Table 6.4   Continued

Study	Exposure	Factors adjusted for*	Outcome	Odds ratio Unadjusted	Odds ratio Adjusted
Community studies of wheeze illnesses					
Gergen et al. 1998	Mother smoked prenatally	Age, gender, ethnicity, birth weight, day care, family history of allergy	Asthma	1.75	1.7
	Mother smoked prenatally	Age, gender, ethnicity, birth weight, day care, family history of allergy	Wheeze	2.15	2.1
	>20 cigarettes/ day in the home vs. none	Age, gender, ethnicity, birth weight, day care, family history of allergy	Asthma	1.63	2.0
	>20 cigarettes/ day in the home vs. none	Age, gender, ethnicity, birth weight, day care, family history of allergy	Wheeze	2.26	2.7
Chen and Millar 1999	Mother was a current smoker	Age, gender, mother's age and education, family type, income, birth weight, gestational age	Asthma	1.56	1.3
Dezateux et al. 1999	NR	None	Wheeze	NR	NR
Gold et al. 1999	Mother smoked prenatally	LRI, low birth weight, maternal asthma, dog exposure, cockroach allergen, ethnicity, income	Wheeze	2.29	1.61
Karaman et al. 1999	NR	None	NR	NR	NR
Mrazek et al. 1999	NR	None	NR	NR	NR
Rusconi et al. 1999	Mother smoked prenatally	(Age), gender, area, father's education, respondent to questionnaire, family history of asthma, birth weight, maternal age, breastfeeding, number of siblings, day care, child's eczema or rhinitis	Transient wheeze	1.48	1.33
	Mother smoked prenatally	(Age), gender, area, father's education, respondent to questionnaire, family history of asthma, birth weight, maternal age, breastfeeding, number of siblings, day care, child's eczema or rhinitis	Persistent wheeze	1.71	1.77
Yau et al. 1999	NR	None	NR	NR	NR

Table 6.4   Continued

Study	Exposure	Factors adjusted for*	Outcome	Odds ratio	
				Unadjusted	Adjusted
Community studies of wheeze illnesses					
Diez et al. 2000	NR	None	NR	NR	NR
Lux et al. 2000⁑	Mother smoked prenatally	(Age), housing tenure, mother's education, persons per room, parity, breastfeeding	Wheeze	1.55	NR
Young et al. 2000a	Mother smoked prenatally	NR	Wheeze	2.7	NR
Community studies of upper and lower respiratory illnesses (U/LRIs)					
Ogston et al. 1987	Both parents vs. none	Mother's age, heating fuel	U/LRIs	1.74	1.54
Woodward et al. 1990	Mother smoked	Gender, siblings, family history of respiratory disease, day care, SES, stress, breastfeeding	U/LRIs	2.43	2.06
Hospitalizations for LRIs					
Harlap and Davies 1974	Mother smoked	Birth weight, SES	BR/PN	NR	NR
Sims et al. 1978	NR	(Age, gender, SES)	BL	NR	NR
Mok and Simpson 1982	NR	(Age, height, school)	BR/PN	NR	NR
Ekwo et al. 1983	NR	Gas cooking	LRI	NR	NR
Hall et al. 1984	NR	(Age, gender, race, season, form of health insurance)	BL	NR	NR
Taylor and Wadsworth 1987	NR	None	LRI	NR	NR
Anderson et al. 1988	NR	(Age, gender)	PN/BL	NR	NR
Stern et al. 1989b	NR	None	LRI	NR	NR
Reese et al. 1992	NR	None	BL	NR	NR
Jin and Rossignol 1993	Others smoked ≥20 cigarettes/ day	Gender, breastfeeding, birth weight, education, maternal age, cooking fuel	BR/PN	2.0	2.4
Victora et al. 1994	NR	(Age)	PN	NR	NR
Rylander et al. 1995	Both parents smoked	(Age), family history of asthma, duration of breastfeeding	Wheeze	2.23	2.0
Gürkan et al. 2000b	NR	None	NR	NR	NR

Table 6.4   Continued

Study	Exposure	Factors adjusted for*	Outcome	Odds ratio Unadjusted	Odds ratio Adjusted
		Hospitalizations for LRIs			
Hjern et al. 2000	Mother smoked prenatally	Age, gender, maternal education, living in apartment, single parent, country of birth, number of siblings	LRI	1.42	1.3
		Hospitalizations for URIs or LRIs			
Rantakallio 1978	NR	None	URI or LRI	NR	NR
Ogston et al. 1985	NR	None	URI or LRI	NR	NR
Chen 1994	Any smoking	Low birth weight	URI or LRI	1.49	1.48

*Matching variables are in parentheses.

[†]NR = Data were not reported.

[‡]An analysis of incidence to 1 year of age (Fergusson et al. 1980) shows that smoking effects are independent of breastfeeding and housing.

[§]No unadjusted relative risk was reported.

[Δ]Additional adjustments for family history of asthma, pets, and SES (in Arshad and Hide 1992); matched for incidence to 1 year of age.

[¶]Same study as Baker et al. 1998 but with different definitions of exposure.

Biomarkers of Exposure

Cotinine was measured as an objective marker of tobacco smoke exposure in four studies that used urine (Reese et al. 1992; Rylander et al. 1995), serum (Gürkan et al. 2000b), or meconium (Nuesslein et al. 1999). In all four studies, cotinine levels were significantly higher in the case group. These results are consistent with another small case-control study of emergency room visits for wheeze illnesses (Duff et al. 1993), which measured urinary cotinine but did not report details of parental smoking patterns.

Specific Respiratory Diagnoses

Some studies assessed the effects of parental smoking on specifically diagnosed illnesses. One study addressed tracheitis and bronchitis (Pedreira et al. 1985), another examined wheeze and pneumonia but not bronchitis or bronchiolitis (Marbury et al. 1996), and the NHANES III study found stronger effects for chronic bronchitis, asthma, and wheeze than for pneumonia (Gergen et al. 1998). One cohort study explicitly distinguished between LRIs with and without wheeze (Wright et al. 1991). The proportion of cases exposed to maternal smoking (defined as

≥20 cigarettes per day) was 14 percent in each subgroup. This finding is not entirely consistent with the pooled ORs obtained from community studies that suggest a stronger effect from maternal smoking specifically in studies of wheeze than in studies that included a broader range of chest illnesses (Table 6.3).

Seven case-control studies that focused specifically on bronchiolitis or illnesses associated with evidence of RSV infection yielded a somewhat stronger effect compared with studies of other outcomes (Sims et al. 1978; Hall et al. 1984; McConnochie and Roghmann 1986b; Anderson et al. 1988; Hayes et al. 1989; Spencer et al. 1996; Gürkan et al. 2000b). This finding, however, may reflect a positive publication bias (see "Publication Bias and Meta-Analyses" later in this chapter).

Parental Smoking at Different Ages

The early report by Colley and colleagues (1974) suggested that the effects of parental smoking on bronchitis and pneumonia incidence were most marked in the first year of life (OR = 1.96 [95 percent CI, 1.30–2.99]), and declined thereafter with the increasing age of the child to an inverse relationship in the fifth year. Results from the Dunedin (New Zealand) cohort showed a similar pattern, with a slightly greater effect in the first year than in the second year (Fergusson et al. 1981) and little evidence of an association with consultation for bronchitis or pneumonia after two years of age (Fergusson and Horwood 1985). One study reported a decline in the risk ratio for pneumonia admissions and maternal smoking during pregnancy from between 1.2 to 1.3 up to three years of age and to 1.0 at three to four years of age, but a formal test of statistical significance was not carried out for the trend (Hjern et al. 2000).

A study in Shanghai documented that the effects of smoking by persons other than the mother on hospitalizations for respiratory diseases were stronger for admissions before 6 months of age than for admissions at 7 through 18 months of age (Chen et al. 1988a). However, a significantly increased risk persisted after six months of age for children exposed to more than 10 cigarettes per day in the home (incidence ratio = 1.83 [95 percent CI, 1.03–3.24]). In the 1970 British cohort, the effects of maternal smoking on hospitalizations for wheeze illnesses, bronchitis, or pneumonia were similar at all ages up to five years (Taylor and Wadsworth 1987).

The ALSPAC is a cohort study that examined and measured both maternal smoking during pregnancy and secondhand smoke exposure during the first six months of life. The study measured the number of hours the infant was exposed as a predictor of wheeze between 6 and 18 months of age and from 18 through 30 months of age (Lux et al. 2000). There was no evidence of any reduction in the ORs across age strata. In the Isle of Wight cohort study (Arshad et al. 1993), ORs of asthmatic wheeze with maternal smoking declined from 2.5 (95 percent CI, 1.7–3.7) at one year of age to 2.2 (95 percent CI, 1.5–3.4) at two years of age and to 1.2 (95 percent CI, 0.3–2.7) at four years of age (Tariq et al. 2000).

In a Swedish study based on record linkage (Table 6.1), the authors reported a clear decrease with increasing age of the child in the OR for hospital admissions for asthma associated with maternal smoking during pregnancy (Hjern et al. 1999). The OR was 1.6 (95 percent CI, 1.4–1.8) at two years of age, but was lower and not significantly different from 1 at three to six years of age. In the NHANES III study (Gergen et al. 1998), patterns of effect by age varied with the outcome. The OR for chronic bronchitis in children under two years of age (2.2 [95 percent CI, 1.6–3.0]) was higher than the OR for children three to five years of age (1.0 [95 percent CI, 0.6–1.8]). ORs for the younger age group were also higher for wheeze (2.1 [95 percent CI, 1.5–2.9] versus 1.3 [95 percent CI,

0.8–2.0], respectively), but not for diagnosed asthma (1.7 [95 percent CI, 1.1–2.6] versus 1.7 [95 percent CI, 1.1–2.8], respectively).

Susceptible Subgroups

Infants born prematurely are one group potentially at an increased risk from parental smoking because of the still immature lungs at birth and, for some, the development of bronchopulmonary dysplasia after birth. The effects of parental smoking on early respiratory illnesses were reported in two controlled trials (Burr et al. 1989; Lucas et al. 1990), three cohort studies (Elder et al. 1996; Gold et al. 1999; Mrazek et al. 1999), and one nested case-control study (Diez et al. 2000) that recruited infants at high risk based on prematurity (Lucas et al. 1990; Elder et al. 1996), a parental history of allergy (Burr et al. 1989; Gold et al. 1999; Mrazek et al. 1999), or both (Diez et al. 2000). The ORs obtained from these studies are within the general range of the data (Table 6.2) and have therefore been included in the meta-analyses.

Only one study permits a direct comparison between high- and low-risk infants (Chen 1994). In two Chinese cohorts, an adverse effect of household smoking on hospitalizations for a respiratory disease was evident among both low birth weight (<2.5 kilograms) (OR = 6.87 [95 percent CI, 0.89–53.0]) and normal birth weight (OR = 1.36 [95 percent CI, 0.96–1.93]) infants. There was an indication of a significant effect modification by birth weight (test for interaction: p = 0.06).

Smoking by Other Household Members

The effects of smoking by other household members when the mother did not smoke are summarized in Tables 6.2 and 6.3. These findings are derived from three studies in China (Chen et al. 1988a; Jin and Rossignol 1993; Chen 1994) that included nonsmoking mothers, and 14 studies from westernized countries with data only for paternal smoking. The results are quantitatively consistent and only two of the OR estimates are less than unity. The pooled OR obtained in the meta-analysis is 1.31 (95 percent CI, 1.19–1.43). In the Chinese studies, this effect is independent of birth weight and a range of other potential confounding factors (Jin and Rossignol 1993; Chen 1994). Another study from Malaysia, which was not included in the meta-analysis because the age range of the participants was one to five years, also found an increased risk when the fathers smoked and the mothers did not report smoking (OR = 1.20 [95 percent CI, 0.86–1.67]) (Quah et al. 2000). A large national survey from Australia with an age range from birth to four years reported a significant risk of asthma associated with maternal smoking (adjusted OR = 1.52 [95 percent CI, 1.19–1.94]); there was evidence of a dose-response relationship, but no effect from paternal smoking (OR = 0.77 [95 percent CI, 0.60–0.98]) when adjusted for maternal smoking (Lister and Jorm 1998).

Prenatal Versus Postnatal Exposure

Few studies have evaluated the effects of prenatal and postnatal maternal smoking in the same sample. In western countries, too few mothers change their smoking habits in the perinatal period to offer the statistical power to reliably separate prenatal from postnatal effects. For example, in a large study based on a national British cohort, half of the children were born to mothers who had smoked during pregnancy (Taylor and Wadsworth 1987). Only 8 percent of those mothers subsequently quit, and 6 percent of the prenatal nonsmokers smoked after the child was born. The rate of having a hospitalization for LRI differed between these two groups, but not significantly (5.9 percent for those whose mothers smoked only during pregnancy versus 3.1 percent for those whose mothers smoked only after the child's birth; OR = 1.94 [95 percent CI, 0.96–3.94]). Postnatal smoking by mothers who did not smoke during pregnancy compared with lifetime nonsmoking mothers increased the risk, but not significantly (OR = 1.36 [95 percent CI, 0.73–2.54]). The magnitude of the effect is consistent with the pooled effect in this study and in other studies when only the father smoked (Table 6.3). More recent evidence for the independent effects of prenatal and postnatal maternal smoking comes from the ALSPAC cohort study (Lux et al. 2000). The effects of maternal smoking during pregnancy were compared with those of secondhand smoke exposure by assessing the number of hours the mother smoked in the child's presence and by including both prenatal and postnatal smoking in the same logistic regression model. For wheeze illnesses occurring between 18 and 30 months of age, independent effects were found for each smoking pattern: ORs of 1.19 (95 percent CI, 1.02–1.39) for prenatal maternal smoking and 1.17 (95 percent CI, 1.03–1.32) for postnatal secondhand smoke exposure. These effects were adjusted for the other exposure as well as for multiple other potential confounding variables.

The reported ORs in the NHANES III survey for diagnosed asthma, chronic bronchitis, wheeze, and pneumonia were similar for prenatal and postnatal maternal smoking (Gergen et al. 1998). The authors noted the difficulty of distinguishing between the two time periods and did not assess the independent effects of smoking by fathers only.

One controlled intervention study (the control arm is included in the meta-analysis) (Margolis et al. 1997) monitored the incidence of acute LRI after an intervention that was designed to reduce postnatal tobacco smoke exposure (Greenberg et al. 1994). Among 581 infants followed to six months of age, there was no difference in the incidence of episodes of cough, wheeze, or rattling in the chest between the intervention group (1.6 episodes per year of observation) and the control group (1.5 episodes per year of observation). However, the effectiveness of the intervention in reducing tobacco smoke exposure was uncertain because the mean cotinine levels did not differ between the study groups despite a reduction in reported tobacco smoke exposure of infants in the intervention group.

Publication Bias and Meta-Analyses

Publication bias might occur if studies were more likely to be published that were "positive" (i.e., with statistically significant increases in risk), or that tended to show greater effect estimates of secondhand smoke ("Use of Meta-Analysis" in Chapter 1). Figure 6.1 suggests evidence of such a bias because there are few small studies with wide confidence limits below the pooled estimate of effect, an interpretation confirmed formally by Begg's test (Begg and Mazumdar 1994) for a nonparametric correlation between effect estimates and their standard errors (p = 0.030 after continuity correction). Egger's test (Egger et al. 1997) provides even stronger evidence for a publication bias (p = 0.002). Maternal smoking data also showed evidence of a publication bias (Begg's test, p = 0.221; Egger's test, p <0.001). For smoking by fathers only, there was no evidence of heterogeneity in the ORs and no evidence of a publication bias (Begg's test, p = 0.880; Egger's test, p = 0.890), perhaps reflecting the fact that publication was unlikely to hinge on the presentation or significance of the data for paternal smoking.

One approach that mitigates the consequences of any publication bias is to restrict analyses to the largest studies; for this sensitivity analysis, all studies with more than 800 cases were selected. For maternal smoking, there were six studies with a pooled random effects estimate of 1.49 (95 percent CI, 1.36–1.64). For smoking by either parent, such an analysis was not possible. Of only three large studies that provided estimates, one Chinese study included only fathers who smoked (Chen et al. 1988a), and the findings of the other two studies were too divergent in their estimated ORs of 1.85 (Ferris et al. 1985) and 1.32 (Lux et al. 2000).

Three studies (Fergusson and Horwood 1985; Chen et al. 1988a; Gergen et al. 1998) appear in more than one row in Table 6.2 and were thus included as separate and independent studies in the meta-analysis. However, a sensitivity analysis confirmed that restricting the inclusion of each study to its most frequent outcome had little effect on the pooled estimates.

Evidence Synthesis

The finding of an association between parental smoking and LRI is consistent across diverse study populations and study designs, methods of case ascertainment, and diagnostic groupings (Table 6.2). The association cannot be attributed to confounding or publication bias. Only two studies found an inverse association. One small study that reported an inverse association for maternal smoking had wide confidence limits and a positive association with cotinine levels in meconium (Nuesslein et al. 1999). A study from Brazil found an inverse association with pneumonia (Victora et al. 1994). Studies in developing countries generally have tended not to find an increased risk associated with exposure of infants and children to parental smoking. This pattern may reflect the different nature of LRIs in developing countries where bacteria are key pathogens and there is a powerful effect from biomass fuel combustion (Smith et al. 2000; Black and Michaelsen 2002), and where levels of secondhand smoke exposure are possibly lower because of housing characteristics and smoking patterns.

Some variation among studies in the magnitude of OR estimates would be anticipated as patterns of smoking differed among countries and over time, and the methods of the studies were not consistent in all respects. This variation is reflected in statistically significant heterogeneity in some of the pooled analyses (Table 6.3). For this reason, the summary ORs derived under the fixed effects assumption should be interpreted with caution. The random effects method may be more appropriate in these circumstances because its wider confidence limits reflect the heterogeneity between studies. This method is, however, more susceptible to the effects of any publication bias because the random effects method gives greater weight to smaller studies. Thus, considering the largest studies only, the fixed effects estimate for maternal smoking

was 1.56 and the random effects estimate was 1.72. Regardless, the pooled estimates were statistically significant and it is highly unlikely that the association emerged by chance.

The papers that have been cited were selected using keywords relevant to passive/involuntary smoking and children in the title or abstract. When cross-checked against previous reviews of involuntary smoking in children, major omissions were not identified (USDHHS 1986; USEPA 1992; DiFranza and Lew 1996; Li et al. 1999), whereas the systematic search identified relevant references not cited elsewhere. There is a possibility that the selection was biased toward studies reporting a positive association; it is more likely that statistically significant findings would be mentioned in the abstract in comparison with nonsignificant or null findings. Three of the higher ORs were derived from small case-control studies in which involuntary smoking was not the focus of the original research (Hall et al. 1984; McConnochie and Roghmann 1986b; Hayes et al. 1989), and for these three studies publication bias may have been operative. The slightly higher pooled ORs obtained by the random effects compared with the fixed effects method (Table 6.3) reflect the greater weight assigned by the random effects approach to these small studies with a relatively large OR. However, inclusion of the large Chinese studies (Chen et al. 1988a; Jin and Rossignol 1993; Chen 1994) in the meta-analysis of the effects of smoking by either parent would have had a conservative effect (i.e., a smaller pooled estimate), because few mothers smoked in these communities.

The biologic basis for the association of paternal smoking with LRI is possibly complex, and may reflect mechanisms of injury that are in play before and after birth. These mechanisms operate to make respiratory infections more severe or to possibly increase the likelihood of infection. Although viral infection is a well-characterized etiologic factor (Graham 1990), there is evidence that the severity of the illness may be determined in part by lung function abnormalities detectable from birth that result from maternal smoking during pregnancy (Dezateux and Stocks 1997). Many early childhood episodes of wheeze, including bronchiolitis, probably form part of this spectrum of viral illnesses, although other episodes may be the first evidence of more persistent childhood asthma with associated atopic manifestations (Silverman 1993; Martinez et al. 1995). The evidence does not indicate that parental smoking increases the rate of infection with respiratory pathogens. Respiratory viruses are isolated with equal frequency among infants in smoking and nonsmoking households (Gardner et al. 1984).

The effect of parental smoking on the incidence of wheeze and nonwheeze illnesses appears similar, suggesting a general increase in susceptibility to clinical illness upon exposure to respiratory infections rather than to influences on mechanisms more specifically related to asthma.

The pooled results from families with nonsmoking mothers suggest that the effects of parental smoking are at least partly attributable to postnatal (i.e., environmental) exposure to tobacco smoke in the home. The somewhat stronger effects of smoking by the mother compared with other household members may be related to the role of the mother as the principal caregiver, which would explain a higher degree of postnatal exposure of the child from the mother's smoking. However, there is also evidence pointing to altered intrauterine lung development as a specific adverse effect of maternal smoking during pregnancy (Tager et al. 1993).

The effect of parental smoking is largely independent of potential confounding variables in studies that have measured and incorporated such variables into the analyses, suggesting that residual confounding by other factors is unlikely. It thus appears that smoking by the parents, rather than characteristics of the family related to smoking, adversely affect children and cause LRIs. The evidence supports the conclusion found in other recent reviews that there is a causal relationship between parental smoking and acute LRIs (USDHHS 1986; USEPA 1992; DiFranza and Lew 1996; WHO 1997; Li et al. 1999; California EPA 2005). The findings are consistent, properly temporal in the exposure-outcome relationship, and biologically plausible. The evidence is strongest for the first two years of life. The studies that were reviewed also suggest a clear reduction in the estimated effect after two to three years of age, particularly for pneumonia and bronchitis. The failure to find statistically significant associations in some studies of older children should not be interpreted, however, as indicative of no effect of secondhand smoke exposure at older ages.

Conclusions

1. The evidence is sufficient to infer a causal relationship between secondhand smoke exposure from parental smoking and lower respiratory illnesses in infants and children.

2. The increased risk for lower respiratory illnesses is greatest from smoking by the mother.

Implications

Respiratory infections remain a leading cause of childhood morbidity in the United States and other developed countries and are a leading cause of childhood deaths worldwide. The effect of parental smoking, particularly maternal smoking, is of a substantial magnitude. Reducing smoking by parents, beginning with maternal smoking during pregnancy, should reduce the occurrence of LRI. Health care practitioners providing care for pregnant women, infants, and children should urge smoking cessation; parents who are unable to quit should be encouraged not to smoke in the home.

Middle Ear Disease and Adenotonsillectomy

A possible link between parental smoking and the risk of otitis media (OM) with effusion (OME) in children was first suggested in 1983 (Kraemer et al. 1983). A number of subsequent epidemiologic studies have investigated the association of secondhand tobacco smoke exposure with diseases of the ear, nose, and throat (ENT), and the evidence has been summarized in narrative reviews (USEPA 1992; Gulya 1994; Blakley and Blakley 1995; NCI 1999) and quantitative meta-analyses (DiFranza and Lew 1996; Uhari et al. 1996). Strachan and Cook (1998a) systematically reviewed the evidence relating parental smoking to acute otitis media (AOM), recurrent otitis media (ROM), OME (glue ear), and ENT surgery in children. This section updates that 1998 review following the methods described earlier. Full journal publications cited in an overview by Thornton and Lee (1999) were also considered, but abstracts and conference proceedings were not included.

Relevant Studies

In combination with the 45 reports included in the previous review, there are now 61 relating to 59 studies of possible associations between parental smoking and AOM, ROM, middle ear disease, and adenotonsillectomy in children: 19 cross-sectional surveys, 20 prospective cohort studies, 17 case-control studies, 2 uncontrolled case-series, and 1 controlled trial of surgical intervention for middle ear effusion.

Studies were grouped according to the outcome measure and whether they were included in the meta-analysis, as shown in Tables 6.5 and 6.6. Some studies contributed data to more than one outcome or age group. In total, there were 17 studies of AOM (5 were included in the meta-analysis); 28 studies of ROM with 1 study (Ståhlberg et al. 1986) that also included adenotonsillectomy (13 in the meta-analysis); 7 studies of ear infections or hearing loss in schoolchildren (all were unsuitable for the meta-analysis); and 6 studies of adenoidectomy, tonsillectomy, or sore throat (4 were included in the meta-analysis). Studies of middle ear effusion were subdivided into 2 studies of incidence (not suitable for the meta-analysis), 8 prevalence studies (reported in 9 papers) based on population surveys (6 were included in the meta-analysis), and 11 clinic-based studies of referral for glue ear surgery (all were included) and postoperative natural history (1 trial was reported in 2 papers).

Evidence Review

Acute Otitis Media

Episodes of acute middle ear infection are common in young children, and a variety of methods have been used to establish the diagnosis and identify the incidence of the condition. For this reason, and because few studies present quantitative information in relation to parental smoking, a quantitative meta-analysis was not included in the previous review (Strachan and Cook 1998a). However, a conclusion was reached that the limited available evidence was consistent with a weak adverse effect of parental smoking on the incidence of AOM in children, with ORs ranging from 1.0 to 1.5.

More recent publications address AOM. Some specifically excluded recurrent episodes (Gryczyńska et al. 1999; Lubianca Neto et al. 1999), but others offered no clear distinction between infrequent and frequent ear infections (Lister and Jorm 1998; Stathis et al. 1999; Tariq and Memon 1999; Rylander and Mégevand 2000). As in the previous review (Strachan

and Cook 1998a), several publications offered insufficient quantitative data for a meta-analysis (Jackson and Mourino 1999; Rylander and Mégevand 2000). In one study of Swiss children attending preschool medical examinations, the OR for ear infection (not clearly defined as single or recurrent) was 1.04 (95 percent CI, 0.54–1.98) for exposures of 1 to 19 cigarettes daily at home, and 1.18 (95 percent CI, 0.58–2.39) for exposures of 20 or more cigarettes per day, with an apparent reference group of unexposed children (Rylander and Mégevand 2000). The other report only stated that parental smoking was not a significant risk factor for AOM (p = 0.52) (Jackson and Mourino 1999).

Several papers compared the effects of parental smoking on AOM and recurrent or subacute OM in the same population sample. Although the effect was stronger for AOM among Inuit children in Greenland, for example, the effect did not reach statistical significance (Table 6.6) (Homøe et al. 1999). In an Australian birth cohort, the risks associated with maternal smoking did not differ significantly across the outcomes considered: AOM, subacute OM, and a history of ear surgery (predominantly grommet insertion) (Table 6.6) (Stathis et al. 1999). In another Australian national health survey, OM (not further specified) was associated with maternal smoking (OR = 1.31 [95 percent CI, 0.95–1.80]), but the OR for health services utilization was weaker (OR = 1.04 [95 percent CI, 0.71–1.53]) (Lister and Jorm 1998).

Stathis and colleagues (1999) examined the independent effects of exposure to prenatal and postnatal maternal cigarette smoking on the three outcomes in their study at different ages. However, results were not presented for the various specific combinations of exposure, thus limiting the interpretation. In general, maternal smoking at the first prenatal visit had a greater effect compared with exposure at older ages. Smoking during the third trimester and at five years of age had few independent effects. These results need to be interpreted cautiously as there is likely to be co-linearity between early prenatal and postnatal smoking patterns.

The pooled OR for the three studies that document the effects of smoking by either parent provides less convincing evidence (OR = 0.99 [95 percent CI, 0.70–1.40]) (see "Respiratory Symptoms and Prevalent Asthma in School-Age Children" later in this chapter; see also Table 6.14).

Recurrent Otitis Media

The epidemiologic evidence is more abundant for ROM, which is usually defined as greater than a

Table 6.5 Design, sample size, and recruitment criteria of studies of illness associated with parental smoking excluded from meta-analyses

Study	Design/population	Sample size	Case definition	Source of cohort or controls	Outcome
Vinther et al. 1979	Cohort Aged 3 years Denmark	494	AOM episodes	Random sample of children	AOM
Pukander 1982	Case-control Aged 0–4 years Finland	200	AOM in the past year	Health center controls	AOM
van Cauwenberge 1984	Survey Aged 2–6 years Belgium	2,065	AOM, tympanogram	"Healthy" kindergarten pupils	AOM, otitis media with effusion (glue ear) (OME)
Vinther et al. 1984	Cohort Aged 3–4 years Denmark	681	History of AOM	Random sample of birth cohort	AOM, OME
Fleming et al. 1987	Survey Aged 0–4 years United States (Georgia)	609	AOM in the past 2 weeks	Random sample of households	AOM
Sipila et al. 1988	Cohort Aged 0–3 years Finland	1,294	AOM episodes	Random sample of urban area	AOM
Harsten et al. 1990	Cohort Aged 0–3 years Sweden	414	AOM, OME, upper respiratory tract illness (URTI), lower respiratory tract illness (LRTI)	Population-based birth cohort	Acute RTI
Alho et al. 1996	Cohort Aged 0–2 years Finland	825	AOM episodes	Population-based birth cohort	AOM
Salazar et al. 1997	Cohort Aged <6 months United States (Minnesota)	414	>1 physician-diagnosed AOM by 6 months of age	Health maintenance organization (HMO)-based birth cohort	AOM
Jackson and Mourino 1999	Survey Aged <1 year United States (Virginia)	200	Physician-diagnosed AOM	General pediatric clinic	AOM
Tariq and Memon 1999	Case-series Aged <2 years Pakistan	75	AOM presented to the outpatient department	1,724 outpatient visits	AOM

Acute otitis media (AOM) in preschool children

Table 6.5   Continued

Study	Design/population	Sample size	Case definition	Source of cohort or controls	Outcome
		AOM in older children			
Tariq and Memon 1999	Case-series Aged 2–14 years Pakistan	38	AOM presented to the outpatient department	5,401 outpatient visits	AOM
Rylander and Megevand 2000	Survey Aged 4–5 years Switzerland	304	Reported ear infection	Routine preschool screening	AOM, recurrent otitis media (ROM)
		ROM			
Daly et al. 1999	Cohort Aged <6 months United States (Minnesota)	596	>1 physician-diagnosed AOM by 6 months of age	HMO-based birth cohort	AOM
		Middle ear effusion (MEE) incidence			
Paradise et al. 1997	Cohort Aged 0–2 years United States (Pennsylvania)	2,253	Tympanometry and otoscopy	Primary care-based birth cohort	OME
Engel et al. 1999	Cohorts Aged 0–2 years Holland	250	Tympanometry and otoscopy	Healthy and high-risk birth cohort	OME
		Ear infections in schoolchildren			
Goren and Goldsmith 1986	Survey Age data were not provided Israel	1,449	Ear infection (ever)	2nd and 5th graders	Infection
Porro et al. 1992	Survey Aged 6–14 years Italy	2,304	Otitis (ever)	Random sample of schoolchildren	"Otitis"
Goren and Hellmann 1995	Survey Age data were not provided Israel	6,302	Ear infection (ever)	2nd and 5th graders	Infection
Chayarpham et al. 1996	Survey Aged 6–10 years Thailand	2,384	History and examination	3 primary schools	AOM or OME
		MEE prevalence			
Reed and Lutz 1988	Survey Age data were not provided United States (Utah)	45	Flat tympanogram	Outpatients (half with AOM)	OME

Table 6.5   Continued

Study	Design/population	Sample size	Case definition	Source of cohort or controls	Outcome
		MEE prevalence			
Zielhuis et al. 1988*	Cohort Aged 3 years Holland	1,439	Flat tympanogram	Population-based birth cohort	OME
Takasaka 1990	Case-control Aged 4–5 years Japan	201	Tympanometry plus examination	Population screening survey	OME
		MEE natural history			
Maw and Bawden 1993	Trial Aged 2–11 years United Kingdom	66	No effusion	Untreated ears with OME	Resolution
Maw and Bawden 1994	Trial Aged 3–9 years United Kingdom	133	No effusion	Trial participants with OME	Resolution
		Hearing loss			
Lyons 1992	Survey Aged 10 months Ireland	87	Distraction test	Routine postnatal screening	Impairment
Bennett and Haggard 1998	Cohort Aged 5 years United Kingdom	10,880	Parental report	Population-based birth cohort	Hearing loss
Stathis et al. 1999	Cohort Aged 5 years Australia	5,627	Physician consultation	Population-based birth cohort	Hearing loss
		Sore throat, tonsils, and adenoids			
Gryczynska et al. 1999	Survey Aged 3–14 years Poland	60	Histology of excised tissue	General population sample	Adenoidectomy
Rylander and Megevand 2000	Survey Aged 4–5 years Switzerland	304	>1 sore throat/year	Routine preschool screening	Sore throat

*Zielhuis et al. 1988 and 1989 analyze the same study, but the 1989 paper provides more details (OME prevalence).

Table 6.6   Design, sample size, and recruitment criteria of studies of illness associated with parental smoking included in meta-analyses

Study	Design/population	Sample size	Case definition	Source of cohort or controls	Outcome
**Acute otitis media (AOM)**					
Lister and Jorm 1998	Survey Aged <5 years Australia	4,281	Definition unclear	Population sample with no AOM	AOM
Daly et al. 1999	Cohort Aged <6 months United States (Minnesota)	596	Physician-diagnosed AOM by 6 months of age	Health maintenance organization-based birth cohort	AOM
Homøe et al. 1999	Survey Aged 3–8 years Greenland	740	Only 1 reported AOM	Population sample with no AOM	AOM
Lubianca Neto et al. 1999	Survey Aged <3 years Brazil	192	>4 physician-diagnosed AOM/year, no otitis media with effusion (glue ear) (OME)	Same hospital outpatient department as cases	AOM
Stathis et al. 1999	Cohort Aged 5 years Australia	5,627	AOM lasting <1 month	Population-based birth cohort	AOM
**Recurrent otitis media (ROM)**					
Pukander et al. 1985	Case-control Aged 2–3 years Finland	395	>3 physician-diagnosed AOM (outpatient clinic)	Same health center as cases	ROM
Ståhlberg et al. 1986*	Survey Aged <4 years Finland	321	≥3 recorded physician-diagnosed AOM	≤3 AOM (population sample)	ROM
Tainio et al. 1988	Cohort Aged <2 years Finland	108	>5 physician-diagnosed AOM by 2 years of age	No physician-diagnosed AOM, same physician	ROM
Teele et al. 1989[†]	Cohort Aged <1 year United States (Massachusetts)	877	>3 physician-diagnosed AOM by 1 year of age	Clinic-based birth cohort	ROM
	Cohort Aged <3 years United States (Massachusetts)	698	>3 physician-diagnosed AOM by 3 years of age	Clinic-based birth cohort	ROM
	Cohort Aged <7 years United States (Massachusetts)	498	>3 physician-diagnosed AOM by 7 years of age	Clinic-based birth cohort	ROM

Table 6.6   Continued

Study	Design/population	Sample size	Case definition	Source of cohort or controls	Outcome
			ROM		
Daigler et al. 1991	Case-control Aged about 4 years United States (New York)	246	>2 physician-diagnosed AOM in 8 months	Private clinic health check	ROM
Alho et al. 1993	Cohort Aged <2 years Finland	2,512	>3 physician-diagnosed AOM by 2 years of age	Population-based birth cohort	ROM
Stenstrom et al. 1993	Case-control Aged <5 years Canada	170	>4 physician-diagnosed AOM in 12 months	Ophthalmology clinic	ROM
Collet et al. 1995	Cohort Aged <4 years Canada	918	>4 recalled AOM	Population-based birth cohort	ROM
Ey et al. 1995	Cohort Aged <1 year United States (Arizona)	1,013	>3 physician-diagnosed AOM in 6 months	Population-based birth cohort	ROM
Stenström and Ingvarsson 1997	Case-control Aged 3–7 years Sweden	484	>4 reported AOM	General pediatric clinic	ROM
Adair-Bischoff and Sauve 1998	Case-control Aged 4–5 years Canada	625	>3 reported AOM or OME	Population survey (nested case-control)	ROM
Homøe et al. 1999	Survey Aged 3–8 years Greenland	740	>4 reported AOM	Population sample with no AOM	ROM
Stathis et al. 1999	Cohort Aged 5 years Australia	5,627	Subacute OM (duration of 1–3 months)	Population-based birth cohort	ROM
		Middle ear effusion (MEE) prevalence			
Iversen et al. 1985	Cohort Aged 3–6 years Denmark	337	Flat tympanogram	Day care center (6 tests)	OME
Zielhuis et al. 1989	Cohort Aged 2–4 years Holland	435	Flat tympanogram	Population sample (9 tests)	OME
Strachan 1990	Survey Aged 7 years United Kingdom	864	Flat tympanogram	Population sample (1 test)	OME
Etzel et al. 1992	Cohort Aged <3 years United States (North Carolina)	132	Otoscopy plus symptoms	Day care center	OME

Table 6.6   Continued

Study	Design/population	Sample size	Case definition	Source of cohort or controls	Outcome
		MEE prevalence			
Saim et al. 1997	Survey Aged 5–6 years Malaysia	1,097	Flat tympanogram and no reflex	Population sample (1 test)	OME
Apostolopoulos et al. 1998	Survey Aged 6–12 years Greece	4,838	Flat or C2 tympanogram and no reflex	Population sample (1 test)	OME
		MEE referral for surgery			
Kraemer et al. 1983	Case-control Age data were not provided United States (Washington state)	152	Operation for OME	General surgical clinic	OME (outpatients)
Black 1985	Case-control Aged 4–9 years United Kingdom	442	Operation for OME	Clinic and community conrols	OME (outpatients)
Hinton and Buckley 1988	Case-control Aged about 6 years United Kingdom	70	Ear, nose, and throat outpatient referrals	Orthoptic clinic	OME (outpatients)
Hinton 1989	Case-control Aged 1–12 years United Kingdom	151	Grommet insertion	Orthoptic clinic	OME (outpatients)
Barr and Coatesworth 1991	Case-control Aged 1–11 years United Kingdom	230	Grommet insertion	Orthopedic and eye clinics	OME (outpatients)
Green and Cooper 1991	Case-control Aged 1–8 years Germany	328	Otalgia and deafness	Various pediatric clinics	OME (outpatients)
Rowe-Jones and Brockbank 1992	Case-control Aged 2–12 years United Kingdom	163	Bilateral OME >3 months	Orthopedic and surgical clinics	OME (outpatients)
Rasmussen 1993	Cohort Aged <7 years Sweden	1,022	Grommet insertion	Population-based birth cohort	OME (outpatients)
Kitchens 1995	Case-control Aged <3 years United States (Alabama)	350	Grommet insertion	General pediatric clinic	OME (outpatients)
Ilicali et al. 1999	Case-control Aged 3–7 years Turkey	332	Grommet insertion	Otorhinolaryngology clinic	OME (outpatients)
Stathis et al. 1999	Cohort Aged 5 years Australia	5,627	Ear surgery (93% grommets)	Population-based birth cohort	OME (outpatients)

Table 6.6   Continued

Study	Design/population	Sample size	Case definition	Source of cohort or controls	Outcome
Tonsillectomy and/or adenoidectomy					
Said et al. 1978	Survey Aged 10–20 years France	3,920	Recall of surgery	General population sample	Adenoidectomy/ tonsillectomy
Ståhlberg et al. 1986*	Case-controls Aged <4 years Finland	425	Adenoidectomy and ROM	General population sample	Adenoidectomy
Willatt 1986	Survey Aged 2–15 years United Kingdom	154	Tonsillectomy	Children of hospital visitors	Tonsillectomy
Hinton et al. 1993	Case-control Aged about 6 years United Kingdom	120	Tonsillectomy	Orthoptic clinic	Tonsillectomy

*Ståhlberg et al. 1986 appears twice but with mutually exclusive comparisons.
†Teele et al. 1989 appears with three potentially overlapping comparisons but with sample attrition.

specified number of episodes of physician-diagnosed AOM in a defined interval (Table 6.6) (Pukander et al. 1985; Ståhlberg et al. 1986; Tainio et al. 1988; Teele et al. 1989; Daigler et al. 1991; Alho et al. 1993; Stenström et al. 1993; Collet et al. 1995; Ey et al. 1995; Stenström and Ingvarsson 1997; Adair-Bischoff and Sauve 1998; Homøe et al. 1999; and Stathis et al. 1999). Studies that tested for the presence of a dose-response relationship generally found significant relationships (Table 6.7). Several studies adjusted for multiple potential confounding factors and found similar ORs before and after adjustment (Table 6.8). These results suggest that uncontrolled confounding is unlikely to be a major issue in the interpretation of the crude ORs.

One birth cohort study documented the relationship of parental smoking to ROM at one, three, and seven years of age (Teele et al. 1989). The size of the cohort differed for each age because of sample attrition, but the case group increased because of an accumulation of children with at least three episodes of OM. For purposes of the meta-analysis, results from the three-year follow-up were used because this age corresponds most closely to the populations in other similar studies.

Four additional studies were included in the updated meta-analysis (Stenström and Ingvarsson 1997; Adair-Bischoff and Sauve 1998; Homøe et al. 1999; Stathis et al. 1999). In the previous review, not enough papers provided results for smoking by each parent separately to derive summary measures for maternal and paternal smoking. All four additional studies contribute to a pooled estimate for maternal smoking and three contribute estimates for paternal smoking. The findings suggest that the effects are stronger for maternal smoking.

Figure 6.4 summarizes the results comparing children from smoking and nonsmoking parents. There was some evidence for heterogeneity among the nine ORs for smoking by either parent ($\chi^2 = 16.3$, degrees of freedom [df] = 8, p = 0.038). Some variation is to be expected given the different age ranges and case definitions in the studies. Under the fixed effects assumption, the pooled OR for ROM if either parent smoked is 1.32 (95 percent CI, 1.14–1.52). Using the random effects model, the pooled estimate is 1.37 (95 percent CI, 1.10–1.70). Under the fixed effects assumption, the pooled OR for ROM is 1.37 (95 percent CI, 1.19–1.59) for an association with maternal smoking and 0.90 (95 percent CI, 0.70–1.15) for an association with paternal smoking.

Middle Ear Effusion: Population Surveys and Birth Cohorts

The 1997 review identified four cross-sectional or longitudinal studies of general population samples

Table 6.7   Unadjusted relative risks for updated meta-analysis of illness associated with parental smoking

Study	Cases/ controls	Dose-response effect	Outcome	Odds ratio for smoking (95% confidence interval)		
				Either parent	Mother	Father
Acute otitis media (AOM)						
Lister and Jorm 1998	232/4,049	NR*	AOM	NR	1.31 (0.95–1.80)	NR
Daly et al. 1999	221/346	NR	AOM	0.98 (0.60–1.59)	NR	NR
Homøe et al. 1999	102/193	NS† (p = 0.51)	AOM	1.64 (0.85–3.19)	NR	NR
Lubianca Neto et al. 1999	71/121	NR	AOM	0.82 (0.67–1.02)	NR	NR
Stathis et al. 1999	722/4,591	Slight (p = 0.054)	AOM	NR	1.23 (1.04–1.44)‡	NR
Recurrent otitis media (ROM)						
Pukander et al. 1985	188/207	NR	ROM	1.96 (1.28–3.0)	NR	NR
Ståhlberg et al. 1986	100/221	NR	ROM	1.54 (0.93–2.56)	NR	NR
Tainio et al. 1988	28/80	NR	ROM	2.40 (0.91–6.33)	NR	NR
Teele et al. 1989	129/748	NR	ROM before 1 year of age	1.42 (0.96–2.11)	NR	NR
	303/395	NR	ROM before 3 years of age	1.04 (0.76–1.43)	NR	NR
	368/130	NR	ROM before 7 years of age	1.18 (0.77–1.80)	NR	NR
Daigler et al. 1991	125/246	NR	ROM	NR	0.90 (0.54–1.50)	0.83 (0.50–1.39)
Alho et al. 1993	960/1,552	NR	ROM	1.0 (0.68–1.48)	NR	NR
Stenstrom et al. 1993	85/85	Yes; total cigarettes/day	ROM	2.54§ (1.23–5.41)	NR	NR
Collet et al. 1995	164/754	Yes; total cigarettes/day	ROM	1.69 (1.19–2.43)	NR	NR
Ey et al. 1995	169/844	Yes; mother smoked >20 cigarettes/day	ROM	NR	1.33 (0.90–1.95)	NR
Stenström and Ingvarsson 1997	179/305	NS (p = 0.71); mother smoked >20 cigarettes/ day	ROM	NR	1.30 (0.89–1.88)	0.73 (0.48–1.10)

Table 6.7   Continued

Study	Cases/ controls	Dose-response effect	Outcome	Odds ratio for smoking (95% confidence interval)		
				Either parent	**Mother**	**Father**
ROM						
Adair-Bischoff and Sauve 1998	227/398	NS; mother smoked >10 cigarettes/day	ROM	1.11 (0.78–1.57)	1.37 (0.93–2.0)	1.11 (0.77–1.63)
Homøe et al. 1999	117/193	NS (p = 0.64)	ROM	0.96 (0.55–1.69)	NR	NR
Stathis et al. 1999	360/4,852	NS (p = 0.56)	ROM	NR	1.53[‡] (1.24–1.91)	NR
Middle ear effusion prevalence (MEE)						
Iversen et al. 1985	183/154	NR	OME	1.55 (0.98–2.46)	NR	NR
Zielhuis et al. 1989	128/307	No; total cigarettes/day	OME	1.11 (0.59–2.09)	NR	NR
Strachan 1990	82/782	Yes; number of smokers[Δ]	OME	1.41 (0.87–2.28)	NR	NR
Etzel et al. 1992	Total = 132	NR	OME	1.38[¶] (1.21–1.56)	NR	NR
Saim et al. 1997	151/946	NR	OME	0.87 (0.61–1.24)	NR	NR
Apostolopoulos et al. 1998	308/4,530	NS (p = 0.85)	OME	1.60 (1.23–2.08)	NR	NR
OME referral for surgery						
Kraemer et al. 1983	76/76	Yes; number of smokers	OME (outpatients)	1.45 (0.72–2.94)	NR	NR
Black 1985	150/292	Yes; cigarettes times years	OME (outpatients)	NR	NR	NR
Hinton and Buckley 1988	26/44	No; total cigarettes/day	OME (outpatients)	1.10 (0.37–3.23)	NR	NR
Hinton 1989	115/36	NR	OME (outpatients)	2.04 (0.89–4.71)	NR	NR
Barr and Coatesworth 1991	115/115	No; total cigarettes/day	OME (outpatients)	0.72[§] (0.41–1.27)	1.23[§] (0.70–2.15)	NR
Green and Cooper 1991	164/164	No; total cigarettes/day	OME (outpatients)	NR	1.92 (1.20–3.06)	1.37 (0.87–2.17)
Rowe-Jones and Brockbank 1992	100/63	NR	OME (outpatients)	1.21 (0.61–2.39)	NR	NR
Rasmussen 1993	176/846	NR	OME (outpatients)	0.87 (0.49–1.55)	NR	NR

Table 6.7   Continued

Study	Cases/ controls	Dose-response effect	Outcome	Odds ratio for smoking (95% confidence interval)		
				Either parent	Mother	Father
OME referral for surgery						
Kitchens 1995	175/175	No; number of smokers	OME (outpatients)	1.65 (1.05–2.59)**	1.28 (0.65–2.54)**	1.54 (0.89–2.66)**
Ilicali et al. 1999	166/166	NS (p = 0.61)	OME (outpatients)	NR	3.93 (2.42–6.41)	1.57 (1.01–2.45)
Stathis et al. 1999	290/4,971	NS (p = 0.13)	OME (outpatients)	NR	1.71 (1.35–2.17)‡	NR
Tonsillectomy and/or adenoidectomy						
Said et al. 1978	1,490/2,430	Yes; cigarettes smoked by each parent	Adenoidectomy/ tonsillectomy	2.07 (1.80–2.38)	1.68 (1.44–1.95)	1.89 (1.64–2.17)
Ståhlberg et al. 1986	114/321	NR	Adenoidectomy	2.06 (1.30–3.26)	NR	NR
Willatt 1986	93/61	NR	Tonsillectomy	2.06 (1.06–4.0)	NR	NR
Hinton et al. 1993	60/60	Yes; estimated secondhand smoke exposure	Tonsillectomy	2.10 (1.01–4.35)	2.29 (1.02–5.13)	1.26 (0.55–2.90)

*NR = Data were not reported.

†NS = Not significant.

‡Maternal smoking during pregnancy at first prenatal visit. For maternal smoking when their children were 5 years of age, odds ratios were 1.14 (0.97–1.34) for AOM, 1.38 (1.11–1.72) for ROM, and 1.47 (1.16–1.87) for middle ear surgery (OME outpatients). OME = Otitis media with effusion (glue ear).

§Matched analysis.

ΔDose-response effect was assessed by salivary cotinine levels that appear in a separate paper (Strachan et al. 1989).

¶Incidence density ratio.

**95% confidence interval was derived from the p value.

that objectively measured the presence of OME by tympanometry (Iversen et al. 1985; Zielhuis et al. 1989; Strachan 1990) or otoscopy (Etzel et al. 1992). Regardless of the diagnostic method, all studies found an increase in the prevalence of OME in children exposed to parental smoking (Table 6.7). Two additional cross-sectional studies, one from Malaysia (Saim et al. 1997) and the other from Greece (Apostolopoulos et al. 1998), were included in this meta-analysis (Figure 6.4, middle). The former study showed no association of OME with household smoking but the latter study found a significant relationship, with an OR of 1.60 (95 percent CI, 1.23–2.08) for smoking by either parent but no dose-response trend in relation to the number of cigarettes smoked daily by the parents (p = 0.85).

The pooled (random effects) OR for smoking by either parent is 1.33 (95 percent CI, 1.12–1.58).

Two more recent studies followed children prospectively from birth with examinations by tympanometry and otoscopy at intervals of three months throughout the first two years of life (Paradise et al. 1997; Engel et al. 1999). These studies are not readily integrated into the earlier meta-analysis, but they do show that OME in infancy is extremely common. For instance, among 2,253 children in Pittsburgh, 48 percent had at least one episode of effusion by 6 months of age, 79 percent by 12 months of age, and 91 percent by 24 months of age (Paradise et al. 1997). In the Netherlands, parental smoking was not a risk factor for early OME (OR = 1.09 [95 percent CI, 0.84–1.41]),

Table 6.8 **Effects of adjusting for potential confounders in each study of illness associated with parental smoking**

Study	Outcome	Odds ratio for smoking			Factors adjusted for or addressed in the text
		Exposure	Unadjusted	Adjusted	
	Acute otitis media (AOM)
Lister and Jorm 1998	AOM	Mother	NR*	1.31	Gender, lived in the capital, income, occupation, no English at home, maternal education, family size, paternal smoking
Daly et al. 1999	AOM	Both parents	1.5	1.3	Family history of OM, birth season, day care, infections, infant feeding, number of siblings
Homøe et al. 1999	AOM	Either parent	NR	NR	NR
Lubianca Neto et al. 1999	AOM	Either parent	0.82	0.80	Gender, age, race, socioeconomic status (SES), infant feeding
Stathis et al. 1999	AOM	Mother smoked 10–19 cigarettes/ day vs. 0†	2.3	2.6	Gender, age, maternal age, SES, infant feeding, day care, number of siblings
	Recurrent otitis media (ROM)
Pukander et al. 1985	ROM	NR	NR	NR	None
Ståhlberg et al. 1986	ROM	NR	NR	NR	None
Tainio et al. 1988	ROM	NR	NR	NR	SES was similar in cases and controls
Teele et al. 1989	ROM before 1 year of age	NR	NR	NR	None
	ROM before 3 years of age	NR	NR	NR	None
	ROM before 5 years of age	NR	NR	NR	None
Daigler et al. 1991	ROM	NR	NR	NR	None
Alho et al. 1993	ROM	Either parent	1.0	0.99	Gender, siblings, day care, breastfeeding
Stenstrom et al. 1993	ROM	Either parent	2.54	2.68	Age, gender, family history of OM, atopy, SES, day care, breastfeeding

Table 6.8   Continued

Study	Outcome	Odds ratio for smoking			Factors adjusted for or addressed in the text
		Exposure	Unadjusted	Adjusted	
		ROM			
Collet et al. 1995	ROM	Both parents	2.08	1.80	Gender, family history of OM, day care, SES
Ey et al. 1995	ROM	Mother smoked >20 cigarettes/day	2.10	1.78	Gender, siblings, day care, breastfeeding, family history of hay fever
Stenström and Ingvarsson 1997	ROM	Both parents	NR	NR	Age was similar in cases and controls
Adair-Bischoff and Sauve 1998	ROM	2 or more household smokers vs. 1 or 0	1.85	1.88	Day care, infant feeding, SES, prenatal and postnatal health service utilization
Homøe et al. 1999	ROM	Both parents	NR	NR	NR
Stathis et al. 1999	ROM	Mother smoked 10–19 cigarettes/ day vs. 0[†]	2.4	2.6	Gender, age, maternal age, SES, infant feeding, day care, number of siblings
		Middle ear effusion prevalence (MEE)			
Iversen et al. 1985	OME[‡]	Either parent	1.55	1.60	Age
Zielhuis et al. 1989	OME	NR	NR	NR	None
Strachan 1990	OME	Both parents	1.89	1.80	SES, crowding, cooking fuel, dampness
Etzel et al. 1992	OME	NR	NR	NR	Gender, race, infection, atopy, breastfeeding, heating
Saim et al. 1997	OME	Either parent	NR	NR	NR
Apostolopoulos et al. 1998	OME	Either parent	NR	NR	Gender, age, SES, area, medical history
		MEE referral for surgery			
Kraemer et al. 1983	OME (outpatients)	Both parents	2.81	2.80	Age, gender
Black 1985	OME (outpatients)	NR	NR	NR	None
Hinton and Buckley 1988	OME (outpatients)	NR	NR	NR	None
Hinton 1989	OME (outpatients)	NR	NR	NR	None

Table 6.8   Continued

Study	Outcome	Odds ratio for smoking			Factors adjusted for or addressed in the text
		Exposure	Unadjusted	Adjusted	
MEE referral for surgery					
Barr and Coatesworth 1991	OME (outpatients)	NR	NR	NR	Age, gender, race, SES (by matching)
Green and Cooper 1991	OME (outpatients)	NR	NR	NR	Age, gender (by matching), SES (all armed forces)
Rowe-Jones and Brockbank 1992	OME (outpatients)	NR	NR	NR	Area and SES were similar in cases and controls
Rasmussen 1993	OME (outpatients)	NR	NR	NR	None
Kitchens 1995	OME (outpatients)	NR	NR	NR	Age, area, and SES were similar in cases and controls
Ilicali et al. 1999	OME (outpatients)	Both parents	NR	NR	Gender, age, and SES were similar in cases and controls
Stathis et al. 1999	OME (outpatients)	Mother smoked 10–19 cigarettes/day vs. 0[†]	1.4	1.7	Gender, age, maternal age, SES, infant feeding, day care, number of siblings
Tonsillectomy or adenoidectomy					
Said et al. 1978	Adenoidectomy/tonsillectomy	NR	NR	NR	Gender, siblings (separate stratified tabulations)
Ståhlberg et al. 1986	Adenoidectomy	NR	NR	NR	None
Willatt 1986	Tonsillectomy	NR	NR	NR	None
Hinton et al. 1993	Tonsillectomy	NR	NR	NR	Age, gender, and SES were similar in cases and controls

*NR = Data were not reported.
[†]Maternal smoking during pregnancy at first prenatal visit, adjusted for smoking prenatally in the third trimester and 6 months and 5 years postnatally.
[‡]OME = Otitis media with effusion (glue ear).

Figure 6.4   Odds ratios for the effect of smoking by either parent on middle ear disease in children

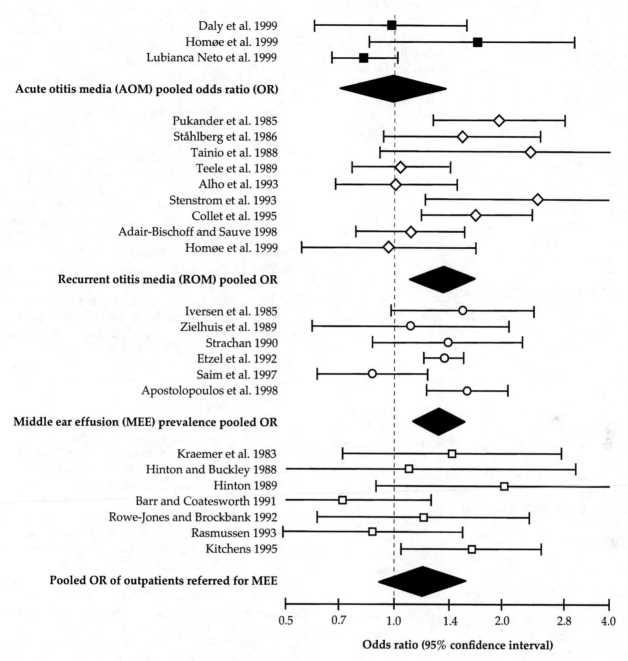

but a more appropriate measure for such a common outcome may be the duration of the effusion (Engel et al. 1999). The Pittsburgh study documented consistent gradients in the cumulative percentage of days with OME during the first year of life, from 18.4 percent among children not exposed to smokers in the home to 24.8 percent among children living with three or more smokers; in the second year of life the gradients ranged from 15.7 percent to 19.4 percent, respectively. Each dose-response trend was statistically significant (p <0.001), but there were no adjustments for potential confounding variables. The effects of secondhand smoke exposure during the first year of life remained significant after adjustment for area of residence, gender, socioeconomic status (SES), family size, day care, and infant feeding. The adjusted effect of having smokers in the home was not significant in the second year of life (Paradise et al. 1997).

Middle Ear Effusion: Clinic Referrals

The 1998 review considered nine studies that examined the relationship between secondhand smoke exposure and outpatient referrals or operative interventions for glue ear (Table 6.6) (Kraemer et al. 1983; Black 1985; Hinton and Buckley 1988; Hinton 1989; Barr and Coatesworth 1991; Green and Cooper 1991; Rowe-Jones and Brockbank 1992; Rasmussen 1993; Kitchens 1995). Seven of these studies that were suitable for the meta-analysis (Figure 6.4, bottom) yielded a pooled OR for smoking by either parent of 1.20 (95 percent CI, 0.90–1.60). Two additional studies from Australia (Stathis et al. 1999) and Turkey (Ilicali et al. 1999) that have also been included strengthen the evidence for an association with parental smoking, particularly by the mother (Table 6.7). The pooled OR for maternal smoking is 1.84 (95 percent CI, 1.54–2.20) compared with 1.49 (95 percent CI, 1.13–1.96) for paternal smoking.

Most of the studies in this category use the case-control design. Only one compared ORs before and after adjusting for confounders but only for age and gender (Kraemer et al. 1983). However, several case-control studies were either matched for age, gender, and SES, or the reports comment that these variables were similarly distributed among cases and controls (Table 6.8). The Australian cohort study controlled for a wider range of covariates and found a stronger association after adjustment compared with the univariate tabulations (Table 6.8) (Stathis et al. 1999). This finding weighs against residual confounding.

Middle Ear Effusion: Natural History

Studies document that OME commonly resolves spontaneously, and about one-third of the cases may remit between outpatient referrals and operative treatments. For example, in a follow-up of a case series in the United Kingdom, the rate of spontaneous resolution in children with at least one smoking parent was 31.5 percent, similar to the rate in children of nonsmoking parents (31 percent) (Hinton 1989).

Insights into the long-term natural history of untreated effusions emerge from controlled trials of operative interventions for glue ear (Maw and Bawden 1993, 1994). Among 133 children followed for five years after adenoidectomy or adenotonsillectomy, the persistence of fluid at the end of the study was three times more likely if either parent smoked (OR = 3.32 [95 percent CI, 1.17–9.41]) (Maw and Bawden 1994). A similar finding emerged using a survival analysis from a trial of unilateral grommet insertion for OME (Maw and Bawden 1993). Among 66 untreated ears followed for five or more years, a spontaneous resolution of fluid was less common among children of smokers (hazard ratio = 0.44 [95 percent CI, 0.22–0.87]), implying a twofold or threefold difference in the rates of resolution between children of smokers and children of nonsmokers.

Hearing Loss

Researchers have related middle ear effusion to hearing loss (Roland et al. 1989; Roberts et al. 1995). However, only one study was found that related parental smoking to objectively confirmed hearing impairments (Lyons 1992). This study was based on a sample of 87 Irish children having routine developmental screening at 10 months of age. A persistently abnormal distraction test was five times more common in infants involuntarily exposed to cigarette smoke, and the authors calculated that 75 percent of the cases of hearing loss were attributable to secondhand smoke exposure.

Parental reports of "suspected or confirmed hearing difficulty" by five years of age were analyzed in a British birth cohort of more than 10,000 children born in 1970 (Bennett and Haggard 1998). The lifetime incidence was 8.4 percent, and was somewhat higher among children five years of age whose mothers had smoked (unadjusted OR = 1.22; no CIs were supplied). After adjustment for gender, SES, day care, and mouth breathing, the adjusted OR for maternal smoking was 1.31 (95 percent CI, 1.14–1.51).

In a birth cohort of more than 5,000 children from Brisbane (Australia), 10 percent of the children had parental reports of consultations with a physician for hearing problems by five years of age (Stathis et al. 1999). There were significant univariate associations with maternal smoking at the first prenatal clinic visit (OR = 1.35 [95 percent CI, 1.13–1.62]) and at five years of age (OR = 1.31 [95 percent CI, 1.09–1.57]).

Adenoidectomy and Tonsillectomy

The 1997 review identified four studies relating to adenoidectomy, tonsillectomy, or adenotonsillectomy without a specific reference to OME as an indicator (Table 6.6) (Said et al. 1978; Ståhlberg et al. 1986; Willatt 1986; Hinton et al. 1993). These studies documented consistent ORs relating to smoking by either parent, with a pooled OR of 2.07 (95 percent CI, 1.82–2.35). However, that pooled analysis was dominated by one large population survey of French secondary schoolchildren (Said et al. 1978). A large British cohort study was identified that showed an OR of 1.0 for parental smoking with tight 95 percent CIs (0.90–1.11) (Strachan et al. 1996) that did not overlap with those of the French study (Said et al. 1978).

More recently published data do not add substantially to this contradictory evidence, but one Polish study reported large differences in adenoid histology between children involuntarily exposed to cigarette smoke and those who were not exposed (Gryczyńska et al. 1999). Epithelial thickening, significantly fewer ciliated cells, and an increase in squamous epithelium were more common in the exposed children. These findings are consistent with chronic inflammatory changes related to cigarette smoke exposure.

Evidence Synthesis

Evidence from different study designs and for different chronic or recurrent disease outcomes related to the middle ear in young children is remarkably consistent in showing a modest elevation in risk associated with parental smoking. Although the outcome measures used are subject to misclassification, the evidence is nonetheless consistent in spite of this heterogeneity.

Subsequent publications over the last four years have not substantially affected the findings of the 1997 meta-analysis (Strachan and Cook 1998a), although quantitative summarization can now be extended to AOM. No single study addresses all of the potential methodologic concerns about selection (referral) bias, information (reporting) bias, or confounding. However, multiple studies that have considered these potential methodologic problems using objective measurements, matched designs, or multivariate analyses have found that the association of secondhand smoke exposure with middle ear disease persists with little alteration in the magnitude of the effect across studies, or within studies that controlled for potential confounding. There are multiple potential pathogenetic mechanisms related to the effects of tobacco smoke components on the upper airway (Samet 2004) (Chapter 2, Toxicology of Secondhand Smoke). A causal association between acute and chronic middle ear disease and secondhand smoke exposure is thus biologically plausible.

Conclusions

1. The evidence is sufficient to infer a causal relationship between parental smoking and middle ear disease in children, including acute and recurrent otitis media and chronic middle ear effusion.

2. The evidence is suggestive but not sufficient to infer a causal relationship between parental smoking and the natural history of middle ear effusion.

3. The evidence is inadequate to infer the presence or absence of a causal relationship between parental smoking and an increase in the risk of adenoidectomy or tonsillectomy among children.

Implications

The etiology of acute and chronic middle ear disease is still a focus of investigation. Nonetheless, the finding that parental smoking causes middle ear disease offers an opportunity for the prevention of this common problem. Health care providers making diagnoses of acute and chronic middle ear disease need to communicate with parents who smoke concerning the consequences for their children.

Respiratory Symptoms and Prevalent Asthma in School-Age Children

The first reports (based on telephone surveys) documenting an adverse effect of parental smoking on the health of children were published in the late 1960s (Cameron 1967; Cameron et al. 1969). By the early 1970s, studies with more formal designs addressed respiratory symptoms (Norman-Taylor and Dickinson 1972; Colley 1974; Colley et al. 1974). Since then, many epidemiologic studies have found an association between parental smoking and respiratory symptoms and diseases throughout childhood. These outcomes were considered in the 1984 and 1986 reports of the Surgeon General (USDHHS 1984, 1986). The narrative review of the 1992 EPA risk assessment (USEPA 1992) concluded that the evidence causally relating secondhand smoke exposure at home to respiratory symptoms was very strong among preschool-age children, but less compelling in school-age children. A subsequent quantitative review did not distinguish between different types of secondhand smoke exposure and their effects at different ages (DiFranza and Lew 1996).

This section summarizes the evidence on the prevalence of respiratory symptoms and asthma in children aged 5 through 16 years, assessed from surveys carried out in schools or populations. This review includes primarily cross-sectional studies and cohorts studied at a single point in time, and updates an earlier 1997 review by Cook and Strachan (1997). A subsequent section of this chapter addresses studies on the onset of asthma and exposure to secondhand smoke. These two sets of outcome measures for asthma—prevalent and incident disease—were separated because disease prevalence reflects not only factors determining incidence, but factors affecting persistence. The studies of asthma prevalence, however, receive further consideration when assessing the evidence related to asthma onset. There are additional complexities in comparisons across studies of varied designs that arise from the different approaches used to ascertain the presence of asthma, and from the heterogeneity of the asthma phenotype by age. Additionally, wheeze, cough, phlegm, and breathlessness are common symptoms for children with asthma.

Relevant Studies

In the 1997 review, 100 articles were identified from their abstracts as possibly containing data that related the prevalence of respiratory symptoms or asthma to secondhand smoke exposure (Cook and Strachan 1997). If a study resulted in additional publications, those publications were used to extract the necessary data. Data from cohort studies were included only if a prevalence estimate for the cohort was available at some point. However, 39 studies were excluded for various reasons.

Out of 47 new studies identified as possibly relevant, 19 were excluded for the following reasons: 7 papers did not present any findings despite having data on symptoms and secondhand smoke (Asgari et al. 1998; Jedrychowski et al. 1998; Goren et al. 1999; Kalyoncu et al. 1999; Suárez-Varela et al. 1999; Hölscher et al. 2000; Moreau et al. 2000); 3 studies presented data that were insufficient for inclusion in a meta-analysis, although there was usually a comment about either the lack of statistical significance (Garcia-Marcos et al. 1999) or the statistical significance of the findings (Faniran et al. 1998; Peters et al. 1999); 1 study presented no separate data on children (Nriagu et al. 1999); 3 were non-English language publications (Galván Fernández et al. 1999; Vitnerova et al. 1999; Kardas-Sobantka et al. 2000); 2 publications related to studies already included (Renzoni et al. 1999; Forastiere et al. 2000); 2 studies presented data on other endpoints (Gomzi 1999; Heinrich et al. 1999); and 1 study was based on sharing a room with a smoker as the exposure indicator (Odhiambo et al. 1998).

Three additional papers presented relevant data but were not considered suitable for inclusion in a meta-analysis: a study in Taiwan (Wu et al. 1998) that merited some attention because of its size but appears to overlap with a study already included that is based on another report (Wang et al. 1999); a Danish study that focused on the underdiagnosis of asthma (Siersted et al. 1998); and a study with cohorts of secondhand smoke-exposed and unexposed children aged nine years. This study addressed postnatal secondhand smoke exposure versus in utero exposure in relation to risk for all respiratory infections, upper and lower combined (Jedrychowski and Flak 1997).

In addition, a publication from 2001 that lies outside the period of the search is also included because it is based on NHANES III data and is therefore relevant to the United States (Mannino et al. 2001).

Table 6.9 summarizes the characteristics of 88 studies that were included in the quantitative overview. Some papers cover more than one study and, because they may present data on different age groups or outcomes, results may be included in several rows in subsequent tables. The rows that are included in any particular meta-analysis are clearly identified.

One study that was not published in the peer-reviewed literature (Florey et al. 1983) is presented separately from the main meta-analyses because of the uniform protocol, the size of the study (approximately 22,000 children), and because only two centers appear to ever have separately published their findings on secondhand smoke in a peer-reviewed journal (Gepts et al. 1978; Melia et al. 1982). Using a standard questionnaire to parents that was based on the WHO questionnaire (Colley and Brasser 1980), the main purpose of this European study was to investigate the relationship between air pollution and respiratory health in schoolchildren; data were also collected on the number of smokers in each home.

Symptom Questionnaires

With a few exceptions, the studies reviewed here are based on data collected from questionnaires filled out by the parents. Inevitably, definitions of asthma and symptoms varied and reflected the state of development of standard questionnaires. Many early studies, particularly in the United Kingdom, used the respiratory questionnaire developed by the Medical Research Council (MRC) for adults as a starting point (MRC 1966). The purpose of this questionnaire was to study chronic respiratory symptoms, and its two most important characteristics are (1) that it did not ask about symptoms in a defined period but asked whether "a person *usually* coughed first thing in the morning" (cough usually in the a.m.), or whether "a child's chest *ever* sounded wheezy or whistling" (wheeze ever); and (2) if the answer was yes, a second question was usually asked to elicit the severity: "Does he/she cough like this on most days or nights for as much as three months each year?" (persistent cough) or "Does he/she get this [wheeze] on *most* days or nights?" (persistent wheeze). In 1978, the American Thoracic Society's Epidemiology Standardization Project published a questionnaire for children based on the adult questionnaires (Ferris 1978). The children's questionnaire determined whether symptoms occurred only with or

apart from colds, and provided information used to distinguish allergic from nonallergic asthma (Ferris 1978). More recently developed questionnaires focus on symptoms in the past 12 months and use a number of methods to assess severity (Asher et al. 1995). One particularly important questionnaire was developed for the International Study of Asthma and Allergy in Childhood (ISAAC) (Asher et al. 1995). This questionnaire has been used in many recent studies. The differences in definitions are explicitly identified in this review where possible, but for some studies a clear definition was not provided in the published report.

Many papers published since the 1997 review have been based on the multicountry ISAAC protocol (Asher et al. 1995). A parental questionnaire was used for younger children in ISAAC while the adolescents themselves completed the questionnaire or, in some locations, were administered a video questionnaire. As a result of the widespread use of the ISAAC study protocol, more of the recent publications relate to asthma (N = 17) and wheeze (N = 21) than to cough (N = 12), phlegm (N = 5), or breathlessness (none).

Evidence Review

Asthma

A total of 41 studies contained quantitative information (Table 6.10); 2 studies presented two separate sets of results (Søyseth et al. 1995; Selçuk et al. 1997). Most studies reported on "asthma ever," which is typically a positive response to "Has this child ever had asthma?" Some studies focused on current asthma, usually defined as in the past year, while other studies specifically asked whether the diagnosis had been made by a physician. One study that reported physician consultations for wheeze is included under asthma for purposes of consistency (Strachan and Elton 1986).

The OR estimates for asthma in children from families in which either parent smoked compared with children of nonsmoking parents were consistently above 1; only three ORs were below 1 (Moyes et al. 1995; Peters et al. 1996; Lam et al. 1999), but the majority of confidence limits included 1. The pooled estimate was 1.23 (95 percent CI, 1.14–1.33), but there is evidence of heterogeneity among the studies ($\chi^2_{30} = 78.8$, p <0.001). The studies reporting the highest ORs were more likely to be early publications that had small study populations and did not adjust for potential confounders Table 6.10 and Figure 6.5. The pooled OR for the unadjusted studies is

Table 6.9   List of secondhand smoke exposure analyses included in the meta-analysis

Study	Population (sample size)	Response rate (%)	Respiratory symptoms
Norman-Taylor and Dickinson 1972	All St. Albans school entrants Aged 5 years (1,119) United Kingdom	NR*	Chronic cough
Colley 1974	7 schools in Aylesbury Aged 6–14 years (2,426) United Kingdom	93	Chronic cough
Lebowitz and Burrows 1976	Stratified cluster sample of Tucson homes Aged 0–15 years (626) United States (Arizona)	72	Asthma, wheeze, chronic cough, chronic phlegm
Schilling et al. 1977	Families from 3 towns Aged 7–18 years (816) United States	NR	Wheeze, chronic cough
Bland et al. 1978	Random sample of Derbyshire schools Aged 11–12 years (5,835) United Kingdom	86	Chronic cough, breathlessness
Kasuga et al. 1979	2 schools Aged 6–11 years (1,896) Japan	99	Wheeze
Stanhope et al. 1979	1 college Aged 12–18 years (715) New Zealand	96	Wheeze
Weiss et al. 1980	Random sample of children aged 5–9 years attending school in East Boston in 1974, plus siblings (383) United States (Massachusetts)	42	Wheeze, chronic cough
Dodge 1982	Schools in 3 Arizona communities Aged 8–12 years (628) United States	76	Asthma, wheeze, chronic cough, chronic phlegm
Ekwo et al. 1983	Primary school in Iowa City Aged 6–12 years (1,138) United States (Iowa)	55	Chronic cough
Schenker et al. 1983[†]	Stratified sample of Pennsylvania schools Aged 5–14 years (4,071) United States	93	Wheeze, chronic cough, chronic phlegm
Charlton 1984	65 schools in northern England Aged 8–19 years (6,988) United Kingdom	NR	Chronic cough
Ware et al. 1984	6 cities Aged 6–9 years (8,380) United States	NR	Wheeze, chronic cough
Burchfiel et al. 1986	Residents of Tecumseh Aged 0–19 years (3,460) United States (Michigan)	NR	Asthma, wheeze, chronic cough, chronic phlegm

Table 6.9   Continued

Study	Population (sample size)	Response rate (%)	Respiratory symptoms
Goren and Goldsmith 1986	Sampling unclear; near coal-fired power station 2nd and 5th graders (sample size not reported) Israel	86	Asthma, wheeze, chronic cough, breathlessness
McConnochie and Roghmann 1986a	Historical birth cohort Aged 6–10 years (223) United States	62	Wheeze
Park and Kim 1986	Households in Wonsung County Aged 0–14 years (3,651) Korea	NR	Chronic cough
Strachan and Elton 1986	Born in 1976 from 1 general practice Aged 7–8 years (165) United Kingdom	83	Asthma, wheeze, chronic cough
Andrae et al. 1988	7 areas near Norrkoping Aged 6 months–16 years (4,990) Sweden	94	Chronic cough
Somerville et al. 1988	Stratified sample from 22 areas in England Aged 5–11 years (5,169) United Kingdom	75	Asthma, wheeze, chronic cough
Strachan 1988[‡]	30 primary schools in Edinburgh Aged 7 years (1,001) United Kingdom	91	Wheeze, chronic cough
Hosein et al. 1989	3 North American towns Aged 7–17 years (1,357) United States	>90	Wheeze, chronic cough, chronic phlegm, breathlessness
Stern et al. 1989a	2 rural communities Aged 7–12 years (1,317) Canada	81	Asthma, wheeze, chronic cough
Stern et al. 1989b[§]	5 rural communities in Ontario and 5 in Saskatchewan Aged 7–12 years (4,003) Canada	81	Asthma, wheeze, chronic cough, chronic phlegm
Dijkstra et al. 1990	9 schools in southeast Holland Aged 6–12 years (1,051) Netherlands	72	Wheeze, chronic cough, breathlessness
Chinn and Rona 1991	National stratified sample Aged 5–11 years (14,256) United Kingdom	>90	Asthma, wheeze, chronic cough
Dekker et al. 1991	30 communities Aged 5–8 years (14,059) Canada	83	Asthma, wheeze
Henry et al. 1991	2 schools: 1 in a polluted area and 1 in a control area Aged 5–12 years (602) Australia	72	Wheeze

Table 6.9   Continued

Study	Population (sample size)	Response rate (%)	Respiratory symptoms
Forastiere et al. 1992	Random sample of schools in 3 areas Aged 7–11 years (2,929) Italy	94	Asthma, chronic cough
Duffy and Mitchell 1993	Stratified sample of 36 schools Aged 8 and 12 years (4,549) Australia	94	Wheeze
Florey et al. 1983	19 European centers Aged 6–10 years (22,078) Europe	62–99	Wheeze
Halliday et al. 1993	2 areas Aged 5–12 years (787) Australia	86	Wheeze
Jenkins et al. 1993	Children born in 1961 (7 years of age) (8,585) Australia (Tasmania)	99	Wheeze
Schmitzberger et al. 1993	3 zones of air pollution Aged 6–15 years (1,626) Austria	88	Asthma
Brabin et al. 1994	15 primary schools in 3 areas around Liverpool Aged 5–11 years (1,872) United Kingdom	92	Asthma, wheeze, breathlessness
Shaw et al. 1994	1 town Aged 8–13 years (708) New Zealand (Kawerau)	82	Wheeze
Soto-Quiros et al. 1994[Δ]	Stratified random sample of 98 schools Aged 5–17 years (2,534) Costa Rica	89	Asthma
Bråbäck et al. 1995	All schools in 1 area Aged 10–12 years (665) Sweden	97	Wheeze, chronic cough
	1 school in Konin Aged 10–12 years (410) Poland	97	Wheeze, chronic cough
	11 schools in Tallin and 4 in Tartu Aged 10–12 years (1,519) Estonia	96	Wheeze, chronic cough
Cuijpers et al. 1995	2 primary schools Aged 6–12 years (470) Netherlands	88	Wheeze, chronic cough, breathlessness
Goren and Hellmann 1995[¶]	3 coastal towns 2nd and 5th graders (6,822) Israel	95	Asthma, wheeze, chronic cough

Table 6.9   Continued

Study	Population (sample size)	Response rate (%)	Respiratory symptoms
Kay et al. 1995	Large, urban general practices Aged 3–11 years (1,077) United Kingdom	98	Asthma
Lau et al. 1995	4 selected Chinese middle-class schools Aged 3–10 years (433) Hong Kong	89	Asthma
Moyes et al. 1995	All children in defined area Aged 6–14 years (2,614) New Zealand	85	Asthma, wheeze, chronic cough
Ninan et al. 1995	Primary schools in Aberdeen Aged 8–13 years (259) United Kingdom	NR	Chronic cough
Søyseth et al. 1995	2 western valleys Aged 7–13 years (620) Norway	96	Asthma
Stoddard and Miller 1995	Stratified cluster sample of all U.S. households Aged <18 years (7,578) United States	NR	Wheeze
Volkmer et al. 1995	All school entries Aged 4–5 years (14,124**) Southern Australia	73	Asthma, wheeze, chronic cough
Abuekteish et al. 1996	Primary schools in and around 1 city Aged 6–12 years (3,186) Jordan (Irbid)	90	Wheeze
Beckett et al. 1996	Older children of mothers who gave birth in hospitals Aged 1–18 years (5,171) United States	91	Asthma
Bener et al. 1996	Sampling unclear Aged 6–14 years (729) United Arab Republic	86	Asthma
Chen et al. 1996	1 town Aged 6–17 years (892) Canada (Humboldt)	NR	Asthma
Peters et al. 1996[††]	17 schools in 2 areas with different air pollution levels Aged 10–13 years (3,521) Hong Kong	96	Asthma, wheeze, chronic phlegm
Wright et al. 1996	Birth cohort from Tucson Aged 6 years (987) United States (Arizona)	78	Wheeze, chronic cough

Table 6.9   Continued

Study	Population (sample size)	Response rate (%)	Respiratory symptoms
Zejda et al. 1996	Cluster sample of primary schools in 2 towns Aged 7–9 years (1,622) Poland	75	Chronic cough
Austin and Russell 1997	Schools in Scottish Highlands Aged 12 and 14 years (1,537) United Kingdom	85	Wheeze, chronic cough
Butland et al. 1997	All children attending school in Croydon Aged 7.5–8.5 years (7,237) United Kingdom	81–87	Wheeze
Dales et al. 1997	Sampling unclear; 1 community (138) Canada	NR	Chronic cough
Farber et al. 1997	The 1992–1994 Bogalusa Heart Study survey Aged 5–17 years (2,975) United States	NR	Asthma
Forsberg et al. 1997	Schools in Oslo, Malmo, Umea, and Kuopio Aged 6–12 years (15,962) Scandinavia	90	Asthma, chronic cough
Hu et al. 1997	13 schools in Illinois with mostly Black students Aged 10–11 years (707) United States	NR	Asthma, wheeze
Leung et al. 1997	13 randomly selected schools Aged 13–14 years (>3,733) Hong Kong	NR	Wheeze
Maier et al. 1997	Schools in Seattle Aged 5–9 years (925) United States (Washington state)	31	Asthma, wheeze
Selçuk et al. 1997	Random sample Aged 7–12 years (5,412) Turkey	86	Asthma, wheeze
Chen et al. 1998	1 town Aged 6–17 years (892) Canada	88	Chronic cough
Chhabra et al. 1998	2 schools in Delhi Aged 4–17 years (2,609) India	91	Wheeze
Kendirli et al. 1998	Random selection of schools in Adana Aged 6–14 years (2,334) Turkey	88	Asthma, wheeze
Lam et al. 1998	2-stage cluster sample from 172 classes in 61 schools Aged 12–15 years (4,482) Hong Kong	88	Asthma, wheeze, chronic cough, chronic phlegm

Table 6.9   Continued

Study	Population (sample size)	Response rate (%)	Respiratory symptoms
Lewis and Britton 1998	Birth cohort born in 1 week in 1970 Aged 16 years (6,000) United Kingdom	NR	Wheeze
Lewis et al. 1998	Primary schoolchildren from industrial and nonindustrial areas Aged 8–11 years (2,340) Australia	77	Wheeze, chronic cough
Peters et al. 1998	27 schools within 2 districts Aged 8–13 years (10,615) Hong Kong	95	Wheeze, chronic cough, chronic phlegm
Rönmark et al. 1998	3 areas in northernmost Sweden Aged 7–8 years (3,431)	97	Asthma
Saraçlar et al. 1998	12 schools in Ankara Aged 7–14 years (2,784) Turkey	88	Wheeze
Withers et al. 1998	86 general practitioners in Southampton Aged 14–16 years (2,289) United Kingdom	75	Asthma, wheeze, chronic cough
Agabiti et al. 1999	School-based sample aged 6–7 years from 10 centers in northern Italy; SIDRIA[##] (children) sample (18,737)	96	Asthma, wheeze
	School-based sample aged 13–14 years from 10 centers in northern Italy; SIDRIA (adolescent) sample (21,068)	93	Asthma, wheeze
Belousova et al. 1999	All primary schools in 7 regions within New South Wales Aged 8–11 years (6,394) Australia	76	Wheeze
Burr et al. 1999	93 schools in Great Britain Aged 12–14 years (25,393) United Kingdom	79	Wheeze, chronic cough, chronic phlegm
Chhabra et al. 1999	9 randomly selected schools in Delhi Aged 5–17 years (18,955) India	NR	Asthma, wheeze
Lam et al. 1999	30 schools in Hong Kong Aged 8–13 years (3,480) China	NR	Wheeze, chronic cough, chronic phlegm
Nilsson et al. 1999	Residents of Ostergotland Aged 13–14 years (1,878) Southwest Sweden	NR	Asthma

Table 6.9   Continued

Study	Population (sample size)	Response rate (%)	Respiratory symptoms
Shamssain and Shamsian 1999	78 schools in northeast England Aged 6–7 years (3,000) United Kingdom	80	Asthma, wheeze, chronic cough
Wang et al. 1999	Cross-sectional study of 2 communities Aged 11–16 years (165,173) Taiwan	97	Wheeze
Csonka et al. 2000	All 40 primary schools in 1 city (Tampere) Aged 6–13 years (1,814) Finland	90	Wheeze
Ponsonby et al. 2000	All children aged 7 years from Tasmania who had participated in an earlier infant health survey (863) Australia	NR	Asthma
Qian et al. 2000	3 large cities Aged 5–14 years (2,060) China	NR	Asthma, wheeze, chronic cough, chronic phlegm
Räsänen et al. 2000	5 consecutive birth cohorts of 16-year-old twins (4,538) Finland	NR	Asthma

*NR = Data were not reported.
†Data for standard errors are from Wright et al. 1996.
‡Data for cotinine are in Strachan et al. 1990.
§Prevalence data are from Beckett et al. 1996.
△Note error in Table 3 in this paper.
¶See also Bener et al. 1996.
**Number of families.
††1991 data were used.
‡‡SIDRIA = Italian Studies on Respiratory Disorders in Childhood and the Environment.

1.26 (95 percent CI, 1.15–1.38, χ^2_{21} = 51.3, p <0.001). In contrast, the relative odds for the 18 studies that adjusted for various potential confounders are quantitatively consistent and slightly lower than those for the unadjusted studies (pooled OR = 1.22 [95 percent CI, 1.12–1.32], χ^2_{17} for heterogeneity = 39.1, p = 0.002). For the 11 studies reporting both adjusted and unadjusted ORs, the adjustment had very little effect (Table 6.10) (Somerville et al. 1988; Dekker et al. 1991; Forastiere et al. 1992; Brabin et al. 1994; Kay et al. 1995; Beckett et al. 1996; Maier et al. 1997; Selçuk et al. 1997; Agabiti et al. 1999; Chhabra et al. 1999; Ponsonby et al. 2000).

Only one of the ORs for asthma where either parent smoked was below 1; the highest ORs were from small studies that had not adjusted for potential confounders (Figure 6.5). There was clear evidence of heterogeneity of effect estimates among the unadjusted studies (pooled OR = 1.30 [95 percent CI, 1.20–1.41], χ^2_{28} for heterogeneity = 152.1, p <0.001). Among the adjusted studies, the pooled OR was only slightly lower at 1.25 (95 percent CI, 1.17–1.33), again with evidence of heterogeneity (χ^2_{24} = 88.4, p <0.001). Studies that provided both adjusted and unadjusted ORs found a similar but very small effect of adjustment (Table 6.11), except for one early Japanese study (Kasuga et al. 1979). The overall pooled OR from all of the studies, using adjusted values if available, was 1.23 (95 percent CI, 1.14–1.33) (see Table 6.14).

One foreign language article published in the *Chinese Journal of Public Health* also merits attention because of the study size: 359,000 children aged 12 through 14 years were screened, making it larger than all other cross-sectional studies combined. There is an overlap between this study in Taiwan and the data presented in another publication included in the meta-analysis (Wang et al. 1999). Disease definitions were based on an ISAAC protocol that included both a written questionnaire to parents and a video questionnaire to children. "Asthma" was based on a somewhat restrictive definition requiring the following three criteria: (1) in the parent's questionnaire, the student's asthma was diagnosed by a physician; (2) after watching the video, the student reported a shortness of breath similar to what was depicted in a particular scene of the video; and (3) in the past 12 months, the student reported a shortness of breath similar to what was shown in the first scene of the video and had also awakened during the night (Crane et al. 2003). "Suspected asthma" was based on a much broader definition that included cough as well as wheeze.

Although the univariate analyses of the larger study did not show an association between either the number of cigarettes per day smoked by household members or the number of household smokers and asthma risk, there was an exposure-response relationship for "suspected asthma" with the number of cigarettes smoked by household members. However, these univariate results were potentially confounded by age, gender, air pollution, and area as well as by correlates of SES. Adjusted ORs were presented only for asthma (not suspected asthma), and were controlled for gender, school grade, air pollution, burning incense, area, and physical activity. Although unadjusted ORs tended to be below 1.0 for students living in smoking households, the adjusted ORs showed an elevated risk that increased with an increasing number of household smokers. Adjusted data for the number of cigarettes smoked by household members are difficult to interpret because the results were adjusted for the number of household members who smoked. The ORs of 1.1, 1.2, and 1.3 in households with one to two, three to four, and four or more smokers, respectively, are compatible with results from the related Taiwanese paper that offers an OR of 1.08 for any exposure after adjustment. An overall effect of household smoking cannot be derived because the number of children exposed in the different groups was not reported. Two other design issues are unclear: consideration does not appear to have been made for active smoking by these 12- through 14-year-olds, although it was controlled in the analysis reported by Wang and colleagues (1999); and secondhand smoke exposure is not specified as to the

source: maternal smoking, paternal smoking, and/or other household members. Data from Taiwan were not presented in the 1997 WHO publication *Tobacco or Health: A Global Status Report* (WHO 1997), but in mainland China it was uncommon for women to smoke. Although the ORs presented in both papers from Taiwan are thus broadly compatible with those in Table 6.14, they are more in keeping with the effects of smoking by fathers or others only, as opposed to maternal smoking or smoking by either parent.

Wheeze

Using a variety of definitions (Table 6.11), 58 studies were identified with data on wheeze that could be broadly grouped under three headings: wheeze ever, current wheeze, and persistent wheeze. Wheeze is a common but nonspecific manifestation of asthma, as it has other underlying causes, including respiratory infection.

Of the 43 studies reporting effects of smoking by either parent, the 2 studies with the highest ORs reported on wheeze that was classified as both current and persistent (Weiss et al. 1980) and on wheeze most days or nights (Lebowitz and Burrows 1976), rather than wheeze ever or current wheeze. These two studies also reported the lowest prevalence rates (Table 6.11), suggesting that the definitions probably reflected more severe wheeze. In two studies that reported on both wheeze ever and wheeze most days or nights, the ORs were greater for wheeze most days or nights (Somerville et al. 1988; Chinn and Rona 1991). More recently, one study in Hong Kong reported a slightly higher OR for current than for severe wheeze (Table 6.11) (Leung et al. 1997). Two large studies from the United Kingdom found higher odds for maternal smoking in relation to frequent attacks than for less frequent attacks (Butland et al. 1997), and for speech-limiting wheeze than for all wheeze in the past year (Table 6.11) (Burr et al. 1999). However, a smaller United Kingdom study reported stronger associations with wheeze ever than for wheeze in the past year or for speech-limiting attacks (Table 6.11) (Shamssain and Shamsian 1999). The overall pooled OR from all studies using adjusted values if available was 1.26 (Figure 6.6) (see also Table 6.14).

Similar to the findings for asthma, all but one of the ORs for smoking by either parent were above 1. The highest ORs were from small studies that had not adjusted for potential confounders (Figure 6.6). There was clear evidence of heterogeneity of effect among the unadjusted studies (pooled OR = 1.30 [95 percent CI, 1.20–1.41], χ^2_{28} for heterogeneity = 152.1,

Table 6.10   Studies of asthma prevalence associated with parental smoking

Study	Population age (years)/ location	Definition of asthma	Prevalence in unexposed (%)	Odds ratio for smoking (95% confidence interval)	
				Either parent (unadjusted)	Either parent (adjusted)
Lebowitz and Burrows 1976	0–15 United States	Physician diagnosis	7.6	3.53 (2.13–5.86)	NR*
Dodge 1982	8–12 United States	NR	4.1	1.61 (0.78–3.33)	NR
Burchfiel et al. 1986	0–19 United States	NR	11.5	NR	1.14 (0.92–1.41)
Goren and Goldsmith 1986	2nd and 5th graders Israel	Ever	8.9	1.07 (0.74–1.56)	NR
Strachan and Elton 1986	5–7 United Kingdom	Wheeze consultations	13	1.60 (0.56–4.60)	NR
Somerville et al. 1988	5–11 United Kingdom	An attack in the past year	4	1.0 (0.78–1.28)	1.18 (0.86–1.62)
Stern et al. 1989a	7–12 Canada	Current	3.6	NR	NR
Stern et al. 1989b	7–12 Canada	Physician diagnosis (ever)	4§	NR	NR
Chinn and Rona 1991	5–11 United Kingdom	In the past year	NR	NR	1.02 (0.86–1.20)
Dekker et al. 1991	5–8 Canada	Current	4.8	1.53 (1.30–1.81)	1.49 (NR)
Forastiere et al. 1992	7–11 Italy	Ever (or symptoms)	6.3	1.4 (NR)	1.3 (0.9–1.8)
Schmitzberger et al. 1993	6–15 Austria	Physician diagnosis	3.4	NR	NR
Brabin et al. 1994	5–11 United Kingdom	Ever	17	1.09 (0.85–1.41)	1.06 (0.83–1.37)
Soto-Quiros et al. 1994	6–12 Costa Rica	NR	NR	NR	NR
Goren and Hellmann 1995	2nd and 5th graders Israel	Ever	9.6	1.19 (1.01–1.41)	NR
Kay et al. 1995	3–11 United Kingdom	Current (definition unclear)	17	1.42 (1.05–1.92)	1.31 (0.96–1.81)

Odds ratio for smoking (95% confidence interval)				
One parent only vs. neither	**Both parents vs. neither**	**Mother only vs. neither**	**Father only vs. neither**	**Confounders adjusted for**
NR	NR	NR	NR	NR
1.36 (0.57–3.21)	1.94 (0.81–4.50)	NR	NR	NR
0.84 (0.63–1.13)	1.62 (1.18–2.22)	1.28 (0.68–2.40)	0.76 (0.56–1.04)	Age, gender, socioeconomic status (SES), family size
NR	NR	1.36 (0.87–2.14)	0.91 (0.59–1.39)	NR
NR	NR	NR	NR	NR
NR	NR	NR	NR	Child's age, gender, birth weight, and triceps skinfold; mother's age and education; number of siblings; and father's social class and job
NR	NR	1.11[†] (0.63–1.98)	1.41[‡] (0.80–2.48)	NR
NR	NR	1.43[Δ] (1.09–1.88)	NR	NR
NR	NR	NR	NR	Birth weight; father's social class and job; mother's age, education, and smoking during pregnancy; and family size and ethnic origin
1.4 (1.13–1.73)	1.59 (1.28–1.98)	NR	NR	Dampness, gas cooking, type of heating, pets
NR	1.50 (1.04–2.20)	1.70 (1.04–2.70)	1.0 (0.70–1.50)	Age, gender, area, SES
NR	NR	2.11[†] (1.22–3.67)	NR	NR
NR	NR	NR	NR	Area
NR	NR	1.53[†] (1.14–2.04)	1.19[‡] (0.97–1.45)	NR
1.13 (0.94–1.36)	1.33 (1.07–1.66)	1.27[†] (1.04–1.55)	1.19[‡] (1.0–1.41)	NR
NR	1.81 (1.16–2.84)	1.13 (0.71–1.80)	1.3 (0.86–1.97)	SES

Table 6.10   Continued

Study	Population age (years)/ location	Definition of asthma	Prevalence in unexposed (%)	Odds ratio for smoking (95% confidence interval)	
				Either parent (unadjusted)	Either parent (adjusted)
Lau et al. 1995	3–10 Hong Kong	Current (definition unclear)	7	1.35 (0.60–3.06)	NR
Moyes et al. 1995	6–7 New Zealand	Ever	25	1.06 (0.89–1.27)	NR
	13–14 New Zealand	Ever	23	0.94 (0.79–1.13)	NR
Søyseth et al. 1995[¶]	7–13 Norway	Ever	7.7	NR	NR
	7–13 Norway	Ever	NR	NR	NR
	7–13 Norway	Ever	NR	NR	NR
Volkmer et al. 1995[¶]	4–5 Australia	Ever	NR	Not significant	Not significant
Beckett et al. 1996	1–18 United States	Physician diagnosis	10.3	1.56 (1.30–1.88)	1.40 (1.13–1.72)
Bener et al. 1996	6–14 United Arab Republic	Ever	12.7	1.28 (0.82–1.99)	NR
Chen et al. 1996[##]	6–17 Canada	Physician diagnosis (ever)	10.0	1.14 (0.72–1.79)	NR
Peters et al. 1996	8–11 Hong Kong	Current physician diagnosis (definition unclear)	6.1[§]	NR	0.90 (0.69–1.17)
Farber et al. 1997	5–17 United States	Ever	15.9[§]	NR	1.39 (1.11–1.72)
Forsberg et al. 1997	6–12 Scandinavia	Treatment by physician in the past 12 months	3.5[§]	NR	1.4 (1.1–1.7)
Hu et al. 1997	10–11 United States (Illinois)	Physician diagnosis (ever)	25.3	NR	NR
Maier et al. 1997	5–9 United States (Washington state)	Physician diagnosis (ever)	11[§]	1.5 (1.0–2.4)	1.6 (0.9–2.7)

Odds ratio for smoking (95% confidence interval)				
One parent only vs. neither	Both parents vs. neither	Mother only vs. neither	Father only vs. neither	Confounders adjusted for
NR	NR	NR	NR	NR
NR	NR	NR	NR	NR
NR	NR	NR	NR	NR
NR	NR	1.17[†] (0.66–2.07)	0.72[‡] (0.39–1.31)	NR
NR	NR	1.26** (0.71–2.25)	NR	NR
NR	NR	1.99[††] (1.08–3.67)	NR	NR
NR	NR	NR	NR	NR
NR	NR	NR	NR	Ethnicity, gas stove, mold, maternal age, maternal allergy, number of children at home
NR	NR	NR	NR	NR
0.92 (0.53–1.63)	1.55 (0.84–2.84)	1.17[†] (0.71–1.95)	1.0[‡] (0.61–1.64)	NR
0.76 (0.55–1.07)	1.22 (0.78–1.92)	NR	NR	NR
NR	NR	NR	NR	Age, gender, ethnicity
NR	NR	NR	NR	Age, gender, area, fitted carpets, pets, mold, stove use, parental asthma, early day care
NR	NR	1.22 (0.79–1.89)	NR	None
NR	NR	NR	NR	Gender, ethnicity, allergy, SES, parental asthma

Table 6.10   Continued

Study	Population age (years)/ location	Definition of asthma	Prevalence in unexposed (%)	Odds ratio for smoking (95% confidence interval) Either parent (unadjusted)	Odds ratio for smoking (95% confidence interval) Either parent (adjusted)
Selçuk et al. 1997	7–12 Turkey	Ever	13.1	1.41 (1.19–1.67)	1.35[¶] (1.12–1.62)
	7–12 Turkey	Current	4.6	1.34 (1.02–1.77)	1.28 (0.94–1.75)
Kendirli et al. 1998	6–14 Turkey	Ever (by questionnaire)	12.9[§]	1.41 (1.16–1.72)	NR
Lam et al. 1998	12–15 Hong Kong	Physician diagnosis (ever)	8.5	NR	NR
Rönmark et al. 1998	7–8 Sweden	Physician diagnosis and current	6.4[§]	NR	NR
Withers et al. 1998	14–16 United Kingdom	Physician diagnosis (ever)	22.3[§]	NR	p >0.05
Agabiti et al. 1999	6–7 Italy	Asthma with symptoms in the past year	5.0	1.33 (1.10–1.60)	1.34 (1.11–1.62)
	13–14 Italy	Asthma with symptoms in the past year	5.9	1.26 (1.07–1.49)	1.17 (0.99–1.39)
Chhabra et al. 1999	5–17 India	Current	10.8	1.61 (NR)	1.51 (1.34–1.69)
Lam et al. 1999	8–13 Hong Kong	Physician diagnosis (ever) (definition unclear)	6.8	NR	0.91[¶¶] (0.69–1.18)
Nilsson et al. 1999	13–14 Sweden	Ever (International Study of Asthma and Allergy in Childhood [ISAAC] child questionnaire)	9.3[§]	1.0 (0.7–1.4)	NR
Shamssain and Shamsian 1999	6–7 United Kingdom	Ever	20.6	NR	NR
Ponsonby et al. 2000	6–7 Australia	Has your child ever had asthma	30.0	1.16 (0.85–1.57)	1.03 (0.83–1.26)

Odds ratio for smoking (95% confidence interval)				
One parent only vs. neither	Both parents vs. neither	Mother only vs. neither	Father only vs. neither	Confounders adjusted for
NR	NR	NR	NR	Age, gender, place, animals, atopic family, breastfeeding
NR	NR	NR	NR	NR
NR	NR	NR	NR	NR
0.89 (0.69–1.12)	NR	1.32 (0.71–2.45)	0.92§§ (0.72–1.17)	Age, gender, area, housing type
NR	NR	1.6ΔΔ (1.1–2.3)	NR	Gender, area, pets, dampness, family history
NR	NR	1.50 (1.14–1.98)	p >0.05	Parent and child atopy, sibling with asthma
NR	1.35 (1.09–1.69)	1.46 (1.13–1.87)	1.26 (1.01–1.58)	Age, gender, area, father's education, crowding, dampness, gas heating, parental asthma, other smokers
NR	1.29 (1.06–1.56)	1.23 (0.98–1.53)	1.04 (0.86–1.27)	Age, gender, area, father's education, crowding, dampness, gas heating, parental asthma, other smokers, active smoking
NR	NR	NR	NR	Age, gender, atopic family
NR	NR	NR	NR	Age, gender, area, active smoking
NR	NR	1.4** (1.0–2.0)	NR	None
1.35 (NR)	1.55 (NR)	1.39† (1.12–1.74)	NR	None
NR	NR	1.08** (0.90–1.30)	NR	Gender, family history, breastfeeding, gas heat, mother's education, number in household

Table 6.10   Continued

Study	Population age (years)/ location	Definition of asthma	Prevalence in unexposed (%)	Odds ratio for smoking (95% confidence interval) Either parent (unadjusted)	Odds ratio for smoking (95% confidence interval) Either parent (adjusted)
Qian et al. 2000	5–14 China	Recall of asthma ever with physician diagnosis	0.8–3.6	NR	2.11 (0.79–5.66)
Räsänen et al. 2000	16 Finland	Physician diagnosis (ever) by questionnaire	3.2	NR	NR

*NR = Data were not reported.
†Mother currently smoked vs. did not smoke.
‡Father currently smoked vs. did not smoke.
§Overall prevalence.
△Mother smoked vs. did not smoke during pregnancy and infancy.
¶Not included in the meta-analysis.
**Mother smoked vs. did not smoke prenatally.
††Mother smoked vs. did not smoke postnatally.
‡‡Estimates were determined by combining data for allergic and nonallergic participants.
§§Father smoked vs. neither parent smoked where only 2.5% of the mothers smoked.
△△Approximate confidence limits were derived from the given p value.
¶¶Analyses excluded active smokers.
***Mother ever vs. never smoked.

p <0.001). Among the adjusted studies, the pooled OR was only slightly lower (OR = 1.25 [95 percent CI, 1.17–1.33]), which again provided evidence of heterogeneity (χ^2_{24} = 88.4, p <0.001). For those studies with both adjusted and unadjusted ORs, there was a similar, very small effect of adjustment except for one early Japanese study (Table 6.11) (Kasuga et al. 1979).

For the 19 centers participating in the European Communities (EC) Study, it was possible to extract data for wheeze ever. There was no evidence of heterogeneity between centers (χ^2_{18} = 18.6, p = 0.42); the pooled OR across the 19 centers was 1.20 (95 percent CI, 1.09–1.32).

Chronic Cough

A total of 44 published studies of cough have used a variety of symptom definitions (Table 6.12). Although most of the studies were based on either the MRC or American Thoracic Society questionnaires, the largest study was based on a study-specific questionnaire (Charlton 1984). Two studies reported raised ORs for cough without wheeze (Ninan et al. 1995; Wright et al. 1996), thus emphasizing the

importance of cough as a symptom. There is no suggestion that the studies reporting the lowest prevalence rates (implying a more restrictive definition) contributed the highest ORs. The pooled OR for the 26 studies with no adjustments for potential confounders was 1.45 (95 percent CI, 1.34–1.58, χ^2_{25} for heterogeneity = 84.0, p <0.001), somewhat greater than for the 16 studies that adjusted for various factors: pooled OR = 1.27 (95 percent CI, 1.21–1.33, χ^2_{15} for heterogeneity = 18.0, p = 0.26) (Figure 6.7). In four studies reporting both adjusted and unadjusted estimates, the adjustments had little impact (Bland et al. 1978; Somerville et al. 1988; Wright et al. 1996; Burr et al. 1999); the study conducted by Forastiere and colleagues (1992) was excluded because CIs were not reported for the unadjusted category. It is worth noting, however, that Wright and colleagues (1996) and Burr and colleagues (1999) adjusted for active smoking.

Chronic Phlegm

Out of 12 studies reporting on phlegm, 4 used a definition of persistent phlegm and 3 were unclear with regard to the definition in the study report

Odds ratio for smoking (95% confidence interval)				
One parent only vs. neither	Both parents vs. neither	Mother only vs. neither	Father only vs. neither	Confounders adjusted for
NR	NR	NR	NR	Age, gender, ventilation, family history, mother's education, coal use, area
NR	NR	1.49*** (1.02–2.18)	NR	Gender, parental asthma and hay fever, number of older siblings, father's occupation

(Table 6.13); 7 out of 10 studies reported significant ORs for smoking by either parent, although all ORs were above 1 (Figure 6.8). The pooled OR for smoking by either parent was 1.35 (95 percent CI, 1.30–1.41), with no evidence of heterogeneity between studies (χ^2_9 for heterogeneity = 4.6, p = 0.87).

Breathlessness

Six studies reported on shortness of breath using various definitions (Table 6.13). Only two studies reported statistically significant effects even though results were above 1 for all but one of the ORs (Figure 6.8). The pooled OR for smoking by either parent was 1.31 (95 percent CI, 1.14–1.50), with no evidence of heterogeneity (χ^2_5 for heterogeneity = 4.6, p = 0.47).

Pooled Odds Ratios

The pooled ORs for smoking by either parent compared with smoking by neither parent are consistent across different outcomes, ranging from 1.23 for asthma to 1.35 for cough and phlegm (Table 6.14). For asthma, wheeze, and cough—for which there are sufficient studies to justify a pooled analysis—there is clear

evidence of an increased risk of respiratory symptoms if only one parent smokes, regardless of whether it is only the mother or the father. Exposure to smoking only by the mother appears to have a greater effect, but a formal comparison of smoking by only the mother or father is not possible because it requires within-study estimates of standard errors for the calculation. Evidence exists of a dose-response relationship with the number of parents who smoke; the summary ORs for smoking by both parents are greater than for one parent only in all cases (Table 6.14).

Restricting Analyses to Preteens

Because a number of the cited studies cover teenagers who may be active smokers, and only some studies have included controls for active smoking, the analyses have been repeatedly restricted to those studies in Table 6.9 with no children older than 11 years of age. The results are presented in Table 6.15. Although the number of studies is markedly reduced and confidence limits are widened, the estimated ORs are similar to those in Table 6.14.

Figure 6.5   Odds ratios for the effect of smoking by either parent on asthma prevalence

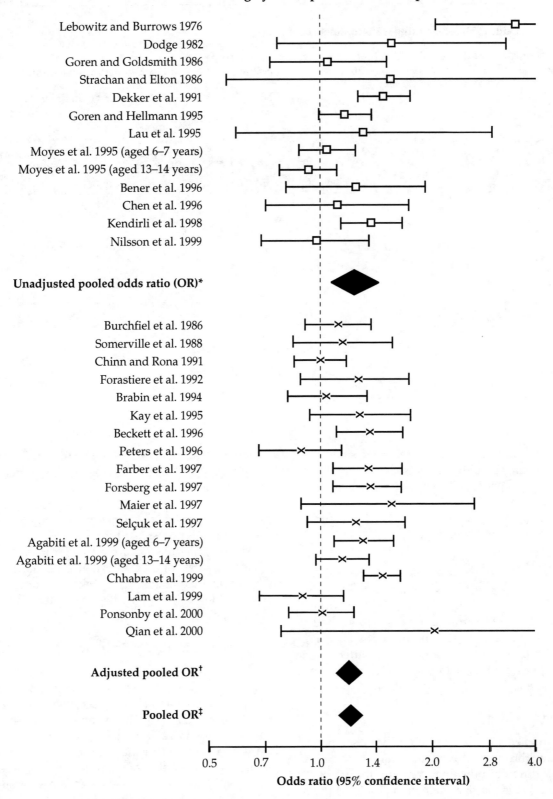

*Studies that did not adjust for potential confounders.
†Studies that adjusted for a variety of potential confounders.
‡Based on all studies.

Effect of Parental Smoking at Different Ages

Modification of the effect of parental smoking as children age is quite plausible. The relationship of parental smoking to the personal exposure of their children may change as the children age, and susceptibility to secondhand smoke may also change. In addition, the constellation of symptoms, signs, and physiologic abnormalities leading to a diagnosis of asthma may vary by age. A comparison across different studies is unlikely to provide a valid assessment of the risks associated with exposure to parental smoking at different ages because of the considerable overlap of age range in many studies, different definitions of symptoms, and the need to control for active smoking in older children. However, within-study comparisons can be made if comparable information is available across age groups. For example, a large U.S. study found evidence of a reduction in the OR associated with maternal smoking and current wheeze from 1.9 among infants to 1.07 among teenagers (Table 6.11) (Stoddard and Miller 1995). Recent analyses of NHANES III data documented similar results, where ORs for current wheeze in the top versus the bottom tertile of cotinine levels declined from 4.8 (95 percent CI, 2.4–9.9) at 4 through 6 years of age to 1.5 (95 percent CI, 0.7–3.3) at 7 through 11 years of age, and to 0.9 (95 percent CI, 0.3–2.2) at 12 through 16 years of age (Mannino et al. 2001). Similarly, a large questionnaire survey in the United Kingdom found a reduction in the OR for cough from 1.60 at 8 through 10 years of age to 1.50 at 11 through 13 years of age, and to 1.12 at 14 through 19 years of age (Table 6.12) (Charlton 1984). A Korean study found that the OR for cough during a two-week period fell from 3.9 for 5-year-olds and younger to 2.6 for 6- through 11-year-olds, and to 2.0 for 12- through 14-year-olds (Park and Kim 1986). The Italian Studies on Respiratory Disorders in Childhood and the Environment reported a reduction in the odds of current asthma from 1.34 at 6 through 7 years of age to 1.17 in adolescents (Table 6.10) (Agabiti et al. 1999). In contrast, a relatively small New Zealand study found slightly higher ORs for current wheeze and cough at 13 through 14 years of age than at 6 through 7 years of age (Tables 6.11 and 6.12) (Moyes et al. 1995).

For a given level of parental smoking, the reported ORs in this review of the effects of parental smoking on LRIs in schoolchildren were somewhat lower than ORs found in infancy and early childhood. For LRIs, the pooled OR for either parent smoking was 1.57 (95 percent CI, 1.42–1.74). This pattern is consistent with previous claims of smaller effects in older

children, but the contrast is less marked than has been suggested (USEPA 1992). Moreover, it is necessary to consider the level of exposure when comparing estimates of the effects, which some earlier reviews did not provide (DiFranza and Lew 1996). For the same level of maternal smoking, biomarker cotinine assessments showed that personal exposure of children to secondhand smoke declined markedly between infancy and school age (Irvine et al. 1997).

Even after entering school, salivary cotinine levels provided evidence that exposure of nonsmoking children to secondhand smoke continues to fall as children grow older; exposures also are affected by gender, geographic area, and time of year (Jarvis et al. 1992; Cook et al. 1994; Pirkle et al. 1996). This decline in cotinine levels with an increase in age is consistent with large, nationwide U.S. study data, and strongly suggests that the adverse effects of parental smoking on respiratory symptoms in their children decline with age even among schoolchildren (Stoddard and Miller 1995).

Prenatal and Postnatal Exposure

Few studies have separately analyzed the effects of past versus current exposure to secondhand smoke. An early study reported a slightly lower prevalence of cough during the day or at night in children of former smokers (14.2 percent of 634) than in the offspring of lifetime nonsmokers (15.6 percent of 320) (Colley 1974). A more recent New Zealand study found that smoking by the current primary caregiver was associated with current wheeze (OR = 1.4 [95 percent CI, 1–2.1]), whereas maternal smoking during pregnancy was not (OR = 0.9 [95 percent CI, 0.7–1.4]) (Shaw et al. 1994). In a Norwegian study, postnatal smoking by the mother was more strongly related to asthma compared with either prenatal or current smoking (Table 6.10) (Søyseth et al. 1995). A recent Scottish study reported slightly stronger effects for current maternal smoking versus prenatal maternal smoking for both wheeze (OR = 1.15 versus 1.10, respectively) and cough (1.93 versus 1.42, respectively) (Beckett et al. 1996).

Findings of an analysis of NHANES III data are relevant to the U.S. experience. In general, the effects of in utero exposure to maternal smoking did not explain the effects of current secondhand smoke exposure (Mannino et al. 2001). Specifically, being in the top tertile of current cotinine levels, after excluding any active smokers, was associated with an increased risk of both current asthma and wheeze, regardless of prenatal maternal smoking. In contrast, a small U.S.

Table 6.11   Studies of wheeze prevalence associated with parental smoking

Study	Population age (years)/ location	Definition of wheeze	Prevalence in unexposed (%)	Odds ratio for smoking (95% confidence interval)	
				Either parent (unadjusted)	Either parent (adjusted)
Lebowitz and Burrows 1976	0–15 United States	Most days	1.4	2.86 (0.92–8.87)	NR*
Schilling et al. 1977	7–15 United States	Ever	11.7	1.99 (1.28–3.10)	NR
Kasuga et al. 1979	6–11 Japan	Current (or asthma)	9.8	2.08 (1.49–2.91)	1.15 (0.83–1.61)
Stanhope et al. 1979	12–18 New Zealand	Current (or asthma)	NR	NR	NR
Weiss et al. 1980	5–9 United States	Current and persistent	1.8	5.89 (0.79–44.1)	NR
Dodge 1982	8–12 United States	Ever	27.9	1.32 (0.94–1.85)	NR
Schenker et al. 1983	5–14 United States	Persistent	7.2	0.93 (0.73–1.19)	NR
Ware et al. 1984	6–9 United States	Persistent	9.9	NR	1.2 (1.05–1.37)
Burchfiel et al. 1986	0–19 United States	NR	18.4	NR	1.28 (1.08–1.52)
Goren and Goldsmith 1986	Grades 2–5 Israel	Wheeze with a cold	12.7	1.27 (0.95–1.70)	NR
McConnochie and Roghmann 1986a	6–10 United States	Current	10.2	NR	NR
Strachan and Elton 1986	7–8 United Kingdom	Ever	20	2.1 (0.87–5.1)	NR
Somerville et al. 1988	5–11 United Kingdom	Ever	11	1.09§ (0.95–1.26)	1.22 (1.02–1.45)
	5–11 United Kingdom	Most days/nights	3	1.66 (1.01–2.12)	1.54 (1.16–2.04)
Strachan 1988	7 United Kingdom	In the past year	12.1	1.04 (0.72–1.52)	NR
Hosein et al. 1989	7–17 United States	Current	13	NR	1.23 (0.88–1.72)
Stern et al. 1989a	7–12 Canada	Ever	22.9	NR	NR
Stern et al. 1989b	7–12 Canada	Persistent	9Δ	NR	NR

Odds ratio for smoking (95% confidence interval)				
One parent only vs. neither	Both parents vs. neither	Mother only vs. neither	Father only vs. neither	Confounders adjusted for
NR	NR	NR	NR	NR
1.47 (0.90–2.4)	4.57 (2.45–8.51)	2.08 (1.14–3.79)	1.07 (0.57–1.99)	NR
NR	NR	NR	NR	Distance from a major road
NR	NR	0.53 (0.26–1.05)[†]	NR	NR
4.12 (0.52–32.9)	7.52 (0.99–57.3)	NR	NR	NR
1.01 (0.67–1.52)	1.8 (1.19–2.73)	NR	NR	NR
1.08 (0.82–1.40)	0.74 (0.53–1.04)	NR	NR	NR
1.11 (0.95–1.29)	1.32 (1.14–1.53)	1.18 (0.95–1.48)	1.08 (0.92–1.28)	Age, gender, city
1.1 (0.87–1.39)	1.53 (1.19–1.97)	1.42 (0.85–2.36)	1.03 (0.80–1.33)	Age, gender, parental education
NR	NR	0.98 (0.66–1.46)	1.44 (1.05–1.98)	NR
NR	NR	2.16[†] (0.97–4.80)	1.20[‡] (0.55–2.62)	NR
NR	NR	NR	NR	NR
NR	NR	NR	NR	Age, gender, birth weight, obesity, socioeconomic status (SES), mother's age, number of siblings
NR	NR	NR	NR	Age, gender, birth weight, obesity, SES, mother's age, number of siblings
1.0 (0.65–1.54)	1.13 (0.67–1.90)	NR	NR	NR
1.32 (0.91–1.91)	1.14 (0.78–1.68)	NR	NR	Gender, active smoking
NR	NR	1.59 (1.24–2.03)	1.03 (0.80–1.31)	NR
NR	NR	1.26 (0.95–1.67)	NR	NR

Table 6.11   Continued

Study	Population age (years)/ location	Definition of wheeze	Prevalence in unexposed (%)	Odds ratio for smoking (95% confidence interval)	
				Either parent (unadjusted)	Either parent (adjusted)
Dijkstra et al. 1990	6–12 Netherlands	In the past year	7.1△	NR	1.86 (0.99–3.49)
Chinn and Rona 1991	5–11 United Kingdom	Ever	NR	NR	1.11§ (1.0–1.22)
	5–11 United Kingdom	Most days or nights	NR	NR	1.31 (1.11–1.55)
Dekker et al. 1991	5–8 Canada	Current	7.2	1.6 (1.39–1.83)	1.55 (NR)
Henry et al. 1991	5–12 Australia	In the past year	17.3	NR	1.4 (0.8–2.3)
Duffy and Mitchell 1993	8 and 12 Australia	Ever	22△	NR	NR
Halliday et al. 1993	5–12 Australia	Current	NR	NR	1.02 (0.71–1.47)
Jenkins et al. 1993	7 Australia	Ever (or asthma)	NR	NR	NR
Brabin et al. 1994	5–11 United Kingdom	Ever	18	1.32 (1.03–1.69)	1.28 (1.0–1.64)
Shaw et al. 1994	8–13 New Zealand	Current	22	1.0 (0.7–1.4)	NR
	8–13 New Zealand	Current	18	NR	NR
	8–13 New Zealand	Current§	22	NR	NR
Bråbäck et al. 1995	10–12 Sweden	NR	11.9	NR	NR
	10–12 Poland	NR	9.4	NR	NR
	10–12 Estonia	NR	7.1	NR	NR
Cuijpers et al. 1995	6–12 Netherlands	Ever (definition unclear)	14.7△	NR	1.08 (0.67–1.74)
Goren and Hellmann 1995	2nd and 5th graders Israel	Wheeze with a cold	13.1	1.25 (1.09–1.44)	NR

Odds ratio for smoking (95% confidence interval)				
One parent only vs. neither	**Both parents vs. neither**	**Mother only vs. neither**	**Father only vs. neither**	**Confounders adjusted for**
NR	NR	NR	NR	Age, parental education
NR	NR	NR	NR	Age, gender, country, birth weight, obesity, SES, mother's age, number of siblings, ethnicity, gas cooking
NR	NR	NR	NR	Age, gender, country, birth weight, obesity, SES, mother's age, number of siblings, ethnicity, gas cooking
1.39 (1.17–1.65)	1.72 (1.44–2.05)	NR	NR	Dampness, gas cooking
NR	NR	NR	NR	Age, gender, area, dust mite allergy
NR	NR	1.36 (0.96–1.93)	0.94 (0.70–1.26)	NR
NR	NR	NR	NR	Age, gender, area, atopy
NR	NR	1.35[†] (1.2–1.52)	1.10[‡] (0.97–1.23)	NR
NR	NR	NR	NR	Area
NR	NR	NR	NR	NR
NR	NR	1.4[¶] (1.0–2.1)	NR	NR
NR	NR	0.9** (0.7–1.4)	NR	NR
NR	NR	0.73 (0.41–1.29)	NR	Gender, atopy, dampness, overcrowding
NR	NR	1.54 (0.91–2.60)	NR	Gender, atopy, dampness, overcrowding
NR	NR	1.45 (0.94–2.24)	NR	Gender, atopy, dampness, overcrowding
NR	NR	NR	NR	Age, gender, dampness, father's education, dog, unvented geyser
1.24 (1.07–1.45)	1.27 (1.06–1.53)	1.25[†] (1.06–1.48)	1.27[‡] (1.10–1.47)	NR

Table 6.11   Continued

Study	Population age (years)/ location	Definition of wheeze	Prevalence in unexposed (%)	Odds ratio for smoking (95% confidence interval)	
				Either parent (unadjusted)	Either parent (adjusted)
Moyes et al. 1995	6–7 New Zealand	Current	23	1.06 (0.88–1.27)	NR
	13–14 New Zealand	Current	28	1.16 (0.98–1.37)	NR
Stoddard and Miller 1995	0–17 United States	Current (or asthma)§	NR	NR	NR
	0–2 United States	Current (or asthma)	11.6	NR	NR
	3–5 United States	Current (or asthma)	8	NR	NR
	6–12 United States	Current (or asthma)	7.5	NR	NR
	13–17 United States	Current (or asthma)	8.5	NR	NR
Volkmer et al. 1995	4–5 Australia	In the past year	NR	1.12 (NR)	Not significant§
	4–5 Australia	Ever	NR	1.24 (NR)	1.18 (1.08–1.30)
Abuekteish et al. 1996	6–12 Jordan	In the past 3 years	12.4Δ	NR	NR
Peters et al. 1996	10–13 Hong Kong	NR	7.1Δ	NR	1.01 (0.79–1.29)
Wright et al. 1996	6 United States	Current	26.4	1.32 (0.98–1.80)	NR
Austin and Russell 1997	12 and 14 United Kingdom	Current	16.6	1.13 (0.87–1.48)	NR
Butland et al. 1997	7.5–8.5 United Kingdom	≤4 attacks in the past year; parent questionnaire	6.6	NR	NR
	7.5–8.5 United Kingdom	>4 attacks in the past year; parent questionnaire	2.6	NR	NR
Hu et al. 1997	10–11 United States (Chicago)	In the past year	29.0	NR	NR

Odds ratio for smoking (95% confidence interval)				
One parent only vs. neither	**Both parents vs. neither**	**Mother only vs. neither**	**Father only vs. neither**	**Confounders adjusted for**
NR	NR	NR	NR	NR
NR	NR	NR	NR	NR
NR	NR	1.36 (1.14–1.62)	0.83 (0.67–1.02)	Gender, race, area, SES, family size
NR	NR	1.90 (1.23–2.94)	NR	Gender, race, area, SES, family size
NR	NR	1.53 (0.99–2.37)	NR	Gender, race, area, SES, family size
NR	NR	1.35 (1.01–1.81)	NR	Gender, race, area, SES, family size
NR	NR	1.07 (0.76–1.49)	NR	Gender, race, area, SES, family size
NR	NR	NR	NR	Method of heating and ventilating
NR	NR	NR	NR	Method of heating and ventilating
NR	NR	1.87[†] (1.28–2.75)	1.31[‡] (1.05–1.63)	NR
0.94 (0.69–1.28)	1.70 (1.15–2.54)	NR	NR	Age, gender, district, father's education, housing
NR	NR	NR	NR	NR
NR	NR	1.15 (0.84–1.56)	NR	NR
NR	NR	1.27** (0.93–1.74)	1.04[††] (0.76–1.43)	Study period
NR	NR	1.55** (1.02–2.34)	1.06[††] (0.69–1.62)	Study period
NR	NR	0.79 (0.51–1.21)	NR	None

Table 6.11   Continued

Study	Population age (years)/ location	Definition of wheeze	Prevalence in unexposed (%)	Odds ratio for smoking (95% confidence interval)	
				Either parent (unadjusted)	Either parent (adjusted)
Leung et al. 1997	13–14 Hong Kong	Current[##]	12[Δ]	1.14 (0.92–1.42)	NR
	13–14 Hong Kong	Severe attack[##]	2.4[Δ]	1.05[§] (0.64–1.74)	NR
Maier et al. 1997	5–9 United States (Washington state)	In the past year (no asthma diagnosis)	7[Δ]	1.7 (1.0–2.9)	1.8 (1.0–3.2)
Selçuk et al. 1997	7–12 Turkey	Ever	16.1	1.29 (1.10–1.51)	1.25[§] (1.05–1.48)
	7–12 Turkey	Current	4.1	1.39 (1.02–1.90)	1.52 (1.10–2.09)
Chhabra et al. 1998	4–17 India	Current wheeze	15.3	1.62 (1.27–2.05)	NR
Kendirli et al. 1998	6–14 Turkey	Wheeze (ever)	8.4	1.63 (1.29–2.08)	NR
Lam et al. 1998	12–15 Hong Kong	In the past 3 months	4.8	NR	NR
Lewis and Britton 1998	16 United Kingdom	Current wheeze	NR	NR	NR
Lewis et al. 1998	8–11 Australia	>3 episodes of wheeze in the past year	8.6	NR	1.16 (0.85–1.59)
Peters et al. 1998	8–13 Hong Kong	Physician consultation for wheeze in the past 3 months	2.2	1.22 (0.96–1.57)	NR
Saraçlar et al. 1998	7–14 Turkey	Ever (International Study of Asthma and Allergy in Childhood [ISAAC])	4.7[Δ]	NR	1.33 (1.03–1.76)
Withers et al. 1998	14–16 United Kingdom	Current wheeze	18.2[Δ]	NR	1.48 (1.17–1.88)
Agabiti et al. 1999	6–7 Italy	Wheeze in the past year (no asthma diagnosis); parent questionnaire	5.2	1.09 (0.90–1.32)	1.13 (0.93–1.37)
	13–14 Italy	Wheeze in the past year (no asthma diagnosis); child questionnaire	8.4	1.42 (1.23–1.63)	1.24 (1.07–1.44)

Odds ratio for smoking (95% confidence interval)				
One parent only vs. neither	Both parents vs. neither	Mother only vs. neither	Father only vs. neither	Confounders adjusted for
NR	NR	NR	NR	NR
NR	NR	NR	NR	NR
NR	NR	NR	NR	Gender, ethnicity, allergy, SES, parental asthma
NR	NR	NR	NR	Age, gender, place, animals, atopic family, breastfeeding
NR	NR	NR	NR	NR
NR	NR	NR	NR	NR
NR	NR	NR	NR	NR
1.21 (0.91–1.60)	NR	1.71 (0.84–3.49)	1.24[††] (0.93–1.64)	Age, gender, area, housing type
NR	NR	1.27** (1.16–1.39)	NR	Gender, SES, breastfeeding, maternal age, parity, birth weight, gestational age
NR	NR	NR	NR	Age, gender, PM_{10}[§§], SO_2[ΔΔ], gas heating, maternal allergy
1.04 (0.76–1.41)	1.57 (1.02–2.43)	NR	NR	Age, gender, housing type, area, father's education
NR	NR	NR	NR	Age, gender, pets, parental atopy, SES
NR	NR	p >0.05	p >0.05	Maternal asthma, child eczema and hay fever, atopic sibling, pets, gas cooking; active smoking was "not significant"
NR	1.24 (0.99–1.56)	1.18 (1.0–1.39)	1.14 (0.97–1.36)	Age, gender, area, father's education, crowding, dampness, gas heating, parental asthma, other smokers
NR	1.31 (1.11–1.56)	1.26 (1.13–1.41)	1.09 (0.96–1.24)	Age, gender, area, father's education, crowding, dampness, gas heating, parental asthma, other smokers, active smoking

Table 6.11   Continued

Study	Population age (years)/ location	Definition of wheeze	Prevalence in unexposed (%)	Odds ratio for smoking (95% confidence interval)	
				Either parent (unadjusted)	Either parent (adjusted)
Belousova et al. 1999	8–11 Australia	Wheeze in the past year	23.8	NR	NR
Burr et al. 1999	12–14 United Kingdom	Wheeze in the past 12 months; child questionnaire	31.8	1.22 (1.15–1.28)	1.14[¶¶] (1.09–1.19)
	12–14 United Kingdom	Speech-limiting wheeze in the past 12 months	7.6	1.40 (1.28–1.52)	1.27[§,¶¶] (1.17–1.36)
Chhabra et al. 1999	5–17 India	Current wheeze (definition unclear)	10.8	1.69 (NR)	1.61 (1.47–1.78)
Lam et al. 1999	8–13 Hong Kong	Wheeze (ever)	9.6	NR	1.12 (0.89–1.41)[¶¶]
Shamssain and Shamsian 1999	6–7 United Kingdom	Wheeze in the past year	15.5	NR	NR
	6–7 United Kingdom	Speech-limiting attack in the past year	2.7	NR	NR
	6–7 United Kingdom	Wheeze (ever)	25.6	NR	NR
Wang et al. 1999	11–16 Taiwan	Wheeze in the past year; video; written questionnaires	13.2	1.02 (0.99–1.05)	1.08 (1.05–1.12)
Csonka et al. 2000	6–13 Finland	Current wheeze or asthma	>9.6	1.6 (1.0–2.6)	NR
Qian et al. 2000	5–14 China	Wheeze (ever)	6.9–17.4	NR	1.31 (0.96–1.78)

*NR = Data were not reported.
[†]Mother currently smoked vs. did not smoke.
[‡]Father currently smoked vs. did not smoke.
[§]Not included in the meta-analysis.
[Δ]Overall prevalence.
[¶]Primary caregiver smoked vs. did not smoke.
**Mother smoked vs. did not smoke prenatally.
[††]Father smoked vs. neither parent smoked where only 2.5% of the mothers smoked.
[‡‡]Based on a written questionnaire.
[§§]PM_{10} = Particulate matter (levels of particles [particulate pollution] with an aerodynamic diameter of less than 10 micrometers).
[ΔΔ]SO_2 = Sulfur dioxide.
[¶¶]Derived from pooled results of all household smokers.

Odds ratio for smoking (95% confidence interval)				
One parent only vs. neither	Both parents vs. neither	Mother only vs. neither	Father only vs. neither	Confounders adjusted for
NR	NR	1.33[†] (1.2–1.5)	NR	Atopy, parental asthma, early life bronchitis
NR	NR	NR	NR	Gender, area, pets, cooking fuel, heating fuel, housing type, active smoking
NR	NR	NR	NR	Gender, area, pets, cooking fuel, heating fuel, housing type, active smoking
NR	NR	NR	NR	Age, gender, family atopy
NR	NR	NR	NR	Age, gender, area, active smoking
1.11 (NR)	1.50 (NR)	1.15 (0.86–1.54)	NR	None
NR	NR	1.12 (0.66–1.90)	NR	None
NR	NR	1.46 (1.19–1.79)	NR	None
NR	NR	NR	NR	Age, gender, parental education, area, Chinese incense, exercise, active smoking, alcohol consumption
NR	NR	NR	NR	NR
NR	NR	NR	NR	Age, gender, ventilation, family history, mother's education, coal use, area

Figure 6.6   Odds ratios for the effect of smoking by either parent on wheeze prevalence

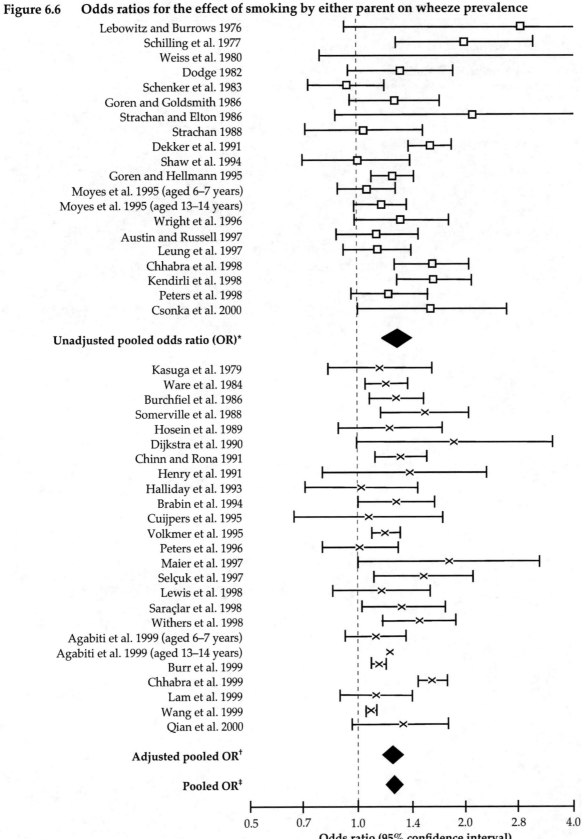

*Studies that did not adjust for potential confounders.
†Studies that adjusted for a variety of potential confounders.
‡Based on all studies.

Figure 6.7   Odds ratios for the effect of smoking by either parent on cough prevalence

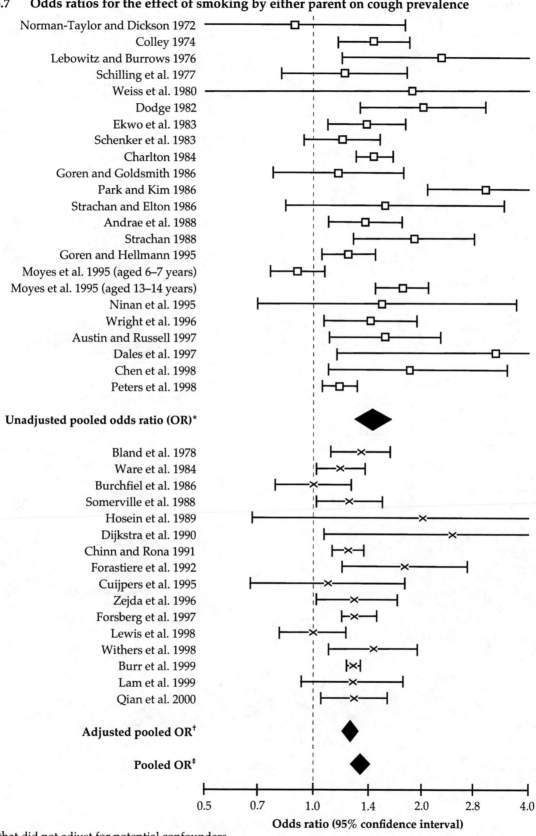

*Studies that did not adjust for potential confounders.
†Studies that adjusted for a variety of potential confounders.
‡Based on all studies.

Table 6.12   Studies of cough prevalence associated with parental smoking

Study	Population age (years)/ location	Definition of cough	Prevalence in unexposed (%)	Odds ratio for smoking (95% confidence interval)	
				Either parent (unadjusted)	Either parent (adjusted)
Norman-Taylor and Dickinson 1972	5 United Kingdom	Recent recurrence	3.1	0.89 (0.44–1.80)	NR*
Colley 1974	6–14 United Kingdom	Usually, in winter	14.7	1.47 (1.17–1.85)	NR
Lebowitz and Burrows 1976	0–15 United States	Persistent	4.8	2.28 (1.20–4.32)	NR
Schilling et al. 1977	7–18 United States	Cough and/or phlegm, usually (definition unclear)	12.8	1.22 (0.82–1.82)	NR
Bland et al. 1978	11–12 United Kingdom	Day or night	19.4	1.56 (1.36–1.79)	1.36 (1.12–1.64)
Weiss et al. 1980	5–9 United States	Cough and phlegm	1.7	1.88 (0.24–15.0)	NR
Dodge 1982	8–12 United States	NR	14.1	2.03 (1.35–3.06)	NR
Ekwo et al. 1983	6–12 United States	With colds	30	1.40 (1.09–1.80)	NR
Schenker et al. 1983	5–14 United States	Chronic	6.3	1.21 (0.95–1.54)	NR
Charlton 1984	8–19 United Kingdom	Frequent recurrences	22	1.47 (1.31–1.66)	NR
	8–10 United Kingdom	Frequent recurrences	33.5	1.60[†] (1.33–1.96)	NR
	11–13 United Kingdom	Frequent recurrences	17.5	1.50[†] (1.26–1.79)	NR
	14–19 United Kingdom	Frequent recurrences	8.5	1.12[†] (0.83–1.52)	NR
Ware et al. 1984	6–9 United States	Persistent	7.7	NR	1.19 (1.02–1.39)
Burchfiel et al. 1986	0–19 United States	NR	8.5	NR	1.0 (0.78–1.27)
Goren and Goldsmith 1986	2nd and 5th graders Israel	With sputum	6	1.17 (0.77–1.78)	NR

Odds ratio for smoking (95% confidence interval)				
One parent only vs. neither	Both parents vs. neither	Mother only vs. neither	Father only vs. neither	Confounders adjusted for
0.62 (0.25–1.46)	1.4 (0.61–3.2)	NR	NR	NR
1.25 (0.94–1.66)	1.66 (1.28–2.16)	NR	NR	NR
NR	NR	NR	NR	NR
1.06 (0.68–1.63)	1.99 (1.06–3.73)	1.1 (0.56–2.15)	1.04 (0.64–1.69)	NR
1.2 (0.96–1.49)	1.57 (1.25–1.94)	NR	NR	Active smoking, gender
1.64 (0.18–15.0)	2.09 (0.25–17.8)	NR	NR	NR
1.84 (1.15–2.95)	2.29 (1.41–3.73)	NR	NR	NR
1.33 (1.0–1.78)	1.50 (1.10–2.04)	1.38 (0.87–2.17)	1.32 (0.96–1.80)	NR
1.12 (0.84–1.49)	1.35 (1.0–1.83)	NR	NR	NR
1.36 (1.19–1.56)	1.64 (1.41–1.91)	1.36 (1.15–1.62)	1.34 (1.13–1.59)	NR
NR	NR	NR	NR	NR
NR	NR	NR	NR	NR
NR	NR	NR	NR	NR
1.09 (0.91–1.30)	1.38 (1.16–1.63)	0.99 (0.75–1.29)	1.13 (0.94–1.36)	Age, gender, city
0.93 (0.67–1.30)	1.27 (0.89–1.81)	0.78 (0.37–1.64)	0.97 (0.67–1.41)	Age, gender, parental education
NR	NR	1.22 (0.72–2.07)	1.15 (0.73–1.81)	NR

Table 6.12   Continued

Study	Population age (years)/ location	Definition of cough	Prevalence in unexposed (%)	Odds ratio for smoking (95% confidence interval) Either parent (unadjusted)	Either parent (adjusted)
Park and Kim 1986	0–14 Korea	In the past 2 weeks	5	3.04 (2.09–4.43)	NR
Strachan and Elton 1986	7–8 United Kingdom	Night	49.1	1.7 (0.85–3.44)	NR
Andrae et al. 1988	6 months–16 years Sweden	Exercise induced	5.1	1.39 (1.10–1.76)	NR
Somerville et al. 1988	5–11 United Kingdom	Usually in the morning	4	1.24 (1.0–1.53)	1.24[†] (0.94–1.65)
	5–11 United Kingdom	Usually day/night	8	1.46 (1.27–1.68)	1.26 (1.02–1.56)
Strachan 1988	7 United Kingdom	At night in the past month	9	1.91 (1.29–2.82)	NR
Hosein et al. 1989	7–17 United States	Persistent	0.9	NR	2.02 (0.68–6.03)
Stern et al. 1989a	7–12 Canada	With phlegm	5.3	NR	NR
Stern et al. 1989b	7–12 Canada	Persistent	8[‡]	NR	NR
Dijkstra et al. 1990	6–12 Netherlands	Persistent	4.6[‡]	NR	2.46 (1.07–5.64)
Chinn and Rona 1991	5–11 United Kingdom	Usually	NR	NR	1.25 (1.13–1.38)
Forastiere et al. 1992	7–11 Italy	With phlegm	5.5	1.3 (NR)	1.3[†] (0.9–1.9)
	7–11 Italy	Night	3.4	1.8 (NR)	1.8 (1.2–2.7)
Bråbäck et al. 1995	10–12 Sweden	Night	8.4	NR	NR
	10–12 Poland	Night	6.7	NR	NR
	10–12 Estonia	Night	7.4	NR	NR

Odds ratio for smoking (95% confidence interval)				
One parent only vs. neither	Both parents vs. neither	Mother only vs. neither	Father only vs. neither	Confounders adjusted for
3.2 (2.11–4.85)	3.0 (2.05–4.38)	NR	NR	NR
NR	NR	NR	NR	NR
NR	NR	NR	NR	NR
NR	NR	NR	NR	Age, gender, birth weight, obesity, socioeconomic status (SES), mother's age, number of siblings
NR	NR	NR	NR	Age, gender, birth weight, obesity, SES, mother's age, number of siblings
1.64 (1.05–2.56)	2.45 (1.5–4.02)	NR	NR	NR
1.84 (0.55–6.18)	2.23 (0.69–7.19)	NR	NR	Gender, active smoking
NR	NR	0.98 (0.60–1.62)	0.85 (0.52–1.39)	NR
NR	NR	1.45§ (1.13–1.87)	NR	NR
NR	NR	NR	NR	Age, parental education
NR	NR	NR	NR	Age, gender, country, birth weight, obesity, SES, mother's age, number of siblings, ethnicity, gas cooking
NR	1.7 (1.1–2.5)	1.2 (0.7–2.0)	1.0 (0.7–1.6)	Age, gender, area, SES
NR	2.5 (1.6–3.9)	1.5 (0.8–2.8)	1.2 (0.8–2.0)	Age, gender, area, SES
NR	NR	2.09Δ (1.51–2.90)	NR	Gender, atopy, dampness, overcrowding
NR	NR	1.10Δ (0.62–1.93)	NR	Gender, atopy, dampness, overcrowding
NR	NR	2.27Δ (1.55–3.32)	NR	Gender, atopy, dampness, overcrowding

Table 6.12   Continued

Study	Population age (years)/ location	Definition of cough	Prevalence in unexposed (%)	Odds ratio for smoking (95% confidence interval)	
				Either parent (unadjusted)	**Either parent (adjusted)**
Cuijpers et al. 1995	6–12 Netherlands	Chronic	12.6[‡]	NR	1.10 (0.67–1.8)
Goren and Hellmann 1995	2nd and 5th graders Israel	With sputum	8.1	1.25 (1.06–1.49)	NR
Moyes et al. 1995	6–7 New Zealand	Night	30	0.91 (0.77–1.08)	NR
	13–14 New Zealand	Night	24	1.78 (1.50–2.11)	NR
Ninan et al. 1995	8–13 United Kingdom	Isolated, persistent, nocturnal	NR	1.61 (0.70–3.70)	NR
Volkmer et al. 1995[†]	4–5 Australia	Dry	NR	Not significant	Not significant
Wright et al. 1996	6 United States	Persistent	27.4	1.44** (1.07–1.94)	NR
	6 United States	Persistent, without wheeze	11.8	1.67[†],** (1.10–2.54)	1.93[†],** (1.09–3.45)
Zejda et al. 1996	7–9 Poland	Chronic	31.9[‡]	NR	1.3 (1.02–1.71)
Austin and Russell 1997	12 and 14 United Kingdom	Chronic	7.2	1.58 (1.11–2.27)	NR
Dales et al. 1997	NR Canada	Recorded night cough	86	3.25 (1.16–9.09)	NR
Forsberg et al. 1997	6–12 Scandinavia	Dry cough at night apart from colds in the past year	8–19[‡]	NR	1.3 (1.2–1.5)
Chen et al. 1998	6–17 Canada	Night	5.5[‡]	1.97 (1.10–3.52)	NR
Lam et al. 1998	12–15 Hong Kong	Saw a physician for cough in the past 3 months	7.3	NR	NR

Odds ratio for smoking (95% confidence interval)				
One parent only vs. neither	Both parents vs. neither	Mother only vs. neither	Father only vs. neither	Confounders adjusted for
NR	NR	NR	NR	NR
1.12 (0.93–1.36)	1.51 (1.22–1.87)	1.42△ (1.17–1.73)	1.25¶ (1.05–1.48)	Age, gender, dampness, father's education, dog, unvented geyser
NR	NR	NR	NR	NR
NR	NR	NR	NR	NR
NR	NR	NR	NR	NR
NR	NR	NR	NR	NR
NR	NR	NR	NR	NR
NR	NR	NR	NR	Gender, hay fever, lower respiratory infection in the first year
NR	NR	NR	NR	Crowding
NR	NR	1.93 (1.30–2.85)	NR	NR
NR	NR	NR	NR	NR
NR	NR	NR	NR	Age, gender, area, fitted carpets, pets, mold, stove use, parental asthma, early day care
2.01 (1.04–3.88)	1.91 (0.84–4.33)	NR	NR	None
1.19 (0.94–1.51)	NR	0.73 (0.32–1.70)	1.31†† (1.03–1.65)	Age, gender, area, housing type

Table 6.12   Continued

Study	Population age (years)/ location	Definition of cough	Prevalence in unexposed (%)	Odds ratio for smoking (95% confidence interval)	
				Either parent (unadjusted)	Either parent (adjusted)
Lewis et al. 1998	8–11 Australia	Dry night cough that lasted >2 weeks in the past 12 months without a cold	19.1	NR	1.0 (0.81–1.23)
Peters et al. 1998	8–13 Hong Kong	Physician consultation for cough in the past 3 months	12.5	1.18 (1.06–1.32)	NR
Withers et al. 1998	14–16 United Kingdom	Current	12.4[‡]	NR	1.47 (1.11–1.95)
Burr et al. 1999	12–14 United Kingdom	Cough without colds in the past 12 months	25.5	1.49 (1.41–1.57)	1.29[ΔΔ] (1.24–1.35)
Lam et al. 1999	8–13 Hong Kong	Cough for 3 months	4.8	NR	1.29[¶¶] (0.93–1.78)
Shamssain and Shamsian 1999	6–7 United Kingdom	Nighttime cough in the past 12 months	NR	NR	NR
Qian et al. 2000	5–14 China	Often, with or without colds	41–84	NR	1.30 (1.05–1.61)

*NR = Data were not reported.
[†]Not included in the meta-analysis.
[‡]Overall prevalence.
[§]Mother smoked vs. did not smoke during pregnancy and infancy.
[Δ]Mother currently smoked vs. did not smoke.
[¶]Father currently smoked vs. did not smoke.
**Reference group = Children without cough or wheeze.
[††]Father smoked vs. neither parent smoked where only 2.5% of the mothers smoked.
[‡‡]PM_{10} = Particulate matter (levels of particles [particulate pollution] with an aerodynamic diameter of less than 10 micrometers).
[§§]SO_2 = Sulfur dioxide.
[ΔΔ]Derived from pooled results of all household smokers.
[¶¶]Analyses excluded active smokers.

Odds ratio for smoking (95% confidence interval)				
One parent only vs. neither	Both parents vs. neither	Mother only vs. neither	Father only vs. neither	Confounders adjusted for
NR	NR	NR	NR	Age, gender, PM_{10}[##], SO_2[§§], gas heating, maternal allergy
1.15 (1.01–1.32)	1.33 (1.08–1.64)	NR	NR	Age, gender, housing type, area, father's education
NR	NR	p >0.05	p >0.05	Maternal hay fever, child's eczema and hay fever, active smoking, single parent
NR	NR	NR	NR	Gender, area, pets, cooking and heating fuel, housing type, active smoking
NR	NR	NR	NR	Age, gender, area, active smoking
1.04 (NR)	1.10 (NR)	1.05 (0.85–1.29)	NR	None
NR	NR	NR	NR	Age, gender, ventilation, family history, mother's education, coal use, area

Table 6.13   Studies of phlegm and breathlessness associated with parental smoking

Study	Population age (years)/ location	Prevalence in unexposed (%)	Odds ratio for smoking (95% confidence interval)		
			Either parent (unadjusted)	Either parent (adjusted)	One parent
Lebowitz and Burrows 1976	0–15 United States	3.1	1.96 (0.88–4.38)	NR*	NR
Bland et al. 1978	11–12 United Kingdom	9.8	1.42 (1.22–1.66)	1.33 (1.08–1.65)	1.26 (0.99–1.60)
Dodge 1982	8–12 United States	6.7	1.85 (1.05–3.25)	NR	1.77 (0.93–3.37)
Schenker et al. 1983	5–14 United States	4.1	1.09 (0.81–1.48)	NR	1.18 (0.84–1.67)
Burchfiel et al. 1986	0–19 United States	11	NR	1.37 (1.12–1.68)	1.25 (0.95–1.65)
Goren and Goldsmith 1986	2nd and 5th graders Israel	10.7	1.07 (0.76–1.43)	NR	NR
Hosein et al. 1989	7–17 United States	1.4	NR	1.05 (0.40–2.79)	0.76 (0.23–2.51)
	7–12 United States	4.6	NR	0.99 (0.57–1.71)	1.05 (0.57–1.95)
Stern et al. 1989b	7–12 Canada	8.0†	NR	NR	NR
Dijkstra et al. 1990	6–12 Netherlands	4.6†	NR	1.95 (0.91–4.19)	NR
Brabin et al. 1994	5–11 United Kingdom	10	1.54 (1.13–2.09)	1.44 (1.06–1.95)	NR
Cuijpers et al. 1995	6–12 Netherlands	11.9†	NR	1.58 (0.98–2.56)	NR
Peters et al. 1996	10–13 Hong Kong	8.7†	NR	1.40 (1.13–1.75)	1.26 (0.96–1.64)
Lam et al. 1998	12–15 Hong Kong	4.8	NR	NR	1.14 (0.86–1.52)
Peters et al. 1998	8–13 Hong Kong	4.7	1.32 (1.12–1.57)	NR	1.26 (1.02–1.54)
Burr et al. 1999	12–14 United Kingdom	17.7	1.58 (1.48–1.67)	1.35Δ (1.30–1.42)	NR
Lam et al. 1999	8–13 Hong Kong	6.7	NR	1.44 (1.09–1.90)	NR
Qian et al. 2000	5–14 China	14–57	NR	1.36 (1.08–1.72)	NR

*NR = Data were not reported.
†Overall prevalence.
‡Mother currently smoked vs. did not smoke.
§Father smoked vs. neither parent smoked where only 2.5% of the mothers smoked.
ΔDerived from pooled results for all household smokers.

Odds ratio for smoking (95% confidence interval)

Both parents	Mother only	Father only	Outcome	Confounders adjusted for
NR	NR	NR	Persistent phlegm	NR
1.42 (1.11–1.83)	NR	NR	Shortness of breath (SOB) on exertion	Gender, active smoking
1.95 (1.0–3.81)	NR	NR	Sputum	NR
0.98 (0.66–1.49)	NR	NR	Chronic phlegm	NR
1.53 (1.14–2.05)	1.3 (0.71–2.39)	1.24 (0.91–1.70)	Phlegm	Age, gender, socioeconomic status, family size
NR	1.26 (0.85–1.87)	0.92 (0.64–1.32)	SOB	NR
1.37 (0.47–4.03)	NR	NR	Persistent phlegm	Gender
0.93 (0.49–1.77)	NR	NR	SOB when hurrying	Gender, active smoking
NR	1.15[‡] (0.90–1.47)	NR	Persistent phlegm	Parental symptoms, gas cooking (not area)
NR	NR	NR	SOB plus wheeze in the past year	Age, parental education (not school)
NR	NR	NR	SOB (ever)	Area
NR	NR	NR	SOB	Age, gender, dampness, father's education, dog, unvented geyser
1.75 (1.19–2.56)	NR	NR	Phlegm	Age, gender, area, housing type, father's education
NR	2.03 (1.05–3.92)	1.22[§] (0.92–1.62)	Phlegm in the past 3 months	Age, gender, area, housing type
1.33 (0.97–1.83)	NR	NR	Physician diagnosis of phlegm in the past 3 months	Age, gender, housing type, area, father's education
1.38 (1.25–1.53)	1.24 (1.12–1.37)	1.26 (1.14–1.38)	Phlegm without colds in the past 12 months	Gender, area, pets, cooking and heating fuel, housing type, active smoking
NR	NR	NR	Phlegm in the past 3 months	Age, gender, area, active smoking
NR	NR	NR	Frequent phlegm	Age, gender, ventilation, family history, mother's education, coal use, area

Figure 6.8   Odds ratios for the effect of smoking by either parent on phlegm and breathlessness

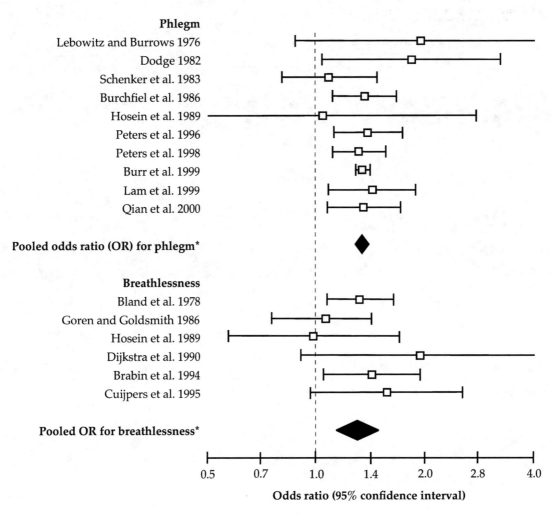

*Adjusted and unadjusted studies.

study found stronger effects of maternal smoking during pregnancy compared with current postnatal maternal smoking (Hu et al. 1997).

A study in Tasmania found that prenatal and postnatal exposure had similar health effects, with some evidence for an effect of smoking in the child's presence (Ponsonby et al. 2000). A Swedish study reported a borderline significant effect from maternal smoking during pregnancy (1.4 [95 percent CI, 1.0–2.0]) but no effect from current parental smoking (1.0 [95 percent CI, 0.7–1.4]) (Nilsson et al. 1999). The Italian collaborative group study tended to find greater ORs in preadolescent children from prenatal maternal smoking than from current maternal smoking, but not among adolescents (Agabiti et al. 1999). Moreover, the authors acknowledged that even in this very large study, disentangling current from past effects was problematic.

Raised ORs for respiratory symptoms in studies from China (Qian et al. 2000), Hong Kong (Lau et al. 1995; Peters et al. 1996, 1998; Leung et al. 1997; Lam et al. 1998, 1999), and Taiwan (Wang et al. 1999), where maternal smoking is uncommon, also suggest a role for postnatal secondhand smoke exposure. One Hong Kong study found that symptoms were more strongly related to smoking by grandparents than by fathers, which fit the role of grandparents as caregivers (Lam et al. 1999).

Table 6.14   Summary of pooled random effects (odds ratios) of respiratory symptoms associated with parental smoking

Symptom	Number of studies	Odds ratio for smoking (95% confidence interval)				
		Either parent	One parent	Both parents	Mother only	Father only
Asthma	31*	1.23 (1.14–1.33)				
	7		1.01 (0.84–1.22)			
	10			1.42 (1.30–1.56)		
	21				1.33 (1.24–1.43)	
	12					1.07 (0.97–1.18)
Wheeze[†]	45*,[‡]	1.26 (1.20–1.33)				
	13		1.18 (1.10–1.26)			
	14			1.41 (1.23–1.63)		
	27[§]				1.28 (1.21–1.35)	
	14					1.13 (1.08–1.20)
Cough	39	1.35 (1.27–1.43)				
	18		1.27 (1.14–1.41)			
	18			1.64 (1.48–1.81)		
	16[§]				1.34 (1.17–1.54)	
	10					1.22 (1.12–1.32)
Phlegm[Δ]	10	1.35 (1.30–1.41)				
	7		1.24 (1.10–1.39)			
	6			1.42 (1.19–1.70)		
Breathlessness[Δ]	6	1.31 (1.14–1.50)				

*Two age groups from Moyes et al. 1995 were included as separate studies.
[†]Excluded the European Communities Study, which had a pooled odds ratio of 1.20.
[‡]Agabiti et al. 1999 was included as two separate studies.
[§]Bråbäck et al. 1995 was included as three separate studies.
[Δ]Data for phlegm and breathlessness are restricted because several comparisons were based on fewer than five studies.

Former Parental Smoking

On balance, limited evidence suggests that there is no increase in the prevalence of respiratory symptoms among children of former smokers (Colley 1974; Shaw et al. 1994). Symptom prevalence seems to be more closely related to current maternal smoking than to prenatal maternal smoking (Søyseth et al. 1995; Beckett et al. 1996; Mannino et al. 2001), although the data are not entirely consistent (Agabiti et al. 1999). Although the data are compatible with the hypothesis that current rather than past exposure makes the predominant contribution to symptoms, the evidence is not strong. There are only a few relevant studies. One major limitation of these studies is that the exposure data were not collected prospectively and consequently, recall bias is a potential problem.

Publication Bias and Wheeze

Researchers have found evidence of publication bias, particularly for wheeze, in small published studies that have higher ORs. Some studies that reported estimated effects and confidence limits only for those exposure and outcome combinations that were statistically significant further suggest publication bias (Withers et al. 1998). However, the effect of this source of bias on the pooled ORs is small because there are so many large published studies. The similarity between the pooled OR for wheeze in published studies and in the unpublished EC Study provides further reassurance that the association is not an artifact of selective publication. Notably, however, the two EC centers whose published data have appeared in journals—Middlesbrough (Melia et al. 1982) and Ardennes

Table 6.15   Summary of pooled random effects (odds ratios) associated with parental smoking restricted to studies of children aged ≤11 years

Symptom	Number of studies	Odds ratio for smoking (95% confidence interval)				
		Either parent	**One parent**	**Both parents**	**Mother only**	**Father only**
Asthma	13	1.18 (1.06–1.31)				
	5		Insufficient studies	1.47 (1.29–1.68)		
	7				1.31 (1.15–1.50)	
	4					1.13 (0.99–1.29)
Wheeze*	15	1.27 (1.16–1.38)				
	4		1.21 (1.10–1.45)			
	5			1.41 (1.16–1.71)		
	8				1.26 (1.15–1.38)	
	5					1.10 (1.02–1.20)
Cough	13	1.28 (1.13–1.44)				
	4		1.17 (0.84–1.61)			
	5			1.85 (1.29–2.64)		
	4				1.07 (0.91–1.24)	
	3					1.12 (0.95–1.38)

Note: The symptoms "phlegm" and "breathlessness" were not included in this table because of an insufficient number of studies.

*Excluded the European Communities Study, which had a pooled odds ratio of 1.20.

(Gepts et al. 1978)—had ORs of 1.36 and 1.37, respectively, which were above the overall average for the EC Study.

Evidence Synthesis

This report has described multiple mechanisms by which secondhand smoke exposure could increase the prevalence of respiratory symptoms and asthma in childhood. Secondhand smoke exposure might increase the prevalence of respiratory symptoms and asthma through in utero effects or through inflammation and an altered lung immunophenotype from postnatal exposure. Multiple studies from diverse countries consistently show that parental smoking is positively associated with the prevalence of asthma and respiratory symptoms (including wheeze) in schoolchildren; the findings of individual studies as well as the pooled analyses show that these associations are unlikely to be attributable to chance alone. The magnitude of the effects is similar for the different outcome measures. The estimated effects, particularly for wheeze, were robust to adjustments for a wide range of potentially confounding environmental and

other factors. This robustness supports the conclusion that residual confounding is unlikely to be an issue and that the associations between parental smoking and the prevalence of asthma and respiratory symptoms in schoolchildren are causal.

The case for a causal interpretation is further strengthened by the trend for the OR to increase with the number of parents who smoke (i.e., none, one, or both). In the meta-analysis, the trends with the number of smoking parents were statistically significant for asthma, wheeze, and cough, and trends were evident in most of the individual studies as well. The effect of maternal smoking is greater than that of paternal smoking, but there is nevertheless evidence for a small effect of paternal smoking. Maternal smoking is associated with higher cotinine levels in school-age children, implying that maternal smoking probably has a greater impact on the exposure of children to secondhand smoke (Cook et al. 1994). These results also imply that the increased risk for asthma and other symptoms reflects postnatal exposure, although prenatal exposure may also be a contributing factor. First, there is an effect of paternal smoking; second, risk tends to rise with the number of household smokers; third, many women who do not smoke while pregnant smoke after the birth of their children; and fourth, limited evidence shows no increase in symptoms in children of former smokers. Few studies have examined dose-response trends with the number of cigarettes smoked in the household per day or dose-response trends among exposed children alone.

The prevalence of symptoms ascertained by cross-sectional surveys is determined by both disease incidence and prognosis, and the pattern of morbidity tends to be dominated by a large number of children with mild symptoms. There are indications that secondhand smoke exposure is associated with more severe wheeze, both in studies where ORs were reported for different severity measures and in studies where ORs were highest when the prevalence of wheeze was low.

Conclusions

1. The evidence is sufficient to infer a causal relationship between parental smoking and cough, phlegm, wheeze, and breathlessness among children of school age.

2. The evidence is sufficient to infer a causal relationship between parental smoking and ever having asthma among children of school age.

Implications

Respiratory symptoms are common among children, even among those without asthma. Secondhand smoke exposure increases the risk for the major symptoms; these symptoms should not be dismissed as minor because they may impact the activities of the affected children. Secondhand smoke exposure is causally associated with asthma prevalence, perhaps reflecting a greater clinical severity associated with exposure. Secondhand smoke exposure, particularly at home, should be addressed by clinicians caring for any child with a respiratory complaint and particularly children with asthma.

Childhood Asthma Onset

As discussed earlier in this chapter (see "Lower Respiratory Illnesses in Infancy and Early Childhood"), parental smoking is causally associated with an increased incidence of acute LRIs, including illnesses with wheeze, in the first one or two years of a child's life. Prevalence surveys of schoolchildren show that wheeze and diagnosed asthma are more common among children of smoking parents, with a greater elevation in risk for outcomes based on definitions of wheeze that reflect a greater severity. Evidence presented in the prior section supported conclusions that parental smoking was causally associated with respiratory symptoms and prevalent asthma; the cross-sectional evidence did not address asthma onset. This section reviews cohort and case-control studies of wheeze illnesses that provide evidence concerning the effects of parental smoking on the incidence, prognosis, and severity of childhood asthma. The design of these studies addresses the temporal relationship between exposure and disease onset. This discussion also considers case-control studies of prevalent asthma

that provide findings complementary to the surveys of schoolchildren. This section represents an update of the 1998 review by Strachan and Cook (1998c).

Relevant Studies

The study findings are separated into categories by outcomes: incidence, natural history, and prevalence. Incidence data come largely from prospective cohort studies that follow groups of children without asthma and monitor the development of wheeze illnesses or a new diagnosis of asthma. Incidence studies provide evidence for factors that cause the development of asthma, including exposure to secondhand smoke. The prevalence of asthma reflects not only the incidence but also the duration of the disease or its natural history. Factors that increase the severity of asthma tend to increase prevalence, particularly if the definition of prevalent asthma incorporates elements of clinical severity.

This review includes cohort and case-control studies of asthma or wheeze that occurred after infancy and includes case series of patients with asthma that investigated parental smoking and disease severity. The literature search identified 66 relevant papers that included 11 cohort studies, 24 case-control studies, 16 uncontrolled case series, and 1 large record-linkage study. Because only a small number of cohort studies were identified, ORs relating parental smoking to the incidence and prognosis of wheeze illnesses were pooled using weights inversely proportional to their variance (the "fixed effects" assumption). The ORs from the larger number of case-control studies were pooled using a "random effects" model. A quantitative meta-analysis was not possible for studies of disease severity.

Evidence Review

Cohort Studies of Incidence

The earlier review by Strachan and Cook (1998c) identified 10 papers based on six cohort studies that documented the incidence of wheeze illnesses after the first two years of life in relation to parental smoking behaviors (Table 6.16) (Taylor et al. 1983; Fergusson and Horwood 1985; Horwood et al. 1985; Anderson et al. 1986; Neuspiel et al. 1989; Sherman et al. 1990; Martinez et al. 1992, 1995; Lewis et al. 1995; Strachan et al. 1996). Five papers addressed mainly wheeze during the preschool years (Taylor et al. 1983; Fergusson and Horwood 1985; Horwood et al. 1985; Lewis et al. 1995; Martinez et al. 1995), two studies focused on the prevalence of wheeze for the first time during the school years (Sherman et al. 1990; Strachan et al. 1996), and three papers included both early and later childhood (Anderson et al. 1986; Neuspiel et al. 1989; Martinez et al. 1992). Only one additional birth cohort study, based on very low birth weight infants, has been published since the 1998 review (Darlow et al. 2000). These studies complement the larger number of studies that address wheeze illness incidence in infancy and are reviewed in the next section. The results are summarized in Table 6.17 and Figure 6.9 and are discussed briefly in the next section.

Investigators in Tucson (Arizona) followed a birth cohort registered with a health maintenance organization (Martinez et al. 1995). Among 762 children followed for the first three years of life and also at six years of age, 403 had no history of wheeze, 147 had wheeze by three years of age but not at six

years of age ("transient" early wheeze), 112 developed wheeze after three years of age ("late-onset" wheeze), and 100 developed wheeze before three years of age and had wheeze at six years of age ("persistent" wheeze). The incidence of wheeze before three years of age—transient and persistent combined—doubled if the mother smoked 10 or more cigarettes per day. The incidence of a later onset of wheeze was less strongly associated with maternal smoking (Table 6.17). These associations were unchanged after adjustment for gender, ethnicity, eczema, noninfective rhinitis, and maternal asthma. For a comparison with other studies of early childhood wheeze, the cumulative incidence of wheeze by six years of age is also presented in Table 6.17. Although these incidence data are presented and analyzed by maternal smoking, another publication from the same cohort study has suggested that for children in day care, smoking by the caregiver may also be of importance as a determinant of the frequency of wheeze illnesses in the third year of life (Holberg et al. 1993).

In a similar population-based birth cohort study in Christchurch, New Zealand, 1,032 children were followed at annual intervals until six years of age (Fergusson and Horwood 1985; Horwood et al. 1985). In contrast to other studies, the cumulative incidence of asthmatic symptoms that parents reported was lower if the mother smoked and higher if the father smoked. The incidence was also lower if both parents smoked versus if neither parent smoked. Analyses that used medical consultations for asthma (Horwood et al. 1985) and the frequency of asthma attacks in the first six years of life (Fergusson and Horwood 1985) showed a similar pattern.

The incidence of all forms of wheeze in the nationwide 1970 British birth cohort was ascertained retrospectively by parental recall at five years of age. The direction and strength of dose-response relationships with smoking during pregnancy (Table 6.17) and when the child was five years of age were almost identical (Lewis et al. 1995). The cumulative incidence of wheeze among children of smoking mothers was elevated and changed little after adjustment for gender, birth weight, and breastfeeding, which may have potentially confounded or modified the association (Lewis et al. 1995). There was also an increased incidence of asthma by five years of age if the mother smoked (Taylor et al. 1983). Another study based on the same birth cohort explicitly excluded wheeze in the first year of life and included information from follow-up data gathered at 5 and 10 years of age

Table 6.16   Design, sample size, and recruitment criteria for studies of asthma incidence and prognosis associated with parental smoking included in this overview

Study	Design/population	Sample size	Case definition	Source of cohort or controls	Outcome
			Incidence studies		
Taylor et al. 1983 Lewis et al. 1995	Cohort Aged 0–5 years United Kingdom	12,530	Reported wheeze	National birth cohort	Wheeze incidence
Fergusson and Horwood 1985 Horwood et al. 1985	Cohort Aged 0–6 years New Zealand	1,032	Reported asthma	Population-based birth cohort	Asthma incidence
Anderson et al. 1986 Strachan et al. 1996	Cohort Aged 0–16 years United Kingdom	4,583	Reported asthma/bronchitis with wheeze	National birth cohort	Asthma/ bronchitis with wheeze incidence
Neuspiel et al. 1989	Cohort Aged 1–10 years United Kingdom	9,670	Reported wheeze	National birth cohort	Wheeze incidence
Sherman et al. 1990	Cohort Aged 5–17 years United States (Massachusetts)	722	Physician-diagnosed asthma	Schools-based cohort	Asthma incidence
Martinez et al. 1992	Cohort Aged 0–11 years United States (Arizona)	739	Physician-diagnosed asthma	Random household sample	Asthma incidence
Holberg et al. 1993 Martinez et al. 1995	Cohort Aged 0–6 years United States (Arizona)	762	Reported wheeze	Health maintenance organization-based birth cohort	Wheeze incidence
Hjern et al. 1999	Cohort Aged 2–6 years Sweden	Approximately 156,000	Hospitalization	Record linkage in 3 cities	Asthma incidence
Darlow et al. 2000	Cohort Aged 0–7 years New Zealand	299	Reported physician-diagnosed asthma	Very low birth weight babies	Asthma incidence
			Natural history studies		
McConnochie and Roghmann 1984	Cohort Aged 0–9 years United States (New York)	236	Wheeze 8 years later	Bronchiolitis before 2 years of age	Early prognosis
Welliver et al. 1986	Cohort Aged 0–2 years United States (New York)	27	Recurrent wheeze	Parainfluenza bronchiolitis	Early prognosis

Table 6.16   Continued

Study	Design/population	Sample size	Case definition	Source of cohort or controls	Outcome
		Natural history studies			
Geller-Bernstein et al. 1987	Cohort Aged 0–5 years Israel	80	Persistent wheeze at 5 years of age	Atopic infants with wheeze	Early prognosis
Toyoshima et al. 1987	Cohort Aged 1–4 years Japan	48	Wheeze 22–44 months later	Infants with wheeze	Early prognosis
Rylander et al. 1988	Cohort Aged 0–7 years Sweden	67	Wheeze 4 years later	Respiratory syncytial virus plus illness before 3 years of age	Early prognosis
Lewis et al. 1995	Cohort Aged 5–16 years United Kingdom	1,477	Wheeze at 16 years of age	Wheeze before 5 years of age	Later prognosis
Martinez et al. 1995	Cohort Aged 0–6 years United States (Arizona)	247	Wheeze at 6 years of age	Wheeze before 3 years of age	Early prognosis
Strachan 1995	Cohort Aged 7–23 years United Kingdom	1,090	Asthma/ bronchitis with wheeze at 11 and 23 years of age	Asthma/ bronchitis with wheeze before 7 years of age	Later prognosis
Wennergren et al. 1997	Cohort Aged 0–10 years Sweden	92	Asthma at 10 years of age	Bronchitis with wheeze before 2 years of age	Early prognosis
Infante-Rivard et al. 1999	Case-control and follow-up Aged 3–10 years Canada	394	Asthma symptoms at 9–10 years of age	First emergency room asthma visit	Early prognosis
Rusconi et al. 1999	Survey Aged 0–7 years Italy	1,892	Wheeze at 6–7 years of age	Lower respiratory illness with wheeze before 2 years of age	Early prognosis
		Case-control studies			
O'Connell and Logan 1974	Aged 2–16 years United States (Minnesota)	628	Outpatients with asthma	Other outpatients (no atopic disease)	Asthma (outpatients)
Palmieri et al. 1990	Aged 1–12 years Italy	735	Outpatients with asthma	Routine health check	Asthma (outpatients)
Daigler et al. 1991	Aged 0–17 years United States (New York)	383	Hospital admission or 2 outpatient visits	Private pediatric practice	Asthma (inpatients/ outpatients)
Willers et al. 1991	Aged 3–15 years Sweden	126	New outpatient referrals	2 local schools	Asthma (outpatients)

Table 6.16   Continued

Study	Design/population	Sample size	Case definition	Source of cohort or controls	Outcome
		Case-control studies			
Butz and Rosenstein 1992	Aged about 9 years United States (Maryland)	346	Outpatients with asthma	Private pediatric practice	Asthma (outpatients)
Ehrlich et al. 1992	Aged 3–14 years United States (New York)	114	Emergency room visit for asthma	Other emergency room patients	Asthma (emergency room)
Infante-Rivard 1993	Aged 3–4 years Canada	914	First emergency room visit for asthma	Population sample	Asthma (inpatients)
Rylander et al. 1993, 1995	Aged 1½–4 years Sweden	212	Bronchitis with wheeze treated in the hospital	Random population sample	Bronchitis with wheeze (inpatients)
Clark et al. 1994	Aged 5–7 years United Kingdom	62	Outpatients with asthma	Surgical outpatients	Asthma (outpatients)
Fagbule and Ekanem 1994	Aged about 5½ years Nigeria	280	Outpatients with wheeze (no family history)	Neighbors	Wheeze (outpatients)
Leen et al. 1994	Aged 5–11 years Ireland	211	Reported asthma	Population survey	Asthma (survey)
Mumcuoglu et al. 1994	Aged 3–15 years Israel	400	Asthma treatment	Neighbors	Wheeze (outpatients)
Azizi et al. 1995	Aged 0–5 years Malaysia	359	First asthma admission	Nonrespiratory admissions	Asthma (inpatients)
Henderson et al. 1995	Aged 7–12 years United States (North Carolina)	342	≥2 wheeze attacks	Pediatric clinic sample	Wheeze (outpatients)
Lindfors et al. 1995	Aged 1–4 years Sweden	511	Asthma outpatient referral	Random population sample	Asthma (outpatients)
Strachan and Carey 1995	Aged 12–18 years United Kingdom	961	Frequent/severe wheeze	Population survey (no wheeze)	Wheeze (survey)
Ehrlich et al. 1996	Aged 7–9 years South Africa	620	Asthma symptoms	Population survey (no wheeze)	Asthma/ wheeze (survey)
Moussa et al. 1996	Aged 6–18 years United Arab Emirates	406	Physician-diagnosed asthma on therapy	School classmates (survey)	Asthma
Oliveti et al. 1996	Aged 4–9 years United States (Ohio)	262	Physician-diagnosed asthma on therapy	Adjacent birth records	Asthma (outpatients)

Table 6.16   Continued

Study	Design/population	Sample size	Case definition	Source of cohort or controls	Outcome
Case-control studies					
Jones et al. 1999	Aged 4–16 years United Kingdom	200	Physician-diagnosed asthma on therapy	General practice population	Asthma (primary care)
Chang et al. 2000	Aged 0–16 years United States (Virginia)	271	Wheeze on auscultation	Nonrespiratory emergencies	Wheeze (emergency room)
Other studies					
Kershaw 1987*	Case-control Aged 0–5 years United Kingdom	1,285	≥3 wheeze attacks	Neonates in locality	Wheeze (outpatients)
Murray and Morrison 1990*	Case-control Aged 1–17 years Canada	620	Asthma diagnosis	Allergy clinic patients	Asthma (outpatients)
Duff et al. 1993*	Case-control Aged 2–16 years United States (Virginia)	114	Emergency room visit for asthma/ bronchiolitis	Other emergency room patients	Wheeze (emergency room)
Chen et al. 1996*	Survey Aged 6–17 years Canada	892	Physician-diagnosed asthma and symptoms	Survey of complete town	Recent asthma (survey)
Knight et al. 1998*	Case-control Aged 2–18 years Canada	152	Physician-diagnosed asthma	General pediatric clinic	Asthma (outpatients)

*Not included in the meta-analysis of case-control studies in Table 6.3.

(Neuspiel et al. 1989). Maternal smoking was associated with wheeze that was labeled as bronchitis with wheeze (incidence ratio 1.44 [95 percent CI, 1.24–1.68]), but not with wheeze that was labeled as asthma (incidence ratio 0.96 [95 percent CI, 0.77–1.22]). Most of the published analyses related only to the former category, which accounted for only 38 percent of all wheeze incidents (Strachan and Cook 1998c). In the absence of maternal smoking, smoking by the father was not associated with an increased risk of bronchitis with wheeze (incidence ratio 0.99 [95 percent CI, 0.76–1.29]) and was not assessed for other forms of wheeze.

An earlier national British birth cohort of persons born in 1958 contributes information on both early and later onset of wheeze illnesses (Anderson et al. 1986; Strachan et al. 1996). As in the 1970 cohort, early wheeze illnesses were ascertained retrospectively, in this case at seven years of age, and were more common if the mother had smoked during pregnancy. This association was independent of other risk factors (Strachan et al. 1996). Among 4,583 children without a history of asthma or bronchitis with wheeze reported by parents at 7 years of age, the incidence from 7 to 16 years of age differed little according to whether the mother had smoked during pregnancy; however, there were weak, nonsignificant, and positive associations with smoking by both the mother and father at the 16-year follow-up (Table 6.17).

A smaller cohort study in Boston also found little evidence for a relationship between parental smoking and asthma incidence (Sherman et al. 1990). The study

Table 6.17   Incidence and prognosis of asthma or wheeze in relation to parental smoking

Study	Population		Age (years) at start/end (length of follow-up period)	Smoking exposure	Outcome	Odds ratio for smoking (95% confidence interval)
	Cases	Non-cases				
				Incidence studies		
Fergusson and Horwood 1985	141	891	0/6	Mother smoked	Asthma	0.88* (0.61–1.27)
	141	891	0/6	Father smoked	Asthma	1.27 (0.89–1.81)
Neuspiel et al. 1989	1,662	8,016	1/10	Mother smoked at any age	Asthma Wheeze	0.96 (0.77–1.22) 1.44 (1.24–1.68)
Sherman et al. 1990	43	679	5–9/NR[†] (9 years)	Mother smoked	Asthma	0.97* (0.51–1.84)
	43	679	5–9/NR (9 years)	Father smoked	Asthma	0.91 (0.49–1.69)
Martinez et al. 1992	86	653	<5/NR (12 years)	Mother smoked ≥10 cigarettes/day	Asthma	1.68* (1.10–2.58)
	78	622	<5/NR (12 years)	Father smoked ≥10 cigarettes/day	Asthma	1.06 (0.67–1.69)
Lewis et al. 1995	2,616	9,914	0–1 years	Mother smoked during pregnancy	Wheeze	1.34* (1.22–1.45)
Martinez et al. 1995	247	515	0/3	Mother smoked ≥10 cigarettes/day	Wheeze	2.07 (1.34–3.19)
	112	403	3/6	Mother smoked ≥10 cigarettes/day	Wheeze	1.59 (0.89–2.84)
	359	403	0/6	Mother smoked ≥10 cigarettes/day	Wheeze	1.91* (1.28–2.86)
Strachan et al. 1996	1,026	4,583	0/7	Mother smoked during pregnancy	Asthma or bronchitis with wheeze	1.25* (1.08–1.44)
	368	4,215	7/16	Mother smoked during pregnancy	Asthma or bronchitis with wheeze	0.99 (0.78–1.25)
	368	4,215	7/16	Mother smoked at 16-year follow-up	Asthma or bronchitis with wheeze	1.14* (0.92–1.41)
	368	4,215	7/16	Father smoked at 16-year follow-up	Asthma or bronchitis with wheeze	1.10 (0.88–1.36)

Table 6.17   Continued

Study	Population Cases	Population Non-cases	Age (years) at start/end (length of follow-up period)	Smoking exposure	Outcome	Odds ratio for smoking (95% confidence interval)
				Natural history studies		
McConnochie and Roghmann 1984	26	33	<2/8	Either parent smoked	Persistent wheeze	1.45* (0.45–4.70)
Geller-Bernstein et al. 1987	26	54	<2/5	Either parent smoked	Persistent wheeze	3.10* (1.08–8.91)
Toyoshima et al. 1987	18	22	<3/NR (22–44 months)	Household members smoked	Recent wheeze	11.80* (1.32–105.0)
Rylander et al. 1988	22	45	<3/NR (4 years)	Either parent smoked	Recent wheeze	0.80* (0.28–2.27)
Lewis et al. 1995	218	1,259	<5/16	Mother smoked during pregnancy	Wheeze in the past year	0.86* (0.64–1.15)
Martinez et al. 1995	100	147	<3/6	Mother smoked ≥10 cigarettes/day	Recent wheeze	0.99* (0.53–1.86)
Strachan 1995	203	887	<7/11	Mother smoked during pregnancy	Asthma/bronchitis with wheeze in the past year	0.56* (0.40–0.78)
	101	989	<7/23	Mother smoked during pregnancy	Asthma/bronchitis with wheeze in the past year	0.70 (0.50–0.98)
Wennergren et al. 1997	28	64	<2/10	Household member(s) smoked during the child's infancy	Asthma symptoms	3.14‡
	28	64	<2/10	Household member(s) smoked when the child was 10 years of age	Asthma symptoms	1.08 (0.69–1.71)
Infante-Rivard et al. 1999	288	105	3–4/9–10	Mother smoked when the child was 3–4 years of age	Asthma symptoms	1.06 (0.67–1.67)
Rusconi et al. 1999	671	1,221	<2/6–7	Mother smoked during pregnancy	Recent wheeze	1.16* (0.92–1.45)

*Odds ratios were used in the meta-analysis.
†NR = Data were not reported.
‡Odds ratios were used in the meta-analysis; confidence intervals were not provided.

Figure 6.9   Odds ratios for the effect of maternal smoking on asthma or wheeze incidence throughout childhood (cohort studies)

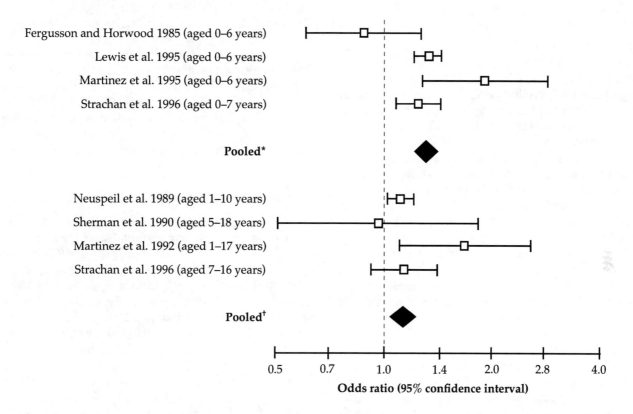

*Studies that included the first year of life (exact incidence period shown on left in parentheses), derived by the fixed effects method.

†Studies that excluded the first year of life (exact incidence period shown on left in parentheses), derived by the fixed effects method.

had a mean annual follow-up of nine years among 722 children with no history of asthma upon entry into the study at five to nine years of age (Table 6.17). In a second cohort study in Tucson (Arizona) that was based on a random sample of households, physician-diagnosed asthma was ascertained at one- to two-year intervals (Martinez et al. 1992). Maternal smoking was associated with an increased risk of asthma, whereas smoking by the father was not (Table 6.17). The effect of maternal smoking was stronger among less educated families, although the effect modification by educational level was not statistically significant.

A national cohort study followed 299 very low birth weight children born in New Zealand in 1986 (96 percent of all survivors) through seven years of age (Darlow et al. 2000). In this potentially vulnerable group, maternal smoking during pregnancy was associated with an increased cumulative incidence of physician-diagnosed asthma (OR = 2.0 [95 percent CI, 1.2–3.3]), but a decreased risk of requiring daily medication for asthma at seven years of age (OR = 0.6 [95 percent CI, 0.3–1.3]). This unique group was not included in the meta-analyses described below.

In quantitative meta-analyses of studies of early and later incidence of asthma and wheeze illnesses, the association with maternal smoking was significantly stronger for the first five to seven years of life (the pooled OR for the four studies = 1.31 [95 percent CI, 1.22–1.41], χ^2 for heterogeneity = 8.58, p = 0.036) (Fergusson and Horwood 1985; Lewis et al. 1995; Martinez et al. 1995; Strachan et al. 1996) than for the school years (Sherman et al. 1990; Strachan et al. 1996) or throughout childhood (Neuspiel et al. 1989; Martinez et al. 1992), excluding infancy (the pooled OR for the four studies = 1.13 [95 percent CI, 1.04–1.22], χ^2 for heterogeneity = 3.71, p = 0.29).

Natural History

Tables 6.16 and 6.17 summarize 11 studies that related parental smoking to the natural history of wheeze illnesses in childhood (McConnochie and Roghmann 1984; Welliver et al. 1986; Geller-Bernstein et al. 1987; Toyoshima et al. 1987; Rylander et al. 1988; Lewis et al. 1995; Martinez et al. 1995; Strachan 1995; Wennergren et al. 1997; Infante-Rivard et al. 1999; Rusconi et al. 1999). Five studies addressed the short-term prognosis of all forms of wheeze from infancy through school age (Geller-Bernstein et al. 1987; Toyoshima et al. 1987; Martinez et al. 1995; Wennergren et al. 1997; Rusconi et al. 1999). Two studies reported specifically on the prognosis of wheeze following RSV infection (Rylander et al. 1988) or bronchiolitis in infancy (McConnochie and Roghmann 1984). The results of these seven studies are all consistent with an association between parental smoking and a small but increased risk of wheeze persisting after early childhood (pooled OR = 1.49 [95 percent CI, 1.24–1.78], χ^2 for heterogeneity = 28.4, p <0.001).

The short-term prognosis of bronchiolitis from a parainfluenza virus infection in infancy was evaluated among 27 children after an approximate follow-up period of three years (ranging from 8 to 51 months) (Welliver et al. 1986). The mean number of subsequent wheeze episodes was significantly higher (p <0.05) in children whose parents smoked compared with children whose parents were nonsmokers (3.0 versus 1.6 episodes, respectively), but the findings cannot be expressed in the form of an OR for a direct comparison with other prognostic studies.

A contrasting pattern of effect of parental smoking on prognosis emerges from a follow-up of a longer duration in two British birth cohort studies (Lewis et al. 1995; Strachan 1995). Among children from the 1958 cohort with a history of asthma or bronchitis with wheeze by 7 years of age, maternal smoking was associated with a significantly reduced risk of these illnesses at 11 and 23 years of age (Strachan 1995), despite the tendency of children of smoking parents to become active smokers, which is strongly associated with the recurrence of symptoms (Strachan et al. 1996). In the 1970 cohort, children younger than 5 years of age with wheeze whose mothers had smoked during pregnancy were less likely to experience wheeze in the past year at 16 years of age. This inverse association was not statistically significant but changed little after adjustment for gender, maternal age, parity, birth weight, and SES (Lewis et al. 1995). The pooled OR for maternal smoking with a follow-up to 11 (1958 cohort) or 16 years of age (1970 cohort) is 0.71 (95 percent CI, 0.57–0.89, χ^2 for heterogeneity = 3.58, p = 0.058).

A study in Canada that initiated a follow-up at three to four years of age found no effect of maternal smoking on the persistence of symptoms six years later (OR = 1.06 [95 percent CI, 0.67–1.67]) (Infante-Rivard et al. 1999). This result is consistent with prevalence studies that found a declining influence of parental smoking on asthmatic symptoms as the child grows older.

Prevalence Case-Control Studies

Tables 6.16 and 6.18 summarize 21 case-control studies that relate parental smoking to asthma or wheeze illnesses after the first year of life (O'Connell and Logan 1974; Palmieri et al. 1990; Daigler et al. 1991; Willers et al. 1991; Butz and Rosenstein 1992; Ehrlich et al. 1992, 1996; Infante-Rivard 1993; Clark et al. 1994; Fagbule and Ekanem 1994; Leen et al. 1994; Mumcuoglu et al. 1994; Azizi et al. 1995; Henderson et al. 1995; Lindfors et al. 1995; Rylander et al. 1995; Strachan and Carey 1995; Moussa et al. 1996; Oliveti et al. 1996; Jones et al. 1999; Chang et al. 2000). The studies are based mostly on outpatient or inpatient cases, although four ascertained more severe forms of wheeze illnesses using a population survey (Leen et al. 1994; Strachan and Carey 1995; Ehrlich et al. 1996; Moussa et al. 1996). These papers complement the results of population surveys of diagnosed asthma or symptoms of wheeze reviewed earlier in this chapter (see "Respiratory Symptoms and Prevalent Asthma in School-Age Children") by more specifically addressing the relationship of parental smoking to the prevalence of more severe forms of asthma that require clinical care.

For asthma, the results for smoking by either parent (from 15 studies) are summarized in Figure 6.10. There is evidence for borderline significant heterogeneity between studies (χ^2 = 23.3, df = 14, p = 0.06), but the size of the effect does not appear to be systematically related to the age ranges studied or to the sources of cases or controls. The pooled OR for smoking by either parent, derived by random effects modeling, is 1.39 (95 percent CI, 1.19–1.64). In a comparison of the effects of maternal and paternal smoking, there is a consistent finding of an association with maternal smoking (pooled OR = 1.54 [95 percent CI, 1.31–1.81]) but not with paternal smoking (pooled OR = 0.93 [95 percent CI, 0.81–1.07]). This finding

Table 6.18   Unadjusted relative risks associated with parental smoking for asthma (meta-analysis of case-control studies)

Study	Population (cases/controls)	Odds ratios for smoking (95% confidence intervals)			Dose-response effect*	Cotinine measured
		Either parent	Mother	Father		
O'Connell and Logan 1974	400/213 Aged 2–16 years	1.30 (0.93–1.83)	NR[†]	NR	NR	NR
Palmieri et al. 1990	302/433 Aged 1–12 years	1.0 (0.70–1.42)	NR	NR	No[‡]	NR
Daigler et al. 1991	137/246 Aged 0–17 years	NR	1.43 (0.92–2.23)	0.71 (0.44–1.15)	NR	NR
Willers et al. 1991	49/77 Aged 3–15 years	1.97 (0.90–4.35)	2.56 (1.23–5.32)	0.87 (0.42–1.80)	Yes	Yes
Butz and Rosenstein 1992	102/105 Aged about 9 years	1.43 (0.75–2.71)	NR	NR	NR	NR
Ehrlich et al. 1992	107/121 Aged 3–14 years	1.13 (0.67–1.90)	2.0 (1.16–3.48)	NR	Yes	Yes
Infante-Rivard 1993	457/457 Aged 3–4 years	NR	1.16 (0.89–1.51)	0.81 (0.62–1.06)	NR	NR
Clark et al. 1994	19/43 Aged 5–7 years	0.71 (0.22–2.22)	NR	NR	NR	Yes
Fagbule and Ekanem 1994	140/140 Aged about 5½ years	2.12 (1.32–3.42)	NR	NR	NR	NR
Leen et al. 1994	115/96 Aged 5–11 years	0.76 (0.44–1.31)	NR	NR	NR	NR
Mumcuoglu et al. 1994	300/100 Aged 3–15 years	0.90 (0.57–1.42)	Few smoked	0.95 (0.60–1.50)	NR	NR
Azizi et al. 1995	158/201 Aged 0–5 years	1.80 (1.20–2.70)	NR	NR	NR	NR
Henderson et al. 1995	193/149 Aged 7–12 years	2.0 (1.22–3.27)	NR	NR	NR	Yes
Lindfors et al. 1995	193/318 Aged 1–4 years	1.62 (1.13–2.32)	NR	NR	NR	NR
Rylander et al. 1995	75/137 Aged 1½–4 years	1.46 (0.83–2.58)	1.70 (0.93–3.14)	1.02 (0.42–2.46)	No	Yes
Strachan and Carey 1995	486/475 Aged 12–18 years	NR	1.38 (1.18–1.61)	0.96 (0.69–1.34)	Yes	NR

Table 6.18   Continued

Study	Population (cases/controls)	Odds ratios for smoking (95% confidence intervals)			Dose-response effect*	Cotinine measured
		Either parent	Mother	Father		
Ehrlich et al. 1996	348/272 Aged 7–9 years	1.57 (1.06–2.33)	1.70 (1.23–2.34)	1.23 (0.90–1.70)	Yes	Yes
Moussa et al. 1996	203/203 Aged 6–18 years	NR	Few smoked	1.03 (0.63–1.70)	NR	NR
Oliveti et al. 1996	131/131 Aged 4–9 years	NR	2.79 (1.66–4.67)	NR	Yes	NR
Jones et al. 1999	100/100 Aged 4–16 years	NR	1.17 (0.62–2.21)	0.85 (0.48–1.49)	NR	NR
Chang et al. 2000	165/106 Aged 0–16 years	1.90 (1.10–3.40)	1.30 (0.70–2.30)	NR	Yes	Yes

*Urinary cotinine was measured (not all such studies reported dose-response relationships).
†NR = Data were not reported.
‡Dose-response relationship was only evident for participants with negative skin pricks.

contrasts with prevalence surveys of asthma and wheeze among schoolchildren that found an effect of paternal smoking.

Six studies provided findings before and after adjustment for potential confounding variables (Fagbule and Ekanem 1994; Henderson et al. 1995; Rylander et al. 1995; Strachan and Carey 1995; Ehrlich et al. 1996; Oliveti et al. 1996). Only one study from Nigeria (Fagbule and Ekanem 1994) reported a substantial reduction in the OR for smoking by either parent (from 2.12 to 1.41) after adjustment for potential confounders that included pet ownership, indoor mold, cockroaches, wood smoke, and the use of mosquito coils. The OR for parental smoking changed little (from 1.32 to 1.3) after adjustment for family history of asthma and duration of breastfeeding in Sweden (Rylander et al. 1995); in the United Kingdom the OR changed from 1.44 to 1.49 after adjustment for age, gender, SES, gas cooking, indoor mold, feather bedding, and pet ownership (Strachan and Carey 1995); in the United States the OR changed from 1.74 to 1.8 after adjustment for family history of asthma and skin-prick positivity to common aeroallergens (Henderson et al. 1995); in South Africa the OR changed from 1.97 to 1.87 after adjustment for personal and family histories of atopic disease, SES, indoor mold, and salt preference (Ehrlich et al. 1996); and in the United States the OR changed from

2.79 to 2.82 after adjustment for maternal asthma, history of bronchiolitis, and a range of obstetric and perinatal variables (Oliveti et al. 1996).

Seven studies included measurements of urinary cotinine as an objective marker of tobacco smoke exposure (Willers et al. 1991; Ehrlich et al. 1992, 1996; Clark et al. 1994; Henderson et al. 1995; Rylander et al. 1995; Chang et al. 2000). Generally, the results of questionnaire and biochemical assessments were similar, although one study (Clark et al. 1994) found a stronger association between asthma and exposure classified by cotinine levels rather than by parental smoking assessed from a questionnaire. At least one study suggested that children with asthma may differ from other children exposed to secondhand tobacco smoke in terms of a lower clearance rate for nicotine metabolites, raising the possibility of a pharmacokinetic predisposition underlying the association between parental smoking and childhood asthma (Knight et al. 1998).

Four studies found a significant dose-response relationship of parental smoking with cotinine concentrations (Willers et al. 1991; Ehrlich et al. 1992, 1996; Chang et al. 2000), but a fifth did not (Rylander et al. 1995). Two other studies with findings for exposure-response trends based on a questionnaire assessment have inconsistent results (Palmieri et al. 1990; Strachan and Carey 1995), whereas a third, based

Figure 6.10 Odds ratios for the effect of smoking by either parent on childhood asthma or wheeze prevalence (case-control studies)

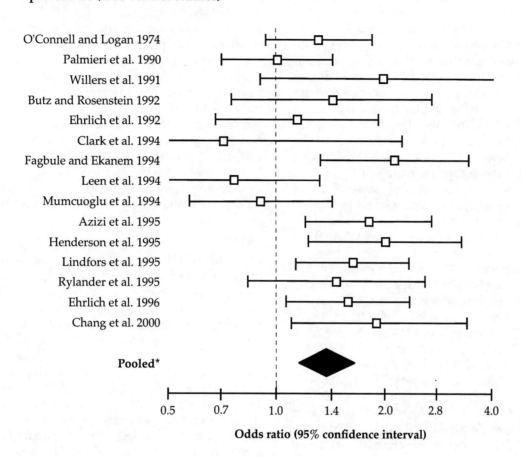

Odds ratio (95% confidence interval)

*Derived by the random effects method.

on obstetric records, reported a strong exposure-response relationship for daily cigarette smoking by the mother during pregnancy (Oliveti et al. 1996).

Three studies compared the effects of parental smoking at different ages. In the Swedish study by Rylander and colleagues (1993, 1995), the effect of parental smoking was greater at 18 months of age than at a younger age. This pattern was the same, regardless of whether exposure was assessed by the number of smoking parents or by urinary cotinine concentrations (Rylander et al. 1995). A U.S. case-control study that measured urinary cotinine concentrations found a positive association with wheeze before two years of age, but a nonsignificant inverse relationship at older ages (Duff et al. 1993). An Italian case-control study compared the effect of parental smoking before and after six years of age (Palmieri et al. 1990). The ORs for smoking by either parent were, respectively,

1.13 (95 percent CI, 0.71–1.80) and 0.83 (95 percent CI, 0.48–1.44).

In this context, it is relevant to note that a large record-linkage study of hospital admissions for asthma in Sweden (see "Respiratory Symptoms and Prevalent Asthma in School-Age Children" earlier in this chapter) found a significant effect of maternal smoking only on hospital admissions for children under three years of age (Hjern et al. 1999).

Atopic and Nonatopic Wheeze

In the 1958 British birth cohort, the increased incidence of bronchitis with wheeze or asthma by 16 years of age among children whose mothers had smoked during pregnancy occurred only among the 3,815 participants with no history of hay fever, allergic rhinitis, or eczema (cumulative incidence was

24.5 percent versus 18.9 percent among those with a history, OR = 1.39 [95 percent CI, 1.18–1.63]) (Strachan et al. 1996). Among the 1,794 participants reporting hay fever, allergic rhinitis, or eczema at one or more follow-up visits, maternal smoking had little effect on disease incidence (cumulative incidence was 32.2 percent among those whose mothers had smoked during pregnancy versus 33.5 percent among those whose mothers had not smoked during pregnancy, OR = 0.95 [95 percent CI, 0.76–1.18]). The difference in the effect of maternal smoking during pregnancy by the presence or absence of hay fever, allergic rhinitis, or eczema was statistically significant (p <0.01).

In the Italian case-control study, cases (but not controls) were tested by skin prick with six locally relevant aeroallergens (Palmieri et al. 1990). Fewer prick-positive cases were exposed to any parental smoking than were prick-negative cases (77 percent versus 82 percent, respectively, OR = 0.72 [95 percent CI, 0.37–1.41]). The association of exposure with a positive skin-prick result was more marked and statistically significant at the 5 percent level with exposure to more than 20 cigarettes a day (44 percent for those exposed to ≤20 cigarettes per day versus 60 percent for those exposed to >20 cigarettes per day, OR = 0.54 [95 percent CI, 0.31–0.92]). Among 70 children with asthma aged younger than six years in a British outpatient series, maternal smoking was less common if the serum IgE was elevated (>1 SD above the population mean): 54 percent versus 69 percent among those who did not have an elevated serum Ig (OR = 0.54 [95 percent CI, 0.21–1.45]) (Kershaw 1987). A cross-sectional survey of Canadian children also identified a stronger association between parental smoking and recent asthma among children with no reported history of an allergy (OR for current smoking by either parent = 2.93 [95 percent CI, 0.83–10.3]) than among children with an allergy (OR = 0.73 [95 percent CI, 0.37–1.46]) (Chen et al. 1996). Although these differences are nonsignificant, they are consistent with the 1958 British birth cohort study results and thus suggest a stronger association between parental smoking and nonatopic "wheezy bronchitis" than with "allergic asthma."

A recent cross-sectional study of six- to seven-year-old children in northern Sweden presented results separately for atopic and nonatopic asthma defined by the presence or absence of positive skin-prick tests (Rönmark et al. 1999). Maternal smoking was significantly associated with nonatopic asthma (OR = 1.67 [95 percent CI, 1.04–2.68]) but not with atopic asthma (OR = 1.17 [95 percent CI, 0.68–2.01]).

Because the study data were not fully displayed, effect modification by atopy cannot be formally evaluated for statistical significance.

A contrasting pattern was found in a study of allergy clinic patients aged 1 through 17 years in Vancouver (Canada) (Murray and Morrison 1990). Among 224 patients with atopic dermatitis, maternal smoking was associated with an increased risk of diagnosed asthma (OR = 3.42 [95 percent CI, 1.60–7.30]), whereas among 396 patients without atopic dermatitis there was no association (OR = 0.93 [95 percent CI, 0.57–1.51]). This interaction is statistically significant at the 1 percent level, but the findings are difficult to interpret biologically without the consideration of possible referral biases in this clinic-based study.

Severity

The severity of an episodic disease such as asthma has several dimensions: frequency of wheeze episodes, persistence of symptoms between "attacks," occurrence of clinically severe or life-threatening bronchospasm, the need for preventive and/or rescue medications, health services utilization, and interference with daily activities. Seven population surveys (Gortmaker et al. 1982; Weitzman et al. 1990a,b; Strachan and Carey 1995; Ehrlich et al. 1996; Chew et al. 1999; Schwartz et al. 2000), 1 case-control study (Henderson et al. 1995), 11 uncontrolled case series (Aderele 1982; Evans et al. 1987; Murray and Morrison 1989, 1993; Chilmonczyk et al. 1993; LeSon and Gershwin 1995; Macarthur et al. 1996; Minkovitz et al. 1999; Wafula et al. 1999; Gürkan et al. 2000a; Sandberg et al. 2000), and 1 record-linkage study (Hjern et al. 1999) present data on asthma severity in relation to parental smoking (Table 6.19). Various dimensions of severity were used and some studies combined a number of indices into a composite "severity score" (Aderele 1982; Murray and Morrison 1989, 1993).

Because each study employed different approaches, a formal quantitative meta-analysis was not carried out, but Table 6.20 presents a qualitative review. These studies suggest greater disease severity in children exposed to smoking at home, a pattern that is more consistently found among persons with asthma who are hospital outpatients or inpatients than among children with asthma identified through population surveys (Table 6.20).

Several studies adjusted for potential confounding variables, and it is possible that some of the associations of parental smoking with health service utilization, in particular, may reflect a common association with a lower SES and correlates of SES that affect

Table 6.19 **Design, sample size, and severity index for studies of asthma severity associated with parental smoking included in this overview**

Study	Design/population	Severity index
Aderele 1982	Case series of 380 outpatients with asthma Aged 1–13 years Nigeria	Severity score
Gortmaker et al. 1982	Survey of 272 patients with reported current asthma Aged 0–17 years United States (Massachusetts/Michigan)	Functional impairment
Evans et al. 1987	Case series of 276 outpatients with asthma Aged 4–17 years United States (New York)	Emergency room visits per year
Murray and Morrison 1989	Case series of 415 outpatients with asthma Aged 1–17 years Canada	Severity score
Weitzman et al. 1990a	Survey of 99 patients with reported current asthma Aged 2–5 years United States (All states)	Asthma medication
Weitzman et al. 1990b	Survey of 117 patients with reported current asthma Aged 0–5 years United States (All states)	Hospitalizations
Chilmonczyk et al. 1993	Case series of 199 outpatients with asthma Aged 0–13 years United States (Maine)	Attack frequency
Murray and Morrison 1993	Case series of 807 outpatients with asthma Aged 1–17 years Canada	Severity score
Henderson et al. 1995	Case-control study of 149 children from a pediatric clinic sample Aged 7–12 years United States (North Carolina)	>1 wheeze attack
LeSon and Gershwin 1995	Case series of 300 inpatients with asthma Aged 5–12 years United States (California)	Intubation
Strachan and Carey 1995	Survey of 486 patients with current wheeze Aged 12–18 years United Kingdom	Frequent/severe wheeze
Ehrlich et al. 1996	Survey of 325 children with current asthma/wheeze Aged 7–9 years South Africa	Asthma symptoms

Table 6.19   Continued

Study	Design/population	Severity index
Macarthur et al. 1996	Case series of 68 inpatients with asthma Aged 1–10 years Canada	Readmission within 1 year
Chew et al. 1999	Survey of 2,222 children with current wheeze Aged 6–13 years Singapore	"Increased morbidity"
Hjern et al. 1999	Routine data of about 2,500 admissions in 3 cities Aged 2–6 years Sweden	Readmission by 6 years of age
Minkovitz et al. 1999	Case series of 107 inpatients with asthma Aged 0–14 years United States (Maryland)	Readmission within 1 year
Wafula et al. 1999	Case series of 150 inpatients and outpatients with wheeze Aged 0–9 years Kenya	>1 attack in 2 months
Gürkan et al. 2000a	Case series of 140 inpatients with asthma Aged 3–15 years Turkey	Readmission within 4 years
Sandberg et al. 2000	Case series of 90 outpatients with asthma Aged 6–13 years United Kingdom	New asthma attacks
Schwartz et al. 2000	Survey of 74 current patients with asthma Aged 7–12 years Finland	Daily medication and peak expiratory flow

utilization. On the other hand, the striking association of secondhand tobacco smoke exposure with near-fatal asthma, evaluated retrospectively in a tertiary medical care center in California, was stronger than a range of psychosocial variables, which suggests that the association cannot be entirely explained by SES confounding (LeSon and Gershwin 1995). However, a mutually adjusted analysis was not possible as only 2 of the 13 patients who required intubation came from nonsmoking households.

Effects of Reducing Tobacco Smoke Exposure

Information on secondhand smoke exposure and asthma severity can also be found in studies that track the consequences of exposure reduction.

According to the early case-control study by O'Connell and Logan (1974), 67 percent of the 265 children who were exposed to parental smoking considered that it had aggravated their symptoms. In addition, tobacco smoke exposure was considered a "significant factor" for symptoms in 10 percent (16/158) of children if one parent smoked and in 20 percent (21/107) if both parents smoked. These 37 children were included in an empirical study of antismoking advice that included a follow-up 6 to 24 months later of 35 of the children. Symptoms improved in 90 percent (18/20) of the children whose parents had stopped smoking, and in 27 percent (4/15) of the children who remained involuntarily exposed to tobacco smoke. These results suggest a benefit from reducing exposure, but interpretation is limited by the nonrandomized nature of the intervention.

Table 6.20   Summary of studies on asthma severity associated with parental smoking

Study	Population age (years)	Index of exposure	Index of severity	Association of disease severity with secondhand smoke exposure		
				Direction	Significance	Comments
Population-based case series						
Gortmaker et al. 1982	0–17	Mother smoked	Functional impairment	Positive	p = 0.47	Functional impairment was reported for 22% of those with asthma whose mothers smoked (n = 144), and for 18% of the remaining population with asthma (n = 128)
Weitzman et al. 1990a	2–5	Mother smoked	Asthma medication	Positive	p = 0.08	Medication was taken by 41% of those with asthma whose mothers smoked ≥10 cigarettes/day (n = 23), and by 19% of others with asthma (n = 76)
Weitzman et al. 1990b	0–5	Mother smoked	Hospitalizations	No trend	p = 0.88	Mean admission rates were 1.1 per year if mother was a nonsmoker, 1.3 if mother smoked <10 cigarettes/day, and 1.0 if mother smoked ≥10 cigarettes/day
Henderson et al. 1995	7–12	Household smoker	Attack frequency	Inverse	p = 0.59	35% (29/82) of those with infrequent wheeze and 30% (20/67) with ≥5 attacks/year were exposed to secondhand smoke; urinary cotinine levels were similar in the 2 groups
Strachan and Carey 1995	12–18	Mother smoked	Frequency and intensity	Positive	p = 0.02	34% (38/113) of children with both frequent and intense attacks, and 23% (84/373) of children with less severe cases had mothers who smoked
Ehrlich et al. 1996	7–9	Mother smoked	Frequency and intensity	Weak positive	NR*	Published odds ratio (OR) of 2.04 (95% confidence interval [CI] ,1.25–3.34) for severe wheeze (179 cases) is similar to the 1.87 (95% CI, 1.25–2.81) for all wheeze cases (325)

Table 6.20   Continued

Study	Population age (years)	Index of exposure	Index of severity	Association of disease severity with secondhand smoke exposure		
				Direction	Significance	Comments
Population-based case series						
Chew et al. 1999	6–13	Father smoked (<1% of the mothers smoked)	"Increased morbidity"	Weak positive	p = 0.34	Father smoked in 14% (122/899) of cases in children with "increased morbidity," and in 12% (160/1,323) of other cases in children with wheeze
Hjern et al. 1999	2–6	Mother smoked during pregnancy	Multiple admissions	No effect	NR	Large record-linkage study; there was no difference in the adjusted OR for any asthma admission (1.3 [95% CI, 1.1–1.4]) and for multiple admissions (1.3 [95% CI, 1.0–1.6])
Schwartz et al. 2000	7–12	Smoking in the home (day-by-day exposure)	Daily medication	Positive	p = 0.02	Secondhand smoke exposure on the previous day increased the use of bronchodilator medication (OR = 10.3 [95% CI, 1.3–83.7]); there was also a dose-dependent effect of secondhand smoke on morning and evening peak flows
Clinic-based case series						
Aderele 1982	1–13	Household smoker	Composite score	Positive	p = 0.15	Exposure (mainly to nonmaternal smoking): 23% (43/186) mild, 26% (23/87) moderate, and 31% (33/107) severe cases
Evans et al. 1987	4–17	Any secondhand smoke exposure	Emergency room visits per year	Positive	p = 0.008	Mean visits of 3.1 per year in 137 smoking homes, 1.8 per year in 122 nonsmoking homes
Murray and Morrison 1989	1–17	Mother smoked	Composite score	Positive	p <0.01	Severity score was related to maternal smoking (p <0.01) but not to paternal smoking (p >0.5)
Chilmonczyk et al. 1993	0–13	Urinary cotinine	Attack frequency	Positive	p <0.05	Mean of 3.6 episodes per year if cotinine was >39 ng/mL[†] (n = 30), 2.8 per year if cotinine was 10–39 ng/mL (n = 53), and 2.1 per year if cotinine was <10 ng/mL (n = 116)

Table 6.20   Continued

Study	Population age (years)	Index of exposure	Index of severity	Association of disease severity with secondhand smoke exposure		
				Direction	Significance	Comments
Clinic-based case series						

Study	Population age (years)	Index of exposure	Index of severity	Direction	Significance	Comments
Murray and Morrison 1993	1–17	Mother smoked	Composite score	Inverse	p <0.01	Reversal of previous relationship in Aderele (1982) after introducing antismoking advice
LeSon and Gershwin 1995	5–12	Any secondhand smoke exposure	Intubation	Positive	p <0.001	85% (11/13) of intubated patients and 20% of 287 nonintubated patients were exposed to secondhand smoke (OR = 22.4 [95% CI, 7.4–68.0])
Macarthur et al. 1996	1–10	Household smoker	Readmission	Positive	p = 0.24	53% (17/32) of children who were readmitted and 36% (13/36) of children not readmitted were from smoking homes (OR = 2.0 [95% CI, 0.8–5.3])
Minkovitz et al. 1999	0–14	Household smoker	Readmission	Inverse	p = 0.19	49% (16/33) of children with multiple admissions compared with 62% (46/74) of single admissions were exposed to smoking in the home
Wafula et al. 1999	0–9	Household smoker	>1 attack in 2 months	Positive	p = 0.09	51% (36/71) of persons with moderate and severe asthma were exposed, compared with 33% of persons with mild asthma cases (OR = 2.1 [95% CI, 0.9–4.7])
Gürkan et al. 2000a	3–15	Household smoker	Readmission	Positive	p = 0.04	Among children with multiple hospitalizations, 53% (16/30) were from smoking households and 23% (7/30) had mothers who smoked; among other children these figures were 31% (34/110) and 7% (8/110), respectively
		Mother smoked			p = 0.02	
Sandberg et al. 2000	6–13	Parents smoked	New asthma attacks	Positive	p = 0.05	Adjusted OR for asthma exacerbation during follow-up in offspring of smoking parents was 1.33 (95% CI, 1.01–1.77)

*NR = Data were not reported.
†ng/mL = Nanograms per milliliter.

A composite score was used to grade severity among 415 children aged 1 through 17 years diagnosed with asthma who attended an allergy clinic in Vancouver (Canada) from 1983 to 1986 (Murray and Morrison 1989). The severity score was significantly higher among children of smoking mothers (p <0.01), but when the analysis was repeated for an additional 387 children attending the same clinic from 1986 to 1990, the relationship between maternal smoking and the asthma severity score was reversed, reflecting a highly significant (p <0.001) decline in severity among children of smoking mothers, and little change in severity for children whose mothers did not smoke (Murray and Morrison 1993). The authors attributed this change to an alteration in parental smoking behaviors following advice from clinicians to avoid smoking in the home or in the presence of the child. However, this interpretation was based on anecdotal reports, and no objective data were presented to confirm the postulated reduction in the personal exposure of the children.

Evidence Synthesis

The results summarized in this discussion and in previous sections present a complex picture of the associations of parental smoking with asthma incidence, prognosis, prevalence, and severity. The rates of incidence and recurrence of wheeze illnesses in early life are greater if there is smoking in the home, particularly by the mother, whereas the incidence of asthma during the school-age years is less strongly affected by parental smoking. A similar age-related decline in the strength of the effect of secondhand smoke exposure is evident in cross-sectional studies. These findings may simply reflect the diminishing level of secondhand tobacco smoke exposure from household sources as children age (Irvine et al. 1997; Chang et al. 2000). Alternatively or additionally, parental smoking may have differential effects on the incidence of various forms of wheeze illnesses; there may be a stronger effect on the viral infection associated with wheeze that is common in early childhood, and a weaker effect on the atopic wheeze that occurs often as a later onset component of asthma (Wilson 1989). Five studies comparing the effect of smoking on wheeze in atopic and nonatopic children lend support to the latter hypothesis (Kershaw 1987; Palmieri et al. 1990; Chen et al. 1996; Strachan et al. 1996; Rönmark et al. 1999), but a sixth does not (Murray and Morrison 1990).

The earlier section on LRIs in infancy presented evidence of an increased risk from postnatal exposure to smoking by the father in households where the mother did not smoke, but there was insufficient evidence to distinguish the separate effects of prenatal and postnatal smoking by the mother. Several of the cohort studies reviewed here have reported findings in relation to maternal smoking during pregnancy. These data are limited, and the potential role of prenatal exposure as an independent cause of asthma is still unclear. The published data are insufficient to assess the independent effect of nonmaternal smoking on the incidence or natural history of childhood asthma after the first few years of life. Most cohort studies show a weak association of asthma incidence with paternal smoking. In case-control studies, maternal smoking has the dominant effect, with little effect from smoking by the father.

Although wheeze in infancy is more likely to recur if both parents smoke, at least maternal smoking alone is associated with seemingly little long-term risk (Table 6.17). This indication could also reflect a stronger association of parental smoking with nonatopic wheeze ("wheezy bronchitis" than with "allergic asthma"), which is associated with a better prognosis. On the other hand, atopic children tend to have more severe and more frequent or persistent wheeze, and case-control studies of ("clinic") children with more severe asthma show a positive association with maternal smoking that again appears to be of greater importance. Indeed, the pooled OR for smoking by either parent from these case-control studies (1.39) is somewhat greater than the corresponding pooled ORs from cross-sectional surveys of wheeze (1.27) and asthma (1.22) among schoolchildren. Furthermore, most studies have found a greater severity of disease among children with asthma if the parents smoke (Table 6.20), and prevalence surveys among schoolchildren suggest a stronger association with more restrictive (presumably more severe) definitions of wheeze than with any recent wheeze.

These findings by age and phenotype are complex to interpret: studies of incidence and prognosis suggest an association of parental smoking primarily with early, nonatopic wheeze that tends to run a mild and transient course, whereas studies of prevalence and severity suggest that secondhand tobacco smoke exposure increases the risk of more severe symptoms and more outpatient clinic visits or emergency hospital admissions. One explanation for this pattern would be to consider secondhand tobacco smoke as a cofactor operating with intercurrent infections as a trigger of wheeze attacks, rather than as a factor initiating or inducing persistent asthma. This distinction between induction (initiation) and exacerbation (provocation) also emerges when considering the role of outdoor air pollution as a cause of asthma (Department of Health Committee on the Medical Effects of Air Pollutants 1995). There is also strong familial aggregation for childhood asthma that certainly has genetic determinants, although research on the genetics of asthma is still inconclusive.

The incidence of both wheeze and nonwheeze LRIs in infancy increases to a similar extent if both parents smoke, and the increase reflects, at least in part, postnatal secondhand (environmental) tobacco smoke exposure. It is likely that the clinical severity of viral respiratory infections in older children is also exacerbated by secondhand smoke exposure, which leads to an increased risk of respiratory symptoms in general, including wheeze. Among children at low risk for wheeze, secondhand smoke exposure at the time of an intercurrent infection may be sufficient to cause occasional episodes of asthmatic symptoms and thus increase the risk of a mild, often transient wheeze tendency that the child outgrows as the airways become larger or less reactive with increasing age. In a previous section of this chapter, the conclusion was reached that secondhand smoke exposure from parental smoking causes LRIs in infants and children. The wheezing that accompanies many of these LRIs may be clinically classified as asthma, although the cohort study findings suggest that this phenotype is not generally persistent as the child ages.

Some previous reviews have concluded that exposure to secondhand smoke is causally associated with an increase in the incidence of childhood asthma (USEPA 1992; Halken et al. 1995). This association has been attributed to chronic (but possibly reversible) effects of parental smoking on bronchial hyperreactivity rather than to the acute effects of cigarette smoke on airway caliber (USEPA 1992). The most relevant evidence for secondhand smoke exposure and onset of asthma comes from studies of older children at an age when there is reasonable diagnostic certainty. This evidence comes from only a small number of studies and their statistical power is limited, particularly within specific age strata. In addition, all studies are inherently limited by the difficulty of classifying the outcome, and there may be variations in the phenotypes that were considered across the studies. Within these constraints, the evidence indicating an association of secondhand smoke exposure from parental smoking with asthma incidence is inconsistent. The evidence for asthma prevalence, by contrast, was sufficient to support an inference of causality.

Conclusions

1. The evidence is sufficient to infer a causal relationship between secondhand smoke exposure from parental smoking and the onset of wheeze illnesses in early childhood.

2. The evidence is suggestive but not sufficient to infer a causal relationship between secondhand smoke exposure from parental smoking and the onset of childhood asthma.

Implications

The etiology of childhood asthma includes the interplay of genetic and environmental factors. The asthma phenotype likely comprises several distinct entities. The evidence is clear in showing that secondhand smoke exposure causes wheeze illnesses in early life and makes asthma more severe clinically. This evidence provides a strong basis for limiting exposure of infants and children to secondhand smoke, even though a causal link with asthma onset is not yet established for asthma incidence.

Atopy

The hypothesis that secondhand tobacco smoke exposure might increase allergic sensitization was first proposed more than 20 years ago (Kjellman 1981). However, the role of secondhand smoke exposure (specifically from maternal smoking) in allergic sensitization remains uncertain despite many investigations since that time. Some studies have documented an association between maternal smoking during pregnancy and elevated cord blood total IgE, as well as an elevated risk for the development of allergic disease (Magnusson 1986; Bergmann et al. 1995). Other studies, however, have not replicated these findings (Halonen et al. 1991; Oryszczyn et al. 1991; Ownby et al. 1991). Many studies have investigated the relationships of secondhand smoke exposure from parental smoking with cord blood IgE concentrations, IgE levels later in childhood, skin-test reactivity, and allergic manifestations such as rhinitis (Strachan and Cook 1998c). The comprehensive, systematic review reported by Strachan and Cook (1998c) of the effects of secondhand smoke exposure from parental smoking covered IgE levels, skin-prick test reactivity, and allergic rhinitis and eczema. The review included 9 studies of IgE levels in neonates, 8 studies of IgE levels in older children, 12 studies of skin-prick tests, and 10 studies of allergic symptoms (Strachan and Cook 1998c). The quantitative summary did not show a significant association of maternal smoking with total serum IgE, allergic rhinitis, or eczema. The meta-analysis for skin-prick test positivity and smoking during infancy and pregnancy yielded a pooled OR estimate of 0.87 (95 percent CI, 0.62–1.24), suggesting no effect of secondhand smoke on skin-prick positivity during these stages of development. The summary estimate supported a conclusion that maternal smoking before birth or parental smoking during infancy is unlikely to increase the risk of allergic sensitization.

This conclusion remains consistent with results from studies conducted since this systematic review, which also found no increase in risk for allergic sensitization from secondhand smoke exposure. The discussion that follows reviews some of the key studies published since 1997 (Table 6.21).

Immunoglobulin E

Evidence for the level of cord blood IgE as a predictor of IgE-mediated disease is inconsistent. Some studies suggest that cord blood IgE predicts the development of allergic disease (Michel et al. 1980; Magnusson 1988), but others do not support that hypothesis (Halonen et al. 1991; Ruiz et al. 1991; Hansen et al. 1992). If maternal smoking during pregnancy influences immune system development and gene expression in the fetus, then the cord blood IgE concentration may be a biomarker for the effects of smoking. However, expression of genes primed in the fetal environment may not be manifest until later in life, so the complete effect of in utero tobacco smoke exposure on allergic phenotypes may not be apparent until adulthood.

A study by Kaan and colleagues (2000) examined cord blood IgE and cotinine levels in a cohort of 62 infants. The infants were part of a randomized trial of primary intervention for the prevention of asthma and allergic disease. As expected, infants of mothers who smoked at the time of study recruitment had significantly higher cotinine levels when compared with unexposed children and with children exposed to secondhand smoke from smoking by the father or other household adults. Although cord blood IgE was a significant predictor of food allergy at 12 months of age, cord blood IgE and cotinine levels were not correlated. The investigators concluded that the cord blood IgE level is not influenced by maternal smoking (Kaan et al. 2000). It should be noted that cord blood IgE values have the weakest relationship with allergy and these data should be considered separate from measures of whole blood IgE obtained at postnatal and childhood time points.

In a cohort study of 342 children followed from birth to early childhood, prenatal and postnatal tobacco smoke exposure was investigated to assess whether secondhand smoke exposure has a role in the development of allergic sensitization to food allergens during infancy and childhood (Kulig et al. 1999). The researchers collected cord blood and used a questionnaire to evaluate secondhand smoke exposure. At three years of age, children with a history of prenatal and postnatal tobacco smoke exposure had a higher risk of food allergen sensitization than children with no exposure (OR = 2.3 [95 percent CI, 1.1–4.6]). There was no association between secondhand smoke exposure and quantitative measures of cord blood IgE (p = 0.58) (Kulig et al. 1999). Another birth cohort study of 1,218 infants measured cord blood IgE levels in 1,064 infants (Tariq et al. 2000). Maternal smoking was evaluated at birth and again when the children were one, two, and four years of age; 20.5 percent of the mothers reported smoking during pregnancy and 25.2 percent reported smoking after childbirth. Maternal smoking during pregnancy was not associated with cord blood IgE levels at birth (Tariq et al. 2000).

Allergic Sensitization During Childhood

Other studies published since 1997 have investigated childhood IgE levels and exposure to secondhand tobacco smoke. Lindfors and colleagues (1999) investigated 189 children with asthma aged one to four years. The researchers explored the association between exposures to dog and cat allergens and the

Table 6.21   Atopy studies of markers for exposure to secondhand smoke

Study	Design/population	Measures	Findings	Comments
Farooqi and Hopkin 1998	Retrospective cohort 1975–1984 birth cohort N = 1,934 United Kingdom (Oxfordshire)	• Log regression of predictors of atopic disease • Maternal atopy • Maternal smoking	• 45.4% (879) developed atopic disorder (OR* = 1.16 [95% CI†, 0.95–1.43]) • 25% developed asthma (OR = 1.29 [95% CI, 1.03–1.63], p <0.05) • 25% developed hay fever (OR = 1.04 [95% CI, 0.82–1.32]) • 19% developed eczema (OR = 0.97 [95% CI, 0.75–1.26])	No significant association was found between maternal smoking and atopic symptoms
Lewis and Britton 1998	1970s birth cohort N = 6,068 with complete follow-up data Follow-up at 5, 10, and 16 years of age United Kingdom	• Wheeze • Eczema • Hay fever	• Wheeze increased at 16 years of age in relation to maternal smoking • There was no evidence to support maternal smoking as a contributing factor to the development of atopy	Suggested that an independent effect of smoking reduced the effect of allergic disease; hay fever was less common with high levels of maternal smoking
Tariq et al. 1998	Birth cohort N = 1,218 Followed to 4 years of age	Serum and cord IgE‡	• 27% had symptoms of allergic disease by 4 years of age • Parental smoking did not increase allergen sensitization among children	Family history of atopy was deemed the most important risk
Kalyoncu et al. 1999	N = 738 358 boys, 380 girls Aged 6–13 years Turkey (Ankara)	• Questionnaire • Prevalence of asthma, wheeze, rhinitis, and atopic dermatitis in the last 12 months	• Secondhand smoke exposure affected occurrence of allergic rhinitis (OR = 1.84 [95% CI, 1.3–3.0]) • Occurrence of any type of allergic disease or symptoms in the past 12 months was associated with secondhand smoke exposure (OR = 1.74 [95% CI, 1.18–2.56])	None

Table 6.21   Continued

Study	Design/population	Measures	Findings	Comments
Kulig et al. 1999	Birth cohort N = 342 of 1,314 from initial cohort Studied from infancy to early childhood Measured at 1, 2, and 3 years of age Children were grouped into 4 exposure categories, depending on parental smoking Germany	• Specific IgE • Questionnaire assessed parental smoking at birth, and at 18 and 36 months	• Allergic sensitization to food and aeroallergens • By 3 years of age with prenatal exposure (OR = 2.3 [95% CI, 1.1–4.6]) and postnatal exposure (OR = 2.2 [95% CI, 0.9–5.9]) to secondhand smoke, there was an increased risk of food allergy • There was no association between secondhand smoke and cord blood IgE	Effect was restricted to food allergens; there were no consistent dose-response patterns; no association between secondhand smoke and sensitization to inhaled allergens was found
Lindfors et al. 1999	N = 189 children with asthma Aged 1–4 years Sweden	• Specific IgE antibody to cat and dog allergens • Questionnaire • House dust analysis	Secondhand smoke increased the risk for sensitization to cat (OR = 2.2 [95% CI, 0.9–4.9]) and dog (OR = 2.0 [95% CI, 0.9–4.5])	There was an interaction between secondhand smoke exposure, window pane condensation, and a high level of cat allergen (OR = 42 [95% CI, 3.7–472.8]); wide CI
Suárez-Varela et al. 1999	Cross-sectional N = 3,948 Aged 6–7 years Spain (Valencia)	• Rhinitis • Atopic dermatitis • Asthma • Secondhand smoke exposure	• Severity of atopic disease increased in lower social classes • Secondhand smoke exposure increased in lower social classes	None
Vinke et al. 1999	N = 20 10 exposed and 10 unexposed	Immunohistochemical staining for Langerhans cells, T cells, B cells, granulocytes, macrophages, mast cells, and eosinophils in the nasal mucosa	There were more IgE-positive cells and eosinophils in the nasal mucosa of children exposed to secondhand smoke	Secondhand smoke leads to a tissue infiltrate that resembles infiltrates in the nasal mucosa of children with allergy; no significant sensitization was found in nasal mucosa with increased IgE on cell surface
Kaan et al. 2000	397 high-risk infants in a controlled trial to prevent asthma and allergic disease Canada (Vancouver and Winnepeg)	• Total IgE • Serum cotinine in cord blood taken at birth	There was no correlation between cord blood IgE and cotinine levels	None

Table 6.21   Continued

Study	Design/population	Measures	Findings	Comments
Tariq et al. 2000	Birth cohort N = 1,218 Tested at 1, 2, and 4 years of age 981 were skin-prick tested Cord IgE from 1,064 United Kingdom (Isle of Wight)	• Skin testing • Cord blood IgE	• Maternal smoking did not increase allergen sensitization at 4 years of age • There was an inverse association between maternal smoking during and after pregnancy and allergen sensitization at 4 years of age	Smoking while pregnant has no effect on cord blood IgE at birth
Ulrik and Backer 2000	408 participants from case histories of 983 children Aged 7–17 years Longitudinal surveys were 6 years apart Denmark (Copenhagen)	• Skin-prick test • Total serum IgE • Pulmonary function • Airway responsiveness	There was an increased risk of a positive skin prick at second survey with exposure to maternal smoking (OR = 2.0 [95% CI, 1.3–3.1], p = 0.002)	None
Zacharasiewicz et al. 2000	N = 18,606 children Aged 6–9 years Austria	Nasal symptoms suggestive of atopic rhinitis	• Maternal smoking during pregnancy and/or breastfeeding increased risks for rhinitis in the last 12 months (OR = 1.28 [95% CI, 1.07–1.52]) • ≥50 cigarettes smoked at home: OR = 2.9 (95% CI, 1.21–6.95)	There was a demonstrated dose-response pattern for allergic symptoms depending on the amount of secondhand smoke exposure

*OR = Odds ratio.

†CI = Confidence interval.

‡IgE = Immunoglobulin E.

risk for allergic sensitization, and assessed whether the risk of allergen sensitization was modified by secondhand smoke exposure (Lindfors et al. 1999). In this study, questionnaires were completed regarding exposures to dogs, cats, home dampness as indicated by window pane condensation, and secondhand smoke, which was evaluated from questions about parental smoking in the home during the child's first two years of life; house dust was also analyzed. Exposure to secondhand tobacco smoke increased the risk for allergic sensitization to cats (Radioallergosorbent Test [RAST] e1 cat ≥0.35 kilounit per liter (kU/L), OR = 2.2 [95 percent CI, 0.9–4.9]; RAST e1 cat ≥0.70 kU/L, OR = 2.1 [95 percent CI, 0.7–6.5]). Exposure to secondhand smoke also increased the risk for sensitization to dogs (RAST e5 dog ≥0.35 kU/L,

OR = 2.0 [95 percent CI, 0.9–4.5]). With joint exposure to cats, secondhand smoke, and home dampness, the OR of 42.0 indicated a very high risk for allergic sensitization to cats, although CIs were broad (95 percent CI, 3.7–472.8). The investigators concluded that secondhand smoke exposure may promote atopic sensitization in children with asthma. The study did not control for in utero exposure to smoking (Lindfors et al. 1999).

A six-year prospective cohort study of 408 Danish children and adolescents aged 7 to 17 years initially included measurements of IgE and skin tests to common allergens. Only a single measurement of IgE was available when the study began. An analysis of individuals who were not atopic at the time of the first examination showed that exposure to secondhand tobacco smoke from maternal smoking increased the risk for a positive skin-prick test at the second evaluation (OR = 2.0 [95 percent CI, 1.3–3.1]), but changes in IgE levels could not be assessed. The authors concluded that exposure to secondhand smoke was associated with an increased risk of sensitization to common aeroallergens in adolescence (Ulrik and Backer 2000).

Other recent investigations have focused on children in the first three to four years of life, a critical time for alveolar and immune system development. In a birth cohort study, 981 children of the original cohort of 1,218 children were tested by skin prick for common aeroallergens at one, two, and four years of age (Tariq et al. 2000). An inverse association was noted for exposure to maternal smoking during pregnancy and childhood and the development of allergic sensitization at four years of age. Among children whose mothers smoked during pregnancy and/or after birth, 31.4 percent were not sensitized to aeroallergens versus 21.2 percent who were (p <0.05). Paternal smoking was not associated with allergen sensitization or skin-test reactivity (17.2 percent of those exposed versus 20.5 percent who were not exposed to paternal smoking). The investigators noted that secondhand smoke exposure from paternal sources may have been underestimated because more mothers than fathers were available for interviews (Tariq et al. 2000). Kulig and colleagues (1999) found that in children three years of age who had been exposed to secondhand smoke prenatally and postnatally, secondhand smoke exposure and sensitization to aeroallergens were not associated.

For the updated meta-analysis of the evidence relating parental smoking to allergic sensitization in children as measured by a skin-prick test (Strachan and Cook 1998b), 50 potentially relevant studies were identified, 3 of which yielded sufficient data to calculate the effect measure of interest. One of these papers was not included in the synthesis (Burr et al. 1997) because it measured allergic sensitization in neonates instead of in children. Two papers (Arshad et al. 1993; Tariq et al. 2000) analyzed the same data, and the more recent results (Tariq et al. 2000) are included here. In both the 1998 synthesis and this meta-analysis, the effect measure compared the relative odds of positive skin-prick reactions in exposed versus unexposed children. Studies were grouped according to the timing of secondhand smoke exposure: perinatal (maternal smoking during pregnancy and parental smoking from infancy to four years of age) and childhood (parental smoking at five or more years of age). The updated meta-analysis includes 10 papers (Table 6.22). There

was significant heterogeneity among the studies. The heterogeneity does not seem to be explained by study characteristics such as design, location, age group, or exposure measure.

The results of studies of perinatal exposure were the least heterogeneous; the pooled ORs suggest a nonsignificant reduction in risk among children exposed to secondhand smoke (Table 6.23 and Figure 6.11). The evidence is less consistent for childhood exposures (Figure 6.12 and Table 6.23). The random effects estimate, which is more appropriate than the fixed effects given the significant heterogeneity, shows a small and nonsignificant increase in risk associated with exposure, although this conclusion is limited by the small number of studies included in this analysis.

Considering all of the studies together, the random effects estimate is 1.10 (95 percent CI, 0.85–1.42), a nonsignificant increase in risk among exposed children (Figure 6.13 and Table 6.23). The results of these studies confirm those of the previous meta-analysis: parental smoking during pregnancy or childhood is not consistently associated with an increased risk of allergic sensitization.

Atopic Disease

Findings from recent investigations of atopic disease indicators such as allergic symptoms, eczema, rhinitis, and dermatitis are generally consistent with the earlier systematic review. Studies document that secondhand smoke exposure affects cellular biomarkers. Vinke and colleagues (1999) demonstrated that IgE-positive cells and eosinophils were higher in the nasal mucous of children exposed to secondhand smoke than in unexposed children. The researchers concluded that although secondhand tobacco smoke exposure led to a tissue infiltrate in biopsy specimens that resembles that in the nasal mucosa of children with allergy, a key difference was the lack of IgE-positive mast cells in biopsy specimens from the nonatopic children exposed to secondhand smoke (Vinke et al. 1999).

In a prospective cohort study of 6,068 children born in 1970, a follow-up for indicators of atopy was carried out at 5, 10, and 16 years of age by questioning parents (Lewis and Britton 1998). Maternal smoking was measured as "maternal smoking during pregnancy" and "current maternal smoking." The findings did not support the hypothesis that maternal smoking during pregnancy or current maternal smoking contributes to the development of atopy. In fact, the occurrence of hay fever at 16 years of age was less

Table 6.22   Studies relating parental smoking to skin-prick positivity in children

Study/location	Design/ population	Exposure measure	Outcome measure	Odds ratio (95% confidence interval)
Perinatal secondhand smoke exposure				
Kuehr et al. 1992 Germany	Survey N = 1,470 Aged 6–8 years	Mother smoked during pregnancy	Any of 7 SPT* ≥3 mm[†]	0.6 (0.3–1.1)
Bråbäck et al. 1995 Estonia	Survey N = 1,519 Aged 10–12 years	Secondhand smoke in home during infancy	Any of 8 SPT ≥0 mm	1.2 (0.9–1.8)
Poland	Survey N = 410 Aged 10–12 years	Secondhand smoke in home during infancy	Any of 8 SPT ≥0 mm	0.6 (0.3–1.1)
Sweden	Survey N = 665 Aged 10–12 years	Secondhand smoke in home during infancy	Any of 8 SPT ≥0 mm	1.3 (0.9–1.8)
Henderson et al. 1995 United States (North Carolina)	Survey N = 219 Aged 7–12 years	Mother smoked during pregnancy	Any of 14 SPT ≥4 mm	0.8 (0.4–2.0)
Søyseth et al. 1995 Norway	Survey N = 529 Aged 7–13 years	Mother smoked during pregnancy	Any of 8 SPT ≥3 mm	0.6 (0.4–1.0)
Tariq et al. 2000 United Kingdom	Cohort N = 1,456 Aged 0–4 years	Mother smoked when child was 4 years of age	Any of 12 SPT ≥3 mm	1.1 (0.6–1.6)
Childhood secondhand smoke exposure				
Weiss et al. 1985 United States (Massachusetts)	Cohort N = 163 Aged 12–16 years	Mother currently smoked	Any of 4 SPT >0 mm	2.2 (1.1–4.4)
Ronchetti et al. 1992 Italy	Cohort N = 142 Aged 13 years	Either parent smoked	Any of 10 positive SPT	1.7 (0.8–3.8)
von Mutius et al. 1994 Germany	Survey N = 8,653 Aged 9–11 years	Mother currently smoked	Any of 6 SPT ≥3 mm	0.8 (0.7–0.9)
Henderson et al. 1995 United States (North Carolina)	Survey N = 219 Aged 7–12 years	Parental smoking when child was 5 years of age	Any of 14 SPT ≥4 mm	1.1 (0.6–1.9)
Søyseth et al. 1995 Norway	Survey N = 529 Aged 7–13 years	Mother currently smoked	Any of 8 SPT ≥3 mm	0.8 (0.5–1.2)

Table 6.22   Continued

Study/location	Design/ population	Exposure measure	Outcome measure	Odds ratio (95% confidence interval)
		Childhood secondhand smoke exposure		
Zeiger and Heller 1995 United States	Trial N = 165 Aged 7 years	Regular smoking at home	Any of 9 positive SPT	2.9 (1.1–7.7)
Ulrik and Backer 2000 Denmark	Cohort N = 408 Aged 7–17 years	Maternal smoking during childhood	Any of 9 SPT ≥3 mm	2 (1.2–3.1)

*SPT = Skin-prick test.
†mm = Millimeter.

Table 6.23   Summary of pooled odds ratios (95% confidence intervals) in skin-prick positivity comparing unexposed children with children exposed to secondhand smoke at various time points

	Perinatal exposure	Childhood exposure	Perinatal or childhood exposure
Number of studies	7	7	12
Fixed effects	0.97 (0.81–1.15)	0.90 (0.81–1.01)	0.92 (0.84–1.02)
Random effects	0.90 (0.68–1.18)	1.35 (0.91–2.01)	1.10 (0.85–1.42)
Q (p value)	13.1 (0.042)	29.5 (0.000)	42.2 (0.000)

Note: Q is the chi-square distributed test statistic for the null hypothesis of no heterogeneity between studies.

common in those with the highest levels smoked by the mother (current smoking OR = 0.78 [95 percent CI, 0.67–0.92]). A risk for eczema at 16 years of age was not associated with current maternal smoking.

Kalyoncu and colleagues (1999) conducted two questionnaire surveys five years apart to evaluate prevalence rates for asthma, allergic disease, and risk factors among primary school-age children. The second survey included 358 boys and 380 girls aged 6 through 13 years. In this sample, smoking at home was associated with the occurrence of allergic rhinitis (OR = 1.84 [95 percent CI, 1.3–3.0]), and the occurrence of allergic symptoms during the past 12 months was associated with secondhand tobacco smoke exposure (OR = 1.74 [95 percent CI, 1.18–2.56]) (Kalyoncu et al. 1999).

In a retrospective cohort study of 1,934 children, there was no significant association between maternal smoking and atopy (OR = 1.16 [95 percent CI, 0.95–1.43]), hay fever (OR = 1.04 [95 percent CI, 0.82–1.32]), or eczema (OR = 0.97 [95 percent CI, 0.75–1.26]) (Farooqi and Hopkin 1998). The authors concluded that genetic factors constitute the main risk for the development of atopy in children. With an OR of 1.97 (95 percent CI, 1.46–2.66), maternal atopy was a predictor of the development of atopy in these children (Farooqi and Hopkin 1998).

As part of ISAAC, parents answered a supplemental questionnaire regarding indoor environmental exposures and childhood symptoms of atopic rhinitis. For participants in Austria, there were questionnaire responses for 18,606 children aged six through nine years (Zacharasiewicz et al. 2000). Multiple indoor environmental exposures were considered in the analyses, including maternal smoking during pregnancy and/or while breastfeeding, secondhand smoke exposure, mattress and bedding type, home dampness, cooking fuels, home heating, and indoor pets. Overall, there was no difference between indoor environmental exposures in children with rhinitis symptoms only during the pollen season versus those with symptoms year round. Maternal smoking during pregnancy and

Figure 6.11   Odds ratios for the association between parental smoking during pregnancy and infancy and skin-prick positivity

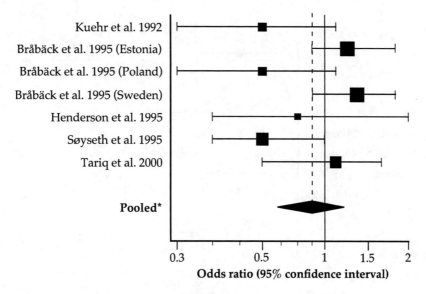

Note: Size of boxes is proportional to the weight of each study in the pooled odds ratio (OR). Solid line represents an OR of 1, dotted line is the combined result.
*From random effects meta-analysis.

Figure 6.12   Odds ratios for the association between parental smoking during childhood and skin-prick positivity

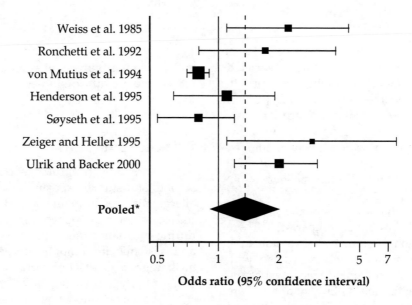

Note: Size of boxes is proportional to the weight of each study in the pooled odds ratio (OR). Solid line represents an OR of 1, dotted line is the combined result.
*From random effects meta-analysis.

Figure 6.13   Odds ratios for the association between parental smoking and skin-prick positivity

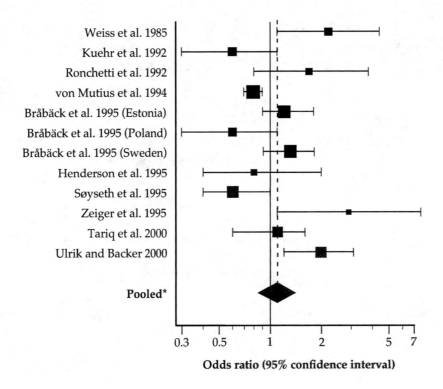

Note: Size of boxes is proportional to the weight of each study in the pooled odds ratio (OR). Solid line represents an OR of 1, dotted line is the combined result.
*From random effects meta-analysis.

after birth while the mother breastfed was associated with an increased risk for atopic rhinitis symptoms in the 12 months before the interview (OR = 1.28 [95 percent CI, 1.07–1.52]). There was also evidence of a dose-response relationship: nasal symptoms in the previous 12 months increased if household smokers smoked 50 or more cigarettes per day in the home (OR = 2.9 [95 percent CI, 1.21–6.95]) (Zacharasiewicz et al. 2000).

Heterogeneity in the measures of allergic sensitization across the studies limits comparisons. There are no prospective cohort studies that demonstrate longitudinal changes in IgE levels associated with prenatal and postnatal secondhand smoke exposure. Assessments of parental and sibling symptoms are critical to these studies, as those children predisposed to the development of allergic sensitization secondary to secondhand smoke exposure may be those most genetically predisposed to the development of atopy,

and gene-environment interactions will need to be considered in future studies of secondhand smoke exposure in children.

Evidence Synthesis

There are multiple mechanisms by which secondhand smoke exposure might alter the risk for allergic diseases in infants and children. Exposure to tobacco smoke components from maternal smoking during pregnancy might have lasting effects on lung and systemic immunophenotypes. Exposures after birth might also affect immunophenotype or increase susceptibility to sensitization by common allergens.

The observational evidence across a range of outcome measures is inconsistent, however. The inconsistency may partially reflect the limited number of studies for any particular outcome and the methodologic complexities of studies on atopic disorders.

Conclusion

1. The evidence is inadequate to infer the presence or absence of a causal relationship between parental smoking and the risk of immunoglobulin E-mediated allergy in their children.

Implications

Studies on secondhand smoke exposure and atopy need to be prospective in design and should track exposures back to the pregnancy. Further studies on secondhand smoke and atopy in childhood are needed, but the studies need to be large enough and need to have sufficient and valid measurements of allergic phenotype. Future studies also need to address potential genetic determinants of susceptibility, particularly as they modify the effect of secondhand smoke.

Lung Growth and Pulmonary Function

Beginning with the 1984 report (USDHHS 1984), the U.S. Surgeon General's reports in this series have covered the adverse effects of exposure to secondhand smoke, including effects from maternal smoking during pregnancy and effects on lung growth from exposure during infancy and childhood. Both cross-sectional and cohort studies on this topic have used lung function level as the primary indicator (Table 6.24). The level of lung function achieved at any particular age and measured cross-sectionally is an indicator of the rate of growth of function up to that age; cohort studies with repeated measurements of lung function directly estimate the rate of growth. The 1986 Surgeon General's report, *The Health Consequences of Involuntary Smoking*, reviewed 18 cross-sectional and cohort studies and concluded that "available data demonstrate that maternal smoking reduced lung function in young children" (USDHHS 1986, p. 54). The report further suggests that although this reduction is small, with an average of 1 to 5 percent, "some children might be affected to a greater extent, and even small differences might be important for children who become active cigarette smokers as adults" (USDHHS 1986, p. 54). The EPA issued its risk assessment in 1992 and concluded that the decline in lung function associated with exposure to secondhand smoke represented a causal effect (USEPA 1992). Similar conclusions were reached by the California Environmental Protection Agency (NCI 1999) and WHO (1999). Thus, for nearly two decades the weight of evidence has been sufficient to conclude that prenatal and postnatal tobacco smoke exposure is associated with a decrease in lung function in childhood. As discussed earlier in this chapter (see "Mechanisms of Health Effects from Secondhand Tobacco Smoke"), lung maturation and growth decrements secondary to exposure are reflected in changes in measured pulmonary function.

A 1998 meta-analysis by Cook and colleagues (1998) concluded that maternal smoking was associated with reduced ventilatory function assessed by spirometry. In a quantitative synthesis of 21 cross-sectional studies, the effects of parental smoking on lung function were reductions of the FVC by 0.2 percent (95 percent CI, -0.4–0.1), the FEV_1 by 0.9 percent (95 percent CI, -1.2 to -0.7), the MEFR by 4.8 percent (95 percent CI, -5.4 to -4.3), and the end-expiratory flow rate (EEFR) by 4.3 percent (95 percent CI, -5.3 to -3.3). The meta-analysis also considered six prospective cohort studies and found only a small effect of current exposure on decreased growth in lung function. The researchers attributed most of the decreased growth to a lasting consequence of in utero exposure from maternal smoking (Cook et al. 1998).

This discussion considers some of the studies included in this 1998 meta-analysis in addition to studies published subsequently. The studies are both cross-sectional and cohort in design, include data on maternal smoking during pregnancy and after birth, and indicate that maternal smoking during pregnancy has a substantially greater adverse effect. As discussed above, maternal smoking affects lung development in utero perhaps by a direct toxic effect, by gene regulation, or by leading to developmental abnormalities. The number of airways in the lung is considered fixed

Table 6.24   Cross-sectional and cohort studies that used lung function level as the primary indicator of adverse effects of exposure to secondhand smoke

Study	Design/population	Measures	Findings	Comments
Cook et al. 1993	Random population-based sample N = 2,511 children Aged 5–7.9 years 10 towns in England and Wales	• Questionnaire • Salivary cotinine • FEV_1* • $FVC^\dagger$ • FEF_{25}‡ • FEF_{50} • FEF_{75}	• PFT§ results were negatively associated with cotinine • FEV_1/FVC^Δ was not correlated with salivary cotinine • FEV_1 decreased linearly with an increase in salivary cotinine	Cannot distinguish as an early effect
Rona and Chinn 1993	Cross-sectional national health survey N = 2,756 children Aged 6.5–12 years Great Britain	Data were not reported	• There was a significant association between maternal smoking and decreased FEF_{25-75}¶ and FEF_{75-85} in boys but not in girls • The FEV_1 decreased in boys exposed to maternal secondhand smoke	Concluded that reduced childhood lung function was associated with maternal smoking
Cunningham et al. 1994	N = 8,863 children Aged 8–12 years 24 cities United States	• Questionnaire • FEV_1 • FVC • FEV_1/FVC • FEV_{75} • PEFR** • FEF_{25-75} • FEF_{65-75}	• FEV_{75} decreased by 1.8% • FEV_1 decreased by 1.4% • FEV_1/FVC decreased by 1.3% • PEFR decreased by 2.1% • FEF_{25-75} decreased by 5.2% (findings are unadjusted for covariates)	When adjusted for prenatal smoking, effects of current smoking decreased; there was no significant association of secondhand smoke exposure with a decrease in lung function between birth and 2 years of age except in the FEF_{25-75}
Haby et al. 1994	N = 2,765 children Aged 7–12 years Australia	• FEV_1 • FVC • PEFR • FEF_{25-75}	Dose-related decrease in FEV_1, PEFR, and FEF_{25-75} but not in FVC with secondhand smoke exposure	Dose was the number of cigarettes smoked in the home; there was no report on gender difference in maternal or paternal smoking

Table 6.24   Continued

Study	Design/population	Measures	Findings	Comments
Wang et al. 1994	N = 8,796 children Aged 6–18 years Exposure was measured in preschool (first 5 years of life), cumulative exposure from 6 years of age to 1 year before the exam China	• Regression splines to model pulmonary function as a function of secondhand smoke exposure were adjusted for age, weight, city, and parental education • Current maternal and paternal smoking	• Preschool exposure was a significant predictor of child pulmonary function • There was no difference in effect for boys vs. girls; there was a small but statistically significant reduction in FEV_1/FVC and FEF_{25-75} through adolescence • Early maternal smoking was associated with a small increase in FVC (statistically significant in children aged 11–18 years) • Children aged 6–10 years exposed to current maternal smoking had slower FVC and FEV_1 growth	Early exposure to secondhand smoke had long-lasting effects on lung growth
Cuijpers et al. 1995	N = 535 children Aged 6–12 years Netherlands	• FVC • FEV_1 • PEF • FEF_{25-75}	• Decreases in FVC, FEV_1, PEF, and FEF_{25-75} in boys were related to lifetime secondhand smoke exposure • A decrease in FEF_{25-75} was significant only in girls	None
Cunningham et al. 1995	N = 876 children Aged 9–11 years United States (Pennsylvania)	• Secondhand smoke exposure was determined by questionnaire • Pulmonary function • FEV_1 • FVC • FEV_1/FVC • FEF_{25-75}	• There was a statistically significant decrease in FEF_{25-75} of -8.1% (95% confidence interval [CI], -12.9 to -3.1), and a decrease in FEV_1/FVC of -2% (95% CI, -3.0 to -0.9) with maternal smoking during pregnancy • There was no statistically significant decrease in FEV_1 • There was no decrease in FVC	Current secondhand smoke exposure was not associated with lung function decrease after adjustment for maternal smoking during pregnancy; effect on boys was greater than effect on girls
Goren and Hellmann 1995	Cross-sectional N = 8,259 children 2nd and 5th graders (ages not provided) Israel	• FVC • FEV_1 • PEF • FEV_1/FVC	There was no relationship between lung volume and secondhand smoke	None

Table 6.24   Continued

Study	Design/population	Measures	Findings	Comments
Søyseth et al. 1995	N = 573 children (out of a birth cohort of 620) Aged 7–13 years Norway	• Parental smoking • Prenatal smoking	There was a slight (but not statistically significant) decrease in FEV_1/FVC in relation to maternal smoking	None
Richards et al. 1996	N = 395 children Aged 14–18 years South Africa	• FEF_{25-75} • FEV_1	There was no significant difference in the FEV_1 or FEF_{25-75} in exposed vs. unexposed adolescents	None
Behera et al. 1998	N = 2,000 children 77 girls, 123 boys Aged 7–15 years Northern India	• FEV_1 • FVC • PEFR • Maximal MEF[++] • FEF_{25} • FEF_{50} • FEF_{75}	• FVC and FEV_1 were lowest in boys whose households used biomass fuels ($p < 0.05$) • All parameters were lower in children exposed to secondhand smoke but were not statistically significant	None
Bono et al. 1998	Longitudinal N = 394 children Aged 14–16 years 2 consecutive years (1992–1993) Northwest Italy	• Questionnaire • Urinary cotinine • FVC • FEV_1 • Maximal MEF_{25} • Maximal MEF_{50} • PEF[++]	Effect for FEV_1 percentage change as measured for natural log of the mean cotinine concentration was -0.66% ($p < 0.05$)	Active and involuntary exposure to tobacco smoke had a significant effect on lung growth measured by linear change in FEV_1; effect was small but dose-related
Demissie et al. 1998	N = 989 children Aged 5–13 years 1990–1992 Canada (Montreal)	• Questionnaire • FVC • FEV_1 • FEV_1/FVC	• FEV_1/FVC decreased (β = -2.13 [95% CI, -4.07–0.19], the estimated effect for a household exposure of 7.25 cigarettes/day vs. none) in boys exposed to secondhand smoke • Maternal smoking during pregnancy was associated with a lower FEV_1 ($p = 0.04$) • Maternal smoking was associated with a lower FEV_1/FVC	Gender difference could be attributable to the difference in maturation rates of lungs in girls vs. in boys
Hoo et al. 1998	108 preterm infants United Kingdom	• $Vmax_{FRC}$[§§] • $T_{PTEF}:T_E$[ΔΔ] • Infant urine cotinine • Passive respiratory compliance	$T_{PTEF}:T_E$ was lower in infants exposed in utero, $p \leq 0.02$	Measured respiratory function in preterm infants only; concluded that an adverse effect was present and was not limited to the last weeks of pregnancy

Table 6.24   Continued

Study	Design/population	Measures	Findings	Comments
Bek et al. 1999	N = 360 children 169 girls, 191 boys Aged 9–13 years Turkey (Ankara)	• Questionnaire • Spirometry for FEV_1/FVC • FEV_1/FVC • PIF^{11}/PEF • FEF_{25-75} • $Vmax_{25}$ • $Vmax_{50}$ • $Vmax_{75}$	• All spirometric indices were lower in those with secondhand smoke exposure • Maternal smoking had no significant effect but paternal smoking was associated with reduced FEF_{25-75} (p = 0.02), PEF (p = 0.03), $Vmax_{50}$ (p = 0.008), and $Vmax_{75}$ (p = 0.009) • There was no significant reduction in peak flow in children whose mothers had smoked during pregnancy	79% of fathers smoked, suggesting that fathers should be targeted, although it may be a sampling issue; there was no significant dose-response pattern
Gilliland et al. 2000	Cross-sectional N = 3,357 children 4th, 7th, and 10th graders United States (Southern California)	• Questionnaire • Current/former smoking while pregnant • PEFR • FVC • FEV_1 • FEV_1/FVC	• In utero exposure • Decreased PEFR: -3% (95% CI, -4.4% to -1.4%) • Decreased maximal MEF: -4.6% (95% CI, -7% to -2.3%) • Decreased FEF_{75}: -6.2% (95% CI, -9.1% to -3.1%) • There was no decrease in FEV_1	In utero exposure to maternal smoking was independently associated with decreased lung function in school-age children, especially for small airway flows
Li et al. 2000	Cross-sectional N = 5,263 children 49% boys, 51% girls Aged 7–19 years Two consecutive years (1992–1993)	• Questionnaire • FVC • FEV_1 • FEV_1/FVC • Maximal MEF	• In utero effects were independently associated with lung function deficits, which were greater in children with asthma • Decreased maximal MEF • Decreased FEV_1/FVC	Used regression splines to account for nonlinear effects; effects of secondhand smoke depend on gender and/or asthma status; in utero exposure leads to persistent lung function deficits, with the greatest effects in those with asthma
O'Connor et al. 2000	N = 2,043 children Aged 10–11 years Boys and girls in 8 U.S. and Canadian communities	• Questionnaire • FVC • FEV_1 • FEV_1/FVC ratio • V_{35M} • V_{30M} • V_{25M}	• V_{30M}/V_{30P} ratio was not related to asthma or maternal smoking • V_{30M}/V_{30P} ratio was slightly higher among girls than boys • FVC was lower with a history of asthma or maternal smoking	Spirometric indices such as FEF_{25-75}/FVC are sensitive to effects of asthma and secondhand smoke exposure; volume history has no benefit

Table 6.24   Continued

Study	Design/population	Measures	Findings	Comments
Mannino et al. 2001	Cross-sectional N = 5,400 children Aged 4–16 years NHANES III*** United States	• Questionnaire • Serum cotinine (stratified by tertiles) • Spirometry on children aged 8 or more years • FEV_1 • FVC • Maximal MEF • FEV_1/FVC	• Children with highest cotinine levels had decreased FEV_1 (mean = -1.8% [95% CI, -3.2% to -0.4%]) • At highest cotinine levels, children were more likely to have FEV_1/FVC <0.8 (odds ratio = 1.8 [95% CI, 1.3–2.4]) • Secondhand smoke was associated with decreased lung function at ages 8–11 years without prenatal secondhand smoke exposure but with secondhand smoke exposure during childhood	Used cotinine to decrease misclassification bias; large sample, but may lack power to detect small increases in odds ratio for some outcomes

*FEV_1 = Forced expiratory volume in 1 second during maximal expiratory effort.

†FVC = Forced vital capacity or total volume of air expired after a full inspiration.

‡FEF_{25} = Amount of air expelled in the first 25% of the total forced vital capacity test. This test is useful when looking for obstructive diseases.

§PFT = Pulmonary function test.

ΔFEV_1/FVC = Percentage of the vital capacity that is expired in the first second of maximal expiration.

¶FEF_{25-75} = Forced mid-expiratory flow rate. Average rate of airflow between 25% and 75% of the FVC, which is reduced in both obstructive and restrictive disorders.

**PEFR = Peak expiratory flow rate.

††MEF = Mid-expiratory flow.

‡‡PEF = Peak expiratory flow or maximum flow achieved after a maximal inhalation and forced exhalation.

§§$Vmax_{FRC}$ = Maximal forced expiratory flow at functional residual capacity.

ΔΔT_{PTEF}:T_E = The ratio of time to peak tidal expiratory flow to expiratory time.

¶¶PIF = Peak inspiratory flow.

***NHANES III = Third National Health and Nutrition Examination Survey.

by the time a child is born, but the number of alveoli in the lung increases until four years of age (Dezateux and Stocks 1997). The period from gestation to four years of age thus represents a vulnerable time for lung growth and development, and exposures during this time are potentially the most critical for structural and functional lung development and performance. This section reviews the evidence that associates different phases of lung growth and development with corresponding ages.

Neonatal and Infant Lung Function and Growth

Evaluating lung function in neonates and infants is challenging because of an inability of the young child to cooperate with testing. However, methods that do not rely on cooperation from the child have been developed and standardized to assess pulmonary function during this period of ongoing lung development. The FRC is the most common measure of lung volumes performed in infants and is an indicator of normal lung volume growth. Measures of FRC can be completed using gas dilution (nitrogen washout) techniques or plethysmography, although plethysmographic measures are more difficult to perform accurately with this age group. Airway resistance can be measured using plethysmography; lung resistance and compliance can be measured using esophageal manometry and forced oscillation methods. The partial forced expiratory maneuver can be used to obtain estimates of the forced expiratory flow rate (FEFR). This maneuver is performed using an inflatable jacket around the thorax of the infant, who is sedated and in the supine position. A rapid mechanical squeeze of the thorax by the jacket accomplishes the expiratory maneuver. With exhalation data from the FRC, partial expiratory flow maneuvers can be normalized and provide information on lung growth and disease in infants. These methods have been used both clinically and in research. The relationship of these infant lung function tests to standard spirometry, which can be measured reproducibly from around five years of age, is still unclear; researchers have published reviews of infant lung function measurements (Stocks et al. 2001; Davis 2003).

Hanrahan and colleagues (1992) conducted a birth cohort study in east Boston that was designed to measure the effect of maternal smoking during and after pregnancy on infant lung function after birth. Maternal reports of smoking during pregnancy were validated against measures of urinary cotinine. In 80 infants studied at a mean age of 4.2 (±1.9) weeks of age, there was a reduced flow in the FRC among infants born to mothers who had smoked during pregnancy (74.3 milliliters [mL] per second) compared with infants whose mothers had not smoked during pregnancy (150.4 mL per second, p = 0.0007). The effects were independent of effects from secondhand smoke on gestational age and birth weight. After stratification by prenatal exposure, the flow rates were not associated with postnatal exposure.

Tager and colleagues (1995) investigated the growth of pulmonary function in 159 infants in the same east Boston cohort. Infant pulmonary function tests were evaluated at 2 to 6 weeks, 4 to 6 months, 9 to 12 months, and 18 months of age using partial expiratory flow volume curves and helium dilution measures for the FVC to evaluate the effects of prenatal tobacco smoke exposure on lung function growth in the first 18 months of life. Maternal smoking during pregnancy was associated with a decrease in the FRC itself (9.4 ± 4.3 mL, p = 0.03) and a decrease in the FRC flow rate (33 ± 12.3 mL per second, p = 0.0008); these estimates were adjusted for the growth of the child. Because of the longitudinal structure of the data, including lung function assessment shortly after birth, the study data could separate the effects of prenatal and postnatal exposure. The study demonstrated an effect of maternal smoking on the FEFR at the FRC, with a multivariate analysis showing that the effect was secondary to prenatal but not to postnatal exposure.

An Australian cohort study that recruited participants from a prenatal care clinic assessed secondhand smoke exposure from a questionnaire and evaluated cotinine levels. The researchers tested lung function in 461 infants by measuring the $T_{PTEF}:T_E$. Measurements at one to six and one-half days of age showed lower values in infants whose mothers smoked more than one-half pack of cigarettes per day (Stick et al. 1996).

Two studies published since the 1998 meta-analysis (Cook et al. 1998) also assessed the effects of maternal smoking during pregnancy on infants (Hoo et al. 1998; Dezateux et al. 1999). Hoo and colleagues (1998) measured the $Vmax_{FRC}$ and $T_{PTEF}:T_E$ in a cohort of preterm infants born at a mean gestational age of 33.5 weeks. Of the 108 infants in the cohort, 40 were born to mothers who had smoked during pregnancy. The $T_{PTEF}:T_E$ was lower in infants exposed to secondhand smoke in utero (mean 0.369, SD 0.109) compared with unexposed infants (mean 0.426, SD 0.135, p ≤0.024). This was the first study to evaluate preterm infants, and the investigators found an effect of maternal smoking on lung development by the 33rd week of gestation.

A study by Dezateux and colleagues (1999) investigated the association of postnatal maternal smoking with measures of specific airway conductance at eight weeks and at one year of age. The initial cohort consisted of 108 term infants with a lung function assessment at eight weeks of age; 100 were available for a longitudinal follow-up at one year of age. Specific airway conductance at end expiration ($sGaw_{EE}$) was used as a measure of airway function with a correction for airway size. In multivariate models that included physician-diagnosed wheeze, a family history of asthma, $sGaw_{EE}$ measured at eight weeks, and a maternal history of postnatal smoking, there was a decrease of 0.40 seconds per kilopascal (unit of pressure) (95 percent CI, -0.71 to -0.10, p = 0.01) in sGaw among infants of mothers who had smoked in the early postnatal period. The authors concluded that early postnatal maternal smoking was an important cause of altered airway function in the infant, with implications for lung growth and development.

Childhood Lung Function and Growth

Researchers have conducted multiple studies of older children to characterize the effects of second-hand smoke exposure on lung growth and development beyond the neonate or infancy stage. Some of these studies evaluated in utero, postnatal, and current tobacco smoke exposures. Although several large, cross-sectional studies (presented below) have been published since the 1998 meta-analysis (Cook et al. 1998), there has been little additional longitudinal evidence since 1997.

One cross-sectional study was carried out in 24 U.S. and Canadian cities to assess the effects of air pollution on child respiratory health. Using data from 8,863 children aged 8 to 12 years in 22 of the cities, Cunningham and colleagues (1994) found that lung function was lower in children whose mothers had smoked during pregnancy. The study recorded maternal smoking histories and pulmonary function measures. Regardless of whether these mothers were still smoking the year before study assessment, their children had lower spirometric measures than children with no in utero or postnatal exposure to maternal smoking. In comparisons of exposed and unexposed children, adjusted findings in exposed children included a 5.7 percent reduction (95 percent CI, -7.7 to -3.6 percent) in the FEF that was between 65 and 75 percent of the FVC, a 4.9 percent reduction (95 percent CI, -6.5 to -3.2 percent) in the FEF measured between 25 and 75 percent of the FVC (FEF_{25-75}), and a 1.7 percent reduction (95 percent CI, -2.4 to -1.0 percent) in the measure of the FEV during the first three-fourths of a second of exhalation ($FEV_{0.75}$). Current maternal smoking was not associated with spirometric decrements. There were 75 children whose mothers had smoked only during the prepartum but not in the postpartum phase. These children had FEF_{25-75} values that were 11 percent lower (95 percent CI, -16.5 to -5.1, p = 0.0004) than those in children of mothers who had never smoked. In this cohort, 6,508 mothers had not smoked during pregnancy. Multivariate models that adjusted for gender, height, age, parental education, place of residence, and current tobacco smoke exposure in the home (maternal, paternal, or other smokers in the home) documented an estimated 2.8 percent decrease (p = 0.026) in the FEF_{25-75} for postpartum maternal smoking up to two years of age of the child. This estimate is about half the size of the effect of smoking during pregnancy. The authors concluded that the decrements in lung function associated with maternal smoking during pregnancy were not explained by current maternal smoking; the observation that these effects were most significant on flow measures suggests involvement, likely inflammation and obstruction, of the small airways.

Several additional cross-sectional studies have been reported since Cunningham and colleagues (1994) conducted their large, cross-sectional analysis. Gilliland and colleagues (2000) investigated 3,357 children in 12 southern California communities and assessed the effects of maternal prenatal and postnatal smoking on pulmonary function measures in children. Current and past secondhand smoke exposures and in utero maternal smoking were assessed from a questionnaire that was completed by parents of fourth-, seventh-, and tenth-grade students. In utero exposure was associated with reduced flow rates measured by spirometry, but not with reductions in the FEV_1. More specifically, the peak expiratory flow rate was reduced by 3 percent (95 percent CI, -4.4 to -1.4 percent), the mean MEF (closely equivalent to the FEF_{25-75}) was reduced by 4.6 percent (95 percent CI, -7.0 to -2.3 percent), and the FEF at 75 percent of vital capacity (FEF_{75}) was reduced by 6.2 percent (95 percent CI, -9.1 to -3.1 percent). Adjustment for confounding factors such as secondhand smoke from the mother, father, or other adult household smokers; gender; race; school grade; income; personal smoking; or parental education levels did not significantly alter the effect estimate for in utero exposure. The researchers concluded that in utero exposure to maternal secondhand smoke was independently associated with a reduction in lung function among school-age children. The authors also suggested that the predominant reduction in flows may reflect an effect of in utero exposure on distal airway maturation and growth during in utero development.

The Children's Health Study evaluated the effects of in utero and postnatal secondhand smoke exposure on lung function in boys and girls with and without a history of asthma. In utero exposure from maternal smoking and secondhand smoke exposure postnatally (from maternal, paternal, or other adult household members) was associated with a measured decrease in lung function in 5,263 children (Li et al. 2000). Children exposed to tobacco smoke in utero from maternal smoking had reductions in maximal MEF and FEV_1/FVC ratios. Specifically, the maximal MEF decreased by 5.9 percent (95 percent CI, -8.4 to -3.4 percent, p <0.001) in boys and by 3.9 percent (95 percent CI, -6.3 to -1.5 percent) in girls (4.2 and 3.0 percent, respectively, when children with asthma were excluded). The FEV_1/FVC ratio decreased by

2.0 percent (95 percent CI, -2.7 to -1.2 percent, p <0.001) in boys and by 1.7 percent (95 percent CI, -2.3 to -1.0 percent) in girls (1.6 and 1.2 percent, respectively, when children with asthma were excluded). In this study, decreased airflow in children without asthma was significantly associated with current secondhand smoke exposure from two or more current smokers.

The NHANES III included a cross-sectional U.S. national sample of 5,400 children aged 4 through 16 years (Mannino et al. 2001). The study data included a respiratory symptoms questionnaire, spirometric measurements, and serum cotinine levels. Participants were stratified by cotinine levels to assess the effects of secondhand tobacco smoke exposure on a variety of health outcomes including lung function. Prenatal secondhand smoke exposure was also retrospectively assessed in the group of children aged 4 to 11 years. Children in the highest cotinine tertile were more likely to have a FEV_1/FVC ratio of less than 0.8 (OR = 1.8 [95 percent CI, 1.3–2.4]). Children exposed to secondhand smoke had reductions in the FEV_1 (-1.8 percent [95 percent CI, -3.2 to -0.4 percent]), the FEV_1/FVC ratio (-1.5 percent [95 percent CI, -2.2 to -0.8 percent]), and the maximal MEF (-5.9 percent [95 percent CI, -8.1 to -3.4 percent]).

Lung Function

To date, prospective cohort studies have not incorporated measurements of lung function along with serial cotinine level measurements. On the other hand, reports of smoking by key household members have high validity and are likely to provide an adequate index of usual exposure to secondhand smoke. One small, prospective cohort study that assessed the effects of tobacco smoke on lung growth in adolescents used urine cotinine levels as a biomarker for active and secondhand tobacco smoke exposure (Bono et al. 1998). Questionnaires, urinary cotinine levels, and spirometric measurements were used to evaluate 394 schoolchildren aged 14 through 16 years. Approximately one year later, data from 333 adolescents were reassessed in multiple regression analyses. The reassessments revealed a trend for reductions in lung growth suggested by spirometry (FEV_1), in association with active and involuntary smoking measured by serum cotinine levels. The effect on FEV_1 growth, although small, demonstrated a dose-related linear trend (Bono et al. 1998).

In a meta-analysis of the cross-sectional evidence relating parental smoking to spirometric indices in children (Cook et al. 1998), new cross-sectional studies (published from 1997 to 2000) were identified by using the same search strategy that the 1998 review had used (Cook et al. 1998). Six additional studies were identified (Behera et al. 1998; Demissie et al. 1998; Bek et al. 1999; Gilliland et al. 2000; O'Connor et al. 2000; Mannino et al. 2001). Three of these studies (Behera et al. 1998; Bek et al. 1999; O'Connor et al. 2000) could not be included in this quantitative synthesis because they did not provide sufficient data to calculate the effect measure of interest (average percentage difference in spirometric index between exposed and unexposed children). The other three papers (Demissie et al. 1998; Gilliland et al. 2000; Mannino et al. 2001) were included in the following updated meta-analysis. One additional paper published before the 1998 synthesis (Rona and Chinn 1993) that was included in the present analysis had not been included in the 1998 quantitative synthesis—the data needed to calculate the effect measure of interest were not available at the time; the data have since become available. The data in this study were presented separately for girls and boys, and a combined estimate was obtained with a random effects method (Egger et al. 2001).

This analysis used the same effect measure that was used in the 1998 synthesis: the average difference in spirometric index between the exposed and unexposed children expressed as a percentage of the level in the unexposed group. Four different spirometric indices were considered: FVC, FEV_1, MEFR, and EEFR. Pooled estimates of the percentage differences were calculated using both fixed and random effects models (Egger et al. 2001).

To determine whether the classification of exposure influenced the relationship between parental smoking and lung function, studies were pooled within exposure groups: both parents did versus did not smoke, mother did versus did not smoke, either parent did versus did not smoke, the highest cotinine category versus the lowest, and high levels of household secondhand tobacco smoke versus none. To test whether adjusting for variables other than age, gender, and body size affected the relationship, studies were pooled separately depending on what adjustments were made for other variables. A final assessment was then made as to whether adjustments for SES measures, such as parental education and social class, were assessed for possible effects on the pooled results.

Of the 26 studies included in the updated quantitative synthesis, 4 were not in the 1998 analysis. There was significant variability among studies for all spirometric measures except the EEFR (Figures 6.14–6.17 and Table 6.25). Heterogeneity was

Figure 6.14   Percentage difference in the forced vital capacity (FVC) between children of smokers and children of nonsmokers in studies included in the meta-analysis

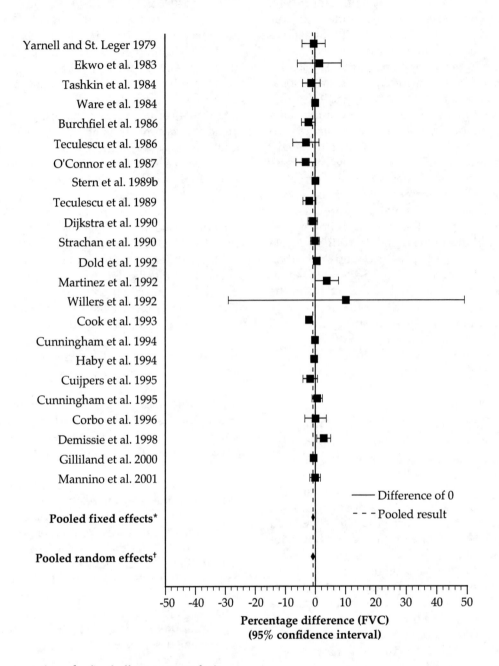

*Pooled difference is from the fixed effects meta-analysis.
†Pooled difference is from the random effects meta-analysis.

Figure 6.15   Percentage difference in the forced expiratory volume in 1 second (FEV₁) between children of smokers and children of nonsmokers in studies included in the meta-analysis

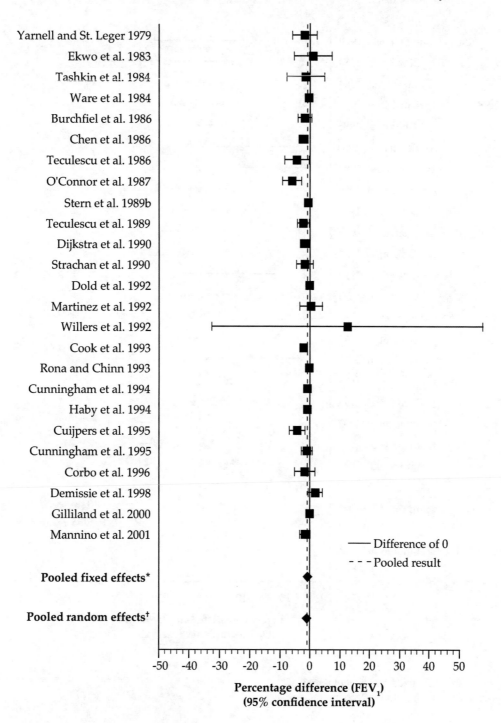

Percentage difference (FEV₁)
(95% confidence interval)

*Pooled difference is from the fixed effects meta-analysis.
†Pooled difference is from the random effects meta-analysis.

Figure 6.16   Percentage difference in the mid-expiratory flow rate (MEFR) between children of smokers and children of nonsmokers in studies included in the meta-analysis

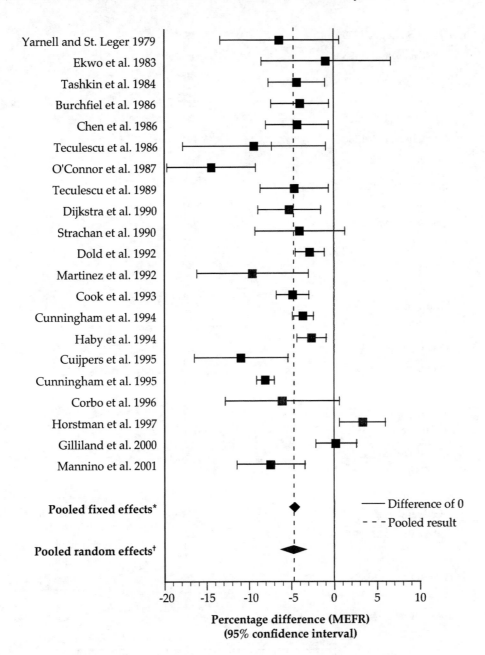

Percentage difference (MEFR)
(95% confidence interval)

*Pooled difference is from the fixed effects meta-analysis.
†Pooled difference is from the random effects meta-analysis.

Figure 6.17 Percentage difference in the end-expiratory flow rate (EEFR) between children of smokers and children of nonsmokers in studies included in the meta-analysis

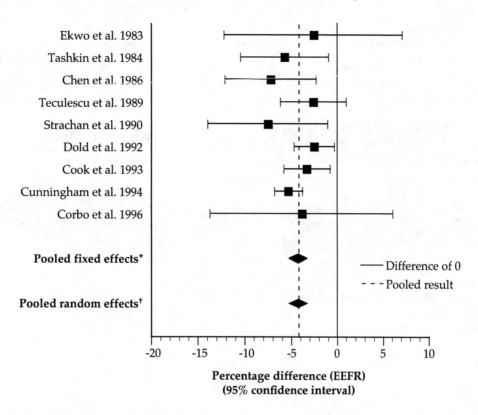

*Pooled difference is from the fixed effects meta-analysis.
†Pooled difference is from the random effects meta-analysis.

Table 6.25 Summary of pooled percentage differences in cross-sectional studies of lung function in children exposed to secondhand smoke compared with unexposed children

	Number of studies	% differences, fixed effects (95% CI*)	% differences, random effects (95% CI)	Q (p value)
FVC†	23	-0.15 (-0.37–0.07)	-0.32 (-0.71–0.08)	40.64 (0.009)
FEV₁‡	25	-0.85 (-1.05 to -0.64)	-1.15 (-1.56 to -0.75)	50.12 (0.001)
MEFR§	21	-4.62 (-5.16 to -4.09)	-4.76 (-6.34 to -3.18)	129.3 (0.000)
EEFRᐃ	9	-4.30 (-5.30 to -3.30)	-4.26 (-5.34 to -3.19)	8.49 (0.387)

Note: Q is the chi-square distributed test statistic for the null hypothesis of no heterogeneity between studies. The corresponding p values indicate significant heterogeneity between studies.
*CI = Confidence interval.
†FVC = Forced vital capacity.
‡FEV₁ = Forced expiratory volume in 1 second.
§MEFR = Mid-expiratory flow rate.
ᐃEEFR = End-expiratory flow rate.

Table 6.26   Pooled percentage differences in lung function according to secondhand smoke exposure category (random effects results)

	FVC*		FEV$_1$†		MEFR‡		EEFR§	
	% difference (95% CI△)	n	% difference (95% CI)	n	% difference (95% CI)	n	% difference (95% CI)	n
Both parents or the mother smoked vs. neither parent smoked	-0.2 (-0.6–0.3)	13	-1.1 (-1.6 to -0.6)	13	-6.0 (-8.1 to -3.9)	10	-4.0 (-5.8 to -2.2)	4
Either parent smoked vs. neither	1.6 (-5.7–8.9)	1	-1.0 (-2.7 to -0.6)	3	-3.7 (-7.0 to -0.4)	2	-6.3 (-10.7 to -1.9)	2
Cotinine (highest vs. lowest level)	-0.9 (-2.5–0.7)	3	-2.1 (-3.0 to -1.2)	3	-4.8 (-6.5 to -3.1)	3	-3.9 (-6.1 to -1.6)	3
Secondhand smoke (highest level vs. none)	-0.2 (-0.9–0.5)	6	-1.0 (-2.0–0.01)	6	-3.3 (-6.6–0.1)	6	Data were not reported	0
All	-0.3 (-0.7–0.0)	23	-1.2 (-1.6 to -0.8)	25	-4.8 (-6.3 to -3.2)	21	-4.3 (-5.3 to -3.2)	9

*FVC = Forced vital capacity.
†FEV$_1$ = Forced expiratory volume in 1 second.
‡MEFR = Mid-expiratory flow rate.
§EEFR = End-expiratory flow rate.
△CI = Confidence interval.

to be expected given the variability in secondhand smoke exposure classifications. Pooling all of the studies found statistically significant reductions in three out of the four measures of lung function (FEV$_1$, MEFR, and EEFR) for children exposed to secondhand smoke in their homes compared with unexposed children. The pooled percentage differences in lung function were smallest for FVC (-0.3 percent) and FEV$_1$ (-1.2 percent) and larger for MEFR (-4.8 percent) and EEFR (-4.3 percent). The MEFR and EEFR are more sensitive indicators of airways function compared with the FVC and the FEV$_1$.

The association between exposure to secondhand smoke and lung function differed according to the exposure classification, but not in a consistent pattern across the four lung function measures (Table 6.26). Adjusting for factors in addition to age, gender, and body size did not significantly affect the associations between secondhand smoke exposure and lung function (Table 6.27). Adjusting for social class had little effect on the FVC, FEV$_1$, and MEFR measures, but nearly doubled the percentage difference in the EEFR (Table 6.27).

The evidence of associations between secondhand smoke exposure and lung function growth and development continues to come largely from cross-sectional studies. The resulting data indicate the level of lung function at only a single age, which at that point is considered indicative of the cumulative consequences of the various factors influencing lung function growth, including prenatal and postnatal maternal smoking. Prospective cohort studies have the advantages of directly measuring lung function over time and directly estimating the rate of change, but few have been carried out because of cost and logistical constraints.

Evidence Synthesis

Smoking during pregnancy exposes the developing lung to a variety of toxins and reduces the delivery of oxygen to the fetus (USDHHS 2001). Animal models indicate structural consequences that may underlie the physiologic effects that are well documented shortly after birth. Secondhand smoke exposure

Table 6.27 Pooled percentage differences in lung function according to confounders adjusted for (random effects results)

	FVC*		FEV$_1$[†]		MEFR[‡]		EEFR[§]	
	% difference (95% CI[Δ])	n	% difference (95% CI)	n	% difference (95% CI)	n	% difference (95% CI)	n
Adjusted only for age, gender, body size	-0.7 (-1.8–0.4)	8	-1.2 (-2.2 to -0.2)	8	-4.3 (-7.0 to -1.6)	8	-2.7 (-5.9–0.5)	3
Adjusted for more than age, gender, body size	-0.3 (-0.6–0.2)	15	-1.2 (-1.6–0.7)	17	-4.9 (-6.8 to -3.0)	13	-4.5 (-5.9 to -3.0)	6
Not adjusted for social class	-0.7 (-1.4–0.1)	14	-1.3 (-2.1 to -0.6)	14	-4.9 (-6.8 to -2.9)	12	-3.1 (-4.5 to -1.7)	6
Adjusted for social class	-0.1 (-0.5–0.3)	9	-1.1 (-1.6 to -0.6)	11	-4.5 (-7.1 to -2.0)	9	-5.6 (-7.0 to -4.1)	3
All	-0.3 (-0.7–0.0)	23	-1.2 (-1.6 to -0.8)	25	-4.8 (-6.3 to -3.2)	21	-4.3 (-5.3 to -3.2)	9

*FVC = Forced vital capacity.
[†]FEV$_1$ = Forced expiratory volume in 1 second.
[‡]MEFR = Mid-expiratory flow rate.
[§]EEFR = End-expiratory flow rate.
[Δ]CI = Confidence interval.

from parents who smoke would be expected to lead to pulmonary inflammation that would be sustained across childhood.

Thus, there is substantial biologic plausibility for causation of reduced lung growth by secondhand smoke exposure. Multiple studies have measured lung function shortly after birth and document the adverse effects on lung function from maternal smoking during pregnancy. The pattern of abnormalities is suggestive of a persistent adverse effect on the airways of the fetus from maternal smoking during pregnancy.

There is also substantial evidence from both cross-sectional and cohort studies of a sustained effect from in utero exposure, as well as an additional adverse effect from postnatal exposure. Multiple studies have shown cumulative consequences of both prenatal and postnatal exposures. Across the set of studies, potentially important confounding factors have been given consideration and the adverse effects of secondhand smoke exposure on lung function cannot be attributed to other factors.

In the context of this body of evidence against causal criteria, the effects of prenatal and postnatal exposures merit separate consideration because they correspond to substantially different phases of development and potential susceptibility. For both exposures, the evidence is substantial and consistent. There are multiple bases for biologic plausibility, and the temporal relationships of exposures with the outcome measures are appropriate.

Conclusions

1. The evidence is sufficient to infer a causal relationship between maternal smoking during pregnancy and persistent adverse effects on lung function across childhood.

2. The evidence is sufficient to infer a causal relationship between exposure to secondhand smoke after birth and a lower level of lung function during childhood.

Implications

Lung growth continues throughout childhood and adolescence and is completed by young adulthood, when lung growth peaks and then begins to decline as a result of aging, smoking, and other environmental factors. The evidence shows that parental smoking reduces the maximum achieved level, although not to a degree (on average) that would impair individuals. Nonetheless, a reduced peak level increases the risk for future chronic lung disease, and there is heterogeneity of the effect so that some exposed children may have a much greater reduction than the mean. In addition, children of smokers are more likely to become smokers and thus face a future risk for impairment from active smoking.

Conclusions

Lower Respiratory Illnesses in Infancy and Early Childhood

1. The evidence is sufficient to infer a causal relationship between secondhand smoke exposure from parental smoking and lower respiratory illnesses in infants and children.

2. The increased risk for lower respiratory illnesses is greatest from smoking by the mother.

Middle Ear Disease and Adenotonsillectomy

3. The evidence is sufficient to infer a causal relationship between parental smoking and middle ear disease in children, including acute and recurrent otitis media and chronic middle ear effusion.

4. The evidence is suggestive but not sufficient to infer a causal relationship between parental smoking and the natural history of middle ear effusion.

5. The evidence is inadequate to infer the presence or absence of a causal relationship between parental smoking and an increase in the risk of adenoidectomy or tonsillectomy among children.

Respiratory Symptoms and Prevalent Asthma in School-Age Children

6. The evidence is sufficient to infer a causal relationship between parental smoking and cough, phlegm, wheeze, and breathlessness among children of school age.

7. The evidence is sufficient to infer a causal relationship between parental smoking and ever having asthma among children of school age.

Childhood Asthma Onset

8. The evidence is sufficient to infer a causal relationship between secondhand smoke exposure from parental smoking and the onset of wheeze illnesses in early childhood.

9. The evidence is suggestive but not sufficient to infer a causal relationship between secondhand smoke exposure from parental smoking and the onset of childhood asthma.

Atopy

10. The evidence is inadequate to infer the presence or absence of a causal relationship between parental smoking and the risk of immunoglobulin E-mediated allergy in their children.

Lung Growth and Pulmonary Function

11. The evidence is sufficient to infer a causal relationship between maternal smoking during pregnancy and persistent adverse effects on lung function across childhood.

12. The evidence is sufficient to infer a causal relationship between exposure to secondhand smoke after birth and a lower level of lung function during childhood.

Overall Implications

The extensive evidence considered in this chapter causally links parental smoking to adverse health effects in children. The association between parental smoking and childhood respiratory disease is stronger at younger ages, a pattern plausibly explained by a higher level of exposure to secondhand smoke among infants and preschool-age children for any given level of parental smoking. In general, associations with maternal smoking are stronger than with paternal smoking, but for several outcomes, associations were found for smoking by the father in homes where the mother does not smoke. This finding argues strongly for an independent adverse effect of a postnatal involuntary (environmental) exposure to secondhand smoke in the home. There may be an additional hazard related to prenatal exposure of the fetus to maternal smoking during pregnancy (USDHHS 2001, 2004). The published evidence does not adequately separate the independent effects on childhood respiratory health of prenatal versus postnatal exposure to maternal smoking. This unresolved research issue should not detract from the public health message that smoking by either parent is potentially damaging to the health of children.

Interpretation of the evidence is perhaps most complex in relation to childhood asthma, which is a term generally applied to a mixed group of clinical phenotypes. Recurrent wheeze illnesses are common among young children, and there is controversy about whether these illnesses should all be classified as "asthma." Cohort studies show that symptoms do not persist for many children beyond the first few years of life. The balance of evidence strongly supports a causal relationship between parental

smoking and the incidence of wheeze illnesses in infancy, the prevalence of wheeze and related symptoms among schoolchildren, and the relative severity of disease among children with physician-diagnosed asthma. These are all important indicators of a substantial and potentially preventable public health burden.

The evidence related to the wheeze illnesses can be separated to an extent from that related to a clearer clinical phenotype of asthma, a chronic condition of variable airflow obstruction with a heightened susceptibility to environmental triggers of bronchospasm. The evidence is less clear as to whether parental smoking initiates the disease among previously healthy children. Because the clinical diagnosis of asthma relies to a large extent upon a history of recurrent wheeze attacks or other chest illnesses, any exposure (including parental smoking) that increases the incidence of such episodes will tend to be associated with an apparent increase in the incidence of diagnosed "asthma," even if secondhand smoke exposure does not contribute to the incidence directly. Studies of nonspecific bronchial responsiveness, a surrogate for the asthma phenotype, offer some insights into the long-term susceptibility that underlies chronic asthma. Secondhand smoke exposure is linked to an increase in responsiveness, beginning with in utero exposure. However, bronchial responsiveness is also nonspecifically and transiently increased following respiratory tract infections. For this reason, the conclusion regarding parental smoking as a cause of childhood asthma has been phrased in less definite terms than the conclusions relating to asthma prevalence and severity.

References

Abuekteish F, Alwash R, Hassan M, Daoud AS. Prevalence of asthma and wheeze in primary school children in Northern Jordan. *Annals of Tropical Paediatrics* 1996;16(3):227–31.

Adair-Bischoff CE, Sauve RS. Environmental tobacco smoke and middle ear disease in preschool-age children. *Archives of Pediatrics & Adolescent Medicine* 1998;152(2):127–33.

Aderele WI. Aetiologic, precipitating and environmental factors in childhood asthma. *Nigerian Journal of Paediatrics* 1982;9(1):26–31.

Agabiti N, Mallone S, Forastiere F, Corbo GM, Ferro S, Renzoni E, Sestini P, Rusconi F, Ciccone G, Viegi G, et al. The impact of parental smoking on asthma and wheezing. *Studi Italiani sui Disturbi Respiratori nell'Infanzia e l'Ambiente. Epidemiology* 1999;10(6):692–8.

Alho OP, Kilkku O, Oja H, Koivu M, Sorri M. Control of the temporal aspect when considering risk factors for acute otitis media. *Archives of Otolaryngology—Head & Neck Surgery* 1993;119(4):444–9.

Alho O-P, Läärä E, Oja H. Public health impact of various risk factors for acute otitis media in northern Finland. *American Journal of Epidemiology* 1996;143(11):1149–56.

Anderson HR, Bland JM, Patel S, Peckham C. The natural history of asthma in childhood. *Journal of Epidemiology and Community Health* 1986;40(2):121–9.

Anderson LJ, Parker RA, Strikas RA, Farrar JA, Gangarosa EJ, Keyserling HL, Sikes RK. Day-care center attendance and hospitalization for lower respiratory tract illness. *Pediatrics* 1988;82(3):300–8.

Andrae S, Axelson O, Björkstén B, Fredriksson M, Kjellman N-IM. Symptoms of bronchial hyperreactivity and asthma in relation to environmental factors. *Archives of Disease in Childhood* 1988;63(5):473–8.

Apostolopoulos K, Xenelis J, Tzagaroulakis A, Kandiloros D, Yiotakis J, Papafragou K. The point prevalence of otitis media with effusion among school children in Greece. *International Journal of Pediatric Otorhinolaryngology* 1998;44(3):207–14.

Arshad SH, Hide DW. Effect of environmental factors on the development of allergic disorders in infancy. *Journal of Allergy and Clinical Immunology* 1992;90(2):235–41.

Arshad SH, Stevens M, Hide DW. The effect of genetic and environmental factors on the prevalence of allergic disorders at the age of two years. *Clinical and Experimental Allergy* 1993;23(6):504–11.

Asgari MM, Dubois A, Asgari M, Gent J, Beckett WS. Association of ambient air quality with children's lung function in urban and rural Iran. *Archives of Environmental Health* 1998;53(3):222–30.

Asher MI, Keil U, Anderson HR, Beasley R, Crane J, Martinez F, Mitchell EA, Pearce N, Sibbald B, Stewart AW, Strachan D, Weiland SK, Williams HC. International study of asthma and allergies in childhood (ISAAC): rationale and methods. *European Respiratory Journal* 1995;8(3):483–91.

Austin JB, Russell G. Wheeze, cough, atopy, and indoor environment in the Scottish Highlands. *Archives of Disease in Childhood* 1997;76(1):22–6.

Azizi BHO, Zulkifli HI, Kasim MS. Indoor air pollution and asthma in hospitalized children in a tropical environment. *Journal of Asthma* 1995;32(6):413–8.

Baker D, Taylor H, Henderson J, ALSPAC Study Team. Inequality in infant morbidity: causes and consequences in England in the 1990s. Avon Longitudinal Study of Pregnancy and Childhood. *Journal of Epidemiology and Community Health* 1998;52(7): 451–8.

Barker K, Mussin E, Taylor DK. Fetal exposure to involuntary maternal smoking and childhood respiratory disease. *Annals of Allergy, Asthma, & Immunology* 1996;76(5):427–30.

Barr GS, Coatesworth AP. Passive smoking and otitis media with effusion. *British Medical Journal* 1991;303(6809):1032–3.

Bassi JA, Rosso P, Moessinger AC, Blanc WA, James LS. Fetal growth retardation due to maternal tobacco smoke exposure in the rat. *Pediatric Research* 1984;18(2):127–30.

Bayne EK, Rupp EA, Limjuco G, Chin J, Schmidt JA. Immunocytochemical detection of interleukin 1 within stimulated human monocytes. *Journal of Experimental Medicine* 1986;163(5):1267–80.

Beckett WS, Belanger K, Gent JF, Holford TR, Leaderer BP. Asthma among Puerto Rican Hispanics: a multi-ethnic comparison study of risk factors. *American Journal of Respiratory and Critical Care Medicine* 1996;154(4 Pt 1):894–9.

Begg CB, Mazumdar M. Operating characteristics of a rank correlation test for publication bias. *Biometrics* 1994;50(4):1088–101.

Behera D, Sood P, Singh S. Passive smoking, domestic fuels and lung function in north Indian children. *Indian Journal of Chest Diseases & Allied Sciences* 1998;40(2):89–98.

Bek K, Tomaç N, Delibas A, Tuna F, Teziç HT, Sungur M. The effect of passive smoking on pulmonary function during childhood. *Postgraduate Medical Journal* 1999;75(884):339–41.

Belousova EG, Toelle BG, Xuan W, Peat JK. The effect of parental smoking on presence of wheeze or airway hyper-responsiveness in New South Wales school children. *Australian and New Zealand Journal of Medicine* 1999;29(6):794–800.

Bener A, Abdulrazzaq YM, Al-Mutawwa J, Debuse P. Genetic and environmental factors associated with asthma. *Human Biology* 1996;68(3):405–14.

Bennett KE, Haggard MP. Accumulation of factors influencing children's middle ear disease: risk factor modelling on a large population cohort. *Journal of Epidemiology and Community Health* 1998; 52(12):786–93.

Bergmann RL, Schulz J, Gunther S, Dudenhausen JW, Bergmann KE, Bauer CP, Dorsch W, Schmidt E, Luck W, Lau S. Determinants of cord-blood IgE concentrations in 6401 German neonates. *Allergy* 1995;50(1):65–71.

Bisgaard H, Dalgaard P, Nyboe J. Risk factors for wheezing during infancy. A study of 5,953 infants. *Acta Paediatrica Scandinavica* 1987;76(5):719–26.

Black N. The aetiology of glue ear—a case-control study. *International Journal of Pediatric Otorhinolaryngology* 1985;9(2):121–33.

Black RE, Michaelsen KF. *Public Health Issues in Infant and Child Nutrition.* Philadelphia: Lippincott Williams & Wilkins, 2002.

Blakley BW, Blakley JE. Smoking and middle ear disease: are they related? A review article. *Otolaryngology—Head & Neck Surgery* 1995;112(3):441–6.

Bland M, Bewley BR, Pollard V, Banks MH. Effect of children's and parents' smoking on respiratory symptoms. *Archives of Disease in Childhood* 1978;53(2):100–5.

Bonham AC, Kott KS, Joad JP. Sidestream smoke exposure enhances rapidly adapting receptor responses to substance P in young guinea pigs. *Journal of Applied Physiology* 1996;81(4):1715–22.

Bonner JC, Rice AB, Lindroos PM, O'Brien PO, Dreher KL, Rosas I, Alfaro-Moreno E, Osornio-Vargas AR. Induction of the lung myofibroblast PDGF receptor system by urban ambient particles from Mexico City. *American Journal of Respiratory Cell and Molecular Biology* 1998;19(4):672–80.

Bono R, Nebiolo F, Bugiani M, Meineri V, Scursatone E, Piccioni P, Caria E, Gilli G, Arossa W. Effects of tobacco smoke exposure on lung growth in adolescents. *Journal of Exposure Analysis and Environmental Epidemiology* 1998;8(3):335–45.

Bråbäck L, Breborowicz A, Julge K, Knutsson A, Riikjärv M-A, Vasar M, Björkstén B. Risk factors for respiratory symptoms and atopic sensitisation in the Baltic area. *Archives of Disease in Childhood* 1995;72(6):487–93.

Brabin B, Smith M, Milligan P, Benjamin C, Dunne E, Pearson M. Respiratory morbidity in Merseyside schoolchildren exposed to coal dust and air pollution. *Archives of Disease in Childhood* 1994;70(4): 305–12.

Braun KM, Cornish T, Valm A, Cundiff J, Pauly JL, Fan S. Immunotoxicology of cigarette smoke condensates: suppression of macrophage responsiveness to interferon γ. *Toxicology and Applied Pharmacology* 1998;149(2):136–43.

Brown RW, Hanrahan JP, Castile RG, Tager IB. Effect of maternal smoking during pregnancy on passive respiratory mechanics in early infancy. *Pediatric Pulmonology* 1995;19(1):23–8.

Burchfiel CM, Higgins MW, Keller JB, Howatt WF, Butler WJ, Higgins ITT. Passive smoking in childhood: respiratory conditions and pulmonary function in Tecumseh, Michigan. *American Review of Respiratory Disease* 1986;133(6):966–73.

Burr ML, Merritt TG, Dunstan FD, Maguire MJ. The development of allergy in high-risk children. *Clinical and Experimental Allergy* 1997;27(11):1247–53.

Burr ML, Anderson HR, Austin JB, Harkins LS, Kaur B, Strachan DP, Warner JO. Respiratory symptoms and home environment in children: a national survey. *Thorax* 1999;54(1):27–32. [See also erratum in *Thorax* 1999;54(4):376.]

Burr ML, Miskelly FG, Butland BK, Merrett TG, Vaughan-Williams E. Environmental factors and symptoms in infants at high risk of allergy. *Journal of Epidemiology and Community Health* 1989;43(2): 125–32.

Butland BK, Strachan DP, Anderson HR. The home environment and asthma symptoms in childhood: two population based case-control studies 13 years apart. *Thorax* 1997;52(7):618–24.

Butz AM, Rosenstein BJ. Passive smoking among children with chronic respiratory disease. *Journal of Asthma* 1992;29(4):265–72.

California Environmental Protection Agency. *Proposed Identification of Environmental Tobacco Smoke as a Toxic Air Contaminant. Part B: Health Effects.*

Sacramento (CA): California Environmental Protection Agency, Office of Environmental Health Hazard Assessment, 2005.

Cameron P. The presence of pets and smoking as correlates of perceived disease. *Journal of Allergy* 1967;40(1):12–5.

Cameron P, Kostin JS, Zaks JM, Wolfe JH, Tighe G, Oselett B, Stocker R, Winton J. The health of smokers' and non-smokers' children. *Journal of Allergy* 1969;43(6):336–41.

Catlin EA, Powell SM, Manganaro TF, Hudson PL, Ragin RC, Epstein J, Donahoe PK. Sex-specific fetal lung development and Müllerian inhibiting substance. *American Review of Respiratory Diseases* 1990;141(2):466–70.

Chang MY, Hogan AD, Rakes GP, Ingram JM, Hoover GE, Platts-Mills TAE, Heymann PW. Salivary cotinine levels in children presenting with wheezing to an emergency department. *Pediatric Pulmonology* 2000;29(4):257–63.

Charlton A. Children's coughs related to parental smoking. *British Medical Journal Clinical Research Ed* 1984;288(6431):1647–9.

Chayarpham S, Stuart J, Chongsuvivatwong V, Chinpairoj S, Lim A. A study of the prevalence of and risk factors for ear diseases and hearing loss in primary school children in Hat Yai, Thailand. *Journal of the Medical Association of Thailand* 1996;79(7):468–72.

Chen Y. Synergistic effect of passive smoking and artificial feeding on hospitalization for respiratory illness in early childhood. *Chest* 1989;95(5):1004–7.

Chen Y. Environmental tobacco smoke, low birth weight, and hospitalization for respiratory disease. *American Journal of Respiratory and Critical Care Medicine* 1994;150(1):54–8.

Chen J, Millar WJ. Birth outcome, the social environment and child health. *Health Reports* 1999;10(4):57–67.

Chen MF, Kimizuka G, Wang NS. Human fetal lung changes associated with maternal smoking during pregnancy. *Pediatric Pulmonology* 1987;3(1):51–8.

Chen Y, Li W, Yu S. Influence of passive smoking on admissions for respiratory illness in early childhood. *British Medical Journal Clinical Research Ed* 1986;293(6542):303–6.

Chen Y, Li WX, Yu SZ, Qian WH. Chang-Ning epidemiological study of children's health. I: passive smoking and children's respiratory diseases. *International Journal of Epidemiology* 1988a;17(2):348–55.

Chen Y, Rennie DC, Dosman JA. Influence of environmental tobacco smoke on asthma in nonallergic and allergic children. *Epidemiology* 1996;7(5):536–9.

Chen Y, Rennie DC, Lockinger LA, Dosman JA. Effect of environmental tobacco smoke on cough in children with a history of tonsillectomy or adenoidectomy. *European Respiratory Journal* 1998;11(6):1319–23.

Chen Y, Yu SZ, Li WX. Artificial feeding and hospitalization in the first 18 months of life. *Pediatrics* 1988b;81(1):58–62.

Chew FT, Teo J, Quak SH, Lee BW. Factors associated with increased respiratory symptoms among asthmatic children in Singapore. *Asian Pacific Journal of Allergy and Immunology* 1999;17(3):143–53.

Chhabra SK, Gupta CK, Chhabra P, Rajpal S. Prevalence of bronchial asthma in schoolchildren in Delhi. *Journal of Asthma* 1998;35(3):291–6.

Chhabra SK, Gupta CK, Chhabra P, Rajpal S. Risk factors for development of bronchial asthma in children in Delhi. *Annals of Allergy, Asthma & Immunology* 1999;83(5):385–90.

Chilmonczyk BA, Salmun LM, Megathlin KN, Neveux LM, Palomaki GE, Knight GJ, Pulkkinen AJ, Haddow JE. Association between exposure to environmental tobacco smoke and exacerbations of asthma in children. *New England Journal of Medicine* 1993;328(23):1665–9.

Chinn S, Rona RJ. Quantifying health aspects of passive smoking in British children aged 5–11 years. *Journal of Epidemiology and Community Health* 1991;45(3):188–94.

Christie G, Helms P. Childhood asthma: what is it and where is it going [review]? *Thorax* 1995;50(10):1027–30.

Clark SJ, Warner JO, Dean TP. Passive smoking amongst asthmatic children: questionnaire or objective assessment? *Clinical and Experimental Allergy* 1994;24(3):276–80.

Collet JP, Larson CP, Boivin JF, Suissa S, Pless IB. Parental smoking and risk of otitis media in preschool children. *Canadian Journal of Public Health* 1995;86(4):269–73.

Colley JRT. Respiratory symptoms in children and parental smoking and phlegm production. *British Medical Journal* 1974;2(912):201–4.

Colley JRT, Brasser LJ, editors. *Chronic Respiratory Disease in Children in Relation to Air Pollution.* Report on a WHO study. Copenhagen: World Health Organization, 1980.

Colley JRT, Holland WW, Corkhill RT. Influence of passive smoking and parental phlegm on pneumonia and bronchitis in early childhood. *Lancet* 1974;2(7888):1031–4.

Collins MH, Moessinger AC, Kleinerman J, Bassi J, Rosso P, Collins AM, James LS, Blanc WA. Fetal lung hypoplasia associated with maternal smoking: a morphometric analysis. *Pediatric Research* 1985;19(4):408–12.

Cook DG, Strachan DP. Health effects of passive smoking: 3. Parental smoking and prevalence of respiratory symptoms and asthma in school age children. *Thorax* 1997;52(12):1081–94.

Cook DG, Strachan DP. Health effects of passive smoking: 7. Parental smoking, bronchial reactivity and peak flow variability in children. *Thorax* 1998;53(4):295–301.

Cook, DG, Strachan DP. Health effects of passive smoking: 10. Summary of effects of parental smoking on the respiratory health of children and implications for research. *Thorax* 1999;54(4):357–66.

Cook DG, Strachan DP, Carey IM. Health effects of passive smoking: 9. Parental smoking and spirometric indices in children. *Thorax* 1998;53(10):884–93.

Cook DG, Whincup PH, Jarvis MJ, Strachan DP, Papacosta O, Bryant A. Passive exposure to tobacco smoke in children aged 5–7: individual, family, and community factors. *British Medical Journal* 1994;308(6925):384–9.

Cook DG, Whincup PH, Papacosta O, Strachan DP, Jarvis MJ, Bryant A. Relation of passive smoking as assessed by salivary cotinine concentration and questionnaire to spirometric indices in children. *Thorax* 1993;48(1):14–20.

Corbo GM, Agabiti N, Forastiere F, Dell'Orco V, Pistelli R, Kriebel D, Pacifici R, Zuccaro P, Ciappi G, Perucci CA. Lung function in children and adolescents with occasional exposure to environmental tobacco smoke. *American Journal of Respiratory and Critical Care Medicine* 1996;154:695–700.

Crane J, Mallol J, Beasley R, Stewart A, Asher MI, International Study of Asthma and Allergies in Childhood Phase I Study Group. Agreement between written and video questions for comparing asthma symptoms in ISAAC. *European Respiratory Journal* 2003;21(3):455–61.

Csonka P, Kaila M, Laippala P, Kuusela A-L, Ashorn P. Wheezing in early life and asthma at school age: predictors of symptom persistence. *Pediatric Allergy and Immunology* 2000;11(4):225–9.

Cuijpers CEJ, Swaen GMH, Wesseling G, Sturmans F, Wouters EFM. Adverse effects of the indoor environment on respiratory health in primary school children. *Environmental Research* 1995;68(1):11–23.

Cunningham J, Dockery DW, Gold DR, Speizer FE. Racial differences in the association between maternal smoking during pregnancy and lung function in children. *American Journal of Respiratory and Critical Care Medicine* 1995;152(2):565–9.

Cunningham J, Dockery DW, Speizer FE. Maternal smoking during pregnancy as a predictor of lung function in children. *American Journal of Epidemiology* 1994;139(12):1139–52.

Daigler GE, Markello SJ, Cummings KM. The effect of indoor air pollutants on otitis media and asthma in children. *Laryngoscope* 1991;101(3):293–6.

Dales RE, White J, Bhumgara C, McMullen E. Parental reporting of childrens' coughing is biased. *European Journal of Epidemiology* 1997;13(5):541–5.

Daly KA, Brown JE, Lindgren BR, Meland MH, Le CT, Giebink GS. Epidemiology of otitis media onset by six months of age. *Pediatrics* 1999;103(6 Pt 1):1158–66.

Darlow BA, Horwood LJ, Mogridge N. Very low birthweight and asthma by age seven years in a national cohort. *Pediatric Pulmonology* 2000;30(4):291–6.

Davis SD. Neonatal and pediatric respiratory diagnostics. *Respiratory Care* 2003;48(4):367–84.

Deb SK. Acute respiratory disease survey in Tripura in case of children below five years of age. *Journal of the Indian Medical Association* 1998;96(4):111–6.

Dejin-Karlsson E, Hanson BS, Ostergren PO, Sjoberg NO, Marsal K. Does passive smoking in early pregnancy increase the risk of small-for-gestational-age infants? *American Journal of Public Health* 1998;88(10):1523–7.

Dekker C, Dales R, Bartlett S, Brunekreef B, Zwanenburg H. Childhood asthma and the indoor environment. *Chest* 1991;100(4):922–6.

Demissie K, Ernst P, Joseph L, Becklake MR. The role of domestic factors and day-care attendance on lung function of primary school children. *Respiratory Medicine* 1998;92(7):928–35.

Department of Health Committee on the Medical Effects of Air Pollutants. *Asthma and Outdoor Air Pollution.* London: HMSO, 1995.

Dezateux C, Stocks J. Lung development and early origins of childhood respiratory illness. *British Medical Bulletin* 1997;53(1):40–57.

Dezateux C, Stocks J, Dundas I, Fletcher ME. Impaired airway function and wheezing in infancy: the influence of maternal smoking and a genetic predisposition to asthma. *American Journal of Respiratory and Critical Care Medicine* 1999;159(2):403–10.

Diez U, Kroessner T, Rehwagen M, Richter M, Wetzig H, Schulz R, Borte M, Metzner G, Krumbiegel P, Herbarth O. Effects of indoor painting and smoking on airway symptoms in atopy risk children in the first year of life results of the LARS-study. *International Journal of Hygiene and Environmental Health* 2000;203(1):23–8.

DiFranza JR, Lew RA. Morbidity and mortality in children associated with the use of tobacco products by other people. *Pediatrics* 1996;97(4):560–8.

Dijkstra L, Houthuijs D, Brunekreef B, Akkerman I, Boleij JSM. Respiratory health effects of the indoor environment in a population of Dutch children. *American Review of Respiratory Disease* 1990;142(5):1172–8.

Divers WA Jr, Wilkes MM, Babaknia A, Yen SS. Maternal smoking and elevation of catecholamines and metabolites in the amniotic fluid. *American Journal of Obstetrics and Gynecology* 1981;141(6):625–8.

Dodge R. The effects of indoor pollution on Arizona children. *Archives of Environmental Health* 1982;37(3):151–5.

Dold S, Reitmeir P, Wjst M, von Mutius E. Effects of passive smoking on the pediatric respiratory tract. *Monatsschrift Kinderheilkunde* 1992;140:763–8.

Duff AL, Pomeranz ES, Gelber LE, Price GW, Farris H, Hayden FG, Platts-Mills TA, Heymann PW. Risk factors for acute wheezing in infants and children: viruses, passive smoke, and IgE antibodies to inhalant allergens. *Pediatrics* 1993;92(4):535–40.

Duffy DL, Mitchell CA. Lower respiratory tract symptoms in Queensland schoolchildren: risk factors for wheeze, cough and diminished ventilatory function. *Thorax* 1993;48(10):1021–4.

Edwards K, Braun KM, Evans G, Sureka AO, Fan S. Mainstream and sidestream cigarette smoke condensates suppress macrophage responsiveness to interferon γ. *Human & Experimental Toxicology* 1999; 18(4):233–40.

Egger M, Davey Smith G, Schneider M, Minder C. Bias in meta-analysis detected by a simple, graphical test. *British Medical Journal* 1997;315(7109):629–34.

Egger M, Smith GD, Altman DG, editors. *Systematic Reviews in Health Care: Meta-analysis in Context*. 2nd ed. London: BMJ Publishing Group, 2001.

Ehrlich R, Kattan M, Godbold J, Saltzberg DS, Grimm KT, Landrigan PJ, Lilienfeld DE. Childhood asthma and passive smoking: urinary cotinine as a biomarker of exposure. *American Review of Respiratory Disease* 1992;145(3):594–9.

Ehrlich RI, Du Toit D, Jordaan E, Zwarenstein M, Potter P, Volmink JA, Weinberg E. Risk factors for childhood asthma and wheezing: importance of maternal and household smoking. *American Journal of Respiratory and Critical Care Medicine* 1996;154 (3 Pt 1):681–8.

Ekwo EE, Weinberger MM, Lachenbruch PA, Huntley WH. Relationship of parental smoking and gas cooking to respiratory disease in children. *Chest* 1983;84(6):662–8.

Elder DE, Hagan R, Evans SF, Benninger HR, French NP. Recurrent wheezing in very preterm infants. *Archives of Disease in Childhood Fetal and Neonatal Edition* 1996;74(3):F165–F171.

Elliot J, Vullermin P, Carroll N, James A, Robinson P. Increased airway smooth muscle in sudden infant death syndrome. *American Journal of Respiratory and Critical Care Medicine* 1999;160(1):313–6.

Engel J, Anteunis L, Volovics A, Hendriks J, Marres E. Risk factors of otitis media with effusion during infancy. *International Journal of Pediatric Otorhinolaryngology* 1999;48(3):239–49.

Etzel RA, Pattishall EN, Haley NJ, Fletcher RH, Henderson FW. Passive smoking and middle ear effusion among children in day care. *Pediatrics* 1992; 90(2 Pt 1):228–32.

Evans D, Levison MJ, Feldman CH, Clark NM, Wasilewski Y, Levin B, Mellins RB. The impact of passive smoking on emergency room visits of urban children with asthma. *American Review of Respiratory Disease* 1987;135(3):567–72.

Ey JL, Holberg CJ, Aldous MB, Wright AL, Martinez FD, Taussig LM, Group Health Medical Associates. Passive smoke exposure and otitis media in the first year of life. *Pediatrics* 1995;95(5):670–7.

Fagbule D, Ekanem EE. Some environmental risk factors for childhood asthma: a case-control study. *Annals of Tropical Paediatrics* 1994;14(1):15–9.

Faniran AO, Peat JK, Woolcock AJ. Persistent cough: is it asthma? *Archives of Disease in Childhood* 1998;79(5):411–4.

Farber HJ, Wattigney W, Berenson G. Trends in asthma prevalence: the Bogalusa Heart Study. *Annals of Allergy, Asthma & Immunology* 1997;78(3):265–9.

Farooqi IS, Hopkin JM. Early childhood infection and atopic disorder. *Thorax* 1998;53(11):927–32.

Fergusson DM, Horwood LJ. Parental smoking and respiratory illness during early childhood: a six-year longitudinal study. *Pediatric Pulmonology* 1985;1(2):99–106.

Fergusson DM, Horwood LJ, Shannon FT. Parental smoking and respiratory illness in infancy. *Archives of Disease in Childhood* 1980;55(5):358–61.

Fergusson DM, Horwood LJ, Shannon FT, Taylor B. Parental smoking and lower respiratory illness in the first three years of life. *Journal of Epidemiology and Community Health* 1981;35(3):180–4.

Ferris BG. Epidemiology Standardization Project. *American Review of Respiratory Disease* 1978;118 (6 Pt 2):1–120.

Ferris BG Jr, Ware JH, Berkey CS, Dockery DW, Spiro A III, Speizer FE. Effects of passive smoking on health of children. *Environmental Health Perspectives* 1985;62:289–95.

Fleming DW, Cochi SL, Hightower AW, Broome CV. Childhood upper respiratory tract infections: to what degree is incidence affected by day-care attendance? *Pediatrics* 1987;79(1):55–60.

Florey C duV, Swan AV, van der Lende R, Holland WW, Berlin A, Di Ferrante E. *Report on the EC Epidemiological Survey on the Relationship Between Air Pollution and Respiratory Health in Primary School Children*. Brussels: Commission of the European Communities Environmental Research Programme, 1983.

Forastiere F, Corbo GM, Michelozzi P, Pistelli R, Agabiti N, Brancato, G, Ciappi G, Perucci CA. Effects of environment and passive smoking on the respiratory health of children. *International Journal of Epidemiology* 1992;21(1):66–73.

Forastiere F, Pistelli R, Sestini P, Fortes C, Renzoni E, Rusconi F, Dell'Orco V, Ciccone G, Bisanti L, SIDRIA (Italian Studies on Respiratory Disorders in Children and the Environment) Collaborative Group, Italy. Consumption of fresh fruit rich in vitamin C and wheezing symptoms in children. *Thorax* 2000;55(4):283–8.

Forsberg B, Pekkanen J, Clench-Aas J, Martensson M-B, Stjernberg N, Bartonova A, Timonen KL, Skerfving S. Childhood asthma in four regions in Scandinavia: risk factors and avoidance effects. *International Journal of Epidemiology* 1997;26(3):610–9.

Forsthuber T, Yip HC, Lehmann PV. Induction of TH1 and TH2 immunity in neonatal mice. *Science* 1996;271(5256):1728–30.

Galván Fernández C, Díaz Gómez NM, Suárez López de Vergara RG. Tobacco exposure and respiratory disease in children. *Revista Española de Pediatría* 1999;55(328):323–7.

Garcia-Marcos L, Guillén JJ, Dinwiddie R, Guillén A, Barbero P. The relative importance of socioeconomic status, parental smoking and air pollution (SO_2) on asthma symptoms, spirometry and bronchodilator response in 11-year-old children. *Pediatric Allergy and Immunology* 1999;10(2):96–100.

Gardner G, Frank AL, Taber LH. Effects of social and family factors on viral respiratory infection and illness in the first year of life. *Journal of Epidemiology and Community Health* 1984;38(1):42–8.

Geller-Bernstein G, Kenett R, Weisglass L, Tsur S, Lahav M, Levin S. Atopic babies with wheezy bronchitis: follow-up study relating prognosis to sequential IgE values, type of early infant feeding, exposure to parental smoking and incidence of lower respiratory tract infections. *Allergy* 1987;42(2):85–91.

Gepts L, Borlee I, Minette A. Prevalence of respiratory symptoms in 1659 school children living in a non polluted area [French]. *Acta Tuberculosea et Pneumologica Belgica* 1978;69(3–4):179–210.

Gergen PJ, Fowler JA, Maurer KR, Davis WW, Overpeck MD. The burden of environmental tobacco smoke exposure on the respiratory health of children 2 months through 5 years of age in the United States: Third National Health and Nutrition Examination Survey, 1988 to 1994. *Pediatrics* 1998; 101(2):E8.

Gilliland FD, Berhane K, McConnell R, Gauderman WJ, Vora H, Rappaport EB, Avol E, Peters JM. Maternal smoking during pregnancy, environmental tobacco smoke exposure and childhood lung function. *Thorax* 2000;55(4):271–6.

Gold DR, Burge HA, Carey V, Milton DK, Platts-Mills T, Weiss ST. Predictors of repeated wheeze in the first year of life: the relative roles of cockroach, birth weight, acute lower respiratory illness, and maternal smoking. *American Journal of Respiratory and Critical Care Medicine* 1999;160(1):227–36.

Gomzi M. Indoor air and respiratory health in preadolescent children. *Atmospheric Environment* 1999;33(24–25):4081–6.

Goren A, Hellmann S, Gabbay Y, Brenner S. Respiratory problems associated with exposure to airborne particles in the community. *Archives of Environmental Health* 1999;54(3):165–71.

Goren AI, Goldsmith JR. Epidemiology of childhood respiratory disease in Israel. *European Journal of Epidemiology* 1986;2(2):139–50.

Goren AI, Hellmann S. Respiratory conditions among schoolchildren and their relationship to environmental tobacco smoke and other combustion products. *Archives of Environmental Health* 1995; 50(2):112–8.

Gortmaker SL, Walker DK, Jacobs FH, Ruch-Ross H. Parental smoking and the risk of childhood asthma. *American Journal of Public Health* 1982;72(6):574–9.

Graham NM. The epidemiology of acute respiratory infections in children and adults: a global perspective. *Epidemiologic Reviews* 1990;12:149–78.

Green RE, Cooper NK. Passive smoking and middle ear effusions in children of British servicemen in West Germany—a point prevalence survey by clinics of outpatient attendance. *Journal of the Royal Army Medical Corps* 1991;137(1):31–3.

Greenberg RA, Strecher VJ, Bauman KE, Boat BW, Fowler MG, Keyes LL, Denny FW, Chapman RS, Stedman HC, LaVange LM, et al. Evaluation of a home-based intervention program to reduce infant passive smoking and lower respiratory illness. *Journal of Behavioral Medicine* 1994;17(3):273–90.

Gryczyńska D, Kobos J, Zakrzewska A. Relationship between passive smoking, recurrent respiratory tract infections and otitis media in children. *International Journal of Pediatric Otorhinolaryngology* 1999;49(Suppl 1):S275–S278.

Gulya AJ. Environmental tobacco smoke and otitis media [review]. *Otolaryngology—Head & Neck Surgery* 1994;111(1):6–8.

Gürkan F, Ece A, Haspolat K, Derman O, Bosnak M. Predictors for multiple hospital admissions in children with asthma. *Canadian Respiratory Journal* 2000a;7(2):163–6.

Gürkan F, Kiral A, Dağli E, Karakoç F. The effect of passive smoking on the development of respiratory syncytial virus bronchiolitis. *European Journal of Epidemiology* 2000b;16(5):465–8.

Haby MM, Peat JK, Woolcock AJ. Effect of passive smoking, asthma, and respiratory infection on lung function in Australian children. *Pediatric Pulmonology* 1994;18(5):323–9.

Håkansson A, Carlsson B. Maternal cigarette smoking, breast-feeding, and respiratory tract infections in infancy: a population-based cohort study. *Scandinavian Journal of Primary Health Care* 1992;10(1):60–5.

Halken S, Høst A, Husby S, Hansen LG, Østerballe O, Nyboe J. Recurrent wheezing in relation to environmental risk factors in infancy: a prospective study of 276 infants. *Allergy* 1991;46(7):507–14.

Halken S, Host A, Nilsson L, Taudorf E. Passive smoking as a risk factor for development of obstructive respiratory disease and allergic sensitization. *Allergy* 1995;50(2):97–105.

Hall CB, Hall WJ, Gala CL, MaGill FB, Leddy JP. Long-term prospective study in children after respiratory syncytial virus infection. *Journal of Pediatrics* 1984;105(3):358–64.

Halliday JA, Henry RL, Hankin RG, Hensley MJ. Increased wheeze but not bronchial hyperreactivity near power stations. *Journal of Epidemiology and Community Health* 1993;47(4):282–6.

Halonen M, Stern D, Lyle S, Wright A, Taussig L, Martinez FD. Relationship of total serum IgE levels in cord and 9-month sera of infants. *Clinical and Experimental Allergy* 1991;21(2):235–41.

Hanke W, Kalinka J, Florek E, Sobala W. Passive smoking and pregnancy outcome in central Poland. *Human & Experimental Toxicology* 1999;18(4):265–71.

Hanrahan JP, Tager IB, Segal MR, Tosteson TD, Castile RG, Van Vunakis H, Weiss ST, Speizer FE. The effect of maternal smoking during pregnancy on early infant lung function. *American Review of Respiratory Diseases* 1992;145(5):129–35.

Hansen LG, Host A, Halken S, Holmskov A, Husby S, Lassen LB, Storm K, Østerballe O. Cord blood IgE: II. Prediction of atopic disease: a follow-up at the age of 18 months. *Allergy* 1992;47(4 Pt 2):397–403.

Harlap S, Davies AM. Infant admissions to hospital and maternal smoking. *Lancet* 1974;1(7857):529–32.

Harsten G, Prellner K, Heldrup J, Kalm O, Kornfalt R. Acute respiratory tract infections in children: a three-year follow-up from birth. *Acta Paediatrica Scandinavica* 1990;79(4):402–9.

Hasday JD, Bascom R, Costa JJ, Fitzgerald T, Dubin W. Bacterial endotoxin is an active component of cigarette smoke. *Chest* 1999;115(3):829–35.

Hayes EB, Hurwitz ES, Schonberger LB, Anderson LJ. Respiratory syncytial virus outbreak on American Samoa: evaluation of risk factors. *American Journal of Diseases of Children* 1989;143(3):316–21.

Heinrich J, Hoelscher B, Jacob B, Wjst M, Wichmann H-E. Trends in allergies among children in a region of former East Germany between 1992–1993 and 1995–1996. *European Journal of Medical Research* 1999;4(3):107–13.

Henderson FW, Henry MM, Ivins SS, Morris R, Neebe EC, Leu S-Y, Stewart PW, the Physicians of Raleigh Pediatric Associates. Correlates of recurrent wheezing in school-age children. *American Journal of Respiratory and Critical Care Medicine* 1995;151(6):1786–93.

Henry RL, Abramson R, Adler JA, Wlodarcyzk J, Hensley MJ. Asthma in the vicinity of power stations: I. A prevalence study. *Pediatric Pulmonology* 1991;11(2):127–33.

Hinton AE. Surgery for otitis media with effusion in children and its relationship to parental smoking. *Journal of Laryngology & Otology* 1989;103(6):559–61.

Hinton AE, Buckley G. Parental smoking and middle ear effusions in children. *Journal of Laryngology and Otology* 1988;102(11):992–6.

Hinton AE, Herdman RCD, Martin-Hirsch D, Saeed SR. Parental cigarette smoking and tonsillectomy in children. *Clinical Otolaryngology and Allied Sciences* 1993;18(3):178–80.

Hjern A, Haglund B, Bremberg S. Lower respiratory tract infections in an ethnic and social context. *Paediatric and Perinatal Epidemiology* 2000;14(1):53–60.

Hjern A, Haglund B, Bremberg S, Ringbäck-Weitoft G. Social adversity, migration and hospital admissions for childhood asthma in Sweden. *Acta Paediatrica* 1999;88(10):1107–12.

Holberg CJ, Wright AL, Martinez FD, Morgan WJ, Taussig LM, Group Health Medical Associates. Child day care, smoking by caregivers, and lower respiratory tract illness in the first 3 years of life. *Pediatrics* 1993;91(5):885–92.

Hölscher B, Heinrich J, Jacob B, Ritz B, Wichmann H-E. Gas cooking, respiratory health and white blood cell counts in children. *International Journal of Hygiene and Environmental Health* 2000;203(1): 29–37.

Homøe P, Christensen RB, Bretlau P. Acute otitis media and sociomedical risk factors among unselected children in Greenland. *International Journal of Pediatric Otorhinolaryngology* 1999;49(1):37–52.

Hoo A-F, Henschen M, Dezateux C, Costeloe K, Stocks J. Respiratory function among preterm infants whose mothers smoked during pregnancy. *American Journal of Respiratory and Critical Care Medicine* 1998;158(3):700–5.

Horstman D, Kotesovec F, Vitnerova N, Leixner M, Nozicka J, Smitkova D, Sram R. Pulmonary functions of school children in highly polluted northern Bohemia. *Archives of Environmental Health* 1997;52(1):56–62.

Horwood LJ, Fergusson DM, Shannon FT. Social and familial factors in the development of early childhood asthma. *Pediatrics* 1985;75(5):859–68.

Hosein HR, Corey P, Robertson JMD. The effect of domestic factors on respiratory symptoms and FEV$_1$. *International Journal of Epidemiology* 1989;18(2):390–6.

Hu FB, Persky V, Flay BR, Zelli A, Cooksey J, Richardson J. Prevalence of asthma and wheezing in public schoolchildren: association with maternal smoking during pregnancy. *Annals of Allergy, Asthma & Immunology* 1997;79(1):80–4.

Hunt LW, Gleich GJ, Ohnishi T, Weiler DA, Mansfield ES, Kita H, Sur S. Endotoxin contamination causes neutrophilia following pulmonary allergen challenge. *American Journal of Respiratory and Critical Care Medicine* 1994;149(6):1471–5.

Ilicali ÖC, Keleş N, Değer K, Savaş I. Relationship of passive cigarette smoking to otitis media. *Archives of Otolaryngology—Head & Neck Surgery* 1999;125(7):758–62.

Infante-Rivard C. Childhood asthma and indoor environmental risk factors. *American Journal of Epidemiology* 1993;137(8):834–44.

Infante-Rivard C, Gautrin D, Malo J-L, Suissa S. Maternal smoking and childhood asthma. *American Journal of Epidemiology* 1999;150(5):528–31.

Ingalls RR, Heine H, Lien E, Yoshimura A, Golenbock D. Lipopolysaccharide recognition, CD14, and lipopolysaccharide receptors. *Infectious Disease Clinics of North America* 1999;13(2):341–53, vii.

Irvine L, Crombie IK, Clark RA, Slane PW, Goodman KE, Feyerabend C, Cater JI. What determines levels of passive smoking in children with asthma? *Thorax* 1997;52(9):766–9.

Iversen M, Birch L, Lundqvist GR, Elbrond O. Middle ear effusion in children and the indoor environment: an epidemiological study. *Archives of Environmental Health* 1985;40(2):74–9.

Jackson JM, Mourino AP. Pacifier use and otitis media in infants twelve months of age or younger. *Pediatric Dentistry* 1999;21(4):255–60.

Jarvis MJ, Strachan DP, Feyerabend C. Determinants of passive smoking in children in Edinburgh, Scotland. *American Journal of Public Health* 1992;82(9):1225–9.

Jedrychowski W, Flak E. Maternal smoking during pregnancy and postnatal exposure to environmental tobacco smoke as predisposition factors to acute respiratory infections. *Environmental Health Perspectives* 1997;105(3):302–6.

Jedrychowski W, Maugeri U, Flak E, Mroz E, Bianchi I. Predisposition to acute respiratory infections among overweight preadolescent children: an epidemiologic study in Poland. *Public Health* 1998;112(3):189–95.

Jenkins MA, Hopper JL, Flander LB, Carlin JB, Giles GG. The associations between childhood asthma and atopy, and parental asthma, hay fever and smoking. *Paediatric and Perinatal Epidemiology* 1993;7(1):67–76.

Jin C, Rossignol AM. Effects of passive smoking on respiratory illness from birth to age eighteen months, in Shanghai, People's Republic of China. *Journal of Pediatrics* 1993;123(4):553–8.

Jones JG, Minty BD, Lawler P, Hulands G, Crawley JC, Veall N. Increased alveolar epithelial permeability in cigarette smokers. *Lancet* 1980;1(8159):66–8.

Jones RC, Hughes CR, Wright D, Baumer JH. Early house moves, indoor air, heating methods and asthma. *Respiratory Medicine* 1999;93(12):919–22.

Kaan A, Dimich-Ward H, Manfreda J, Becker A, Watson W, Ferguson A, Chan H, Chan-Yeung M. Cord blood IgE: its determinants and prediction of development of asthma and other allergic disorders at 12 months. *Annals of Allergy, Asthma & Immunology* 2000;84(1):37–42.

Kalyoncu AF, Selçuk ZT, Enünlü T, Demir AU, Çöplü L, Şahin AA, Artvinli M. Prevalence of asthma and allergic diseases in primary school children in Ankara, Turkey: two cross-sectional studies, five years apart. *Pediatric Allergy and Immunology* 1999;10(4):261–5.

Karaman Ö, Uguz A, Uzuner N. Risk factors in wheezing infants. *Pediatrics International* 1999;41(2): 147–50.

Kardas-Sobantka D, Stańczyk A, Kubik M. Prevalence of asthma symptoms among adolescents in Łódź. *Alergia Astma Immunologia* 2000;5(1):51–5.

Kasuga H, Hasebe A, Osaka F, Matsuki H. Respiratory symptoms in school children and the role of passive smoking. *Tokai Journal of Experimental and Clinical Medicine* 1979;4(2):101–14.

Kay J, Mortimer MJ, Jaron AG. Do both paternal and maternal smoking influence the prevalence of childhood asthma: a study into the prevalence of asthma in children and the effects of parental smoking. *Journal of Asthma* 1995;32(1):47–55.

Kendirli GS, Altintaş DU, Alparslan N, Akmanlar N, Yurdakul Z, Bolat B. Prevalence of childhood allergic diseases in Adana, Southern Turkey. *European Journal of Epidemiology* 1998;14(4):347–50.

Kershaw CR. Passive smoking, potential atopy and asthma in the first five years. *Journal of the Royal Society of Medicine* 1987;80(11):683–8.

Kitchens GG. Relationship of environmental tobacco smoke to otitis media in young children [review]. *Laryngoscope* 1995;105(5 Pt 2 Suppl 69):1–13.

Kjellman NI. Effect of parental smoking on IgE levels in children [letter]. *Lancet* 1981;1(8227):993–4.

Klig JE, Chen L. Lower respiratory infections in children. *Current Opinion in Pediatrics* 2003;15(1):121–6.

Knight JM, Eliopoulos C, Klein J, Greenwald M, Koren G. Pharmacokinetic predisposition to nicotine from environmental tobacco smoke: a risk factor for pediatric asthma. *Journal of Asthma* 1998;35(1):113–7.

Kossove D. Smoke-filled rooms and lower respiratory disease in infants. *South African Medical Journal* 1982;61(17):622–4.

Kraemer MJ, Richardson MA, Weiss NS, Furukawa CT, Shapiro GG, Pierson WE, Bierman CW. Risk factors for persistent middle-ear effusions: otitis media, catarrh, cigarette smoke exposure, and atopy. *Journal of the American Medical Association* 1983;249(8):1022–5.

Kuehr J, Frischer T, Karmaus W, Meinert R, Barth R, Herrman-Kunz E, Forster J, Urbanek R. Early childhood risk factors for sensitization at school age. *Journal of Allergy and Clinical Immunology* 1992; 90(3 Pt 1):358–63.

Kulig M, Luck W, Lau S, Niggemann B, Bergmann R, Klettke U, Guggenmoos-Holzmann I, Wahn U, Multicenter Allergy Study Group, Germany. Effect of pre- and postnatal tobacco smoke exposure on specific sensitization to food and inhalant allergens during the first 3 years of life. *Allergy* 1999;54(3):220–8.

Lam TH, Chung SF, Betson CL, Wong CM, Hedley AJ. Respiratory symptoms due to active and passive smoking in junior secondary school students in Hong Kong. *International Journal of Epidemiology* 1998;27(1):41–8.

Lam TH, Hedley AJ, Chung SF, Macfarlane DJ, Child Health and Activity Research Group (CHARG). Passive smoking and respiratory symptoms in primary school children in Hong Kong. *Human & Experimental Toxicology* 1999;18(4):218–23.

Lau YL, Karlberg J, Yeung CY. Prevalence of and factors associated with childhood asthma in Hong Kong. *Acta Paediatrica* 1995;84(7):820–2.

Lebowitz MD, Burrows B. Respiratory symptoms related to smoking habits of family adults. *Chest* 1976;69(1):48–50.

Lee LY, Widdicombe JG. Modulation of airway sensitivity to inhaled irritants: role of inflammatory mediators. *Environmental Health Perspectives* 2001;109(Suppl 4):585–9.

Leeder SR, Corkhill R, Irwig LM, Holland WW, Colley JRT. Influence of family factors on the incidence of lower respiratory illness during the first year of life. *British Journal of Preventive & Social Medicine* 1976;30(4):203–12.

Leen MG, O'Connor T, Kelleher C, Mitchell EB, Loftus BG. Home environment and childhood asthma. *Irish Medical Journal* 1994;87(5):142–4.

LeSon S, Gershwin ME. Risk factors for asthmatic patients requiring intubation. I: observations in children. *Journal of Asthma* 1995;32(4):285–94.

Leung R, Wong G, Lau J, Ho A, Chan JKW, Choy D, Douglass C, Lai CKW. Prevalence of asthma and allergy in Hong Kong schoolchildren: an ISAAC study. *European Respiratory Journal* 1997;10(2): 354–60.

Lewis KW, Bosque EM. Deficient hypoxia awakening response in infants of smoking mothers: possible relationship to sudden infant death syndrome. *Journal of Pediatrics* 1995;127(5):691–9.

Lewis PR, Hensley MJ, Wlodarczyk J, Toneguzzi RC, Westley-Wise VJ, Dunn T, Calvert D. Outdoor air pollution and children's respiratory symptoms in the steel cities of New South Wales. *Medical Journal of Australia* 1998;169(9):459–63.

Lewis S, Richards D, Bynner J, Butler N, Britton J. Prospective study of risk factors for early and persistent wheezing in childhood. *European Respiratory Journal* 1995;8(3):349–56.

Lewis SA, Britton JR. Consistent effects of high socioeconomic status and low birth order, and the modifying effect of maternal smoking on the risk of allergic disease during childhood. *Respiratory Medicine* 1998;92(10):1237–44.

Li JSM, Peat JK, Xuan W, Berry G. Meta-analysis on the association between environmental tobacco smoke (ETS) exposure and the prevalence of lower respiratory tract infection in early childhood. *Pediatric Pulmonology* 1999;27(1):5–13.

Li Y-F, Gilliland FD, Berhane K, McConnell R, Gauderman WJ, Rappaport EB, Peters JM. Effects of *in utero* and environmental tobacco smoke exposure on lung function in boys and girls with and without asthma. *American Journal of Respiratory and Critical Care Medicine* 2000;162(6):2097–104.

Lieberman E, Torday J, Barbieri R, Cohen A, Van Vunakis H, Weiss ST. Association of intrauterine cigarette smoke exposure with indices of fetal lung maturation. *Obstetrics and Gynecology* 1992;79(4):564–70.

Lindfors A, van Hage-Hamsten M, Rietz H, Wickman M, Nordvall SL. Influence of interaction of environmental risk factors and sensitization in young asthmatic children. *Journal of Allergy and Clinical Immunology* 1999;104(4 Pt 1):755–62.

Lindfors A, Wickman M, Hedlin G, Pershagen G, Rietz H, Nordvall SL. Indoor environmental risk factors in young asthmatics: a case-control study. *Archives of Disease in Childhood* 1995;73(5):408–12.

Lister SM, Jorm LR. Parental smoking and respiratory illnesses in Australian children aged 0–4 years: ABS 1989–90 National Health Survey results. *Australian and New Zealand Journal of Public Health* 1998;22(7):781–6.

Lodrup Carlsen KC, Jaakkola JJ, Nafstad P, Carlsen KH. In utero exposure to cigarette smoking influences lung function at birth. *European Respiratory Journal* 1997;10(8):1774–9.

Lubianca Neto JF, Burns AG, Lu L, Mombach R, Saffer M. Passive smoking and nonrecurrent acute otitis media in children. *Otolaryngology—Head & Neck Surgery* 1999;121(6):805–8.

Lucas A, Brooke OG, Cole TJ, Morley R, Bamford MF. Food and drug reactions, wheezing, and eczema in preterm infants. *Archives of Disease in Childhood* 1990;65(4):411–5.

Lux AL, Henderson AJ, Pocock SJ, ALSPAC Study Team. Wheeze associated with prenatal tobacco smoke exposure: a prospective, longitudinal study. *Archives of Disease in Childhood* 2000;83(4):307–12.

Lyons RA. Passive smoking and hearing loss in infants. *Irish Medical Journal* 1992;85(3):111–2.

Macarthur C, Calpin C, Parkin PC, Feldman W. Factors associated with pediatric asthma readmissions. *Journal of Allergy and Clinical Immunology* 1996; 98(5 Pt 1):992–3.

Magnusson CG. Maternal smoking influences cord serum IgE and IgD levels and increases the risk for subsequent infant allergy. *Journal of Allergy and Clinical Immunology* 1986;78(5 Pt 1):898–904.

Magnusson CG. Cord serum IgE in relation to family history and as predictor of atopic disease in early infancy. *Allergy* 1988;43(4):241–51.

Maier WC, Arrighi HM, Morray B, Llewellyn C, Redding GJ. Indoor risk factors for asthma and wheezing among Seattle school children. *Environmental Health Perspectives* 1997;105(2):208–14.

Mainous AG 3rd, Hueston WJ. Passive smoke and low birth weight: evidence of a threshold effect. *Archives of Family Medicine* 1994;3(10):875–8.

Mannino DM, Moorman JE, Kingsley B, Rose D, Repace J. Health effects related to environmental tobacco smoke exposure in children in the United States: data from the Third National Health and Nutrition Examination Survey. *Archives of Pediatrics & Adolescent Medicine* 2001;155(1):36–41.

Marbury MC, Maldonado G, Waller L. The Indoor Air and Children's Health Study: methods and incidence rates. *Epidemiology* 1996;7(2):166–74.

Margolis PA, Keyes LL, Greenberg RA, Bauman KE, LaVange LM. Urinary cotinine and parent history (questionnaire) as indicators of passive smoking and predictors of lower respiratory illness in infants. *Pediatric Pulmonology* 1997;23(6):417–23.

Martinez FD, Antognoni G, Macri F, Bonci E, Midulla F, De Castro G, Ronchetti R. Parental smoking enhances bronchial responsiveness in nine-year-old children. *American Review of Respiratory Diseases* 1988;138(3):518–23.

Martinez FD, Cline M, Burrows B. Increased incidence of asthma in children of smoking mothers. *Pediatrics* 1992;89(1):21–6.

Martinez FD, Wright AL, Taussig LM, Holberg CJ, Halonen M, Morgan WJ. Asthma and wheezing in the first six years of life: the Group Health Medical Associates. *New England Journal of Medicine* 1995;332(3):133–8.

Maw AR, Bawden R. Factors affecting resolution of otitis media with effusion in children. *Clinical Otolaryngology and Allied Sciences* 1994;19(2):125–30.

Maw R, Bawden R. Spontaneous resolution of severe chronic glue ear in children and the effect of adenoidectomy, tonsillectomy, and insertion of ventilation tubes (grommets). *British Medical Journal* 1993;306(6880):756–60.

McConnochie KM, Roghmann KJ. Bronchiolitis as a possible cause of wheezing in childhood: new evidence. *Pediatrics* 1984;74(1):1–10.

McConnochie KM, Roghmann KJ. Breast feeding and maternal smoking as predictors of wheezing in children age 6 to 10 years. *Pediatric Pulmonology* 1986a;2(5):260–8.

McConnochie KM, Roghmann KJ. Parental smoking, presence of older siblings, and family history of asthma increase risk of bronchiolitis. *American Journal of Diseases of Children* 1986b;140(8):806–12.

Medical Research Council. Questionnaire on Respiratory Symptoms (1966). London: Medical Research Council, 1966.

Melia RJ, Florey CV, Morris RW, Goldstein BD, John HH, Clark D, Craighead IB, Mackinlay JC. Childhood respiratory illness and the home environment. II: association between respiratory illness and nitrogen dioxide, temperature and relative humidity. *International Journal of Epidemiology* 1982;11(2):164–9.

Michel FB, Bousquet J, Greillier P, Robinet-Levy M, Coulomb Y. Comparison of cord blood immunoglobulin E concentrations and maternal allergy for the prediction of atopic diseases in infancy. *Journal of Allergy and Clinical Immunology* 1980;65(6):422–30.

Michel O, Kips J, Duchateau J, Vertongen F, Robert L, Collet H, Pauwels R, Sergysels R. Severity of asthma is related to endotoxin in house dust. *American Journal of Respiratory and Critical Care Medicine* 1996;154(6 Pt 1):1641–6.

Michie C. Th1 and Th2 cytokines in pregnancy, from a fetal viewpoint [letter]. *Immunology Today* 1998;19(7):333–4.

Michie HR, Manogue KR, Spriggs DR, Revhaug A, O'Dwyer S, Dinarello CA, Cerami A, Wolff SM, Wilmore DW. Detection of circulating tumor necrosis factor after endotoxin administration. *New England Journal of Medicine* 1988;318(23):1481–6.

Minkovitz CS, Andrews JS, Serwint JR. Rehospitalization of children with asthma. *Archives of Pediatrics & Adolescent Medicine* 1999;153(7):727–30.

Misra DP, Nguyen RHN. Environmental tobacco smoke and low birth weight: a hazard in the workplace? *Environmental Health Perspectives* 1999;107(Suppl 6):879–904.

Mok JY, Simpson H. Outcome of acute lower respiratory tract infection in infants: preliminary report of seven-year follow-up study. *British Medical Journal Clinical Research Edition* 1982;285(6338):333–7.

Monto AS. Epidemiology of viral respiratory infections. *American Journal of Medicine* 2002;112(6A):4S–12S.

Moreau D, Ledoux S, Choquet M, Annesi-Maesano I. Prevalence and severity of asthma in adolescents in France: cross-sectional and retrospective analyses of a large population-based sample. *International Journal of Tuberculosis and Lung Disease* 2000;4(7):639–48.

Moussa MAA, Skaik MB, Yaghy OY, Salwanes SB, Bin-Othman SA. Factors associated with asthma in school children. *European Journal of Epidemiology* 1996;12(6):583–8.

Moyes CD, Waldon J, Ramadas D, Crane J, Pearce N. Respiratory symptoms and environmental factors in schoolchildren in the Bay of Plenty. *New Zealand Medical Journal* 1995;108(1007):358–61.

Mrazek DA, Klinnert M, Mrazek PJ, Brower A, McCormick D, Rubin B, Ikle D, Kastner W, Larsen G, Harbeck R, et al. Prediction of early-onset asthma in genetically at-risk children. *Pediatric Pulmonology* 1999;27(2):85–94.

Mumcuoglu KY, Abed Y, Armenios B, Shaheen S, Jacobs J, Bar-Sela S, Richter E. Asthma in Gaza refugee camp children and its relationship with house dust mites. *Annals of Allergy* 1994;72(2):163–6.

Murray AB, Morrison BJ. Passive smoking by asthmatics: its greater effect on boys than on girls and on older than on younger children. *Pediatrics* 1989;84(3):451–9.

Murray AB, Morrison BJ. It is children with atopic dermatitis who develop asthma more frequently if the mother smokes. *Journal of Allergy and Clinical Immunology* 1990;86(5):732–9.

Murray AB, Morrison BJ. The decrease in severity of asthma in children of parents who smoke since the parents have been exposing them to less cigarette smoke. *Journal of Allergy and Clinical Immunology* 1993;91(1 Pt 1):102–10.

Mutoh T, Bonham AC, Kott KS, Joad JP. Chronic exposure to sidestream tobacco smoke augments lung C-fiber responsiveness in young guinea pigs. *Journal of Applied Physiology* 1999;87(2):757–68.

Nafstad P, Kongerud J, Botten G, Hagen JA, Jaakkola JJ. The role of passive smoking in the development of bronchial obstruction during the first 2 years of life. *Epidemiology* 1997;8(3):293–7.

National Cancer Institute. *Health Effects of Exposure to Environmental Tobacco Smoke: The Report of the California Environmental Protection Agency.* Smoking and Tobacco Control Monograph No. 10. Bethesda

(MD): U.S. Department of Health and Human Services, National Institutes of Health, National Cancer Institute, 1999. NIH Publication No. 99-4645.

National Research Council. *Research Priorities for Airborne Particulate Matter. IV: Continuing Research Progress*. Washington: National Academies Press, 2004.

Neuspiel DR, Rush D, Butler NR, Golding J, Bijur PE, Kurzon M. Parental smoking and post-infancy wheezing in children: a prospective cohort study. *American Journal of Public Health* 1989;79(2):168–71.

Niewoehner DE, Kleinerman J, Rice DB. Pathologic changes in the peripheral airways of young cigarette smokers. *New England Journal of Medicine* 1974;291(15):755–8.

Nilsson L, Castor O, Löfman O, Magnusson A, Kjellman N-IM. Allergic disease in teenagers in relation to urban or rural residence at various stages of childhood. *Allergy* 1999;54(7):716–21.

Ninan TK, Macdonald L, Russell G. Persistent nocturnal cough in childhood: a population based study. *Archives of Disease in Childhood* 1995;73(5):403–7.

Norman-Taylor W, Dickinson VA. Danger for children in smoking families. *Community Medicine* 1972;128(1):32–3.

Nriagu J, Robins T, Gary L, Liggans G, Davila R, Supuwood K, Harvey C, Jinabhai CC, Naidoo R. Prevalence of asthma and respiratory symptoms in south-central Durban, South Africa. *European Journal of Epidemiology* 1999;15(8):747–55.

Nuesslein TG, Beckers D, Rieger CHL. Cotinine in meconium indicates risk for early respiratory tract infections. *Human & Experimental Toxicology* 1999;18(4):283–90.

O'Connell EJ, Logan GB. Parental smoking in childhood asthma. *Annals of Allergy* 1974;32(3):142–5.

O'Connor GT, Sparrow D, Demolles D, Dockery D, Raizenne M, Fay M, Ingram RH, Speizer FE. Maximal and partial expiratory flow rates in a population sample of 10- to 11-yr-old schoolchildren: effect of volume history and relation to asthma and maternal smoking. *American Journal of Respiratory and Critical Care Medicine* 2000;162(2 Pt 1):436–9.

O'Connor GT, Weiss ST, Tager IB, Speizer FE. The effect of passive smoking on pulmonary function and nonspecific bronchial responsiveness in a population-based sample of children and young adults. *American Review of Respiratory Disease* 1987;135:800–4.

Odhiambo JA, Ng'ang'a LW, Mungai MW, Gicheha CM, Nyamwaya JK, Karimi F, Macklem PT, Becklake MR. Urban-rural differences in questionnaire-derived markers of asthma in Kenyan school children. *European Respiratory Journal* 1998;12(5):1105–12.

Ogston SA, Florey CDV, Walker CHM. The Tayside infant morbidity and mortality study: effect on health of using gas for cooking. *British Medical Journal (Clinical Research Edition)* 1985;290(6473):957–60.

Ogston SA, Florey CDV, Walker CHM. Association of infant alimentary and respiratory illness with parental smoking and other environmental factors. *Journal of Epidemiology and Community Health* 1987;41(1):21–5.

Oliveti JF, Kercsmar CM, Redline S. Pre- and perinatal risk factors for asthma in inner city African-American children. *American Journal of Epidemiology* 1996;143(6):570–7.

Oryszczyn MP, Godin J, Annesi I, Hellier G, Kauffmann F. In utero exposure to parental smoking, cotinine measurements, and cord blood IgE. *Journal of Allergy and Clinical Immunology* 1991;87(6):1169–74.

Ownby DR, Johnson CC, Peterson EL. Maternal smoking does not influence cord serum IgE or IgD concentrations. *Journal of Allergy and Clinical Immunology* 1991;88(4):555–60.

Ownby DR, McCullough J. Passive exposure to cigarette smoke does not increase allergic sensitization in children. *Journal of Allergy and Clinical Immunology* 1988;82(4):634–8.

Palmieri M, Longobardi G, Napolitano G, Simonetti DML. Parental smoking and asthma in childhood. *European Journal of Pediatrics* 1990;149(10):738–40.

Paradise JL, Rockette HE, Colborn DK, Bernard BS, Smith CG, Kurs-Lasky M, Janosky JE. Otitis media in 2253 Pittsburgh-area infants: prevalence and risk factors during the first two years of life. *Pediatrics* 1997;99(3):318–33.

Park J-H, Gold DR, Spiegelman DL, Burge HA, Milton DK. House dust endotoxin and wheeze in the first year of life. *American Journal of Respiratory and Critical Care Medicine* 2001;163(2):322–8.

Park JK, Kim IS. Effects of family smoking on acute respiratory disease in children. *Yonsei Medical Journal* 1986;27(4):261–70.

Pedreira FA, Guandolo VL, Feroli EJ, Mella GW, Weiss IP. Involuntary smoking and incidence of respiratory illness during the first year of life. *Pediatrics* 1985;75(3):594–7.

Peters J, Hedley AJ, Wong CM, Lam TH, Ong SG, Liu J, Spiegelhalter DJ. Effects of an ambient air pollution intervention and environmental tobacco smoke on children's respiratory health in Hong Kong. *International Journal of Epidemiology* 1996;25(4):821–8.

Peters J, McCabe CJ, Hedley AJ, Lam TH, Wong CM. Economic burden of environmental tobacco smoke on Hong Kong families: scale and impact. *Journal of Epidemiology and Community Health* 1998;52(1):53–8.

Peters JM, Avol E, Navidi W, London SJ, Gauderman WJ, Lurmann F, Linn WS, Margolis H, Rappaport E, Gong H Jr, et al. A study of twelve southern California communities with differing levels and types of air pollution. I: prevalence of respiratory morbidity. *American Journal of Respiratory and Critical Care Medicine* 1999;159(3):760–7.

Philipp K, Pateisky N, Endler M. Effects of smoking on uteroplacental blood flow. *Gynecologic and Obstetric Investigation* 1984;17(4):179–82.

Pierce RA, Nguyen NM. Prenatal nicotine exposure and abnormal lung function. *American Journal of Respiratory Cell and Molecular Biology* 2002;26(1):31–41.

Pirkle JL, Flegal KM, Bernert JT, Brody DJ, Etzel RA, Maurer KR. Exposure of the US population to environmental tobacco smoke: the Third National Health and Nutrition Examination Survey, 1988 to 1991. *Journal of the American Medical Association* 1996;275(16):1233–40.

Ponsonby A-L, Couper D, Dwyer T, Carmichael A, Kemp A, Cochrane J. The relation between infant indoor environment and subsequent asthma. *Epidemiology* 2000;11(2):128–35.

Porro E, Calamita P, Rana I, Montini L, Criscione S. Atopy and environmental factors in upper respiratory infections: an epidemiological survey on 2304 school children. *International Journal of Pediatric Otorhinolaryngology* 1992;24(2):111–20.

Pukander J. Acute otitis media among rural children in Finland. *International Journal of Pediatric Otorhinolaryngology* 1982;4(4):325–32.

Pukander J, Luotonen J, Timonen M, Karma P. Risk factors affecting the occurrence of acute otitis media among 2–3-year-old urban children. *Acta Oto-Laryngologica* 1985;100(3–4):260–5.

Qian Z, Chapman RS, Tian Q, Chen Y, Lioy PJ, Zhang J. Effects of air pollution on children's respiratory health in three Chinese cities. *Archives of Environmental Health* 2000;55(2):126–33.

Quah BS, Mazidah AR, Simpson H. Risk factors for wheeze in the last 12 months in preschool children. *Asian Pacific Journal of Allergy and Immunology* 2000;18(2):73–9.

Rantakallio P. Relationship of maternal smoking to morbidity and mortality of the child up to the age of five. *Acta Paediatrica Scandinavica* 1978;67(5):621–31.

Räsänen M, Kaprio J, Laitinen T, Winter T, Koskenvuo M, Laitinen LA. Perinatal risk factors for asthma in Finnish adolescent twins. *Thorax* 2000;55(1):25–31.

Rasmussen F. Protracted secretory otitis media: the impact of familial factors and day-care center attendance. *International Journal of Pediatric Otorhinolaryngology* 1993;26(1):29–37.

Reed BD, Lutz LJ. Household smoking exposure—association with middle ear effusions. *Family Medicine* 1988;20(6):426–30.

Reese AC, James IR, Landau LI, Lesouëf PN. Relationship between urinary cotinine level and diagnosis in children admitted to hospital. *American Review of Respiratory Disease* 1992;146(1):66–70.

Renzoni E, Forastiere F, Biggeri A, Viegi G, Bisanti L, Chellini E, Ciccone G, Corbo G, Galassi C, Rusconi F, et al. Differences in parental- and self-report of asthma, rhinitis and eczema among Italian adolescents. *European Respiratory Journal* 1999;14(3):597–604.

Richards GA, Terblanche APS, Theron AJ, Opperman L, Crowther G, Myer MS, Steenkamp KJ, Smith FCA, Dowdeswell R, van der Merwe CA, et al. Health effects of passive smoking in adolescent children. *South African Medical Journal* 1996;86(2):143–7.

Roberts JE, Burchinal MR, Medley LP, Zeisel SA, Mundy M, Roush J, Hooper S, Bryant D, Henderson FW. Otitis media, hearing sensitivity, and maternal responsiveness in relation to language during infancy. *Journal of Pediatrics* 1995;126(3):481–9.

Roland PS, Finitzo T, Friel-Patti S, Brown KC, Stephens KT, Brown O, Coleman JM. Otitis media: incidence, duration, and hearing status. *Archives of Otolaryngology—Head & Neck Surgery* 1989;115(9):1049–53.

Rona RJ, Chinn S. Lung function, respiratory illness, and passive smoking in British primary school children. *Thorax* 1993;48(1):21–5.

Ronchetti R, Bonci E, Cutrera R, De Castro G, Indinnimeo L, Midulla F, Tancredi G, Martinez FD. Enhanced allergic sensitisation related to parental smoking. *Archives of Disease in Childhood* 1992;67(4):496–500.

Ronchetti R, Macri F, Ciofetta G, Indinnimeo L, Cutrera R, Bonci E, Antognoni G, Martinez FD. Increased serum IgE and increased prevalence of eosinophilia in 9-year-old children of smoking parents. *Journal of Allergy and Clinical Immunology* 1990;86(3 Pt 1):400–7.

Rönmark E, Jönsson E, Platts-Mills T, Lundbäck B. Different pattern of risk factors for atopic and non-atopic asthma among children—report from the Obstructive Lung Disease in Northern Sweden Study. *Allergy* 1999;54(9):926–35.

Rönmark E, Lundbäck B, Jönsson E, Platts-Mills T. Asthma, type-1 allergy and related conditions in 7- and 8-year-old children in Northern Sweden: prevalence rates and risk factor pattern. *Respiratory Medicine* 1998;92(2):316–24.

Rowe-Jones JM, Brockbank MJ. Parental smoking and persistent otitis media with effusion in children. *International Journal of Pediatric Otorhinolaryngology* 1992;24(1):19–24.

Ruiz RG, Richards D, Kemeny DM, Price JF. Neonatal IgE: a poor screen for atopic disease. *Clinical and Experimental Allergy* 1991;21(4):467–72.

Rumold R, Jyrala M, Diaz-Sanchez D. Secondhand smoke induces allergic sensitization in mice. *Journal of Immunology* 2001;167(8):4765–70.

Rusconi F, Galassi C, Corbo GM, Forastiere F, Biggeri A, Ciccone G, Renzoni E, SIDRIA Collaborative Group. Risk factors for early, persistent, and late-onset wheezing in young children. *American Journal of Respiratory and Critical Care Medicine* 1999;160 (5 Pt 1):1617–22.

Rylander E, Eriksson M, Freyschuss U. Risk factors for occasional and recurrent wheezing after RSV infection in infancy. *Acta Paediatrica Scandinavica* 1988;77(5):711–5.

Rylander E, Pershagen G, Eriksson M, Bermann G. Parental smoking, urinary cotinine, and wheezing bronchitis in children. *Epidemiology* 1995;6(3):289–93.

Rylander E, Pershagen G, Eriksson M, Nordvall L. Parental smoking and other risk factors for wheezing bronchitis in children. *European Journal of Epidemiology* 1993;9(5):517–26.

Rylander R, Mégevand Y. Environmental risk factors for respiratory infections. *Archives of Environmental Health* 2000;55(5):300–3.

Said G, Zalokar J, Lellouch J, Patois E. Parental smoking related to adenoidectomy and tonsillectomy in children. *Journal of Epidemiology and Community Health* 1978;32(2):97–101.

Saim A, Saim L, Saim S, Ruszymah BHI, Sani A. Prevalence of otitis media with effusion amongst pre-school children in Malaysia. *International Journal of Pediatric Otorhinolaryngology* 1997;41(1):21–8.

Salazar JC, Daly KA, Giebink GS, Lindgren BR, Liebeler CL, Meland M, Le CT. Low cord blood pneumococcal immunoglobulin G (IgG) antibodies predict early onset acute otitis media in infancy. *American Journal of Epidemiology* 1997;145(11):1048–56.

Samet JM. Adverse effects of smoke exposure on the upper airway. *Tobacco Control* 2004;13(Suppl 1):i57–i60.

Samet JM, Tager IB, Speizer FE. The relationship between respiratory illness in childhood and chronic air-flow obstruction in adulthood. *American Review of Respiratory Disease* 1983;127(4):508–23.

Sandberg S, Paton JY, Ahola S, McCann DC, McGuinness D, Hillary CR, Oja H. The role of acute and chronic stress in asthma attacks in children. *Lancet* 2000;356(9234):982–7.

Saraçlar Y, Şekerel BE, Kalayci Ö, Çetinkaya F, Adalioğlu G, Tuncer A, Tezcan S. Prevalence of asthma symptoms in school children in Ankara, Turkey. *Respiratory Medicine* 1998;92(2):203–7.

Schenker MB, Samet JM, Speizer FE. Risk factors for childhood respiratory disease: the effect of host factors and home environmental exposures. *American Review of Respiratory Disease* 1983;128(6):1038–43.

Schilling RSF, Letai AD, Hui SL, Beck GJ, Schoenberg JB, Bouhuys A. Lung function, respiratory disease, and smoking in families. *American Journal of Epidemiology* 1977;106(4):274–83.

Schmitzberger R, Rhomberg K, Büchele H, Puchegger R, Schmitzberger-Natzmer D, Kemmler G, Panosch B. Effects of air pollution on the respiratory tract of children. *Pediatric Pulmonology* 1993;15(2):68–74.

Schwartz J, Timonen KL, Pekkanen J. Respiratory effects of environmental tobacco smoke in a panel study of asthmatic and symptomatic children. *American Journal of Respiratory and Critical Care Medicine* 2000;161(3 Pt 1):802–6.

Scientific Committee on Tobacco and Health. *Report of the Scientific Committee on Tobacco and Health*. London: The Stationary Office, 1998.

Sekhon HS, Jia Y, Raab R, Kuryatov A, Pankow JF, Whitsett JA, Lindstrom J, Spindel ER. Prenatal nicotine increases pulmonary α7 nicotine receptor expression and alters fetal lung development in monkeys. *Journal of Clinical Investigation* 1999;103(5):637–47.

Sekhon HS, Keller JA, Proskocil BJ, Martin EL, Spindler ER. Maternal nicotine exposure upregulates collagen gene expression in fetal monkey lung: associated with α7 nicotine acetylcholine receptors. *American Journal of Respiratory Cell and Molecular Biology* 2002;26(1):10–3.

Selçuk ZT, Çaglar T, Enünlü T, Topal T. The prevalence of allergic diseases in primary school children in Edirne, Turkey. *Clinical & Experimental Allergy* 1997;27(3):262–9.

Seymour BW, Pinkerton KE, Friebertshauser KE, Coffman RL, Gershwin LJ. Second-hand smoke is an adjuvant for T helper-2 responses in a murine model of allergy. *Journal of Immunology* 1997;159(12):6169–75.

Shamssain MH, Shamsian N. Prevalence and severity of asthma, rhinitis, and atopic eczema: the north east study. *Archives of Disease in Childhood* 1999;81(4):313–7.

Shaw R, Woodman K, Crane J, Moyes C, Kennedy J, Pearce N. Risk factors for asthma symptoms in Kawerau children. *New Zealand Medical Journal* 1994;107(987):387–91.

Sherman CB, Tosteson TD, Tager IB, Speizer FE, Weiss ST. Early childhood predictors of asthma. *American Journal of Epidemiology* 1990;132(1):83–95.

Siersted HC, Boldsen J, Hansen HS, Mostgaard G, Hyldebrandt N. Population based study of risk factors for underdiagnosis of asthma in adolescence: Odense schoolchild study. *British Medical Journal* 1998;316(7132):651–5.

Silverman M. Out of the mouths of babes and sucklings: lessons from early childhood asthma. *Thorax* 1993;48(12):1200–4.

Simani AS, Inoue S, Hogg JC. Penetration of the respiratory epithelium of guinea pigs following exposure to cigarette smoke. *Laboratory Investigation* 1974;31(1):75–81.

Sims DG, Downham MAPS, Gardner PS, Webb JKG, Weightman D. Study of 8-year-old children with a history of respiratory syncytial virus bronchiolitis in infancy. *British Medical Journal* 1978;1(6104):11–4.

Sipila M, Karma P, Pukander J, Timonen M, Kataja M. The Bayesian approach to the evaluation of risk factors in acute and recurrent acute otitis media. *Acta Oto-Laryngologica* 1988;106(1–2):94–101.

Smith KR, Samet JM, Romieu I, Bruce N. Indoor air pollution in developing countries and acute lower respiratory infections in children. *Thorax* 2000;55(6):518–32.

Somerville SM, Rona RJ, Chinn S. Passive smoking and respiratory conditions in primary school children. *Journal of Epidemiology and Community Health* 1988;42(2):105–10.

Soto-Quiros M, Bustamante M, Gutierrez I, Hanson LC, Strannegard I-L, Karlberg J. The prevalence of childhood asthma in Costa Rica. *Clinical & Experimental Allergy* 1994;24(12):1130–6.

Søyseth V, Kongerud J, Boe J. Postnatal maternal smoking increases the prevalence of asthma but not of bronchial hyperresponsiveness or atopy in their children. *Chest* 1995;107(2):389–94.

Spencer N, Logan S, Scholey S, Gentle S. Deprivation and bronchiolitis. *Archives of Disease in Childhood* 1996;74(1):50–2.

Ståhlberg M-R, Ruuskanen O, Virolainen E. Risk factors for recurrent otitis media. *Pediatric Infectious Disease* 1986;5(1):30–2.

Stanhope JM, Rees RO, Mangan AJ. Asthma and wheeze in New Zealand adolescents. *New Zealand Medical Journal* 1979;90(645):279–82.

Stankus RP, Menon PK, Rando RJ, Glindmeyer H, Salvaggio JE, Lehrer SB. Cigarette smoke-sensitive asthma: challenge studies. *Journal of Allergy and Clinical Immunology* 1988;82(3 Pt 1):331–8.

Stathis SL, O'Callaghan DM, Williams GM, Najman JM, Andersen MJ, Bor W. Maternal cigarette smoking during pregnancy is an independent predictor for symptoms of middle ear disease at five years' postdelivery. *Pediatrics* 1999;104(2):e16.

Stein RT, Holberg CJ, Morgan WJ, Wright AL, Lombardi E, Taussig L, Martinez FD. Peak flow variability, methacholine responsiveness and atopy as markers for detecting different wheezing phenotypes in childhood. *Thorax* 1997;52(11):946–52.

Stenström C, Ingvarsson L. Otitis-prone children and controls: a study of possible predisposing factors. 2: physical findings, frequency of illness, allergy, day care and parental smoking. *Acta Oto-Laryngologica* 1997;117(5):696–703.

Stenstrom R, Bernard PAM, Ben-Simhon H. Exposure to environmental tobacco smoke as a risk factor for recurrent acute otitis media in children under the age of five years. *International Journal of Pediatric Otorhinolaryngology* 1993;27(2):127–36.

Stern B, Jones L, Raizenne M, Burnett R, Meranger JC, Franklin CA. Respiratory health effects associated with ambient sulfates and ozone in two rural Canadian communities. *Environmental Research* 1989a;49(1):20–39.

Stern B, Raizenne M, Burnett R. Respiratory effects of early childhood exposure to passive smoke. *Environment International* 1989b;15(1–6):29–34.

Stick SM, Burton PR, Gurrin L, Sly PD, LeSouef PN. Effects of maternal smoking during pregnancy and a family history of asthma on respiratory function in newborn infants. *Lancet* 1996;348(9034):1060–4.

Stocks J, Godfrey S, Beardsmore C, Bar-Yishay E, Castile R, ERS/ATS Task Force on Standards for Infant Respiratory Function Testing. Plethysmographic measurements of lung volume and airway resistance. *European Respiratory Journal* 2001;17(2):302–12.

Stoddard JJ, Miller T. Impact of parental smoking on the prevalence of wheezing respiratory illness in children. *American Journal of Epidemiology* 1995;141(2):96–102.

Strachan DP. Damp housing and childhood asthma: validation of reporting of symptoms. *British Medical Journal* 1988;297(6658):1223–6.

Strachan DP. Impedance tympanometry and the home environment in seven-year-old children. *Journal of Laryngology and Otology* 1990;104(1):4–8.

Strachan DP. Epidemiology. In: Silverman M, editor. *Childhood Asthma and Other Wheezing Disorders*. New York: Chapman & Hall, 1995:7–31.

Strachan DP, Butland BK, Anderson HR. Incidence and prognosis of asthma and wheezing illness from early childhood to age 33 in a national British cohort. *British Medical Journal* 1996;312(7040):1195–9.

Strachan DP, Carey IM. Home environment and severe asthma in adolescence: a population based case-control study. *British Medical Journal* 1995;311(7012):1053–6.

Strachan DP, Cook DG. Health effects of passive smoking. 1: parental smoking and lower respiratory illness in infancy and early childhood. *Thorax* 1997;52(10):905–14.

Strachan DP, Cook DG. Health effects of passive smoking. 4: parental smoking, middle ear disease and adenotonsillectomy in children. *Thorax* 1998a;53(1):50–6.

Strachan DP, Cook DG. Health effects of passive smoking. 5: parental smoking and allergic sensitisation in children. *Thorax* 1998b;53(2):117–23.

Strachan DP, Cook DG. Health effects of passive smoking. 6: parental smoking and childhood asthma: longitudinal and case-control studies. *Thorax* 1998c;53(3):204–12.

Strachan DP, Elton RA. Relationship between respiratory morbidity in children and the home environment. *Family Practice* 1986;3(3):137–42.

Strachan DP, Jarvis MJ, Feyerabend C. Passive smoking, salivary cotinine concentrations, and middle ear effusion in 7 year old children. *British Medical Journal* 1989;298(6687):1549–52.

Strachan DP, Jarvis MJ, Feyerabend C. The relationship of salivary cotinine to respiratory symptoms, spirometry, and exercise-induced bronchospasm in seven-year-old children. *American Review of Respiratory Disease* 1990;142(1):147–51.

Suárez-Varela MM, González AL, Martínez Selva MI. Socioeconomic risk factors in the prevalence of asthma and other atopic diseases in children 6 to 7 years old in Valencia, Spain. *European Journal of Epidemiology* 1999;15(1):35–40.

Tager IB, Hanrahan JP, Tosteson TD, Castile RG, Brown RW, Weiss ST, Speizer FE. Lung function, pre- and post-natal smoke exposure, and wheezing in the first year of life. *American Review of Respiratory Disease* 1993;147(4):811–7.

Tager IB, Ngo L, Hanrahan JP. Maternal smoking during pregnancy: effects on lung function during the first 18 months of life. *American Journal of Respiratory and Critical Care Medicine* 1995;152(3):977–83.

Tainio V-M, Savilahti E, Salmenperä L, Arjomaa P, Siimes MA, Perheentupa J. Risk factors for infantile recurrent otitis media: atopy but not type of feeding. *Pediatric Research* 1988;23(5):509–12.

Takasaka T. Incidence, prevalence and natural history of otitis media in different geographic areas and populations: epidemiology of otitis media with effusion in Japan. *Annals of Otology, Rhinology and Laryngology* 1990;99(7 Pt 2 Suppl 149):13–4.

Tariq S, Memon IA. Acute otitis media in children. *Journal of the College of Physicians and Surgeons Pakistan* 1999;9(12):507–10.

Tariq SM, Hakim EA, Matthews SM, Arshad SH. Influence of smoking on asthmatic symptoms and allergen sensitisation in early childhood. *Postgraduate Medical Journal* 2000;76(901):694–9.

Tariq SM, Matthews SM, Hakim EA, Stevens M, Arshad SH, Hide DW. The prevalence of and risk factors for atopy in early childhood: a whole population birth cohort study. *Journal of Allergy and Clinical Immunology* 1998;101(5):587–93.

Tashkin DP, Clark VA, Simmons M, Reems C, Coulson AH, Bourque LB, Sayre JW, Detels R, Rokaw S. The UCLA population studies of chronic obstructive respiratory disease. VII: relationship between parental smoking and children's lung function. *American Review of Respiratory Disease* 1984;129(6):891–7.

Taylor B, Wadsworth J. Maternal smoking during pregnancy and lower respiratory tract illness in early life. *Archives of Disease in Childhood* 1987;62(8):786–91.

Taylor B, Wadsworth J, Golding J, Butler N. Breast feeding, eczema, asthma, and hayfever. *Journal of Epidemiology and Community Health* 1983;37(2):95–9.

Teele DW, Klein JO, Rosner B, Greater Boston Otitis Media Study Group. Epidemiology of otitis media during the first seven years of life in children in greater Boston: a prospective, cohort study. *Journal of Infectious Diseases* 1989;160(1):83–94.

Teculescu D, Pham QT, Aubry C, Chau N, Viaggi MN, Henquel JC, Manciaux M. Respiratory health of children and atmospheric pollution: II. Ventilatory function. *Revue Des Maladies Respiratoires* 1989;6:221–8.

Teculescu DB, Pham QT, Varona-Lopez W, Deschamps JP, Marchand M, Henquel JC, Manciaux M. The single-breath nitrogen test does not detect functional impairment in children with passive exposure to tobacco smoke. *Bulletin Europeen De Physiopathologie Respiratoire* 1986;22:605–7.

Thaler I, Goodman JD, Dawes GS. Effects of maternal cigarette smoking on fetal breathing and fetal movements. *American Journal of Obstetrics and Gynecology* 1980;138(3):282–7.

Thornton AJ, Lee PN. Parental smoking and middle ear disease in children: a review of the evidence. *Indoor and Built Environment* 1999;8(1):21–39.

Toyoshima K, Hayashida M, Yasunami J, Takamatsu I, Niwa H, Muraoka T. Factors influencing the prognosis of wheezy infants. *Journal of Asthma* 1987;24(5):267–70.

Tulić MK, Wale JL, Holt PG, Sly PD. Modification of the inflammatory response to allergen challenge after exposure to bacterial lipopolysaccharide. *American Journal of Respiratory Cell and Molecular Biology* 2000;22(5):604–12.

Uhari M, Mäntysaari K, Niemelä M. A meta-analytic review of the risk factors for acute otitis media. *Clinical Infectious Diseases* 1996;22(6):1079–83.

Ulrik CS, Backer V. Atopy in Danish children and adolescents: results from a longitudinal population study. *Annals of Allergy, Asthma and Immunology* 2000;85(4):293–7.

U.S. Department of Health and Human Services. *The Health Consequences of Smoking: Chronic Obstructive Lung Disease. A Report of the Surgeon General*. Rockville (MD): U.S. Department of Health and Human Services, Public Health Service, Office on Smoking and Health, 1984. DHHS Publication No. (PHS) 84-50205.

U.S. Department of Health and Human Services. *The Health Consequences of Involuntary Smoking. A Report of the Surgeon General*. Rockville (MD): U.S. Department of Health and Human Services, Public Health Service, Centers for Disease Control, Center for Health Promotion and Education, Office on Smoking and Health, 1986. DHHS Publication No. (CDC) 87-8398.

U.S. Department of Health and Human Services. *Reducing the Health Consequences of Smoking: 25 Years of Progress. A Report of the Surgeon General*. Rockville (MD): U.S. Department of Health and Human Services, Public Health Service, Centers for Disease Control, National Center for Chronic Disease Prevention and Health Promotion, Office on Smoking and Health, 1989. DHHS Publication No. (CDC) 89-8411.

U.S. Department of Health and Human Services. *Women and Smoking. A Report of the Surgeon General*. Rockville (MD): U.S. Department of Health and Human Services, Public Health Service, Office of the Surgeon General, 2001.

U.S. Department of Health and Human Services. *The Health Consequences of Smoking: A Report of the Surgeon General*. Atlanta: U.S. Department of Health and Human Services, Centers for Disease Control and Prevention, National Center for Chronic Disease Prevention and Health Promotion, Office on Smoking and Health, 2004.

U.S. Environmental Protection Agency. *Respiratory Health Effects of Passive Smoking: Lung Cancer and Other Disorders*. Washington: U.S. Environmental Protection Agency, Office of Research and Development, Office of Air and Radiation, 1992. Publication No. EPA/600/6-90/006F.

van Cauwenberge PB. Relevant and irrelevant predisposing factors in secretory otitis media. *Acta Oto-Laryngologica* 1984;414:147–53.

Victora CG, Fuchs SC, Flores JAC, Fonseca W, Kirkwood B. Risk factors for pneumonia among children in a Brazilian metropolitan area. *Pediatrics* 1994;93(6 Pt 1):977–85.

Vidic B. Transplacental effect of environmental pollutants on interstitial composition and diffusion capacity for exchange of gases of pulmonary parenchyma in neonatal rat. *Bulletin de l'Association des Anatomistes (Nancy)* 1991;75(229):153–5.

Vinke JG, KleinJan A, Severijnen LW, Fokkens WJ. Passive smoking causes an 'allergic' cell infiltrate in the nasal mucosa of non-atopic children. *International Journal of Pediatric Otorhinolaryngology* 1999;51(2):73–81.

Vinther B, Brahe Pedersen C, Elbrrnd O. Otitis media in childhood: sociomedical aspects with special reference to day-care conditions. *Clinical Otolaryngology and Allied Sciences* 1984;9(1):3–8.

Vinther B, Elbrond O, Pedersen CB. A population study of otitis media in childhood. *Acta Oto-Laryngologica* 1979;360(Suppl):135–7.

Vitnerova N, Horstman D, Hnizdova E. Prevalence of symptoms of airway diseases in schoolchildren living in areas with different atmospheric contamination. *Hygiena* 1999;44(Suppl 2):30–9.

Volkmer RE, Ruffin RE, Wigg NR, Davies N. The prevalence of respiratory symptoms in South Australian preschool children. II: factors associated with indoor air quality. *Journal of Paediatrics and Child Health* 1995;31(2):116–20.

von Mutius E, Martinez FD, Fritzsch C, Nicolai T, Reitmeir R, Thiemann HH. Skin test reactivity and number of siblings. *British Medical Journal* 1994;308(6930):692–5.

Wafula EM, Limbe MS, Onyango FE, Nduati R. Effects of passive smoking and breastfeeding on childhood bronchial asthma. *East African Medical Journal* 1999;76(11):606–9.

Wang FL, Love EJ, Liu N, Dai XD. Childhood and adolescent passive smoking and the risk of female lung cancer. *International Journal of Epidemiology* 1994;23(2):223–30.

Wang T-N, Ko Y-C, Chao Y-Y, Huang C-C, Lin R-S. Association between indoor and outdoor air pollution and adolescent asthma from 1995 to 1996 in Taiwan. *Environmental Research* 1999;81(3):239–47.

Ware JH, Dockery DW, Spiro A III, Speizer FE, Ferris BG Jr. Passive smoking, gas cooking, and respiratory health of children living in six cities. *American Review of Respiratory Disease* 1984;129(3):366–74.

Weber MW, Milligan P, Hilton S, Lahai G, Whittle H, Mulholland EK, Greenwood BM. Risk factors for severe respiratory syncytial virus infection leading to hospital admission in children in the western region of The Gambia. *International Journal of Epidemiology* 1999;28(1):157–62.

Weiss ST, Tager IB, Munoz A, Speizer FE. The relationship of respiratory infections in early childhood to the occurrence of increased levels of bronchial responsiveness and atopy. *American Review of Respiratory Diseases* 1985;131(4):573–8.

Weiss ST, Tager IB, Speizer FE, Rosner B. Persistent wheeze: its relation to respiratory illness, cigarette smoking, and level of pulmonary function in a population sample of children. *American Review of Respiratory Disease* 1980;122(5):697–707.

Weitzman M, Gortmaker S, Sobol A. Racial, social, and environmental risks for childhood asthma. *American Journal of Diseases of Children* 1990a;144(11):1189–94.

Weitzman M, Gortmaker S, Walker DK, Sobol A. Maternal smoking and childhood asthma. *Pediatrics* 1990b;85(4):505–11.

Welliver RC, Wong DT, Sun M, McCarthy N. Parainfluenza virus bronchiolitis: epidemiology and pathogenesis. *American Journal of Diseases of Children* 1986;140(1):34–40.

Wennergren G, Cmark M, Cmark K, Óskarsdóttir S, Sten G, Redfors S. Wheezing bronchitis reinvestigated at the age of 10 years. *Acta Paediatrica* 1997;86(4):351–5.

Willatt DJ. Children's sore throats related to parental smoking. *Clinical Otolaryngology and Allied Sciences* 1986;11(5):317–21.

Willers S, Attewell R, Bensryd I, Schutz A, Skarping G, Vahter M. Exposure to environmental tobacco smoke in the household and urinary cotinine excretion, heavy metals retention, and lung function. *Archives of Environmental Health* 1992;47:357–63.

Willers S, Svenonius E, Skarping G. Passive smoking and childhood asthma: urinary cotinine levels in children with asthma and in referents. *Allergy* 1991;46(5):330–4.

Wilson NM. Wheezy bronchitis revisited. *Archives of Disease in Childhood* 1989;64(8):1194–9.

Wilson NM. The significance of early wheezing. *Clinical and Experimental Allergy* 1994;24(6):522–9.

Wisborg K, Henriksen TB, Obel C, Skajaa E, Østergaard JR. Smoking during pregnancy and hospitalization of the child. *Pediatrics* 1999;104(4):e46.

Withers NJ, Low L, Holgate ST, Clough JB. The natural history of respiratory symptoms in a cohort of adolescents. *American Journal of Respiratory and Critical Care Medicine* 1998;158(2):352–7.

Woodward A, Douglas RM, Graham NM, Miles H. Acute respiratory illness in Adelaide children: breast feeding modifies the effect of passive smoking. *Journal of Epidemiology and Community Health* 1990;44(3):224–30.

World Health Organization. *Tobacco or Health: A Global Status Report*. Geneva: World Health Organization, 1997.

World Health Organization. *International Consultation on Environmental Tobacco Smoke (ETS) and Child Health: Consultation Report*. Geneva: World Health Organization, Tobacco Free Initiative, 1999. Report No. WHO/NCD/TFI/99.10.

Wright AL, Holberg C, Martinez FD, Taussig LM, Group Health Medical Associates. Relationship of parental smoking to wheezing and nonwheezing lower respiratory tract illnesses in infancy. *Journal of Pediatrics* 1991;118(2):207–14.

Wright AL, Holberg CJ, Morgan WJ, Taussig LM, Halonen M, Martinez FD. Recurrent cough in childhood and its relation to asthma. *American Journal of Respiratory and Critical Care Medicine* 1996;153(4 Pt 1):1259–65.

Wu J-H, Lin RS, Hsieh K-H, Chiu W-T, Chen L-M, Chiou S-T, Huang K-C, Liu W-L, Chiu HI, Hsiao H-C, et al. Adolescent asthma in Northern Taiwan. *Chinese Journal of Public Health* 1998;17(3):214–25.

Yarnell JWG, St Leger AS. Respiratory illness, maternal smoking habit and lung function in children. *British Journal of Diseases of the Chest* 1979;73(3):230–6.

Yau K-I, Fang L-J, Shieh K-H. Factors predisposing infants to lower respiratory infection with wheezing in the first two years of life. *Annals of Allergy, Asthma & Immunology* 1999;82(2):165–70.

Young S, Arnott J, O'Keeffe PT, Le Souef PN, Landau LI. The association between early life lung function and wheezing during the first 2 yrs of life. *European Respiratory Journal* 2000a;15(1):151–7.

Young S, Sherrill DL, Arnott J, Diepeveen D, LeSouëf PN, Landau LI. Parental factors affecting respiratory function during the first year of life. *Pediatric Pulmonology* 2000b;29(5):331–40.

Zacharasiewicz A, Zidek T, Haidinger G, Waldhör T, Vutuc C, Zacharasiewicz A, Goetz M, Pearce N. Symptoms suggestive of atopic rhinitis in children aged 6–9 years and the indoor environment. *Allergy* 2000;55(10):945–50.

Zeiger RS, Heller S. The development and prediction of atopy in high-risk children: follow-up at age seven years in a prospective randomized study of combined maternal and infant food allergen avoidance. *Journal of Allergy and Clinical Immunology* 1995;95(6):1179–90.

Zejda JE, Skiba M, Orawiec A, Dybowska T, Cimander B. Respiratory symptoms in children of Upper Silesia, Poland: cross-sectional study in two towns of different air pollution levels. *European Journal of Epidemiology* 1996;12(1):115–20.

Zielhuis GA, Heuvelmans-Heinen EW, Rach GH, van den Broek P. Environmental risk factors for otitis media with effusion in preschool children. *Scandinavian Journal of Primary Health Care* 1989;7(1):33–8.

Zielhuis GA, Rach GH, van den Broek P. Predisposing factors for otitis media with effusion in young children. *Advances in Oto-Rhino-Laryngology* 1988;40:65–9.

Chapter 7
Cancer Among Adults from Exposure to Secondhand Smoke

Introduction

Active cigarette smoking causes cancer in multiple organs (U.S. Department of Health and Human Services [USDHHS] 2004). Secondhand tobacco smoke contains the same carcinogens that are inhaled by smokers and consequently, there been a concern for a long time that involuntary smoking also causes cancer. Secondhand smoke was first determined to be causally associated with lung cancer (USDHHS 1986), and research on secondhand smoke exposure and cancer risk has been extended to other sites for which there are multiple studies, including the breast, nasal sinuses, and the cervix. This chapter returns to the topic of lung cancer and updates the 1986 evaluation; reviews of the evidence on secondhand smoke exposure and risk for cancer of other sites are also included.

Lung Cancer

The first Surgeon General's report in 1964 identified active smoking as a cause of lung cancer (U.S. Department of Health, Education, and Welfare 1964). Researchers have identified more than 50 carcinogenic compounds and many other toxic substances in tobacco smoke (USDHHS 1986; Hoffmann and Hecht 1990; Hecht 1999) (see "Carcinogens in Sidestream Smoke and Secondhand Smoke" in Chapter 2). Smoking tobacco is acknowledged as the leading cause of lung cancer. Because the compounds that are inhaled by the active smoker are also present in the mixture of sidestream and exhaled mainstream smoke inhaled by involuntary smokers, it is biologically plausible that secondhand smoke is also a cause of lung cancer among nonsmokers, a conclusion reached 20 years ago in the 1986 report (USDHHS 1986).

In 1981, the first major epidemiologic studies of secondhand smoke and lung cancer showed that nonsmoking women married to smokers had a higher risk of lung cancer than did nonsmoking women married to nonsmokers (Garfinkel 1981; Hirayama 1981; Trichopoulos et al. 1981). These three initial studies were followed by numerous investigations that were specifically conducted to evaluate secondhand smoke exposure and the risk of lung cancer among nonsmokers. The combined evidence from more than 50 additional epidemiologic studies on this topic has confirmed and expanded the 1981 findings of an association between secondhand smoke exposure and lung cancer. These more recent studies were conducted within and outside of the United States, and several authoritative scientific panels in the United States and elsewhere have reviewed the findings (Table 7.1). These reviews have carefully considered the possibility of whether the association of secondhand smoke with lung cancer risk could reflect solely uncontrolled bias or confounding. This possibility has been set aside by each group. The number of studies has increased since 1986, but the conclusions of each major review and each of the pooled relative risk (RR) estimates have remained consistent—exposure to secondhand smoke causally increases the risk for lung cancer.

This chapter considers the full body of evidence on secondhand smoke exposure and lung cancer published through 2002, the ending date for the systematic review of the epidemiologic studies. The chapter includes details of more recent studies and provides results of an updated meta-analysis of published studies.

Methods

This chapter includes an updated literature review for lung cancer that focused on studies published since the release of prior major reports. Medline was used to identify the studies included in this review by searching for the following terms: environmental tobacco smoke, secondhand smoke, passive smoking, and lung cancer. Reference lists from each study were also reviewed. These later studies include 3 cohort studies (Table 7.2) (de Waard et al. 1995; Jee et

Table 7.1   Conclusions of selected authoritative scientific bodies on the role of secondhand smoke and the risk of lung cancer among lifetime nonsmokers

Year of publication/agency	Studies reviewed	Conclusions and summary comments
1982 Office of the Surgeon General, U.S. Department of Health and Human Services (USDHHS) *The Health Consequences of Smoking: Cancer*	The first 3 epidemiologic studies on secondhand smoke and lung cancer (Garfinkel 1981; Hirayama 1981; Trichopoulos et al. 1981)	"Although the currently available evidence is not sufficient to conclude that passive or involuntary smoking causes lung cancer in nonsmokers, the evidence does raise concern about a possible serious public health problem." (p. 9)
1986 International Agency for Research on Cancer *Monographs on the Evaluation of the Carcinogenic Risk of Chemicals to Humans: Tobacco Smoking*	7 epidemiologic studies on secondhand smoke and lung cancer published between 1981 and 1984 (Garfinkel 1981; Hirayama 1981 [Japan]; Trichopoulos et al. 1981 [Greece]; Chan and Fung 1982 [Hong Kong]; Correa et al. 1983; Kabat and Wynder 1984; Koo et al. 1984)	"Knowledge of the nature of sidestream and mainstream smoke, of the materials absorbed during 'passive' smoking, and of the quantitative relationships between dose and effect that are commonly observed from exposure to carcinogens, however, leads to the conclusion that passive smoking gives rise to some risk of cancer." (p. 314)
1986 National Research Council *Environmental Tobacco Smoke: Measuring Exposures and Assessing Health Effects*	12 studies on secondhand smoke and lung cancer published since 1981 (Chan and Fung 1982; Correa et al. 1983; Tricholoupos et al. 1983; Buffler et al. 1984; Gillis et al. 1984; Hirayama 1984; Kabat and Wynder 1984; Garfinkel et al. 1985; Akiba et al. 1986; Lee et al. 1986; Koo et al. 1987; Pershagen et al. 1987)	"The weight of evidence derived from epidemiologic studies shows an association between ETS [environmental tobacco smoke] exposure of nonsmokers and lung cancer that, taken as a whole, is unlikely to be due to chance or systematic bias. The observed estimate of increased risk is 34%, largely for spouses of smokers compared with spouses of nonsmokers." (p. 245)
1986 Office of the Surgeon General, USDHHS *The Health Consequences of Involuntary Smoking*	12 studies on spousal secondhand smoke and lung cancer published since 1981 (Chan and Fung 1982; Correa et al. 1983; Trichopoulos et al. 1983; Gillis et al. 1984; Hirayama 1984; Kabat and Wynder 1984; Koo et al. 1984; Garfinkel et al. 1985; Wu et al. 1985; Akiba et al. 1986; Lee et al. 1986; Pershagen et al. 1987)	"Involuntary smoking can cause lung cancer in nonsmokers." (p. 13)

Table 7.1   Continued

Year of publication/agency	Studies reviewed	Conclusions and summary comments
1992 U.S. Environmental Protection Agency (USEPA) *Respiratory Health Effects of Passive Smoking: Lung Cancer and Other Disorders*	32 epidemiologic studies on secondhand smoke and lung cancer; 24 of 32 showed a positive association (Garfinkel 1981; Trichopoulos et al. 1981, 1983; Chan and Fung 1982; Correa et al. 1983; Buffler et al. 1984; Hirayama 1984; Kabat and Wynder 1984; Garfinkel et al. 1985; Lam 1985; Wu et al. 1985; Akiba et al. 1986; Lee et al. 1986; Brownson et al. 1987; Gao et al. 1987; Humble et al. 1987; Koo et al. 1987; Lam et al. 1987; Pershagen et al. 1987; Butler 1988; Geng et al. 1988; Inoue and Hirayama 1988; Katada et al. 1988; Shimizu et al. 1988; Hole et al. 1989; Svensson et al. 1989; Janerich et al. 1990; Kalandidi et al. 1990; Sobue 1990; Wu-Williams and Samet 1990; Fontham et al. 1991; Liu et al. 1991); the association between exposure levels (amount smoked by spouses) and the risk of lung cancer was also examined	"ETS constituents include essentially all of the same carcinogens found in [mainstream tobacco smoke], and many of these appear in greater amounts in [sidestream tobacco smoke]. . . . This quantitative comparison is consistent with the observation noted above that [sidestream] condensates apparently have even greater carcinogenic potential than [mainstream] condensates." (p. 4-28) "The unequivocal causal association between tobacco smoking and lung cancer in humans with dose-response relationships extending down to the lowest exposure categories, as well as the corroborative evidence of the carcinogenicity of both [mainstream] and ETS provided by animal bioassays and in vitro studies and the chemical similarity between [mainstream] and ETS, clearly establish the plausibility that ETS is also a human lung carcinogen. In addition, biomarker studies verify that passive smoking results in detectable uptake of tobacco smoke constituents by nonsmokers, affirming that ETS exposure is a public health concern. In fact, these observations are sufficient in their own right to establish the carcinogenicity of ETS to humans." (p. 4-28) "ETS is a human lung carcinogen, responsible for approximately 3,000 lung cancer deaths annually in U.S. nonsmokers." (p. 1-1)
1999 National Cancer Institute *Health Effects of Exposure to Environmental Tobacco Smoke: The Report of the California EPA.* Smoking and Tobacco Control Monograph No. 10	• 8 epidemiologic studies published since the 1992 U.S. EPA report that have information on secondhand smoke exposure and lung cancer (Brownson et al. 1992; Stockwell et al. 1992; Liu et al. 1993; Fontham et al. 1994; Kabat et al. 1995; Schwartz et al. 1996; Cardenas et al. 1997; Ko et al. 1997) • 13 epidemiologic studies with data on secondhand smoke workplace exposures and 14 studies with data on other household members	"The 1986 Report of the Surgeon General, the 1986 National Research Council report. . . and the 1992 U.S. EPA report. . . have established that ETS exposure causes lung cancer. Results from recent epidemiological studies are compatible with the causal association already established." (p. ES-12)
2001 Office of the Surgeon General, USDHHS *Women and Smoking*	• 9 studies on spousal secondhand smoke and lung cancer (Brownson et al. 1992; Stockwell et al. 1992; Liu et al. 1993; Fontham et al. 1994; Wang et al. 1994; Kabat et al. 1995; Cardenas et al. 1997; Boffetta et al. 1998; Jöckel et al. 1998) • 16 epidemiologic studies with data on secondhand smoke workplace exposures	"Exposure to ETS is a cause of lung cancer among women who have never smoked." (p. 16)

Table 7.2   Cohort studies of the associations between adult exposure to secondhand smoke and the relative risks for lung cancer incidence and mortality among women who had never smoked

Study	Population/follow-up	Number of lung cancer events	Data collection
de Waard et al. 1995	2 population-based breast screening cohorts, 12,000–13,000 women in each cohort Netherlands 15 years	23 incident cases and deaths	Active smoking histories were collected at the time of urine collection; no information was collected on secondhand smoke exposure
Jee et al. 1999	157,436 married women aged >40 years Health insurance subscribers Korea 3.5 years	79 incident and prevalent cases	Questionnaires and medical exams of the husbands in 1992 and 1994; women completed questionnaires in 1993
Nishino et al. 2001	9,675 women aged >40 years Miyagi Prefecture, Japan 9 years	24 incident cases	Self-completed questionnaire by 31,345 (13,992 men and 17,353 women)

al. 1999; Nishino et al. 2001) and 13 case-control studies from around the world (Table 7.3) (Lei et al. 1996; Shen et al. 1996, 1998; Wang et al. 1996, 2000; Jöckel et al. 1998; Nyberg et al. 1998a; Zaridze et al. 1998; Rapiti et al. 1999; Zhong et al. 1999; Kreuzer et al. 2000; Lee et al. 2000; Zhou et al. 2000; Johnson et al. 2001; Seow et al. 2002). The case-control studies are organized by geographic areas because the relative importance of different sources of secondhand smoke exposure and the prevalence of other risk factors of lung cancer (such as occupational exposures, other sources of indoor air pollutants, and previous lung diseases) may differ from one country to another. Study design issues such as the reliance on pathologic confirmation and the proportion of surrogate respondents also differ by study area.

Researchers have conducted several meta-analyses on secondhand smoke exposure and the risk of lung cancer (National Research Council [NRC] 1986; Dockery and Trichopoulos 1997; Hackshaw et al. 1997; Zhong et al. 2000). This chapter also contains a meta-analysis that includes the more recent studies through 2002 in the pooled estimates, and in the estimates from the stratification of the studies by parameters such as gender and geographic area. Pooled estimates associated with secondhand smoke exposure from spouses, at the workplace, and during childhood are specifically presented (see "Pooled Analyses" later in this chapter).

Cohort Studies

A total of eight cohort studies have evaluated secondhand smoke and the risk of lung cancer: three in the United States (Garfinkel 1981; Butler 1988; Cardenas et al. 1997), two in Japan (Hirayama 1981; Nishino et al. 2001), one in Scotland (Hole et al. 1989), one in Korea (Jee et al. 1999), and one in the Netherlands (de Waard et al. 1995). These cohort studies used questionnaires that asked about spousal smoking behaviors and used spousal smoking as the

Findings	Measure of secondhand smoke	Relative risk (95% confidence interval)	Comments

• Urinary nicotine and cotinine levels were significantly associated with lung cancer risk
• Risk increased with increasing urinary cotinine levels
	Cotinine levels (nanograms/milligram):
	  <9.2
	  9.2–23.4
	  23.4–100
		
		1.0
		2.7 (0.8–9.1)
		2.4 (0.7–8.3)
			Crude risk estimates; the only published study with an objective measure of secondhand smoke exposure

• Risk increased with increasing duration and amount smoked by the husband	Husband's smoking status:
	  Lifetime nonsmokers
	  Former smokers
	  Current smokers
		
		1.0
		1.30 (0.6–2.7)
		1.90 (1.0–3.5)
			Controlled for age of husbands and wives, social class, residency, and husbands' occupation and vegetable intake; husbands' smoking was associated with an increased risk of breast cancer but not with cancers at other sites (cervix, stomach, liver)

• No increased risk was associated with secondhand smoke exposure from other household members	Husband smoked:
	  No
	  Yes
		
		1.0
		1.8 (0.7–4.6)
			Controlled for age; study area; intake of alcohol, green and yellow vegetables, fruit, and meat; and history of lung disease; husbands' smoking was associated with an increased risk of rectum and smoking-related cancers combined; there was no increased risk of breast cancer

exposure variable to examine the relationship between secondhand smoke and either incidence (Hole et al. 1989; Jee et al. 1999; Nishino et al. 2001) or mortality from lung cancer (Garfinkel 1981; Hirayama 1981; Butler 1988; Cardenas et al. 1997) among nonsmokers. All of the studies reported a higher risk among women whose husbands smoked than among women whose husbands did not smoke. The RR ranged from 1.18 to 2.02 among women whose husbands smoked. Two studies included data for men (Hirayama 1981; Cardenas et al. 1997), and one study found a higher risk of lung cancer among men married to women who smoked (Hirayama 1981). One nested case-control study using urinary cotinine as a marker of secondhand smoke exposure found that cotinine levels were associated with the risk of lung cancer among nonsmoking women (de Waard et al. 1995). Appendix 7.1 (at the end of this chapter) provides detailed information on the more recent cohort studies reviewed in this chapter on the association between exposure to secondhand smoke and lung cancer.

Case-Control Studies

More than 40 case-control studies have examined the relationship of exposure to secondhand smoke and lung cancer. The studies are almost equally divided between hospital-based and population-based. Methodologic differences across the studies include sources of the cases, types of controls, the use of surrogate respondents, the degree of pathologic confirmation of lung cancer diagnoses, and data collection, such as the assessment of secondhand smoke exposure and other relevant covariates. The first studies tended to be small and classified secondhand smoke exposures largely or solely on the basis of spousal smoking habits (Correa et al. 1983; Kabat and Wynder 1984; Wu et al. 1985; Brownson et al. 1987; Humble et al. 1987). Many larger studies have since been conducted in the United States (Brownson et al. 1992; Stockwell et al. 1992; Fontham et al. 1994) and elsewhere (Wu-Williams et al. 1990; Boffetta et al. 1998; Nyberg et al.

Table 7.3 Case-control studies by geographic area of exposure to secondhand smoke and the relative risks for lung cancer among lifetime nonsmokers

Study	Population/date of study	Cases/histologic confirmation and cell type (%)*	Controls	Data collection
Canada				
Johnson et al. 2001	Women aged 20–74 years from 8 Canadian Tumor Registries Frequency was matched for age and province of residence Canada 1994–1997	161 100% histologic confirmation No cell type information	1,271 selected from insurance/ property assessment databases or by random-digit telephone dialing (RDD)	Mailed questionnaire Response rate Cases: 70% Controls: 70% Approximately all self-respondents
Europe				
Jöckel et al. 1998	Men and women well enough to be interviewed from all hospitals in the study area Germany (Bremen, Frankfurt) 1988–1993	55 lifetime nonsmokers 100% histologic or cytologic confirmation	160 lifetime nonsmokers selected from population registries (general population)	In-person interview 100% self-respondents
Nyberg et al. 1998a	Men and women aged >30 years from 3 main local hospitals 2 controls per case Frequency matched for gender, age, and area of residence Sweden (Stockholm county) 1989–1995	124 (35 men, 89 women) 96% histologic confirmation Squamous cell carcinoma: 10% Small cell carcinoma: 2% Adenocarcinoma: 67%	235 (72 men, 163 women) selected from population register	In-person interview or by telephone Response rate Cases: 86% Controls: 83% 100% self-respondents
Zaridze et al. 1998	2 main cancer treatment hospitals Controls were from the same hospital as cases Russia (Local Moscow residents only)	189 women 100% histologic confirmation Squamous cell carcinoma: 22% Small cell carcinoma: 5% Adenocarcinoma: 56%	358 other cancer patients	In-person interview within 3 days of hospital admission Response rate was not reported 100% self-respondents

Findings	Measure of secondhand smoke	Relative risk (95% confidence interval)	Comments (covariates considered, definition of lifetime nonsmokers)
	Canada		
• Significant trend with smoker-years[†] of workplace and residential/workplace (i.e., total) secondhand smoke exposures	Any secondhand smoke exposure (childhood and adulthood): No Yes Total (smoker-years): None 1–36 37–77 ≥78	1.0 1.63 (0.8–3.5) 1.0 0.83 (0.3–2.1) 1.54 (0.7–3.5) 1.82 (0.8–4.2)	Controlled for age (10-year age group), education, province, fruit and vegetable intake; these results were based on 71 cases and 761 controls who had a more complete secondhand smoke exposure history; lifetime nonsmokers had smoked <100 cigarettes per lifetime
	Europe		
• Risk increased with high secondhand smoke exposure during childhood and adulthood from spouse and other sources (all sources combined = total)	Secondhand smoke exposure from spouse: No Yes Total secondhand smoke exposure by intensity: None Medium High	1.0 1.12 (0.54–2.32) 1.0 0.87 (0.36–2.07) 3.24 (1.44–7.32)	Controlled for gender, age, fruit and vegetable intake, and region; lifetime nonsmokers smoked regularly for <6 months (regular = 1 cigarette/day); intensity of the secondhand smoke exposure was based on hours and years of exposure and the degree of smokiness[‡]
• Significant trends of increasing risk with increasing years of workplace secondhand smoke exposure • Strongest association with recent secondhand smoke exposure	Men Spousal secondhand smoke: No Yes Workplace secondhand smoke: No Yes Women Spousal secondhand smoke: No Yes Workplace secondhand smoke: No Yes	1.0 1.96 (0.72–5.36) 1.0 1.89 (0.53–6.67) 1.0 1.05 (0.60–1.86) 1.0 1.57 (0.80–3.06)	Controlled for age, gender, catchment area, occasional smoking, vegetable intake, degree of urban residence, and occupation; lifetime nonsmokers smoked <1 cigarette/day or <10 cigarettes/week and other equivalences for cigars, pipes, and cigarillos
• Increased risk with husband's smoking was stronger when restricted to controls with nonsmoking-related cancers • Stronger association with squamous cell cancers	Husband smoked: No Yes Workplace secondhand smoke: No Yes	1.0 1.53 (1.06–2.21) 1.0 0.88 (0.55–1.41)	Controlled for age and education; lifetime nonsmokers were not defined; age of participants and the study period were not reported

Table 7.3   Continued

Study	Population/date of study	Cases/histologic confirmation and cell type (%)	Controls	Data collection
		Europe		
Kreuzer et al. 2000	Men and women aged <76 years from 15 clinics/hospitals Area residents for at least 25 years Frequency matched for gender, age, region, and length of residence East/West Germany 1990–1996	292 (234 women, 58 men) 100% histologic confirmation Squamous cell carcinoma: 20% Adenocarcinoma: 59% (n = 173)	1,338 (535 women, 803 men) RDD and local residential registries	In-person interview within 3 months of diagnosis Response rate: Cases: 76% Controls: 41% 100% self-respondents
		Asia		
Du et al. 1996; Lei et al. 1996	Reviewed death certificates of local residents Matched for gender, age, year of death, and block of residence Guangzhou, China 1986	75 women No histologic confirmation or cell type information	128 women Excluded those with history of respiratory disease/tumors	In-person interview with next of kin Response rate was not reported No self-respondents
Shen et al. 1996, 1998	Hospital-based Local residents ≥20 years Matched for age, gender, neighborhood, and occupation Nanjing, China 1986–1993	70 women 100% histologic confirmation Included only adenocarcinoma	70 women General population	In-person interview Response rate was not reported 100% self-respondents
Wang et al. 1996; Zhou et al. 2000	18 hospitals Aged 35–69 years Matched for age and lifetime nonsmoking status Shenyang, China 1991–1995	135 women, 72 with adenocarcinoma Approximately 50% histologic confirmation Squamous cell carcinoma: 16% Small cell carcinoma: 20% Adenocarcinoma: 55%	135 women, 72 designated specifically for adenocarcinoma patients General population	In-person interview within 2 weeks of case diagnosis Response rate was not reported 100% self-respondents
Rapiti et al. 1999	1 hospital Men and women Excluded some diseases among hospital controls No matching Chandigarh, India 1991–1992	58 (17 men, 41 women) 100% histologic confirmation Squamous cell carcinoma: 28% Small cell carcinoma: 19% Adenocarcinoma: 51%	123 (56 men, 67 women) 2 sources: other hospital patients and visitors	In-person interview Response rate was not reported 100% self-respondents

Findings	Measure of secondhand smoke	Relative risk (95% confidence interval)	Comments (covariates considered, definition of lifetime nonsmokers)
Europe			

• No significant association with any secondhand smoke exposure from spouse, work, or childhood
• Increased risk with weighted duration of secondhand smoke exposures from all sources
	Men and women
	  Spouse smoked:
	    No
	    Yes
	  Secondhand smoke from all sources with weighted duration:
	    None
	    Low
	    Medium
		
		1.0
		0.99 (0.73–1.34)
		
		1.0
		1.29 (0.79–2.09)
		1.78 (1.05–3.04)
			Controlled for gender, age, region, occupation, education, radon, family history, previous lung diseases, length of residence, and selected vegetable intake; lifetime nonsmokers had smoked <400 cigarettes/lifetime; secondhand smoke from all sources combined included exposures inside and outside the home (weighted duration = hours times smokiness)

Asia			

• No significant increased risk was associated with husband's smoking by amount or duration	Husband smoked:
	  No
	  Yes
		
		1.0
		1.19 (0.66–2.16)
			Crude risk estimate; definition of lifetime nonsmokers was not reported; there were many limitations in the study methods

• No significant trend with amount and duration of secondhand smoke exposure at home	Daily household secondhand smoke exposure:
	  No
	  Yes
		
		1.0
		1.63 (0.68–3.89)
			Controlled for neighborhood, gender, age, and occupation; possible overmatching

• No significant trend with years/amount smoked by husband
• Results in analyses restricted to adenocarcinoma were similar
	Husband smoked:
	  No
	  Yes
	Workplace exposure:
	  No
	  Yes
		
		1.0
		1.11 (0.65–1.88)
		
		1.0
		0.89 (0.45–1.77)
			Crude risk estimates; histologic cell type classification is questionable

• No significant association with years of spousal smoking
• Increased risk with secondhand smoke exposure during childhood
	Husband smoked:
	  No
	  Yes
		
		1.0
		1.1 (0.5–2.6)
			Controlled for gender, age, religion, and residence; lifetime nonsmokers had smoked <400 cigarettes/lifetime

Table 7.3   Continued

Study	Population/date of study	Cases/histologic confirmation and cell type (%)*	Controls	Data collection
Asia				
Zhong et al. 1999	Women aged 35–69 years Permanent residents of the area Frequency matched for age Shanghai, China Cancer Registry 1992–1994	504 Approximately 77% histologic confirmation Squamous cell carcinoma: 12.4% Small cell carcinoma: 2% Adenocarcinoma: 76.5%	601 General population	In-person interview at home, hospital, or work Response rate: Cases: 92% Controls: 84% Self-respondents: Cases: 80% Controls: 98%
Lee et al. 2000	1 hospital Women only Matched for age, lifetime nonsmoking status, date of admission Kaohsiung (Taiwan) 1992–1998	268 100% histologic confirmation Squamous cell carcinoma: 18% Small cell carcinoma: 11% Adenocarcinoma: 68%	445 hospital controls Eye or orthopedic patients, or in for check-ups	In-person interview Response rate: Cases: 91% Controls: 90% 100% self-respondents
Wang et al. 2000	Local hospitals and clinics Aged 30–75 years Frequency matched for age, gender, and prefecture of residence Gansu Province (China) 1994–1998	233 (33 men, 200 women) 30% histologic confirmation Cell type distribution was not reported	521 (114 men, 407 women) General population	In-person interview at home/hospital Response rate: Cases: 95% Controls: 90% Self-respondents: Cases: 46% Controls: 96%
Seow et al. 2002	3 major hospitals Aged <90 years (alert enough for interview) Frequency matched for age, hospital, and date of admission Singapore 1996–1998	176 women 100% histologic confirmation Squamous cell carcinoma: 10% Small cell carcinoma: 1.1% Adenocarcinoma: 72%	663 No history of cancer, heart or chronic respiratory disease, or renal failure	In-person interview within 3 months of diagnosis Response rate: Cases: 95% Controls: 97% 100% self-respondents

*Percentages do not add up to 100%.
†Smoker-years = The number of years of exposure weighted by the number of smokers.
‡Smokiness = Subjective index: (1) not visible but smellable, (2) visible, and (3) very smoky.

Findings	Measure of secondhand smoke	Relative risk (95% confidence interval)	Comments (covariates considered, definition of lifetime nonsmokers)
	Asia		
• Significant association between secondhand smoke exposure at work and risk when stratified by various intensity measures	Secondhand smoke at home: No Yes Workplace exposure: No Yes	 1.0 1.2 (0.8–1.7) 1.0 1.9 (0.9–3.7)	Controlled for age, income, vitamin C intake, respondent status, smokiness of kitchen, family history of lung cancer, and high-risk occupations; lifetime nonsmokers had smoked <1 cigarette/day for 6 months
• Significant associations between various sources of secondhand smoke exposure and risk (husband, work, and paternal smoking)	Husband smoked: No In wife's absence In wife's presence Lifetime exposure: None 1–20 smoker-years 21–40 smoker-years 41–60 smoker-years >60 smoker-years	 1.0 1.2 (0.7–2.0) 2.2 (1.5–3.3) 1.0 1.3 (0.6–2.6) 1.6 (0.9–2.6) 2.0 (1.2–3.5) 2.8 (1.6–4.8)	Controlled for area of residence, education, occupation, tuberculosis, cooking fuels, and fume extractor; lifetime nonsmokers had smoked <1 cigarette/day for 1 year or <365 cigarettes/lifetime
• No significant association with secondhand smoke exposure in adulthood • Significant association with secondhand smoke exposure in childhood	Secondhand smoke in adulthood: No Yes Secondhand smoke in childhood: No Yes Lifetime secondhand smoke: No Yes	 1.0 0.90 (0.6–1.4) 1.0 1.52 (1.1–2.2) 1.0 1.19 (0.7–2.0)	Controlled for age, social class, prefecture, and other potential confounders; lifetime nonsmokers smoked cigarettes or pipes regularly for ≤6 months
• Increased risk with any household secondhand smoke exposure	Any secondhand smoke: No Yes	 1.0 1.3 (0.9–1.8)	Controlled for age, birthplace, family history of cancer, soy intake, length of menstrual cycle; lifetime nonsmokers had smoked <1 cigarette/day for 1 year; there was a single question on secondhand smoke exposure

1998a; Zaridze et al. 1998; Zhong et al. 1999; Kreuzer et al. 2000; Lee et al. 2000; Wang et al. 2000; Seow et al. 2002) that expanded the assessment of the exposure to include smoking habits of other household members during childhood and adulthood, and exposure at work and in other social settings. Recent studies based largely on interviews with the index participants also attempted to determine intensity measures of exposure by assessing hours of exposure, the number of smokers, and whether the exposure occurred in the presence of the participants (Jöckel et al. 1998; Nyberg et al. 1998a; Kreuzer et al. 2000; Lee et al. 2000). These newer studies have demonstrated that under certain circumstances, investigators may be able to classify exposure at least semiquantitatively. Appendix 7.1 provides detailed information on the more recent case-control studies reviewed in this chapter on the association between exposure to secondhand smoke and lung cancer.

Summary of New Epidemiologic Studies on Lung Cancer and Secondhand Smoke Exposure

Between 1996 and 2001, 15 epidemiologic studies were published that further expand the evidence supporting a causal association between secondhand smoke exposure and the risk of lung cancer among lifetime nonsmokers. Recent cohort studies from Korea (Jee et al. 1999) and Japan (Nishino et al. 2001) have improved the assessment of secondhand smoke exposure by obtaining information on the husband's smoking on two occasions during medical examinations approximately two years apart (Jee et al. 1999), or by asking about smoking by other household members (Nishino et al. 2001). Potential confounders were considered in both studies and their results were very similar to those reported by Hirayama (1981). By design, five hospital-based European studies (Jöckel et al. 1998; Nyberg et al. 1998a; Zaridze et al. 1998; Kreuzer et al. 2000, 2001) and one study from Taiwan (Lee et al. 2000) restricted the study population to patients diagnosed with lung cancer who were well enough to participate in an in-person interview shortly after diagnosis. Thus, these investigators were able to obtain more information regarding the intensity of secondhand smoke exposure than was previously available in most population-based, case-control studies. The higher RR estimates in these studies are likely due to the incorporation of intensity measures of exposure that separated those who were highly exposed to secondhand smoke from those who were less highly exposed.

Six additional studies were conducted among Chinese persons who resided in China or other countries in Asia. Although some of these studies were small and the quality of the methods uncertain, three studies are large and well-designed. Conducted in Shanghai, China; Kaohsiung, Taiwan; and Gansu Province, China (Zhong et al. 1999; Lee et al. 2000; Wang et al. 2000), these larger studies showed that secondhand smoke exposures at home and at work during adulthood were associated with an increased risk of lung cancer among lifetime nonsmokers. This association remained consistent even in populations where other sources of indoor and outdoor air pollution were also prevalent. In addition to the questionnaire-based studies, de Waard and colleagues (1995) conducted a small nested case-control study that provided supportive evidence based on urinary cotinine for an association between secondhand smoke exposure and an increased risk of lung cancer among lifetime nonsmokers.

Pooled Analyses

Secondhand Smoke Exposure from Spouses: An Update of the Literature

Of the published meta-analyses on secondhand smoke and lung cancer, only two recent comprehensive meta-analyses are mentioned here, as their findings subsume those of earlier reports. Hackshaw and colleagues (1997) pooled 37 published studies and obtained an estimated RR of 1.24 (95 percent confidence interval [CI], 1.13–1.36) for nonsmokers who lived with a smoker. The results were remarkably consistent with analyses stratified by gender, geographic region, year of publication, and study design. Zhong and colleagues (2000) reached similar conclusions when they updated that same pooled analysis to include 40 published studies. They obtained a RR of 1.20 (95 percent CI, 1.12–1.29) for lung cancer risk among nonsmoking women with exposure to secondhand smoke from their husbands' smoking. The increased RR was observed for case-control and cohort studies and separately by gender, study location, year of publication, and other parameters.

The update of the pooled analyses that follows was prepared by reviewing published studies already included in the meta-analyses conducted by Hackshaw and colleagues (1997) and Zhong and colleagues (2000), as well as the new studies discussed in the Appendix at the end of this chapter. Results of the meta-analyses were calculated with the method of DerSimonian and Laird (1986). Random-effects analyses were used to account for heterogeneity between studies. The statistical program Stata was used for the calculations. For studies that reported both crude (or minimally adjusted) and more adjusted RR estimates, the more adjusted risk estimate was selected for the meta-analysis. Table 7.4 provides the findings.

There are 52 studies in this analysis on spousal secondhand smoke exposure (8 cohort, 44 case-control studies). Those studies that lacked specific information on spousal smoking were not included (Svensson et al. 1989; Wang et al. 1994; de Waard et al. 1995; Seow et al. 2002). Three studies (Jöckel et al. 1998; Nyberg et al. 1998b; Kreuzer et al. 2000) that were part of the International Agency for Research on Cancer (IARC) European multicenter study (Boffetta et al. 1998) were also published as separate reports. The study by Jöckel and colleagues (1998) was not included because almost all of the lifetime nonsmokers in this report (71 of the 76 cases and 229 of the 236 controls) were already included in the IARC European multicenter study (Boffetta et al. 1998). However, because the study by Nyberg and colleagues (1998b) included an additional 54 cases and 123 controls and the study by Kreuzer and colleagues (2000) included an additional 119 cases and 1,123 controls who were not included in the European multicenter study, these two studies were included in the meta-analysis presented here.

When RR estimates from prospective cohort and case-control studies were combined, the RR of lung cancer among male and female nonsmokers who were ever exposed to secondhand smoke from their spouses was 1.21 (95 percent CI, 1.13–1.30). The RR estimates were 1.20 (95 percent CI, 1.11–1.29) from case-control studies and 1.29 (95 percent CI, 1.125–1.49) from cohort studies. The magnitude of the effect associated with spousal secondhand smoke exposure was comparable for men (odds ratio [OR] = 1.37 [95 percent CI, 1.05–1.79]) and women (OR = 1.22 [95 percent CI, 1.13–1.31]). There were no significant differences in the RR estimates by geographic area; the point estimate was 1.15 (95 percent CI, 1.04–1.26) for studies conducted in the United States and Canada, 1.16 (95 percent CI, 1.03–1.30) for studies conducted in Europe, and 1.43 (95 percent CI, 1.24–1.66) for studies conducted in Asia. The pooled RR estimates were 1.30 (95 percent CI, 1.13–1.50) for studies published between 1981 and 1986, 1.20 (95 percent CI, 1.05–1.38) for studies published between 1987 and 1994, and 1.20 (95 percent CI, 1.09–1.31) for studies published

since 1994. Significantly increased risks were observed regardless of the sample size: the pooled RR estimate was 1.44 (95 percent CI, 1.16–1.78) for studies with 55 or fewer lung cancer cases, 1.25 (95 percent CI, 1.08–1.46) for studies with 56 to 99 cases, and 1.18 (95 percent CI, 1.08–1.29) for studies with 100 or more lung cancer cases.

Secondhand Smoke Exposure in the Workplace

In addition to the home, the workplace has been a location where significant exposure takes place (see Chapter 4, Prevalence of Exposure to Secondhand Smoke) (Jaakkola and Samet 1999). Large cross-sectional studies have consistently demonstrated the prevalence of secondhand smoke exposure in the workplace and in other settings outside the home (National Cancer Institute [NCI] 1999). In the Third National Health and Nutrition Examination Survey, which included a large representative sample of the U.S. population, nearly 40 percent of working people who were nontobacco users reported secondhand smoke exposure in the workplace (Pirkle et al. 1996). Reviews of indoor air nicotine and/or respirable suspended particulate concentrations in different micro-environments show that the levels were essentially comparable between work and residential environments in the United States and other countries. Secondhand smoke exposures in homes and workplaces were not only qualitatively similar in chemical composition but also in concentrations (Guerin et al. 1992; U.S. Environmental Protection Agency [USEPA] 1992; Hammond 1999).

A total of 25 epidemiologic studies (7 from the United States, 1 from Canada, 7 from Europe, and 10 from Asia) have provided information on workplace secondhand smoke exposure and the risk of lung cancer among lifetime nonsmokers (Table 7.5). The questions on workplace secondhand smoke exposure are heterogeneous among the studies (Wu 1999), and nine of the studies have assessed individual lifetime workplace secondhand smoke exposure. Almost all of the controls in these studies were self-respondents, so differences in exposure prevalences may reflect the heterogeneous questions that were asked, different workplace smoking policies, and/ or different demographic characteristics of the controls, such as social class. Of the studies conducted in the United States and Canada, an estimated 38 to 66 percent of the controls reported any exposure at the workplace; the prevalence of exposure was similar for men and women (Kabat and Wynder 1984; Kabat et al. 1995). The prevalence of workplace secondhand

Table 7.4   Quantitative estimate of lung cancer risk with differing sources of exposure to secondhand smoke

Study	Data source	Exposure vs. referent	Relative risk	95% confidence interval
Previous meta-analyses				
Hackshaw et al. 1997	37 studies	Smoking vs. nonsmoking spouse	1.24	1.13–1.36
Zhong et al. 2000	40 studies (including 37 from Hackshaw et al. 1997)	Smoking vs. nonsmoking husband	1.20	1.12–1.29
Spousal smoking (52 studies)				
Meta-analysis conducted for this 2006 Surgeon General's report	Case-control (44 studies)	Smoking vs. nonsmoking spouse	1.21	1.13–1.30
	Cohort (8 studies)	Smoking vs. nonsmoking spouse	1.29	1.125–1.49
	Men	Smoking vs. nonsmoking wife	1.37	1.05–1.79
	Women	Smoking vs. nonsmoking husband	1.22	1.13–1.31
	United States and Canada	Smoking vs. nonsmoking spouse	1.15	1.04–1.26
	Europe	Smoking vs. nonsmoking spouse	1.16	1.03–1.30
	Asia	Smoking vs. nonsmoking spouse	1.43	1.24–1.66
Workplace exposure (25 studies)				
Meta-analysis conducted for this 2006 Surgeon General's report	Nonsmokers (25 studies)	Workplace secondhand smoke vs. none	1.22	1.13–1.33
	Nonsmoking men (11 studies)	Workplace secondhand smoke vs. none	1.12	0.86–1.50
	Nonsmoking women (25 studies)	Workplace secondhand smoke vs. none	1.22	1.10–1.35
	Nonsmokers in the United States and Canada (8 studies)	Workplace secondhand smoke vs. none	1.24	1.03–1.49
	Nonsmokers in Europe (7 studies)	Workplace secondhand smoke vs. none	1.13	0.96–1.34
	Nonsmokers in Asia (10 studies)	Workplace secondhand smoke vs. none	1.32	1.13–1.55
Childhood exposure (24 studies)				
Meta-analysis conducted for this 2006 Surgeon General's report	Men and women	Maternal smoking	1.15	0.86–1.52
	Men and women	Paternal smoking	1.10	0.89–1.36
	Men and women	Smoking by either parent	1.11	0.94–1.31
	Women	Maternal smoking	1.28	0.93–1.78
	Women	Paternal smoking	1.17	0.91–1.50
	United States and Canada (8 studies)	Smoking by either parent	0.93	0.81–1.07
	Europe (6 studies)	Smoking by either parent	0.81	0.71–0.92
	Asia (10 studies)	Smoking by either parent	1.59	1.18–2.15

Table 7.5   Relative risks for lung cancer associated with any workplace exposure to secondhand smoke among lifetime nonsmokers

Study	Population	Types of questions asked regarding workplace secondhand smoke exposure	Percentage with workplace secondhand smoke exposure		Relative risk (95% confidence interval)
			Cases	Controls	
United States					
Kabat and Wynder 1984	Men Women U.S. cities	Exposure at current or last job	72 49	44 58	3.3 (1.0–10.4) 0.7 (0.3–1.5)
Garfinkel et al. 1985	Women New Jersey and Ohio	Exposure—past 5 years past 25 years	45	47	0.88 (0.7–1.2) 0.93 (0.7–1.2)
Wu et al. 1985	Women Los Angeles	Exposure at all jobs	55	50	1.3 (0.5–3.3)
Butler 1988	Men Women	Years worked with smokers	29 33	38 43	0.98 (0.2–5.4) 1.0 (0.2–5.4)
Brownson et al. 1992	Women Missouri	Exposure at current/last job	NR*	NR	0.98 (0.74–1.32)[†]
Kabat et al. 1995	Men Women 4 U.S. cities	Exposure at 4 jobs lasting >1 year	56 60	56 57	1.02 (0.50–2.09) 1.15 (0.62–2.13)
Reynolds et al. 1996	Women 5 U.S. cities	Exposure at all jobs	73	66	1.6 (1.2–2.0)
Schwartz et al. 1996	Men and women Detroit	Not specified	53	46	1.5 (1.0–2.2)
Canada					
Johnson et al. 2001	Women	Exposure at all jobs	54	49	1.20 (0.74–1.95)[‡]
Europe					
Lee et al. 1986	Men Women United Kingdom	Not specified	70 20	59 29	1.61 (0.39–6.6) 0.63 (0.17–2.33)
Kalandidi et al. 1990	Women Greece	Exposure at current/last job	73	66	1.39 (0.76–2.54)
Boffetta et al. 1998	Men Women 7 European countries	Exposure at all jobs	74 53	71 47	1.13 (0.68–1.86) 1.19 (0.94–1.51)
Nyberg et al. 1998a	Men Women Sweden	Exposure at all jobs	86 75	81 66	1.89 (0.53–6.67) 1.57 (0.80–3.06)
Zaridze et al. 1998	Women Russia	Exposure—past 20 years	19	19	0.88 (0.55–1.41)

Table 7.5   Continued

Study	Population	Types of questions asked regarding workplace secondhand smoke exposure	Percentage with workplace secondhand smoke exposure		Relative risk (95% confidence interval)
			Cases	Controls	
Europe					
Boffetta et al. 1999	Men and women 7 European countries	Exposure at all jobs	55	54	1.0 (0.5–1.8)
Kreuzer et al. 2000, 2001	Men Women Germany	Exposure at all jobs	66 53	71 52	0.78 (0.44–1.38) 1.14 (0.83–1.57)
Asia					
Koo et al. 1984	Women Hong Kong	Exposure at all jobs	NR	NR	1.19 (0.48–2.95)
Shimizu et al. 1988	Women Japan	Most recent/current job, any smokers at work	NR	NR	1.2 (0.7–2.04)
Wu-Williams et al. 1990	Women Northern China	Exposure at all jobs	55	50	1.2 (1.0–1.6)
Sun et al. 1996	Women Northern China	Not specified	NR	NR	1.38 (0.94–2.04)
Wang et al. 1996	Women Shenyang, China	Not specified	84	85	0.89 (0.45–1.77)
Rapiti et al. 1999	Men and women India	Not specified	NR	NR	1.1 (0.3–4.1)
Zhong et al. 1999	Women Shanghai, China	Exposure at each job held for ≥2 years	27	21	1.7 (1.3–2.3)
Lee et al. 2000	Women Taiwan	Exposure at each job held for ≥5 years	10	7	1.2 (0.5–2.4)
Wang et al. 2000	Men and women Gansu Province	Any workplace exposure	NR	NR	1.56 (0.7–3.3)
Zhou et al. 2000	Women Shenyang, China	Not specified	85	82	0.89 (0.25–3.16)

*NR = Data were not reported.
†Relative risk from calculations presented by Wells 1998 (Table 2).
‡Calculations based on the numbers presented in Table 2 of Johnson et al. 2001.

smoke exposure was more varied among controls in European countries: women in Moscow had the lowest prevalence (Zaridze et al. 1998) and Swedish men in Stockholm had the highest (Nyberg et al. 1998a). Similarly, there was a wide range of prevalences in workplace secondhand smoke exposure in Asia.

Despite these geographic differences in exposure prevalences, the effect of secondhand smoke exposure in the workplace on the risk of lung cancer among lifetime nonsmokers is remarkably consistent. On the basis of these 25 studies, the pooled RR estimate associated with reported workplace secondhand smoke exposure was 1.22 (95 percent CI, 1.13–1.33) for all studies combined, 1.12 (95 percent CI, 0.86–1.50) for men, and 1.22 (95 percent CI, 1.10–1.35) for women. When the pooled analysis was conducted separately by geographic area, the pooled RR estimate was 1.24 (95 percent CI, 1.03–1.49) for the United States and Canada, 1.13 (95 percent CI, 0.96–1.34) for European countries, and 1.32 (95 percent CI, 1.13–1.55) for Asia.

Studies have also assessed dose-response relationships between secondhand smoke exposure in the workplace and lung cancer risk among lifetime nonsmokers (Table 7.6). At least six studies have reported RR estimates stratified by years of exposure (Fontham et al. 1994; Boffetta et al. 1998; Nyberg et al. 1998a; Zhong et al. 1999; Wang et al. 2000; Johnson et al. 2001), and these studies concur that there is a trend of an increase in risk with an increased duration of exposure. In addition, studies that used a combined index incorporating years and intensity of exposure, such as the number of hours of exposure and the number of smokers in the work environment (Boffetta et al. 1998; Nyberg et al. 1998a; Zhong et al. 1999; Kreuzer et al. 2000; Johnson et al. 2001), found up to a threefold increase in risk associated with the highest intensity levels of workplace exposure (Table 7.6).

Secondhand Smoke Exposure During Childhood

At least 24 epidemiologic studies have investigated secondhand smoke exposure during childhood (Table 7.7). The prevalence of secondhand smoke exposure during childhood varied and depended on whether the source of the exposure was from mothers, fathers, both parents, other household members, or a combined index that incorporated all sources of exposure. Although some studies found suggestions of a significantly increased risk of lung cancer in association with childhood exposures (Janerich et al. 1990; Sun et al. 1996; Rapiti et al. 1999; Wang et al. 2000), most studies did not find significant associations. When a pooled RR estimate in association with maternal and paternal smoking was calculated, in addition to a calculated combined index that represented childhood exposure from either parent, there was some increase in risk in association with secondhand smoke exposure to maternal smoking (OR = 1.15 [95 percent CI, 0.86–1.52]), paternal smoking (OR = 1.10 [95 percent CI, 0.89–1.36]), or smoking by either parent (OR = 1.11 [95 percent CI, 0.94–1.31]). The risk pattern was slightly stronger in analyses restricted to women (maternal smoking OR = 1.28 [95 percent CI, 0.93–1.78]; paternal smoking OR = 1.17 [95 percent CI, 0.91–1.50]). The pooled RR

estimate associated with childhood secondhand smoke exposure was 0.93 (95 percent CI, 0.81–1.07) for studies conducted in the United States, 0.81 (95 percent CI, 0.71–0.92) for studies conducted in European countries, and 1.59 (95 percent CI, 1.18–2.15) for studies conducted in Asian countries.

There are several alternative explanations for the generally weaker association between childhood exposures and lung cancer risk compared with exposure during adulthood. Nyberg and colleagues (1998a) found that recent secondhand smoke exposures had the greatest impact on overall lung cancer risk among lifetime nonsmoking adults. If more recent exposures convey a greater risk, then remote childhood exposures would be anticipated to have little effect. In addition, assessments of childhood exposure may also have higher rates of misclassification than assessments of exposure during adulthood. In some studies, interviews with next of kin were conducted when the case patient was ill or deceased (Janerich et al. 1990; Brownson et al. 1992; Stockwell et al. 1992; Fontham et al. 1994; Wang et al. 2000). Next of kin, particularly spouses, who may not be knowledgeable about childhood events and exposures could provide incomplete and/or misclassified exposure histories. But most of these studies included few or no interviews with next of kin among the controls. Thus, differential misclassification of secondhand smoke exposures during childhood may have occurred in some studies.

Evidence Synthesis

Twenty years after secondhand smoke was first classified as a cause of lung cancer in lifetime nonsmokers, the evidence supporting causation continues to mount (USDHHS 1986). More than 50 epidemiologic studies have addressed the association between secondhand smoke exposure and the risk of lung cancer among lifetime nonsmokers. These studies included men and women of diverse racial and ethnic backgrounds and were conducted using heterogeneous study designs in some 20 countries of North America, Europe, and Asia. An increased risk of lung cancer associated with secondhand smoke exposure was found in most of the studies, with few exceptions (Chan et al. 1982; Buffler et al. 1984; Kabat and Wynder 1984; Lee et al. 1986; Wu-Williams et al. 1990; Liu et al. 1991; Brownson et al. 1992; Wang et al. 1996). A consistent association obtained in different populations under diverse circumstances strengthens a causal interpretation because different patterns of potential bias and confounding would be expected across different populations. Not surprisingly,

Table 7.6   Dose-response relationships between workplace secondhand smoke exposure and lung cancer risk among lifetime nonsmokers

| Study/gender | Exposure level | | Weighted exposure level | |
	Duration	Relative risk (95% confidence interval)	Intensity	Relative risk (95% confidence interval)
Fontham et al. 1994 Women	In years: None 1–15 16–30 ≥31 p for trend	1.0 1.30 (1.01–1.67) 1.40 (1.04–1.88) 1.86 (1.24–2.78) 0.001	NR*	NR
Boffetta et al. 1998 Men and women	In years: None 1–29 30–38 ≥39 p for trend	1.0 1.15 (0.91–1.44) 1.26 (0.85–1.85) 1.19 (0.77–1.86) 0.21	Level × hours/day × years: None 0.1–46.1 46.2–88.9 ≥89 p for trend	 1.0 0.97 (0.76–1.25) 1.41 (0.93–2.12) 2.07 (1.33–3.21) <0.01
Nyberg et al. 1998a Men and women	In years: None <30 ≥30 p for trend[†]	1.0 1.40 (0.76–2.56) 2.21 (1.08–4.52) 0.03	Hour-years[‡]: None <30 ≥30 p for trend[†]	1.0 1.27 (0.69–2.34) 2.51 (1.28–4.93) 0.01
Zhong et al. 1999 Women	In years: None 1–12 13–24 >24 p for trend	1.0 2.0 (1.2–3.3) 1.4 (0.9–2.3) 1.8 (1.1–2.8) 0.50	Number of hours per day: None 1–2 3–4 >4 p for trend	 1.0 1.0 (0.6–1.7) 1.6 (1.0–2.5) 2.9 (1.8–4.7) <0.001
Kreuzer et al. 2000 Men and women	In hours: 0–29,000 >29,000–61,000 >61,000 p for trend	1.0 1.57 (0.97–2.54) 1.36 (0.71–2.61) 0.10	Hours times smokiness[§] level: 0–56,200 >56,200–100,600 >100,600 p for trend	 1.0 1.09 (0.55–2.19) 1.93 (1.04–3.58) 0.06
Wang et al. 2000 Men and women	In years: None <20 ≥20 p for trend	1.0 1.29 (0.5–3.3) 1.76 (0.5–5.6) 0.19	NR	NR
Johnson et al. 2001 Women	In years: None Residential only: 1–7 8–19 ≥20 p for trend	1.0 1.21 (0.5–2.8) 1.24 (0.5–3.3) 1.71 (0.7–4.3) 1.71 (0.7–4.3) NS[Δ]	Smoker-years[¶]: None Residential only: 1–25 26–64 ≥65 p for trend	1.0 1.21 (0.5–2.8) 1.16 (0.4–3.1) 1.98 (0.8–4.9) 1.58 (0.6–4.0) NS

*NR = Data were not reported.
[†]Calculations are based on the data presented.
[‡]Hour-years = 365 hours or the equivalent of 1 hour per day per year.
[§]Smokiness = Subjective index: (1) not visible but smellable, (2) visible, and (3) very smoky.
[Δ]NS = Not statistically significant.
[¶]Smoker-years = The number of years of exposure weighted by the number of smokers.

Table 7.7 **Relative risks for lung cancer associated with exposure to secondhand smoke during childhood among lifetime nonsmokers**

Study	Population	Childhood secondhand smoke exposure	Percentage with childhood secondhand smoke exposure		Relative risk (95% confidence interval) with any exposure from a family member
			Cases	Controls	
United States					
Garfinkel et al. 1985	Women 4 U.S. hospitals	Any childhood exposure	NR*	NR	0.91 (0.74–1.12)
Wu et al. 1985	Women Los Angeles	Parents	40	53	0.6 (0.2–1.7)
Janerich et al. 1990	Men and women New York	Any childhood exposure†	70	54	1.3 (0.85–1.99)
Brownson et al. 1992	Women Missouri	Parents	17	25	0.7 (0.5–0.9)
		Other household members	25	31	0.8 (0.6–1.1)
Stockwell et al. 1992	Women Central Florida	Mother‡	NR	NR	1.6 (0.6–4.3)
		Father	NR	NR	1.2 (0.6–2.3)
		Siblings	NR	NR	1.7 (0.8–3.9)
Fontham et al. 1994	Women 5 U.S. cities	Father	50	55	0.83 (0.67–1.02)
		Mother	12	13	0.86 (0.62–1.18)
		Other household members	21	21	1.03 (0.80–1.32)
		Any household member during childhood	62	65	0.89 (0.72–1.10)
Kabat et al. 1995	Men Women 4 U.S. cities	Any childhood exposure	62 68	65 57	0.90 (0.43–1.89) 1.55 (0.95–2.79)
Canada					
Johnson et al. 2001	Women National cancer registry	Any childhood exposure	83	78	1.39 (0.8–2.2)
Europe					
Pershagen et al. 1987	Women Sweden	1 or both parents smoked	19	NR	1.0 (0.4–2.3)
Svensson et al. 1989	Women Sweden	Father	12	71	0.9 (0.4–2.3)
		Mother	3	5	3.3 (0.5–18.8)
Boffetta et al. 1998	Men and women 7 European countries	Father	NR	NR	0.76 (0.61–0.94)
		Mother	NR	NR	0.92 (0.57–1.49)
		Any childhood exposure	60	66	0.78 (0.64–0.96)
Nyberg et al. 1998a	Men	Father	69	52	1.90 (0.69–5.23)
		Mother	40	21	0.90 (0.14–6.00)
	Women Sweden	Father	46	49	0.76 (0.42–1.37)
		Mother	8	15	0.29 (0.07–1.14)

Table 7.7   Continued

Study	Population	Childhood secondhand smoke exposure	Percentage with childhood secondhand smoke exposure		Relative risk (95% confidence interval) with any exposure from a family member
			Cases	Controls	
Europe					
Zaridze et al. 1998	Women Russia	Father (assumed during childhood)	49	50	0.92 (0.64–1.32)
Kreuzer et al. 2000	Men and women Germany	Any exposure	62	64	0.84 (0.63–1.11)
Asia					
Koo et al. 1987	Women Hong Kong	During childhood	NR	NR	2.07 (0.51–95.17)
Shimizu et al. 1988	Women Japan	Father	NR	41	1.1 (p >0.05)
		Mother	NR	3	4.0 (p <0.05)
		Brothers or sisters	NR	32	0.8 (p >0.05)
Sobue 1990	Women Japan	Father	76	80	0.79 (0.52–1.21)
		Mother	12	9	1.33 (0.74–2.37)
		Other household member	22	16	1.18 (0.76–1.84)
Wu-Williams et al. 1990	Women Northern China	Father	44	42	1.1 (0.8–1.4)
		Mother	29	32	0.9 (0.6–1.1)
Sun et al. 1996	Women Northern China	Father	NR	NR	2.4 (1.6–3.5)
		Mother	NR	NR	2.1 (1.3–3.3)
Wang et al. 1996	Women Shenyang (China)	During childhood	59	61	0.91 (0.55–1.49)
Rapiti et al. 1999	Women India	Father	73	18	12.6 (4.9–32.7)
		Mother	31	6	7.7 (1.6–37.2)
Zhong et al. 1999	Women Shanghai (China)	During childhood	34	36	0.9 (0.5–1.6)
Lee et al. 2000	Women Taiwan	Father	49	45	1.2 (0.9–1.6)
		Mother	3	2	1.5 (0.6–3.9)
Wang et al. 2000	Men Women Gansu (China) (nonindustrial)	During childhood	63 67	49 61	1.46 (0.6–3.7) 1.51 (1.0–2.2)

*NR = Data were not reported.
†The respective relative risks were 1.0, 1.1, and 2.1 associated with 0, 1–24, and ≥25 smoker-years, in childhood and adolescence. (Smoker-years = The number of years of exposure weighted by the number of smokers.)
‡The respective relative risks were 1.0, 1.6, 1.1, and 2.4 associated with 0, <18, 18–21, and >21 years, in childhood and adolescence.

associations did not reach statistical significance in all studies because of variations in the sample sizes; some had modest sample sizes with low statistical power. The pooled analyses of earlier reports (Hackshaw et al. 1997; Zhong et al. 2000) and of this report document a 20 to 30 percent increase in RR of lung cancer in association with secondhand smoke exposures during adulthood; the effects are comparable in cohort and case-control studies, among men and women, in different geographic areas, by year of publication, and by study population size (Table 7.4). In addition, the pooled analyses showed comparable increases in risk in association with secondhand smoke exposures from spousal smoking and from smoking in the workplace, thus emphasizing that all sources of exposure increase the risk for lung cancer. Most of the studies published during the 1990s were designed to address weaknesses that previous studies on secondhand smoke and lung cancer were criticized for, including small sample size, possible selection bias, possible misclassification biases, and inadequate adjustments for potential confounders. With the improved designs, therefore, bias becomes an unlikely explanation for the observed increase in risk.

There is strong biologic support for a role of secondhand smoke in the etiology of lung cancer in nonsmokers, and the association is coherent based on the total weight of the evidence (see "Human Carcinogen Uptake from Secondhand Smoke" in Chapter 2). Exposure to secondhand smoke has been repetitively linked to elevation of biomarker levels in nonsmokers, including the tobacco-specific biomarkers nicotine, cotinine, and 4-(methylnitrosamino)-1-(3-pyridyl)-1-butanone (NNK), and nonspecific biomarkers such as white blood cell adducts. As reviewed in Chapter 2, mechanistic understanding related to tobacco smoke and lung cancer has advanced greatly since the 1986 report of the Surgeon General. The development of a cancer is considered to result from multiple genetic changes, and exposure to secondhand smoke involves exposure to the same carcinogens that are linked to genetic changes in active smokers. The genetic basis of susceptibility to these carcinogens is an active area of investigation.

The risk associated with involuntary smoking is consistent with the dose-response relationship observed with active smoking and lung cancer. Hackshaw and colleagues (1997) demonstrated that the risk estimate obtained directly from a meta-analysis of epidemiologic studies was compatible with the risk estimate calculated indirectly from a linear extrapolation of risk among active current smokers. This concept is considered to have limitations (USDHHS 1986).

Lubin's (1999) calculations led to a similar conclusion. Thus, the strength of the secondhand smoke and lung cancer association is consistent with current knowledge of dosimetry and exposure-response relationships among active smokers. Studies of active smoking and lung cancer risk have consistently demonstrated compelling exposure-response relationships (Blot and Fraumeni 1986). As already discussed (see "Secondhand Smoke Exposure in the Workplace" earlier in this chapter), investigators have demonstrated exposure-response relationships with various aspects of secondhand smoke exposure, including duration (e.g., years of spousal smoking and years of exposure at work) and intensity (e.g., number of cigarettes smoked by spouse, number of coworkers who smoked, or hours of exposure per day) (Hackshaw et al. 1997; Zhong et al. 2000). Most of the studies that reported results separately on secondhand smoke and different lung cancer histologic types show a stronger increase in the risk of squamous cell and small cell carcinomas than in the risk of adenocarcinoma. These findings are compatible with the pattern of association found in active smoking and lung cancer by histologic type (Boffetta et al. 1999; Zhong et al. 2000).

The criterion of temporality requires that secondhand smoke exposure antedate the onset of cancer. Support for this criterion is provided by prospective studies in which men and women initially free of lung cancer were followed over varying time intervals, and their risk differed in accordance with a secondhand smoke exposure that was either self-reported (e.g., spousal smoking history) or determined by a biologic marker of exposure (e.g., urinary cotinine levels) (de Waard et al. 1995).

Despite the extent of the evidence and its consistency, coherence, and temporality, the causal association between secondhand smoke exposure and lung cancer risk has been continuously questioned because of concerns related to various biases (see "Use of Meta-Analysis" in Chapter 1). Much of the criticism has come from the tobacco industry around the association of secondhand smoke with lung cancer (Drope and Chapman 2001; Muggli et al. 2001). Public health researchers recognize the difficulties inherent in studying exposures such as secondhand smoke, where the RR associated with the exposure is anticipated to be small and the exposure is common. Two comprehensive commentaries on this topic reviewed four primary concerns related to studies of secondhand smoke and lung cancer: confounding, measurement error, misclassification, and publication bias (Kawachi and Colditz 1996; Smith and Phillips 1996), and several reports have addressed publication bias specifically (Bero et al. 1994; Misakian and Bero 1998). These investigators independently concluded that the observed increase in risk of lung cancer associated with secondhand smoke exposure cannot be "explained" by these inherent methodologic limitations.

One concern raised has been that secondhand smoke itself may not be causally related to lung cancer, but that the association reflects confounding by factors that are causally linked to lung cancer. In cross-sectional studies of nonsmoking women, some investigators observed a higher risk profile for potential confounding factors such as a higher alcohol intake, a lower intake of vitamin supplements and dietary sources of various antioxidants, and a higher body mass index among women exposed to secondhand smoke compared with unexposed women (Koo et al. 1987; Matanoski et al. 1995; Kawachi and Colditz 1996). Other investigators, however, have not found these differences (Cardenas et al. 1997; Steenland et al. 1998; Curtin et al. 1999; Forastiere et al. 2000), and the relevance of these studies that investigated current patterns of association of possible confounders with secondhand smoke exposure to patterns from previous decades is uncertain. More important, unlike studies of heart disease where numerous risk factors have been identified, there are few true potential confounders for studies of secondhand smoke and lung cancer (Kawachi and Colditz 1996). Although many of the earlier studies of secondhand smoke and lung cancer did not consider lifestyle variables such as diet in the statistical analysis, most of the larger studies published since the 1990s have accounted for these factors and have found that the effect of secondhand smoke remained after adjusting for them (Stockwell et al. 1992; Fontham et al. 1994; Cardenas et al. 1997; Boffetta et al. 1998; Jöckel et al. 1998; Nyberg et al. 1998a; Zhong et al. 1999; Kreuzer et al. 2000; Lee et al. 2000; Wang et al. 2000; Seow et al. 2002). Finally, in a comprehensive investigation of the possible confounding effect of dietary factors (intake of fruits, vegetables, and dietary fat) that included data from nearly 20 studies on this topic, Fry and Lee (2001) concluded that the pooled RR for secondhand smoke exposure and lung cancer was negligibly altered after allowing for these potential dietary confounders.

In analyses of workplace secondhand smoke exposures, occupational exposures to other carcinogens may also confound this association. However, Zhong and colleagues (1999) documented that the strong association between workplace secondhand smoke exposure and lung cancer risk remained even after making additional adjustments for other occupational exposures. The comparable effects of secondhand smoke exposure from spouses and from the workplace on risk also argue against uncontrolled potential confounding as an explanation for the observed association, because the same set of confounders is unlikely to be operative for both exposure settings.

Because secondhand smoke exposure is ubiquitous, some investigators have expressed concern that exposure measurement error (or misclassification) affects estimates, particularly in studies that do not ascertain exposures outside the home. In fact, ideally, the exposure assessment would cover all environments where exposures occur so the total exposure could be estimated. Although a questionnaire remains the only feasible method for assessing these long-term exposures, some investigators have made concerted international efforts to validate and test the reliability of other instruments (Riboli et al. 1990). For example, many of the questions and approaches used in the IARC collaborative study have been adopted, modified, and used in subsequent case-control studies on secondhand smoke and lung cancer (Riboli et al. 1990). Almost all of the studies reviewed (see "Cohort Studies" earlier in this chapter), and other studies published since the 1990s, have included a comprehensive assessment of all sources of secondhand smoke exposure during childhood and adulthood. Of the more than 20 studies investigating secondhand smoke and lung cancer that included assessments of exposures at work and in social settings, most found an increased risk of lung cancer comparable to the risk associated with spousal smoking (NCI 1999; USDHHS 2001). Thus, the total risk of exposure was likely underestimated in studies that investigated only spousal smoking or single sources of exposures. The increased risk of lung cancer in relation to increased urinary cotinine levels among nonsmokers was documented in a Dutch cohort study (de Waard et al. 1995). Using a biomarker to classify past exposure, the investigators confirmed that secondhand smoke exposure is causally related to lung cancer risk among nonsmokers. Interestingly, results from this single study suggest a twofold increased risk of lung cancer among nonsmokers associated with an objective marker of exposure. The lower risk estimate associated with secondhand smoke exposure in questionnaire-based, case-control studies may be attributable to a misclassification of exposures from self-reports, although a single cotinine measurement is an imprecise measure of exposure. Overall, random misclassification of exposure in a particular environment or of an overall estimate would tend to bias estimates of risk from the true value toward the null.

A second type of misclassification error, frequently cited by tobacco industry-funded experts (Lee 1992), is potential misclassification from the claim by some current or former smokers that they are lifetime nonsmokers and that the observed increase in risk from involuntary smoking is really attributable to their former (or current) smoking. This potential bias has been repeatedly considered and found not to explain the association of lung cancer with secondhand smoke (Wu 1999). Recent studies have confirmed that the proportion of former smokers who classify themselves as lifetime nonsmokers is low (Nyberg et al. 1997). Several investigators have also demonstrated that the proportion of nonsmokers misclassified as those who had ever smoked (based on cotinine measurements) is low (Riboli et al. 1990; Wu 1999). In the only case-control study of secondhand smoke and lung cancer among reported lifetime nonsmokers that also determined urinary cotinine levels as a marker of recent exposure to tobacco smoke, 0.6 percent of cases and 2.3 percent of controls were considered to be misclassified as lifetime nonsmokers because their urinary cotinine levels exceeded the designated limit for involuntary smoking only (Fontham et al. 1994). Nyberg and colleagues (1998a) also showed that the risk of lung cancer among misclassified smokers was low. These findings are consistent with the conclusion of the NRC that smoker misclassification cannot explain the secondhand smoke effect on lung cancer risk among lifetime nonsmokers (NRC 1986). The EPA reached a similar conclusion in its risk assessment analysis (USEPA 1992).

Publication bias, or the failure to publish findings construed as "negative" or that are not statistically significant, has also been raised as a concern. For example, if the apparent association between secondhand smoke and lung cancer reflects the failure of investigators to publish negative findings from studies that do not find an increased risk associated with secondhand smoke, the omission of such unpublished findings can skew the conclusions of meta-analyses (Copas and Shi 2000). Vandenbroucke (1988) conducted a formal statistical analysis and found no evidence of a selective publication bias. Woodward and McMichael (1991) searched for unpublished data on secondhand smoke by contacting the tobacco industry and investigators listed in the *Directory of Ongoing Research in Cancer Epidemiology* and found few unpublished studies on secondhand smoke. Other investigators who reached similar conclusions reported a publication delay for studies with nonsignificant results, but with no evidence of a publication bias in the peer-reviewed literature (Bero et al. 1994; Misakian and Bero 1998). Copas and Shi (2000) again raised the question of publication bias in their analysis. They estimated that allowing for a publication bias could reduce a pooled RR of 1.25 associated with exposure to secondhand smoke and lung cancer to 1.15. However, this calculation assumes that 40 percent of all studies on lung cancer have not been published. As already mentioned, because unpublished studies have yet to be identified, this assumption is inappropriate.

This report, published 20 years after the 1986 report, again concludes that involuntary smoking causes lung cancer in lifetime nonsmokers. The evidence was judged sufficient in 1986, and there is even greater certainty now, reflecting the substantial new research published since 1986 that has reduced uncertainties related to mechanistic considerations and to methodologic issues in the epidemiologic studies. The body of epidemiologic research now includes a number of large studies that were designed specifically to limit misclassification and confounding. The estimated risk for lung cancer associated with involuntary smoking has changed little as new evidence has become available.

Conclusions

1. The evidence is sufficient to infer a causal relationship between secondhand smoke exposure and lung cancer among lifetime nonsmokers. This conclusion extends to all secondhand smoke exposure, regardless of location.

2. The pooled evidence indicates a 20 to 30 percent increase in the risk of lung cancer from secondhand smoke exposure associated with living with a smoker.

Implications

Eliminating or reducing secondhand smoke exposure at home, in the workplace, and in other public settings will reduce the risk of lung cancer among lifetime nonsmokers.

Other Cancer Sites

Active smoking is firmly established as a causal factor of cancer for a large number of sites including lung, urinary tract, upper aerodigestive tract, liver, stomach, pancreas, and many others (USDHHS 2004; Vineis et al. 2004). The absence of a threshold for carcinogenesis in active smoking (i.e., a level of smoking that does not increase the risk of cancer), the presence of the same carcinogens in mainstream and sidestream smoke, and the demonstrated uptake of tobacco smoke constituents by involuntary smokers are compelling arguments for the hypothesis that secondhand smoke would increase the risk of cancer in other smoking-related sites in nonsmokers. The role of secondhand smoke in the risk of cancers among nonsmokers has been investigated mainly for lung cancer, with considerably less data on other cancer sites. However, for some sites the evidence is now sufficient to warrant review and evaluation. The discussion that follows reviews studies on involuntary smoking and three adult cancers for which the evidence are most abundant: breast cancer, cervical cancer, and nasal sinus/nasopharyngeal cancer. The chapter covers all investigations of secondhand smoke in relation to breast cancer, a site that was also addressed in the 2001 report (USDHHS 2001).

Breast Cancer

The role of tobacco smoke in the etiology of breast cancer has been investigated in numerous epidemiologic studies since the 1960s (USDHHS 2001). Studies have addressed the risk of active smoking in current and former smokers and the risk of involuntary smoking in lifetime nonsmokers. Several recent reports have considered the evidence on active and involuntary smoking and breast cancer risk (USDHHS 2001, 2004; Cal/EPA 2005).

There is substantial evidence that active smoking is not associated with an increased risk of breast cancer in studies that compare active smokers with persons who have never smoked (Hamajima et al. 2002). In a pooled analysis of data from 53 studies, the RR for women who were current smokers versus lifetime nonsmokers was 0.99 (95 percent CI, 0.92–1.05) for 22,255 cases and 40,832 controls who reported not drinking alcohol. The effect of smoking did not vary by menopausal status.

In spite of this overall null finding, active smoking could be involved in breast cancer risk. Active smoking may have effects on breast cancer development that tend to increase and decrease risk; tissues of smokers are exposed to carcinogens but smoking has antiestrogenic effects (USDHHS 2004). Carcinogens in tobacco smoke, such as 3-4 benzo[a]pyrene, and their metabolites are distributed systemically, and many known tobacco carcinogens, including heterocyclic aromatic amines, polycyclic aromatic hydrocarbons, and arylamines, are also mammary mutagens and carcinogens (Nagao et al. 1994; Dunnick et al. 1995; El-Bayoumy et al. 1995). Convincing data document that constituents of cigarette smoke reach tissues outside of the respiratory system, including the breast. For example, mutagens from cigarette smoke have been found in nipple aspirates of nonlactating female smokers, and nicotine levels in breast fluid tend to increase with the daily amount smoked (Petrakis et al. 1978, 1988). Aromatic DNA adducts that are characteristic of tobacco smoke exposure have been found in normal breast tissues of breast cancer patients but not in healthy women without cancer (Li et al. 1996).

However, tobacco smoking also has antiestrogenic consequences; it is consistently associated with an earlier age at menopause and a lower risk of endometrial cancer (USDHHS 2001, 2004). Smokers have lower urinary estrogen levels (MacMahon et al. 1982) and increased estradiol 2-hydroxylation, resulting in less urinary excretion of estriol relative to estrone in smokers compared with nonsmokers (Michnovicz et al. 1986). However, uncertainty remains concerning the influence of tobacco smoke on blood estrogen levels, and the evidence is not consistent (Key et al. 1991, 1996; Terry and Rohan 2002). Nonetheless, the information on smoking and hormones has led to the hypothesis that the antiestrogenic effects of active smoking, but not of involuntary smoking, may obscure an increase in breast cancer risk that would otherwise result from the carcinogens in tobacco smoke. Thus, researchers have hypothesized that the dual carcinogenic and antiestrogenic effects of tobacco smoking may counteract and potentially balance influences on breast cancer risk (Palmer and Rosenberg 1993).

When considering the biologic plausibility of a causal association of secondhand smoke exposure with breast cancer, the evidence on active smoking is critical. The absence of an established and consistent relationship between active smoking and breast cancer in epidemiologic studies weakens the biologic plausibility of a possible causal association of involuntary smoking with breast cancer. Other conditions caused by secondhand smoke exposure, such as lung cancer and coronary heart disease (CHD), are strongly and causally related to active smoking. Evidence on the association between active smoking and breast cancer risk was reviewed thoroughly in the Surgeon General's reports of 2001 and 2004 (USDHHS 2001, 2004). The reports addressed both the biologic basis for a possible association and the findings of epidemiologic studies. These reviews considered large, well-designed studies published in the 1990s that investigated risk patterns among various meaningful subgroups and carefully considered the role of potential confounders. These reports concluded that the weight of epidemiologic evidence strongly suggests that active smoking is not causally related to breast cancer risk. A similar conclusion was reached by IARC in its 2004 monograph on smoking (IARC 2004). Possibly, the dose-response relationship for tobacco smoke and breast cancer might be complex and nonlinear, such that the doses associated with secondhand smoke cause breast cancer and the far greater doses from active smoking do not. There is neither mechanistic nor empiric evidence supporting this possibility.

The absence of a net increase in breast cancer risk among active, female smokers does not exclude the possibility that certain subgroups of women may be at an increased risk because of genetic or other factors. However, such groups have yet to be consistently identified (USDHHS 2004). Studies continue on active smoking and breast cancer risk. There are recent reports of elevated RRs in smokers in some recent studies, notably in two large prospective cohort studies. In the Nurses Health Study II (NHS-II) cohort of young women (aged 25 through 42 years at the time of enrollment), there was an association between 20 or more years of active smoking and a significant 21 percent increase in risk (Al-Delaimy et al. 2004). In the California Teachers Study, current smokers showed a statistically significant increase in risk of 30 percent compared with lifetime nonsmokers (Reynolds et al. 2004). Nonetheless, sufficient evidence has not accumulated since 2004 to suggest that the conclusions of the Surgeon General's report and the IARC monograph should be revised, and the possibility of selective reporting of positive associations for active smoking needs to be considered when interpreting these recent reports.

Since the 1980s, studies have also examined the relationship between secondhand smoke exposure and breast cancer risk. One of the first reports was based on Hirayama's (1984) cohort study in Japan—the same cohort that provided evidence on involuntary smoking and lung cancer. Horton (1988) hypothesized a role for secondhand smoke in the etiology of breast cancer on the basis that countries with high male mortality rates of lung cancer generally had high rates of breast cancer, and countries with low rates of lung cancer had low rates of breast cancer. Another ecologic study that investigated the relationship between female breast cancer and male lung cancer in five countries found little support for this hypothesis (Williams and Lloyd 1989). Substantial data from cohort and case-control studies that directly address the hypothesis have now been published. Seven prospective cohort studies (Hirayama 1984; Jee et al. 1999; Wartenberg et al. 2000; Nishino et al. 2001; Egan et al. 2002; Reynolds et al. 2004; Hanaoka et al. 2005) and 14 case-control studies (Sandler et al. 1985a,b; Smith et al. 1994; Morabia et al. 1996, 2000; Millikan et al. 1998; Lash and Aschengrau 1999, 2002; Zhao et al. 1999; Delfino et al. 2000; Johnson et al. 2000; Liu et al. 2000; Kropp and Chang-Claude 2002; Gammon et al. 2004; Shrubsole et al. 2004; Bonner 2005) offer information on secondhand smoke and breast cancer. Several reports described findings using different measures of secondhand smoke exposure and breast cancer risk (Hirayama 1984; Wells 1991; Sandler et al. 1985a,b; Morabia et al. 1996, 2000; Millikan et al. 1998; Marcus et al. 2000). As for secondhand smoke and lung cancer, studies of breast cancer should include a comprehensive assessment of lifetime secondhand smoke exposure and adequate controls for potential confounders. However, the approaches to exposure assessment vary among the studies, and consideration of confounding has also been variable.

Several reports have evaluated the evidence on secondhand smoke exposure and breast cancer risk. The 1986 IARC monograph commented on the general issue of causation of cancer by secondhand smoke: "It is unlikely that any effects will be produced in passive smokers that are not produced to a greater extent in smokers and that types of effects that are not seen in smokers will not be seen in passive smokers" (IARC 1986, p. 314). The IARC monograph on involuntary smoking, published in 2004, concluded that the evidence did not support a causal association between breast cancer and secondhand smoke (IARC 2004). The 2001 Surgeon General's report also addressed the topic. The report considered cohort and case-control studies on involuntary smoking and breast cancer and found that the issue had not been "resolved" (USDHHS 2001, p. 217). Most recently, the 2005 report of the California EPA (Cal/EPA) found the evidence to be conclusive for secondhand smoke as a cause of premenopausal breast cancer (Cal/EPA 2005).

The following section describes the prospective cohort and case-control studies on involuntary smoking and breast cancer. Whenever available, results on active smoking and breast cancer in the same study population are shown so the findings on involuntary and active smoking can be compared.

Prospective Cohort Studies

There are seven published prospective cohort studies on secondhand smoke exposure and the risk of breast cancer among lifetime nonsmoking women (Table 7.8) (Hirayama 1984; Wells 1991; Jee et al. 1999; Wartenberg et al. 2000; Nishino et al. 2001; Egan et al. 2002; Reynolds et al. 2004; Hanaoka et al. 2005). In these studies, exposure was classified based on information collected at the start of follow-up. Because this information was not updated in most of the studies, exposure misclassification may have increased as duration of the follow-up lengthened and the exposure status of the participants changed. Some studies only assessed spousal smoking; other studies covered additional sources of exposure, including during childhood. Secondhand smoke exposure was not significantly associated with breast cancer risk in these studies, although two studies did find increased point estimates of RR (Hirayama 1984; Jee et al. 1999), and a third study found an increased risk in premenopausal women (Hanaoka et al. 2005).

Hirayama (1984) published the first report based on a population-based, prospective cohort in Japan. Active and involuntary smoking statuses were based on information supplied on enrollment and were not updated. After 15 years of follow-up, this study identified 115 breast cancer deaths among women who had never smoked. Lifetime nonsmoking women whose husbands smoked had an increase in the RR compared with women married to nonsmokers (RR = 1.26 [95 percent CI, 0.8–2.0]) (Table 7.8). In a further analysis of this data set, Wells (1991) reported that the increased risk associated with the husband's smoking was more marked among women who were younger than 60 years of age. The effect of active smoking on breast cancer risk was similar to that of involuntary smoking (RR = 1.28 [95 percent CI, 0.93–1.73]).

A similar increase in risk of breast cancer associated with the husband's smoking was reported

in a Korean cohort study (Jee et al. 1999) (see "Lung Cancer" earlier in this chapter). During three and one-half years of follow-up, 138 women with breast cancer were identified. The exposure status was fixed based on baseline information. The risks of breast cancer were 1.2 (95 percent CI, 0.8–1.8) for nonsmoking women married to former smokers and 1.3 (95 percent CI, 0.9–1.8) for nonsmoking women married to current smokers compared with nonsmoking women married to nonsmokers. These investigators reported that the RR increased significantly with the duration of the husband's smoking (>30 years), but details were not provided. Information on active smoking and breast cancer risk was also not reported in this study, but smoking by women in Korea is still uncommon (Jee et al. 1999, 2004).

The relationship between secondhand smoke and breast cancer was investigated in the Japan Public Health Center (JPHC)-based prospective cohort study of 21,805 middle-aged women of whom 20,169 were lifetime nonsmokers (Hanaoka et al. 2005). Participants completed a self-administered questionnaire and provided information about exposure to secondhand smoke at home before and after 20 years of age. For exposure outside the home, such as at work and other settings, participants were asked about exposures of at least one hour per day, including the frequency of exposure (e.g., almost never, one to three days per month, one to four days per week, almost every day). During the nine years of follow-up, this information was not updated. After the nine years, the investigators identified 180 breast cancers; 162 occurred in lifetime nonsmokers (Table 7.8). Compared with lifetime nonsmokers who were not exposed to secondhand smoke, women who were exposed did not show a significant increase in the RR (adjusted RR = 1.1 [95 percent CI, 0.8–1.6]). The RR was 1.0 (95 percent CI, 0.7–1.4) for exposure at home and 1.3 (95 percent CI, 0.9–1.9) for exposure outside of the home (i.e., occupational and/or public exposure). However, risk patterns differed by menopausal status. Secondhand smoke exposure (residential or occupational) was not associated with breast cancer risk in postmenopausal women (n = 83) (adjusted RR = 0.7 [95 percent CI, 0.4–1.0]) but it was associated with an increased RR in premenopausal women (n = 77) (adjusted RR = 2.6 [95 percent CI, 1.3–5.2]). Exposures at home (adjusted RR = 1.6 [95 percent CI, 0.9–2.7]) and outside of the home (adjusted RR = 2.3 [95 percent CI, 1.4–3.8]) were both associated with risk in premenopausal women. Active smoking was associated with an increased risk in this study population. The RR of breast cancer among current smokers was 1.9 (95 percent CI, 1.0–3.6) compared with lifetime nonsmokers without secondhand smoke exposure. Researchers found an association between active smoking and breast cancer only in premenopausal women (adjusted RR = 3.9 [95 percent CI, 1.5–9.9]) and not in postmenopausal women (adjusted RR = 1.1 [95 percent CI, 0.5–2.5]).

This study included a comprehensive assessment of secondhand smoke exposure. Childhood exposures were not explored, but both residential and workplace exposures were considered. There were differences in the profiles of breast cancer risk factors across the smoking exposure groups, but these profiles were not explored by menopausal status. However, the estimates of breast cancer risk associated with active and involuntary smoking were adjusted for these factors.

In contrast, secondhand smoke exposure was not associated with breast cancer risk in four other cohort studies, including another study conducted in Japan (Nishino et al. 2001) and three in the United States (Wartenberg et al. 2000; Egan et al. 2002; Reynolds et al. 2004). The third Japanese cohort study was conducted in Miyagi Prefecture (see "Lung Cancer" earlier in this chapter). During nine years of follow-up, Nishino and colleagues (2001) identified 67 women with breast cancer. The age-adjusted RR for breast cancer was 0.58 (95 percent CI, 0.34–0.99) for women whose husbands were smokers at baseline compared with women married to nonsmokers. The reduced risk in association with the husbands' smoking was unchanged but no longer statistically significant after further adjustment for reproductive history and lifestyle factors (multivariate-adjusted RR = 0.58 [95 percent CI, 0.32–1.11]) (Table 7.8) (Nishino et al. 2001). Smoking by other household members was also not associated with breast cancer risk in this same population (multivariate-adjusted RR = 0.81 [95 percent CI, 0.44–1.5]); an association between active smoking and breast cancer risk was not reported.

Studies also investigated the relationship between secondhand smoke and breast cancer risk in a group of women in the American Cancer Society's (ACS's) Cancer Prevention Study II (CPS-II) cohort; this study included 146,488 lifetime nonsmoking women who were married only once and who were free of cancer when they entered the study in 1982 (Wartenberg et al. 2000). Exposures classified at baseline were based on index participant and spousal reports and were considered to be fixed. Breast cancer mortal-

ity, not incidence, was the outcome measure in this study. Mortality from breast cancer reflects not only incidence, but factors determining survival. A total of 669 women who had died of breast cancer were identified after 12 years of follow-up. All of the RRs associated with different categories of secondhand smoke exposure, including husbands' current and former smoking patterns, tobacco products used, number of years and pack-years[1], and timing of the exposure, were close to unity with or without adjustment for numerous dietary and nondietary covariates. Compared with lifetime nonsmokers married to nonsmokers, lifetime nonsmokers whose husbands were current smokers (adjusted RR =1.0 [95 percent CI, 0.8–1.2]) or former smokers (adjusted RR = 1.0 [95 percent CI, 0.8–1.2]) did not have increased risks (Table 7.8). The RR for breast cancer was not significantly associated with secondhand smoke exposures at home (RR = 1.1 [95 percent CI, 0.9–1.3]), at work (RR = 0.8 [95 percent CI, 0.6–1.0]), or in other places (RR = 0.9 [95 percent CI, 0.7–1.2]). Exposures from all sources combined were also not associated with breast cancer mortality (RR = 1.0 [95 percent CI, 0.8–1.2]). The only observed elevated risk was among women who were younger than 20 years of age when they married smokers (RR = 1.2 [95 percent CI, 0.8–1.8]). Using the results from six years of follow-up of CPS-II participants, Calle and colleagues (1994) observed that current active smoking was associated with an increased risk for breast cancer mortality. Women who were current smokers at baseline showed an increased risk (RR = 1.26 [95 percent CI, 1.05–1.50]) compared with lifetime nonsmokers, but the RR did not increase among former smokers (RR = 0.85 [95 percent CI, 0.70–1.03]).

Using data from the NHS, Egan and colleagues (2002) investigated the relationship between secondhand smoke exposure and breast cancer risk. Persons who were eligible (n = 78,206) for participation in the study included women who responded to the baseline and subsequent questionnaires that assessed dietary habits and secondhand smoke exposures, including childhood and current adult exposures at home, at work, and in other settings, as well as other factors. Involuntary smoking was assessed at only one time point (1982), while other information on other risk factors was updated every two years. After 14 years of follow-up, the investigators identified 3,140 women with invasive breast cancer, of whom 1,359 were lifetime nonsmokers (Table 7.8) (Egan et

---

[1]Pack-years = The number of years of smoking multiplied by the number of packs of cigarettes smoked per day.

Table 7.8 Cohort studies of associations between exposures to secondhand smoke and the relative risks for breast cancer incidence and mortality among women who had never smoked

Study	Population/follow-up	Number of breast cancer events	Data collection
Hirayama 1984 Wells 1991	91,540 wives who had never smoked 6 prefectures in Japan 16 years	115 breast cancer deaths	Brief in-person interview at the time of study enrollment
Jee et al. 1999	157,436 married women who had never smoked Health insurance subscribers Korea 3.5 years	138 (incident and prevalent cases)	Husbands of women who had never smoked completed medical exams and questionnaires on active smoking in 1992 and 1994 Women who had never smoked completed questionnaires in 1993
Wartenberg et al. 2000	146,488 single-marriage women who had never smoked American Cancer Society 12 years	669 breast cancer deaths	Secondhand smoke questions were based on active smoking histories reported by spouses Women reported the number of hours per day they were exposed to the smoke of others at home, at work, and in other settings
Nishino et al. 2001	9,675 women who had never smoked Aged ≥40 years Miyagi Prefecture (Japan) 9 years	67 incident cases	Self-completed questionnaires on lifestyle habits Secondhand smoke questions asked about smokers in the household and, if so, whether husband, father, mother, children, or other household members smoked
Egan et al. 2002	78,206 women (35,193 who had never smoked, 22,258 former smokers, 20,755 current smokers) Nurses Health Study United States 14 years	3,140 invasive breast cancer (1,359 lifetime nonsmokers)	Completed a 1976 baseline questionnaire on reproductive factors and active smoking, and follow-up questionnaires every 2 years The 1980 and 1982 questionnaires asked about diet and secondhand smoke exposure

Findings	Measure of secondhand smoke	Relative risk (95% confidence interval)	Comments

• Effect of secondhand smoke was similar to the effect of active smoking	Husband's smoking:
	    Lifetime nonsmoker
	    Ever smoked
		
		1.0
		1.26 (0.8–2.0)
			Controlled for age

• Risk increased significantly with duration of husband's smoking (>30 years)	Husband's smoking:
	    Lifetime nonsmoker
	    Former smoker
	    Current smoker
		
		1.0
		1.2 (0.8–1.8)
		1.3 (0.9–1.8)
			Controlled for age of husbands and wives, social class, residence, and husband's vegetable intake and occupation; data on duration of smoking were not reported; analyses included incident and prevalent cases

• No increased risk with any source of secondhand smoke exposure
• No dose-response relationships
• Current active smokers showed an increase in risk but former smokers did not
	Husband's smoking:
	    Lifetime nonsmoker
	    Former smoker
	    Current smoker
	Duration of smoking (years):
	    None
	    1–10
	    11–20
	    21–30
	    ≥31
		
		1.0
		1.0 (0.8–1.2)
		1.0 (0.8–1.2)
		
		1.0
		0.8 (0.6–1.2)
		0.7 (0.5–1.0)
		1.0 (0.7–1.3)
		1.1 (0.9–1.4)
			Controlled for age, race, education, family history, age at first live birth, age at menarche, menopause, number of spontaneous abortions, use of oral contraceptives and hormone replacement therapy, body size, history of breast cysts, alcohol use, intake of dietary fat and vegetables, and the occupation of the wife and her spouse; there were no changes in results with or without adjustments

• Inverse association between risk and secondhand smoke exposure based on the smoking habits of the husband and other household members
• No active smoking data
	Husband's:
	    Nonsmoker
	    Smoker
	Other household members:
	    Nonsmoker
	    Smoker
		
		1.0
		0.58 (0.32–1.1)
		
		1.0
		0.81 (0.44–1.5)
			Controlled for age; study area; alcohol, fruit, and green/yellow vegetable intake; age at first birth; number of live births; age at menarche; and body mass index (BMI)

• No association with any sources of secondhand smoke exposure—results were similar in premenopausal and postmenopausal women
• Very weak association with active smoking
	Parental smoking:
	    Neither
	    Mother only
	    Father only
	    Both parents
	Current home/work secondhand smoke exposure:
	    None
	    Occasional
	    Regular (home or work)
	    Regular (home and work)
		
		1.0
		0.98 (0.70–1.38)
		1.12 (0.99–1.27)
		0.92 (0.76–1.13)
		
		1.0
		1.16 (0.98–1.36)
		1.0 (0.83–1.20)
		0.90 (0.67–1.22)
			Controlled for age, age at menarche, age at first birth and parity, history of benign breast disease, family history of breast cancer, menopausal status, age at menopause, weight at 18 years of age, adult weight change, adult height, alcohol use, total carotenoid intake, and use of menopausal hormones

Table 7.8   Continued

Study	Population/follow-up	Number of breast cancer events	Data collection
Reynolds et al. 2004	76,189 lifetime nonsmokers from the California Teachers Study Cohort 5 years	1,150 incident breast cancer	Self-administered questionnaire at the time of study enrollment to determine household secondhand smoke exposure during childhood and adulthood
Hanaoka et al. 2005*	20,169 women who had never smoked* Recruited from 4 public health centers in Japan Japan Public Health Center Cohort Aged 40–59 years 9 years	162 incident breast cancer	Self-administered questionnaire at the time of study enrollment to determine household secondhand smoke exposure before and after 20 years of age; exposure at the workplace and in other settings (≥1 hour/day) and frequency of exposure

*The number 20,169 was listed in Table 1 of this paper. However, the number of lifetime nonsmokers in Table 2 added up to 20,193. (It is unclear why the numbers in the two tables differ.)

al. 2002). Almost all estimated RRs associated with childhood and adulthood secondhand smoke exposures were close to 1.0. The estimates were unchanged with and without adjustment for a large number of covariates. There was a small increase in the RR associated with paternal smoking (adjusted RR = 1.12 [95 percent CI, 0.99–1.27]) but not with maternal smoking (adjusted RR = 0.98 [95 percent CI, 0.70–1.38]) (Table 7.8). Current secondhand smoke exposures were also unrelated to risk; the RR was 1.0 (95 percent CI, 0.83–1.20) in association with regular secondhand smoke exposure at home or at work and 0.90 (95 percent CI, 0.67–1.22) for regular exposures in both settings (Table 7.8). Similarly, the investigators found no evidence that long-term adult exposures to household smoke increased breast cancer risk (p for trend = 0.87); the RR for living with a smoker as an adult for 30 or

more years was 1.03 (95 percent CI, 0.86–1.24). The RR of breast cancer among women with the highest levels of secondhand smoke exposure as adults was similar to that of women who reported no current exposure to secondhand smoke (RR = 1.01 [95 percent CI, 0.80–1.29]). The results were similar in premenopausal and postmenopausal women. Active smoking was weakly associated with a risk of breast cancer in this study. Compared with lifetime nonsmokers, Egan and colleagues (2002) reported that the RR of breast cancer was 1.04 (95 percent CI, 0.94–1.15) among current smokers and 1.09 (95 percent CI, 1.00–1.18) among former smokers. A modest increase in the RR was confined to women who initiated active smoking before 17 years of age (RR = 1.19 [95 percent CI, 1.03–1.37]). This large prospective study assessed childhood and adulthood household and workplace secondhand

Findings	Measure of secondhand smoke	Relative risk (95% confidence interval)	Comments

• No significant positive association between breast cancer risk and secondhand smoke exposure during childhood and/or adulthood
• Results were similar in premenopausal, perimenopausal, and postmenopausal women
	Household:
	  Never exposed
	  Childhood only
	  Adulthood only
	  Childhood and adulthood
		
		1.0
		0.92 (0.78–1.07)
		0.94 (0.79–1.12)
		0.93 (0.79–1.09)
			Controlled for age, race, family history of breast cancer, age at menarche, parity, age at first full-term pregnancy, physical activity, alcohol use, BMI, menopausal status, and use of hormone therapy

• No significant positive association between household and/or workplace exposure and breast cancer risk in all participants combined
• Household and workplace exposures were associated with a significantly increased risk in premenopausal women; a reduced risk in postmenopausal women was nonsignificant
	All participants
	Household/work:
	  No
	  Household
	  Workplace
	
	Premenopausal:
	  No
	  Household
	  Workplace
	
	Postmenopausal:
	  No
	  Household
	  Workplace
		
		1.0
		1.0 (0.7–1.4)
		1.3 (0.9–1.9)
		
		1.0
		1.6 (0.9–2.7)
		2.3 (1.4–3.8)
		
		1.0
		0.7 (0.4–1.1)
		0.4 (0.2–1.0)
			Controlled for study area, age, employment status, education, BMI, family history of breast cancer, parity, age at menarche, alcohol intake, menopausal status (in a combined analysis), history of benign breast disease, and hormone use

smoke exposures. Almost all of the risk estimates associated with adulthood exposure were near unity, regardless of the duration of exposure.

The relationship between secondhand smoke and breast cancer risk was investigated in the California Teachers Study, which included 116,544 women who had no personal history of breast cancer and who completed a baseline questionnaire in 1995 to determine their active and involuntary smoking status (Reynolds et al. 2004). That analysis was limited to the 77,708 members who were lifetime nonsmokers (i.e., smoked fewer than 100 cigarettes during their lifetime) and who responded to questions on household secondhand smoke that covered both childhood and adulthood. A total of 1,150 breast cancers were identified in lifetime nonsmokers after five years of follow-up. Lifetime nonsmokers were categorized

as unexposed, only exposed during childhood, only exposed during adulthood, or exposed during both childhood and adulthood. All of the RRs associated with secondhand smoke exposure were close to unity after adjustment for various reproductive factors and nondietary covariates. The RR of breast cancer was 0.92 (95 percent CI, 0.78–1.07) among women with only childhood household secondhand smoke exposure, 0.94 (95 percent CI, 0.79–1.12) among women with only adulthood household secondhand smoke exposure, and 0.93 (95 percent CI, 0.79–1.09) among women with both exposures compared with unexposed lifetime nonsmokers. Results were very similar for premenopausal/perimenopausal (n = 254) and postmenopausal (n = 778) women (Table 7.8). In contrast, active smoking was associated with breast cancer risk. Compared with lifetime nonsmokers with no secondhand smoke exposure, the RR of breast cancer was 1.03 (95 percent CI, 0.89–1.18) among former smokers and 1.25 (95 percent CI, 1.02–1.53) among current smokers. However, the increased risk among current smokers was restricted to women who were postmenopausal at baseline (adjusted RR = 1.21 [95 percent CI, 0.95–1.54]) and was not observed among women who were premenopausal or peri-menopausal at baseline (adjusted RR = 0.96 [95 percent CI, 0.55–1.68]). One limitation of this large, prospective cohort study is that information on work place secondhand smoke exposure was not assessed. In addition, this analysis was limited to relatively crude measures of childhood and adulthood house-hold secondhand smoke exposures.

Case-Control Studies

Fourteen case-control studies have investigated the association between secondhand smoke exposure and a risk of breast cancer among lifetime nonsmokers. These studies were conducted in the United Kingdom (Smith et al. 1994), Switzerland (Morabia et al. 1996, 2000), Germany (Kropp and Chang-Claude 2002), the United States (Sandler et al. 1985a; Millikan et al. 1998; Lash and Aschengrau 1999, 2002; Delfino et al. 2000; Marcus et al. 2000; Gammon et al. 2004; Bonner et al. 2005), Canada (Johnson et al. 2000), and China (Zhao 1999; Liu et al. 2000; Shrubsole et al. 2004) (Table 7.9).

The first study that included data on secondhand smoke exposures during childhood and adulthood and the risk of breast cancer among lifetime non-smokers was a hospital-based, multicancer site study conducted in North Carolina (Sandler et al. 1985a). The analysis on adult secondhand smoke exposures was based on 59 breast cancer cases and 330 controls; 32 cases and 178 controls were nonsmokers. Second-hand smoke exposure based on the husbands' smoking was associated with an increased RR of breast cancer among nonsmokers (OR = 2.0 [95 percent CI, 0.9–4.3]) (Sandler et al. 1985a). The risk of breast cancer in relation to secondhand smoke exposure during childhood was investigated using a slightly smaller set of participants (52 breast cancer cases, 312 controls) (Sandler et al. 1985b). The risk of breast cancer among nonsmokers was not associated with maternal (OR = 0.9) or paternal (OR = 0.9) smoking. On the basis that 27 out of 59 breast cancer patients and 152 out of 330 controls were active smokers, the crude OR for active smoking calculated in one report was

1.0 (Sandler et al. 1985b). Methodologic limitations of the study included the use of a control group of friends and acquaintances with no adjustment for reproductive factors (only age, race, and education were considered), and the small number of nonsmokers among the breast cancer cases.

A second study on this topic was conducted as part of the United Kingdom National Case-Control Study Group, which was originally designed to investigate the relationship between oral contraceptive use and breast cancer risk in young women (Smith et al. 1994). Although the original study (755 case-control pairs) was not designed to evaluate the role of second-hand smoke, Smith and colleagues (1994) were able to successfully recontact approximately one-third of the participants (208 cases with breast cancer and 201 healthy controls) who completed a questionnaire on exposures to secondhand smoke during childhood and adulthood (partner/spouse, cohabitant, work-place). Complete data for 204 cases and 199 controls from the original 755 pairs were available for the exposure analysis. The association between second-hand smoke exposure and breast cancer risk was investigated among nonsmokers (94 cases, 99 controls) after controlling for various potential confounders. The investigators estimated an associated OR of 1.32 (95 percent CI, 0.16–10.8) for childhood exposure only, 3.13 (95 percent CI, 0.73–13.31) for adulthood exposure only, and 2.63 (95 percent CI, 0.73–9.44) for both time periods combined compared with unexposed nonsmokers (Table 7.9) (Smith et al. 1994). There was no evidence of an exposure-response relationship with cigarette-years[2] of exposure during childhood, from partners in adulthood, or at work. In the parent case-control study, active smoking was not associated with a risk of breast cancer (adjusted OR = 1.01 [95 percent CI, 0.81–1.26]) (Smith et al. 1994).

Morabia and colleagues conducted a study of secondhand smoke and breast cancer risk in Switzerland (Morabia et al. 1996; USDHHS 2001). The study included 244 women with breast cancer (cases) and 1,032 healthy controls from the general population, of whom 126 cases and 620 controls were lifetime non-smokers (Table 7.9). The data collection attempted a complete assessment of active smoking and secondhand smoke exposure. Specifically, active smoking and secondhand smoke exposure histories were recorded year by year from 10 years of age to the date of the interview. Those who were classified as active smokers were women who had smoked at least

---

[2]Cigarette-years = The number of years of smoking multiplied by the number of cigarettes smoked per day.

100 cigarettes in their lifetime; those who had smoked regularly during the two years before the study interview were categorized as current smokers. Secondhand smoke exposure was defined as an exposure lasting at least one hour per day during one year or more either at home, at work, or during leisure time (Morabia et al. 1996).

This study showed that several measures of secondhand smoke exposure were associated with at least a doubling of breast cancer risk after adjusting for relevant covariates. Morabia and colleagues (1996) found that compared with lifetime nonsmokers who had never been exposed to secondhand smoke in this classification approach (28 cases, 241 controls), nonsmokers with exposure from spousal smoking (adjusted OR = 2.6 [95 percent CI, 1.6–4.3]) or from all sources combined including at home, at work, or during leisure time (adjusted OR = 2.3 [95 percent CI, 1.5–3.7]) had an increased risk of breast cancer. However, there was little difference in risk between those with high exposures (>50 hours per day-years[3] adjusted OR = 2.5 [95 percent CI, 1.5–4.2]) and those with lower exposures (1 to 50 hours per day-years adjusted OR = 2.2 [95 percent CI, 1.3–3.7]). The RRs associated with active smoking were stronger than those associated with secondhand smoke when lifetime nonsmokers with no secondhand smoke exposure served as the baseline comparison group: for active smokers, the ORs were 2.4 (1 to 9 cigarettes per day), 3.6 (10 to 19 cigarettes per day), and 3.7 (≥20 cigarettes per day, p trend = 0.09).

Using this parental case-control study, Morabia and colleagues (2000) conducted a substudy to investigate whether the *N-acetyltransferase 2* (*NAT2*) genotype influenced the effects of smoking on breast cancer risk. The investigators hypothesized that the association between secondhand smoke and breast cancer would be modified by the *NAT2* genotype, which some studies of active smoking have found to be associated with cancer risk. Researchers contacted cases and a subset of controls who were still alive in 1996–1997 (n = 205) and asked them to provide a buccal cell swab for DNA analysis. Data were available on active smoking, secondhand smoke exposure, and the *NAT2* genotyping for 160 cases and 162 controls (Morabia et al. 2000).

Morabia and colleagues (2000) showed that, compared with lifetime nonsmokers with no exposure to secondhand smoke, lifetime nonsmokers exposed to secondhand smoke had an increased risk of breast cancer regardless of the *NAT2* genotype. The OR was 1.9 (95 percent CI, 0.7–4.6) for persons with the *NAT2* slow acetylation genotype and 5.9 (95 percent CI, 2.0–17.4) for those with the *NAT2* fast acetylation genotype. Compared with unexposed lifetime nonsmokers, current active smokers with the *NAT2* slow acetylator genotype had an OR of 2.7 (95 percent CI, 1.1–6.6), and those with the fast genotype had an OR of 4.2 (95 percent CI, 1.5–12.0). The researchers interpreted these findings as supportive of a role for secondhand smoke in causing breast cancer because the increased risks associated with both active smoking and secondhand smoke exposure were more apparent among *NAT2* fast acetylators. However, the evidence that the *NAT2* genotype influences breast cancer risk among active smokers is weak. Although one small study suggested an increased risk of breast cancer among women who were both active smokers and slow *NAT2* acetylators (Ambrosone et al. 1996), this finding has not been confirmed in subsequent, larger studies (Hunter et al. 1997, 1998; Millikan et al. 1998).

Lash and Aschengrau (1999) investigated the role of secondhand smoke and breast cancer using a population-based case-control study that was originally designed to evaluate the role of various environmental contaminants on the risk of multiple cancers, including breast cancer (Aschengrau et al. 1996). A total of 265 women with breast cancer and 765 controls were included in the study that investigated an association between active and involuntary smoking and breast cancer risk (Lash and Aschengrau 1999). Of the parental study participants, 120 cases and 406 controls were lifetime nonsmokers.

Cases and controls were categorized by their active cigarette smoking history and, among lifetime nonsmokers, by residential secondhand smoke exposure with consideration of age at first exposure (secondhand smoke exposures outside of the home were not assessed). Compared with lifetime nonsmokers who reported no secondhand smoke exposure (40 cases, 139 controls), those with any secondhand smoke exposure had a significantly increased risk of breast cancer (adjusted OR = 2.0 [95 percent CI, 1.1–3.7]) (Table 7.9) (Lash and Aschengrau 1999). Risk did not increase with an increase in the duration of exposure (adjusted OR = 3.2 [95 percent CI, 1.5–7.1] for 1 to 20 years and 2.1 [95 percent CI, 1.0–4.1] for

---

[3]Day-years = The sum of hours per day exposed to secondhand smoke multiplied by the number of years of all episodes of secondhand smoke exposure, whether at home, at work, or during leisure time.

Table 7.9 Case-control studies of the association between exposures to secondhand smoke and relative risks for breast cancer incidence and mortality among women who had never smoked

Study	Population	Cases	Controls	Data collection
Sandler et al. 1985a	Hospital based Aged 15 and 59 years United States (North Carolina) 1979–1981	59 32 lifetime nonsmokers	330 friends or from telephone lists 178 lifetime nonsmokers	Mailed questionnaire
Smith et al. 1994	Aged ≥36 years Only 3 out of 11 health regions were included in the study United Kingdom 1982–1985	204 94 lifetime nonsmokers	199 99 lifetime nonsmokers	In-person interview for all lifestyle factors; mailed questionnaire on secondhand smoke exposure
Morabia et al. 1996	Population-based Aged 30–74 years Resident of Geneva in Switzerland 1992–1993	244 126 lifetime nonsmokers	1,032 620 lifetime nonsmokers	In-person interview, detailed lifetime history on active smoking and secondhand smoke exposure
Millikan et al. 1998	Population-based registry Aged 20–74 years United States (North Carolina) Included only persons enrolled between 1993 and 1996 who granted home interviews and gave blood samples	498 248 lifetime nonsmokers	473 253 lifetime nonsmokers (sources were drivers' licenses or HCFA[+])	In-person interviews Classified as exposed if the participant was >18 years of age when living with a smoker
Lash and Aschengrau 1999	State cancer registry 5 Massachusetts towns United States 1983–1986	265 120 lifetime nonsmokers	765 406 lifetime nonsmokers 3 sources: RDD[Δ], HCFA, and deceased	Mix of in-person and telephone interviews 33% of cases and 45% of controls were interviews with next of kin

Findings	Measure of secondhand smoke	Relative risk (95% confidence interval)	Comments

• Husband's smoking increased the risk; stronger among premenopausal women
• No association with parental smoking
• No association with active smoking
	Husband smoked:
	  No
	  Yes
		
		1.0
		2.0 (0.9–4.3)
			Controlled for age, race, and education

• Partner's and workplace smoking were associated with increased risk
• No exposure-response relationship
• No association with active smoking
	Partner (cigarette-years*):
	  None
	  ≥1
	Workplace exposure (duration):
	  None
	  1–5 years
	  ≥6 years
	Exposure by period:
	  None
	  Childhood only
	  Adulthood only
	  Childhood plus adulthood
		
		1.0
		1.58 (0.81–3.10)
		
		1.0
		1.66 (0.72–3.83)
		1.35 (0.59–3.07)
		
		1.0
		1.32 (0.16–10.8)
		3.13 (0.73–13.3)
		2.63 (0.73–9.4)
			Controlled for age (<32 years and ≥32 years), region, menstrual and reproductive factors, family history, biopsy for breast disease, and alcohol intake; role of secondhand smoke was studied in a subset of the total number of cases (n = 755) and controls (n = 755)

• Increased risk associated with husband's smoking
• Risk estimates were very similar to those for all sources of secondhand smoke
• Little difference in risk from intensity of exposure
	None
	All sources
	Hours/day/years+ (all sources):
	  1–50
	  >50
		1.0
		2.3 (1.5–3.7)
		
		2.2 (1.3–3.7)
		2.5 (1.5–4.2)
			Controlled for age, education, body mass index (BMI), age at menarche, age at first live birth, oral contraceptive use, family history of breast cancer, and history of a breast biopsy

• This analysis was based on secondhand smoke exposures occurring after 18 years of age
• No association with active smoking
• No association with N-acetyltransferase (NAT) 1 or NAT2 genotype and risk
	All lifetime nonsmokers:
	  No exposure
	  Exposed
	By menopausal status:
	  Premenopausal
	    No
	    Yes
	  Postmenopausal
	    No
	    Yes
		
		1.0
		1.3 (0.9–1.9)
		
		1.0
		1.5 (0.8–2.8)
		
		1.0
		1.2 (0.7–2.2)
			Controlled for age, race, age at menarche, AFTP§, parity, family history, benign breast biopsy, and alcohol intake; 889 cases and 841 controls were interviewed, but this analysis included only those who also gave blood samples

• Risk associated with any secondhand smoke exposure was as strong or stronger than the association with active smoking	Residential exposure:
	  Never
	  Any
	By duration (years):
	  ≤20
	  >20
		
		1.0
		2.0 (1.1–3.7)
		
		3.2 (1.5–7.1)
		2.1 (1.0–4.1)
			Controlled for age, BMI, family history of breast cancer, history of breast cancer other than the index diagnosis and history of radiation therapy, parity, and history of benign breast disease; the number of cases with previous breast cancer and the number of cases/controls with previous cancer and radiation therapy were not specified

Table 7.9   Continued

Study	Population	Cases	Controls	Data collection
Zhao et al. 1999	Hospital-based Aged 26–82 years Clinical diagnosis of breast cancer China (Chengdu) 1994–1997	265 265 nonsmokers	265 265 nonsmokers (included family members, visitors, friends, neighbors, other outpatients), matched for age, residence, occupation, and education	No information was presented except questions about a history of cigarette smoking and exposure to secondhand smoke
		Active smoking status was given for 272 cases (259 did not smoke); the discrepancy was not explained	Active smoking status was given for 258 controls (252 did not smoke); the discrepancy was not explained	
Delfino et al. 2000	3 breast cancer centers Recruitment was based on moderate/high clinical suspicion of breast cancer United States (Orange county, California)	113 64 lifetime nonsmokers	278 147 lifetime nonsmokers who had benign masses histopathologically	All participants completed a self-administered risk factor questionnaire before the biopsy test
Johnson et al. 2000	Aged 25–74 years 8 Canadian provincial tumor registries Canada 1994–1997	Premenopausal women: 520 222 lifetime nonsmokers Postmenopausal women: 895 386 lifetime nonsmokers	Premenopausal women: 512 229 lifetime nonsmokers Postmenopausal women: 1,012 498 lifetime nonsmokers	Mailed questionnaire Role of secondhand smoke was investigated among those with information on residential secondhand smoke exposure for at least 90% of their lifetimes and for whom menopausal status and active smoking status were provided

Findings	Measure of secondhand smoke	Relative risk (95% confidence interval)	Comments

• Significant positive association with any secondhand smoke exposure	Any exposure:
	  No
	  Yes
		
		1.0
		2.49 (1.65–3.77)
			Controlled for history of benign breast disease, breastfeeding, and intake of soybean products

• No association with active smoking
• No association between *NAT2* genotype and breast cancer risk overall or by smoking
	All participants:
	  No exposure
	  Any exposure
	Premenopausal:
	  No exposure
	  Exposed
	Postmenopausal:
	  No exposure
	  Exposed
		
		1.0
		1.32 (0.69–2.52)
		
		1.0
		2.69 (0.91–8.0)
		
		1.0
		1.01 (0.45–2.27)
			Controlled for age, age at menarche, menopausal status, AFTP, parity, total months of pregnancy, lactation history, education, race, ethnicity, family history of breast cancer among first- and second-degree relatives, and BMI

• Active smoking/breast cancer association was weaker than the secondhand smoke effect in premenopausal women	Premenopausal:
	  None
	  Secondhand smoke only
	  Former smokers only
	  Current smokers
	Postmenopausal:
	  None
	  Secondhand smoke only
	  Former smokers
	  Current smokers
		
		1.0
		2.3 (1.2–4.6)
		2.6 (1.3–5.3)
		1.9 (0.9–3.8)
		
		1.0
		1.2 (0.8–1.8)
		1.4 (0.9–2.1)
		1.6 (1.0–2.5)
			Controlled for 10-year age groups, province, education, BMI, alcohol use, age at menarche, age at end of first pregnancy of 5 months or later, number of live births, months of breastfeeding, and height

Table 7.9   Continued

Study	Population	Cases	Controls	Data collection
Liu et al. 2000	Hospital-based Aged 24–55 years Chongqing, China	186 lifetime nonsmokers	186 lifetime nonsmokers free of cancer Matched for age (±2 years) and date of admission (Women's Health Care and Breast Surgery Department)	In-person interview Household secondhand smoke exposure during childhood (aged <10 years), adolescence (aged 10–16 years), and adulthood; asked about the number of smokers and amount smoked during each time period; workplace exposure: if worked around smokers, number of smokers, and amount smoked
Marcus et al. 2000	Population-based registry (same study population as Millikan et al. 1998) United States (North Carolina) Included all participants enrolled between 1993 and 1996	864 445 lifetime nonsmokers	790 423 lifetime nonsmokers	Exposures to secondhand smoke before and after 18 years of age were investigated in all participants and in lifetime nonsmokers
Kropp and Chang-Claude 2002	Population-based Aged <51 years Two regions in Southern Germany Original study 1992–1996 Participants were recontacted in 1999–2000	468 197 lifetime nonsmokers 76.9% premenopausal	1,093 459 lifetime nonsmokers (resident listing) 2 controls matched to each case by age and study region in original study 81.1% premenopausal	Telephone interviews (blinded to case/control status) Household exposure during childhood and adulthood, and workplace exposure; many details collected included number of smokers, duration of exposure (amount/day), and years of exposure Definition of "exposed" was 1 hour a day for at least 1 year

Findings	Measure of secondhand smoke	Relative risk (95% confidence interval)	Comments

• Significant positive association with household exposure during childhood and adulthood; similar results during youth but not significant
• Significant positive association with workplace exposure
	Household exposure
	  Childhood:
	    None
	    Light
	    Medium
	    Heavy
	    Very heavy
	  p trend
	
	  Adulthood:
	    None
	    Light
	    Medium
	    Heavy
	    Very heavy
	  p trend
	
	Workplace exposure:
	    None
	    1–4 smokers
	    5–9 smokers
	    ≥10 smokers
	  p trend
		
		1.0
		0.69 (0.36–1.31)
		1.31 (0.73–2.33)
		1.64 (0.83–3.23)
		1.74 (0.70–4.36)
		p <0.05
		
		1.0
		0.47 (0.18–1.20)
		1.64 (0.96–2.79)
		2.14 (0.88–5.25)
		3.09 (0.98–10.3)
		p <0.01
		
		1.0
		1.56 (0.95–2.56)
		0.77 (0.33–1.78)
		2.94 (1.26–6.99)
		p <0.05
			Results remained statistically significant in multivariate analyses (see text); analyses controlled for secondhand smoke variables simultaneously and other variables that included age at menarche, body weight in childhood and adulthood, family income during youth, history of hospitalization, benign breast disease, and stress

• No active smoking association
• Little change in findings when secondhand smoke exposures occurring after 18 years of age were considered
	Lifetime nonsmokers <18 years of age:
	    No
	    Yes
		
		1.0
		0.8 (0.6–1.1)
			Controlled for race, age, age at diagnosis and selection, and sampling design

• Significant positive association with lifetime exposure
• No significant association with childhood exposure
• No significant effects from the timing of exposure (before or after first pregnancy)
	Any:
	    No
	    Yes
	    Former smoker
	    Current smoker
	
	Timing in life:
	    None
	    Childhood only
	    Adulthood only
	    Childhood and adulthood
	
	Lifetime (hours/day; years):
	    1–50
	    ≥51
	  p trend
		
		1.0
		1.59 (1.06–2.39)
		1.61 (1.08–2.39)
		1.55 (1.00–2.40)
		
		1.0
		1.11 (0.55–2.27)
		1.86 (1.16–2.98)
		1.63 (1.03–2.57)
		
		1.42 (0.90–2.26)
		1.83 (1.16–2.87)
		p = 0.009
			Stratified by age (5 years); controlled for education, alcohol intake, breastfeeding, family history of breast cancer, menopausal status, and BMI

Table 7.9   Continued

Study	Population	Cases	Controls	Data collection
Lash and Aschengrau 2002	Population-based Aged ≥65 years 8 Cape Cod towns that reported to the Massachusetts Cancer Registry 1987–1993	666 305 lifetime nonsmokers	615 249 lifetime nonsmokers from (RDD and HCFA)	Interviews were conducted with self-respondents and proxies; no description except that the methods were similar to those used in Lash and Aschengrau 1999
Gammon et al. 2004	Population-based Aged 24–98 years Nassau and Suffolk counties of Long Island (New York) (Long Island Breast Cancer Study) United States 1996–1997	1,356 598 lifetime nonsmokers 211 premenopausal and 387 postmeno-pausal women	1,383 627 lifetime nonsmokers 231 premenopausal and 396 postmeno-pausal women RDD and Medicare records	In-person interview; residential history; history of active smoking and exposure to secondhand smoke, including living with smokers, age at exposure, and duration of exposure
Shrubsole et al. 2004	Population-based Aged 25–64 years China (Shanghai) 1996–1998	1,119 1,013 married lifetime non-smokers 684 premenopausal and 329 postmeno-pausal	1,231 1,117 lifetime married nonsmokers 763 premenopausal and 354 postmeno-pausal women (selected from Shanghai Resident Registry listing)	In-person interview Sources: (1) Husband's smoking (amount and years smoked) (2) Exposure at work for the 5 years before interview/ diagnosis (minutes of exposure per day)

Findings	Measure of secondhand smoke	Relative risk (95% confidence interval)	Comments

• No association between lifetime exposure and risk
• No association when duration or timing of exposure (before or after first birth) was considered
	Lifetime exposure:
	  No
	  Yes
	
	Duration (years):
	  Never
	  0 to <20
	  20 to <40
	  ≥40
		
		1.0
		0.85 (0.63–1.1)
		
		1.0
		0.87 (0.59–1.3)
		0.94 (0.66–1.3)
		0.75 (0.47–1.2)
			Controlled for parity, age at first birth, alcohol use, family history and personal history of breast cancer, history of benign breast disease, use of medical radiation, and BMI

• No significant association between any exposure or duration of household exposure before 18 years of age or adulthood (all or from spouses)
• Some suggestion of an increased risk with ≥27 years of exposure to spousal smoking was not significant
• No significant association in subgroup analyses considering menopausal status, weight, family history, and other factors
	Household exposure:
	  No
	  Yes
	
	Total duration (months):
	  None
	  1–192
	  193–360
	  ≥361
	
	Total duration (months) of spousal exposure:
	  None
	  1–181
	  182–325
	  ≥326
	  p trend
		
		1.0
		1.04 (0.81–1.35)
		
		1.0
		1.07 (0.73–1.57)
		0.84 (0.62–1.14)
		1.22 (0.90–1.66)
		
		1.0
		1.50 (1.05–2.14)
		1.01 (0.70–1.47)
		2.10 (1.47–3.02)
		p >0.05
			Controlled for age, number of pregnancies, menopausal status, history of benign breast disease, BMI at 20 years of age and at reference date, family history of breast cancer, history of fertility problems, use of oral conraceptives, and alcohol use

• No association with husbands' smoking among premenopausal and postmenopausal women
• No association with any workplace exposure but a suggestion of an increased risk with ≥5 hours of daily exposure; results were stronger in premenopausal women
	Husband:
	  No
	  Yes
	Workplace:
	  No
	  Yes
	Adult life:
	  None
	  Workplace only
	  Husband only
	  Work and husband
	Workplace (minutes/day):
	  None
	  1–59
	  60–179
	  180–299
	  ≥300
	p trend
		
		1.0
		1.0 (0.8–1.2)
		
		1.0
		1.1 (0.9–1.4)
		
		1.0
		1.1 (0.8–1.5)
		0.9 (0.7–1.2)
		1.1 (0.8–1.4)
		
		1.0
		0.9 (0.6–1.3)
		1.1 (0.8–1.6)
		1.1 (0.8–1.7)
		1.6 (1.0–2.4)
		p = 0.02
			Controlled for age, education, household income, age at menarche, age at first live birth, age at menopause, body size, physical activity, breast cancer in first-degree relatives, history of fibroadenoma; no information on household exposure during childhood; workplace exposure was limited to previous 5 years

Table 7.9   Continued

Study	Population	Cases	Controls	Data collection
Bonner et al. 2005	Population-based Aged 35–79 years Erie and Niagara counties in western New York United States 1996–2001	1,122 525 lifetime nonsmokers 149 premenopausal and 376 postmeno-pausal	2,036 1,012 lifetime 326 nonsmokers were premenopausal and 686 post-menopausal Frequency was matched to cases by age, race, and county of residence; Department of Motor Vehicles and HCFA	In-person interview Household exposure for 7 age periods (<21 years of age, 21–30, 31–40, 41–50, 51–60, 61–70, >70); number of smokers, years of exposure; workplace exposure: number of hours and years of exposure to coworkers who smoked Lifetime residential history of number of smokers at each residence for 334 cases and 609 controls

*Cigarette years = The number of years of smoking multiplied by the number of cigarettes smoked per day.
†Hours/day/year = The sum of hours per day of exposure to secondhand smoke multiplied by the number of years of all episodes of secondhand smoke exposure whether at home, at work, or during leisure time.
‡HCFA = Health Care Financing Administration.
§AFTP = Age at first full-term pregnancy.
ᴬRDD = Random-digit telephone dialing.

>20 years) (Table 7.9). In this study, the effect of active smoking (adjusted OR = 2.0 [95 percent CI, 1.1–3.6]) was quantitatively similar to that of secondhand smoke exposure when compared with lifetime non-smokers with no secondhand smoke exposure. However, when active smokers were compared with all nonsmokers, regardless of secondhand smoke exposure, the effect of active smoking was weaker (the calculated crude OR was 1.34) than the effect of secondhand smoke exposure. Age, history of radiation therapy, a history of breast cancer other than the index diagnoses, parity, and several other covariates were included in the analyses (Lash and Aschengrau 1999).

The study has several limitations. First, multiple cancer sites (the largest three sites were lung, breast, and colorectal) were included in the parental case-control study, and it was unclear whether controls in the breast cancer analysis were appropriate and "matched" to the breast cancer cases. Information bias

cannot be dismissed because a substantial proportion of control (45 percent) and case (33 percent) interviews were conducted with surrogate respondents, and the accuracy and completeness of the information on secondhand smoke exposure may differ by respondent type. Presumably, some proportion of the breast cancer controls had a history of breast cancer and other cancers because a history of breast cancer, other than the index diagnosis, and a history of radiation therapy were included as covariates in the secondhand smoke analysis. The inclusion of persons with previous breast or other cancers further limits this study because it is unclear whether information on secondhand smoke exposure and other factors was assessed up to the first cancer diagnosis or to the index cancer diagnosis.

Lash and Aschengrau (2002) conducted a second case-control study using similar study methods in the same study area (Table 7.9). They included cases of invasive breast cancers diagnosed between 1987 and 1993 among residents of eight Cape Cod towns,

Findings	Measure of secondhand smoke	Relative risk (95% confidence interval)	Comments
• No significant associations between risk and household (lifetime or before 21 years of age) or workplace exposure	Premenopausal Household (person-years):		Controlled for age, education, race, history of benign breast disease, age at menarche, age at first birth, BMI, family history of breast cancer, alcohol intake, and age at menopause in analyses for postmenopausal women
	0	1.0	
	>0 to ≤20	1.31 (0.70–2.44)	
	>20 to ≤33	1.56 (0.77–3.14)	
• Using data from lifetime residential histories, there were no significant associations between risk and exposure at other times (birth, menarche, and first birth)	>33 to ≤49	1.35 (0.69–2.63)	
	>49	1.16 (0.51–2.62)	
	p trend	p = 0.60	
	Postmenopausal Household (person-years):		
	0	1.0	
• Results were similar in premenopausal and postmenopausal women	>0 to ≤20	1.24 (0.79–1.95)	
	>20 to ≤33	0.82 (0.50–1.36)	
	>33 to ≤49	1.03 (0.64–1.66)	
	>49	1.25 (0.79–1.96)	
	p trend	p = 0.38	

which were reported to the Massachusetts Cancer Registry. Controls were women who were matched to cases on age and vital status and were selected by random-digit dialing or from rosters of Medicare beneficiaries. Interviews were conducted with the study participants or their proxies (the number of proxy interviews was not specified). This analysis included 305 cases and 249 controls who were lifetime nonsmokers. Compared with lifetime nonsmokers who reported no secondhand smoke exposure (80 cases, 53 controls), those with any exposure showed no increased risk of breast cancer (adjusted OR = 0.85 [95 percent CI, 0.63–1.1]). The null finding persisted with consideration of the duration of secondhand smoke exposure, age at exposure, and timing of exposure relative to age at pregnancy (Table 7.9). Active smokers also showed no increased risk of breast cancer relative to unexposed lifetime nonsmokers (adjusted OR = 0.81 [95 percent CI, 0.64–1.0]).

The differences in results in these two case-control studies, both conducted in the Cape Cod area, cannot be readily explained. Comparison of demographic and other relevant characteristics of lifetime nonsmoking cases and controls from the first study (Lash and Aschengrau 1999) with this series of cases and controls may provide some clues regarding the differences in results. Selection bias and the use of proxies for deceased participants in the two studies may have contributed to the differences in results. Duration of secondhand smoke exposure and timing of exposure were missing for 20 to 30 percent of the participants in the two studies, raising additional concerns regarding the quality of the information.

A role of secondhand smoke and breast cancer risk was investigated in a large, population-based study of cancer that included 19,453 Canadians who were diagnosed with 1 of 18 types of cancer and 4,523 population controls (Johnson et al. 2000). The influence of secondhand smoke on the risk of lung cancer in this population (Johnson et al. 2001) was described above (see "Lung Cancer" earlier in this chapter for study methods). In brief, 8 of the 10 provinces in the National Enhanced Cancer Surveillance System participated in this study and identified 3,310 women aged 25 through 74 years with histologically confirmed invasive primary breast cancer. Controls were selected from provincial health insurance plans, property assessment databases, or random-digit telephone dialing. A total of 2,340 women with breast cancer (77.4 percent of 3,023 women contacted) and 2,531 controls (71.3 percent of 3,550 women contacted) responded to a mailed questionnaire that asked about lifestyle factors, including a lifetime history of residential and occupational secondhand smoke exposure.

The association of secondhand smoke with breast cancer risk was investigated among 1,415 cases (520 premenopausal and 895 postmenopausal) and 1,524 controls (512 premenopausal and 1,012 postmenopausal) who provided information on residential secondhand smoke exposure for at least 90 percent of their lifetimes, in addition to menopausal and active smoking information. After adjusting for various covariates, Johnson and colleagues (2000) found that premenopausal lifetime nonsmokers exposed to secondhand smoke showed an increased risk of breast cancer (OR = 2.3 [95 percent CI, 1.2–4.6]) compared with those who had not been exposed to secondhand smoke. This increased risk was comparable to the risk of former smokers (OR = 2.6 [95 percent CI, 1.3–5.3]) and was higher than that of current smokers (OR = 1.9 [95 percent CI, 0.9–3.8]) compared with unexposed nonsmokers. Associations between secondhand smoke exposure and breast cancer risk were weaker among postmenopausal women. The investigators found that the RR of breast cancer was 1.2 (95 percent CI, 0.8–1.8) among lifetime nonsmokers exposed to secondhand smoke, 1.4 (95 percent CI, 0.9–2.1) for former smokers, and 1.6 (95 percent CI, 1.0–2.5) for current smokers compared with unexposed nonsmoking postmenopausal women (Johnson et al. 2000). There was also a significant trend of an increase in RR with increasing years and increasing smoker-years[4] of exposure (residential plus occupational years) for premenopausal women; these trends were weaker among postmenopausal women (Johnson et al. 2000). For perimenopausal breast cancer, ORs were 1.5 (95 percent CI, 0.5–4.4), 2.0 (95 percent CI, 0.9–4.5), 2.9 (95 percent CI, 1.3–6.6), and 3.0 (95 percent CI, 1.3–6.6) for increasing levels of total secondhand smoke

exposure (p for trend = 0.03). The postmenopausal dose-response results with increasing exposures were ORs of 1.1, 1.3, and 1.4 (95 percent CI, 0.9–2.3).

When interpreting these findings, researchers need to consider the substantial amount of missing information. Complete information on secondhand smoke exposure was not available for 919 women with breast cancer (cases) and 1,006 controls, and they were subsequently excluded from the analysis, leaving those women who provided information for at least 90 percent of their lifetimes. For the premenopausal women with breast cancer, complete information about secondhand smoke exposure and potential confounders was available for 59 percent of the lifetime nonsmokers, 73 percent of the former smokers, and 67 percent of the current smokers. Corresponding figures for the premenopausal controls were 62 percent, 71 percent, and 67 percent, respectively. Among postmenopausal women with breast cancer, information about secondhand smoke was available for 55 percent of the lifetime nonsmokers, 62 percent of the former smokers, and 65 percent of the current smokers. Corresponding figures for the postmenopausal controls were 59 percent, 62 percent, and 66 percent, respectively. The high proportion of incomplete data on residential secondhand smoke exposure is a concern. The authors noted that 314 cases and 347 controls were missing exposure data. The consequences of these exclusions are uncertain without additional information about those persons with missing exposure histories. It should be noted that the role of secondhand smoke in the risk of lung cancer was analyzed using the same large population-based study that did find an association with secondhand smoke exposure (Johnson et al. 2001). It is unclear whether the controls in the breast cancer analysis were also in the lung cancer analysis.

Another case-control study on secondhand smoke exposure and breast cancer identified participants from one of three breast cancer centers in Orange County, California (Delfino et al. 2000). Persons (n = 535) diagnosed with a suspicious breast mass that was detected clinically or by mammography were considered eligible. A total of 391 women were recruited, and 374 completed a self-administered risk factor questionnaire before having a breast biopsy. Participants were asked about active smoking (current or former smokers, smoking duration, and average number of cigarettes smoked per day) and secondhand smoke exposure. Of the 374 women, 113 were

---

[4]Smoker-years = The number of years of exposure weighted by the number of smokers.

diagnosed with histopathologically confirmed malignant tumors (cases), and 278 women were diagnosed with benign masses (controls). The controls were further categorized as "high-risk" (n = 148) if they had breast lesions that displayed hyperplasia with no atypia, atypical hyperplasia, or complex fibroadenomas; they were classified as "low-risk" (n = 107) if they had no proliferative changes in the breast. There were 23 controls with insufficient tissue surrounding the fibroadenocarcinoma who were not classified by their proliferative state. A total of 64 cases and 147 controls had never smoked.

Compared with lifetime nonsmokers classified as having "low" exposure (33 cases, 96 controls), lifetime nonsmokers with "high" secondhand smoke exposure had an increased risk (adjusted OR = 1.32 [95 percent CI, 0.69–2.52]) of breast cancer after adjusting for age, menopausal status, and family history of breast cancer (Table 7.9) (Delfino et al. 2000). In contrast to lifetime nonsmokers with low secondhand smoke exposure, former smokers (adjusted OR = 0.94 [95 percent CI, 0.53–1.68]) and current smokers (OR = 0.55 [95 percent CI, 0.18–1.67]) showed no increase in risk. In subgroup analyses stratified by risk for breast cancer based on the biopsy findings, the increased RR associated with secondhand smoke exposure was observed among women in the "low-risk" controls (OR = 1.78 [95 percent CI, 0.77–4.11]) but not among those in the "high-risk" controls (OR = 1.03 [95 percent CI, 0.50–2.12]). The RR of secondhand smoke exposure was greater among premenopausal women (OR = 2.69 [95 percent CI, 0.91–8.01]) than among postmenopausal women (OR = 1.01 [95 percent CI, 0.45–2.27]) (Table 7.9) (Delfino et al. 2000). This study was small and the exposure assessment was limited. With regard to the potential for information bias, the risk factor questionnaires on secondhand smoke and other lifestyle factors were obtained before the biopsy test or before the diagnosis of breast cancer, thus minimizing concerns regarding selective recall.

Secondhand smoke exposure and breast cancer risk was investigated in a population-based case-control study in North Carolina that included women aged 20 through 74 years who had been diagnosed with invasive primary breast cancer between 1993 and 1996 (Millikan et al. 1998; Marcus et al. 2000). All cases in African Americans younger than 50 years of age and about an equal number of cases in African Americans and Whites 50 years of age and older were included in the study. Controls were identified from listings of drivers' licenses or Medicare beneficiaries (if participants were aged ≥65 years). During the in-person interview, participants were asked about age

at initiation of cigarette smoking, alcohol use, and exposure to secondhand smoke at home.

The first report on active smoking and secondhand smoke exposure from this case-control study was based on 498 cases and 473 controls who participated in the interview and who also donated blood specimens (Table 7.9) (Millikan et al. 1998). Compared with lifetime nonsmokers (248 cases, 253 controls), the RR of breast cancer was 1.3 (95 percent CI, 0.9–1.8) for former smokers and 1.0 (95 percent CI, 0.7–1.4) for current smokers. Compared with lifetime nonsmokers who were not exposed to secondhand smoke, women who reported secondhand smoke exposure after 18 years of age (based on living with a smoker at age 18 years or older) had a RR of 1.3 (95 percent CI, 0.9–1.9); this association was stronger among premenopausal women (OR = 1.5 [95 percent CI, 0.8–2.8]) than among postmenopausal women (OR = 1.2 [95 percent CI, 0.7–2.2]).

A second report on active smoking and secondhand smoke exposure from this population was based on all participants (864 cases, 790 controls) who were interviewed between 1993 and 1996, including 445 cases and 423 controls who had never smoked (Table 7.9) (Marcus et al. 2000). Lifetime nonsmokers who reported secondhand smoke exposures before 18 years of age did not show an elevated risk of breast cancer (OR = 0.8 [95 percent CI, 0.6–1.1]) compared with women who reported no exposures. The association with secondhand smoke exposures before 18 years of age did not change after adjusting for exposures after 18 years of age. In both reports, Millikan and colleagues (1998) and Marcus and colleagues (2000) adjusted the results on secondhand smoke exposure for race, age at diagnosis/selection, and sampling design, but not for other covariates. Questions on secondhand smoke exposure were not comprehensive, but focused primarily on exposures in the home before and after the women were 18 years of age.

Kropp and Chang-Claude (2002) conducted a case-control study of breast cancer in women 51 years of age or less in two study areas in Germany (Table 7.9). Active smoking, but not involuntary smoking, was assessed in the original study, which was conducted between 1992 and 1995. In 1999, the 706 women with in situ or invasive breast cancer and the 1,381 controls who were interviewed in the original study were recontacted. A total of 468 cases (66.3 percent) and 1,093 (79.2 percent) controls participated in the second interview; 115 cases and 3 controls were deceased by the time of the attempted recontact. Participants were asked extensive questions regarding active smoking and involuntary smoking that included household exposure during childhood and adulthood, as well as workplace exposure. Information on age at exposure, duration of exposure, and intensity of exposure (i.e., number of smokers, hours of daily exposure) was obtained. Compared with lifetime nonsmokers with no secondhand smoke exposure, lifetime nonsmokers who were exposed showed a significantly increased risk (adjusted OR = 1.61 [95 percent CI, 1.08–2.39]). The increased risk was associated with exposure during adulthood (adjusted OR = 1.80 [95 percent CI, 1.12–2.89]) but not with exposure only during childhood (adjusted OR = 1.07 [95 percent CI, 0.52–2.19]). There was little difference in risk by duration of exposure; the adjusted OR was 1.85 (95 percent CI, 1.15–2.98) for a shorter duration (1 to 10 years) and 1.51 (95 percent CI, 0.89–2.56) for a longer duration of exposure (≥21 years). Risk patterns were also similar for current versus former secondhand smoke exposure. There was a trend of increasing risk with lifetime exposure (childhood and adulthood combined) when an index of lifetime hours per day-years of exposure was used: the ORs were 1.83 (95 percent CI, 1.16–2.87) for high exposures (≥51 hours per day-years) and 1.42 (95 percent CI, 0.90–2.26) for lower exposures (1 to 50 hours per day-years). However, in this study, the estimated OR for secondhand smoke exposure (OR = 1.61) was higher than for former (OR = 1.15) or current active smokers (OR = 1.47).

This study has several limitations. First, the women were recontacted specifically regarding a secondhand smoke exposure history, raising the possibility of information bias. Second, a substantial proportion of both cases and controls did not participate, indicating a potential for the introduction of selection bias.

Gammon and colleagues (2004) investigated the role of secondhand smoke and breast cancer using the Long Island Breast Cancer Study, which was conducted among residents of Nassau and Suffolk counties. The study included 1,356 women with breast cancer and 1,383 controls from the general population; 598 cases and 627 controls were lifetime nonsmokers (Table 7.9). Lifetime exposure to residential secondhand smoke was assessed, including exposure to smoking by parents, spouses, and other household members. Compared with lifetime nonsmokers who were not exposed to secondhand smoke (155 cases, 170 controls), lifetime nonsmokers who were exposed showed no increased risk (adjusted OR = 1.04 [95 percent CI, 0.81–1.35]). The risk of breast cancer was not increased in association with exposure to parental smoking before 18 years of age or exposure before a first full-term pregnancy. When the total duration of exposure was considered, there was little indication that long-term exposure to household tobacco smoke increased breast cancer risk; the OR for living with a smoker for 361 or more months was 1.22 (95 percent CI, 0.90–1.66). When the analysis was restricted to household exposure from spouses, the OR for living with a spouse who smoked for 361 or more months was 2.10 (95 percent CI, 1.47–3.02), but there was not a significant trend of increasing risk with increasing duration. Analysis by menopausal status showed a small increased risk associated with secondhand smoke exposure in premenopausal women (adjusted OR = 1.21 [95 percent CI, 0.78–1.90]), but not in postmenopausal women (adjusted OR = 0.93 [95 percent CI, 0.68–1.29]). Exposure to secondhand smoke was not significantly associated with risk in analyses that were stratified by other parameters of interest including age, body mass index, use of alcohol, use of hormone replacement therapy, use of oral contraceptives, and family history of breast cancer.

A risk of breast cancer was not related to active smoking in this study. Compared with lifetime nonsmokers who were not exposed to secondhand smoke, the adjusted OR was 1.06 (95 percent CI, 0.76–1.48) for active smokers and 1.15 (95 percent CI, 0.90–1.48) for active smokers who were also exposed to secondhand smoke. The study did not assess exposure in the workplace.

Bonner and colleagues (2005) investigated the role of secondhand smoke and breast cancer among residents in Erie and Niagara counties as part of the Western New York Exposures and Breast Cancer Study. This population-based, case-control study included women aged 35 to 79 years who were diagnosed with histologically confirmed, primary incident breast cancer. Population controls from the study areas were selected from Department of Motor Vehicles driver's license list or from the Centers for Medicare and Medicaid Services lists. There were questions about exposure to secondhand smoke from other household residents and coworkers for seven time periods (<21 years of age and for each subsequent decade of life). The questions asked for the number of smokers in the household and how long they lived in the same residence. Workplace exposure was estimated by the number of hours per week study participants were exposed to coworkers' smoking. The main analysis on lifetime household and workplace exposure included 525 cases (149 premenopausal, 376 postmenopausal) and 1,012 controls (326 premenopausal, 686 postmenopausal) who were lifetime nonsmokers. In addition, secondhand smoke exposure was determined as part of the residential history assessment. Participants listed every residence for their entire life with corresponding information on the number of smokers at each residence. On the basis of this information, exposures at birth, at menarche, and at the time of first birth were evaluated. Residential history assessment was obtained from a subset of lifetime nonsmoking cases (106 premenopausal, 228 postmenopausal) and controls (238 premenopausal, 371 postmenopausal).

Breast cancer risk increased, but not significantly, in association with lifetime household exposure to secondhand smoke; there were no significant trends of increasing risks with increasing duration of exposure in premenopausal (p trend = 0.60) and postmenopausal (p trend = 0.38) women (Table 7.9). In an analysis restricted to household smoking before 21 years of age, risk did not increase significantly in premenopauasal (p trend = 0.99) and postmenopausal (p trend = 0.09) women. Breast cancer risk was unrelated to workplace secondhand smoke exposure in premenopausal (p trend = 0.38) and postmenopausal (p trend = 0.41) women; almost all of the RR estimates were below unity. In premenopausal women, exposures to smoking at birth, at menarche, and at the time of first birth were associated with an 11 to 49 percent increase in risk, but none of the associations was statistically significant. In postmenopausal women, all the RR estimates were close to or below unity.

This case-control study obtained extensive information on lifetime household and workplace exposure. In addition, exposure to household smoking was collected using a second method as part of a residential history assessment. Risk of breast cancer was not significantly associated with any of the measures of secondhand smoke exposure in premenopausal and postmenopausal women. This is one of the few studies that presented data on lifetime nonsmoking cases and controls by menopausal status, so comparability of the case and control groups can be assessed.

Three Chinese studies have addressed the role of secondhand smoke exposure and breast cancer risk in lifetime nonsmokers (Zhao et al. 1999; Liu et al. 2000; Shrubsole 2004). As discussed below, there is concern regarding the design of two of the studies (Zhao et al. 1999; Liu et al. 2000). Zhao and colleagues (1999) conducted a hospital-based study of breast cancer in Chengdu, China, between 1994 and 1997. The study included 265 women who were clinically determined to have breast cancer and an equal number of female controls who were individually matched to cases for age, area of residence, similar occupation, and similar education (the nature of this matching was not specified). The sources of controls were heterogeneous and included family members, visitors, neighbors, friends, or outpatients with benign conditions. Although 259 breast cancer patients and 252 controls were identified as nonsmokers of cigarettes, information on secondhand smoke was presented on 265 cases and 265 controls who were presumably nonsmokers, although this difference was not specifically mentioned in the text. The authors reported a significantly increased risk associated with secondhand smoke exposure (adjusted OR = 2.49 [95 percent CI, 1.65–3.77]) after adjustment for various covariates including breastfeeding, history of benign breast disease, and intake of soybean products. On the basis of 13 cases and 6 controls who were cigarette smokers (it is not known whether these were current smokers or former smokers), breast cancer risk increased more than twofold among smokers (OR = 2.75 [95 percent CI, 0.87–8.65]) compared with nonsmokers (Table 7.9). Methodologic limitations of this study include the uncertain selection criteria of the cases (i.e., incident versus prevalent cases, clinical diagnosis of breast cancer), the suitability of the control groups, and a lack of information regarding the questions on secondhand smoke exposure (e.g., sources and timing of exposure).

Liu and colleagues (2000) conducted a hospital-based, case-control study of breast cancer in Chongqing, China, that included 186 women with incident breast cancer and 186 controls who were outpatients in the same hospital and were individually matched to cases for age (±2 years), date of hospitalization/admission, and marital status, and were lifetime nonsmokers. Cases and controls were 24 to 55 years of age. Questions related to secondhand smoke exposure for three time periods: childhood (aged <10 years), youth (aged 10 through 16 years), and adulthood (including exposures at home and at work). Two variables were used to describe exposures at home: number of smokers and a combined exposure index that included the number of smokers and the amount they smoked (light, medium, heavy, and very heavy). The risk of breast cancer increased significantly in association with the number of smokers in the household during childhood (p trend <0.05) but not during youth (p trend >0.05) or adulthood (p trend >0.05). When the amount smoked was also considered (i.e., using the combined exposure index), there was a significant trend of increasing risk with increasing levels of exposure during childhood (p trend <0.05) and adulthood (p trend <0.01) but not during youth. When household exposures during childhood, youth, and adulthood and workplace exposure were considered simultaneously, the researchers found a significantly increased risk associated with childhood household exposure (adjusted OR = 1.24 [95 percent CI, 1.07–1.43]), adulthood household exposure (adjusted OR = 4.07 [95 percent CI, 2.21–7.50]), and workplace exposure (adjusted OR = 1.27 [95 percent CI, 1.04–1.55]).

Cases and controls differed considerably in terms of education, occupation, and social class. Cases had less education than controls (26 percent of cases versus 9 percent of controls had less than high school). A significant excess of cases also reported below average family socioeconomic status (SES) during each of the three time periods (childhood, youth, adulthood) than controls. However, cases were more likely to be professionals (46 percent) than controls (25 percent) and were less likely to be workers (29 percent) than controls (66 percent). Exposure to secondhand smoke at home and in the workplace may vary by education, occupation, and family SES. In the multivariate analysis, only socioeconomic class during youth was considered. Thus, potential confounding by these social class and occupational variables cannot be ruled out in this study.

Shrubsole and colleagues (2004) investigated the role of secondhand smoke exposure in the Shanghai Breast Cancer Study, a large population-based study of 1,459 breast cancer cases and 1,556 population controls aged 25 to 64 years. Questions about secondhand smoke exposure were added to the study seven months after data collection began, and 1,119 cases and 1,231 controls responded. Analyses on secondhand smoke exposure and risk were restricted to lifetime nonsmokers who were currently married (1,103 cases and 1,117 controls). Two sources of secondhand smoke exposure were assessed: husband's smoking and exposure at work the during the five years before diagnosis/interview. A risk of breast cancer was unrelated to the husband's smoking (adjusted OR = 1.0 [95 percent CI, 0.8–1.2]); all of the ORs associated with different categories of the husband's smoking, including the number of cigarettes smoked and the number of years and pack-years of smoking, were close to unity. Breast cancer risk was also unrelated to secondhand smoke exposure in the workplace (adjusted OR = 1.1 [95 percent CI, 0.9–1.4]). The RRs were also close to unity when both sources of exposure were considered together (i.e., none, workplace only, husband's smoking only, and both exposures); these results were similar in premenopausal and postmenopausal women (Table 7.9). However, breast cancer risk tended to increase with an intense exposure at work. When women with workplace secondhand smoke exposure (457 cases, 463 controls) were compared with those with no exposure at work or from their husbands (176 cases, 184 controls), there was a significant trend of an increase in risk with an increase in duration of daily workplace secondhand smoke exposure (p trend = 0.02). In premenopausal women, the ORs were 1.0, 0.9, 1.1, 1.1, and 1.6, respectively, in association with none, 1 to 59, 60 to 179, 180 to 299, and 300 or more minutes of exposure per day (p trend = 0.03). The corresponding ORs were 1.0, 1.1, 1.3, 1.4, and 1.4, respectively (p trend = 0.37), in postmenopausal women. To date, this is the largest case-control study of breast cancer in lifetime nonsmokers that assessed information on household and workplace exposures. One limitation is that information on workplace exposures was limited to the five years before the interview. In addition, there was no information on childhood exposures.

Quantitative Meta-Analysis

To synthesize the observational evidence, the technique of quantitative meta-analysis was used. The RR estimates for the various exposure measures from reports on cohort and case-control studies were abstracted and then combined using the statistical software package Stata. The studies used a variety of exposure measures to assess childhood or adulthood exposures, sources of exposure, and location of exposure. A documented set of decisions was made as to the selection of estimates from the studies. Additionally, some of the studies provided results by menopausal status.

Pooled estimates were calculated for three population samples: all women in a study (regardless of menopausal status), premenopausal women, and postmenopausal women. Eight exposure categories were considered: (1) any source during adulthood (adult all sources), (2) adult spousal/partner (adult spousal), (3) adult at home (includes smoking from any cohabitant), (4) adult at work, (5) child at home (usually parental), (6) both childhood and adulthood exposure (either at home or work or both), (7) ever exposure in studies that measured child and adult exposures (either at home or at work or both), and (8) the most comprehensive exposure for each study. For all categories, estimates of independent effects were selected over estimates of "ever" effects. In other words, if a study presented results for "ever exposed as a child" (regardless of adulthood exposure) as well as "exposed during childhood only" (no adulthood exposure), the latter was used in the analysis of childhood exposure because it represents a more unbiased estimate of the effect of childhood exposure independent of exposure during adulthood.

Whenever possible, the studies used adjusted estimates. The researchers performed subanalyses to investigate the influence of adjustment on the results. Studies were categorized according to whether they adjusted for reproductive factors (age at menarche, age at first birth, and parity) and for alcohol consumption. These factors were the focus of attention because they were the most important potential confounders.

Table 7.10 provides the main findings of the meta-analysis, including the pooled estimates and 95 percent CIs. Overall, breast cancer risk in lifetime nonsmokers was significantly associated with secondhand smoke exposure, but with stratification by menopausal status, the association was limited to premenopausal women, and estimates for postmenopausal women for adult exposure were below unity, although not statistically significant (Table 7.10, Figures 7.1–7.4). The pattern was similar when spousal smoking alone was considered (Table 7.10) and the estimate for workplace exposure was also higher for women with premenopausal breast cancer than for those with postmenopausal breast cancer. Exposure in childhood was not associated with increased risk.

Sensitivity analyses were carried out that explored variations in the pooled estimates by the type of study, the extent of the exposure information available, and consideration of confounding (Table 7.10). Findings from the cohort studies showed no association overall of breast cancer risk with secondhand smoke exposure, although the pooled estimate from the case-control studies was positive and statistically significant. The estimate was particularly high for hospital-based case-control studies. Comparing estimates for studies with and without consideration of confounding, the estimate was lower for those studies that included adjustment for potential confounding.

In Figure 7.5, the 21 studies are evaluated for potential publication bias using a funnel plot and a test developed by Begg and Mazumdar (1994). The funnel plot shows that less precise studies tended to have more strongly positive results, a pattern indicative of possible publication bias. The formal test for such bias was statistically significant (p <0.05).

Table 7.10   Pooled risk estimates and 95% confidence intervals (CI) for breast cancer meta-analysis

Exposure	n*	All women Relative risk (95% CI)	n	Premenopausal Relative risk (95% CI)	n	Postmenopausal Relative risk (95% CI)
Adulthood						
All sources	18	1.15 (1.02–1.29) [0.000][†]	10	1.45 (1.04–2.01) [0.000]	9	0.90 (0.81–1.01) [0.691]
Spouse	9	1.17 (0.96–1.44) [0.002]	4	1.40 (0.92–2.12) [0.1]	3	0.86 (0.67–1.12) [0.645]
Home	8	1.01 (0.85–1.19) [0.006]	4	1.28 (0.94–1.74) [0.355]	3	0.92 (0.76–1.11) [0.591]
Work	6	1.06 (0.84–1.35) [0.008]	4	1.21 (0.70–2.09) [0.000]	3	0.83 (0.53–1.29) [0.086]
Childhood (parent)	9	1.01 (0.90–1.12) [0.101]	4	1.14 (0.90–1.45) [0.342]	3	1.04 (0.86–1.26) [0.242]
Both childhood and adulthood	4	1.39 (0.88–2.18) [0.021]	3	1.63 (0.68–3.91) [0.016]	2	1.02 (0.74–1.42) [0.160]
Ever exposed (in studies measuring lifetime exposure)	10	1.40 (1.12–1.76) [0.000]	6	1.85 (1.19–2.87) [0.001]	5	1.04 (0.84–1.30) [0.048]
"Best" of each study[‡]	21	1.20 (1.08–1.35) [0.000]	11	1.64 (1.25–2.14) [0.001]	10	1.00 (0.88–1.12) [0.321]
Cohort studies	7	1.02 (0.92–1.13) [0.162]				
Case-control studies	14	1.40 (1.17–1.67) [0.000]				

*n = Number of studies included in each analysis.
[†][in brackets] = p value for test of heterogeneity (null hypothesis is no heterogeneity).
[‡]"Best" of each study includes the most comprehensive measure of association from each study: ever being exposed in any setting was preferred over all sources during adulthood, which was preferred over spousal exposure.

Figure 7.1 Relative risks (with 95% confidence intervals) of breast cancer associated with all sources of adult exposure to secondhand smoke

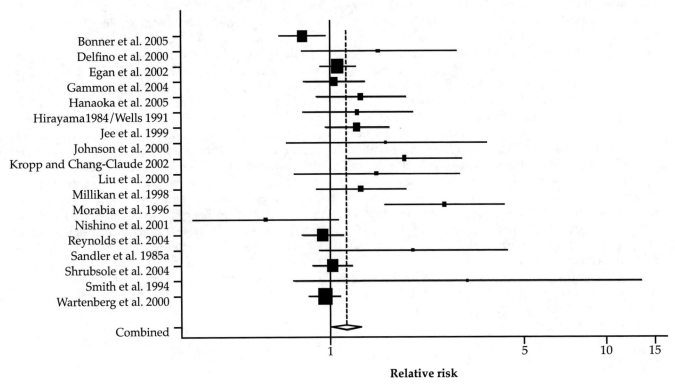

Note: Different sized squares represent the weights of each study's relative risks in the combined estimates.

Evidence Synthesis

The full body of evidence on secondhand smoke and breast cancer was evaluated with the criteria for causality, which have been used in this series of reports for a long time (Chapter 1, Introduction, Summary, and Conclusions). Consideration was also given to the extensive information on active smoking and breast cancer. Issues related to sources of secondhand smoke exposure, dose-response relationships, and differences in findings by menopausal status were also considered.

Consistency

Consistency refers to the replication of findings across studies with different designs, in different populations, and conducted by different investigators (USDHHS 2004). To the extent that findings are comparable across a range of study characteristics, alternative explanations to causation in explaining associations become less tenable, particularly bias arising from methodologic limitations of particular designs.

There are currently 21 epidemiologic studies (7 cohort, 14 case-control) that have directly investigated the association between secondhand smoke exposure and the risk of breast cancer among lifetime nonsmokers. The overall evidence does not consistently show an increased risk of breast cancer in association with secondhand smoke, although the pooled estimate of all the evidence is above unity, the level of no effect (Table 7.10); the evidence is not consistent by study design. Three well-established U.S. cohort studies each include a large number of breast cancer events: 669 breast cancer deaths in the ACS cohort; 1,359 incident invasive breast cancers in the NHS cohort; and 1,174 incident invasive breast cancers in the California Teachers Study cohort. These studies did not find an association between exposure to secondhand smoke and breast cancer risk; all RR estimates were around unity (Wartenberg et al. 2000; Egan et al. 2002; Reynolds et al. 2004).

Figure 7.2   Relative risks (with 95% confidence intervals) of breast cancer associated with adult exposure to secondhand smoke from spouses' smoking

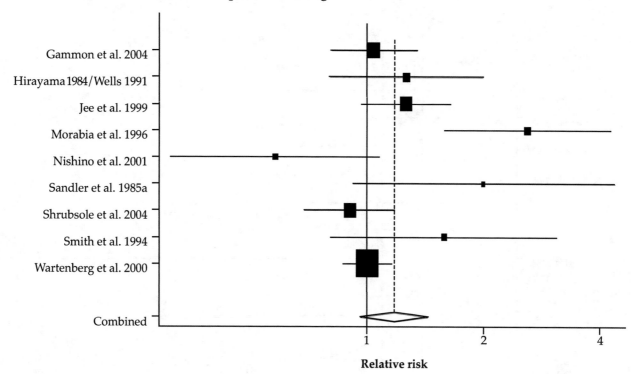

Note: Different sized squares represent the weights of each study's relative risks in the combined estimates.

Results from the four cohort studies from Asia are based on fewer breast cancer events (<200 breast cancer incident cases/deaths) and are more varied, but also do not provide consistent evidence for an association. Small RR increases of 10 to 30 percent were reported in three of the studies (Hirayama 1984; Jee et al. 1999; Hanaoka et al. 2005), whereas a RR less than unity was reported in the fourth study, which is from Japan (Nishino et al. 2001). The only significant finding came from a subgroup analysis in a cohort study in Japan with stratification by menopausal status (Hanaoka et al. 2005). This finding was based on 77 breast cancers in premenopausal women. The pooled estimate for the cohort studies is 1.02 overall. This null finding from the cohort studies cannot be set aside as a result of methodologic limitations, because some of these studies have shown an increased risk for lung cancer and CHD associated with secondhand smoke.

Results from the 14 case-control studies are more supportive of an increased risk associated with secondhand smoke exposure, but there is considerable heterogeneity in the study results. Five studies found at least a twofold increase in RRs associated with secondhand smoke exposure (Smith et al. 1994; Morabia et al. 1996; Lash and Aschengrau 1999; Johnson et al. 2000; Kropp and Chang-Claude 2002); results were statistically significant in four of these studies. As described above, the study conducted by Lash and Aschengrau (1999) had design limitations, and a subsequent study in the same area conducted by the same investigators using a comparable design did not confirm the earlier results (all RR estimates were <1.0) (Lash and Aschengrau 2002). The other four studies (Smith et al. 1994; Morabia et al. 1996; Johnson et al. 2000; Kropp and Chang-Claude 2002) considered by Johnson (2005) to be more complete in assessing lifetime secondhand smoke exposures had other study limitations, including the potential for differential recall bias, misclassification due to missing data, and selection bias. In the study by Kropp and Chang-Claude (2002), participants were

Figure 7.3   Relative risks (with 95% confidence intervals) of breast cancer associated with all sources of adult exposure to secondhand smoke among premenopausal women

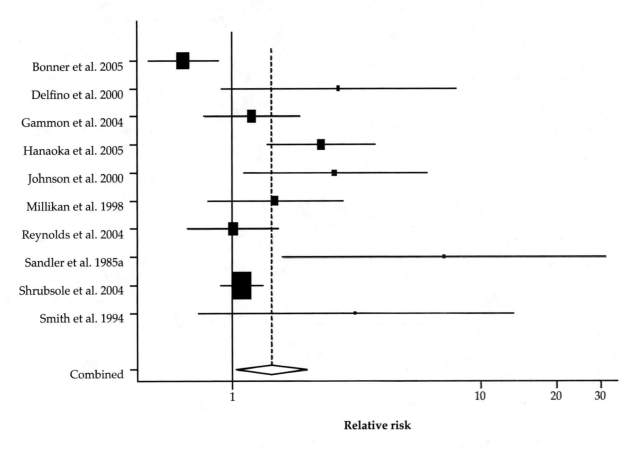

Relative risk

Note: Different sized squares represent the weights of each study's relative risks in the combined estimates.

recontacted four to seven years after the initial interview, and the reinterview response rate was lower in cases (66 percent) than in controls (79 percent). Given that the focus of the reinterview was to determine the history of active smoking and exposure to secondhand smoke, it would have been difficult to "blind" participants as to the study hypothesis, and the possibility of differential recall bias by case/control status exists and may have led to an overestimate of the risk. Smith and colleagues (1994) also recontacted study participants to determine histories of secondhand smoke exposure, and thus the findings of this study are subject to the limitations discussed in regard to the study by Kropp and Chang-Claude (2002). In the study by Johnson and colleagues (2000), information on secondhand smoke exposure was obtained via a mailed questionnaire and was incomplete for 37 percent of

the lifetime nonsmoking cases and 40 percent of the controls. Consequently, 470 (1,078 minus 608) lifetime nonsmoking cases and 487 (1,214 minus 727) lifetime nonsmoking controls were not included in the analysis. In the study by Morabia and colleagues (1996), controls were younger (21 percent were younger than 45 years of age) than cases (11 percent were younger than 45 years of age), and variables related to menopause status were not considered in the analysis. There were also methodologic limitations of the studies carried out in China.

In contrast, no significant increase in risk was found in four large population-based, case-control studies (Millikan et al. 1998; Gammon et al. 2004; Shrubsole et al. 2004; Bonner et al. 2005). According to Johnson (2005), results from three of these studies are less credible because exposure assessment was

Figure 7.4   Relative risks (with 95% confidence intervals) of breast cancer associated with all sources of adult exposure to secondhand smoke among postmenopausal women

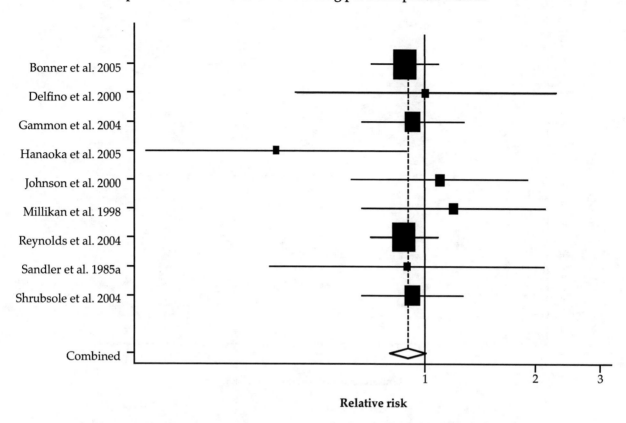

Note: Different sized squares represent the weights of each study's relative risks in the combined estimates.

incomplete (Millikan et al. 1998; Gammon et al. 2004; Shrubsole et al. 2004) (the study by Bonner et al. [2005] was published after Johnson's 2005 review). In fact, major lifetime sources of secondhand smoke exposure (childhood exposure from parents, adult residential exposure, and adult occupational exposure) were assessed in the western New York study, and there was no association between risk and each source of exposure nor with lifetime exposure across these different sources (Bonner et al. 2005). Two of the studies did not assess workplace exposure (Millikan et al. 1998; Gammon et al. 2004), and one study limited workplace secondhand smoke exposure assessment to the most recent job, and did not obtain information on childhood exposure (Shrubsole et al. 2004).

A strength of the epidemiologic evidence on secondhand smoke and lung cancer has been the consistency across prospective cohort and case-control studies. Cohort and case-control studies are generally subject to somewhat differing sources of bias, and a comparability of findings in the two designs weighs against bias as the source of association. The findings of the two designs differ for secondhand smoke exposure and breast cancer, raising a concern that bias affected the findings of the case-control studies. The hospital-based, case-control studies show the strongest association and are particularly prone to bias from the noncomparability of cases and controls, and from the differential reporting of exposures by cases and controls.

To further assess the consistency of the association between secondhand smoke exposure and risk of breast cancer, risk patterns were examined by the sources of exposure. There are three major classes of exposure (childhood exposure from parental smoking, adult residential exposures, and occupational exposures). To date, all studies have characterized adulthood household exposure. Information on

Figure 7.5   Begg's funnel plot with pseudo 95% confidence limits for 21 studies of breast cancer and secondhand smoke exposure

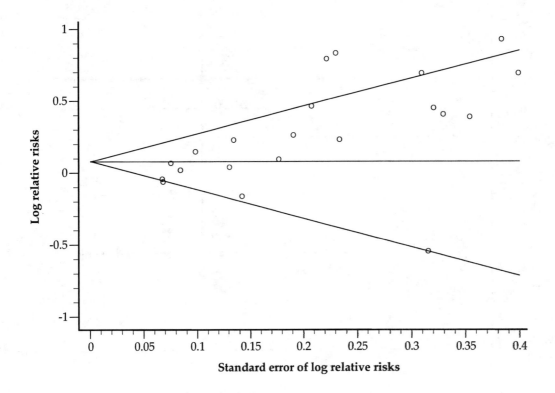

Note: Asymmetry on the right side of the graph (where studies with high standard errors are plotted) provides evidence of publication bias.

childhood secondhand smoke exposure is available in three cohort (Egan et al. 2002; Reynolds et al. 2004; Hanaoka et al. 2005) and seven case-control studies (Smith et al. 1994; Morabia et al. 1996; Johnson et al. 2000; Marcus et al. 2000; Kropp and Chang-Claude 2002; Gammon et al. 2004; Bonner et al. 2005). Workplace exposure was captured in three cohort (Wartenberg et al. 2000; Egan et al. 2002; Hanaoka et al. 2005) and six case-control studies (Smith et al. 1994; Morabia et al. 1996; Johnson et al. 2000; Kropp and Chang-Claude 2002; Gammon et al. 2004; Bonner et al. 2005).

Those studies that have obtained lifetime secondhand smoke exposure histories are also informative because risk patterns by source of exposure may provide information regarding the timing and intensity of exposure. There are different exposure assessment approaches in the studies, however, and results have not been consistently reported for all epochs of exposure, thus complicating comparisons

across studies. Researchers have considered exposure to secondhand smoke early in life to be particularly important for premenopausal breast cancer. In two U.S. cohort studies, breast cancer risk did not increase in association with childhood exposure from parents (Egan et al. 2002; Reynolds et al. 2004). Similarly, a risk of breast cancer was not significantly associated with childhood secondhand smoke exposure in case-control studies (Smith et al. 1994; Johnson et al. 2000; Kropp and Chang-Claude 2002; Gammon et al. 2004; Bonner et al. 2005) (risk patterns were presented for childhood and adulthood exposures combined in two studies [Marcus et al. 2000; Hanaoka et al. 2005]). There is also little support for the hypothesis that secondhand smoke exposure before a first pregnancy is associated with breast cancer risk (Kropp and Chang-Claude 2002; Lash and Aschengrau 2002; Gammon et al. 2004; Bonner et al. 2005). Thus, the collective evidence does not consistently show an association of secondhand smoke exposure during childhood/adolescence or before a first pregnancy—a period of time when the breast may be particularly susceptible to carcinogen exposure, as in the case of ionizing radiation (NRC 2005).

The risk of breast cancer was not significantly related to workplace secondhand smoke exposure in two U.S. cohort studies (Wartenberg et al. 2000; Egan et al. 2002) and in two case-control studies (Smith et al. 1994; Bonner et al. 2005); lifetime workplace exposure was assessed in the case-control studies. In a cohort study conducted in Japan, the risk of breast cancer in premenopausal women was increased in association with workplace secondhand smoke exposure, but no increased risk was observed in postmenopausal women (Hanaoka et al. 2005). In Shanghai, China, an intense (>300 minutes per day), daily, and recent workplace exposure was associated with an increased risk of breast cancer in both premenopausal and post-menopausal women, although the estimate was statistically significant only in premenopausal women (Shrubsole et al. 2004). In the three studies that found a significantly increased risk associated with adulthood exposure (Morabia et al. 1996; Johnson et al. 2000; Kropp and Chang-Claude 2002), RR estimates were not shown separately for occupational versus household exposures. However, in the study by Morabia and colleagues (1996), the risk estimates for spousal smoking were slightly stronger than for all sources of exposure during adulthood combined. Thus, some (but not all) studies offer evidence that breast cancer risk may be increased in association with workplace secondhand smoke exposure.

Temporality

The criterion of temporality requires that exposure to secondhand smoke antedate the onset of cancer, so information from prospective cohort studies is particularly relevant. In prospective cohort studies, women initially free of breast cancer are followed over varying time intervals, and their risk is estimated in relation to secondhand smoke exposure. As described above, there is currently little evidence indicating an increased breast cancer risk from prospective cohort studies, including the three large, well-established cohorts in the United States (Wartenberg et al. 2000; Egan et al. 2002; Reynolds et al. 2004). The risk of breast cancer was unrelated to adulthood secondhand smoke exposure in the ACS study (Wartenberg et al. 2000), the NHS (Egan et al. 2002), and the California Teachers Study (Reynolds et al. 2004) (information on workplace secondhand smoke was available in

the NHS and ACS studies). Similarly, a risk of breast cancer was not related to exposure during childhood in the NHS and the California Teachers Study (Egan et al. 2002; Reynolds et al. 2004). One of the Japanese cohort studies (JPHC study) collected information on household secondhand smoke exposure during childhood and adulthood and on workplace exposure; this study also showed no overall association between secondhand smoke exposure and risk in all subjects combined (Hanaoka et al. 2005). In general, second-hand smoke exposure extends across the life span and typically would have begun long before the onset of breast cancer.

Strength of Association

Increasing the strength of association weighs more heavily against alternatives to causal association (USDHHS 2004). For involuntary smoking and breast cancer risk, the overall association in the pooled estimates for premenopausal breast cancer indicate elevations of 40 to 60 percent (Table 7.10). However, the highlighted limitations of the case-control studies of passive smoking and breast cancer, particularly selection bias and information bias, may be responsible, at least in part, for the increased risk. The inconsistent findings of the case-control and cohort studies for the association of passive smoking with premenopausal breast cancer also raise concerns about potential bias or unmeasured confounding, since consistency of risk estimates across varying study designs would weigh against such bias.

Assessment of dose-response relationships is another aspect of this criterion. Duration of exposure to spousal and household smoking was used in most studies for assessing exposure-response relationships (Smith et al. 1994; Jee et al. 1999; Lash and Aschengrau 1999, 2002; Wartenberg et al. 2000; Egan et al. 2002; Gammon et al. 2004; Shrubsole et al. 2004; Bonner et al. 2005). A few studies also collected information on intensity of exposure (i.e., hours and days of second-hand smoke exposure), and on estimated risk patterns by hours per day-years (Morabia et al. 1996; Kropp and Chang-Claude 2002) or minutes of secondhand smoke exposure per day (Shrubsole et al. 2004). Of the four studies showing a strong positive association between exposure and breast cancer risk (Smith et al. 1994; Morabia et al. 1996; Johnson et al. 2000; Kropp and Chang-Claude 2002), only one showed a trend of increasing risk with increasing duration of exposure and only among premenopausal women (Johnson et al. 2000). Among premenopausal women, the ORs were 1.2, 1.8, 2.0, 3.3, and 2.9, respectively, in association with 1 to 6, 7 to 16, 17 to 21, 22 to 35, and 36 or more years of residential and occupational exposures. The pattern of association is much weaker in postmenopausal women (ORs were 1.1, 1.3, and 1.3, respectively, in association with 1 to 30, 31 to 56, and more than 56 years) (Johnson et al. 2000). However, in three other studies, RR estimates were similar for varying durations of exposure and for current versus former exposures. In the study by Morabia and colleagues (1996), the ORs were 2.2 and 2.5 in association with 1 to 50 and more than 50 hours per day-year of exposure, respectively. In the study by Kropp and Chang-Claude (2002), the ORs were 1.85, 1.59, and 1.51 with 1 to 10, 11 to 20, and 21 or more years of exposure, respectively. In the same study, the risks were 1.55 for former and 1.67 for current exposures to secondhand smoke. In the study by Smith and colleagues (1994), the ORs were 2.82 and 2.24 in association with 1 to 200 and more than 200 cigarette-years, respectively.

Of the studies not showing any overall association between secondhand smoke and breast cancer risk, one showed a twofold increase among women exposed to 326 or more months of spousal smoking, but there was no evidence of an exposure-response gradient (Gammon et al. 2004). Another study showed a 70 percent increase in risk among women married to current smokers of 30 or more years (Jee et al. 1999). However, in several larger cohort (Wartenberg et al. 2000; Egan et al. 2002) and case-control studies (Shrubsole et al. 2004; Bonner et al. 2005), there is little evidence of elevated risks even with the highest duration of household exposure.

Biologic Plausibility

There is substantial literature on carcinogenesis in relation to breast cancer, but with more limited information directly relevant to tobacco smoke. One key aspect of biologic plausibility of secondhand smoke as a cause of breast cancer is the finding on active smoking and breast cancer. Additionally, the potential heterogeneity of breast cancer in relation to etiologic risk factors merits consideration. Epidemiologic research has only recently been directed at subgroups of breast cancer cases, defined by phenotype, such as estrogen and progesterone receptor status and genotype (e.g., susceptibility [*BRCA1* or *BRCA2*] or carcinogen metabolism [*NAT2*]). To date, the evidence has not consistently shown active smoking to be associated with an increased risk in a particular subgroup (Althuis et al. 2004; Ghadirian et al. 2004; USDHHS 2004).

The weight of epidemiologic evidence suggests that active smoking is not causally related to breast cancer risk overall (USDHHS 2001, 2004; IARC 2004). In 2002, an international pooled analysis of 53 studies examining alcohol and active smoking and breast cancer risk found that the association between smoking and breast cancer was substantially confounded by alcohol intake. When the analysis was limited to nondrinkers, to exclude potential confounding by alcohol consumption, no relationship was found between active (former or current) smoking and breast cancer risk (Hamajima et al. 2002). However, this combined analysis did not examine relationships by dose/duration of smoking or timing of tobacco use—parameters of tobacco use that are potentially relevant (Terry et al. 2002). Results from several recent cohort studies show a 20 to 60 percent increase in the RR with 20 or more years of active smoking (Terry et al. 2002; Al-Delaminy et al. 2004; Reynolds et al. 2004; Gram et al. 2005), suggesting that the risk of breast cancer from long-term active smoking cannot be definitively excluded. However, the participants in the pooled analysis had an average age of approximately 52 years, implying more than 30 years of smoking on average, and the overall findings were null. There may now be selective publications of reports with positive findings. Possible consequences of smoking at an early age (i.e., during teenage years) for breast cancer risk continue to be investigated (Gram et al. 2005), although a meta-analysis of 11 studies showed that smoking before the birth of a first child was not associated with an increased risk (Lawlor et al. 2004). Because most of the published studies on active smoking and breast cancer risk examined the association using lifetime non-smokers as the baseline group, thus including those involuntarily exposed, there has been concern that the effect of active smoking is underestimated (Morabia et al. 1996). Several recent studies have examined the association between active smoking and breast cancer risk after the removal of involuntary smokers from the referent category, and the effect of active smoking continues to be weak (Gammon et al. 2004; Reynolds et al. 2004; Gram et al. 2005).

Some case-control studies report a twofold increase in the RR of breast cancer in association with secondhand smoke exposure (Morabia et al. 1996; Johnson et al. 2000; Kropp and Chang-Claude 2002). This high point estimate, higher than for some well-established risk factors for breast cancer, appears biologically implausible because the weight of the evidence does not support a causal association between active smoking and breast cancer. A recent study reported that nonsmoking women exposed to secondhand smoke displayed significantly decreased levels of urinary estrone conjugates (the major metabolite of estrogen) throughout their menstrual cycles, suggesting that secondhand smoke exposure may have antiestrogenic effects (Chen et al. 2005). These results, which need to be confirmed, suggest that both involuntary smoking and active smoking have some antiestrogenic consequences (Baron et al. 1990; USDHHS 2004). There is presently no evidence to support the hypothesis that secondhand smoke exposure may have direct harmful effects on the breast that are not balanced by opposing antiestrogenic effects of involuntary smoking (Johnson 2005).

The findings were heterogeneous by menopausal status. In four case-control studies (Millikan et al. 1998; Gammon et al. 2004; Shrubsole et al. 2004; Bonner et al. 2005) and one cohort study (Reynolds et al. 2004), breast cancer risk was not significantly associated with secondhand smoke exposure in both premenopausal and postmenopausal women (Figure 7.1). All five studies examined adult household exposures; workplace (Shrubsole et al. 2004; Bonner et al. 2005) and childhood (Reynolds et al. 2004; Bonner et al. 2005) secondhand smoke exposures were investigated in fewer studies. In contrast, in a case-control study conducted in Canada (Johnson et al. 2000) and in a cohort study conducted in Japan (Hanaoka et al. 2005), exposure to secondhand smoke was associated with a significant twofold to threefold increased risk in premenopausal women, whereas the RR in postmenopausal women was around unity (Johnson et al. 2000; Hanaoka et al. 2005). The stronger association in premenopausal women in these two studies cannot readily be explained. Although both studies assessed secondhand smoke exposure during childhood, risk patterns associated with childhood versus adulthood exposure were not presented. Thus, it is not known whether secondhand smoke exposure during different time periods contributed to differing risks in premenopausal and postmenopausal women in these studies. However, in two other studies of primarily premenopausal women (Smith et al. 1994; Kropp and Chang-Claude 2002), breast cancer risk was not significantly influenced by secondhand smoke exposure during childhood. Three other studies reported higher (approximately threefold to sevenfold) RR estimates in premenopausal women than in all women combined (Sandler et al. 1985a; Morabia et al. 1996; Delfino et al. 2000), but the CIs were wide, and the actual number of premenopausal lifetime nonsmoking cases and controls that were involved were not

presented in these studies. Thus, the overall evidence on secondhand smoke exposure and breast cancer risk is consistent in postmenopausal women, showing no association (Table 7.10). However, findings are not consistent in premenopausal women.

To an extent, characteristics of premenopausal and postmenopausal breast cancer differ. Although the reproductive risk factors have similar effects in premenopausal and postmenopausal cases, the effects of obesity and physical activity vary by menopausal status (van den Brandt et al. 2000; Friedenreich 2004). Integrated models for breast cancer risk have been proposed that acknowledge the potential interplay of environmental and genetic factors across the life course (Hankinson et al. 2004; Colditz 2005). Such varying effects of risk factors with age would seem most plausible for those related to endogenous estrogens, as well as for exogenous estrogen (Hankinson et al. 2004). There is not yet an established biologic rationale for similarly considering that the effect of involuntary smoking would vary by menopausal status. Consequently, the differing findings by menopausal status cannot yet be interpreted within an established biologic framework, and the findings by menopausal status need to be interpreted with consideration of this constraint.

For one environmental carcinogen, ionizing radiation, there is greater susceptibility with exposure in adolescence (Preston et al. 2002; NRC 2005). By analogy, a greater RR might be anticipated for secondhand smoke exposure during childhood, on the assumption that exposure persists across adolescence. There was no increased risk in association with childhood exposure.

Summary

The overall evidence is mixed and does not strongly or consistently support a causal relationship between secondhand smoke and breast cancer. Findings from prospective cohort studies and case-control studies differ to an extent that cannot plausibly be explained by differences in the quality of exposure measurements. The positive association is largely observed in case-control studies among women with premenopausal breast cancer. While greater susceptibility to tobacco smoke carcinogens during adolescence or at an early age has been hypothesized, there is still considerable uncertainty as to why secondhand smoke would only affect risk for premenopausal breast cancer. The overall pooled estimate is elevated, but the elevation largely comes from the increased risks estimated for premenopausal women in selected case-control studies. With regard to biologic plausibility, involuntary smoking would be expected to expose breast tissue to the carcinogens in secondhand smoke, as would active smoking. However, the evidence that active smoking causes no overall increase in breast cancer risks weighs against a causal role for involuntary smoking.

Conclusion

1. The evidence is suggestive but not sufficient to infer a causal relationship between secondhand smoke and breast cancer.

Implications

Because breast cancer remains one of the most frequent cancers, research should be continued on its potential causes, including secondhand smoke exposure. While awaiting further evidence, women should be encouraged to avoid involuntary exposures to secondhand smoke because of the many documented adverse effects of inhaling secondhand smoke.

Nasal Sinus Cavity and Nasopharyngeal Carcinoma

Nasal Sinus Cavity

Cancers of the nasal cavity and paranasal sinuses are extremely rare; they account for less than 1 percent of all invasive incident cancers and for less than 2 percent of all newly diagnosed respiratory cancers in the United States (Rousch 1996). Occupational exposures such as wood dust, use of tobacco products, history of nasal polyps, and certain dietary factors, including a low intake of plant foods and a high intake of salted preserved foods, have been implicated as risk factors for these tumors (Elwood 1981; Brinton et al. 1984; Hayes et al. 1987; Zheng et al. 1993; Demers et al. 1995; Rousch 1996; Mannetje et al. 1999). In different studies, investigators have observed a 1.5- to 5-fold greater risk in association with heavy smoking. Because the association between active smoking and nasal sinus cancers is strongest for squamous cell carcinomas, the strength of the association between active smoking (and secondhand smoke exposure) and all nasal sinus cancers combined is likely to depend on the proportion of squamous cell carcinomas that is included in different studies.

A few studies have investigated the relationship between secondhand smoke exposure and the risk of cancers in the upper respiratory tract, including nasal sinus cavity and nasopharyngeal carcinoma (NPC), among lifetime nonsmokers. These sites are potentially at risk because both gases and particles in secondhand smoke are removed to some extent in the upper airway. In one cohort study (Hirayama 1984) and two case-control studies (Fukuda and Shibata 1990; Zheng et al. 1993) conducted among Caucasian men in the United States (Zheng et al. 1993) and among women in Japan (Fukuda and Shibata 1990; Zheng et al. 1993), secondhand smoke exposure was associated with up to a threefold increase in risk of nasal sinus cancer after adjusting for potential confounders. These studies were reviewed in detail in the Cal/EPA report (NCI 1999), which concluded that the positive association between risk and secondhand smoke exposure was consistent and suggestive of a causal association. The positive association with secondhand smoke exposure is consistent with the relationship between active smoking and the risk of nasal sinus cancers. However, because the published studies were based on very modest sample sizes, further studies are needed to confirm the magnitude of risk associated with secondhand smoke exposure, to establish dose-response relationships, and to characterize the risk by the source (e.g., spouse, other household members, or coworkers) and by the timing of the exposure (current versus past exposure). The role of potential confounders, particularly occupational exposures, should be considered. Future studies should examine the association between secondhand smoke and nasal sinus cancer by histology type and subsite because the effects of tobacco smoke on nasal sinus cancers vary by both of those characteristics (Rousch 1996).

Nasopharyngeal Carcinoma

In addition to studies on the nasal sinus cavity, three case-control studies investigated the role of secondhand smoke in the etiology of NPC among lifetime nonsmokers (Yu et al. 1990; Cheng et al. 1999; Yuan et al. 2000). NPC is rare in most populations (rates below 1 per 100,000); an exception is the high rate among Chinese, particularly southern Chinese (Yu et al. 1990). Ingestion of Chinese salted fish is an important risk factor for NPC among both high-risk and low-risk Chinese populations. Among nondietary environmental exposures, tobacco smoking has been associated with a modest increase in risk (OR = 1.3 [95 percent CI, 0.9–1.9]) (Yu et al. 1990). An association between active smoking and secondhand smoke exposure and NPC is biologically plausible because the inhalation of cigarette smoke directly exposes the nasopharynx to carcinogens present in tobacco smoke.

Secondhand smoke exposure was not associated with a risk of NPC among nonsmokers in two case-control studies (Yu et al. 1990; Cheng et al. 1999). Yu and colleagues (1990) conducted a case-control study of NPC in Guangzhou (Canton city), China, a high-risk NPC area. In the local primary treatment facility for NPC, 329 histologically confirmed incident cases diagnosed in persons under 50 years of age were identified between 1983 and 1985. A total of 306 NPC cases (209 men, 97 women) were interviewed along with an equal number of age-, gender-, and neighborhood-matched controls. In 1989, Yu and colleagues investigated dietary factors, and in 1990 they investigated nondietary environmental exposures that included active and involuntary smoking, the lifetime use of cigarettes and water pipes by study participants and their spouses, and the smoking patterns of parents and other household members at the time of birth and at 10 years of age (Yu et al. 1989, 1990).

These studies found that active smoking was a risk factor for NPC: persons who had ever smoked cigarettes had a risk of 1.3 (95 percent CI, 0.9–1.9) after adjusting for relevant dietary factors such as salted fish. There was also a significant trend of an increase in risk with increasing amounts of tobacco smoked (adjusted OR = 1.0 [0 pack-years], 1.2 [1 to 14 pack-years], 1.6 [15 to 29 pack-years], and 2.9 [≥30 pack-years], p <0.05). Among the lifetime nonsmokers (142 cases, 154 controls), however, secondhand smoke exposure was not associated with any increased risk of NPC. After adjusting for age and gender, there was no increase in risk associated with secondhand smoke exposure from spousal (OR = 0.8 [95 percent CI, 0.3–1.2]), paternal (OR = 0.6 [95 percent CI, 0.3–1.2]), or maternal smoking (OR = 0.7 [95 percent CI, 0.3–1.5]) (Yu et al. 1989, 1990).

A second study on active smoking, secondhand smoke exposure, and the risk of NPC was conducted in Taiwan, where the risk for NPC falls between that of low- and high-risk countries (Cheng et al. 1999). Incident cases of histologically confirmed NPC (n = 378) among individuals who were younger than 75 years of age at diagnosis were prospectively ascertained from two teaching hospitals in Taipei between 1991 and 1994. Efforts were made to individually match controls for age, gender, and residence. A total of 375 NPC patients (260 men, 115 women) and 327 community controls (223 men, 104 women) were interviewed using a structured interview that asked about secondhand smoke exposures during childhood

and adulthood, including the number of smokers in the household, duration of the exposures (person-years), and cumulative exposures (pack-years and person-years). The last two variables, duration and cumulative exposures, were derived from information obtained on smoking intensity and duration for each member reported to have smoked in the household.

Participants who had ever smoked cigarettes showed a small increase in risk (OR = 1.4 [95 percent CI, 0.9–2.0]) after adjusting for age, gender, race, education, family history of NPC, and drinking status. The risk of NPC tended to increase with an increase in the duration of cigarette smoking (OR = 1.0 [0 years of smoking], 1.1 [1 to 24 years of smoking], and 1.7 [≥25 years of smoking], p for trend = 0.03). Among lifetime nonsmokers (178 cases, 173 controls), Cheng and colleagues (1999) observed no increased risks in association with secondhand smoke exposure during childhood (adjusted OR = 0.6 [95 percent CI, 0.4–1.0]) or adulthood (adjusted OR = 0.7 [95 percent CI, 0.5–1.2]). These results did not change when the duration and amount of secondhand smoke exposures during childhood and adulthood were considered.

A third case-control study on secondhand smoke and NPC was conducted in Shanghai, China (Yuan et al. 2000). Similar to Taiwan, this area is also at an intermediate risk of NPC. Between January 1987 and September 1991, the Shanghai Cancer Registry identified 1,110 patients aged 15 through 74 years with histologically confirmed NPC. A total of 935 eligible patients (668 men, 267 women) were interviewed in person and compared with 1,032 age- and gender-matched controls randomly selected from the urban Shanghai population. Yuan and colleagues (2000) collected information on demographic characteristics, usual dietary habits during adulthood, use of tobacco and alcohol, lifetime exposure to secondhand smoke, type of oils and fuels used for cooking, lifetime occupational history, history of chronic ear and nose conditions, and family history of NPC. They also assessed secondhand smoke exposures during childhood (up to 18 years of age) and adulthood (home and workplace). If the person interviewed reported secondhand smoke exposure from a specific household member, then the participants were asked additional questions about the average daily amount smoked and the number of years of smoking. Similarly, if the response was positive to a workplace exposure, then the participants were asked questions about the number of hours of exposure (per day, week, or month) and duration (in years). For each exposed participant, a summary exposure index was constructed by computing a weighted average of job-specific exposures (number of hours exposed to secondhand smoke per working day). The weighting factor was the number of years at a given job divided by the total number of years holding jobs where secondhand smoke exposure occurred.

The investigators found that active smoking was a significant risk factor for NPC among men and women combined (OR = 1.28 [95 percent CI, 1.02–1.61]). Although the increased risk was statistically significant only for men (OR = 1.28 [95 percent CI, 1.01–1.63]), the magnitude of the effect was comparable for women (OR = 1.28 [95 percent CI, 0.67–2.45]). The association between exposure to secondhand smoke and the risk of NPC was investigated in 429 cases (187 men, 242 women) and 546 controls (240 men, 306 women) who were lifetime nonsmokers only. Yuan and colleagues (2000) observed a significantly increased risk among nonsmoking women associated with the husbands' smoking (adjusted OR = 3.09 [95 percent CI, 1.48–6.46]), any household smoking (OR = 2.88 [95 percent CI, 1.39–5.96]), and coworkers' smoking (OR = 2.47 [95 percent CI, 1.12–5.44] for <3 hours and 3.28 [95 percent CI, 1.48–7.27] for ≥3 hours). However, the association between secondhand smoke exposure and a risk of NPC among men was substantially weaker. There was some increase in risk among men whose wives smoked (OR = 1.53 [95 percent CI, 0.26–8.93]) but no increase associated with other smokers in the household (OR = 0.92 [95 percent CI, 0.41–2.04]). A small, nonsignificant increase in risk was associated with workplace secondhand smoke exposure (OR = 1.32 [95 percent CI, 0.63–2.76]). These results were found in men and women and were adjusted for several potential confounders including dietary factors, exposure to cooking fuels, occupational exposures, and family history.

The gender differences in secondhand smoke associations with NPC among lifetime nonsmokers were of borderline statistical significance. Because there were comparable risk estimates between men and women for active smoking and NPC, the investigators expected to find similar associations with secondhand smoke exposure. However, this was not the case. In addition, the researchers expected the magnitude of risks associated with secondhand smoke exposure to be no higher than the risks associated with active smoking, and this also was not the case.

Conclusions

1. The evidence is suggestive but not sufficient to infer a causal relationship between secondhand

smoke exposure and a risk of nasal sinus cancer among nonsmokers.

2. The evidence is inadequate to infer the presence or absence of a causal relationship between secondhand smoke exposure and a risk of nasopharyngeal carcinoma among nonsmokers.

Implications

Larger studies with more complete information on secondhand smoke exposure are needed, with data on exposures at home and outside the home, timing of the exposure, other potential confounders (occupational factors), and tumor characteristics (histology, subsite) to definitively establish the relationship between secondhand smoke exposure and nasal sinus cancer. Studies that are designed to investigate the mechanism(s) of action of active smoking and secondhand smoke exposure will help to elucidate their respective roles in the development of nasal sinus cancer.

Further studies that include adequate numbers of men and women are needed to clarify whether the significant positive association between secondhand smoke exposure and a risk of NPC among women might reflect a chance finding.

Cervical Cancer

Several reviews have addressed effects of exposures from secondhand smoke on the risk for cervical cancer (NCI 1999; USDHHS 2001). Since these reviews, two studies with data on cervical cancer or abnormalities of the cervix have been published (Jee et al. 1999; Scholes et al. 1999).

Some supportive evidence from epidemiologic and biochemical studies does exist that implicates a role for secondhand smoke exposure in the etiology of cervical cancer among nonsmokers. In a Japanese cohort study, the investigators observed a nonsignificant 15 percent increase in risk of cervical cancer among nonsmoking wives associated with the husbands' smoking (Hirayama 1981). However, no association was found between the husbands' smoking and a risk of cervical cancer among participants in a Korean cohort study (adjusted OR = 0.9 [95 percent CI, 0.6–1.2]) (Jee et al. 1999). Among the case-control studies, a significant positive association was observed in two studies (Sandler et al. 1985b; Slattery et al. 1989). In the third case-control study, Coker and colleagues (1992) found that spousal secondhand smoke was associated with an increased risk of cervical cancer and intraepithelial neoplasia among nonsmokers that was of borderline statistical significance.

In the United States, Scholes and colleagues (1999) investigated the role of active smoking and secondhand smoke exposure in the etiology of lower grade cervical abnormalities at the Group Health Cooperative of Puget Sound in western Washington state. Between 1995 and 1996, a population-based automated cervical cytology database was used to identify women 18 years of age or older who had had cervical cytologic testing. Women with severe dysplastic changes (cervical intraepithelial neoplasia [CIN] 3) or invasive cervical cancer (Class 5 and 6 Pap smear results) were excluded from the study. Women with mild or moderate dysplastic cytologic changes (Class 3 or 4 Pap smear results, also known as CIN 1 or 2) or Class 2 changes with epithelial cell abnormalities were classified as cases, and women with normal or Class 1 cytology results served as the control group.

Women aged 18 through 44 years who were not pregnant and did not have a history of hysterectomy were contacted and interviewed by telephone using a behavioral survey that included questions on active smoking and secondhand smoke exposure. Participants were specifically asked whether they had ever smoked as many as 100 cigarettes in their lifetime. Smokers who averaged one cigarette or more per day during the past 12 months were classified as current smokers. Women who had smoked at least 100 cigarettes in their lifetime but did not smoke daily now were classified as former smokers. Exposure to secondhand smoke was based on the smoking patterns of husbands or partners or other household members (Scholes et al. 1999).

A total of 2,448 women—582 cases (i.e., 465 had Class 2 and 117 had Class 3 to 4 Pap smear results) and 1,866 controls (i.e., normal cytology)—were included in this analysis. Fifty-four percent (n = 315) of cases and 62 percent (n = 1,158) of controls were lifetime nonsmokers. Compared with lifetime nonsmokers, current smokers had an increased risk of an abnormal Pap smear (adjusted OR = 1.4 [95 percent CI, 1.1–1.8]) but former smokers did not (adjusted OR = 1.0 [95 percent CI, 0.8–1.3]). Compared with unexposed lifetime nonsmokers, nonsmokers who were exposed to secondhand smoke also showed an increased risk of abnormal Pap smear results of Class 2 to 4 (adjusted OR = 1.4 [95 percent CI, 1.0–2.0]). These results were adjusted for the lifetime number of sexual partners, age, and age at first sexual intercourse.

Conclusion

1. The evidence is inadequate to infer the presence or absence of a causal relationship between secondhand smoke exposure and the risk of cervical cancer among lifetime nonsmokers.

Implications

There is a need for additional studies with adequate sample sizes and more complete information on secondhand smoke exposures, including exposures at home and outside the home and the timing of the exposure, and other potential confounders to definitively establish an association between secondhand smoke exposure and the risk for cervical cancer and cervical abnormalities.

Conclusions

Lung Cancer

1. The evidence is sufficient to infer a causal relationship between secondhand smoke exposure and lung cancer among lifetime nonsmokers. This conclusion extends to all secondhand smoke exposure, regardless of location.

2. The pooled evidence indicates a 20 to 30 percent increase in the risk of lung cancer from secondhand smoke exposure associated with living with a smoker.

Breast Cancer

3. The evidence is suggestive but not sufficient to infer a causal relationship between secondhand smoke and breast cancer.

Nasal Sinus Cavity and Nasopharyngeal Carcinoma

4. The evidence is suggestive but not sufficient to infer a causal relationship between secondhand smoke exposure and a risk of nasal sinus cancer among nonsmokers.

5. The evidence is inadequate to infer the presence or absence of a causal relationship between secondhand smoke exposure and a risk of nasopharyngeal carcinoma among nonsmokers.

Cervical Cancer

6. The evidence is inadequate to infer the presence or absence of a causal relationship between secondhand smoke exposure and the risk of cervical cancer among lifetime nonsmokers.

Overall Implications

The California Environmental Protection Agency (Cal/EPA) has estimated that more than 3,000 (a range of 3,423 to 8,866) lung cancer deaths in the United States each year are attributable to secondhand smoke exposure (Cal/EPA 2005). The estimated number of lung cancer deaths for men (a range of 863 to 3,498) was lower than the estimated number of deaths for women (a range of 2,560 to 5,368), because a lower proportion of nonsmoking men are exposed to spousal smoking. However, the estimate for men did not consider the potential risk from secondhand smoke exposure at work or in other venues where exposures may be higher for men than for women (Cal/EPA 2005).

There is a need for additional research on the risks of other cancers related to secondhand smoke exposure, particularly nasal sinus cancer, breast cancer in both premenopausal and postmenopausal women, nasopharyngeal carcinoma, and cervical cancer.

Appendix 7.1
Details of Recent Lung Cancer Studies

Cohort Studies on the Relationship of Exposure to Secondhand Smoke and Lung Cancer

Nishino and colleagues (2001) investigated the relationship between secondhand smoke exposure at home and the incidence of lung and other cancers in a population-based, prospective study of lifetime nonsmoking women who lived in Miyagi Prefecture, Japan. At the time of enrollment in 1984, 31,345 persons (13,992 men and 17,353 women) completed a baseline questionnaire on smoking, drinking and dietary habits, and reproductive history. To assess residential secondhand smoke exposure, the participants were asked to identify any smokers in their households (husband, wife, father, mother, children, or other household members).

Of the 10,334 lifetime nonsmoking women, 9,675 had no history of cancer and had a complete history of secondhand smoke exposure that included the smoking status of the husband and other household members. Nishino and colleagues (2001) used the population-based cancer registry of Miyagi Prefecture to identify 24 nonsmoking women who had developed lung cancer during the nine-year follow-up period. These investigators also found that the relative risk (RR) for lung cancer was higher among women whose husbands were smokers (1.9 [95 percent confidence interval (CI), 0.8–4.4]) than among women married to nonsmokers. This risk estimate was slightly weakened (RR = 1.8 [95 percent CI, 0.7–4.6]) after further adjustment for demographic characteristics and fruit and vegetable intake. When the smoking status of the husbands and other household members were considered jointly, the risk of lung cancer was 1.2 (95 percent CI, 0.3–4.0) among women who were exposed to secondhand smoke. The very small number of persons with lung cancer in each category of secondhand smoke exposure limits the interpretation of this study.

Jee and colleagues (1999) evaluated the relationship between smoking by the husbands and lung cancer incidence among 157,436 nonsmoking women in Korea whose husbands were enrolled in a health insurance plan. At the time of enrollment in 1992, information on the smoking patterns of the husbands (never, former, current smoker) was obtained during routine medical examinations, and was reassessed

two years later. The classification of exposure to secondhand smoke was based on smoking intensity (the number of cigarettes currently smoked) and duration (the number of years of continuous smoking to date). During the three and one-half years of follow-up, Jee and colleagues (1999) identified 79 persons with lung cancer both existing and newly incident during follow-up.

The adjusted lung cancer incidence rates were 30 percent higher (RR = 1.3 [95 percent CI, 0.6–2.7]) among women whose husbands were former smokers and 90 percent higher (RR = 1.9 [95 percent CI, 1.0–3.5]) among women whose husbands were current smokers compared with women married to nonsmokers. Jee and colleagues (1999) also noted a significant trend in risk with an increase in the duration of exposure. For example, the RR for women who were exposed to secondhand smoke for 1 to 29 years was 1.6, and the RR for those who were exposed for 30 or more years was 3.1 (p trend <0.01). There was not a similar trend with an increase in the amount smoked: the RR for women whose husbands smoked 1 to 19 cigarettes per day was 2.0, and the RR for women whose husbands smoked 20 or more cigarettes per day was 1.5 (p trend <0.1). Other characteristics of husbands who smoked, such as occupation, alcohol intake, and vegetable consumption, did not significantly influence the risk of lung cancer in their wives (Jee et al. 1999). Although a risk of breast cancer was also significantly associated with the husbands' smoking patterns (see "Breast Cancer" earlier in this chapter), there was no significant influence on the wives' risk of developing other cancers, including cancers of the cervix, stomach, and liver.

de Waard and colleagues (1995) conducted a nested case-control study of lung cancer that used the urinary cotinine level as a marker of secondhand smoke exposure. In 1975, the investigators established a cohort of 14,697 women from Utrecht, Netherlands, to study breast cancer risk factors. There was a second screening one year later and baseline urine samples were collected from 12,865 women. In 1982 and 1983, the same investigators enrolled another breast screening cohort and collected urine specimens from more than 12,000 women aged 40 through 49 years. In 1989, 1991, and 1992, these cohorts were linked to the Netherlands Cancer Registry, and the researchers identified 92 women who had died of lung cancer (69 smokers, 23 nonsmokers). From the same cohorts, two to four comparably age-matched controls donated urine specimens on the same day that the cases were selected. Smoking status was assessed from self-reports at the time of urine collection. A total of 448 participants (257 smokers, 191 nonsmokers) participated in an evaluation of the risk of lung cancer in relation to urinary cotinine levels and self-reported smoking status (de Waard et al. 1995).

All self-reported nonsmokers had urinary cotinine levels of less than 100 nanograms per milligram (ng/mg) of creatinine; all active smokers had levels above that amount. The RR of lung cancer was 1.0 for the reference group (persons whose urinary cotinine levels were less than 100 ng/mg of creatinine), 1.3 for persons with levels of 100 to 900 ng/mg, 10.3 for those with levels of 901 to 2,251 ng/mg, and 9.8 for those with levels greater than 2,251 ng/mg. For nonsmokers (23 persons with lung cancer and 191 persons without lung cancer), the RR of lung cancer was 1.0 for persons with urinary cotinine levels of less than 9.2 ng/mg of creatinine, 2.7 for those with levels of 9.2 to 23.4 ng/mg, and 2.4 for those with levels greater than 23.4 ng/mg. Using a biomarker as an exposure classification, de Waard and colleagues (1995) confirmed that secondhand smoke exposure is a risk factor for lung cancer among nonsmokers. These results established a relationship between exposure to secondhand smoke and cotinine levels measured in urine samples from a cohort of women followed for up to 15 years. Because information on self-reported secondhand smoke exposure was not available, the investigators could not compare risk estimates in relation to both urinary cotinine and self-reported secondhand smoke exposure in this study population.

Speizer and colleagues (1999) investigated the relationship between secondhand smoke exposure and lung cancer risk using data from the Nurses Health Study (NHS). Women who were eligible (n = 118,251) for inclusion in this analysis were free from cancer (except nonmelanoma skin cancer) at baseline and had responded to the 1982 questionnaire that assessed childhood and current adult tobacco smoke exposures at home, at work, and in other settings. After 16 years of follow-up, 593 confirmed cases of lung cancer were identified; 58 cases occurred among lifetime nonsmokers. Thirty-five of the 58 lung cancers were diagnosed after 1982 and provided information on secondhand smoke exposure. All but two of the 35 women reported adult secondhand smoke exposure at home and/or work; the age-adjusted RR

for secondhand smoke exposure in adulthood was 1.5 (95 percent CI, 0.3–6.3).

This report on secondhand smoke exposure and lung cancer in the NHS is limited by the small number of lung cancers among lifetime nonsmokers—only a subset could be included in the analysis. Although information on exposure during childhood was obtained, these results were not presented. In addition, only age was considered in the analysis.

Case-Control Studies on the Relationship of Exposure to Secondhand Smoke and Lung Cancer

Canada and the United States

Of the 1 Canadian and 12 U.S. published case-control studies with data on secondhand smoke exposure and lung cancer risk in lifetime nonsmokers, 5 larger studies conducted in the 1990s were designed to address potential methodologic concerns such as misclassification of lifetime nonsmoking status, assessment of secondhand smoke exposure, and inclusion of potential confounders (Table 7.1) (Brownson et al. 1992; Stockwell et al. 1992; Fontham et al. 1994; Kabat et al. 1995; Schwartz et al. 1996; National Cancer Institute [NCI] 1999). One population-based, case-control study included female lung cancer patients who were identified through 8 of the 10 Canadian provincial cancer registries (Table 7.3) (Johnson et al. 2001). A total of 4,089 women responded to the mailed questionnaire. Of these respondents, 1,558 had histologically confirmed primary lung cancer and 2,531 did not have lung cancer. Of those who were eligible and who agreed to participate, 161 cases and 1,271 controls were identified; all were lifetime nonsmokers (i.e., they had smoked fewer than 100 cigarettes in a lifetime). Each respondent answered questions about the number of regular smokers in the household, the duration of residence, and a lifetime occupational history (for each job of at least one year) that included the number of regular smokers in the participant's immediate work area and the number of years at that job. This study investigated (1) the duration and smoker-years (the number of years of exposure weighted by the number of smokers) of residential secondhand smoke, which was defined as residential years multiplied by the number of regular smokers in the residence; and (2) occupational secondhand smoke exposure, which was defined as years worked multiplied by the number of regular smokers in the workplace.

For 71 women with lung cancer and 761 healthy controls, all lifetime nonsmokers, Johnson and colleagues (2001) obtained a complete residential history of secondhand smoke exposure that covered at least 90 percent of their lifetime. There was less information on residential exposure to secondhand smoke for the rest of the women. Using data from these 71 lifetime nonsmokers and 761 controls, Johnson and colleagues (2001) found that any secondhand smoke exposure during childhood and adulthood was associated with an increased risk of lung cancer (odds ratio [OR] =1.63 [95 percent CI, 0.8–3.5]) after adjusting for age, province, education, and total fruit and vegetable consumption. The total number of years of combined residential and occupational secondhand smoke exposure was not associated with a significant trend of increased risks for lung cancer. The ORs were 1.00, 1.46, 1.40, and 1.35 in association with 0, 1 to 24, 25 to 45, and 46 or more years, respectively, of combined exposure (p for trend = 0.36). The association between secondhand smoke exposure and risk for lung cancer was strengthened when the total number of smoker-years was considered. For lifetime nonsmokers, the ORs were 1.00, 0.83, 1.54, and 1.82 in association with 0, 1 to 36, 37 to 77, and 78 or more smoker-years, respectively, of residential and workplace secondhand smoke exposure (p for trend = 0.05) (Table 7.3) (Johnson et al. 2001).

This study was limited because assessments of secondhand smoke exposures were available only for 44 percent (71 out of 161) of the lifetime nonsmoking cases and 60 percent (761 of 1,271) of the lifetime nonsmoking controls. The positive associations between lung cancer risk and residential and occupational secondhand smoke exposures weakened substantially when the analyses included participants with less complete information on their exposures (137 cases and 1,178 controls), or when the participants were all lifetime nonsmokers (161 cases and 1,271 controls). Although the diluted secondhand smoke effect in all lifetime nonsmokers may be due to random (nondifferential) misclassification, the investigators acknowledged the modest overall response rate (70 percent) from the persons who had received the mailed questionnaire, and the relatively high proportion of respondents with incomplete exposure information. It is unclear whether all of the missing data for lifetime nonsmoking cases (56 percent) and controls (40 percent) was attributable to living outside of Canada. Comparisons of demographic characteristics (such as social class, age, and birthplace) and characteristics of persons with complete and incomplete secondhand smoke exposure histories may provide some clues regarding the nature of bias (if any) as a result of the missing information.

European Countries

Case-control studies from Greece (Trichopoulos et al. 1981; Kalandidi et al. 1990), the United Kingdom (Lee et al. 1986), Sweden (Pershagen et al. 1987; Svensson et al. 1989; Nyberg et al. 1998a), Germany (Jöckel et al. 1998; Kreuzer et al. 2000, 2001), Russia (Zaridze et al. 1998), and a multicenter European study (Boffetta et al. 1998) have investigated the relationship between secondhand smoke and lung cancer risk among nonsmokers. As with the U.S. studies, those studies published before 1992 were generally small (Trichopoulos et al. 1981; Lee et al. 1986; Pershagen et al. 1987; Svensson et al. 1989), and the exposure assessments were based largely on the husband's smoking habits (Trichopoulos et al. 1981; Pershagen et al. 1987). Three studies (Jöckel et al. 1998; Nyberg et al. 1998a; Kreuzer et al. 2000, 2001) that were part of the European multicenter study (Boffetta et al. 1998) were also published as separate reports. These investigators not only examined the usual measures of secondhand smoke exposure, such as ever exposed, years of exposure, and amount of exposure, but they also evaluated risk patterns in association with measures of the intensity of the exposure, including the number of hours, the number of smokers, how recently the exposure occurred, and a subjective index of smokiness defined as (1) not visible but smellable, (2) visible, and (3) very smoky (Jöckel et al. 1998; Nyberg et al. 1998a; Kreuzer et al. 2000). Updated results from Sweden (Nyberg et al. 1998a) and Germany (Kreuzer et al. 2000) showed significant increases in the numbers of cases and controls than were in the multicenter European study (Boffetta et al. 1998). The discussion that follows describes studies from Russia (Zaridze et al. 1998), Sweden (Nyberg et al. 1998a), and Germany (Jöckel et al. 1998; Kreuzer et al. 2000).

The results of the first large, multicenter study of secondhand smoke and lung cancer that was conducted at 12 centers in seven European countries by the International Agency for Research on Cancer were published in 1998 (Boffetta et al. 1998). Five centers were hospital-based, one was hospital- and community-based, and six were community-based. Instead of a single protocol, this study incorporated a core of common questions used by all 12 centers. The selection of controls varied by center: controls were individually matched to cases by gender and age in some centers and by frequency matching in others. Nonsmoking status was defined as smoking no more than 400 cigarettes in a lifetime. For men and women combined, the overall RR for lung cancer associated with ever having had a childhood exposure to secondhand smoke was 0.78 (95 percent CI, 0.64–0.96). The RR was 1.16 (95 percent CI, 0.93–1.44) among those with spousal secondhand smoke exposure and 1.17 (95 percent CI, 0.94–1.45) among those with workplace secondhand smoke exposure. The investigators found no significant trends of an increase in risk with increasing years of exposure to spousal or workplace secondhand smoke. However, they did observe significant trends of an increase in risk with increasing intensity-years (hours per day times years) of exposure to spousal (p = 0.02) and workplace (p <0.01) secondhand smoke.

Russia

This section focuses on a hospital-based, case-control study conducted in Moscow that compared female lifetime nonsmokers with histologically confirmed lung cancer (n = 189) and other oncology patients (n = 358) admitted to the same hospital (Table 7.3) (Zaridze et al. 1998). Cases and controls were interviewed within days of their hospital admission or before starting treatment. The investigators based secondhand smoke exposure on the smoking habits of parents during childhood, and of husbands, other household members, and coworkers during adulthood.

Smoking by the husbands was associated with a significantly increased risk of lung cancer (OR = 1.53 [95 percent CI, 1.06–2.21]) (Table 7.3). Having a husband who smoked papirosy, a special high-tar (>30 mg/cigarette) and high-nicotine (>1.8 mg/ cigarette) Russian cigarette, was strongly associated with risk (OR = 2.12 [95 percent CI, 1.32–3.40]). For lifetime nonsmoking women with lung cancer, the risk of lung cancer increased with the number of years a woman had lived with a husband who smoked (duration), although there was not a clear dose-response trend. For example, the OR was 1.86 for women who were exposed to secondhand smoke for 1 to 15 years and 1.42 for those who were exposed for more than 15 years (p trend = 0.07). In relation to the number of cigarettes smoked by the husbands, the OR was 1.66 for women married to men who smoked 1 to 10 cigarettes per day and 1.35 for those married to men who smoked more than 10 cigarettes per day (p trend = 0.10). However, Zaridze and colleagues (1998) found no associated risk of secondhand smoke and lung cancer with exposure during adulthood from household members (OR = 0.91 [95 percent

CI, 0.58–1.42]) or from exposure at work (OR = 0.88 [95 percent CI, 0.55–1.41]) (Table 7.3). There was also no associated risk among women who were exposed to secondhand smoke from fathers during childhood (OR = 0.92 [95 percent CI, 0.64–1.32]).

For women with husbands who smoked, Zaridze and colleagues (1998) found that the risks for both squamous cell carcinoma (OR = 1.94 [95 percent CI, 0.99–3.81]) and adenocarcinoma of the lung (OR = 1.52 [95 percent CI, 0.96–2.39]) were associated with exposure to secondhand smoke. An association between husbands who smoked and lung cancer risk was more pronounced when the controls in the analyses were restricted to women who had cancer diagnosed in sites where cancer is not associated with active smoking, including breast and endometrial cancer (OR = 1.82 [95 percent CI, 1.18–2.80]). This association was weaker when the analyses included only women who had cancer diagnosed in sites where cancer is associated with smoking, such as cervical and gastric cancers (OR = 1.22 [95 percent CI, 0.79–1.88]).

Although a strength of this study was that all of the interviews were conducted with self-respondents, limitations in the methods included selection of controls and the failure to biochemically validate secondhand smoke exposure. The definition of a lifetime nonsmoker and the process used to determine and verify this status were not described, and the investigators only adjusted for age and education (Zaridze et al. 1998).

Sweden

This section discusses a hospital-based, case-control study of secondhand smoke exposure and lung cancer conducted among male and female lifetime nonsmokers in Stockholm county, Sweden, between 1989 and 1995 (Nyberg et al. 1998a,b). The researchers interviewed 124 lifetime nonsmokers (35 men, 89 women) with histologically confirmed lung cancer, and 235 frequency-matched population controls of lifetime nonsmokers without lung cancer (72 men, 163 women).

Nyberg and colleagues (1998a) conducted a thorough review process to determine the lifetime nonsmoking status of study participants. Specifically, they contacted the next of kin of all cases (n = 124) and of every second control (n = 118 of 235) to confirm the lifetime nonsmoking status for 99.1 percent of the lifetime nonsmokers with lung cancer and 97.2 percent of the lifetime nonsmokers without lung cancer (Nyberg et al. 1998a). The authors assessed exposure to secondhand smoke using questions developed in a study on urinary cotinine and secondhand smoke exposure (Riboli et al. 1990) that covered childhood exposure, domestic exposure from the spouse and other cohabitants, exposure at all workplaces and other places, and exposure in vehicles.

The investigators used gender, age, catchment area, and other covariates to adjust the results on secondhand smoke (Nyberg et al. 1998a). The researchers found that secondhand smoke exposure from spouses was associated with a small increase in risk. This association was stronger among men (OR = 1.96 [95 percent CI, 0.72–5.36]) than among women (OR = 1.05 [95 percent CI, 0.60–1.86]) (Table 7.3). Any secondhand smoke exposure in the workplace was associated with increased risks among both men (OR = 1.89 [95 percent CI, 0.53–6.67]) and women (OR = 1.57 [95 percent CI, 0.80–3.06]) (Table 7.3). In men and women combined, a significant trend of an increase in risk of lung cancer was evident with more years of secondhand smoke exposure at work. For example, adults who were exposed to less than 30 years of secondhand smoke at work had an OR of 1.40, and those who had been exposed for 30 or more years had an OR of 2.21 (p for trend = 0.03). When they considered hours of exposure per day in the workplace, the investigators found that the trends in risks associated with secondhand smoke exposure were strengthened slightly: the OR was 1.27 for persons who were exposed for less than 30 hour-years[1], and the OR was 2.51 for those who were exposed for 30 or more hour-years (p for trend = 0.01). Lung cancer risk in women was not associated with secondhand smoke exposure in other indoor locations or in vehicles (OR = 0.41 [95 percent CI, 0.09–1.75]), but the risks increased nonsignificantly among men (OR = 1.71 [95 percent CI, 0.49–5.98]) (Nyberg et al. 1998a). When secondhand smoke exposures from spouses and coworkers were considered together, those who were currently exposed (within the past two years) had more than a twofold increase in risk (OR = 2.12 [95 percent CI, 0.91–4.92]). The risk was highest (OR = 2.52 [95 percent CI, 1.08–5.85]) among individuals with the highest levels of exposure or in the top 90th percentile of hour-years of exposure. Paternal smoking was associated with an increased risk among men (OR = 1.90 [95 percent CI, 0.69–5.23]) but not among women (OR = 0.76 [95 percent CI, 0.42–1.37]), whereas maternal smoking was not associated with risk in either group (Nyberg et al. 1998a).

One weakness of this study is that 36 participants (12 cases and 24 controls) were occasional smokers (lifetime total of 20 to 408 packs); 11 had smoked during the 10 years before the study. Although the investigators reported no evidence that these occasional smokers confounded the secondhand smoke association, results excluding this group of participants were not presented. An important strength of this study is that a next of kin validation substudy was conducted using all cases and a subset of controls (Nyberg et al. 1998a). There was high concordance exhibited between next of kin and lung cancer cases and controls with the reported lifetime nonsmoking status of cases and controls and their exposures to spousal secondhand smoke. Because interviews were conducted with self-respondents, measures of intensity such as hours of exposure at work and at home (from spouses) were also documented and appeared to be more sensitive markers of exposure than duration of exposure or amount smoked. The stronger effects associated with current secondhand smoke exposure in this study may partially explain the more heterogeneous results associated with childhood secondhand smoke exposure (Nyberg et al. 1998a).

Germany

One hospital-based, case-control study investigated the role of occupational exposure by including 1,004 persons with incident lung cancer (839 men, 165 women) and an equal number of individually matched population controls from Frankfurt, Bremen, and surrounding areas in Germany (Jöckel et al. 1998). An analysis of secondhand smoke exposure was based on 55 cases and 160 controls who reported that they had never smoked regularly, which was defined as smoking for less than six months (Jöckel et al. 1998). Almost all were also included in the European multicenter study (Boffetta et al. 1998), but the results are described separately because of additional data on the intensity of the exposures.

For each source of secondhand smoke exposure (childhood, spouse, workplace, transportation, and other public places), variables of exposure were defined based on hours of exposure, years of exposure, and the degree of smokiness (defined as [1] not visible but smellable, [2] visible, and [3] very smoky). Participants were classified into three exposure categories: no or low exposures from a specific source

---

[1]One hour-year equals 365 hours per year, or 1 hour per day for one year.

if all exposure variables were below the respective 75th percentile, intermediate or medium if at least one variable was above the respective 75th percentile but below the 90th percentile, and high if at least one variable was above the respective 90th percentile. Because secondhand smoke exposure is ubiquitous, this approach focused on those who were highly exposed. The results from an earlier validation study that used urinary cotinine among healthy women in the Bremen area showed that the misclassification of questionnaire-based secondhand smoke exposure tends to be greater in the lower three quartiles of exposure than in the top quartile (Becher et al. 1992).

After adjusting for gender, age, and region, there was a small increased risk associated with ever having lived with a smoking spouse (OR = 1.12 [95 percent CI, 0.54–2.32]) (Table 7.3) (Jöckel et al. 1998). When persons were reclassified to no or low spousal secondhand smoke exposure, or to medium and high exposure (low = all exposure variables below the 75th percentile, medium = at least one variable above the 75th percentile but below the 90th percentile, and high = at least one variable above the 90th percentile), the investigators found that those with a medium exposure showed a risk of 0.22 (95 percent CI, 0.05–1.07) and those with a high exposure showed a risk of 1.87 (95 percent CI, 0.45–7.74). Persons with a high secondhand smoke exposure during childhood, with exposures from other sources during adulthood including workplace, public transportation, and other public places, and persons with a high total of associated secondhand smoke exposures in childhood and in adulthood had a twofold to threefold increase in risk. The investigators also noted that individuals with high combined exposures during childhood and adulthood had a significantly increased risk (OR = 3.24 [95 percent CI, 1.44–7.32]) of lung cancer than did those with no or low secondhand smoke exposure (Table 7.3) (Jöckel et al. 1998). In this and another study from Germany (Kreuzer et al. 2000, 2001), any effect of secondhand smoke exposure on lung cancer risk was stronger among those who were highly exposed.

One clinic-based, case-control study was designed to investigate the role of radon in the etiology of lung cancer in East and West Germany (Kreuzer et al. 2000). Persons with histologically confirmed lung cancer and frequency-matched population controls were interviewed. The analysis included 292 adults (234 women, 58 men) and 1,338 controls (535 women, 803 men) who had smoked fewer than 400 cigarettes during their life (lifetime nonsmokers) (Table 7.3). A subset of these lifetime nonsmokers (173 cases and 215 controls) was previously included in the European multicenter study (Boffetta et al. 1998) as part of the data collected in Germany (referred to as Germany 2 and Germany 3 in the report by Boffetta et al. 1998). The interviews with the participants included questions on secondhand smoke exposure during childhood, from spouses and other cohabitants, at all workplaces and other public places, and in vehicles. Besides classifying persons by ever or never having an exposure to various sources of secondhand smoke, the study determined several measures of intensity that included the duration of exposure (in hours) during childhood; spousal and workplace exposures; pack-years[2] of exposure from spouses; and a weighted duration of exposure (based on hours of exposure and the level of smokiness) at work, in other indoor settings, and in vehicles (Kreuzer et al. 2000).

After the investigators adjusted for age and region, they found that the risk of lung cancer among female lifetime nonsmokers was not significantly associated with secondhand smoke exposure during childhood (OR = 0.78 [95 percent CI, 0.56–1.08]) or adulthood, including exposure from husbands (OR = 0.96 [95 percent CI, 0.70–1.33]), in the workplace (OR = 1.14 [95 percent CI, 0.83–1.57]), in vehicles (OR = 0.96 [95 percent CI, 0.57–1.60]), and in other indoor settings (OR = 0.95 [95 percent CI, 0.66–1.38]). Similar results were obtained when they considered cumulative pack-years of exposure from husbands, or duration of exposure (in hours) during childhood and from spouses (Kreuzer et al. 2000). However, the risk was substantially higher when they considered weighted duration of secondhand smoke exposure (hours times the level of smokiness) at the workplace. There were statistically significant risks (twofold greater) in association with the highest levels of duration (i.e., hours) and with weighted duration of workplace exposures. The risk of lung cancer among women also increased in relation to the weighted duration of secondhand smoke from all sources (hours times the level of smokiness): the ORs were 0.87 (95 percent CI, 0.57–1.34) for those with no or low exposure and

---

[2]Pack-years = The number of years of smoking multiplied by the number of packs of cigarettes smoked per day.

The Health Consequences of Involuntary Exposure to Tobacco Smoke

1.51 (95 percent CI, 0.97–2.33) for those with medium or high secondhand smoke exposures (p trend = 0.21). When the investigators considered the weighted duration of the exposure outside the home, the ORs were 1.38 (95 percent CI, 0.74–2.57) for those with low or no exposure and 1.99 (95 percent CI, 0.95–4.15) for those with medium or high exposures (p trend = 0.11) (Kreuzer et al. 2000). Because of the smaller numbers of male lifetime nonsmokers in the study, the investigators noted that a risk of lung cancer among men was not significantly associated with secondhand smoke exposures from their wives' smoking (OR = 0.8 [95 percent CI, 0.11–6.38] for a high exposure) or in the workplace (OR = 1.1 [95 percent CI, 0.47–2.70] for a high exposure) (Kreuzer et al. 2001). In this study, effects were not confounded by social class; a family history of lung cancer; occupational exposure to carcinogens; radon in their residence; previous lung disease; and consumption of carrots, salad, or fresh fruits. The risk estimate associated with a high exposure from all sources combined remained essentially unchanged when each covariate was included in the regression model.

Adenocarcinoma of the lung accounted for 59 percent (n = 173) of the lung cancers among lifetime nonsmokers in this study population (Table 7.3) (Kreuzer et al. 2000). Results were generally similar in cell-type specific analyses (adenocarcinoma versus nonadenocarcinoma) among women and with both genders combined. Spousal smoking was not associated with a risk for adenocarcinoma or for other types of lung cancer. Secondhand smoke exposure at work was associated with increased risks for both adenocarcinoma and nonadenocarcinoma that were qualitatively similar, but the result was statistically significant only for the latter group.

Using a combined index of exposures during childhood and adulthood, Jöckel and colleagues (1998) found increased risks of lung cancer in association with high secondhand smoke exposures. Kreuzer and colleagues (2000, 2001) found that high levels of secondhand smoke exposure at the workplace in terms of hours or weighted duration (hours times smokiness) were associated with an increased risk of lung cancer. Although this exposure measure cannot be validated because it is self-reported, it appears to identify a highly exposed group that is at an increased risk. Undoubtedly, questions such as hours of exposure, number of smokers, and level of smokiness can be asked directly only when conducting interviews with both cases and controls. Because these two studies included only self-respondents who were well enough to participate in an interview

lasting at least an hour, the information may be valid and useful for identifying an at-risk subgroup: those in the highest category of exposure.

A hospital-based study of lung cancer was conducted among Czech women in Prague to investigate the role of active smoking and secondhand smoke (Kubik et al. 2001). The researchers interviewed females diagnosed with a histologically confirmed lung cancer (n = 140) and control participants who were spouses, relatives, or friends of other patients in the hospital (n = 462). The investigators based secondhand smoke exposure on the smoking behaviors of parents, husbands, cohabitants, and coworkers. Specifically, participants were asked to assess the number of hours per day spent in smoky rooms (at home, at work, and elsewhere) as adults and exposure during childhood before 16 years of age. Using data from 24 cases and 176 controls who were lifetime nonsmokers (i.e., they had smoked fewer than 100 cigarettes in a lifetime), these investigators found that any secondhand smoke exposure during childhood was associated with an increased risk of lung cancer (OR = 2.02 [95 percent CI, 0.8–4.9]) after adjusting for age, residence, and education. The OR was 1.17 (95 percent CI, 0.2–5.6) among women exposed to secondhand smoke as adults (defined as >3 hours per day). For women with both childhood and adulthood exposures, the OR was 3.68 (95 percent CI, 0.6–21.9).

Although this study attempted to obtain information on secondhand smoke exposure at home and outside of the home during childhood and adulthood, the sample size of lifetime nonsmoking lung cancer patients was limited, and the appropriateness of the control groups was uncertain. Information on potential confounders was also lacking.

Chinese in Taiwan, Singapore, Hong Kong, and the People's Republic of China

Chinese women have a high incidence of lung cancer despite a low prevalence of active smoking (Wu-Williams et al. 1990). This elevated incidence, particularly of adenocarcinoma of the lung, has been noted for Chinese women residing in Singapore (Law et al. 1976), Hong Kong (Kung et al. 1984), Shanghai (Gao et al. 1988), and northern China (Xu et al. 1989). A number of case-control studies have investigated secondhand smoke and other sources of indoor air pollution as possible explanations for the high lung cancer rates among Chinese women. Some of the study locations were selected specifically because of local cooking or heating practices considered to be possible sources of carcinogenic indoor pollutants

Cancer Among Adults from Exposure to Secondhand Smoke 491

(Wu-Williams et al. 1990; Liu et al. 1991; Wang et al. 2000). These locations were Hong Kong (Chan and Fung 1982; Koo et al. 1987; Lam et al. 1987), Taiwan (Ko et al. 1997; Lee et al. 2000), Singapore (Seow et al. 2000), and the People's Republic of China: Guangdong Province in the south (Liu et al. 1993; Du et al. 1996; Lei et al. 1996), Xuanwei County in Yunnan Province (Liu et al. 1991), urban regions including Shanghai (Gao et al. 1987; Zhong et al. 1999), Nanjing (Shen et al. 1998), Tianjin (Geng et al. 1988), Harbin and Shenyang in northeastern China (Wu-Williams et al. 1990; Wang et al. 1994, 1996), and Gansu Province in northwestern China (Wang et al. 2000). Study methods and data quality were quite varied. Six of these studies had large sample sizes (Gao et al. 1987; Wu-Williams et al. 1990; Zhong et al. 1999; Lee et al. 2000; Seow et al. 2000; Wang et al. 2000), four were population-based (Gao et al. 1987; Wu-Williams et al. 1990; Zhong et al. 1999; Wang et al. 2000), and two were hospital-based (Lee et al. 2000; Seow et al. 2000). In the four largest studies, exposure to secondhand smoke was assessed from smoking by spouses, by other household members during childhood and adulthood, and by others in the workplace (Wu-Williams et al. 1990; Zhong et al. 1999; Lee et al. 2000; Wang et al. 2000). Although these four studies provided detailed information on secondhand smoke exposures and potential confounders, other studies included no information on key features such as age range of participants (Lei et al. 1996; Shen et al. 1996), the definition of lifetime nonsmokers (Wang et al. 1994, 1996; Lei et al. 1996; Shen et al. 1996, 1998), and response rates (Wang et al. 1994, 1996; Shen et al. 1996, 1998). In an early study conducted in Shanghai (Gao et al. 1987), secondhand smoke exposure was based only on smoking habits of the husbands. The study conducted in Singapore asked a single question about secondhand smoke exposure at home (Seow et al. 2000). Four studies presented crude risk estimates associated with secondhand smoke exposure (Wang et al. 1994; Lei et al. 1996; Shen et al. 1996, 1998). Studies also varied in the degree of pathologic confirmation, particularly those conducted in the People's Republic of China, and the proportion of histologically confirmed participants was generally considerably lower than in studies conducted in western countries or elsewhere in Asia (Table 7.3).

Taiwan

A hospital-based study of lung cancer conducted in Kaohsiung, an industrialized city in southern Taiwan, investigated the role of secondhand smoke, previous lung diseases, cooking practices, and the indoor environment (Ko et al. 1997; Lee et al. 2000). The investigators compared secondhand smoke exposure and other lifestyle factors of female lifetime nonsmokers who had a histologically confirmed lung cancer (n = 268), and of hospital controls who were ophthalmic or orthopedic patients or who were admitted to the same hospital for physical check-ups (n = 445) (Table 7.3) (Lee et al. 2000). Information on secondhand smoke exposure during childhood (aged <19 years) and adulthood (aged ≥19 years) at home and at work was obtained from a structured interview with the study participants. Secondhand smoke exposures were classified as no exposure, absence (secondhand smoke exposure but not in the presence of the participant), and presence of secondhand smoke exposure in the presence of the study participant.

In their analysis, Lee and colleagues (2000) adjusted for demographic characteristics and other potential confounders. These investigators found that husbands who smoked in the presence of participants significantly increased participants' risk of lung cancer (OR = 2.2 [95 percent CI, 1.5–3.3]). The study also noted a significant trend of an increase in risk among wives with increasing pack-years smoked by the husbands: the OR was 1.5 for 1 to 20 pack-years, 2.5 for 21 to 40 pack-years, and 3.3 for more than 40 pack-years.

There were nonsignificant increases in risks of 1.2 to 1.5 in association with other sources of secondhand smoke exposure during adulthood, including exposures from other family members at home and from coworkers at work (Lee et al. 2000). The risk of lung cancer increased significantly in association with a combined index of all sources of exposure during adulthood. For those with no reported exposure in the reference category, the OR was 1; for those with cumulative exposures of 1 to 20 smoker-years, the OR was 1.2; for 21 to 40 smoker-years, the OR was 1.4; and for 41 or more smoker-years, the OR was 2.2 (p trend = 0.002). The risk of lung cancer increased in association with smoking in the presence of the study participant during childhood by fathers (OR = 1.7 [95 percent CI, 1.1–2.6]) and other family members (OR = 1.4 [95 percent CI, 0.8–2.2]) but not by mothers (OR = 0.9 [95 percent CI, 0.3–3.1]). The investigators also observed a significant trend of an increase in risk among women with increasing secondhand smoke exposures during childhood: the ORs were 1.5 for exposures of 1 to 20 smoker-years and 1.8 for exposures of more than 20 smoker-years (p for trend = 0.01). When exposures during childhood and adulthood were considered together, individuals with childhood exposures and with the highest levels of exposure during adulthood, defined as 40 or more smoker-years, showed more than a fourfold increase in risk (OR = 4.7 [95 percent CI, 2.4–9.4]) compared with individuals with no exposures.

One strength of this study is the assessment of smoking by family members and coworkers in the presence of the study participants. In fact, the risks associated with secondhand smoke exposure during childhood, from husbands, and from coworkers were invariably higher when the exposure was in the presence of the study participants. The risk estimates were reduced when the comparison was between women with no exposure and those with any exposure (combining absence and presence). The ORs associated with smoking by fathers (1.19), by other family members during childhood (1.11), by husbands (1.72), by other family members during adulthood (1.27), and by coworkers (1.24) showed weaker effects. These effects were similar to the risk estimates reported in other studies when secondhand smoke exposure in the presence of the study participants was not specifically distinguished.

Singapore

A hospital-based, case-control study in Singapore included women who had pathologically confirmed primary lung cancer (n = 303), and controls who were admitted to the same hospital (n = 756) but did not have a history of malignant or chronic respiratory disease, heart disease, or renal failure (Seow et al. 2000, 2002). All participants were interviewed in person using a standardized questionnaire that asked extensively about diet, reproductive history, and cooking practices, but the question on secondhand smoke exposure was crude. Persons were asked a single question regarding secondhand smoke exposure: whether any household members (spouse, parents, children, or any other relative or friend) had smoked in their presence more often than once a week.

Of the total cases and controls interviewed, 176 cases and 663 controls were lifetime nonsmokers, defined as fewer than one cigarette a day for a year (Table 7.3). Based on the single question on secondhand smoke exposure during childhood and adulthood, an estimated 52 percent of cases and 45 percent of controls had been exposed to secondhand smoke at home at least weekly. The OR was 1.3 (95 percent CI, 0.9–1.8) after adjusting for dietary and nondietary factors (Table 7.3) (Seow et al. 2002). Although this study is well-designed, information on secondhand smoke exposure was extremely limited.

Hong Kong and Southern China

Three studies from Hong Kong (Chan and Fung 1982; Koo et al. 1987; Lam et al. 1987) and three from southern China (Liu et al. 1991, 1993; Lei et al. 1996) have investigated the role of spousal smoking and lung cancer risk among women who had never smoked. Only one study (Lei et al. 1996) had not been previously reviewed (U.S. Environmental Protection Agency [USEPA] 1992; NCI 1999). Two studies found that exposure to smoking by the husbands was associated with a statistically significant increase in the risk of lung cancer among lifetime nonsmokers (Lam et al. 1987; Liu et al. 1993).

The role of secondhand smoke exposure in the risk of lung cancer mortality was investigated in a case-control study in Guangzhou, China (Table 7.3) (Du et al. 1996; Lei et al. 1996). The investigators reviewed death records maintained by the local police stations in the study area. All registered deaths from primary lung cancer (n = 831) of persons who had resided in Guangzhou for at least 10 years were considered eligible for the study. After excluding persons with a history of respiratory diseases or tumors, the investigators successfully identified controls for 792 of the 831 lung cancer deaths that were then matched by gender, age, same year of death, and block of residence. A standardized interview asked spouses or cohabiting relatives of the decedents about active smoking, exposure to secondhand smoke, living conditions, cooking facilities, exposure to coal dust, and dietary habits.

A total of 126 adults with a registered death of lung cancer (85 women, 41 men) and 270 matched adults who had died of causes other than lung cancer (147 women, 123 men) were classified as nonsmokers, but the analysis was based on 75 women who had died of lung cancer and 128 women who had died of other causes. Nonsmoking women married to smokers had a small increase in risk of lung cancer (OR = 1.19 [95 percent CI, 0.66–2.16]) (Table 7.3) (Du et al. 1996; Lei et al. 1996). Compared with nonsmoking women married to nonsmokers, women exposed to 1 to 19 cigarettes per day had an OR of 0.72 and women exposed to 20 or more cigarettes per day an OR of 1.62 (p for trend = 0.20). Risk did not significantly increase in association with duration of the husbands' smoking. For example, the OR for an exposure of 1 to 29 years was 1.39 compared with an OR of 1.17 for an exposure of 30 or more years (Du et al. 1996; Lei et al. 1996).

There are noted limitations in the study methods (see "Chinese in Taiwan, Singapore, Hong Kong, and the People's Republic of China" earlier in this chapter). Some of the adults who died of causes other than lung cancer may have had smoking-related diseases, because only those with respiratory diseases or other tumors were excluded from the analyses. In addition, the accuracy of a diagnosis of lung cancer based on reviewed death records is not known for China, and the quality and completeness of information on secondhand smoke exposures obtained from next of kin were not described.

Urban Areas in Central and Northern China

Six studies were conducted in central and northern China (Gao et al. 1987; Geng et al. 1988; USEPA 1992; Shen et al. 1996, 1998; Zhong et al. 1999). Secondhand smoke exposure from the husbands' smoking was implicated as a risk factor in the studies conducted in Shanghai (Gao et al. 1987) and in Tianjin (Geng et al. 1988; USEPA 1992). Shen and colleagues (1996) examined lung cancer among long-term (at least 20 years) female residents of Nanjing in a hospital-based, case-control study. Shen and colleagues (1998) then investigated the role of secondhand smoke exposure among nonsmoking women diagnosed with adenocarcinoma of the lung (n = 70) and among "healthy" women individually matched for age, neighborhood of residence, and occupation to the women with lung cancer. A standardized questionnaire administered to study participants included questions on secondhand smoke exposures and other lifestyle factors.

Exposure to secondhand smoke was associated with a nonsignificant increase in the risk of adenocarcinoma of the lung (OR = 1.63 [95 percent CI, 0.68–3.89]) (Table 7.3) (Shen et al. 1998). No significant trends were observed in risk with increased numbers of cigarettes per day or increased duration (in years) of the exposure. The investigators noted that the risk associated with any secondhand smoke exposure was weakened after adjusting for other factors that included chronic lung diseases, conditions of living quarters, type of fuel used for cooking and heating, and cooking practices. It was unclear whether the study participants were specifically asked about secondhand smoke exposure from spouses and other household members. The investigators also matched the study participants for occupation, which may have led to overmatching on certain exposures including secondhand smoke (Shen et al. 1996, 1998).

A population-based study of female lung cancer patients was designed to investigate the role of secondhand smoke exposure and other lung cancer risk factors in Shanghai (Zhong et al. 1999). Interviews that asked about active smoking, exposures to secondhand smoke, lifetime occupational history, residential history, family history of lung cancer, cooking activities, and dietary habits were conducted with 649 women diagnosed with lung cancer (cases) and 675 women from the general population (controls). Exposures to secondhand smoke in the home during childhood and adulthood were assessed by asking about all household members who smoked: the type of tobacco product used, the average number of cigarettes smoked per day, and the number of years of smoking while the participant lived in the household. Workplace exposure to secondhand smoke for jobs that lasted at least two years were also assessed. For each job, questions included the number of coworkers who smoked, and the total number of years and average number of hours per day spent with smoking coworkers (Zhong et al. 1999).

The analysis on secondhand smoke and lung cancer among lifetime nonsmokers was based on 504 women diagnosed with lung cancer (cases) and 601 women from the general population (controls); 145 cases and 74 controls reported smoking at least one cigarette per day for at least six months. The investigators adjusted demographic variables and other relevant covariates in the analyses on secondhand smoke exposure and found that compared with nonsmoking women married to nonsmoking husbands, nonsmoking women married to smokers showed a small increased risk (OR = 1.1 [95 percent CI, 0.8–1.5]). The study documented little variation in risk when the amount or duration of the husbands' smoking was considered: increased risks were 1.2 (95 percent CI, 0.8–1.7) and 1.9 (95 percent CI, 0.9–3.7) in association with secondhand smoke exposures during adulthood at home and at work, respectively (Table 7.3) (Zhong et al. 1999). Persons with secondhand smoke exposures both at home and at work as adults showed a significant increase in risk (OR = 1.9 [95 percent CI, 1.1–3.5]). Further investigation of workplace secondhand smoke exposures revealed statistically significant trends of an increase in risk with an increase in the number of hours of daily exposure. (For example, the OR for women exposed to secondhand smoke 1 to 2 hours per day was 1.0; 1.6 for those exposed 3 to 4 hours per day; and 2.9 for those exposed >4 hours per day [p trend <0.001].) A similar trend was noted with an increase in the number of coworkers who smoked (OR = 1.0 [1 to 2 coworkers who smoked], 1.7 [3 to 4 coworkers who smoked], and 3.0 [>4 coworkers] [p trend <0.001]). However, the trend for risk with an increasing number of years of secondhand smoke exposure at work was not significant (OR = 1.0 [0 years], 2.0 [1 to 12 years], 1.4 [13 to 24 years], and 1.8 [>24 years] [p trend = 0.50]). Women with only a childhood exposure to secondhand smoke did not show any increased risk (OR = 0.9 [95 percent CI, 0.5–1.6]); the results remained similar when the investigators considered the duration (number of years) of exposure (Zhong et al. 1999).

Although some of the numbers became quite sparse, Zhong and colleagues (1999) conducted separate analyses among the 387 pathologically or cytologically confirmed lung cancer cases for adenocarcinoma (n = 297), for nonadenocarcinoma (n = 55), and for unknown cell types such as those diagnosed radiologically or clinically. Results associated with any workplace secondhand smoke exposure and the husbands' smoking were generally similar in these cell-type specific analyses. For example, the ORs associated with workplace secondhand smoke exposure were 1.8 (95 percent CI, 1.3–2.6) for adenocarcinoma, 1.7 (95 percent CI, 1.0–2.9) for nonadenocarcinoma, and 1.3 (95 percent CI, 0.7–2.3) for an unknown cell type. All three risk estimates associated with the husbands' smoking were between 1.1 and 1.2. However, the risks associated with secondhand smoke exposure during childhood were only substantially (but not significantly) higher for nonadenocarcinoma (OR = 2.4 [95 percent CI, 0.9–6.4]) than for adenocarcinoma (OR = 0.8 [95 percent CI, 0.3–1.9]), or for those with unknown cell types (OR = 0.8). Because of this risk difference by cell type, a cumulative index of secondhand smoke exposure during childhood and adulthood was more strongly associated with a risk of nonadenocarcinoma (OR = 2.1 [95 percent CI, 0.9–4.8]) than with adenocarcinoma (OR = 1.2 [95 percent CI, 0.7–1.8]), or with those of unknown cell types (OR = 1.0 [95 percent CI, 0.5–1.8]).

Strengths of this study include the population-based design, high response rates, high percentage of completed interviews with self-respondents, a comprehensive assessment of lifetime exposure to secondhand smoke that included various measures of intensity of exposure, and other potential confounding factors. Although only approximately three-fourths of the women diagnosed with lung cancer (i.e., cases) were histologically or cytologically confirmed, the investigators were able to conduct cell-type specific analyses because of the large sample size (Zhong et al. 1999).

Four case-control studies conducted in northern China investigated the role of secondhand smoke in the etiology of lung cancer among women. The locations included a large population-based study in Heilongjiang Province (Wu-Williams et al. 1990) and Gansu Province (Wang et al. 2000), and smaller hospital-based studies in Harbin (Wang et al. 1994) and Shenyang (Wang et al. 1996; Zhou et al. 2000). The RR of lung cancer was below 1.0 in association with secondhand smoke exposure in a large case-control study conducted in northern China (Wu-Williams et al. 1990). This observation should be considered anomalous as this result differs from the collective evidence of studies conducted in other Chinese populations as well as from the overall evidence (see "Pooled Analyses" earlier in this chapter). The effects of secondhand smoke may have been obscured in this study because other sources of indoor air pollution, such as coal-burning stoves and *kang* (brick beds that are typically heated either directly by a stove underneath them or by pipes connected to the cooking stove), were associated with an increased risk.

The role of secondhand smoke and the risk of lung cancer among lifetime nonsmoking women was investigated in a hospital-based, case-control study conducted in Shenyang, China (Table 7.3) (Wang et al. 1996; Zhou et al. 2000). The investigators compared female lifetime nonsmokers diagnosed with primary lung cancer (a total of 135) and an equal number of age-matched lifetime nonsmoking women (controls) selected from the general population of Shenyang. A structured questionnaire was administered to obtain information on demographic characteristics, exposure to tobacco, dietary and cooking practices, the type of fuel used, general medical conditions, history of previous lung diseases, history of cancer, menstrual and pregnancy history, and job history.

Lung cancer risk was not associated with any secondhand smoke exposure during childhood (OR = 0.91 [95 percent CI, 0.55–1.49]) or in the workplace during adulthood (OR = 0.89 [95 percent CI, 0.45–1.77]). Adult exposures to husbands' smoking were associated with a small increase in risk (OR = 1.11 [95 percent CI, 0.65–1.88]), but there were no significant trends of an increase in risk with an increase in duration of exposure (OR = 1.41 [<20 years], 1.08 [20 to 29 years], 1.08 [30 to 39 years], and 1.08 [≥40 years]) or in the amount smoked by the husbands (OR = 1.0 [0 cigarettes per day], 0.35 [1 to 9 cigarettes per day], 1.35 [10 to 19 cigarettes per day], and 1.40 [≥20 cigarettes per day]) (Wang et al. 1996).

A second report investigated the role of secondhand smoke exposure among persons diagnosed with adenocarcinoma of the lung (n = 72) and an equal number of persons from the general population (controls) (Wang et al. 1996; Zhou et al. 2000). A risk of adenocarcinoma of the lung was not associated with secondhand smoke exposures from parents during childhood (OR = 0.89 [95 percent CI, 0.43–1.84]), from husbands (OR = 0.94 [95 percent CI, 0.45–1.97]), or from the workplace (OR = 0.89 [95 percent CI, 0.25–3.16]). There was little variation in risk with years of exposure during childhood or from husbands who smoked (Zhou et al. 2000).

The validity of a diagnosis of adenocarcinoma can be questioned because Wang and colleagues (1996) stated that determining the histologic cell type was "based on review of relevant medical records, chest X-ray and CT films, and cytologic and histologic slides" (p. S94). The cases presented in these two reports overlap. All of the adenocarcinoma cases and their corresponding controls from the general population included in the study by Wang and colleagues (1996) were also included in the study by Zhou and colleagues (2000).

A population-based, case-control study investigated the role of secondhand smoke exposure and other risk factors for lung cancer in Gansu Province, a nonindustrial area in northwestern China (Wang et al. 2000). A total of 886 lung cancer cases (656 men and 230 women) and 1,765 general population controls (1,310 men and 455 women) were interviewed. Cases (or next of kin, n = 481) and controls all completed a structured questionnaire on demographic characteristics; smoking habits of the participant, spouse, and other cohabitants; diet and cooking practices; and occupational, residential, and medical histories. The analysis was based on 233 lung cancer cases (33 men, 200 women) and 521 controls (114 men, 407 women) who had never smoked (Table 7.3) (Wang et al. 2000).

Wang and colleagues (2000) found that secondhand smoke exposure in adulthood, defined as ever having an exposure (OR = 0.90), or the number of pack-years of exposure (OR = 0.81 [1 to 9 pack-years], 0.90 [10 to 19 pack-years], and 0.86 [≥20 pack-years]) was not associated with risk. For men and women combined, there was a statistically significant increase in risk (OR = 1.52 [95 percent CI, 1.1– 2.2]) associated with any childhood exposure to secondhand smoke; the ORs increased with increasing pack-years of exposure (OR = 1.43 [1 to 9 pack-years], 1.81 [10 to 19 pack-years], and 2.95 [≥20 pack-years]; p for trend = 0.02). Overall, there was a nonsignificant increase in risk (OR = 1.19 [95 percent CI, 0.7–2.0]) from a lifetime exposure to secondhand smoke with some suggestion of increased risks with more pack-years of exposure (OR = 1.04 [1 to 9 pack-years], 1.13 [10 to 19 pack-years],

and 1.51 [≥20 pack-years]). The patterns of association were generally similar among men and women and in the analyses restricted to self-respondents or those with histologically confirmed tumors. For example, among the 115 adults with lung cancer (cases) compared with the 501 adult controls from the general population who were self-respondents and who had never smoked, the ORs for ever having an exposure to secondhand smoke were 1.75 (95 percent CI, 1.1–2.8) in childhood and 0.76 (95 percent CI, 0.4–1.3) in adulthood. Among the histologically confirmed lung cancer cases, the risks associated with secondhand smoke were 1.55 (95 percent CI, 0.9–2.8) in childhood and 0.99 (95 percent CI, 0.5–2.0) in adulthood.

Other Asian Populations

Japan

In addition to the case-control studies conducted in various Chinese populations, case-control studies conducted in Japan (Akiba et al. 1986; Inoue and Hirayama 1988; Shimizu et al. 1988; Sobue 1990) generally support the finding that exposure to secondhand smoke is associated with an increased risk of lung cancer in nonsmokers. These studies have been included and discussed in previous reviews.

India

A small hospital-based, case-control study of lifetime nonsmokers in Chandigarh, India, compared 58 nonsmoking adults (17 men and 41 women) diagnosed with lung cancer (histologically confirmed cases) and 123 nonsmoking controls (56 men and 67 women). Controls were either other adult patients admitted to the hospital or visitors in the hospital. Although the conditions of the patients who were admitted to the hospital were not described, the investigators excluded patients with diseases related to smoking, alcohol, or diet. No attempt was made to match cases and controls by gender, age, or other variables (Table 7.3) (Rapiti et al. 1999).

Participants were interviewed in the hospital and responded to a questionnaire designed to assess demographic factors, active smoking, and lifetime secondhand smoke exposure. Questions on secondhand smoke were modeled after those used in a European multicenter case-control study (Boffetta et al. 1998). Among all participants combined, Rapiti and colleagues (1999) found a significantly increased risk associated with secondhand smoke exposure during childhood (OR = 3.9 [95 percent CI, 1.9–8.2]) after adjusting for gender, age, residence, and religion. A significantly increased risk was not observed in association with secondhand smoke from spouses (OR = 1.1 [95 percent CI, 0.5–2.6]) when all sources of tobacco products were considered. Indian smokers use not only cigarettes but bidis, tobacco wrapped in a leaf, and chilum, similar to a pipe. However, the risk of lung cancer increased significantly in association with cigarette smoking by spouses (OR = 5.1 [95 percent CI, 1.5–17]) but was reduced in association with bidi smoking (OR = 0.1 [95 percent CI, 0.01–1.2]). These results among men and women combined were also observed in the analyses that were restricted to women only (Rapiti et al. 1999).

The study was small and the appropriateness of the control groups is uncertain. Information on potential confounders was also lacking. The very high estimate of risk associated with secondhand smoke exposure in childhood may be a chance finding because results from most published studies show either no risk or a much weaker effect on risk. The results observed in association with cigarettes versus bidis smoked by the spouses were also divergent. Although the investigators explained that a bidi is smaller in size and may emit less smoke than a cigarette, they found no basis for anticipating a protective effect from bidis.

References

Akiba S, Kato H, Blot WJ. Passive smoking and lung cancer among Japanese women. *Cancer Research* 1986;46(9):4804–7.

Al-Delaimy WK, Cho E, Chen WY, Colditz G, Willet WC. A prospective study of smoking and risk of breast cancer in young adult women. *Cancer Epidemiology, Biomarkers & Prevention* 2004;13(3): 398–404.

Althuis MD, Fergenbaum JH, Garcia-Closas M, Brinton LA, Madigan MP, Sherman ME. Etiology of hormone receptor–defined breast cancer: a systematic review of the literature. *Cancer Epidemiology, Biomarkers & Prevention* 2004;13(10):1558–68.

Ambrosone CB, Freudenheim JL, Graham S, Marshall JR, Vena JE, Brasure JR, Michalek AM, Laughlin R, Nemoto T, Gillenwater KA, et al. Cigarette smoking, N-acetyltransferase 2 genetic polymorphisms, and breast cancer risk. *Journal of the American Medical Association* 1996;276(18):1494–501.

Aschengrau A, Ozonoff D, Coogan P, Vezina R, Heeren T, Zhang Y. Cancer risk and residential proximity to cranberry cultivation in Massachusetts. *American Journal of Public Health* 1996;86(9):1289–96.

Baron JA, La Vecchia C, Levi F. The antiestrogenic effect of cigarette smoking in women. *American Journal of Obstetrics and Gynecology* 1990;162(2): 502–14.

Becher H, Zatonski W, Jöckel K-H. Passive smoking in Germany and Poland: comparison of exposure levels, sources of exposure, validity, and perception. *Epidemiology* 1992;3(6):509–14.

Begg CB, Mazumdar M. Operating characteristics of a rank correlation test for publication bias. *Biometrics* 1994;50(4):1088–101.

Bero LA, Glantz SA, Rennie D. Publication bias and public health policy on environmental tobacco smoke. *Journal of the American Medical Association* 1994;272(2):133–6.

Blot WJ, Fraumeni JF Jr. Passive smoking and lung cancer [editorial]. *Journal of the National Cancer Institute* 1986;77(5):993–1000.

Boffetta P, Agudo A, Ahrens W, Benhamou E, Benhamou S, Darby SC, Ferro G, Fortes C, Gonzalez CA, Jöckel K-H, et al. Multicenter case-control study of exposure to environmental tobacco smoke and lung cancer in Europe. *Journal of the National Cancer Institute* 1998;90(19):1440–50.

Boffetta P, Ahrens W, Nyberg F, Mukeria A, Brüske-Hohlfeld I, Fortes C, Constantinescu V, Simonato L, Batura-Gabryel H, Lea S, et al. Exposure to environmental tobacco smoke and risk of adenocarcinoma of the lung. *International Journal of Cancer* 1999;83(5):635–9.

Bonner MR, Nie J, Han D, Vena JE, Rogerson P, Muti P, Trevisan M, Edge SB, Freudenheim JL. Secondhand smoke exposure in early life and the risk of breast cancer among never smokers (United States). *Cancer Causes and Control* 2005;16(6):683–9.

Brinton LA, Blot WJ, Becker JA, Winn DM, Browder JP, Farmer JC Jr, Fraumeni JF Jr. A case-control study of cancers of the nasal cavity and paranasal sinuses. *American Journal of Epidemiology* 1984;119(6): 896–906.

Brownson RC, Alavanja MCR, Hock ET, Loy TS. Passive smoking and lung cancer in nonsmoking women. *American Journal of Public Health* 1992; 82(11):1525–30.

Brownson RC, Reif JS, Keefe TJ, Ferguson SW, Pritzl JA. Risk factors for adenocarcinoma of the lung. *American Journal of Epidemiology* 1987;125(1):25–34.

Buffler PA, Pickle LW, Mason TJ, Contant C. The causes of lung cancer in Texas. In: Mizell M, Correa P, editors. *Lung Cancer: Causes and Prevention*. Deerfield Beach (FL): Verlag Chemie International, 1984:83–99.

Butler TL. The relationship of passive smoking to various health outcomes among Seventh-day Adventists in California [dissertation]. Los Angeles: University of California, 1988.

California Environmental Protection Agency. *Proposed Identification of Environmental Tobacco Smoke as a Toxic Air Contaminant. Part B: Health Effects*. Sacramento (CA): California Environmental Protection Agency, Office of Environmental Health Hazard Assessment, 2005.

Calle EE, Miracle-McMahill HL, Thun MJ, Heath CW Jr. Cigarette smoking and risk of fatal breast cancer. *American Journal of Epidemiology* 1994;139(10): 1001–17.

Cardenas VM, Thun MJ, Austin H, Lally CA, Clark WS, Greenberg RS, Heath CW Jr. Environmental tobacco smoke and lung cancer mortality in the American Cancer Society's Cancer Prevention Study II. *Cancer Causes and Control* 1997;8(1):57–64.

Chan WC, Fung SC. Lung cancer in non-smokers in Hong Kong. In: Grundmann E, Clemmesen J, Muir CS, editors. *Geographical Pathology in Cancer Epidemiology*. Cancer Campaign. Vol. 6. New York: Gustav Fischer Verlag, 1982:199–202.

Chen C, Wang X, Wang L, Yang F, Tang G, Xing H, Ryan L, Lasley B, Overstreet JW, Stanford JB, Xu X. Effect of environmental tobacco smoke on levels of urinary hormone markers. *Environmental Health Perspectives* 2005;113(4):412–7.

Cheng Y-J, Hildesheim A, Hsu M-M, Chen I-H, Brinton LA, Levine PH, Chen C-J, Yang C-S. Cigarette smoking, alcohol consumption and risk of nasopharyngeal carcinoma in Taiwan. *Cancer Causes and Control* 1999;10(3):201–7.

Coker AL, Rosenberg AJ, McCann MF, Hulka BS. Active and passive cigarette smoke exposure and cervical intraepithelial neoplasia. *Cancer Epidemiology, Biomarkers & Prevention* 1992;1(5):349–56.

Colditz GA. Epidemiology and prevention of breast cancer. *Cancer Epidemiology, Biomarkers & Prevention* 2005;14(4):768–72.

Copas JB, Shi JQ. Reanalysis of epidemiological evidence on lung cancer and passive smoking. *British Medical Journal* 2000;320(7232):417–8.

Correa P, Pickle LW, Fontham E, Lin Y, Haenszel W. Passive smoking and lung cancer. *Lancet* 1983;2(8350):595–7.

Curtin F, Morabia A, Bernstein MS. Relation of environmental tobacco smoke to diet and health habits: variations according to the site of exposure. *Journal of Clinical Epidemiology* 1999;52(11):1055–62.

de Waard F, Kemmeren JM, van Ginkel LA, Stolker AAM. Urinary cotinine and lung cancer risk in a female cohort. *British Journal of Cancer* 1995;72(3):784–7.

Delfino RJ, Smith C, West JG, Lin HJ, White E, Liao S-Y, Gim JSY, Ma HL, Butler J, Anton-Culver H. Breast cancer, passive and active cigarette smoking and *N*-acetyltransferase 2 genotype. *Pharmacogenetics* 2000;10(5):461–9.

Demers PA, Kogevinas M, Boffetta P, Leclerc A, Luce D, Gérin M, Battista G, Belli S, Bolm-Audorf U, Brinton LA, et al. Wood dust and sino-nasal cancer: pooled reanalysis of twelve case-control studies. *American Journal of Industrial Medicine* 1995;28(2):151–66.

DerSimonian R, Laird N. Meta-analysis in clinical trials. *Controlled Clinical Trials* 1986;7(3):177–88.

Dockery DW, Trichopoulos D. Risk of lung cancer from environmental exposures to tobacco smoke. *Cancer Causes and Control* 1997;8(3):333–45.

Drope J, Chapman S. Tobacco industry efforts at discrediting scientific knowledge of environmental tobacco smoke: a review of internal industry documents. *Journal of Epidemiology and Community Health* 2001;55(8):588–94.

Du Y-X, Cha Q, Chen X-W, Chen Y-Z, Huang L-F, Feng Z-Z, Wu X-F, Wu JM. An epidemiological study of risk factors for lung cancer in Guangzhou, China. *Lung Cancer* 1996;14(Suppl 1):S9–S37.

Dunnick JK, Elwell MR, Huff J, Barrett JC. Chemically induced mammary gland cancer in the National Toxicology Program's carcinogenesis bioassay. *Carcinogenesis* 1995;16(2):173–9.

Egan KM, Stampfer MJ, Hunter D, Hankinson S, Rosner BA, Holmes M, Willett WC, Colditz GA. Active and passive smoking in breast cancer: prospective results from the Nurses' Health Study. *Epidemiology* 2002;13(2):138–45.

El-Bayoumy K, Chae Y-H, Upadhyaya P, Rivenson A, Kurtzke C, Reddy B, Hecht SS. Comparative tumorigenicity of benzo[*a*]pyrene, 1-nitropyrene and 2-amino-1-methyl-6-phenylimidazo[4,5-*b*]pyridine administered by gavage to female CD rats. *Carcinogenesis* 1995;16(2):431–4.

Elwood JM. Wood exposure and smoking: association with cancer of the nasal cavity and paranasal sinuses in British Columbia. *Canadian Medical Association Journal* 1981;124(12):1573–7.

Fontham ETH, Correa P, Reynolds P, Wu-Williams A, Buffler PA, Greenberg RS, Chen VW, Alterman T, Boyd P, Austin DF, et al. Environmental tobacco smoke and lung cancer in nonsmoking women: a multicenter study. *Journal of the American Medical Association* 1994;271(22):1752–9.

Fontham ETH, Correa P, Wu-Williams A, Reynolds P, Greenberg RS, Buffler PA, Chen VW, Boyd P, Alterman T, Austin DF, et al. Lung cancer in nonsmoking women: a multicenter case-control study. *Cancer Epidemiology, Biomarkers & Prevention* 1991;1(1):35–43.

Forastiere F, Mallone S, Lo Presti E, Baldacci S, Pistelli F, Simoni M, Scalera A, Pedreschi M, Pistelli R, Corbo G, et al. Characteristics of nonsmoking women exposed to spouses who smoke: epidemiologic study on environment and health in women from four Italian areas. *Environmental Health Perspectives* 2000;108(12):1171–7.

Friedenreich CM. Physical activity and breast cancer risk: the effect of menopausal status. *Exercise and Sport Science Reviews* 2004;32(4):180–4.

Fry JS, Lee PN. Revisiting the association between environmental tobacco smoke exposure and lung cancer risk. IV. Adjustments for the potential confounding effects of fruit, vegetables, and dietary fat. *Indoor Built Environment* 2001;10(1):20–39.

Fukuda K, Shibata A. Exposure-response relationships between woodworking, smoking or passive smoking, and squamous cell neoplasms of the maxillary sinus. *Cancer Causes and Control* 1990;1(2):165–8.

Gammon MD, Eng SM, Teitelbaum SL, Britton JA, Kabat GC, Hatch M, Paykin AB, Neugut AI, Santella RM. Environmental tobacco smoke and breast cancer incidence. *Environmental Research* 2004;96(2):176–85.

Gao Y-T, Blot WJ, Zheng W, Ershow AG, Hsu CW, Levin LI, Zhang R, Fraumeni JF Jr. Lung cancer among Chinese women. *International Journal of Cancer* 1987;40(5):604–9.

Gao YT, Blot WJ, Zheng W, Fraumeni JF, Hsu CW. Lung cancer and smoking in Shanghai. *International Journal of Epidemiology* 1988;17(2):277–80.

Garfinkel L. Time trends in lung cancer among nonsmokers and a note on passive smoking. *Journal of the National Cancer Institute* 1981;66(6):1061–6.

Garfinkel L, Auerbach O, Joubert L. Involuntary smoking and lung cancer: a case-control study. *Journal of the National Cancer Institute* 1985;75(3):463–9.

Geng G-Y, Liang ZH, Zhang A-Y, Wu GL. On the relationship between smoking and female lung cancer. In: Aoki M, Hisamichi S, Tominaga S, editors. *Smoking and Health 1987*. Proceedings of the 6th World Conference on Smoking and Health, Nov 9–12, 1987; Tokyo. Amsterdam: Elsevier Science, 1988:483–6.

Ghadirian P, Lubinski J, Lynch H, Neuhausen SL, Weber B, Isaacs C, Baruch R-G, Randall S, Ainsworth P, Freidman E, et al. Smoking and the risk of breast cancer among carriers of BRCA mutations. *International Journal of Cancer* 2004;110(3):413–6.

Gillis CR, Hole DJ, Hawthorne VM, Boyle P. The effect of environmental tobacco smoke in two urban communities in the west of Scotland. *European Journal of Respiratory Diseases* 1984;65(Suppl 133):121–6.

Gram IT, Braaten T, Terry PD, Sasco AJ, Adami HO, Lund E, Weiderpass E. Breast cancer risk among women who start smoking as teenagers. *Cancer Epidemiology, Biomarkers & Prevention* 2005;14(1):61–6.

Guerin MR, Jenkins RA, Tomkins BA. *The Chemistry of Environmental Tobacco Smoke: Composition and Measurement*. Chelsea (MI): Lewis Publishers, 1992.

Hackshaw AK, Law MR, Wald NJ. The accumulated evidence on lung cancer and environmental tobacco smoke. *British Medical Journal* 1997;315(7114):980–8.

Hamajima N, Hirose K, Tajima K, Rohan T, Calle EE, Heath CW Jr, Coates RJ, Liff JM, Talamini R, Chantarakul N, et al. Alcohol, tobacco and breast cancer—collaborative reanalysis of individual data from 53 epidemiological studies, including 58,515 women with breast cancer and 95,067 women without the disease. *British Journal of Cancer* 2002;87(11):1234–45.

Hammond SK. Exposure of U.S. workers to environmental tobacco smoke. *Environmental Health Perspectives* 1999;107(Suppl 2):329–40.

Hanaoka T, Yamamoto S, Sobue T, Sasaki S, Tsugane S, the Japan Public Health Center-Based Prospective Study on Cancer and Cardiovascular Disease Study Group. Active and passive smoking and breast cancer risk in middle-aged Japanese women. *International Journal of Cancer* 2005;114:317–22.

Hankinson SE, Colditz GA, Willett WC. Towards an integrated model for breast cancer etiology: the lifelong interplay of genes, lifestyle, and hormones. *Breast Cancer Research* 2004;6(5):213–8.

Hayes RB, Kardaun JWPF, de Bruyn A. Tobacco use and sinonasal cancer: a case-control study. *British Journal of Cancer* 1987;56(6):843–6.

Hecht SS. Tobacco smoke carcinogens and lung cancer. *Journal of the National Cancer Institute* 1999;91(14):1194–210.

Hirayama T. Non-smoking wives of heavy smokers have a higher risk of lung cancer: a study from Japan. *British Medical Journal* 1981;282(6259):183–5.

Hirayama T. Cancer mortality in nonsmoking women with smoking husbands based on a large scale cohort study in Japan. *Preventive Medicine* 1984;13(6):680–90.

Hoffmann D, Hecht SS. Advances in tobacco carcinogenesis. In: Cooper CS, Grover PL, editors. *Handbook of Experimental Pharmacology*. 94/I ed. Heidelberg: Springer-Verlag, 1990:63–102.

Hole DJ, Gillis CR, Chopra C, Hawthorne VM. Passive smoking and cardiorespiratory health in a general population in the west of Scotland. *British Medical Journal* 1989;299(6696):423–7.

Horton AW. Indoor tobacco smoke pollution: a major risk factor for both breast and lung cancer. *Cancer* 1988;62(1):6–14.

Humble CG, Samet JM, Pathak DR. Marriage to a smoker and lung cancer risk. *American Journal of Public Health* 1987;77(5):598–602.

Hunter D, Gertig D, Speigelman D. Response [letter]. *Carcinogenesis* 1998;19(9):1705.

Hunter DJ, Hankinson SE, Hough H, Gertig DM, Garcia-Closas M, Spiegelman D, Manson JE, Colditz GA, Willett WC, Speizer FE, Kelsey K. A prospective study of NAT2 acetylation genotype, cigarette smoking, and risk of breast cancer. *Carcinogenesis* 1997;18(11):2127–32.

Inoue R, Hirayama T. Passive smoking and lung cancer in women. In: Aoki M, Hisamichi S, Tominaga S, editors. *Smoking and Health 1987.* Proceedings of the 6th World Conference on Smoking and Health, Nov 9–12, 1987; Tokyo. Amsterdam: Elsevier Science, 1988:283–5.

International Agency for Research on Cancer. *IARC Monographs on the Evaluation of the Carcinogenic Risk of Chemicals to Humans: Tobacco Smoking.* Vol. 38. Lyon (France): World Health Organization, International Agency for Research on Cancer, 1986.

International Agency for Research on Cancer. *IARC Monographs on the Evaluation of Carcinogenic Risks to Humans: Tobacco Smoke and Involuntary Smoking.* Vol. 83. Lyon (France): International Agency for Research on Cancer, 2004.

Jaakkola MS, Samet JM. Summary: workshop on health risks attributable to ETS exposure in the workplace. *Environmental Health Perspectives* 1999;107(Suppl 6): 823–8.

Janerich DT, Thompson WD, Varela LR, Greenwald P, Chorost S, Tucci C, Zaman MB, Melamed MR, Kiely M, McKneally MF. Lung cancer and exposure to tobacco smoke in the household. *New England Journal of Medicine* 1990;323(10):632–6.

Jee SH, Ohrr H, Kim IS. Effects of husbands' smoking on the incidence of lung cancer in Korean women. *International Journal of Epidemiology* 1999;28(5): 824–8.

Jee SH, Samet JM, Ohrr H, Kim JH, Kim IS. Smoking and cancer risk in Korean men and women. *Cancer Causes and Control* 2004;15(4):341–8.

Jöckel K-H, Pohlabeln H, Ahrens W, Krauss M. Environmental tobacco smoke and lung cancer. *Epidemiology* 1998;9(6):672–5.

Johnson KC. Accumulating evidence on passive and active smoking and breast cancer risk. *International Journal of Cancer* 2005;117(4):619–28.

Johnson KC, Hu J, Mao Y, the Canadian Cancer Registries Epidemiology Research Group. Passive and active smoking and breast cancer risk in Canada, 1994–97. *Cancer Causes and Control* 2000;11(3): 211–21.

Johnson KC, Hu J, Mao Y, the Canadian Cancer Registries Epidemiology Research Group. Lifetime residential and workplace exposure to environmental tobacco smoke and lung cancer in never-smoking women, Canada 1994–97. *International Journal of Cancer* 2001;93(6):902–6.

Kabat GC, Stellman SD, Wynder EL. Relation between exposure to environmental tobacco smoke and lung cancer in lifetime nonsmokers. *American Journal of Epidemiology* 1995;142(2):141–8.

Kabat GC, Wynder EL. Lung cancer in nonsmokers. *Cancer* 1984;53(5):1214–21.

Kalandidi A, Katsouyanni K, Voropoulou N, Bastas G, Saracci R, Trichopoulos D. Passive smoking and diet in the etiology of lung cancer among nonsmokers. *Cancer Causes and Control* 1990;1(1):15–21.

Katada H, Mikami R, Konishi M, Koyama Y, Narita N. The effects of passive smoking in the development of female lung cancer in the Nara district [Japanese]. *Gan No Rinsho* 1988;34(1):21–7.

Kawachi I, Colditz GA. Invited commentary: confounding, measurement error, and publication bias in studies of passive smoking. *American Journal of Epidemiology* 1996;144(10):909–15.

Key TJA, Pike MC, Baron JA, Moore JW, Wang DY, Thomas BS, Bulbrook RD. Cigarette smoking and steroid hormones in women. *Journal of Steroid Biochemistry and Molecular Biology* 1991;39(4A):529–34.

Key TJA, Pike MC, Brown JB, Hermon C, Allen DS, Wang DY. Cigarette smoking and urinary oestrogen excretion in premenopausal and post-menopausal women. *British Journal of Cancer* 1996;74(8):1313–6.

Ko Y-C, Lee CH, Chen MJ, Huang CC, Chang WY, Lin HJ, Wang HZ, Chang PY. Risk factors for primary lung cancer among non-smoking women in Taiwan. *International Journal of Epidemiology* 1997; 26(1):24–31.

Koo LC, Ho JH-C, Saw D. Is passive smoking and [sic] added risk factor for lung cancer in Chinese women? *Journal of Experimental and Clinical Cancer Research* 1984;3(3):277–83.

Koo LC, Ho JH-C, Saw D, Ho C-Y. Measurements of passive smoking and estimates of lung cancer risk among non-smoking Chinese females. *International Journal of Cancer* 1987;39(2):162–9.

Kreuzer M, Gerken M, Kreienbrock L, Wellmann J, Wichmann HE. Lung cancer in lifetime nonsmoking men—results of a case-control study in Germany. *British Journal of Cancer* 2001;84(1):134–40.

Kreuzer M, Krauss M, Kreienbrock L, Jöckel K-H, Wichmann H-E. Environmental tobacco smoke and lung cancer: a case-control study in Germany. *American Journal of Epidemiology* 2000;151(3):241–50.

Kropp S, Chang-Claude J. Active and passive smoking and risk of breast cancer by age 50 years among German women. *American Journal of Epidemiology* 2002;156(7):616–26.

Kubik A, Zatloukal P, Boyle P, Robertson C, Gandini S, Tomasek L, Gray N, Havel L. A case-control study of lung cancer among Czech women. *Lung Cancer* 2001;31(2–3):111–22.

Kung IT, So KF, Lam TH. Lung cancer in Hong Kong Chinese: mortality and histological types, 1973–1982. *British Journal of Cancer* 1984;50(3):381–8.

Lam WK. A clinical and epidemiological study of carcinoma of lung in Hong Kong [dissertation]. Hong Kong: University of Hong Kong, 1985.

Lam TH, Kung ITM, Wong CM, Lam WK, Kleevens JWL, Saw D, Hsu C, Seneviratne S, Lam SY, Lo KK, et al. Smoking, passive smoking and histological types in lung cancer in Hong Kong Chinese women. *British Journal of Cancer* 1987;56(5):673–8.

Lash TL, Aschengrau A. Active and passive cigarette smoking and the occurrence of breast cancer. *American Journal of Epidemiology* 1999;149(1):5–12.

Lash TL, Aschengrau A. A null association between active or passive cigarette smoking and breast cancer risk. *Breast Cancer Research and Treatment* 2002;75(2):181–4.

Law CH, Day NE, Shanmugaratnam K. Incidence rates of specific histological types of lung cancer in Singapore Chinese dialect groups, and their aetiological significance. *International Journal of Cancer* 1976;17(3):304–9.

Lawlor DA, Ebrahim S, Smith GD. Smoking before the birth of a first child is not associated with increased risk of breast cancer: findings from the British Women's Heart and Health Cohort Study and a meta-analysis. *British Journal of Cancer* 2004;91(3):512–8.

Lee PN. *Environmental Tobacco Smoke and Mortality: A Detailed Review of Epidemiological Evidence Relating Environmental Tobacco Smoke to the Risk of Cancer, Heart Disease, and Other Causes of Death in Adults Who Have Never Smoked.* New York: Karger, 1992.

Lee C-H, Ko Y-C, Goggins W, Huang J-J, Huang M-S, Kao E-L, Wang H-Z. Lifetime environmental exposure to tobacco smoke and primary lung cancer of non-smoking Taiwanese women. *International Journal of Epidemiology* 2000;29(2):224–31.

Lee PN, Chamberlain J, Alderson MR. Relationship of passive smoking to risk of lung cancer and other smoking-associated diseases. *British Journal of Cancer* 1986;54(1):97–105.

Lei Y-X, Cai W-C, Chen Y-Z, Du Y-X. Some lifestyle factors in human lung cancer: a case-control study of 792 lung cancer cases. *Lung Cancer* 1996;14(Suppl 1):S121–S136.

Li D, Wang M, Dhingra K, Hittelman WN. Aromatic DNA adducts in adjacent tissues of breast cancer patients: clues to breast cancer etiology. *Cancer Research* 1996;56(2):287–93.

Liu L, Wu K, Lin X, Yin W, Zheng X, Tang X, Mu L, Hu Z, Wang J. Passive smoking and other factors at different periods of life and breast cancer risk in Chinese women who have never smoked—a case-control study in Chongqing, People's Republic of China. *Asian Pacific Journal of Cancer Prevention* 2000;1(2):131–7.

Liu Q, Sasco AJ, Riboli E, Hu MX. Indoor air pollution and lung cancer in Guangzhou, People's Republic of China. *American Journal of Epidemiology* 1993;137(2):145–54.

Liu Z, He X, Chapman RS. Smoking and other risk factors for lung cancer in Xuanwei, China. *International Journal of Epidemiology* 1991;20(1):26–31.

Lubin JH. Estimating lung cancer risk with exposure to environmental tobacco smoke. *Environmental Health Perspectives* 1999;107(Suppl 6):879–83.

MacMahon B, Trichopoulos D, Cole P, Brown J. Cigarette smoking and urinary estrogens. *New England Journal of Medicine* 1982;307(17):1062–5.

Mannetje A, Kogevinas M, Luce D, Demers PA, Bégin D, Bolm-Audorff U, Comba P, Gérin M, Hardell L, Hayes RB, et al. Sinonasal cancer, occupation, and tobacco smoking in European women and men. *American Journal of Industrial Medicine* 1999;36(1):101–7.

Marcus PM, Newman B, Millikan RC, Moorman PG, Baird DD, Qaqish B. The associations of adolescent cigarette smoking, alcoholic beverage consumption, environmental tobacco smoke, and ionizing radiation with subsequent breast cancer risk (United States). *Cancer Causes and Control* 2000;11(3):271–87.

Matanoski G, Kanchanaraksa S, Lantry D, Chang Y. Characteristics of nonsmoking women in NHANES I and NHANES I Epidemiological Follow-up Study with exposure to spouses who smoke. *American Journal of Epidemiology* 1995;142(2):149–57.

Michnovicz JJ, Hershcopf RJ, Naganuma H, Bradlow HL, Fishman J. Increased 2-hydroxylation of estradiol as a possible mechanism for the anti-estrogenic effect of cigarette smoking. *New England Journal of Medicine* 1986;315(21):1305–9.

Millikan RC, Pittman GS, Newman B, Tse C-KJ, Selmin O, Rockhill B, Savitz D, Moorman PG, Bell DA. Cigarette smoking, *N*-acetyltransferases 1 and

2, and breast cancer risk. *Cancer Epidemiology, Biomarkers & Prevention* 1998;7(5):371–8.

Misakian AL, Bero LA. Publication bias and research on passive smoking: comparison of published and unpublished studies. *Journal of the American Medical Association* 1998;280(3):250–3.

Morabia A, Bernstein M, Héritier S, Khatchatrian N. Relation of breast cancer with passive and active exposure to tobacco smoke. *American Journal of Epidemiology* 1996;143(9);918–28.

Morabia A, Bernstein MS, Bouchardy I, Kurtz J, Morris MA. Breast cancer and active and passive smoking: the role of the N-acetyltransferase 2 genotype. *American Journal of Epidemiology* 2000;152(3): 226–32.

Muggli ME, Forster JL, Hurt RD, Repace JL. The smoke you don't see: uncovering tobacco industry scientific strategies aimed against environmental tobacco smoke policies. *American Journal of Public Health* 2001;91(9):1419–23.

Nagao M, Ushijima T, Wakabayashi K, Ochiai M, Kushida H, Sugimura T, Hasegawa R, Shirai T, Ito N. Dietary carcinogens and mammary carcinogens: induction of rat mammary carcinomas by administration of heterocyclicamines in cooked foods. *Cancer* 1994;74(Suppl):1063–9.

National Cancer Institute. *Health Effects of Exposure to Environmental Tobacco Smoke: The Report of the California Environmental Protection Agency.* Smoking and Tobacco Control Monograph No. 10. Bethesda (MD): U.S. Department of Health and Human Services, National Institutes of Health, National Cancer Institute, 1999. NIH Publication No. 99-4645.

National Research Council. *Environmental Tobacco Smoke: Measuring Exposures and Assessing Health Effects.* Washington: National Academy Press, 1986.

National Research Council. *Health Risks from Exposure to Low Levels of Ionizing Radiation: BEIR VII–Phase 2.* Washington: National Academy Press, 2005.

Nishino Y, Tsubono Y, Tsuji I, Komatsu S, Kanemura S, Nakatsuka H, Fukao A, Satoh H, Hisamichi S. Passive smoking at home and cancer risk: a population-based prospective study in Japanese nonsmoking women. *Cancer Causes and Control* 2001;12(9):797–802.

Nyberg F, Agrenius V, Svartengren K, Svensson C, Pershagen G. Environmental tobacco smoke and lung cancer in nonsmokers: does time since exposure play a role? *Epidemiology* 1998a;9(3):301–8.

Nyberg F, Agudo A, Boffetta P, Fortes C, González CA, Pershagen G. A European validation study of smoking and environmental tobacco smoke exposure in nonsmoking lung cancer cases and controls. *Cancer Causes and Control* 1998b;9(2):173–82.

Nyberg F, Isaksson I, Harris JR, Pershagen G. Misclassification of smoking status and lung cancer risk from environmental tobacco smoke in never-smokers. *Epidemiology* 1997;8(3):304–9.

Palmer JR, Rosenberg L. Cigarette smoking and the risk of breast cancer. *Epidemiologic Reviews* 1993:15(1):145–56.

Pershagen G, Hrubec Z, Svensson C. Passive smoking and lung cancer in Swedish women. *American Journal of Epidemiology* 1987;125(1):17–24.

Petrakis NL, Gruenke LD, Beelen TC, Castagnoli N Jr, Craig JC. Nicotine in breast fluid of nonlactating women. *Science* 1978;199(4326):303–5.

Petrakis NL, Miike R, King EB, Lee L, Mason L, Chang-Lee B. Association of breast fluid coloration with age, ethnicity, and cigarette smoking. *Breast Cancer Research and Treatment* 1988;11(3):255–62.

Pirkle JL, Flegal KM, Bernert JT, Brody DJ, Etzel RA, Maurer KR. Exposure of the US population to environmental tobacco smoke: the Third National Health and Nutrition Examination Survey, 1988 to 1991. *Journal of the American Medical Association* 1996;275(16):1233–40.

Preston DL, Mattsson A, Holmberg E, Shore R, Hildreth NG, Boice JD Jr. Radiation effects on breast cancer risk: a pooled analysis of eight cohorts. *Radiation Research* 2002;158(2):220–35.

Rapiti E, Jindal SK, Gupta D, Boffetta P. Passive smoking and lung cancer in Chandigarh, India. *Lung Cancer* 1999;23(3):183–9.

Reynolds P, Hurley S, Goldberg DE, Anton-Culver H, Bernstein L, Deapen D, Horn-Ross PL, Peel D, Pinder R, Ross RK, et al. Active smoking, household passive smoking, and breast cancer: evidence from the California Teachers Study. *Journal of the National Cancer Institute* 2004;96(1):29–37.

Reynolds P, Von Behren J, Fontham ETH, Correra P, Wu A, Buffler PA, Greenberg RS. Occupational exposure to environmental tobacco smoke [letter]. *Journal of the American Medical Association* 1996;275(6):441–2.

Riboli E, Preston-Martin S, Saracci R, Haley NJ, Trichopoulos D, Becher H, Burch D, Fontham ET, Gao Y-T, Jindal SK, et al. Exposure of nonsmoking women to environmental tobacco smoke: a 10-country collaborative study. *Cancer Causes and Control* 1990;1(3):243–52.

Rousch GC. Cancers of the nasal cavity and paranasal sinuses. In: Schottenfeld D, Fraumeni J Jr, editors.

Cancer Epidemiology and Prevention. 2nd edition. New York: Oxford University Press, 1996:587–602.

Sandler DP, Everson RB, Wilcox AJ. Passive smoking in adulthood and cancer risk. *American Journal of Epidemiology* 1985a;121(1):37–48.

Sandler DP, Wilcox AJ, Everson RB. Cumulative effects of lifetime passive smoking on cancer risk. *Lancet* 1985b;1(8424):312–4.

Scholes D, McBride C, Grothaus L, Curry S, Albright J, Ludman E. The association between cigarette smoking and low-grade cervical abnormalities in reproductive-age women. *Cancer Causes and Control* 1999;10(5):339–44.

Schwartz AG, Yang P, Swanson GM. Familial risk of lung cancer among nonsmokers and their relatives. *American Journal of Epidemiology* 1996;144(6): 554–62.

Seow A, Poh WT, Teh M, Eng P, Wang YT, Tan WC, Chia KS, Yu MC, Lee HP. Diet, reproductive factors and lung cancer risk among Chinese women in Singapore: evidence for a protective effect of soy in nonsmokers. *International Journal of Cancer* 2002;97(3):365–71.

Seow A, Poh W-T, Teh M, Eng P, Wang Y-T, Tan W-C, Yu MC, Lee H-P. Fumes from meat cooking and lung cancer risk in Chinese women. *Cancer Epidemiology, Biomarkers & Prevention* 2000;9(11): 1215–21.

Shen X-B, Wang G-X, Huang Y-Z, Xiang L-S, Wang X-H. Analysis and estimates of attributable risk factors for lung cancer in Nanjing, China. *Lung Cancer* 1996;14(Suppl 1):S107–S112.

Shen X-B, Wang G-X, Zhou B-S. Relation of exposure to environmental tobacco smoke and pulmonary adenocarcinoma in non-smoking women: a case control study in Nanjing. *Oncology Reports* 1998;5(5):1221–3.

Shimizu H, Morishita M, Mizuno K, Masuda T, Ogura Y, Santo M, Nishimura M, Kunishima K, Karasawa K, Nishiwaki K, et al. A case-control study of lung cancer in nonsmoking women. *Tohoku Journal of Experimental Medicine* 1988;154(4):389–97.

Shrubsole MJ, Gao YT, Dai Q, Shu XO, Ruan ZX, Jin F, Zheng W. Passive smoking and breast cancer risk among non-smoking Chinese women. *International Journal of Cancer* 2004;110(4):605–9.

Slattery ML, Robison LM, Schuman KL, French TK, Abbott TM, Overall JC Jr, Gardner JW. Cigarette smoking and exposure to passive smoke are risk factors for cervical cancer. *Journal of the American Medical Association* 1989;261(11):1593–8.

Smith GD, Phillips AN. Passive smoking and health: should we believe Philip Morris's "experts"? *British Medical Journal* 1996;313(7062):929–33.

Smith SJ, Deacon JM, Chilvers CED, members of the UK National Case–Control Study Group. Alcohol, smoking, passive smoking and caffeine in relation to breast cancer risk in young women. *British Journal of Cancer* 1994;70(1):112–9.

Sobue T. Association of indoor pollution and passive smoking with lung cancer in Osaka, Japan. *International Journal of Epidemiology* 1990;19(Suppl 1): S62–S66.

Speizer FE, Colditz GA, Hunter DJ, Rosner B, Hennekens C. Prospective study of smoking, antioxidant intake, and lung cancer in middle-aged women (USA). *Cancer Causes and Control* 1999;10(5):475–82.

Steenland K, Sieber K, Etzel RA, Pechacek T, Maurer K. Exposure to environmental tobacco smoke and risk factors for heart disease among never smokers in the Third National Health and Nutritional Examination Survey. *American Journal of Epidemiology* 1998;147(10):932–9.

Stockwell HG, Goldman AL, Lyman GH, Noss CI, Armstrong AW, Pinkham PA, Candelora EC, Brusa MR. Environmental tobacco smoke and lung cancer risk in nonsmoking women. *Journal of the National Cancer Institute* 1992;84(18):1417–22.

Sun X-W, Dai X-D, Lin C-Y, Shi Y-B, Ma Y-Y, Li W. Lung cancer among nonsmoking women in Harbin, China [abstract]. *Lung Cancer* 1996;14(Suppl 1): S237.

Svensson C, Pershagen G, Klominek J. Smoking and passive smoking in relation to lung cancer in women. *Acta Oncologica* 1989;28(5):623–9.

Terry PD, Rohan TE. Cigarette smoking and the risk of breast cancer in women: a review of the literature. *Cancer Epidemiology, Biomarkers & Prevention* 2002;11(10 Pt 1):953–71.

Trichopoulos D, Kalandidi A, Sparros L. Lung cancer and passive smoking: conclusion of Greek study [letter]. *Lancet* 1983;2(8351):677–8.

Trichopoulos D, Kalandidi A, Sparros L, MacMahon B. Lung cancer and passive smoking. *International Journal of Cancer* 1981;27(1):1–4.

U.S. Department of Health and Human Services. *The Health Consequences of Smoking: Cancer. A Report of the Surgeon General.* Rockville (MD): U.S. Department of Health and Human Services, Public Health Service, Office on Smoking and Health, 1982. DHHS Publication No. (PHS) 82-50179.

U.S. Department of Health and Human Services. *The Health Consequences of Involuntary Smoking. A Report of the Surgeon General*. Rockville (MD): U.S. Department of Health and Human Services, Public Health Service, Centers for Disease Control, Center for Health Promotion and Education, Office on Smoking and Health, 1986. DHHS Publication No. (CDC) 87-8398.

U.S. Department of Health and Human Services. *Women and Smoking. A Report of the Surgeon General*. Rockville (MD): U.S. Department of Health and Human Services, Public Health Service, Office of the Surgeon General, 2001.

U.S. Department of Health and Human Services. *The Health Consequences of Smoking: A Report of the Surgeon General*. Atlanta: U.S. Department of Health and Human Services, Centers for Disease Control and Prevention, National Center for Chronic Disease Prevention and Health Promotion, Office on Smoking and Health, 2004.

U.S. Department of Health, Education, and Welfare. *Smoking and Health: Report of the Advisory Committee to the Surgeon General of the Public Health Service*. Washington: U.S. Department of Health, Education, and Welfare, Public Health Service, Center for Disease Control, 1964. PHS Publication No. 1103.

U.S. Environmental Protection Agency. *Respiratory Health Effects of Passive Smoking: Lung Cancer and Other Disorders*. Washington: U.S. Environmental Protection Agency, Office of Research and Development, Office of Air and Radiation, 1992. EPA/600/6-90/006F.

van den Brandt PA, Spiegelman D, Yaun SS, Adami HO, Beeson L, Folsom AR, Fraser G, Goldbohm RA, Graham S, Kushi L, et al. Pooled analysis of prospective cohort studies on height, weight, and breast cancer risk. *American Journal of Epidemiology* 2000;152(6):514–27.

Vandenbroucke JP. Passive smoking and lung cancer: a publication bias? *British Medical Journal Clinical Research Edition* 1988;296(6619):391–2.

Vineis P, Alavanja M, Buffler P, Fontham E, Franceschi S, Gao YT, Gupta PC, Hackshaw A, Matos E, Samet J, et al. Tobacco and cancer: recent epidemiological evidence. *Journal of the National Cancer Institute* 2004;96(2):99–106.

Wang F-L, Love EJ, Liu N, Dai X-D. Childhood and adolescent passive smoking and the risk of female lung cancer. *International Journal of Epidemiology* 1994:23(2):223–30.

Wang L, Lubin JH, Zhang SR, Metayer C, Xia Y, Brenner A, Shang B, Wang Z, Kleinerman RA. Lung cancer and environmental tobacco smoke in a non-industrial area of China. *International Journal of Cancer* 2000;88(1):139–45.

Wang T-J, Zhou B-S, Shi J-P. Lung cancer in nonsmoking Chinese women: a case-control study. *Lung Cancer* 1996;14(Suppl 1):S93–S98.

Wartenberg D, Calle EE, Thun MJ, Heath CW Jr, Lally C, Woodruff T. Passive smoking exposure and female breast cancer mortality. *Journal of the National Cancer Institute* 2000;92(20):1666–73.

Wells AJ. Breast cancer, cigarette smoking, and passive smoking [letter]. *American Journal of Epidemiology* 1991;133(2):208–10.

Wells AJ. Lung cancer from passive smoking at work. *American Journal of Public Health* 1998;88(7):1025–9.

Williams FLR, Lloyd OL. Associations between data for male lung cancer and female breast cancer within five countries. *Cancer* 1989;64(8):1764–8.

Woodward A, McMichael AJ. Passive smoking and cancer risk: the nature and uses of epidemiological evidence. *European Journal of Cancer* 1991;27(11):1472–9.

Wu AH. Exposure misclassification bias in studies of environmental tobacco smoke and lung cancer. *Environmental Health Perspectives* 1999;107(Suppl 6):873–77.

Wu AH, Henderson BE, Pike MC, Yu MC. Smoking and other risk factors for lung cancer in women. *Journal of the National Cancer Institute* 1985;74(4):747–51.

Wu-Williams AH, Dai XD, Blot W, Xu ZY, Sun XW, Xiao HP, Stone BJ, Yu SF, Feng YP, Ershow AG, et al. Lung cancer among women in north-east China. *British Journal of Cancer* 1990;62(6):982–7.

Wu-Williams AH, Samet JH. Environmental tobacco smoke: exposure-response relationships in epidemiolgic studies. *Risk Analysis* 1990;10(1):39–48.

Xu ZY, Blot WJ, Xiao HP, Wu A, Feng YP, Stone BJ, Sun J, Ershow AG, Henderson BE, Fraumeni JF Jr. Smoking, air pollution, and the high rates of lung cancer in Shenyang, China. *Journal of the National Cancer Institute* 1989;81(23):1800–6.

Yu MC, Garabrant DH, Huang T-B, Henderson BE. Occupational and other non-dietary risk factors for nasopharyngeal carcinoma in Guangzhou, China. *International Journal of Cancer* 1990;45(6):1033–9.

Yu MC, Huang TB, Henderson BE. Diet and nasopharyngeal carcinoma: a case-control study in Guangzhou, China. *International Journal of Cancer* 1989;43(6):1077–82.

Yuan J-M, Wang X-L, Xiang Y-B, Gao Y-T, Ross RK, Yu MC. Non-dietary risk factors for nasopharyngeal carcinoma in Shanghai, China. *International Journal of Cancer* 2000;85(3):364–9.

Zaridze D, Maximovitch D, Zemlyanaya G, Aitakov ZN, Boffetta P. Exposure to environmental tobacco smoke and risk of lung cancer in non-smoking women from Moscow, Russia. *International Journal of Cancer* 1998;75(3):335–8.

Zhao Y, Shi Z, Liu L. Matched case-control study for detecting risk factors of breast cancer in women living in Chengdu [Chinese]. *Zhonghua Liu Xing Bing Xue Za Zhi* 1999;20(2):91–4.

Zheng W, McLaughlin JK, Chow W-H, Chien HTC, Blot WJ. Risk factors for cancers of the nasal cavity and paranasal sinuses among white men in the United States. *American Journal of Epidemiology* 1993;138(11):965–72.

Zhong L, Goldberg MS, Gao Y-T, Jin F. A case-control study of lung cancer and environmental tobacco smoke among nonsmoking women living in Shanghai, China. *Cancer Causes and Control* 1999;10(6):607–16.

Zhong L, Goldberg MS, Parent M-E, Hanley JA. Exposure to environmental tobacco smoke and the risk of lung cancer: a meta-analysis. *Lung Cancer* 2000;27(1):3–18.

Zhou B-S, Wang T-J, Guan P, Wu JM. Indoor air pollution and pulmonary adenocarcinoma among females: a case-control study in Shenyang, China. *Oncology Reports* 2000;7(6):1253–9.

Chapter 8
Cardiovascular Diseases from Exposure to Secondhand Smoke

Introduction

Cardiovascular disease is the leading cause of death in the United States (Hoyert et al. 2006). Cardiovascular disease includes coronary heart disease (CHD), which causes the most deaths, and stroke, which ranks as the third leading cause of death (Hoyert et al. 2006). In 2003, CHD was responsible for approximately 480,000 deaths and stroke was responsible for approximately 158,000 deaths (Hoyert et al. 2006). Each year, an estimated 1.2 million Americans experience a new or recurrent heart attack, and an estimated 700,000 people suffer a new or recurrent stroke (American Heart Association 2005). Active smoking is one of the most important modifiable risk factors for both CHD and stroke (U.S. Department of Health and Human Services [USDHHS] 2004). This chapter considers the evidence that links secondhand smoke to these two major outcomes as well as to carotid arterial wall thickness, an indicator of the degree of atherosclerosis. Chapter 2 of this report (Toxicology of Secondhand Smoke) sets out the biologic basis by which exposure to secondhand smoke could increase the risk for CHD and stroke.

The topic of secondhand smoke and CHD was not addressed in the 1986 Surgeon General's report *The Health Consequences of Involuntary Smoking* (USDHHS 1986). At the time, only a few studies had been published on the association of secondhand smoke with CHD, and the evidence was regarded as too limited to review. Since then, many epidemiologic investigations have been carried out on secondhand smoke exposure and its relationship to CHD and stroke. In fact, both animal and human experimental data, along with clinical studies directed at physiologic consequences of exposure to secondhand smoke, have provided a biologic foundation for interpreting the epidemiologic data (Chapter 2, Toxicology of Secondhand Smoke). The evidence linking secondhand smoke and cardiovascular disease was considered in the 2001 Surgeon General's report *Women and Smoking* (USDHHS 2001). Several earlier reports, including those of the California Environmental Protection Agency (Cal/EPA) (National Cancer Institute [NCI] 1999) and the Australian National Health and Medical Research Council Working Party (NHMRC 1997), had comprehensively reviewed the evidence and concluded that exposure to secondhand smoke does cause CHD.

Coronary Heart Disease

The 2001 Surgeon General's Report

The 2001 report *Women and Smoking* reviewed the 10 cohort and 10 case-control studies on secondhand smoke and CHD that had been published up to 1998 (USDHHS 2001). Since then, additional studies have been published (Tables 8.1 and 8.2). The mean duration of follow-up in the cohort studies ranged from 6 to 20 years. Of the 20 earlier studies, 5 cohort and 4 case-control studies found a statistically significant increase in the risk of CHD from secondhand smoke. Most of the remaining 11 studies also showed an increased risk.

Based on the review of the epidemiologic evidence, the 2001 report reached the following conclusions:

- The data from the existing cohort and case-control studies "...support a causal association between ETS [environmental tobacco smoke] exposure and coronary heart disease mortality and morbidity among nonsmokers" (p. 356).

- Secondhand smoke "...is associated with risk for CHD mortality (fatal events), morbidity (nonfatal events), and symptoms. Most of the data on the association with mortality were from cohort studies, but most of the data on the association with morbidity were from case-control investigations. Nonetheless, the magnitude of association is similar in both sets of results" (p. 356).

Table 8.1   Cohort studies of secondhand smoke exposure and the risk of coronary heart disease (CHD) among nonsmokers

Study	Design/population	Duration of follow-up (years)	Exposure	Findings
Hirayama 1984, 1990	91,540 women Nonsmokers Aged ≥40 years 1966–1981 Japan	16	Husband smoked	Death from ischemic heart disease (IHD)
Garland et al. 1985	695 women Lifetime nonsmokers Aged 50–79 years 1974–1983 United States (California)	10	Husband smoked (self-reported)	Death from CHD
Svendsen et al. 1987	1,245 married men Lifetime nonsmokers Aged 35–57 years Free of CHD at baseline but at high risk Enrolled in the Multiple Risk Factor Intervention Trial 1973–1982 United States (18 cities)	Average of 7	Wife smoked	Death from CHD
Butler 1988	6,507 Seventh-Day Adventist women married to men also enrolled in the study Aged ≥25 years 1976–1982 United States (California)	6	Husband smoked	Death from CHD
Helsing et al. 1988 (not included in the meta-analysis conducted for this 2006 Surgeon General's report)	3,488 men and 12,348 women Lifetime nonsmokers Aged ≥25 years 1963 United States (Western Maryland)	12	Cohabitant smoked	Death from CHD
Hole et al. 1989	671 men and 1,784 women Lifetime nonsmokers Aged 45–64 years at baseline 1972–1985 Scotland	Average of 11.5	Cohabitant smoked	Death from IHD
Sandler et al. 1989 (not included in 2001 review)	4,162 White men and 14,873 White women Lifetime nonsmokers in 1963 Aged ≥25 years 1963–1975 United States (Maryland)	12	Home exposure from any household member who smoked	Death from CHD
Humble et al. 1990	513 women Lifetime nonsmokers Aged 40–74 years 1960–1980 United States (Georgia)	20	Husband smoked at baseline	Death from CHD

Relative risk (95% confidence interval)	Variables controlled for
1.18 (0.98–1.41)	Age
2.7 (0.59–12.33)	Age, systolic blood pressure, serum cholesterol level, body mass index (BMI), years of marriage
2.23 (0.72–6.92)	Age, blood pressure, serum cholesterol level, body weight, alcohol consumption, level of education
1.4 (0.51–3.84)	Age
Men: 1.31 (1.1–1.6) Women: 1.24 (1.1–1.4)	Age, education, marital status, housing quality
2.01 (1.21–3.35)	Age, gender, social class, diastolic blood pressure, serum cholesterol level, BMI
1.22 (1.09–1.37)	Age, marital status, years of schooling, quality of housing
1.59 (0.99–2.57)	Age, serum cholesterol level, diastolic blood pressure, BMI, and square of BMI

- Higher intensity exposures to secondhand smoke were "associated with a higher risk for CHD in some of these studies, but the differences in risk between levels of ETS exposure were not large" (p. 353).

Since the preparation of the 2001 report, two additional case-control studies of secondhand smoke exposure and CHD have been published (McElduff et al. 1998; Rosenlund et al. 2001), which are also included in Table 8.2. McElduff and colleagues (1998) pooled the CHD cases from two population-based, case-control studies carried out in Newcastle, Australia, and Auckland, New Zealand. The New Zealand component of the study (Jackson 1989) and a portion of the Australian data (Dobson et al. 1991) had been published previously and were included in the 2001 Surgeon General's report (USDHHS 2001). At both study sites, exposures to secondhand smoke at home and at work were assessed from self-reports. The study included 953 persons with CHD: 670 nonfatal myocardial infarction [MI] patients and 283 persons who had died of coronary disease. After adjusting for age, education, history of heart disease, and body mass index (BMI), McElduff and colleagues (1998) found that women had an increased risk of CHD associated with secondhand smoke (odds ratio [OR] = 1.99 [95 percent confidence interval (CI), 1.40–2.81]). For men, however, the investigators found no association between secondhand smoke and CHD (OR = 1.02 [95 percent CI, 0.81–1.28]).

The case-control study conducted by Rosenlund and colleagues (2001) examined the risk of nonfatal MI associated with secondhand smoke exposure among men and women enrolled in the Stockholm Heart Epidemiology Program—334 lifetime nonsmoking cases and 677 population controls aged 45 through 70 years who resided in Stockholm county. Assessments of exposures to secondhand smoke both at home and at work were based on a mailed questionnaire that also asked about the cumulative time-weighted duration of exposures in both settings, which were expressed as hour-years.[1] After adjusting for age, gender, BMI, hospital catchment area, socioeconomic status (SES), job strain, hypertension, diet, and diabetes mellitus, the OR for MI from an average daily exposure of 20 or more cigarettes smoked by the spouse was 1.58 (95 percent CI, 0.97–2.56). In both men and women,

---

[1] One hour-year equals 365 hours per year, or 1 hour per day for one year.

Table 8.1   Continued

Study	Design/population	Duration of follow-up (years)	Exposure	Findings
LeVois and Layard 1995 (not included in the meta-analysis conducted for this 2006 Surgeon General's report)	88,458 men and 247,412 women Lifetime nonsmokers CPS-I* data 1960 United States	13	Spouse smoked	Death from CHD
	108,772 men and 226,067 women Lifetime nonsmokers CPS-II† data 1983 United States	6	Spouse smoked	Death from CHD
Steenland et al. 1996	126,500 men and 353,180 women Lifetime nonsmokers Aged ≥30 years CPS-II data 1982–1989 United States	8	Home and workplace exposures and spousal smoking (self-reported)	Death from CHD
Kawachi et al. 1997	32,046 female nurses Lifetime nonsmokers Aged 36–61 years 300,325 person-years‡ 1982–1992 United States	10	Home or workplace exposure in 1982	Myocardial infarction and death from CHD

Note: All studies appear in both the original review and updated meta-analysis unless otherwise indicated.
*CPS-I = Cancer Prevention Study I, American Cancer Society cohort.
†CPS-II = Cancer Prevention Study II, American Cancer Society cohort.
‡Person-years = Duration of exposure to secondhand smoke (cumulative).

current exposures were associated with a higher risk of MI compared with past exposures. Moreover, the risk of MI decreased consistently with an increase in time since the last exposure.

Compared with persons who had never been exposed to secondhand smoke, persons with combined exposures from home and work showed an OR for MI of 1.55 (95 percent CI, 1.02–2.34) in the highest category of exposure (more than 90 hour-years) (Rosenlund et al. 2001).

Evaluating the Epidemiologic Evidence

Before evidence is accepted for the purpose of drawing a causal inference from epidemiologic studies, several methodologic issues must be addressed. These include, but are not limited to, the possibility of misclassified exposures, the potential for uncontrolled confounding, and publication bias. The biologic plausibility of a causal association should also be addressed. These issues are considered separately in this chapter.

Relative risk (95% confidence interval)	Variables controlled for
1.0 (0.97–1.04)	Age, race
Women: 1.0 (0.98–1.1) Men: 0.97 (0.9–1.1)	Age, race
1.21 (1.06–1.39)	Age, heart disease history, hypertension, diabetes mellitus, arthritis, BMI, level of education, aspirin use, diuretic use, estrogen use, alcohol consumption, exercise, employment status
1.71 (1.03–2.84)	Age, follow-up period, alcohol consumption, BMI, hypertension, diabetes mellitus, hypercholesterolemia, menopausal status, current use of postmenopausal hormones, past use of oral contraceptives, vigorous exercise, saturated fat intake, vitamin E intake, average aspirin use, parental history of myocardial infarction before 60 years of age, father's occupation when participant was 16 years of age

Misclassifying Exposures

Chapter 1 (see "Methodologic Issues") of this report discussed the need to consider the misclassification of exposures in studies that investigated the effects of secondhand smoke exposure, including CHD and stroke. To validate the questionnaire measures used in the CHD studies, epidemiologic and experimental literature have suggested that exposure biomarkers that are used as the "gold standard" should

reflect both recent and more remote exposures. The 2004 study by Whincup and colleagues (2004) incorporated an independent biochemical validation of secondhand smoke exposures—the current available biomarkers reflect only relatively short-term exposures over a period of days (see "Biomarkers of Exposure to Secondhand Smoke" in Chapter 3). Although short-term exposures may be relevant to CHD, investigators have argued that patterns of risk among active smokers suggest that exposures over the longer term may also be relevant (Wells 1994). Both experimental and epidemiologic findings indicate adverse cardiovascular consequences of immediate and sustained exposures.

Bailar (1999) noted that nonsmokers who develop heart disease may have selectively recalled their exposures to secondhand smoke. However, this criticism applies to case-control studies that relied on retrospective recall rather than to cohort studies. In their meta-analysis, He and colleagues (1999) found that the pooled OR estimate from eight case-control studies was slightly higher (OR = 1.51 [95 percent CI, 1.26–1.81]) than the pooled relative risk (RR) estimate from 10 cohort studies (RR = 1.21 [95 percent CI, 1.14–1.30]). The somewhat higher risks in the case-control studies may reflect recall bias, at least in part, but the pooled estimate is also elevated in the cohort study data, which would not generally be subject to this form of bias.

In addition to the possibility of recall bias in case-control studies, several other types of exposure misclassification may have occurred in the case-control and cohort published studies. For example, Ong and Glantz (2000) suggest that the most important measurement error is likely to be a failure to correct for background exposure to secondhand smoke, as truly unexposed populations are essentially unavailable. Several studies, including Garfinkel (1981), have assessed secondhand smoke exposures from a single source (such as spouses) without considering total exposures in different environments. The effects of secondhand smoke exposures from different sources are likely to be additive because of the qualitative similarity of secondhand smoke in different environments. Thus, not accounting for exposures to background secondhand smoke will bias associations with disease toward the null (Ong and Glantz 2000). In general, nonsmokers are likely to underestimate their true secondhand smoke exposures (Emmons et al. 1992; Bonita et al. 1999). For example, in a study of 663 lifetime nonsmokers and former smokers who attended a cancer screening clinic, Cummings and

Table 8.2   Case-control studies of exposure to secondhand smoke and the risk of coronary heart disease (CHD) among nonsmokers

| Study | Year and location of study | Population | | Exposure |
		Cases	Controls	
Lee et al. 1986	1979–1982 England	41 male and 77 female patients with ischemic heart disease Lifetime nonsmokers and married	133 male and 318 female hospital patients with diseases probably or definitely not related to smoking Lifetime nonsmokers and married	Spouse smoked
He 1989 (not included in the meta-analysis conducted for this 2006 Surgeon General's report)	Years were not reported China	34 female hospital patients Nonsmokers	34 female hospital patients 34 females, population based All nonsmokers	Husband smoked
Jackson 1989 (data included in McElduff et al. 1998 study in the 2006 meta-analysis conducted for this 2006 Surgeon General's report)	1987–1988 New Zealand	44 male and 22 female hospital patients All nonsmokers Myocardial infarction (MI) or death from CHD	84 male and 174 female hospital patients All nonsmokers MI or death from CHD	Home and work exposures combined
Dobson et al. 1991 (data included in McElduff et al. 1998 study in the meta-analysis conducted for this 2006 Surgeon General's report)	1988–1989 Australia (New South Wales)	183 male and 160 female hospital patients MI or death from CHD Nonsmokers	293 male and 174 female hospital patients Nonsmokers Participants in a risk factor prevalence survey	Home and work exposures
La Vecchia et al. 1993	1988–1989 Italy	69 men and 44 women with acute incident MI Lifetime nonsmokers and married Enrolled in the Gruppo Italiano per lo Studio della Sopravvivenza nell'Infarto-2 Median age: 63 years	217 married hospital controls (161 men, 56 women) Lifetime nonsmokers Admitted for acute diseases not related to any potential cardiovascular disease risk factors in the same network of hospitals Median age: 57 years	Spouse smoked
He et al. 1994	1989–1992 China	59 female patients with nonfatal incident CHD in 3 hospitals Nonsmokers Average age: 58 years	126 patients in the same hospitals or from the community Lifetime nonsmokers Average age: 55 years	Husband smoked and workplace exposure for ≥5 years

Relative risk (95% confidence interval)	Variables controlled for
1.03 (0.65–1.62)	Age, gender, hospital region
1.5 (1.3–1.8)	Alcohol consumption, exercise, personal and family history of CHD, hypertension, hyperlipidemia
MI 　Men: 1.0 (0.3–3.0) 　Women: 2.7 (0.6–12.3) Death from CHD 　Men: 1.1 (0.2–5.3) 　Women: 5.8 (1.0–35.2)	Age, social status, history of CHD
Men: 1.0 (0.5–1.8) Women: 2.5 (1.5–4.1)	Age, history of MI
1.21 (0.57–2.52)	Age, gender, level of education, coffee consumption, body mass index (BMI), serum cholesterol level, hypertension, diabetes mellitus, family history of acute MI
2.36 (1.01–5.55)	Age, hypertension, personality type, total serum and high-density lipoprotein cholesterol level

colleagues (1990) found that 91 percent had detectable levels of cotinine in their urine, even though only 76 percent had reported being exposed to secondhand smoke in the previous four days.

Other types of exposure misclassification than those described above have also been noted in epidemiologic studies (see "Misclassification of Secondhand Smoke Exposure" in Chapter 1). Some self-reported lifetime nonsmokers may have been smokers in the past, and persons more exposed to secondhand smoke may be more likely to have been active smokers in the past. This bias has been considered in relation to lung cancer. Hackshaw and colleagues (1997) found this kind of bias to be of minor importance in studies of secondhand smoke and lung cancer. They also noted that this bias was likely to have a negligible effect on studies of secondhand smoke and CHD because the RR of CHD among active smokers is so much smaller than the RR of lung cancer in active smokers: about a 2-fold to 4-fold increase in risk for CHD and a 20-fold increase in risk for lung cancer compared with the risk among nonsmokers. Moreover, researchers have found the actual extent of this type of misclassification to be minor (Kawachi and Colditz 1996; Howard and Thun 1999). In the Coronary Artery Risk Development in Young Adults Study, a cohort study that involved 5,115 community-dwelling adults aged 18 through 30 years, Wagenknecht and colleagues (1992) confirmed self-reported active smoking with a serum cotinine assay and found that these active smoking rates underestimated the true smoking rate by only 1.3 percent.

However, self-reported exposure to secondhand smoke is also subject to misclassification, which is likely to result in a bias toward the null in estimates of dose-response associations between the intensity of the exposure and CHD risk (Kawachi and Colditz 1996). Over time, the prevalence of secondhand smoke exposure has declined within the United States and in other countries as more people stopped smoking and as workplace restrictions on smoking became more widespread (see "Exposure in the Workplace" in Chapter 4). Cohort studies that assessed secondhand smoke exposures in the 1970s and 1980s, and only once at baseline, would have continued to classify individuals as exposed even though the exposure may have diminished or even ceased during the follow-up period. Some investigators have noted that this type of misclassification tends to result in a bias toward the null in estimates of the relationship between secondhand smoke and CHD (Kawachi and Colditz 1996).

Table 8.2   Continued

Study	Year and location of study	Population Cases	Population Controls	Exposure
Layard 1995 (not included in the meta-analysis conducted for this 2006 Surgeon General's report)	1986 National Followback Survey United States	475 men and 914 women who died from heart disease	998 men and 1,930 women who died from other causes	Spouse smoked
Muscat and Wynder 1995	1980–1990 United States	68 men and 46 women hospitalized with incident MI in 4 cities Lifetime nonsmokers Average age: 59 years	108 men and 50 women in the same hospitals Lifetime nonsmokers Frequency matched for age, race, year of diagnosis Average age: 58 years	Home, current workplace, and childhood exposures
Tunstall-Pedoe et al. 1995 (not included in the meta-analysis conducted for this 2006 Surgeon General's report)	1984–1986 Scotland	70 men and women aged 40–59 years from general practitioner list Self-reported CHD diagnosis Nonsmokers	2,278 men and women aged 40–59 years from general practitioner list Self-reported CHD diagnosis	Any exposure from someone else in the 3 days before the survey
Ciruzzi et al. 1998	1991–1994 Argentina	336 male and female patients with acute incident MI in 35 coronary care units Median age: 66 years	446 patients in the same hospitals Matched for age, gender, medical center Median age: 65 years	Spouse and children smoked
McElduff et al. 1998 (not included in 2001 review)	1986–1994 Australia and New Zealand	686 male and 267 female patients with fatal or nonfatal MI or unclassifiable coronary death from population register of coronary events Lifetime nonsmokers or former smokers for >10 years	3,189 residents of the same communities participating in independent community-based survey	Home and workplace exposures combined
Rosenlund et al. 2001 (not included in 2001 review)	1992–1994 Sweden	All nonfatal MIs among nonsmoking Swedish citizens aged 45–70 years, residing in study area during 1992–1993 (n = 334; 199 men) Average age: 62 years	401 males and 276 females Lifetime nonsmokers Matched for gender, age, and hospital catchment area	Spouse smoked

Note: All studies appear in both the original review and the meta-analysis conducted for this 2006 Surgeon General's report unless otherwise indicated.

Relative risk (95% confidence interval)	Variables controlled for
Men: 1.0 (0.7–1.3) Women: 1.0 (0.8–1.2)	Age, race
2.4 (1.1–4.8)	Age, housing, tenure, cholesterol level, diastolic blood pressure
1.5 (0.9–2.6)	Age, gender, race, level of education, hypertension, year of diagnosis
1.68 (1.2–2.37)	Age, gender, race, level of education, BMI, hyperlipidemia, history of diabetes or hypertension, family history of CHD, exercise
1.41 (0.73–2.71)	Age, education, history of CHD, BMI
1.37 (0.9–2.09)	Age, gender, hospital catchment area, BMI, socioeconomic status, job strain, hypertension, diet, diabetes mellitus

Controlling for Confounding

If individuals who are exposed to secondhand smoke have greater exposures to other factors that increase their risk of CHD, then potential confounding by these risk factors has to be taken into account. This section reviews the studies that examined the distribution of coronary risk factors between exposed and unexposed persons. The differences found between the two groups in cardiovascular risk factors, such as diet, were not large enough to explain the observed associations between secondhand smoke and CHD risk.

Using data from the First National Health and Nutrition Examination Survey (NHANES I) and the NHANES I Epidemiologic Follow-up Study, Matanoski and colleagues (1995) examined the dietary and behavioral characteristics of 3,896 nonsmoking women in relation to secondhand smoke exposures. These investigators found that women exposed to secondhand smoke from their spouses were more likely than women whose husbands did not smoke to report lower levels of education, higher alcohol consumption, a lower intake of vitamin supplements, and a lower dietary intake of vitamin A, vitamin C, and calcium. A limitation of this study was that the dietary assessment (from the 1971 to 1975 NHANES I) preceded the secondhand smoke exposure assessment (1982–1984 NHANES I Follow-up Study) by about 10 years.

Thornton and colleagues (1994) studied 9,003 British adults from the Health and Lifestyle Survey and found that compared with unexposed nonsmokers, nonsmokers exposed to secondhand smoke in the home were more likely to report low educational qualifications and employment in blue-collar manual occupations. Nonsmokers exposed to secondhand smoke were also more likely than unexposed nonsmokers to consume fried foods, to be more overweight, and to report a lower intake of fruits, salads, and breakfast cereals.

Koo and colleagues (1997) carried out an international study to examine the characteristics of women who were lifetime nonsmokers with or without smoking husbands. The authors studied 530 women from Hong Kong, 13,047 from Japan, 87 from Sweden, and 144 from the United States. In all four locations, wives of smoking husbands generally ate less healthy diets, with a tendency toward more fried foods and less fresh fruit, compared with wives of nonsmoking husbands. The investigators also noted that wives with nonsmoking spouses had other lifestyle traits, including the avoidance of obesity, dietary cholesterol, and alcohol. Emmons and colleagues (1995) examined the dietary behaviors of 10,833 nonsmoking men and women who were surveyed as part of the Working Well Trial, and found that secondhand smoke exposure in the workplace was associated with lower intakes of vitamin C, fruits, and vegetables (but not of other micronutrients).

In contrast to the studies mentioned above, three other reports—one in the United States and two in Europe—have suggested a more limited potential for confounding in studies of secondhand smoke and heart disease (Steenland et al. 1998; Curtin et al. 1999; Forastiere et al. 2000). Steenland and colleagues (1998) studied the distribution of coronary risk factors among 3,338 lifetime nonsmokers aged 17 years or older who were representative of all U.S. lifetime nonsmokers in the 1988–1991 NHANES (NHANES III). The study examined the following cardiovascular risk factors: diabetes, sedentary behavior, alcohol consumption, serum cholesterol, high-density lipoprotein (HDL) serum cholesterol, systolic and diastolic blood pressure, blood pressure medication, serum triglycerides, BMI, estimated daily grams of dietary fat, the estimated percentage of daily kilocalories from fat, and a log of estimated dietary carotene (Steenland et al. 1998). After adjusting for age, gender, race, and education, the investigators found no significant differences between exposed and unexposed persons in any of the 13 cardiovascular risk factors. The only exception was dietary carotene, which was lower among the exposed group than among the unexposed group. One strength of this study was the availability of serum cotinine measurements, which had a geometric mean value of 0.48 nanograms per milliliter (ng/mL) in the exposed group and 0.12 ng/mL in the unexposed group. For adults aged 40 years or older (the highest risk category for heart disease), the study also noted an inverse linear trend between serum cotinine levels and HDL cholesterol (p <0.001), indicating one possible mechanism for an effect of secondhand smoke exposure.

Curtin and colleagues (1999) carried out a survey of 914 female lifetime nonsmokers in Geneva, Switzerland, that included the administration of a semiquantitative food frequency questionnaire. The authors found that the association between secondhand smoke and dietary habits varied according to the source of the exposure. When women exposed to secondhand smoke at home were compared with unexposed women, the investigators found that dietary patterns did not differ. However, women exposed to secondhand smoke at work ate smaller amounts of fiber, cereals, vegetables, and lean meat, and had a lower intake of iron and beta-carotene than did unexposed women (Curtin et al. 1999).

Forastiere and colleagues (2000) conducted a cross-sectional study of 1,938 nonsmoking women in four areas of Italy. Medical examinations were carried out and urinary cotinine levels were measured. Nonsmoking women married to smokers were compared with unexposed women across a variety of factors, including SES, physician-diagnosed hypertension, hypercholesterolemia, diabetes, diet, BMI, waist:hip ratio, triceps skinfold thickness, systolic and diastolic blood pressure, plasma antioxidant vitamins (alpha- and beta-carotene, retinol, L-ascorbic acid, alpha-tocopherol, and lycopene), total serum and HDL cholesterol, and triglycerides. The investigators found that women married to smokers were more likely to be less educated than women married to nonsmokers, and the husbands of exposed women were also less educated than the husbands of unexposed women (Forastiere et al. 2000). Compared with women married to nonsmokers, women married to smokers were also significantly less likely to eat cooked (OR = 0.72 [95 percent CI, 0.55–0.93]) or fresh (OR = 0.63 [95 percent CI, 0.49–0.82]) vegetables more than once a day. The prevalence of all other variables did not differ. Overall, the investigators concluded that once studies on the health effects of secondhand smoke control for socioeconomic differences, the possibility of confounding is minimal.

Even in studies that found differences in dietary habits between exposed and unexposed nonsmokers, the actual magnitude of the differences was quite modest (Law et al. 1997). Several epidemiologic studies of secondhand smoke exposure and CHD, however, were able to adjust for a range of potential confounding factors. Seven out of 11 published cohort studies were able to control for major cardiovascular risk factors, including blood pressure (or hypertension), serum cholesterol (or hyperlipidemia), and BMI (Table 8.1); only 4 out of the 10 case-control studies controlled for blood pressure and cholesterol (Table 8.2).

Because of the differences in these potential confounding factors between exposed and unexposed lifetime nonsmokers, some investigators have observed that adjusting for other cardiovascular risk factors leads to a modest attenuation of the RR of CHD. In one meta-analysis, He and colleagues (1999) obtained an overall RR of 1.26 when they confined their pooling procedure to the 10 studies that adjusted for major CHD risk factors (blood pressure, serum cholesterol, and BMI). In some studies, such as the Nurses Health Study, investigators controlled for a wide range of potential confounders, including age, alcohol consumption, BMI, physical activity, hypertension, diabetes mellitus, hypercholesterolemia, menopausal status, use of estrogen replacement therapy, past use of oral contraceptives, parental history of heart disease, use of aspirin, and vitamin E and saturated fat intake (Kawachi et al. 1997). After adjusting for the major CHD risk factors, Kawachi and colleagues (1997) found only a modest effect on the RR of CHD from secondhand smoke (a reduction from 1.97 to 1.71). Similarly, in the American Cancer Society Cancer Prevention Study II (CPS-II) cohort, Steenland and colleagues (1996) compared adjustments for age, education, high blood pressure, diabetes, diet, physical activity, and BMI with age adjustment alone and found that the RR estimate for age adjustment alone was reduced from 1.31 to 1.19 in men, and from 1.25 to 1.23 in women.

The studies on secondhand smoke and CHD risk have been reported over a span of several decades and have been carried out in multiple countries. The observed increase in risks is likely attributable to exposures across most of the last century, a time period when the epidemiologic characteristics of CHD changed sharply. Recent cross-sectional studies indicate that persons exposed to secondhand smoke tend to have a less favorable CHD risk factor profile than persons with fewer or no exposures. The relevance of these current patterns of correlation to past exposures is uncertain and the studies may not be readily generalizable to other populations (e.g., Hirayama's cohort in Japan).

Studies that have considered potential confounding factors have observed small reductions in the RR. Some residual confounding can never be excluded, but uncontrolled confounding can be set aside as the sole explanation for the increased RR observed with secondhand smoke exposure.

Workplace Secondhand Smoke Exposure and Risk of Coronary Heart Disease

There is no biologically plausible reason to hypothesize that the risk of CHD from exposures to secondhand smoke would differ across exposure settings (Kawachi and Colditz 1999). The effects of home and workplace exposures are expected to be additive. Workplace exposures also represent background exposures for studies that only inquired about home exposures (and vice versa), and the failure to account for the totality of exposures in different settings would

bias associations with CHD in the direction of the null, as noted earlier in this discussion.

Of the published studies on secondhand smoke and CHD, four case-control studies (Dobson et al. 1991; He et al. 1994; Muscat and Wynder 1995; Rosenlund et al. 2001) and three cohort studies (Svendsen et al. 1987; Steenland et al. 1996; Kawachi et al. 1997) examined the relationship between secondhand smoke exposure in the workplace and CHD risk. The point estimates of the RR for CHD in these studies exceeded 1.0 in six of the seven studies (ranging from 1.2 to 1.9), but the estimates were not statistically significant.

Wells (1998) carried out a meta-analysis of the same six published studies reviewed by Kawachi and Colditz (1999), along with two additional unpublished doctoral dissertations (Butler 1988; Jackson 1989). These eight studies yielded a pooled RR estimate of 1.18 (95 percent CI, 1.04–1.34) for secondhand smoke exposures at work. Two more studies of secondhand smoke and CHD followed these reviews by Wells (1998) and Kawachi and Colditz (1999). The case-control study by McElduff and colleagues (1998) summarized earlier in this chapter reported ORs for CHD from workplace secondhand smoke exposures of 1.31 (95 percent CI, 0.95–1.80) for men and 0.58 (95 percent CI, 0.27–1.24) for women. The case-control study by Rosenlund and colleagues (2001) reported ORs for MI from workplace secondhand smoke exposures of 1.39 for men (95 percent CI, 0.86–2.25) and 1.31 for women (95 percent CI, 0.62–2.79).

Biologic Plausibility of the Magnitude of the Association

Despite estimated exposure levels equivalent to smoking only one-half or one cigarette per day, the estimated increase in risk of CHD from exposure to secondhand smoke is 25 to 30 percent above that of unexposed persons. The magnitude of this association may seem surprisingly large compared with the known association between active smoking and CHD, which is between a twofold and fourfold increase in risk among current smokers of 20 cigarettes per day (Bailar 1999; Howard and Thun 1999).

However, extrapolations from published studies of active smoking yield estimates of CHD risk from exposure to secondhand smoke that are not substantially different from observed risks in epidemiologic studies of secondhand smoke and CHD (Law et al. 1997; Howard and Thun 1999). For example, Howard and Thun (1999) used linear regression to describe the relationship between daily cigarette use and CHD mortality, based on seven studies summarized in the

1983 Surgeon General's report *The Health Consequences of Smoking: Cardiovascular Disease* (USDHHS 1983) that documented CHD risk in relation to the number of cigarettes smoked per day. Assuming that involuntary smokers had been exposed to the equivalent of 0.75 cigarettes per day (the midpoint of the interval between one-half and one cigarette per day), the authors found that the expected CHD mortality ratio ranged from 1.13 to 1.47 across the seven studies, with an overall average of 1.32 (Howard and Thun 1999). This finding was similar to the pooled RR estimated from the published studies of secondhand smoke and CHD.

Some investigators, however, have argued that quantitative extrapolations based on risks for CHD in active smokers are uncertain (Howard and Thun 1999; Steenland 1999). The underlying concept of deriving a "cigarette equivalent" risk factor for CHD from secondhand smoke exposure by linear extrapolation appears biologically inappropriate, particularly in the context of the experimental evidence reviewed in Chapter 2 (see "Heart Rate Variability"). Furthermore, calculating equivalence based on relative exposures to nicotine or to its metabolite cotinine may not be biologically appropriate because the particular components of secondhand smoke that are most relevant for an increased risk of CHD have not yet been identified. For example, an experimental study conducted by Sun and colleagues (2001) found that rabbits exposed to smoke from standard nicotine-containing cigarettes versus smoke from nicotine-free cigarettes during a 10-week period had a similar extent of arterial lipid deposits. Thus, constituents besides nicotine may play a more important role in the damaging effects of secondhand smoke.

Additionally, some of the mechanisms linking tobacco smoke exposure to CHD risk appear to have nonlinear relationships with dose. The effect of tobacco smoke on platelet aggregation provides one plausible and quantitatively consistent mechanism for the association between secondhand smoke and CHD, but the findings on active and involuntary smoking imply a nonlinear relationship (Glantz and Parmley 1991, 1995; Law et al. 1997). In a summary of the experimental evidence on smoking and platelet aggregation, Law and colleagues (1997) found that the acute effects of secondhand smoke were similar to the effects of active smoking. Based on extrapolations from epidemiologic evidence relating a given increase in platelet aggregation to a risk of CHD, the estimated immediate increases in risk attributable to the effects on platelet aggregation were 43 percent for active smoking and 24 percent for involuntary smoking (Law et al. 1997).

An additional plausible mechanism of damage caused by secondhand smoke involves acute endothelial dysfunction (Glantz and Parmley 2001; Otsuka et al. 2001). Normal endothelial cells promote vasodilation and inhibit atherosclerosis and thrombosis, partly mediated by the release of nitric oxide (Glantz and Parmley 2001). Dysfunctional cells, on the other hand, contribute to vasoconstriction, atherogenesis, and thrombosis. Otsuka and colleagues (2001) demonstrated that just 30 minutes of exposure to secondhand smoke compromised the endothelial function in the coronary arteries of healthy nonsmokers, as indexed by the coronary flow velocity reserve, to an extent that was indistinguishable from habitual smokers.

Publication Bias

Publication bias refers to the tendency for investigators to submit manuscripts and for editors to accept them based on the statistical significance and direction of the association (positive rather than negative) found in study results. Overall, there is little evidence to suggest that publication bias attributable to the omission of unpublished data significantly affected the conclusions of the published reviews or meta-analyses of the evidence on CHD. Comprehensive reviews of the evidence linking secondhand smoke to CHD, including the 1997 Cal/EPA report on *Health Effects of Exposure to Environmental Tobacco Smoke* (NCI 1999), the 2001 Surgeon General's report (USDHHS 2001), and the meta-analysis by He and colleagues (1999), have included unpublished studies. In some cases, investigators provided a quantitative estimate of the likelihood of publication bias. For example, of the 19 studies reviewed by Law and colleagues (1997) on secondhand smoke and CHD, 8 indicated a statistically significant association (a probability for each of less than 1 in 40 if there were no association). The total number of studies needed to generate this result by chance would be more than 300 (8×40); that is, the number of unpublished studies would need to be improbably large. In their meta-analysis, He and colleagues (1999) summarized 18 cohort and case-control studies and performed a rank correlation analysis of the association between standard error and log RR. If small studies with negative results were less likely to be published, the correlation between the standard error and log RR would be high, suggesting publication bias. The Kendall tau correlation coefficient for the standard error and the standardized log RR was 0.24 ($p = 0.16$) for all 18 studies, providing little evidence for publication bias. When one study with an extreme value was excluded (Garland et al. 1985), the Kendall tau correlation coefficient for the standard error and the standardized log RR was further reduced to 0.19 (p = 0.28).

The possibility that publication bias has affected meta-analyses of the literature on CHD has also been raised because two meta-analyses excluded studies conducted by consultants to the tobacco industry (Lee 1998; LeVois and Layard 1998). Specifically, several meta-analyses of secondhand smoke and CHD carried out by Law and colleagues (1997), Wells (1998), He and colleagues (1999), and Thun and colleagues (1999) excluded the CPS-I and CPS-II analyses by LeVois and Layard (1995) and the National Mortality Followback Survey (NMFS) analyses by Layard (1995). Both studies suffer from serious methodologic flaws (USDHHS 2001). In the case-control study by Layard (1995), the quality of information on spousal secondhand smoke exposure was uncertain because the exposure categories did not capture whether the spousal exposure was a current or former exposure or whether the spousal exposure was from a current or previous marriage. In addition, all of the NMFS participants had died and exposure data for both case and control groups were obtained from next of kin; 18 percent of the surrogate respondents were not even first-degree relatives. Another flaw was that an estimated 50 percent of the deaths in this study that were attributable to CHD were excluded because of missing information on marital status or spousal smoking behaviors or both.

Methodologic flaws in the cohort analyses of CPS-I and CPS-II data by LeVois and Layard (1995) were also noted in the 2001 Surgeon General's report (USDHHS 2001). The investigators did not distinguish between current exposures from spousal secondhand smoke and former exposures, nor did they separately report the effect of current spousal smoking on the risk of CHD. In a more careful analysis of the CPS-II data, Steenland and colleagues (1996) showed that exposure to current spousal smoking was associated with an increased risk of CHD among both men and women. Using the same data set, Law and colleagues (1997) noted that the estimated RR of CHD from spousal smoking reported by LeVois and Layard (1995) (RR = 1.0 [95 percent CI, 0.87–1.04]) was inconsistent with the estimate reported by Steenland and colleagues (1996) (RR = 1.21 [95 percent CI, 1.06–1.38]). Because both results cannot be correct, Law and colleagues (1997), He and colleagues (1999), and others

rejected the analyses by LeVois and Layard (1995) as less valid than the analysis by Steenland and colleagues (1996).

Previous Reviews of the Evidence

Numerous published reviews, including meta-analyses, summarize the epidemiologic studies of secondhand smoke and CHD (Table 8.3). As the 2001 Surgeon General's report stated, "Although few of the risk estimates in individual studies were statistically significant, pooled estimates from meta-analyses showed a significant, 30-percent increase in risk for CHD in relation to ETS exposure" (USDHHS 2001, p. 356). Two additional reviews of secondhand smoke exposure and CHD were published during the review process preceding the publication of the 2001 Surgeon General's report but were not mentioned in that report: the 1997 Cal/EPA report (NCI 1999) and the 1997 Australian NHMRC Working Party Report (NHMRC 1997) on the health effects of involuntary smoking.

The Cal/EPA report reviewed 10 cohort studies and 8 case-control studies of secondhand smoke and CHD. Although the report did not provide a pooled estimate of RR across the published studies, it concluded that the "epidemiological data...in males and in females, in western and eastern countries, are supportive of a causal association between ETS exposure from spouses and CHD mortality in nonsmokers" (NCI 1999, p. 425). Furthermore, the report concluded that "an overall risk of about 30 percent is supported by the collective evidence and is within range of risk estimates observed for active smoking and CHD" (NCI 1999, p. 425).

The 1997 NHMRC Working Party report considered 22 analyses from 16 studies of secondhand smoke and CHD, with 17 of the 22 analyses indicating some increase in the risk of coronary events among nonsmokers exposed to secondhand smoke; in 8 of the studies, the results were statistically significant. Rather than conducting a quantitative meta-analysis, the NHMRC Working Party report summarized the data using a median RR corresponding to the interquartile range (NHMRC 1997). The median estimate of 1.24 (interquartile range, 1.02 to 1.62) was consistent with the pooled estimate of a 25 to 30 percent increase in risk of CHD reported in other comprehensive meta-analyses (Table 8.3).

Table 8.3   Meta-analyses of secondhand smoke exposure and coronary heart disease

Study	Design	Findings	
		Outcome	Pooled relative risk (95% confidence interval)
Wells 1994	7 cohort studies (Garland et al. 1985; Svendsen et al. 1987; Butler 1988; Hole et al. 1989; Sandler et al. 1989; Hirayama 1990; Humble et al. 1990)	Nonfatal coronary events	Women 1.51 (1.16–1.97) Men 1.28 (0.91–1.81) Combined 1.42 (1.15–1.75)
	5 case-control studies (Lee et al. 1986; He 1989; Jackson 1989; Dobson et al. 1991; He et al. 1994)	Fatal coronary events	Women 1.23 (1.11–1.36) Men 1.25 (1.03–1.51) Combined 1.23 (1.12–1.35)
Law et al. 1997	9 cohort studies (Garland et al. 1985; Svendsen et al. 1987; Butler 1988; Hole et al. 1989; Sandler et al. 1989; Hirayama 1990; Humble et al. 1990; Steenland et al. 1996; Kawachi et al. 1997)	All coronary events	Combined women/men 1.30 (1.22–1.38)
	10 case-control studies (Lee et al. 1986; He 1989; Jackson 1989; Dobson et al. 1991; Lee 1992; La Vecchia et al. 1993; He et al. 1994; Muscat and Wynder 1995; Tunstall-Pedoe et al. 1995; Ciruzzi et al. 1998)		
Wells 1998	9 cohort studies (Garland et al. 1985; Svendsen et al. 1987; Butler 1988; Hole et al. 1989; Sandler et al. 1989; Hirayama 1990; Humble et al. 1990; Steenland et al. 1996; Kawachi et al. 1997)	Nonfatal coronary events	Home exposure only 1.50 (1.23–1.83) Spousal exposure only 1.38 (1.02–1.61) Workplace exposure 1.32 (1.01–1.72)
	9 case-control studies (Lee et al. 1986; He 1989; Jackson 1989; Dobson et al. 1991; La Vecchia et al. 1993; He et al. 1994; Muscat and Wynder 1995; Tunstall-Pedoe et al. 1995; Ciruzzi et al. 1998)	Fatal coronary events	Home exposure only 1.25 (1.12–1.40) Spousal exposure only 1.21 (1.09–1.35) Workplace exposure 1.14 (0.99–1.32)
He et al. 1999	10 cohort studies (Hirayama 1984; Garland et al. 1985; Svendsen et al. 1987; Butler 1988; Hole et al. 1989; Sandler et al. 1989; Hirayama 1990; Humble et al. 1990; Steenland et al. 1996; Kawachi et al. 1997)	All coronary events	Women 1.24 (1.15–1.34) Men 1.22 (1.15–1.34) Combined 1.25 (1.17–1.32) Cohort data 1.21 (1.14–1.30)
	8 case-control studies (Lee et al. 1986; He 1989; Jackson 1989; Dobson et al. 1991; La Vecchia et al. 1993; He et al. 1994; Muscat and Wynder 1995; Ciruzzi et al. 1998)		Case-control data 1.51 (1.26–1.81) Home exposure 1.17 (1.11–1.24) Workplace exposure 1.11 (1.0–1.23)
Thun et al. 1999	10 cohort studies (Hirayama 1984; Garland et al. 1985; Svendsen et al. 1987; Butler 1988; Hole et al. 1989; Sandler et al. 1989; Hirayama 1990; Humble et al. 1990; LeVois and Layard 1995; Steenland et al. 1996)	All coronary events	Women 1.23 (1.15–1.32) Men 1.24 (1.15–1.32) Combined 1.25 (1.17–1.33)
	8 case-control studies (Lee et al. 1986; He 1989; Jackson 1989; Dobson et al. 1991; La Vecchia et al. 1993; He et al. 1994; Muscat and Wynder 1995; Ciruzzi et al. 1998)	Nonfatal coronary events	Combined women/men 1.32 (1.04–1.67)
		Fatal coronary events	Combined women/men 1.22 (1.14–1.30)

Updated Meta-Analysis of Exposure to Secondhand Smoke and Cardiovascular Disease

This meta-analysis updates the 1999 synthesis by He and colleagues (1999) of the literature covering the association between secondhand smoke exposure and cardiovascular disease. Articles on this association in nonsmokers published between June 1998 (the cutoff date for the He and colleagues [1999] paper) and April 2002 were identified through a search of PubMed using the Medical Subject Headings (MeSH) terms tobacco smoke pollution, CHD, and myocardial infarction and the keywords passive smoking and environmental tobacco smoke. The search was limited to English-language studies and yielded two additional studies compared with the previous meta-analysis.

All of the English-language studies included in previous meta-analyses, along with the two new studies, were abstracted and reviewed for inclusion in this meta-analysis. Five papers were excluded from the analysis (Jackson 1989; Dobson et al. 1991; Layard 1995; LeVois and Layard 1995; Tunstall-Pedoe et al. 1995). The articles by Jackson (1989) and Dobson and colleagues (1991) were excluded because they reported data that were reanalyzed in one of the more recent papers (McElduff et al. 1998). The paper by Tunstall-Pedoe and colleagues (1995) was excluded because of its cross-sectional design. The analyses by Layard (1995) and LeVois and Layard (1995) were excluded because of methodologic issues in exposure measurement. Layard's (1995) analysis of data from the 1986 NMFS was based on surrogate reports of exposure. LeVois and Layard (1995) used data from CPS-I and CPS-II; the CPS-II data were analyzed by Steenland and colleagues (1996) and the CPS-I data were insufficient for classifying exposure. The sensitivity of the results when these last three studies were excluded was tested and found not to produce significant differences.

For all of the studies, the estimates used were after adjustments for major cardiovascular disease risk factors, if available. If data were presented separately for women and men or for different exposure levels, they were pooled using random effects models. All quantitative pooling was carried out with Stata (version 7); results presented are for random effects models.

The meta-analysis included nine cohort studies (Table 8.1) and seven case-control studies (Table 8.2). All but two of the cohort studies were conducted in the United States; in contrast, only one of the case-control studies was conducted in the United States.

Six studies included only women, nine studies included both genders, and one study included only men. All study participants were nonsmokers, and in all but three studies they were lifetime nonsmokers. Those three studies either explicitly included former smokers or did not specify whether the nonsmokers had ever smoked (Hirayama 1984; Butler 1988; McElduff et al. 1998). Most of the studies (15) used in the updated meta-analysis documented self-reported exposures to secondhand smoke in the home either from a spouse or a cohabitant. Four studies also reported exposures at work separately from other settings, whereas two studies did not specify the different exposure sources. All but one of the cohort studies reported on the effect of exposure to secondhand smoke on fatal CHD (five) or on ischemic heart disease (IHD) (three). In addition, one cohort study combined fatal CHD and nonfatal acute MI. Four of the case-control studies used nonfatal acute MI as their outcome, one used nonfatal CHD, one used fatal and nonfatal acute MI, and one used nonfatal IHD.

Figure 8.1 provides the findings of the 16 studies included in the meta-analysis, along with the overall pooled estimate (RR = 1.27 [95 percent CI, 1.19–1.36]). The individual RR estimates cover a relatively narrow range, but the CIs are quite wide for the smaller studies.

Variations in the pooled estimates were examined by place of exposure, gender, outcome, study design, and level of adjustment for potential confounding factors (Figure 8.2). Interpretation of these stratified analyses is limited by the precision of the estimates. Nonetheless, point estimates are similar for men and women and by exposure venue. The stringency of adjustment for potential confounding also has little effect on the estimates. The pooled estimate for the case-control studies is somewhat higher than for the cohort studies.

Dose-Response Analysis

Methods

Studies from the overall meta-analysis that provided measures of association stratified by the intensity of exposure to secondhand smoke, determined by the number of cigarettes smoked per day by a cohabitant, were used to generate pooled estimates for the dose-response analysis (Table 8.4). Although most studies categorized the daily number of cigarettes as none, 1 to 19, and 20 or more, several studies used the categories none, 1 to 14, and 15 or more.

Figure 8.1   Relative risks of coronary heart disease associated with secondhand smoke exposure among nonsmokers*

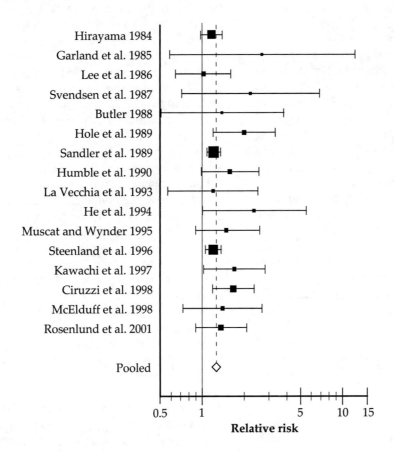

Note: The horizontal bars represent the 95% confidence intervals (CIs), and the size of the box for each study reflects each study's weight in the pooled estimate, with a larger box indicating a larger weight.
*Pooled estimate = 1.27 (95% CI, 1.19–1.36), the dashed line.

For the purpose of pooling as many studies as possible in this analysis, levels of exposure were categorized as none, low to moderate, and moderate to high. Categories of 1 to 19 and 1 to 14 cigarettes per day were therefore combined, as were categories of 20 or more and 15 or more cigarettes per day. Similar to the main analysis, adjusted measures of association were used when available. If confidence limits were not provided in a paper, they were estimated using standard methods appropriate for the study design. Papers that presented separate estimates for men and women were combined using random effects models. Pooled estimates were also calculated using random effects models. All calculations were carried out in Stata (version 7).

Results

Of the 19 studies, 8 included measures of association determined by the number of cigarettes smoked per day by a cohabitant, usually a spouse (Table 8.4). There were four cohort studies (Svendsen et al. 1987; Hole et al. 1989; Hirayama 1990; Steenland et al. 1996) and four case-control studies (La Vecchia et al. 1993; He et al. 1994; Ciruzzi et al. 1998; Rosenlund et al. 2001). The RR of CHD increased slightly with exposure to a higher level of secondhand smoke (Figure 8.3). Compared with unexposed nonsmokers, nonsmokers exposed to levels of secondhand smoke ranging from low to moderate (1 to 14 or 1 to 19 cigarettes per day) had a RR of 1.16 (95 percent

Figure 8.2   Pooled relative risks of coronary heart disease (CHD) associated with secondhand smoke exposure among nonsmokers in various subgroups

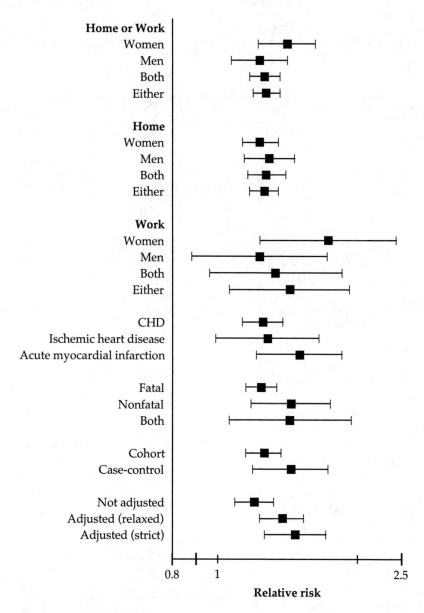

Note: Data are provided in detail in Tables 8.1 and 8.2. Stratified by gender for any exposure and for home and work exposures separately, by diagnosis (CHD, ischemic heart disease, acute myocardial infarction), by outcome (fatal or nonfatal), by study design (cohort or case-control), and whether the estimates were adjusted for important CHD risk factors (strict included several CHD risk factors, relaxed included at least one risk factor).

Sources: Hirayama 1984, 1990; Garland et al. 1985; Lee et al. 1986; Svendsen et al. 1987; Butler 1988; Helsing et al. 1988; He 1989; Hole et al. 1989; Jackson 1989; Sandler et al. 1989; Humble et al. 1990; Dobson et al. 1991; La Vecchia et al. 1993; He et al. 1994; Layard 1995; LeVois and Layard 1995; Muscat and Wynder 1995; Tunstall-Pedoe et al. 1995; Steenland et al. 1996; Kawachi et al. 1997; Ciruzzi et al. 1998; McElduff et al. 1998; Rosenlund et al. 2001.

Table 8.4   Studies included in the dose-response meta-analysis and pooled results

| Study | Low to moderate exposure | | Moderate to high exposure | |
	Cigarettes/day	Relative risk (95% confidence interval)	Cigarettes/day	Relative risk (95% confidence interval)
Svendsen et al. 1987	1–19	0.90 (0.02–6.70)	>19	3.21 (0.71–11.98)
Hole et al. 1989	1–15	2.09 (0.60–7.23)	>15	4.12 (1.21–14.05)
Hirayama et al. 1990	1–19	1.08 (0.9–1.3)	>19	1.3 (1.06–1.6)
La Vecchia et al. 1993	1–14	1.13 (0.45–2.82)	>14	1.3 (0.5–3.4)
He et al. 1994	6–20	1.61 (0.49–5.34)	>20	3.56 (0.81–15.58)
Steenland et al. 1996	1–19	1.31 (1.06–1.62)	>19	1.14 (0.97–1.34)
Ciruzzi et al. 1998	1–20	1.24 (0.61–2.52)	>20	4.03 (0.99–16.32)
Rosenlund et al. 2001	1–19	1.02 (0.73–1.42)	>19	1.58 (0.97–2.56)
Pooled results	Fixed effects:	1.16 (1.03–1.32)		1.26 (1.12–1.42)
	Random effects:	1.16 (1.03–1.32)		1.44 (1.13–1.82)

CI, 1.03–1.32). Nonsmokers exposed to levels ranging from moderate to high (≥15 or ≥20 cigarettes per day) had a RR of 1.44 (95 percent CI, 1.13–1.82) compared with unexposed nonsmokers. These estimates are similar to those of He and colleagues (1999), who found that nonsmokers exposed to 1 to 19 cigarettes per day had a RR of 1.23 (95 percent CI, 1.13–1.34), and nonsmokers exposed to 20 or more cigarettes per day had a RR of 1.31 (95 percent CI, 1.21–1.42). The differences between the two results are attributed to the studies used in the pooling and to the use of random effects models for this report. (He and colleagues [1999] reported results of fixed effects models.)

Figure 8.3   Pooled relative risks of coronary heart disease associated with various levels of exposure to secondhand smoke among nonsmokers

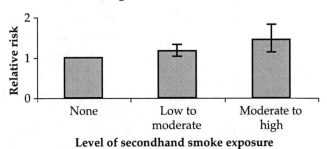

Note: None, low to moderate (1–14 or 1–19 cigarettes per day), and moderate to high (≥15 or ≥20 cigarettes per day).

Stroke

Six studies (four case-control, one cross-sectional, and one cohort) have examined the association between secondhand smoke and risk of stroke (Table 8.5). These studies did not address the risk for specific types of stroke. Two of the six published studies found a statistically significant increase for the risk of stroke among involuntary smokers (Sandler et al. 1989; Bonita et al. 1999).

Lee and colleagues (1986) carried out a hospital-based, case-control study in 10 regions in the United Kingdom. Involuntary smoking was classified according to self-reported secondhand smoke exposures at home, at work, during travel, and during leisure time. A secondhand smoke exposure score (ranging from 0 to 12) was based on a linear summation of the self-reported intensity of an exposure in each setting (0 = not at all; 1 = little; 2 = average; 3 = a lot). Participants were also asked whether their spouses had smoked cigarettes for the duration of their marriage (yes/no). The study included 92 persons who had suffered a stroke, but the authors did not define the diagnostic criteria used for stroke. Persons recruited as controls were hospitalized patients treated in medical, thoracic surgery, and radiotherapy wards and were matched to stroke patients for gender, age, and hospital region. Overall, the study did not find an association between exposure to spousal secondhand smoke and stroke (OR = 0.90 [95 percent CI, 0.53–1.52]). The OR of stroke among patients with a high secondhand smoke exposure score (ranging from 5 to 12) was 2.18 (95 percent CI, 0.86–5.48) compared with those with a low score (0 or 1).

Donnan and colleagues (1989) carried out a case-control study in four hospitals in Melbourne, Australia; a strength of this study was that 98 percent of the stroke cases were confirmed by a computerized tomography (CT) scan. Cases with a first-ever stroke (256 men, 166 women), including transient ischemic attack (TIA), were matched to 422 neighborhood controls. Self-reported exposures to spousal or parental smoking of at least a one-year duration were used to classify the exposure. Eighty-eight cases of stroke occurred among lifetime nonsmokers. The OR of stroke for lifetime nonsmokers with a smoking spouse was 1.6 (95 percent CI, 0.6–3.9). No association was found between exposures to parental smoking and stroke (OR = 1.0 [95 percent CI, 0.5–2.1]). The ORs were adjusted for hypertension, high cholesterol,

alcohol intake, history of MI, and any use of oral contraceptives.

Sandler and colleagues (1989) carried out a 12-year follow-up study of a cohort of 19,035 lifetime nonsmokers who had been identified through a 1963 private census of households in Washington county, Maryland. Investigators ascertained deaths that occurred in the cohort by matching the census to death certificates, with causes of death on the death certificate coded according to the *International Classification of Diseases*, 7th revision (World Health Organization [WHO] 1957). No further information was available to confirm cases of stroke. Investigators calculated the sum of smoking histories of all smokers in the household for a household tobacco smoke exposure score that was used to assess secondhand smoke exposures. The score did not measure the total secondhand smoke exposure because the number of cigarettes smoked per day outside of the home was not specified. Of the 14,873 female and 4,162 male lifetime nonsmokers in the study, 64.2 percent of the women and 30.0 percent of the men reported secondhand smoke exposures. After adjusting for age, marital status, housing quality, and education, the RRs of stroke mortality were 0.97 for men (95 percent CI, 0.65–1.46; based on 33 exposed cases) and 1.24 for women (95 percent CI, 1.03–1.49; based on 297 exposed cases) (Sandler et al. 1989).

Howard and colleagues (1998b) analyzed findings of magnetic resonance imaging (MRI) scans on 1,737 participants aged 55 through 70 years who had been selected from two of the four U.S. communities in the Atherosclerosis Risk in Communities (ARIC) Study. The study included 444 lifetime nonsmokers who were classified as not exposed to secondhand smoke by the definition used and 348 exposed lifetime nonsmokers. The disease outcome in this cross-sectional study was the prevalence of silent cerebral infarction (SCI), which was defined by standardized criteria on the MRI scans; SCI is an indicator of cerebrovascular disease. Acceptable interrater reliability was reported for the detection of lesions and the interpretation of scans. Involuntary smoking was defined as self-reported current exposure to secondhand smoke for one or more hours per week. The authors adjusted their risk estimates for a number of potential confounding factors, including hypertension, HDL cholesterol and triglyceride levels,

Table 8.5   Epidemiologic studies of secondhand smoke exposure and stroke

Study	Design	Population	Case definition	Relative risk (95% confidence interval)	Variables controlled for
Lee et al. 1986	Case-control Hospital-based	Men 4 cases 33 controls Women 8 cases 18 controls United Kingdom	Data were not reported	Spousal secondhand smoke 0.90 (0.53–1.52) All sources of secondhand smoke 2.18* (0.86–5.48)	Age, gender, marital status
Donnan et al. 1989	Case-control Hospital cases and community controls	88 cases and 88 matched controls Lifetime nonsmoking men and women Australia	Incident stroke and transient ischemic attack (98% confirmation by computerized tomography [CT] scan)	Spousal secondhand smoke 1.6 (0.6–3.9) Parental secondhand smoke 1.0 (0.5–2.1)	Age, gender, hypertension, high cholesterol, alcohol intake, history of heart attack, any use of oral contraceptives
Sandler et al. 1989	Cohort study with 12-year follow-up	4,162 men and 14,873 women Lifetime nonsmokers United States	*International Classification of Diseases* codes from death certificates, 7th revision	Secondhand smoke exposure in the home Men 0.97 (0.65–1.46) Women 1.24 (1.03–1.49)	Age, marital status, housing quality, education
Howard et al. 1998b	Cross-sectional study of Atherosclerosis Risk in Communities Study participants	444 lifetime nonsmokers not exposed to secondhand smoke and 348 lifetime nonsmokers exposed to secondhand smoke United States	Prevalent silent cerebral infarction	All sources of secondhand smoke Prevalence odds ratio = 1.06 (0.64–1.75)	Age, gender, race, hypertension, high-density lipoprotein cholesterol and triglyceride levels, diabetes mellitus, dietary fat, exercise, body mass index, alcohol consumption
Bonita et al. 1999	Case-control Hospital cases and community controls	215 cases and 1,336 controls among nonsmokers, including former smokers who quit >10 years ago New Zealand	Incident stroke based on World Health Organization criteria	Secondhand smoke exposure in the home Men 2.10 (1.33–3.32) Women 1.66 (1.07–2.57) Combined 1.82 (1.34–2.49)	Age, gender, hypertension, diabetes, history of heart disease
You et al. 1999	Case-control Hospital cases and community controls	149 cases and 210 controls Lifetime nonsmoking men and women Australia	Incident stroke verified by CT scan	Spousal secondhand smoke 1.70 (0.98–2.92) Parental secondhand smoke 0.78 (0.48–1.26)	Age, gender, education, hypertension, diabetes mellitus, history of heart disease

*Comparing the highest level of exposure with the lowest (see Lee et al. 1986, Table V, p. 102).

diabetes mellitus, dietary fat intake, leisure time physical activity, BMI, and alcohol intake. The investigators calculated an adjusted prevalence OR of 1.06 for SCI for those classified as exposed to secondhand smoke (95 percent CI, 0.64–1.75) compared with unexposed nonsmokers. There was no relationship between hours of exposure to secondhand smoke and SCI (Howard et al. 1998b).

Bonita and colleagues (1999) carried out a population-based, case-control study of secondhand smoke and stroke in Auckland, New Zealand. Diagnostic criteria and methods for the 215 nonsmoking persons aged 35 through 74 years with first-ever acute stroke were defined according to WHO guidelines. The 1,336 nonsmoking controls were community-dwelling participants drawn from a 1993–1994 cross-sectional survey of cardiovascular risk factors carried out in the same city. The investigators determined exposures to secondhand smoke by asking patients and controls the same questions and characterized an exposure as a household member who regularly smoked cigarettes in their presence, or a coworker who smoked in the same indoor room in their presence for more than 1 year during the past 10 years. Risks were assessed among lifetime nonsmokers combined with long-term former smokers. Exposure to secondhand smoke was associated with an increased risk among men (crude OR = 2.10 [95 percent CI, 1.33–3.32]) and women (crude OR = 1.66 [95 percent CI, 1.07–2.57]). Overall, the risk of stroke was 1.82 (95 percent CI, 1.34–2.49)

for involuntary smokers with adjustment for several potential confounding factors. The nonsmokers in this study (both cases and controls) included former smokers who had stopped smoking for more than 10 years. No attempt was made in this study to distinguish secondhand smoke exposures at home, at work, or elsewhere (Bonita et al. 1999).

One case-control study in Australia compared 452 hospitalized cases of first-ever ischemic stroke and 452 gender-matched neighborhood controls (You et al. 1999). Ischemic stroke was defined as the acute onset of a focal neurologic deficit that lasted more than 24 hours and that was verified by CT (excluding hemorrhage). Involuntary smoking was defined as living with a father, mother, or spouse who smoked at least one cigarette per day. To estimate the OR, You and colleagues (1999) controlled for educational attainment, history of CHD, hypertension, and diabetes mellitus, and then excluded current and former smokers. There were 154 participants who had suffered a stroke and 213 with no history of a stroke among the lifetime nonsmokers; missing values in either cases or controls bring the numbers to 149 cases and 210 controls used in the analysis. The adjusted OR of stroke for lifetime nonsmokers exposed to spousal smoking was 1.70 (95 percent CI, 0.98–2.92). No association was found for exposures to parental smoking (OR = 0.78 [95 percent CI, 0.48–1.26]) (Table 8.5). These studies were not pooled in this report because of their small number and the heterogeneity of their methods.

Subclinical Vascular Disease

A number of studies have been published linking secondhand smoke exposure to measures of subclinical vascular disease. These studies offer insights into the mechanisms underlying the relationship between exposures to secondhand smoke and the development of clinical coronary and cerebrovascular events (Howard and Wagenknecht 1999). Five different types of subclinical vascular outcomes that have been studied in humans in relation to secondhand smoke include the following:

- assessing intimal-medial thickness (IMT) of the carotid artery using B-mode ultrasound as an

index of systemic atherosclerosis (Howard et al. 1994, 1998a; Diez-Roux et al. 1995);

- assessing flow-mediated arterial endothelial function using B-mode ultrasound of the brachial artery as an index of vascular damage (Celermajer et al. 1996; Lekakis et al. 1997; Raitakari et al. 1999);

- assessing coronary endothelial dysfunction using a quantitative coronary angiography to measure the extent of impairment of acetylcholine-induced coronary artery dilatation (Sumida et al. 1998);

- assessing coronary flow velocity reserve using noninvasive transthoracic Doppler echocardiography (Otsuka et al. 2001); and

- assessing aortic elastic properties before and after involuntary smoking with the aortic pressure-diameter relation (Stefanadis et al. 1998, 1999).

Published evidence suggests that exposure to secondhand smoke is damaging for each type of subclinical vascular outcome. This section reviews the evidence on secondhand smoke in relation to carotid arterial wall thickness.

Carotid Intimal-Medial Thickness

Carotid IMT, assessed by B-mode ultrasound, is an established predictor of clinical events, including MI and stroke (Bots et al. 1997; Chambless et al. 1997; O'Leary et al. 1999). All three published studies linking secondhand smoke to an increased carotid IMT have used data from the ARIC Study (Howard et al. 1994, 1998a; Diez-Roux et al. 1995). In a cross-sectional analysis of data from the baseline ARIC assessment of 5,113 nonsmokers, Howard and colleagues (1994) found a difference of 11 micrometers (μm) in the average IMT of unexposed compared with exposed nonsmokers. This difference increased to 13 μm (p = 0.003) after adjusting for age, race, gender, education, hypertension, diabetes mellitus, low-density lipoprotein cholesterol level, fat intake, alcohol consumption, BMI, and leisure time physical activity. Among exposed male nonsmokers, there was a statistically significant dose-response relationship between the number of hours of the exposure and carotid IMT (p = 0.03). No dose-response relationship was observed among unexposed female nonsmokers.

Diez-Roux and colleagues (1995) assessed IMT in relation to current and past exposures to secondhand smoke in a cohort of 2,073 persons who were included in the ARIC Study. The participants had information available on secondhand smoke exposure in 1975 and in 1987–1989. The authors defined four groups of lifetime nonsmokers: (1) those not exposed to secondhand smoke at either exam, (2) those exposed at the first but not at the second exam, (3) those exposed at the second but not at the first exam, and (4) those exposed at both exams. Exposure at one or both exams was associated with a nearly identical increase in IMT. This finding suggests that secondhand smoke has long-term harmful effects on atherosclerosis. The average IMT was 706 μm (±13 μm) for those not exposed in either period, 731 μm (±22 μm) for those exposed in the first period only, 738 μm (±11 μm) for those exposed in the second period only, and 734 μm (±12 μm) for those exposed in both periods (Diez-Roux et al. 1995).

Finally, the ARIC Study examined the longitudinal association between secondhand smoke and the progression of IMT (Howard et al. 1998a). During a three-year follow-up period, the IMT progression rate was 31.6 μm for exposed lifetime nonsmokers and 25.9 μm for unexposed lifetime nonsmokers. The estimates of IMT progression were adjusted for the same demographic and coronary risk factors as in the cross-sectional report by the same investigators (Howard et al. 1994). Among lifetime nonsmokers and former smokers combined, exposure to secondhand smoke was associated with an adjusted IMT progression rate of 5.9 μm over three years (±2.3 μm; p = 0.01). In proportional terms, this rate amounted to a 20 percent increase in IMT, which was nearly one-third of the size of the corresponding rate of progression among current smokers. No dose-response pattern was detected, however, between an increase in weekly hours of exposure and increased IMT progression rates.

The evidence on CHD and stroke are considered separately in this section; however, the underlying pathogenetic mechanisms by which involuntary smoking increases risk are shared. For both outcomes, progression of atherosclerosis and increased risk for thrombosis are relevant. The finding that exposure to secondhand smoke increases IMT is supportive of a causal role for secondhand smoke exposure for both CHD and stroke.

Evidence Synthesis

Secondhand Smoke and Coronary Heart Disease

Epidemiologic studies published since the 1986 Surgeon General's report (USDHHS 1986) demonstrate convincingly that secondhand smoke is associated with an increased risk for CHD. The results of both case-control and cohort studies carried out in multiple populations consistently indicate about a 25 to 30 percent increase in risk of CHD from exposure to secondhand smoke. Additionally, cross-sectional and prospective studies convincingly demonstrate an association between exposure to secondhand smoke and the progression of carotid arterial IMT. The excess risk is unlikely to be explained by a measurement error with resulting exposure misclassification or uncontrolled confounding. One type of measurement error, the failure to correct for background secondhand smoke exposure, would lead to an underestimation of the association. Because exposures to secondhand smoke in different environments are presumed to be additive, studies that assess exposures in only one setting will underestimate the true, overall association. Although few studies have addressed CHD risk from secondhand smoke exposure in the workplace, there is no biologically plausible reason to suppose that the effect of secondhand smoke exposure at work differs from the effect of exposures in the home environment.

When interpreting the epidemiologic data, researchers must also consider the possibility that the association reflects uncontrolled confounding. Several cross-sectional studies show differing profiles of cardiovascular risk factors in secondhand smoke-exposed versus unexposed persons. However, an association has been consistently observed in multiple populations, and a number of studies have considered potential confounding factors in the analysis. Whereas some degree of residual confounding can never be fully excluded, the consistency of the association of secondhand smoke exposure with CHD risk and the persistence of an association with controls for confounding weigh heavily against residual confounding as the sole explanation.

A substantial body of experimental evidence supports the biologic plausibility of an association of CHD risk with secondhand smoke exposure. Secondhand smoke exposure adversely affects platelet function and endothelial function. In animal models, secondhand smoke exposure produces atherosclerosis in the coronary arteries.

Current exposures to secondhand smoke appear to be more harmful than past exposures, and several studies suggest a higher risk of CHD from exposures of higher intensities. At least one study suggests that the risk declines as more time elapses since the last exposure.

Compared with the effects of active smoking, the magnitude of the association between secondhand smoke and CHD seems large. This finding can be reconciled, however, with experimental data from both human and animal studies showing that acute effects of secondhand smoke on platelet aggregation as well as on endothelial dysfunction are nonlinear (Chapter 2, Toxicology of Secondhand Smoke).

Secondhand Smoke and Stroke

The evidence is more limited for an association between secondhand smoke and stroke, although the biologic plausibility of an association with stroke risk is supported by the same evidence considered for CHD. The findings of the epidemiologic studies of CHD are complementary to those of stroke. Four case-control studies, one cross-sectional study, and one cohort study have addressed the association between secondhand smoke and the risk of stroke. In these studies, exposures to secondhand smoke were assessed either through self-reports (Lee et al. 1986; Donnan et al. 1989; Howard et al. 1998b; Bonita et al. 1999), or through the use of living in a household with other smokers as an indicator (Sandler et al. 1989; You et al. 1999). In addition to the possibility of measurement error, recall bias may be a problem in case-control studies that assess involuntary smoking with participant reports.

Four of the six studies measured and adjusted for potential confounding variables such as hypertension and diabetes (Donnan et al. 1989; Howard et al. 1998b; Bonita et al. 1999; You et al. 1999). Measures of exposure differed across the studies. Of the six studies, two reported a statistically significant increase in the risk of stroke among involuntary smokers (Sandler et al. 1989; Bonita et al. 1999). Two other studies reported elevated risks of stroke from exposures to spousal smoking, but the lower 95 percent CI was below unity for both studies (Donnan et al. 1989; You et al. 1999).

The six published studies also varied in their definition of stroke. Lee and colleagues (1986) did not define diagnostic criteria, whereas Donnan and colleagues (1989) included cases of TIA. Sandler and colleagues (1989) studied only stroke deaths based on death certificates; Howard and colleagues (1998b) examined SCI using MRI scans. The published studies of secondhand smoke exposure and stroke are still too few and too heterogeneous in their methods and their exposure and outcome measures to warrant a pooled analysis.

Given the established causal associations between active cigarette smoking and stroke and between involuntary smoking and CHD, an association between secondhand smoke and stroke is biologically plausible. There is a need for further research, especially more cohort studies, before a causal association can be inferred.

Conclusions

1. The evidence is sufficient to infer a causal relationship between exposure to secondhand smoke and increased risks of coronary heart disease morbidity and mortality among both men and women.

2. Pooled relative risks from meta-analyses indicate a 25 to 30 percent increase in the risk of coronary heart disease from exposure to secondhand smoke.

3. The evidence is suggestive but not sufficient to infer a causal relationship between exposure to secondhand smoke and an increased risk of stroke.

4. Studies of secondhand smoke and subclinical vascular disease, particularly carotid arterial wall thickening, are suggestive but not sufficient to infer a causal relationship between exposure to secondhand smoke and atherosclerosis.

Overall Implications

Cal/EPA has estimated that 46,000 (a range of 22,700 to 69,600) cardiac deaths in the United States each year are attributable to secondhand smoke exposures at home and in the workplace (Cal/EPA 2005). Thus, the estimated exposures in these two environments can potentially produce a substantial burden of avoidable deaths. Because researchers have identified workplaces as predominant sites for exposure to secondhand smoke (Chapter 4, Prevalence of Exposure to Secondhand Smoke), the estimated pooled RR for workplace exposures suggests that secondhand smoke represents a significant occupational hazard. Following a modified risk assessment approach adopted in 1994 by the U.S. Occupational Safety and Health Administration, Steenland (1999) estimated that as a result of secondhand smoke exposures in the workplace, the excess risk of death from heart disease by 70 years of age was 7 per 1,000 (95 percent CI, 1–13 per 1,000). On the basis of current estimates of exposures to secondhand smoke in U.S. workplaces, Steenland further estimated that these exposures had caused 1,710 excess deaths from CHD annually among nonsmoking workers aged 35 through 69 years.

This review identified several areas for further research. Mechanistic studies that further refine the dose-response relationships and mechanisms of acute responses of the cardiovascular system to secondhand smoke exposure should be carried out. Additional epidemiologic studies of stroke are also needed.

References

American Heart Association. *Heart and Stroke Statistics—2005 Update.* Dallas: American Heart Association, 2005.

Bailar JC III. Passive smoking, coronary heart disease, and meta-analysis [editorial]. *New England Journal of Medicine* 1999;340(12):958–9.

Bonita R, Duncan J, Truelsen T, Jackson RT, Beaglehole R. Passive smoking as well as active smoking increases the risk of acute stroke. *Tobacco Control* 1999;8(2):156–60.

Bots ML, Hoes AW, Koudstaal PJ, Hofman A, Grobbee DE. Common carotid intima-media thickness and risk of stroke and myocardial infarction: the Rotterdam Study. *Circulation* 1997;96(5):1432–7.

Butler TL. The relationship of passive smoking to various health outcomes among Seventh-day Adventists in California [dissertation]. Los Angeles: University of California, 1988.

California Environmental Protection Agency. *Proposed Identification of Environmental Tobacco Smoke as a Toxic Air Contaminant. Part B: Health Effects.* Sacramento (CA): California Environmental Protection Agency, Office of Environmental Health Hazard Assessment, 2005.

Celermajer DS, Adams MR, Clarkson P, Robinson J, McCredie R, Donald A, Deanfield JE. Passive smoking and impaired endothelium-dependent arterial dilatation in healthy young adults. *New England Journal of Medicine* 1996;334(3):150–5.

Chambless LE, Heiss G, Folsom AR, Rosamond W, Szklo M, Sharrett AR, Clegg LX. Association of coronary heart disease incidence with carotid arterial wall thickness and major risk factors: the Atherosclerosis Risk in Communities (ARIC) Study, 1987–1993. *American Journal of Epidemiology* 1997;146(6):483–94.

Ciruzzi M, Pramparo P, Esteban O, Rozlosnik J, Tartaglione J, Abecasis B, César J, De Rosa J, Paterno C, Schargrodsky H. Case-control study of passive smoking at home and risk of acute myocardial infarction. *Journal of the American College of Cardiology* 1998;31(4):797–803.

Cummings KM, Markello SJ, Mahoney M, Bhargava AK, McElroy PD, Marshall JR. Measurement of current exposure to environmental tobacco smoke. *Archives of Environmental Health* 1990;45(2):74–9.

Curtin F, Morabia A, Bernstein MS. Relation of environmental tobacco smoke to diet and health habits: variations according to the site of exposure. *Journal of Clinical Epidemiology* 1999;52(11):1055–62.

Diez-Roux AV, Nieto FJ, Comstock GW, Howard G, Szklo M. The relationship of active and passive smoking to carotid wall thickness 12–14 years later. *Preventive Medicine* 1995;24(1):48–55.

Dobson AJ, Alexander HM, Heller RF, Lloyd DM. Passive smoking and the risk of heart attack or coronary death. *Medical Journal of Australia* 1991;154(12): 793–7.

Donnan GA, McNeil JJ, Adena MA, Doyle AE, O'Malley HM, Neill GC. Smoking as a risk factor for cerebral ischaemia. *Lancet* 1989;2(8664):643–7.

Emmons KM, Abrams DB, Marshall RJ, Etzel RA, Novotny TE, Marcus BH, Kane ME. Exposure to environmental tobacco smoke in naturalistic settings. *American Journal of Public Health* 1992;82(1): 24–8.

Emmons KM, Thompson B, Feng Z, Hebert JR, Heimendinger J, Linnan L. Dietary intake and exposure to environmental tobacco smoke in a worksite population. *European Journal of Clinical Nutrition* 1995;49(5):336–45.

Forastiere F, Mallone S, Lo Presti E, Baldacci S, Pistelli F, Simoni M, Scalera A, Pedreschi M, Pistelli R, Corbo G, et al. Characteristics of nonsmoking women exposed to spouses who smoke: epidemiologic study on environment and health in women from four Italian areas. *Environmental Health Perspectives* 2000;108(12):1171–7.

Garfinkel L. Time trends in lung cancer mortality among nonsmokers and a note on passive smoking. *Journal of the National Cancer Institute* 1981; 66(6):1061–6.

Garland C, Barrett-Connor E, Suarez L, Criqui MH, Wingard DL. Effects of passive smoking on ischemic heart disease mortality of nonsmokers: a prospective study. *American Journal of Epidemiology* 1985;121(5):645–50. [See also erratum in *American Journal of Epidemiology* 1985;122(6):1112.]

Glantz SA, Parmley WW. Passive smoking and heart disease: epidemiology, physiology, and biochemistry. *Circulation* 1991;83(1):1–12.

Glantz SA, Parmley WW. Passive smoking and heart disease: mechanisms and risk. *Journal of the American Medical Association* 1995;273(13):1047–53.

Glantz SA, Parmley WW. Even a little secondhand smoke is dangerous. *Journal of the American Medical Association* 2001;286(4):462–3.

Hackshaw AK, Law MR, Wald NJ. The accumulated evidence on lung cancer and environmental tobacco smoke. *British Medical Journal* 1997;315(7114):980–8.

He J, Vupputuri S, Allen K, Prerost MR, Hughes J, Whelton PK. Passive smoking and the risk of coronary heart disease: a meta-analysis of epidemiologic studies. *New England Journal of Medicine* 1999;340(12):920–6.

He Y. Women's passive smoking and coronary heart disease. *Chinese Journal of Preventive Medicine* 1989;23(1):19–22.

He Y, Lam TH, Li LS, Du RY, Jia GL, Huang JY, Zheng JS. Passive smoking at work as a risk factor for coronary heart disease in Chinese women who have never smoked. *British Medical Journal* 1994;308(6925):380–4.

Helsing KJ, Sandler DP, Comstock GW, Chee E. Heart disease mortality in nonsmokers living with smokers. *American Journal of Epidemiology* 1988;127(5):915–22.

Hirayama T. Lung cancer in Japan: effects of nutrition and passive smoking. In: Mizell M, Correa P, editors. *Lung Cancer: Causes and Prevention.* Deerfield Beach (MA): Verlag Chemie International, 1984:175–95.

Hirayama T. Passive smoking [letter]. *New Zealand Medical Journal* 1990;103(883):54.

Hole DJ, Gillis CR, Chopra C, Hawthorne VM. Passive smoking and cardiorespiratory health in a general population in the west of Scotland. *British Medical Journal* 1989;299(6696):423–7.

Howard G, Burke GL, Szklo M, Tell GS, Eckfeldt J, Evans G, Heiss G. Active and passive smoking are associated with increased carotid wall thickness: the Atherosclerosis Risk in Communities Study. *Archives of Internal Medicine* 1994;154(11):1277–82.

Howard G, Thun MJ. Why is environmental tobacco smoke more strongly associated with coronary heart disease than expected: a review of potential biases and experimental data. *Environmental Health Perspectives* 1999;107(Suppl 6):853–8.

Howard G, Wagenknecht LE. Environmental tobacco smoke and measures of subclinical vascular disease. *Environmental Health Perspectives* 1999;107(Suppl 6):837–40.

Howard G, Wagenknecht LE, Burke GL, Diez-Roux A, Evans GW, McGovern P, Nieto FJ, Tell GS. Cigarette smoking and progression of atherosclerosis: the Atherosclerosis Risk in Communities (ARIC) Study. *Journal of the American Medical Association* 1998a;279(2):119–24.

Howard G, Wagenknecht L, Cai J, Cooper L, Kraut M, Toole JF. Cigarette smoking and other risk factors for silent cerebral infarction in the general population. *Stroke* 1998b;29(5):913–7.

Hoyert DL, Heron M, Murphy SL, Kung H-C. Deaths: final data for 2003, January 19, 2006; <http://www.cdc.gov/nchs/products/pubs/pubd/hestats/finaldeaths03/finaldeaths03.htm>; accessed: February 14, 2006.

Humble C, Croft J, Gerber A, Casper M, Hames CG, Tyroler HA. Passive smoking and 20-year cardiovascular disease mortality among nonsmoking wives, Evans County, Georgia. *American Journal of Public Health* 1990;80(5):599–601.

Jackson R. The Auckland Heart Study: a case-control study of coronary heart disease [dissertation]. Auckland (New Zealand): University of Auckland, 1989.

Kawachi I, Colditz GA. Confounding, measurement error, and publication bias in studies of passive smoking [commentary]. *American Journal of Epidemiology* 1996;144(10):909–15.

Kawachi I, Colditz GA. Workplace exposure to passive smoking and risk of cardiovascular disease: summary of epidemiologic studies. *Environmental Health Perspectives* 1999;107(Suppl 6):847–51.

Kawachi I, Colditz GA, Speizer FE, Manson JE, Stampfer MJ, Willett WC, Hennekens CH. A prospective study of passive smoking and coronary heart disease. *Circulation* 1997;95(10):2374–9.

Koo LC, Kabat GC, Rylander R, Tominaga S, Kato I, Ho JH. Dietary and lifestyle correlates of passive smoking in Hong Kong, Japan, Sweden, and the U.S.A. *Social Science & Medicine* 1997;45(1):159–69.

La Vecchia C, D'Avanzo B, Franzosi MG, Tognoni G. Passive smoking and the risk of acute myocardial infarction. *Lancet* 1993;341(8843):505–6.

Law MR, Morris JK, Wald NJ. Environmental tobacco smoke exposure and ischaemic heart disease: an evaluation of the evidence. *British Medical Journal* 1997;315(7114):973–80.

Layard MW. Ischemic heart disease and spousal smoking in the National Mortality Followback Survey. *Regulatory Toxicology and Pharmacology* 1995;21(1):180–3.

Lee P. Passive smoking and heart disease [letter]. *British Medical Journal* 1998;317(7154):344–5.

Lee PN. *Environmental Tobacco Smoke and Mortality.* Basel: Karger, 1992.

Lee PN, Chamberlain J, Alderson MR. Relationship of passive smoking to risk of lung cancer and other smoking-associated diseases. *British Journal of Cancer* 1986;54(1):97–105.

Lekakis J, Papamichael C, Vemmos C, Nanas I, Kontoyannis D, Stamatelopoulos S, Moulopoulos S. Effect of acute cigarette smoking on endothelium-dependent brachial artery dilatation in healthy individuals. *American Journal of Cardiology* 1997;79(4):529–31.

LeVois ME, Layard MW. Publication bias in the environmental tobacco smoke/coronary heart disease epidemiologic literature. *Regulatory Toxicology and Pharmacology* 1995;21(1):184–91.

LeVois ME, Layard MW. Passive smoking and heart disease: authors need to analyse the data [letter]. *British Medical Journal* 1998;317(7154):344.

Matanoski G, Kanchanaraska S, Lantry D, Chang Y. Characteristics of nonsmoking women in NHANES I and NHANES I Epidemiologic Follow-up Study with exposure to spouses who smoke. *American Journal of Epidemiology* 1995;142(2): 149–57.

McElduff P, Dobson AJ, Jackson R, Beaglehole R, Heller RF, Lay-Yee R. Coronary events and exposure to environmental tobacco smoke: a case-control study from Australia and New Zealand. *Tobacco Control* 1998;7(1):41–6.

Muscat JE, Wynder EL. Exposure to environmental tobacco smoke and the risk of heart attack. *International Journal of Epidemiology* 1995;24(4):715–9.

National Cancer Institute. *Health Effects of Exposure to Environmental Tobacco Smoke: The Report of the California Environmental Protection Agency.* Smoking and Tobacco Monograph No. 10. Bethesda (MD): U.S. Department of Health and Human Services, National Institutes of Health, National Cancer Institute, 1999. NIH Publication No. 99-4645.

National Health and Medical Research Council Working Party. *The Health Effects of Passive Smoking: a Scientific Information Paper.* Canberra (Australia): National Health and Medical Research Council, 1997.

O'Leary DH, Polak JF, Kronmal RA, Maniolo TA, Burke GL, Wolfson SK. Carotid-artery intima and media thickness as a risk factor for myocardial infarction and stroke in older adults: Cardiovascular Health Study Collaborative Research Group. *New England Journal of Medicine* 1999;340(1): 14–22.

Ong EK, Glantz SA. Tobacco industry efforts subverting International Agency for Research on Cancer's second-hand smoke study. *Lancet* 2000;355(9211):1253–9.

Otsuka R, Watanabe H, Hirata K, Tokai K, Muro T, Yoshiyama M, Takeuchi K, Yoshikawa J. Acute effects of passive smoking on the coronary circulation in healthy young adults. *Journal of the American Medical Association* 2001;286(4):436–41.

Raitakari OT, Adams MR, McCredie RJ, Griffiths KA, Celermajer DS. Arterial endothelial dysfunction related to passive smoking is potentially reversible in healthy young adults. *Annals of Internal Medicine* 1999;130(7):578–81.

Rosenlund M, Berglind N, Gustavsson A, Reuterwall C, Hallqvist J, Nyberg F, Pershagen G. Environmental tobacco smoke and myocardial infarction among never-smokers in the Stockholm Heart Epidemiology Program (SHEEP). *Epidemiology* 2001; 12(5):558–64.

Sandler DP, Comstock GW, Helsing KJ, Shore DL. Deaths from all causes in non-smokers who lived with smokers. *American Journal of Public Health* 1989; 79(2):163–7.

Steenland K. Risk assessment for heart disease and workplace ETS exposure among nonsmokers. *Environmental Health Perspectives* 1999;107(Suppl 6): 859–63.

Steenland K, Sieber K, Etzel RA, Pechacek T, Maurer K. Exposure to environmental tobacco smoke and risk factors for heart disease among never smokers in the Third National Health and Nutrition Examination Survey. *American Journal of Epidemiology* 1998;147(10):932–9.

Steenland K, Thun M, Lally C, Heath C Jr. Environmental tobacco smoke and coronary heart disease in the American Cancer Society CPS-II cohort. *Circulation* 1996;94(4):622–8.

Stefanadis C, Dernellis J, Toutouzas P. Mechanical properties of the aorta determined by the pressure-diameter relation. *Pathologie-Biologie* 1999;47(7): 696–704.

Stefanadis C, Vlachopoulos C, Tsiamis E, Diamantopoulos L, Toutouzas K, Giatrakos N, Vaina S, Tsekoura D, Toutouzas P. Unfavorable effects of passive smoking on aortic function in men. *Annals of Internal Medicine* 1998;128(6):426–34.

Sumida H, Watanabe H, Kugiyama K, Ohgushi M, Matsumura T, Yasue H. Does passive smoking impair endothelium-dependent coronary artery dilation in women? *Journal of the American College of Cardiology* 1998;31(4):811–5.

Sun Y, Zhu B, Browne AE, Sievers RE, Bekker JM, Chatterjee K, Parmley WW, Glantz SA. Nicotine does not influence arterial lipid deposits in rabbits exposed to second-hand smoke. *Circulation* 2001;104(7):810–4.

Svendsen KH, Kuller LH, Martin MJ, Ockene JK. Effects of passive smoking in the Multiple Risk Factor Intervention Trial. *American Journal of Epidemiology* 1987;126(5):783–95.

Thornton A, Lee P, Fry J. Difference between smokers, ex-smokers, passive smokers and non-smokers. *Journal of Clinical Epidemiology* 1994;47(10):1143–62.

Thun M, Henley J, Apicella L. Epidemiologic studies of fatal and nonfatal cardiovascular disease and ETS exposure from spousal smoking. *Environmental Health Perspectives* 1999;107(Suppl 6):841–6.

Tunstall-Pedoe H, Brown CA, Woodward M, Tavendale R. Passive smoking by self-report and serum cotinine and the prevalence of respiratory and coronary heart disease in the Scottish heart health study. *Journal of Epidemiology and Community Health* 1995;49(2):139–43.

U.S. Department of Health and Human Services. *The Health Consequences of Smoking: Cardiovascular Disease. A Report of the Surgeon General.* Rockville (MD): U.S. Department of Health and Human Services, Public Health Service, Office on Smoking and Health, 1983. DHHS Publication No. (PHS) 84-50204.

U.S. Department of Health and Human Services. *The Health Consequences of Involuntary Smoking. A Report of the Surgeon General.* Rockville (MD): U.S. Department of Health and Human Services, Public Health Service, Centers for Disease Control, Center for Health Promotion and Education, Office on Smoking and Health, 1986. DHHS Publication No. (CDC) 87-8398.

U.S. Department of Health and Human Services. *Women and Smoking. A Report of the Surgeon General.* Rockville (MD): U.S. Department of Health and Human Services, Public Health Service, Office of the Surgeon General, 2001.

U.S. Department of Health and Human Services. *The Health Consequences of Smoking: A Report of the Surgeon General.* Atlanta: U.S. Department of Health and Human Services, Centers for Disease Control and Prevention, National Center for Chronic Disease Prevention and Health Promotion, Office on Smoking and Health, 2004.

Wagenknecht LE, Burke GL, Perkings LL, Haley NJ, Friedman GD. Misclassification of smoking status in the CARDIA Study: a comparison of self-report with serum cotinine levels. *American Journal of Public Health* 1992;82(1):33–8.

Wells AJ. Passive smoking as a cause of heart disease. *Journal of the American College of Cardiology* 1994;24(2):546–54.

Wells AJ. Heart disease from passive smoking in the workplace. *Journal of the American College of Cardiology* 1998;31(1):1–9.

Whincup PH, Gilg JA, Emberson JR, Jarvis MJ, Feyerabend C, Bryant A, Walker M, Cook DG. Passive smoking and risk of coronary heart disease and stroke: prospective study with cotinine measurement. *British Medical Journal* 2004;329(7459):200–5.

World Health Organization. *Seventh Revision of the International Classification of Diseases.* Geneva: World Health Organization, 1957.

You RX, Thrift AG, McNeil JJ, Davis SM, Donnan GA, and the Melbourne Stroke Risk Factor Study (MSRFS) Group. Ischemic stroke risk and passive exposure to spouses' cigarette smoking. *American Journal of Public Health* 1999;89(4):572–5.

Chapter 9
Respiratory Effects in Adults from Exposure to Secondhand Smoke

Introduction

There have been far fewer studies of involuntary smoking and adverse respiratory effects on adults compared with the number of studies on children. In fact, the evidence for children has causally linked secondhand smoke exposure to a number of adverse respiratory effects (Chapter 6, Respiratory Effects in Children from Exposure to Secondhand Smoke). The more limited research on adults may partly reflect the methodologic challenges in designing studies of nonmalignant respiratory diseases in adults, who are exposed in multiple and often complex environments: the home, the workplace, transportation environments, and additional public and other places. The potential for misclassifying smoking status, with former or current smokers categorized as involuntary smokers, has been a concern in studies that rely on self-reports of former smoking. Measuring past secondhand smoke exposure presents a challenge in studies of chronic effects and diseases that may become clinically apparent only after 20 or more years of exposure. Bias in the reporting of symptoms attributed to involuntary smoking is increasingly possible as public awareness of involuntary smoking and its health consequences increases. It may also be difficult to measure exposures to potential confounding or modifying agents (e.g., infectious agents and dusty occupations) that may need to be considered in studies of involuntary smoking.

Despite these challenges, the literature has been growing since the 1986 reports released by the Surgeon General (U.S. Department of Health and Human Services [USDHHS] 1986) and the National Research Council (NRC 1986). Subsequently, the literature has been summarized by federal and state agencies including the U.S. Environmental Protection Agency (USEPA 1992) and the California Environmental Protection Agency (Cal/EPA) (National Cancer Institute [NCI] 1999), and by several authors in peer-reviewed publications (Trédaniel et al. 1994; Coultas 1998; Weiss et al. 1999). Major reviews of the health effects of involuntary smoking in adults published between 1986 and 1999 examined respiratory health outcomes such as odor and irritation, respiratory symptoms, pulmonary function, and respiratory diseases (e.g., asthma and chronic obstructive pulmonary disease [COPD]) (Table 9.1). This table includes agency reviews as well as systematic reviews carried out by individual authors (Trédaniel et al. 1994; Coultas 1998). The evidence documented a strong link between secondhand smoke exposure and odor annoyance and irritation of mucous membranes of the eyes and nose. Weaker evidence suggested that involuntary smoking is associated with respiratory symptoms and small decrements in lung function among adults. Although experimental studies suggested that some persons with asthma may be susceptible to the effects of secondhand smoke exposure, only scant epidemiologic data consisting of a small number of studies on involuntary smoking and COPD were available on this issue at the time. This chapter reexamines the literature from these earlier reviews (Table 9.1), updates the literature with more recent publications, and evaluates the evidence supporting causal inferences. This discussion does not specifically review sinonasal disease because the evidence remains limited (Samet 2004).

The research strategy for this chapter consisted of searching the Medline database to identify references between 1990 and 2001 using any of five terms for secondhand smoke: environmental tobacco smoke (ETS), tobacco smoke pollution, sidestream smoke, second hand smoke, or secondhand smoke. These terms were then linked to a series of terms: (1) respiratory symptoms (i.e., respiratory symptom, cough, coughing, wheeze, or dyspnea [difficulty breathing]); (2) lung function; (3) lung diseases (i.e., lung diseases, obstructive, asthma, emphysema, and bronchitis); (4) etiology (i.e., cause or risk factor) and morbidity; (5) irritation or irritating of eye or nose or throat; and (6) tobacco smoke sensitivity or odor. In addition, bibliographies from recent studies were reviewed for additional references (Trédaniel et al. 1994; Coultas 1998; NCI 1999; Weiss et al. 1999).

Table 9.1   Major conclusions from reports on adverse respiratory effects of secondhand smoke exposure in adults

Odor and Irritation

U.S. Department of Health and Human Services (USDHHS) 1986

"The main effects of the irritants present in ETS [environmental tobacco smoke] occur in the conjunctiva of the eyes and the mucous membranes of the nose, throat, and lower respiratory tract. These irritant effects are a frequent cause of complaints about poor air quality due to environmental tobacco smoke." (p. 252)

National Research Council (NRC) 1986

"ETS arouses odor responses. The objectionable odor generated by ETS greatly exceeds that generated by simple occupancy under comparable conditions of occupancy, density, temperature, and relative humidity, and is more persistent." (p. 178)

"Whereas odor will govern the reactions of visitors to a smoking space, irritation will largely govern the reactions of occupants. Over time, eye irritation grows to become the most important negative response of the occupant. Dissatisfaction observed in chamber studies is commensurate with that found in field studies." (p. 178)

Trédaniel et al. 1994

"The acute irritating effect of ETS on respiratory mucous membranes is well-established." (p. 180)

California Environmental Protection Agency (Cal/EPA) 1997 (National Cancer Institute [NCI] 1999)

"Eye and nasal irritation are the most commonly reported symptoms among adult nonsmokers exposed to ETS; in addition, odor annoyance from indoor exposure to ETS has been shown in several studies." (p. 253)

Respiratory Symptoms

USDHHS 1986

"The implications of chronic respiratory symptoms for respiratory health as an adult are unknown and deserve further study." (p. 107)

NRC 1986

"The extent to which normal and asthmatic adults are affected by short-term exposures to ETS needs to be studied further." (p. 217)

USEPA 1992

". . .new evidence also has emerged suggesting that exposure to ETS may increase the frequency of respiratory symptoms in adults. These latter effects are estimated to be 30% to 60% higher in ETS-exposed nonsmokers compared to unexposed nonsmokers." (pp. 7-68–7-69)

Trédaniel et al. 1994

". . .no definite conclusion can be drawn from the studies that have investigated chronic respiratory symptoms in relation to ETS exposure." (p. 181)

Cal/EPA 1997 (NCI 1999)

". . .regular ETS exposure in adults has been reported to increase the risk of occurrence of a variety of lower respiratory symptoms." (p. 255)

Pulmonary Function

USDHHS 1986

"Healthy adults exposed to environmental tobacco smoke may have small changes on pulmonary function testing, but are unlikely to experience clinically significant deficits in pulmonary function as a result of exposure to environmental tobacco smoke alone." (p. 107)

Table 9.1   Continued

NRC 1986

"Future cross-sectional studies of ETS exposure and lung function in adults need to be designed to control for other factors that may affect lung function." (p. 217)

"Little information is available from long-term longitudinal studies of the effect of exposure to ETS by nonsmokers on lung function in either children or adults." (p. 217)

USEPA 1992

"Recent studies have confirmed the conclusion by the Surgeon General's report (U.S. DHHS, 1986) that adult nonsmokers exposed to ETS may have small reductions in lung function (approximately 2.5% lower mean FEV_1 [forced expiratory volume in 1 second]). . . ." (p. 7-68)

Trédaniel et al. 1994

"It remains controversial whether acute passive smoking is associated with important pulmonary physiological hazards. . . . Most of the available studies are cross-sectional, and the relationship to long-term changes in lung function is not established." (p. 181)

Cal/EPA 1997 (NCI 1999)

"The effect of chronic ETS exposure upon pulmonary function in otherwise healthy adults is likely to be small, and is unlikely by itself to result in clinically significant chronic disease." (p. 255)

Respiratory Diseases

NRC 1986

"It is unlikely that exposure to ETS can cause much emphysema." (p. 212)

Trédaniel et al. 1994

"Conflicting evidence exists on the association in asthmatic patients between ETS exposure and appearance of symptoms and functional abnormalities (including change in bronchial responsiveness)." (p. 181)

"Four out of five studies offer support to the hypothesis of an association between ETS exposure and risk of COPD [chronic obstructive pulmonary disease]." (p. 181)

Coultas 1998

"While growing evidence suggests that passive smoking is a risk factor for adult onset asthma and COPD, the magnitude of the associations is small. However, additional evidence on the relationship between passive smoking and asthma and COPD is needed to fulfill the criteria for causality, particularly the criteria of temporality and dose-response." (p. 386)

"Although the available literature is limited, it does show that exposure to ETS is associated. . .with worsening of respiratory symptoms and lung function in adult asthmatics." (p. 383)

". . .little is known about the effects of ETS exposure on respiratory symptoms or lung function among patients with COPD." (p. 385)

Cal/EPA 1997 (NCI 1999)

"There is suggestive evidence that ETS exposure may exacerbate adult asthma." (p. 194)

". . .chamber studies. . .suggest that there is likely to be a subpopulation of asthmatics who are especially susceptible to ETS exposure." (p. 203)

Biologic Basis

Chapter 2 (Toxicology of Secondhand Smoke) reviews mechanisms by which secondhand smoke exposure may generally cause respiratory disease in populations. This section focuses more specifically on adults. Active cigarette smoking causes inflammatory injury throughout the respiratory tract, leading to chronic airway and alveolar injury and chronic respiratory symptoms and diseases (Floreani and Rennard 1999; Saetta et al. 2001; USDHHS 2004). Although the evidence on active smoking provides a strong basis of support for the plausibility of adverse respiratory effects from involuntary smoking, differences in the dose from involuntary versus active smoking limit direct inferences from active to involuntary smoking. Experimental studies in animals (Escolar et al. 1995; Joad et al. 1995; Seymour et al. 1997) and humans (Anderson et al. 1991; Yates et al. 1996, 2001; NCI 1999) provide relevant evidence of and insights into underlying mechanisms for the effects of involuntary smoking on the respiratory tract.

The biologic outcomes examined in animal models of involuntary smoking have included antibody responses (Seymour et al. 1997), alterations of airway defense receptors (Joad et al. 1995), and pathologic changes of emphysema (Escolar et al. 1995). Using a mouse allergy model, Seymour and colleagues (1997) exposed the animals to secondhand smoke for 43 days (6 hours per day, 5 days per week, mean total suspended particulates at 1.04 milligrams per cubic meter [mg/m³], mean carbon monoxide [CO] at 6.1 parts per million [ppm]). Secondhand smoke exposure resulted in elevated levels of antibodies to allergens delivered by aerosol challenge, suggesting that such exposures enhance allergic inflammatory responses. Joad and colleagues (1995) exposed 29 developing guinea pigs aged 8 through 43 days to sidestream smoke (CO = 5.6 ± 0.7 ppm) for six hours per day, five days a week. Although lung morphology was unchanged, responsiveness of airway C-fiber receptors (a component of lung defense mechanisms) was reduced, which may facilitate further exposure and injury over time. Escolar and colleagues (1995) exposed 60 rats to secondhand smoke (mean CO at 35 ppm) for 90 minutes per day for three months. Morphometry showed changes in the alveoli consistent with emphysema, including the loss of elasticity in the lung tissue.

Human experimental studies have involved short-term exposures of volunteers to known concentrations of sidestream smoke measured by CO and/or particulate levels in exposure chambers. The effects examined included eye and nasal irritation, nasal mucociliary clearance, respiratory symptoms, pulmonary function changes, and systemic inflammation. Although controlled human exposure studies have the advantages of accurate measurements and controlled levels of exposure, such studies have inherent limitations. Because the duration of exposure must be brief, only short-term effects can be measured. Exposure to sidestream smoke under controlled conditions may not accurately reflect exposure-response relationships associated with multiple exposures found in real-world conditions such as the workplace. These studies are necessarily restricted to a small number of volunteers, thus limiting the generalizability of the findings and the statistical power to detect effects. Moreover, variations in the duration of the exposures limit the comparability of the results.

Controlled human exposures to sidestream smoke have been used to characterize effects on the nose such as odor detection, nasal symptoms, and physiologic changes (USDHHS 1986; Bascom et al. 1991, 1995, 1996; Cummings et al. 1991; Willes et al. 1992, 1998; Nowak et al. 1997a). In general, these exposures have been at the upper end of the range of measured secondhand smoke concentrations in various environments (Chapter 3, Assessment of Exposure to Secondhand Smoke, and Chapter 4, Prevalence of Exposure to Secondhand Smoke). Bascom and colleagues (1991, 1995, 1996) and Willes and colleagues (1992, 1998) conducted a series of chamber studies to characterize nasal responses to sidestream smoke. In an early investigation, Bascom and colleagues (1991) found that posterior nasal resistance (a measurement of nasal sensitivity in the bottom of the passageway) increased after 15 minutes of exposure to sidestream smoke (45 ppm of CO) among 10 healthy persons without asthma who reported nasal sensitivity to secondhand smoke (congestion, rhinorrhea, or sneezing), but not among 11 participants who did not report nasal sensitivity. However, assay of nasal secretions for histamine, kinin, esterase, or albumin provided no evidence for allergic inflammation or increased vascular permeability, indicating a nonallergic mechanism for the physiologic response. Nowak and colleagues (1997a) reported similar findings after examining nasal fluid for markers of inflammation 30 minutes before and 30 minutes after exposing 10 persons with mild asthma to secondhand smoke at 22.4 ppm of CO. Bascom and colleagues (1996) examined exposure-response relationships among 13 persons with reported secondhand smoke sensitivity and 16 persons who were not sensitive; the experiment involved two hours of sidestream smoke exposure at 1 ppm, 5 ppm, and 15 ppm of CO. Nasal resistance increased significantly in both groups after exposure to the highest level of sidestream smoke (15 ppm of CO). Bascom and colleagues (1995) also assessed the effect of sidestream smoke exposure on nasal mucociliary clearance in 12 volunteers. The rate of clearance increased in some participants but slowed in three others; all three had a history of rhinitis associated with secondhand smoke exposure.

Human volunteers, including healthy nonsmokers and persons with asthma, have been exposed to secondhand smoke under controlled conditions to examine symptoms, pulmonary function changes, inflammatory markers, and lung injury (Trédaniel et al. 1994; Yates et al. 1996, 2001; Nowak et al. 1997a,b; NCI 1999; Weiss et al. 1999). The 1997 Cal/EPA report reviewed results from 10 studies of persons with asthma and concluded that "although the design constraints of the chamber studies limit the interpretation of the results, they do suggest that there is likely to be a subpopulation of asthmatics who are especially susceptible to ETS exposure. The physiological responses observed in these investigations appear to be reproducible in both 'reactors' and 'nonreactors.' It is unlikely that the physiological and symptomatic responses reported are due exclusively to either stress or suggestion" (NCI 1999, p. 203). Nowak and colleagues (1997b) provided additional evidence for this conclusion by exposing 17 persons with mild asthma to secondhand smoke (20 ppm of CO) or ambient air ("sham") for three hours. The investigators measured spirometry and bronchial responsiveness one hour, five hours, and nine hours after the exposure. The overall average decline in forced expiratory volume in one second (FEV_1) levels was 9.1 percent after the secondhand smoke exposure and 5.9 percent after the sham exposure. However, the mean FEV_1 decline largely reflected declines in three persons, and secondhand smoke-induced symptoms were not associated with the FEV_1 decline. In a separate study of 10 persons with mild asthma who were exposed to secondhand smoke at 22.4 ppm of CO for three hours, the FEV_1 level and the levels of markers of inflammation obtained by bronchoalveolar lavage were unchanged by the exposure (Nowak et al. 1997a).

Studies have associated nonspecific bronchial hyperresponsiveness with an accelerated decline in lung function, which may thus be a marker for susceptibility to the development of COPD (Kanner et al. 1994; Paoletti et al. 1995; Rijcken et al. 1995; Tracey et al. 1995). Menon and colleagues (1992) exposed 31 smoke-sensitive persons with asthma and 39 smoke-sensitive persons without asthma to secondhand smoke at relatively high levels (suspended particles >1,000 micrograms/m³) for four hours in a test chamber. Compared with pre-exposure bronchial reactivity among those without asthma, bronchial reactivity to methacholine increased in 18 percent of the participants 6 hours after exposure, in 10 percent of the participants 24 hours after exposure, and in 8 percent of the participants three weeks after exposure. These results suggest that secondhand smoke exposure may increase bronchial hyperreactivity even in asymptomatic persons who do not have asthma. In contrast to these results, a study of 17 secondhand smoke-exposed persons with mild asthma did not find an increase in airway responsiveness when measured by the methacholine challenge (Nowak et al. 1997b). Jindal and colleagues (1999) measured bronchial hyperresponsiveness in a sample of 50 women aged 20 through 40 years with asthma who were from a chest clinic in India. Exposure to secondhand smoke was assessed with a questionnaire that included questions on smoking by the husband, smoking by other family members, and smoking by coworkers. Women exposed to secondhand smoke had significantly greater bronchial hyperreactivity than did unexposed women; the mean provocative dose of histamine used to produce a 20 percent drop in FEV_1 was 50 percent lower in the exposed group compared with the unexposed group.

In active smokers, the uptake of inhaled technetium[99m] (labeled diethylenetriamine pentaacetate [^{99m}Tc-DTPA]) was increased, suggesting an increase in alveolar permeability (Jones et al. 1980). Yates and colleagues (1996) applied this technique to 20 healthy nonsmokers and assessed whether exposure to secondhand smoke for one hour in a chamber affected alveolar permeability. The exposure was followed by an increase in the time for ^{99m}Tc-DTPA clearance, from 69.1 to 77.4 minutes. In contrast to active smoking, these results imply a decrease in alveolar permeability following exposure. The findings do, however, provide evidence of a physiologic response to even a very brief exposure to secondhand smoke.

Nowak and colleagues (1997a) also provided indirect evidence for a decrease in epithelial permeability associated with secondhand smoke exposure in a study of 10 persons with mild asthma. Albumin levels from nasal and bronchoalveolar lavage were lower after three hours in a chamber at 22.4 ppm CO compared with a sham exposure. An increase in permeability would be expected to increase albumin leakage into the alveoli.

Nitric oxide (NO) regulates a number of airway and vascular functions and can be measured in exhaled air. Compared with nonsmokers, active smokers had lower exhaled NO levels, and intermediate decrements were found in exhaled NO levels from nonsmokers exposed to secondhand smoke (Yates et al. 2001). Fifteen healthy nonsmoking volunteers were exposed to secondhand smoke at 23 ppm CO in a chamber for one hour, and exhaled NO was measured before and every 15 minutes during the exposure (Yates et al. 2001). Secondhand smoke exposure was associated with a significant decline in exhaled NO (134 parts per billion [ppb] before and 99 ppb 60 minutes after the exposure).

Only limited information is available on the systemic effects of secondhand smoke exposure (Anderson et al. 1991; Oryszczyn et al. 2000). Anderson and colleagues (1991) exposed 16 healthy nonsmokers (mean age 29 years) to cigarette smoke from 6 smokers in a poorly ventilated room for three hours with hourly respirable particulate levels averaging 2.3 to 2.6 mg/m³. This exposure was associated with significant increases in peripheral blood leukocyte counts, chemotaxis, and the release of reactive oxidants; these findings are consistent with the mechanisms of respiratory tract injury in active smokers (Saetta et al. 2001; USDHHS 2004). Oryszczyn and colleagues (2000) examined the relationship between self-reported secondhand smoke exposure (i.e., currently living with one or more smokers) and the total serum immunoglobulin E (IgE) level, which is higher in persons with asthma than in those without asthma. The study included 122 persons with asthma, 430 of their first-degree relatives, and 190 controls. Among lifetime nonsmokers with and without asthma, involuntary smoking was associated with higher IgE levels. The highest levels were among those with asthma who had been exposed to secondhand smoke. However, significant differences in IgE levels were observed only in women after adjusting for asthma.

In summary, compared with research on active smoking, the literature on respiratory tract injury from involuntary smoking is limited. There are only a few animal investigations, and they examined different outcomes (e.g., antibody response to allergens, responsiveness of C-fiber receptors, and morphologic signs of emphysema). Most human studies have examined inflammatory and physiologic effects of short-term secondhand smoke exposure in chambers. The few studies that investigated markers of local inflammation in the nose and lower respiratory tract did not find any evidence of an increased inflammatory response to brief secondhand smoke exposures. Exhaled NO, which has a number of physiologic functions including inflammatory regulation, decreased in persons exposed to secondhand smoke, an effect also found in active smokers. Two studies suggest that there may be an enhanced systemic inflammatory and antibody response to secondhand smoke exposure. Similarly, one human study and one animal study provide complementary evidence that secondhand smoke exposure may enhance antibody responses to allergens. Two other investigations provide evidence that short-term secondhand smoke exposure may actually result in a protective physiologic response based on a decrease in epithelial permeability in the nose and alveoli. Another study paired variable effects with nasal mucociliary clearance.

The physiologic responses to secondhand smoke exposure were examined by measuring lung function in healthy persons and in patients with asthma. These studies documented inconsistent results, but the small number of participants and the types of exposures may not accurately reflect secondhand smoke exposure in the "real" world. Despite these limitations, available evidence suggests that some people, regardless of whether they are healthy or have asthma, experience a short-term decline in lung function from secondhand smoke exposures.

Odor and Irritation

Secondhand smoke contains compounds such as pyridine that produce unpleasant odors (NCI 1999), and other agents such as particles, nicotine, acrolein, and formaldehyde, which may cause mucosal irritation (Lee et al. 1993). The topics of odor, odor annoyance, and mucosal irritation from secondhand smoke were reviewed in the 1986 Surgeon General's report (USDHHS 1986), in the 1986 NRC report (1986), and by Samet and colleagues (1991). Controlled chamber studies (USDHHS 1986; NCI 1999) and epidemiologic studies (USDHHS 1986) have assessed the association of these symptoms with secondhand smoke exposure. The 1986 Surgeon General's report reviewed results of 13 experimental studies and 5 field studies. The conclusions from that review have remained consistent with subsequent reviews of the topic (Table 9.1).

In addition to the level of secondhand smoke exposure, other factors that may determine an odor response to secondhand smoke include the age of the exposed person as it relates to olfactory acuity and visual contact with the smoker (Moschandreas and Relwani 1992), and individual traits such as annoyance thresholds and coping styles (Winneke and Neuf 1996). Limited data suggest that olfactory acuity decreases with age, and seeing a smoker increases the perceived odor intensity and annoyance of secondhand smoke (Moschandreas and Relwani 1992). Although these factors are relevant to designing and interpreting studies of odor responses to secondhand smoke, available studies provide little information on these factors.

Both experimental (Bascom et al. 1991, 1996; Willes et al. 1992, 1998; Nowak et al. 1997a) and observational studies (Cummings et al. 1991; Norback and Edling 1991; Ng and Tan 1994) have assessed nasal symptoms (e.g., congestion, excessive secretions, or sneezing) as measures of upper respiratory tract irritation. In a survey of 77 healthy, nonsmoking adults 18 through 45 years of age, Bascom and colleagues (1991) found that 34 percent reported one or more nasal symptoms following secondhand smoke exposure. Allergen sensitivity, measured by skin-prick testing in 21 persons, was more frequent among secondhand smoke-sensitive persons (70 percent) compared with persons not sensitive to secondhand smoke (27 percent). Bascom and colleagues (1991) then exposed 10 sensitive and 11 persons not sensitive to secondhand smoke (45 ppm of CO for

15 minutes) in a chamber; significant increases in nasal secretions and nose-throat irritation were reported by both groups. Only the secondhand smoke-sensitive persons reported significant increases in nasal congestion, headache, and cough. In a subsequent investigation, Bascom and colleagues (1996) examined exposure-response relationships between secondhand smoke exposure and nasal symptoms among 13 persons with a history of secondhand smoke sensitivity and 16 persons without secondhand smoke sensitivity. Compared with no exposure, the lowest level of secondhand smoke exposure at 1 ppm of CO was associated with a significant increase in selected symptoms (eye irritation, nose irritation, and odor perception) reported by both groups. After the exposure, three of the nine symptoms (headache, eye irritation, and odor perception) increased significantly among persons sensitive to secondhand smoke compared with those who were not sensitive. Nasal congestion, increased nasal secretions, and cough increased significantly in both groups at 15 ppm of CO. Nowak and colleagues (1997a) exposed 10 persons with mild asthma to secondhand smoke (22.4 ± 1.2 ppm of CO) in a chamber and measured nose and mouth symptoms (dry nose, running nose, blocked nose, dry mouth, and mucus accumulation). Three hours of exposure produced increases in nose and mouth symptoms.

The 1986 Surgeon General's report reviewed five cross-sectional studies that described the prevalence of annoyance and symptoms of irritation associated with secondhand smoke exposure, but only one study included an unexposed comparison group (USDHHS 1986). The main indicators of annoyance and irritation were self-reported annoyances (e.g., disturbed by tobacco smoke, poor air quality, frustration, and hostility) and symptoms (e.g., eye, nose, and throat irritation; rhinorrhea; headache; fatigue; nausea; dizziness; and wheeze).

Since that report, a limited number of new observational studies have specifically examined odor annoyance and nasal irritation associated with secondhand smoke exposure (Cummings et al. 1991; Ng and Tan 1994). A larger number of investigations with conflicting results examined the role of secondhand smoke in building-related illnesses that included irritation of the skin and mucous membranes of the eyes, nose, and throat; headache; fatigue; and difficulty concentrating (Norback and Edling 1991;

Menzies and Bourbeau 1997). The inconsistent findings in these studies may be explained by several methodologic challenges (Menzies and Bourbeau 1997) that severely compromise the usefulness of examining the role of indoor secondhand smoke exposures at work, specifically in associations with odor annoyance and nasal irritation. These challenges include the multifactorial basis of building-related symptoms and illnesses, the potential for multiple pollutants to contribute to symptom risk, and limitations of the designs of many of the epidemiologic studies on this issue. Therefore, there is no further discussion of secondhand smoke and nonspecific building-related illnesses in this chapter.

Cummings and colleagues (1991) conducted a cross-sectional survey of 723 volunteers aged 18 through 84 years who attended a free cancer screening at a cancer center in New York. Overall, a high proportion of lifetime nonsmokers reported being bothered by tobacco smoke, with the highest rates among people who were atopic (81 percent) or who had a history of a respiratory illness (82 percent), compared with all others (74 percent). A similar pattern was found for reports of nose irritation (54 percent among those who were atopic, 48 percent among those who had a history of respiratory illnesses, and 30 percent among all others) and sneezing (23 percent among those who were atopic, 17 percent among those who had a history of respiratory illnesses, and 12 percent among all others) associated with secondhand smoke exposure.

To assess risk factors for allergic rhinitis in Singapore, Ng and Tan (1994) conducted a population-based cross-sectional study of 2,868 adults aged 20 through 74 years. Overall, 4.5 percent of the participants had allergic rhinitis defined by self-reports during the previous year of usual nasal blockage and discharge apart from colds or the flu, provoked by allergens, with or without conjunctivitis. Compared with having no household exposure to smokers, exposure to one or more light smokers was not associated with allergic rhinitis (odds ratio [OR] = 0.96 [95 percent confidence interval (CI), 0.6–1.53]), whereas exposure to one or more heavy smokers was weakly associated with allergic rhinitis (OR = 1.43 [95 percent CI, 0.94–2.18]).

Evidence Synthesis

Prior reviews have led to the conclusion that secondhand smoke exposure causes odor annoyance (Table 9.1). Coherent and consistent results from experimental and observational studies provide a strong basis for inferring a causal link between secondhand smoke exposure and odor annoyance and symptoms of nasal irritation. Moreover, experimental studies established both the temporal and dose-response relationships of odor annoyance and nasal irritation with secondhand smoke exposure. The intensity of odor annoyance and nasal irritation increased with increased levels of secondhand smoke exposure. In addition, persons with nasal allergies or a history of respiratory illnesses may be more susceptible to nasal irritation from secondhand smoke exposure compared with persons without these conditions. However, because few observational studies have included unexposed comparison groups, the strength of the association is more difficult to evaluate. Moreover, methodologic limitations, including exposure misclassification and nonspecificity of symptoms, may result in underestimates of the strength of the association.

Conclusions

1. The evidence is sufficient to infer a causal relationship between secondhand smoke exposure and odor annoyance.

2. The evidence is sufficient to infer a causal relationship between secondhand smoke exposure and nasal irritation.

3. The evidence is suggestive but not sufficient to conclude that persons with nasal allergies or a history of respiratory illnesses are more susceptible to developing nasal irritation from secondhand smoke exposure.

Implications

Although the symptoms of odor annoyance and nasal irritation may appear to be minor adverse health consequences, they have the potential to negatively affect daily functioning and quality of life. For example, studies have documented for a long time the potential of secondhand smoke to cause annoyance and irritation. This acute and adverse response is possibly only avoidable in smoke-free environments.

Respiratory Symptoms

The 1986 Surgeon General's report included only a few studies on secondhand smoke exposure and respiratory symptoms in adults (Table 9.1). Although a number of investigations since 1986 have studied this relationship, conclusions from major reviews of this topic (Table 9.1) have been inconsistent. The sources of information on respiratory symptoms include experimental studies of acute exposures and symptoms (Table 9.2) and observational studies of chronic symptoms (Table 9.3).

Experimental Studies

Persons with and without asthma were exposed to secondhand smoke in exposure chambers in efforts to characterize physiologic responses (see "Biologic Basis" earlier in this chapter) and acute symptom responses to secondhand smoke (Table 9.2). Most of the studies are small and provide limited information as to how the participants were recruited. Some were recruited through hospital-based asthma and allergy clinics (Shephard et al. 1979; Danuser et al. 1993) and others through advertisements to students (Bascom et al. 1996).

Out of 10 studies (Table 9.2), 5 were restricted to persons with asthma and did not have a control group (Knight and Breslin 1985; Wiedemann et al. 1986; Stankus et al. 1988; Magnussen et al. 1992; Nowak et al. 1997a), 3 included persons with asthma and a control group without asthma (Shephard et al. 1979; Dahms et al. 1981; Danuser et al. 1993), and 2 were limited to persons without asthma (Bascom et al. 1991, 1996). The investigations using only persons with asthma and no control group provided only limited information on the occurrence of respiratory symptoms with secondhand smoke exposure. In one of these investigations (Magnussen et al. 1992), there was no difference in respiratory symptom responses between the sham and the secondhand smoke exposures. In the three studies that included persons with asthma and controls without asthma, results suggest that acute respiratory symptoms occur with a similar or slightly increased frequency with secondhand smoke exposure among persons with mild to moderate asthma compared with healthy controls. Moreover, the dose-response relationship that was found in persons with asthma (Danuser et al. 1993) and in healthy persons

without asthma (Bascom et al. 1996) strengthens the argument for a causal link between secondhand smoke exposure and acute respiratory symptoms. However, the generalizability of these results may be questioned because of the small numbers in the studies and the use of volunteers. Persons who volunteer may do so because of a perceived sensitivity to secondhand smoke, and may thus overreport symptoms compared with persons randomly selected from the general population.

Observational Studies

Chronic respiratory symptoms of cough, phlegm, wheeze, and dyspnea (difficulty breathing) associated with secondhand smoke exposure have been investigated largely in cross-sectional studies; there have been only a few longitudinal investigations (Schwartz and Zeger 1990; Robbins et al. 1993; Jaakkola et al. 1996). Table 9.3 describes these studies and their results. The documented symptoms are heterogeneous in etiology and vary with gender, age, associated diseases (e.g., allergy or respiratory illness), and smoking status (e.g., never versus former) (Cummings et al. 1991). For example, cough may result from irritation or inflammation of the upper and lower respiratory tract, but it may also be caused by gastroesophageal reflux disease. Similarly, dyspnea is often attributed to a respiratory disease, but it may also result from a cardiovascular disease. It is not feasible in observational studies to separate respiratory from nonrespiratory causes of these symptoms. However, variations in the distribution of the determinants of these symptoms among populations may contribute in part to the inconsistent findings. Moreover, numerous other environmental factors such as outdoor and indoor air pollution, allergens, and occupational exposures may vary among populations and may cause respiratory symptoms. Studies evaluating the relationship between secondhand smoke exposure and respiratory symptoms have not consistently included some of these other environmental factors (Table 9.3).

Although not all of the available observational studies have found significant associations of secondhand smoke exposure with cough (Table 9.3) (Schwartz and Zeger 1990; Jaakkola et al. 1996; Zhang et al. 1999), the point estimates of risk with exposure

Table 9.2   Chamber studies of exposure to secondhand smoke and acute respiratory symptoms

Study	Population	Exposure	Symptoms				Comments
Shephard et al. 1979	14 patients with mild to moderate asthma Aged 19–65 years No controls without asthma	Average CO* = 24 ppm[†], 2 hours	<u>Persons with asthma (%)</u> Wheeze 36 Chest tightness 43 Cough 36 Dyspnea 21	<u>Normal controls (%)</u> Rest 10 5 45 15	 Exercise 0 0 58 17		Regular asthma medications were not withheld before the test in 13 out of 14 patients; 1 or more may have been smokers; normal controls were from another study
Dahms et al. 1981	10 persons with asthma (5 smoke-sensitive) Aged 18–26 years 10 healthy controls Aged 24–53 years	Estimated CO = 15–20 ppm (based on carboxy-hemoglobin levels), 1 hour	All had similar degrees of eye and nasal irritation				Exposure levels were not measured directly; no individual data were reported
Knight and Breslin 1985	6 patients with mild to moderate asthma	CO level was not determined, 1 hour	Wheeze was reported by 33% of participants; increase in chest tightness was reported by 50% of participants				Participants and methods were not well described
Wiedemann et al. 1986	9 asymptomatic persons with asthma Aged 19–30 years	CO = 40–50 ppm, 1 hour	Cough was reported by 33% of participants				None
Stankus et al. 1988	21 smoke-sensitive persons with asthma Aged 21–50 years	Average CO = 8.7 ppm, 2 hours; if no change occurred in lung function, exposure was then increased to average CO = 13.3 ppm, 2 hours	Cough, chest tightness, and dyspnea were reported by 7 participants who had a >20% decline in forced expiratory volume in 1 second				No information was provided on symptoms among those who did not have a decline in lung function
Bascom et al. 1991	21 healthy nonsmokers	45 ppm CO for 15 minutes	Cough and chest tightness were greater among sensitive participants				11 not sensitive and 10 sensitive participants by questionnaire
Magnussen et al. 1992	18 persons with mild to moderate asthma Aged 21–51 years	Average CO = 20.5 ppm, 1 hour	Cough and chest tightness symptom scores were not significantly different for the secondhand smoke exposure compared with the sham exposure				None

Table 9.2   Continued

Study	Population	Exposure	Symptoms	Comments
Danuser et al. 1993	10 persons with hyperreactive airways (5 asthma, 3 suggestive of asthma) Aged 24–51 years 10 healthy controls Aged 24–52 years	Average CO = 0, 2, 4, 8, 16, and 32 ppm; 2 minutes at each level	Over the entire exposure, 7 hyperreactive persons and 6 healthy controls reported cough, chest tightness, or dyspnea	Small likelihood of "suggestibility" because of the mode of secondhand smoke delivery; symptom severity was mild for both groups, even at the highest level of exposure; there was a dose-response relationship between symptom scores and CO levels
Bascom et al. 1996	29 healthy nonsmokers Aged 22–31 years	Average CO = 0, 1, 5, and 15 ppm; 2 hours at each level	Cough and chest tightness scores increased with increasing CO levels	None
Nowak et al. 1997a	10 persons with mild asthma Aged 22–29 years	Average CO = 22.4 ppm, 3 hours	Throat and chest symptom scores (breathing difficulty, chest tightness, dyspnea, and chest pain) significantly increased with exposure	Unable to determine an effect on chest symptoms alone because throat and chest symptoms were combined

*CO = Carbon monoxide.

†ppm = Parts per million.

compared with no exposure have been greater than one (Schwartz and Zeger 1990; White et al. 1991; Pope and Xu 1993; Lam et al. 1995; Jaakkola et al. 1996; Zhang et al. 1999). The studies range in size and in the precision of their estimates; however, many did not consider other factors (e.g., other indoor and outdoor pollutants, allergy, asthma, and occupation) that may influence the occurrence of cough. Pope and Xu (1993) highlight the complexity of investigating the relationship between secondhand smoke exposure and respiratory symptoms. Among 973 Chinese women aged 20 through 40 years who had never smoked, there was a dose-response relationship between cough and the number of smokers at home (OR = 1.02 for 1 smoker and 1.87 for ≥2 smokers). In addition, the combination of heating with coal, a source of indoor smoke, and two or more smokers in the home was associated with a further increase in the occurrence of cough (OR = 3.07). This finding indicates the potential for a joint effect of secondhand smoke exposure with other environmental exposures. Similarly, the findings of Cummings and colleagues (1991) (Table 9.3) suggest that associated illnesses, such as allergy and respiratory illnesses, increase the

occurrence of cough with secondhand smoke exposure compared with persons without these conditions. Phlegm production is a symptom often associated with cough, and findings for this symptom are similar to those for cough (Table 9.3) (Schwartz and Zeger 1990; White et al. 1991; Pope and Xu 1993; Lam et al. 1995; Jaakkola et al. 1996; Zhang et al. 1999). The point estimates for the association between secondhand smoke exposure and phlegm production have ranged from 0.69 to 8.3 (Table 9.3).

Out of five studies that examined the association between secondhand smoke exposure and wheeze, two found significant associations (Leuenberger et al. 1994; Baker and Henderson 1999) and three did not (Pope and Xu 1993; Jaakkola et al. 1996; Zhang et al. 1999). The point estimates ranged from 0.62 to 1.94 (Table 9.3). Although Leuenberger and colleagues (1994) found a dose-response relationship between wheeze and the amount of the exposure, Pope and Xu (1993) did not. Moreover, Pope and Xu (1993) did not find an interaction for wheeze between the number of smokers at home and the use of coal heat as they did find for cough and phlegm.

Table 9.3   Observational studies of exposure to secondhand smoke and chronic respiratory symptoms

Study	Population	Period of study	Findings				Comments
Schwartz and Zeger 1990	Approximately 100 nursing students Los Angeles	Follow-up for up to 3 years	<u>Exposure</u> Roommate smoked	<u>Phlegm OR* (95% CI[†])</u> 1.41 (1.08–1.85)			There was no association with an increased risk of cough
Cummings et al. 1991	723 volunteers attending a free cancer screening, 56% women, 90% White Aged 18–84 years United States	1986			Lifetime nonsmokers		None
			<u>Symptom</u>	<u>Atopic (%)</u>	<u>Respiratory illness (%)</u>	<u>All Others (%)</u>	
			Bothered by tobacco smoke	81	82	74	
			Watery eyes	57	60	43	
			Nose irritation	54	48	30	
			Cough episodes	36	37	21	
			Sore throat	23	19	13	
			Sneezing	23	17	12	
					Former smokers		
			<u>Symptom</u>	<u>Atopic (%)</u>	<u>Respiratory illness (%)</u>	<u>All Others (%)</u>	
			Bothered by tobacco smoke	68	77	65	
			Watery eyes	48	39	35	
			Nose irritation	38	40	21	
			Cough episodes	32	25	17	
			Sore throat	24	14	12	
			Sneezing	14	17	10	
Norback and Edling 1991	466 persons from the general population Aged 20–65 years Sweden	1989	<u>Symptom</u> Eye irratation or swollen eyelids Nasal catarrh, blocked-up nose, dry/sore throat, irritative cough	<u>Adjusted OR (95% CI)</u> 1.3 (0.8–2.2) 1.1 (0.7–1.8)			Secondhand smoke exposure at work
White et al. 1991	40 persons exposed to secondhand smoke at work and 40 nonsmokers evaluated as part of a fitness profile Aged 38–65 years United States	1979–1985	<u>Symptom</u> Cough Phlegm Breathlessness Colds	<u>Secondhand smoke exposure at work (OR)</u> 7.0 8.3 11.8 22.7			None

Table 9.3   Continued

Study	Population	Period of study	Findings			Comments
Pope and Xu 1993	973 lifetime nonsmoking women Aged 20–40 years China	1992	No coal heat			Adjusted for age, job title, and mill employment
			Symptom	1 smoker in home	≥2 smokers in home	
			Chest illness	0.98 (0.50–1.94)	NR‡	
			Cough	1.02 (0.60–1.75)	1.87 (0.71–4.88)	
			Phlegm	1.43 (0.85–2.40)	2.07 (0.85–5.01)	
			Dyspnea	1.17 (0.61–2.25)	1.46 (0.39–5.52)	
			Wheeze	0.93 (0.50–1.75)	1.00 (0.27–3.71)	
			Coal heat			
			Symptom	1 smoker in home	≥2 smokers in home	
			Chest illness	1.57 (0.74–1.39)	3.79 (1.28–11.2)	
			Cough	1.03 (0.97–1.10)	3.07 (1.23–7.65)	
			Phlegm	1.89 (1.07–3.35)	3.64 (1.56–8.52)	
			Dyspnea	1.88 (0.93–3.81)	3.55 (1.2–10.5)	
			Wheeze	1.20 (0.60–2.41)	1.07 (0.29–4.00)	
Robbins et al. 1993	3,914 participants Aged ≥25 years at completion of baseline questionnaire United States	Baseline: 1977 Follow-up: 1987	Obstructive airway disease symptoms			None
			Age of participant at exposure		OR (95% CI)	
			Childhood only		1.09 (0.69–1.79)	
			Adulthood only		1.28 (0.90–1.79)	
			Childhood and adulthood		1.72 (1.31–2.23)	
Leuenberger et al. 1994	4,197 lifetime nonsmokers Aged 18–60 years Switzerland	NR	Symptom		OR (95% CI)	There was a positive dose-response relationship
			Wheeze apart from colds		1.94 (1.39–2.70)	
			Dyspnea on exertion		1.45 (1.20–1.76)	
			Bronchitis		1.59 (1.17–2.15)	
Ng and Tan 1994	2,868 participants Aged 20–74 years Singapore	1989	Unadjusted OR (95% CI)			None
			Secondhand smoke exposure		Allergic rhinitis	
			≥1 light smoker		0.96 (0.60–1.53)	
			≥1 heavy smoker		1.43 (0.94–2.18)	
Lam et al. 1995	2,558 lifetime nonsmoking women Hong Kong	1989	Symptom		Adjusted OR (95% CI)	Exposure to husband's smoking; adjusted for area of residence, education, type of housing, others smoking at home, use of fuel, and use of incense/ mosquito coil
			Sore throat		1.20 (0.89–1.64)	
			Cough, morning		1.72 (1.06–2.79)	
			Cough, evening		1.61 (0.97–2.68)	
			Phlegm, morning		1.43 (1.04–1.98)	
			Phlegm, day or night		1.67 (1.11–2.50)	
			Phlegm for 3 months		1.27 (0.82–1.95)	
			Any symptom		1.26 (0.99–1.59)	

Table 9.3   Continued

Study	Population	Period of study	Findings		Comments
Jaakkola et al. 1996	117 lifetime nonsmokers Aged 15–40 years Montreal, Canada	Baseline: 1980–1981 Follow-up: 1988–1989	Per 10 cigarettes of secondhand smoke exposure/day		None
			Symptom	OR (95% CI)	
			Wheeze	1.15 (0.64–2.06)	
			Dyspnea	2.37 (1.25–4.51)	
			Cough	1.55 (0.61–3.90)	
			Phlegm	0.69 (0.21–2.26)	
			Any symptom	1.48 (0.88–2.49)	
Baker and Henderson 1999	1,954 randomly selected women who gave birth England	1991–1992	Wheeze		None
			Secondhand smoke exposure	OR (95% CI)	
			Partner smoked	1.73 (1.05–2.85)	
Zhang et al. 1999	4,108 adults China	1988	Women exposed to secondhand smoke by ≥1 household member		None
			Symptom	OR (95% CI)	
			Cough	1.18 (0.95–1.46)	
			Phlegm	0.96 (0.75–1.24)	
			Wheeze	0.62 (0.44–0.87)	
Trinder et al. 2000	2,996 randomly selected patients from two general practices Aged ≥16 years England	NR	Reported severe respiratory symptoms		10 respiratory symptoms were reported during the previous month
			Smoking status	OR (95% CI)	
			Involuntary smokers	1.4 (1.0–1.8)	
			Former smokers	1.5 (1.2–1.8)	
			Current smokers	2.9 (2.3–3.6)	

*OR = Odds ratio.

†CI = Confidence interval.

‡NR = Data were not reported.

Although dyspnea is nonspecific with many causes, studies have consistently associated it with secondhand smoke exposure (White et al. 1991; Pope and Xu 1993; Leuenberger et al. 1994; Jaakkola et al. 1996). Leuenberger and colleagues (1994) also found a dose-response relationship between secondhand smoke exposure and dyspnea.

In addition to specific respiratory symptoms, several investigators have examined the association between secondhand smoke exposure and the presence of any respiratory symptom (Robbins et al. 1993; Lam et al. 1995; Jaakkola et al. 1996), the severity of respiratory symptoms (Trinder et al. 2000), chest illness (Pope and Xu 1993), or colds (White et al. 1991). Although not statistically significant, the magnitudes of the associations between secondhand smoke exposure and having any respiratory symptom have been

similar and the relative risk (RR) estimates are above one (Lam et al. 1995; Jaakkola et al. 1996). Among 2,996 randomly selected patients from general practices in England, Trinder and colleagues (2000) found an association between secondhand smoke exposure and reports of severe respiratory symptoms (OR = 1.4 [95 percent CI, 1.0–1.8]).

Evidence Synthesis

Since the 1986 Surgeon General's report (USDHHS 1986), there have been numerous experimental and observational studies on the relationship between secondhand smoke exposure and acute and chronic respiratory symptoms, respectively. Overall, the experimental studies provide consistent evidence for a link between secondhand smoke exposure and acute respiratory symptoms. Furthermore, these studies document that secondhand smoke exposure produced symptoms that meet the criterion of temporality and weigh against the possibility that secondhand smoke exposure leads to a heightened perception of already present symptoms. A limited number of investigations have also documented dose-response relationships. However, the experimental studies are limited by the small number of participants and by the use of volunteers.

Of the chronic respiratory symptoms, cough and dyspnea have been most consistently associated with secondhand smoke exposure in the observational studies. In contrast, this association has been less consistently observed for phlegm and wheeze. Partly because exposures and symptoms often are misclassified in observational studies, the magnitude of the association with chronic respiratory symptoms probably has been underestimated, with weak ORs generally less than 2.0. Little information is available on the temporal or dose-response relationships between chronic symptoms and secondhand smoke exposure.

Conclusions

1. The evidence is suggestive but not sufficient to infer a causal relationship between secondhand smoke exposure and acute respiratory symptoms including cough, wheeze, chest tightness, and difficulty breathing among persons with asthma.

2. The evidence is suggestive but not sufficient to infer a causal relationship between secondhand smoke exposure and acute respiratory symptoms including cough, wheeze, chest tightness, and difficulty breathing among healthy persons.

3. The evidence is suggestive but not sufficient to infer a causal relationship between secondhand smoke exposure and chronic respiratory symptoms.

Implications

These new conclusions strengthen prior statements with regard to respiratory symptoms and secondhand smoke exposure. Because respiratory symptoms are common and may adversely affect functional status, quality of life, and the use of health care resources, the relationship between respiratory symptoms and secondhand smoke exposure has substantial relevance to clinical care, to public health, and to the general comfort of nonsmokers. Eliminating or reducing secondhand smoke exposure will likely decrease the occurrence of acute respiratory symptoms. However, further research on the relationship between secondhand smoke exposure and chronic respiratory symptoms needs to overcome the methodologic limitations of the available observational studies. To overcome these limitations, future studies should be population-based, longitudinal, restricted to lifetime nonsmokers, and should have sufficient power to comprehensively address confounding factors.

Lung Function

Studies of volunteers exposed experimentally to secondhand smoke have examined short-term effects on lung function. Observational studies of real-world exposures have addressed the long-term effects. Acute effects of secondhand smoke exposure on lung function have been examined primarily in patients with mild asthma (see "Biologic Basis" earlier in this chapter). As stated previously, the Cal/EPA report reviewed results from 10 experimental studies of persons with asthma and concluded that despite constraints in interpreting the results of the chamber studies, "they do suggest that there is likely to

be a subpopulation of asthmatics who are especially susceptible to ETS exposure" (NCI 1999, p. 203). Nowak and colleagues (1997b) subsequently provided further support for this conclusion by finding greater average declines in FEV_1 levels compared with baseline FEV_1 levels after a secondhand smoke versus a sham exposure. Nowak and colleagues (1997a) found no changes in FEV_1 levels, but the small number of participants severely limited the statistical power. Bascom and colleagues (1991) recruited 77 healthy nonsmoking adults and exposed 21 to sidestream smoke for 15 minutes at a CO concentration of 45 ppm. In the

11 participants not sensitive to secondhand smoke, spirometric test results before and after exposure were unchanged; small, but statistically significant, effects were found in the 10 participants sensitive to secondhand smoke.

In the only study of the dose-response relationship between secondhand smoke exposure and lung function, Danuser and colleagues (1993) exposed 10 persons with hyperreactive airways and 10 healthy persons matched for age and gender to five increasing levels of secondhand smoke at 2, 4, 8, 16, and 32 ppm of CO for two minutes each. Among participants with hyperreactive airways, the FEV_1 fell an average of 6.5 percent after a 2 ppm exposure of CO, and fell further with higher levels of exposure (-5.6 percent at 4 ppm of CO, -7.1 percent at 8 ppm, -8.2 percent at 16 ppm, and -8.7 percent at 32 ppm). The FEV_1 level did not drop among the healthy participants at any level of exposure.

Chronic effects of secondhand smoke exposure on lung function have been examined primarily in cross-sectional studies (Trédaniel et al. 1994; Coultas 1998; Carey et al. 1999; Chen et al. 2001) and in a few cohort studies (Jaakkola et al. 1995; Abbey et al. 1998; Carey et al. 1999). Carey and colleagues (1999) published a meta-analysis of 15 cross-sectional studies and found a 1.7 percent mean deficit (95 percent CI, -2.8 to -0.6) in the FEV_1 level associated with secondhand smoke exposure. In addition, they conducted a cross-sectional investigation of secondhand smoke exposure, classified by salivary cotinine and FEV_1 levels, among 1,623 British adults aged 18 through 73 years (Carey et al. 1999). Comparing the top with the bottom quintiles of cotinine levels among lifetime nonsmokers, the researchers observed small decrements in FEV_1 levels that were larger in men than in women, -90 milliliters (mL) (95 percent CI, -276–96) and -61 mL (95 percent CI, -154–32), respectively. Chen and colleagues (2001) examined the effects of secondhand smoke exposure among 301 Scottish lifetime nonsmokers and found an inverse dose-response relationship between self-reported levels of secondhand smoke exposure at work ("none, little, some, a lot") and FEV_1 levels. Compared with persons who were unexposed at work, "a lot" (Chen et al. 2001, p. 564 [the term was not defined by the authors]) of secondhand smoke exposure was significantly associated with a lower FEV_1 (-254 mL [95 percent CI, -420 to -84]).

Only three cohort studies have assessed secondhand smoke exposure and lung function (Jaakkola et al. 1995; Abbey et al. 1998; Carey et al. 1999). In 1980, Canadian researchers enrolled 117 lifetime nonsmokers from Montreal aged 15 through 40 years and followed them through 1989 (Jaakkola et al. 1995). The investigators assessed cumulative exposures at enrollment, exposures at follow-up, and exposures at home and at work during the three days before completing the questionnaire. During the eight years of follow-up, the researchers did not find a significant association between secondhand smoke exposure and the rates of decline of FEV_1 and forced expiratory flow between 25 and 75 percent of the forced vital capacity (FVC). Researchers also did not find significant associations for cumulative secondhand smoke exposures up to the start of the study.

In a study of the effects of ambient air pollution on lung function, Abbey and colleagues (1998) followed 1,391 lifetime nonsmokers and former smokers from California for 16 years who were 25 years of age and older at enrollment in 1977. Secondhand smoke exposure was assessed from self-reports of the number of years the participants had lived or worked with a smoker. Among women, a small but nonsignificant decline in the ratio of FEV_1 to FVC (-0.2 percent [95 percent CI, -0.5–0.1]) was associated with living with a smoker for 10 years through 1993. A similar decline was observed for men who had worked with a smoker for 10 years through 1993 (-0.5 percent [95 percent CI, -1.2–0.1]). Moreover, although quantitative data were not reported, the authors stated that concomitant secondhand smoke exposures (≥1 hour per day for at least one year at work or at home in 1987, 1992, or 1993) resulted in stronger effects of particulate pollution on lung function in men but not in women.

In a population-based sample from Britain in 1984 and 1985, Carey and colleagues (1999) enrolled 1,623 lifetime nonsmokers and former smokers aged 18 through 73 years and followed them for 7 years. Living with a smoker at enrollment and at follow-up was not associated with an accelerated FEV_1 decline (25 mL [95 percent CI, -20–70]).

Evidence Synthesis

The effects of acute and chronic secondhand smoke exposure on lung function have been examined in experimental and observational studies, respectively. In experimental studies, some persons with asthma consistently had a small decline in the FEV_1 following secondhand smoke exposure. Small decrements in lung function are coherent with the far greater impairment of lung function observed with active smoking (USDHHS 2004). However, evidence for the dose-response relationship between secondhand smoke exposure and the FEV_1 decline is limited. In the only relevant study, a dose-response relationship was not found (Danuser et al. 1993). The available evidence from experimental studies on the relationship between acute exposure to secondhand smoke and a decline in the FEV_1 suggests that the subgroup of persons with asthma is at risk from secondhand smoke.

The cross-sectional studies documented an association between chronic secondhand smoke exposure and a small decrement in lung function (Carey et al. 1999). However, these findings provide limited support for a causal relationship because the temporality between exposure and lung function decrement cannot be established with this study design, and most of these studies lack information on dose-response relationships. Although the small effect in these observational studies is coherent with larger decrements in lung function level associated with active smoking (USDHHS 2004), the small overall effect may actually reflect a larger decrement in a susceptible subpopulation. However, this hypothesis has received limited attention (Chen et al. 2001). The lack of an effect of secondhand smoke exposure on lung function decline in a small number of longitudinal studies further suggests that chronic secondhand smoke exposure may have little or no effect on lung function in the general population, but the effect in possibly susceptible subgroups has not been examined.

Conclusions

1. The evidence is suggestive but not sufficient to infer a causal relationship between short-term secondhand smoke exposure and an acute decline in lung function in persons with asthma.

2. The evidence is inadequate to infer the presence or absence of a causal relationship between short-term secondhand smoke exposure and an acute decline in lung function in healthy persons.

3. The evidence is suggestive but not sufficient to infer a causal relationship between chronic secondhand smoke exposure and a small decrement in lung function in the general population.

4. The evidence is inadequate to infer the presence or absence of a causal relationship between chronic secondhand smoke exposure and an accelerated decline in lung function.

Implications

Although acute secondhand smoke exposure is associated with small decrements in lung function among persons with asthma, the magnitude of the effect is, on average, small. Moreover, the characteristics of a one-time exposure in the experimental studies do not reflect a real-life exposure repeated over months and years. Future experimental studies of the effects of secondhand smoke exposure need to create better simulations of real-world situations, but these studies cannot address chronic effects on lung function, functional status, quality of life, and health care utilization.

Experimental and observational studies document small decrements in lung function. These findings provide a rationale for conducting observational studies to examine the larger effects of secondhand smoke exposure on lung function in potentially susceptible subgroups, such as persons with asthma (see "Respiratory Diseases" in the next section).

Respiratory Diseases

Asthma

Asthma is a heterogenous and complex disorder characterized by chronic airway inflammation and reversible airflow obstruction (National Heart, Lung, and Blood Institute 1997; Floreani and Rennard 1999). Since the 1992 U.S. EPA risk assessment report (USEPA 1992), a number of published studies have

examined the role of involuntary smoking in causing asthma (etiologic) and in exacerbating asthma (morbidity) among adults. These studies have been reviewed for this report (Coultas 1998; NCI 1999; Weiss et al. 1999). The aim of the etiologic studies has been to determine the association between involuntary smoking and the new diagnosis of asthma among adults. However, because asthma often begins during infancy or childhood (Chapter 6, Respiratory Effects in Children from Exposure to Secondhand Smoke), it may be difficult to truly establish adult-onset asthma and distinguish it from a failure to recall the onset of childhood asthma (see the next section). In contrast to studies of causation, morbidity studies have examined the role of involuntary smoking in causing symptoms, worsening lung function, causing or increasing the use of medication, increasing health care utilization, and worsening the quality of life in persons with asthma.

Etiologic Studies

Asthma is diagnosed by six years of age in approximately 80 percent of the cases (Yunginger et al. 1992), and available data suggest that by early adulthood, 30 to 50 percent of persons with childhood asthma become asymptomatic (Barbee and Murphy 1998). In etiologic investigations of adult-onset asthma, it may thus be difficult to differentiate adult-onset asthma from childhood asthma that is recurrent in adulthood because of exposure to secondhand smoke or to another environmental agent (Weiss et al. 1999). Investigation of the relationship between secondhand smoke exposure and adult-onset asthma may be further complicated by the "healthy smoker effect" (Weiss et al. 1999, p. 891), that is, the self-selection of persons with better respiratory health to be active smokers compared with those who remain nonsmokers. This effect might explain the avoidance of exposure to secondhand smoke by some persons susceptible to the development of asthma. The resulting bias would tend to underestimate the association between secondhand smoke exposure and adult-onset asthma.

Greer and colleagues (1993) examined the association between workplace exposure to secondhand smoke and a new onset of asthma among a nonsmoking population of 3,577 Seventh-Day Adventists from southern California followed between 1977 and 1987. The mean age at enrollment was 56.5 years. During the 10-year follow-up period 78 participants developed asthma, and workplace exposure to secondhand smoke was a significant risk factor (RR = 1.5 [95 percent CI, 1.2–1.8]) after controlling for gender, education, a history of obstructive airway disease before 16 years of age, and ambient ozone levels.

In a cross-sectional study of 4,197 lifetime nonsmoking Swiss adults 18 through 60 years of age, Leuenberger and colleagues (1994) found that self-reports of physician-diagnosed asthma were associated with involuntary smoking (OR = 1.39 [95 percent CI, 1.04–1.86]), defined as any secondhand smoke exposure in the past 12 months. They also found a dose-response relationship between the total number of hours of secondhand smoke exposure per day and a risk of physician-diagnosed asthma.

Flodin and colleagues (1995) conducted a population-based, case-control study in Sweden that included 79 persons with adult-onset asthma, defined as the onset of symptoms consistent with asthma after 20 years of age and bronchial reactivity measured by methacholine challenge or bronchodilator responsiveness. Secondhand smoke exposure at work was associated with an increase in the risk of asthma (OR = 1.5 [95 percent CI, 0.8–2.5]) similar in magnitude to the findings of Greer and colleagues (1993) and Leuenberger and colleagues (1994).

Because active cigarette smoking has been associated with an increased risk of developing occupational asthma attributable to IgE-inducing agents (Venables and Chan-Yeung 1997), and secondhand smoke exposure has been associated with higher IgE levels (Oryszczyn et al. 2000), it is plausible to hypothesize that involuntary smoking may also contribute to the development of occupational asthma in nonsmokers. Although workplace exposures to secondhand smoke have been associated with asthma among adults (Greer et al. 1993; Flodin et al. 1995), no investigations have reported on the interaction of secondhand smoke exposure at the workplace with specific occupational agents.

In 1993, Hu and colleagues (1997) surveyed 1,469 young adults aged 20 through 22 years from Los Angeles and San Diego (California) to determine the prevalence of asthma in this population. Parental reports obtained in 1986 as part of a school-based smoking prevention program were used to determine exposures to secondhand smoke. Maternal and paternal smoking were associated with the young adults ever having had physician-diagnosed asthma (OR = 1.6 [95 percent CI, 1.1–2.3] and 1.3 [95 percent CI, 0.9–1.8], respectively). Similar results were found for current asthma with maternal smoking (OR = 1.6 [95 percent CI, 1.0–2.1]). Hu and colleagues (1997) also found a dose-response relationship with the amount smoked and the number of parents who smoked. The highest risk of having a physician-diagnosed asthma (OR = 2.9 [95 percent CI, 1.6–5.6]) and current asthma (OR = 3.3 [95 percent CI, 1.7–6.4]) was associated with smoking by both parents compared with smoking by neither parent.

Morbidity Studies

Trédaniel and colleagues (1994) summarized results of the effects of secondhand smoke exposure on respiratory symptoms and lung function from four observational studies of patients with respiratory allergies and from five experimental studies of patients with asthma. The authors concluded that "Conflicting evidence exists on the association in asthmatic patients between ETS exposure and appearance of symptoms and functional abnormalities (including change in bronchial responsiveness)" (p. 181). Weiss and colleagues (1999) reached similar conclusions in their review of 2 observational studies and 12 experimental studies of secondhand smoke exposure and an exacerbation of asthma.

Experimental Studies

Results of 10 chamber studies of secondhand smoke exposure in persons with asthma were extensively reviewed in the Cal/EPA report (NCI 1999) and summarized earlier in this chapter (see "Biologic Basis" and "Lung Function"). Methodologic limitations of experimental studies examining the relationship between secondhand smoke exposure and asthma morbidity reflect the inability to replicate real-life exposure conditions and the failure of health outcome measures (e.g., symptoms or lung function) to adequately assess asthma morbidity. Consequently, observational studies provide the best evidence for assessing asthma morbidity associated with secondhand smoke exposure.

Observational Studies

Study designs that have been used to examine secondhand smoke exposure and asthma morbidity include population-based, cross-sectional surveys (Mannino et al. 1997); clinic-based, cross-sectional studies (Jindal et al. 1999); case-control studies (Tarlo et al. 2000); and prospective cohort studies (Jindal et al. 1994; Ostro et al. 1994; Sippel et al. 1999). In a nationally representative sample of 43,732 U.S. adults who participated in the 1991 National Health Interview Survey (NHIS), Mannino and colleagues (1997) examined the relationship between any self-reported secondhand smoke exposure during the previous two weeks and the exacerbation of any chronic respiratory disease (asthma, chronic bronchitis, emphysema, and chronic sinusitis) in the two weeks before the survey. In a multiple logistic regression model that adjusted for age, gender, race, socioeconomic status (SES), living alone, season, and region of the country, exposure

to secondhand smoke was significantly associated with the exacerbation of any chronic respiratory condition among lifetime nonsmokers (OR = 1.44 [95 percent CI, 1.07–1.95]).

Jindal and colleagues (1999) measured bronchial hyperresponsiveness and bronchodilator use in a sample of 50 women with asthma aged 20 through 40 years followed at a chest clinic in India. Exposure to secondhand smoke was assessed with questions on smoking by the husband, by other family members, and by coworkers. Compared with no exposure, secondhand smoke exposure was associated with significantly greater bronchial hyperreactivity and with continuous bronchodilator use (39 percent of exposed women and 26 percent of unexposed women [p <0.05]).

Tarlo and colleagues (2000) conducted a case-control study of 36 patients with an asthma exacerbation within 24 hours of completing the study questionnaire, and 36 persons similar in age with asthma but without an exacerbation. Of the 36 patients with an exacerbation, 21 were adolescents or adults (aged 13 through 55 years) and 15 were children (aged 7 through 12 years). The study documented that exposures to secondhand smoke during the previous year were reported more frequently by cases (39 percent) than by controls (17 percent) (p <0.03).

To assess the clinical consequences of secondhand smoke exposure on patients with asthma, Jindal and colleagues (1994) enrolled 200 lifetime nonsmoking patients with asthma aged 15 through 50 years from a chest outpatient clinic in India, and then followed them for one year. Patients were categorized by whether or not they had been exposed to secondhand smoke. Exposed patients had more acute episodes of asthma, emergency department visits, absences from work, parenteral bronchodilator use, and steroid use. In addition, exposed patients had a greater impairment of lung function (FEV_1/FVC = 68.7 percent) than unexposed patients (FEV_1/FVC = 78.4 percent).

Ostro and colleagues (1994) studied 164 persons with asthma with a mean age of 45.5 years from a clinic in Denver, Colorado. For up to three months, they recorded daily information about symptoms, medication use, physician and emergency room visits, and indoor exposures to secondhand smoke. Using a statistical approach appropriate for these daily data, the researchers estimated risks for symptoms resulting from exposure to secondhand smoke: moderate or worse shortness of breath (OR = 1.35 [95 percent CI, 0.84–2.15]), moderate or worse cough (OR = 1.15 [95 percent CI, 0.97–1.36]), and restricted activity (OR = 1.61 [95 percent CI, 1.06–2.46]).

Sippel and colleagues (1999) enrolled 619 patients with asthma aged 15 through 55 years who were members of a large health maintenance organization. Health outcome data were collected during a 30-month period. Compared with patients without secondhand smoke exposure, exposed persons with asthma had a greater utilization of hospital services (i.e., urgent care, emergency room, and hospitalization) (OR = 2.34 [95 percent CI, 1.80–3.05]). In addition, persons with asthma who were exposed to secondhand smoke had lower quality of life scores compared with unexposed patients.

Evidence Synthesis

Earlier reviews of secondhand smoke exposure and the etiology of adult-onset asthma found the evidence for causality to be inconclusive because of methodologic limitations and the small number of studies (Trédaniel et al. 1994; Coultas 1998; Weiss et al. 1999). Although only a few new studies have been published since these reviews, there is a consistent (albeit weak) association between secondhand smoke exposures at home or in the workplace and a 40 to 60 percent increase in the risk of asthma in exposed adults compared with unexposed adults. Moreover, cross-sectional and longitudinal studies have consistently found this association, and results from longitudinal studies provide support for the temporality criterion of causality. One study documented a dose-response relationship between the number of parents smoking in the home and the risk of asthma among young adults. Because a causal link between active smoking and adult-onset asthma has not been established (USDHHS 2004), the coherence criterion for secondhand smoke currently cannot be fulfilled. However, because the pathogenesis of asthma is complex and coherence between active smoking and secondhand smoke exposure may be too restrictive, researchers should not expect a full parallel between the effects of active and involuntary smoking in asthma.

Both experimental and observational study designs have examined secondhand smoke exposure and asthma morbidity. The small particles and irritant gases in secondhand smoke would be anticipated to adversely affect the hyperresponsive airways of persons with asthma and contribute to lung inflammation, as postulated for air pollution generally (Bascom et al. 1995, 1996). Inconsistent results from experimental studies may be explained in part by a number of methodologic differences and limitations (Weiss et al. 1999). However, these studies provide "evidence that individual asthmatics and groups of asthmatics do respond to levels of ETS that do not elicit responses in healthy volunteers" (Weiss et al. 1999, p. 894). Several published observational studies of secondhand smoke exposure and asthma morbidity were not included in earlier reviews (Trédaniel et al. 1994; Coultas 1998; Weiss et al. 1999). Taken together, these observational studies provide evidence that exposure to secondhand smoke worsens asthma in adults, findings that are consistent with the effects of active smoking (USDHHS 2004).

Conclusions

1. The evidence is suggestive but not sufficient to infer a causal relationship between secondhand smoke exposure and adult-onset asthma.

2. The evidence is suggestive but not sufficient to infer a causal relationship between secondhand smoke exposure and a worsening of asthma control.

Implications

There is a need for additional research on the etiologic relationship between secondhand smoke exposure and adult-onset asthma. Although the available evidence for asthma morbidity suggests that the elimination of secondhand smoke exposure would improve asthma control in adults, no clinical trials have addressed this issue. Despite the evidence on secondhand smoke exposure and poor asthma control, a substantial proportion (43 percent) of persons with asthma presenting for emergency care were exposed to secondhand smoke at home (Dales et al. 1992), suggesting a need for greater awareness among patients and physicians of this relationship.

Chronic Obstructive Pulmonary Disease

COPD is a nonspecific term, defined differently by clinicians, pathologists, and epidemiologists, each using different criteria based on symptoms, physiologic impairment, and pathologic abnormalities (Samet 1989). The hallmark of COPD is the slowing of expiratory airflow measured by spirometric testing, with a persistently low FEV_1 and a low ratio of FEV_1 to FVC despite treatment. Although chronic bronchitis and emphysema are classically associated with the term COPD, they do not invariably involve chronic airways obstruction. Recent evidence suggests that changes in the structure and function of the bronchioles may be fundamental to the development of smoking-induced COPD (Wright 1992; Thurlbeck 1994). Active cigarette smoking is the single most important risk factor for COPD (USDHHS 2004), with 85 to 90 percent of COPD-related mortality attributable to active cigarette smoking (Thun et al. 1997a,b). However, other risk factors such as second-hand smoke, occupational exposures, and genetic factors may also contribute to COPD.

Using survey data from three national health and nutrition examination surveys, Whittemore and colleagues (1995) determined the prevalence of COPD (self-reports of physician-diagnosed chronic bronchitis or emphysema) among 12,980 lifetime non-smokers aged 18 through 74 years. Overall, 3.7 percent of men and 5.1 percent of women reported physician-diagnosed COPD, and the prevalence increased with age and with a low SES. Although this study was limited to self-reports of COPD and lacked information on secondhand smoke exposure, these results provide evidence that COPD occurs among nonsmokers, and that risk factors other than active cigarette smoking (such as secondhand smoke exposure) may contribute to the development of COPD in nonsmoking adults.

Results from the Third National Health and Nutrition Examination Survey provide further evidence that COPD occurs in nonsmokers (Coultas et al. 2001). Among 5,743 persons aged 45 years and older, 3.1 percent reported having physician-diagnosed COPD; of these, 1.6 percent of the men and 12.2 percent of the women were lifetime non-smokers. Furthermore, 12 percent of the entire sample had spirometric evidence of airflow obstruction that was undiagnosed; 10.5 percent of the men and 27.5 percent of the women with undiagnosed airflow obstruction were lifetime nonsmokers. The factors contributing to airflow obstruction in nonsmokers are uncertain, and secondhand smoke exposure may have a role.

The presence of COPD can be measured in numerous ways, including self-reported measures (e.g., symptoms and physician diagnoses), physician diagnoses (e.g., hospitalizations and mortality), and spirometric criteria. All of these measures have been used to investigate the relationship between second-hand smoke exposure and the etiology of COPD. The discussion that follows summarizes the results from each type of investigation.

Etiologic Studies

Published investigations examining the etiologic role of secondhand smoke exposure in COPD use different definitions of COPD, including self-reports

(Robbins et al. 1993; Dayal et al. 1994; Leuenberger et al. 1994; Piitulainen et al. 1998; Forastiere et al. 2000), hospitalizations for COPD (Lee et al. 1986; Kalandidi et al. 1987), COPD mortality (Hirayama 1981; Sandler et al. 1989), and lung function (Dennis et al. 1996; Berglund et al. 1999). Most of the studies that used self-reports relied on recalled physician diagnoses, and all but one (Forastiere et al. 2000) combined asthma, chronic bronchitis, and emphysema to define COPD.

In a cohort study conducted from 1977 to 1987 of 3,914 adults aged 25 years and older, Robbins and colleagues (1993) used self-reported symptoms and physician diagnoses (asthma, chronic bronchitis, and emphysema) to define airway obstructive disease (AOD). They found that secondhand smoke exposures at home and at work during both childhood and adulthood were significantly associated with AOD (RR = 1.7 [95 percent CI, 1.3–2.2]).

Leuenberger and colleagues (1994) conducted a cross-sectional survey of 4,197 Swiss adults 18 through 60 years of age. The investigators examined the relationship of respiratory symptoms and diseases to self-reports of secondhand smoke exposure at home and at work during the previous 12 months. Reports of chronic bronchitis were significantly associated with secondhand smoke exposure (OR = 1.7 [95 percent CI, 1.3–2.2]).

In a population-based study of air pollution, Dayal and colleagues (1994) used a case-control design to examine the association between second-hand smoke exposure and obstructive respiratory disease. A total of 219 lifetime nonsmokers reported a history of physician-diagnosed asthma, chronic bronchitis, or emphysema, and were matched by age, gender, and neighborhood to 657 persons without these diagnoses. Although exposure to less than one pack of cigarettes per day was not significantly associated with obstructive respiratory disease (OR = 1.2 [95 percent CI, 0.8–1.7]), exposure to one or more packs per day was significantly associated with obstructive respiratory disease (OR = 1.9 [95 percent CI, 1.2–2.9]).

Forastiere and colleagues (2000) conducted a cross-sectional survey of 1,938 nonsmoking women from four areas in Italy. Out of 1,212 women who reported that they had ever been married to a smoker, 711 were still exposed to the husband's smoking. After adjusting for age, area, and education, the husband's smoking was not significantly associated with self-reported COPD (OR = 1.75 [95 percent CI, 0.88–3.47]).

In contrast to the general population studies, Piitulainen and colleagues (1998) examined the effects of secondhand smoke exposure in a group susceptible to developing emphysema: 205 non-smokers with a severe alpha-1-antitrypsin deficiency. The researchers found that exposures of 10 or more years to secondhand smoke, compared with no exposure, were significantly associated with chronic bronchitis (OR = 1.6 [95 percent CI, 1.3–2.4]), defined as a daily cough with phlegm at least three months per year.

There have been two case-control studies of hospital admissions for COPD and secondhand smoke exposure (Lee et al. 1986; Kalandidi et al. 1987). In a hospital-based, case-control study of 10 hospital regions in England conducted from 1977 to 1982, Lee and colleagues (1986) found a small increase (OR = 1.3 [95 percent CI was not provided]) in risk for chronic bronchitis with the highest category of second-hand smoke exposure, but this estimate was based on only two cases. Kalandidi and colleagues (1987) studied 103 ever-married women aged 40 through 79 years who, on two separate occasions—first, during routine history-taking, and again categorically at the study interview—denied ever smoking and who were admitted to an Athens, Greece, hospital with a diagnosis of chronic obstructive lung disease. The control group comprised 179 ever-married non-smoking women who were visiting the hospital. Compared with women whose husbands had never smoked, women whose husbands smoked one pack per day or less had an increased risk of COPD (OR = 2.6 [90 percent CI, 1.3–5.0]); those whose husbands smoked more than one pack per day had an OR of 1.5 (90 percent CI, 0.8–2.7).

Two cohort studies examined the association between COPD mortality and involuntary smoking (Hirayama 1981; Sandler et al. 1989). In a population-based cohort of 91,540 nonsmoking Japanese housewives aged 40 years and older, Hirayama (1981) determined that from 1966 to 1979, there were 66 deaths from emphysema and asthma. Compared with women married to nonsmokers, women whose husbands were former smokers or smokers of 19 cigarettes or fewer per day had a 29 percent increased risk of death from emphysema or asthma, and women whose husbands smoked 20 or more cigarettes per day had a 49 percent increased risk. The gradient of risk from smoking by the husbands was not statistically significant. Because the number of deaths was small, these results were not statistically significant. Another study (Sandler et al. 1989) determined the causes of death for White residents of Washington county, Maryland (United States), who had died between 1963 and 1975. The researchers examined associations with secondhand smoke exposure

among 10,799 residents who had reported in 1963 that they were lifetime nonsmokers with household smoking exposures. There was an increased risk of death from emphysema and bronchitis in women (RR = 5.7 [95 percent CI, 1.2–26.8], n = 13) but not in men (RR = 0.9 [95 percent CI, 0.2–5.3], n = 6).

Some studies on involuntary smoking and COPD examined the relationship between lung function level and involuntary smoking (Trédaniel et al. 1994; Kerstjens et al. 1997). Results of several cohort studies published since 1994 (and reviewed in the section on "Lung Function" earlier in this chapter) suggest that secondhand smoke exposure does not increase the average rate of lung function decline (Jaakkola et al. 1995; Abbey et al. 1998; Carey et al. 1999). Although longitudinal data on the effects of active or involuntary smoking and the development of COPD are not available from childhood through adulthood, evidence suggests that the development of COPD in adults may result from impaired lung development and growth and a premature onset of and/or an accelerated decline in lung function (Fletcher et al. 1976; Samet and Lange 1996; Kerstjens et al. 1997). In utero airway development and alveolar proliferation until 12 years of age are critical to the mechanical functioning of the lungs, and impaired lung growth in utero from an exposure to maternal smoking may begin a process that leads to the development of COPD. Exposure to secondhand smoke in infancy and childhood and active smoking during childhood and adolescence contribute to impaired lung growth, which in turn limits the maximum level of lung function attained (Kerstjens et al. 1997; USDHHS 2004) and may increase the risk for developing COPD. The impact of involuntary smoking during adulthood on lung function and the risk for developing COPD remain controversial (Trédaniel et al. 1994). However, because studies have established that active cigarette smoking in adulthood leads to an accelerated decline in the FEV_1 and ultimately to the development of clinically apparent COPD among susceptible smokers, involuntary smoking is considered a biologically plausible risk factor.

Trédaniel and colleagues (1994) reviewed the available evidence on exposure to secondhand smoke and adult non-neoplastic respiratory diseases, citing 18 publications on lung function and secondhand smoke exposure published between 1977 and 1992. Of these 18 publications, 8 found no effect of secondhand smoke exposure on lung function and 10 demonstrated small decrements in lung function. Noted limitations of the available studies include a lack of information on potential confounders and on childhood exposures to secondhand smoke. Further, when detected, the magnitude of the decrement associated with secondhand smoke exposure was small (see the section on "Lung Function" earlier in this chapter), raising questions about the clinical relevance to COPD. This conclusion is further strengthened by the results from Piitulainen and colleagues (1998), who found no effect of secondhand smoke exposure on lung function level among 205 participants with a severe alpha-1-antitrypsin deficiency.

Spirometry is the main physiologic measure of airway obstruction and was used as a measure of COPD in some investigations (Dennis et al. 1996; Berglund et al. 1999). To investigate selected indoor air pollutants and their association with AOD, Dennis and colleagues (1996) conducted a case-control study of 104 women with airways obstruction (mean age 63 years) and 104 controls from three hospitals in Bogota, Colombia. Airways obstruction was defined as a FEV_1/FVC of less than 70 percent and a FEV_1 of less than 70 percent of predicted value. In a multiple logistic regression model that adjusted for smoking and wood and gasoline use, exposure to smoking by the husband was significantly associated with airway obstruction (OR = 2.04 [95 percent CI, 1.1–3.9]).

In a cohort study, Berglund and colleagues (1999) conducted spirometry on 1,391 adult lifetime nonsmokers and former smokers from California who were younger than 80 years of age. Obstructive impairment was defined as a FEV_1/maximum vital capacity of less than 65 percent or a FEV_1 of less than 75 percent of predicted value. Secondhand smoke exposure was based on self-reports and defined as at least one hour per day for at least one year. Ever having a secondhand smoke exposure was significantly associated with airways obstruction (RR = 1.44 [95 percent CI, 1.02–2.01]).

Morbidity Studies

Compared with the numerous investigations of the health effects of secondhand smoke exposure in persons with asthma, there are only a few investigations of the health effects in persons with COPD. One study used a nationally representative sample of 43,732 U.S. adults who participated in the 1991 NHIS (Mannino et al. 1997). These researchers examined the relationship between secondhand smoke exposure and any chronic respiratory disease exacerbation (asthma, chronic bronchitis, emphysema, and chronic sinusitis) in the two weeks before the survey. In a multiple logistic regression model that adjusted for age, gender, race, SES, living alone, season, and region of the country, there was a significant association among lifetime nonsmokers exposed to secondhand smoke with the exacerbation of any chronic respiratory condition (OR = 1.44 [95 percent CI, 1.07–1.95]).

Evidence Synthesis

Investigations of COPD in nonsmokers are limited. Results from a nationwide, population-based survey in the United States suggest that 3 to 5 percent of nonsmokers may be affected (Whittemore et al. 1995). However, these results were based on self-reports of COPD and smoking status, and thus may be overestimates. In another U.S. survey, only 0.5 percent of nonsmokers reported a physician-diagnosed history of COPD, but 5.2 percent had undiagnosed airflow obstruction measured by spirometry (Coultas et al. 2001).

Using diverse methods to define COPD (including self-reported physician diagnoses, hospitalizations, mortality, and lung function diagnoses), a number of studies have consistently identified involuntary smoking as a risk factor for COPD among nonsmokers. Active smoking is a well-established cause of COPD, and there is a substantial understanding of the mechanisms by which tobacco smoke damages the lung to produce COPD. However, studies that have relied on self-reported diagnoses are limited by the inclusion of physician-diagnosed asthma in their definition of COPD. Furthermore, self-reports of smoking status may misclassify current and former smokers as lifetime nonsmokers, resulting in a biased association between secondhand smoke exposure and COPD. The magnitude of these reported associations has been consistent but the risk estimates are weak, ranging from 1.2 to about 2.0, which is a plausible range of association given the exposure levels. Few investigations have examined the dose-response relationship between secondhand smoke exposure and the risk of COPD. Evidence from a limited number of cohort studies documents that secondhand smoke exposure precedes the COPD diagnosis, thus meeting the temporality criterion.

Finally, little is known about the effects of secondhand smoke exposure on respiratory symptoms, lung function, health care utilization, or the quality of life of patients with COPD. An analysis of the 1991 NHIS data showed that among lifetime nonsmokers and current smokers, secondhand smoke exposure was associated with exacerbations of chronic respiratory diseases during the two weeks before their interview (Mannino et al. 1997). The analysis did not specifically separate COPD from the other chronic respiratory diseases that were considered.

This review indicates a surprisingly high prevalence of airflow obstruction among nonsmokers and associations of indicators of airflow obstruction with secondhand smoke exposure. These findings need a targeted follow-up with designs that incorporate state-of-the-art approaches for exposure assessment and longitudinal tracking of lung function.

Conclusions

1. The evidence is suggestive but not sufficient to infer a causal relationship between secondhand smoke exposure and risk for chronic obstructive pulmonary disease.

2. The evidence is inadequate to infer the presence or absence of a causal relationship between secondhand smoke exposure and morbidity in persons with chronic obstructive pulmonary disease.

Implications

Although limited data suggest that COPD is not uncommon among nonsmokers, there is a need for epidemiologic studies that use objective measures of airflow obstruction to establish the prevalence of this condition in nonsmokers. Excluding persons with asthma and using methods to minimize diagnostic misclassification (e.g., questionnaires and spirometric measures) will strengthen future etiologic studies. Investigations need to explore the association between secondhand smoke exposure and health outcomes such as symptoms, functional status, quality of life, and health care utilization in patients with COPD.

Conclusions

Odor and Irritation

1. The evidence is sufficient to infer a causal relationship between secondhand smoke exposure and odor annoyance.

2. The evidence is sufficient to infer a causal relationship between secondhand smoke exposure and nasal irritation.

3. The evidence is suggestive but not sufficient to conclude that persons with nasal allergies or a history of respiratory illnesses are more susceptible to developing nasal irritation from secondhand smoke exposure.

Respiratory Symptoms

4. The evidence is suggestive but not sufficient to infer a causal relationship between secondhand smoke exposure and acute respiratory symptoms including cough, wheeze, chest tightness, and difficulty breathing among persons with asthma.

5. The evidence is suggestive but not sufficient to infer a causal relationship between secondhand smoke exposure and acute respiratory symptoms including cough, wheeze, chest tightness, and difficulty breathing among healthy persons.

6. The evidence is suggestive but not sufficient to infer a causal relationship between secondhand smoke exposure and chronic respiratory symptoms.

Lung Function

7. The evidence is suggestive but not sufficient to infer a causal relationship between short-term secondhand smoke exposure and an acute decline in lung function in persons with asthma.

8. The evidence is inadequate to infer the presence or absence of a causal relationship between short-term secondhand smoke exposure and an acute decline in lung function in healthy persons.

9. The evidence is suggestive but not sufficient to infer a causal relationship between chronic secondhand smoke exposure and a small decrement in lung function in the general population.

10. The evidence is inadequate to infer the presence or absence of a causal relationship between chronic secondhand smoke exposure and an accelerated decline in lung function.

Asthma

11. The evidence is suggestive but not sufficient to infer a causal relationship between secondhand smoke exposure and adult-onset asthma.

12. The evidence is suggestive but not sufficient to infer a causal relationship between second-hand smoke exposure and a worsening of asthma control.

Chronic Obstructive Pulmonary Disease

13. The evidence is suggestive but not sufficient to infer a causal relationship between secondhand smoke exposure and risk for chronic obstructive pulmonary disease.

14. The evidence is inadequate to infer the presence or absence of a causal relationship between secondhand smoke exposure and morbidity in persons with chronic obstructive pulmonary disease.

Overall Implications

This review clearly points to the need for further research. The evidence for adverse respiratory effects in adults has identified a large number of health outcomes for which the data are suggestive of but not sufficient to infer a causal relationship attributable to secondhand smoke exposure. The evidence reviewed in Chapter 2 (Toxicology of Secondhand Smoke) indicates multiple mechanisms by which exposure to secondhand smoke causes injury to the respiratory tract. In addition, researchers have established active smoking as a primary cause of many adverse respiratory effects in adults. However, the number of studies on secondhand smoke is limited, and there is a need for research that examines the types and magnitude of risk for adverse respiratory health effects caused by exposure to secondhand smoke.

References

Abbey DE, Burchette RJ, Knutsen SF, McDonnell WF, Lebowitz MD, Enright PL. Long-term particulate and other air pollutants and lung function in non-smokers. *American Journal of Respiratory and Critical Care Medicine* 1998;158(1):289–98.

Anderson R, Theron AJ, Richards GA, Myer MS, van Rensburg AJ. Passive smoking by humans sensitizes circulating neutrophils. *American Review of Respiratory Disease* 1991;144(3 Pt 1):570–4.

Baker D, Henderson J. Differences between infants and adults in the social aetiology of wheeze. The ALSPAC Study Team. Avon Longitudinal Study of Pregnancy and Childhood. *Journal of Epidemiology and Community Health* 1999;53(10):636–42.

Barbee RA, Murphy S. The natural history of asthma. *Supplement to the Journal of Allergy and Clinical Immunology* 1998;102(4 Pt 2):S65–S72.

Bascom R, Kesavanathan J, Fitzgerald TK, Cheng K-H, Swift DL. Sidestream tobacco smoke exposure acutely alters human nasal mucociliary clearance. *Environmental Health Perspectives* 1995;103(11): 1026–30.

Bascom R, Kesavanathan J, Permutt T, Fitzgerald TK, Sauder L, Swift DL. Tobacco smoke upper respiratory response relationships in healthy non-smokers. *Fundamental and Applied Toxicology* 1996; 29(1):86–93.

Bascom R, Kulle T, Kagey-Sobotka A, Proud D. Upper respiratory tract environmental tobacco smoke sensitivity. *American Review of Respiratory Disease* 1991;143(6):1304–11.

Berglund DJ, Abbey DE, Lebowitz MD, Knutsen SF, McDonnell WF. Respiratory symptoms and pulmonary function in an elderly nonsmoking population. *Chest* 1999;115(1):49–59.

Carey IM, Cook DG, Strachan DP. The effects of environmental tobacco smoke exposure on lung function in a longitudinal study of British adults. *Epidemiology* 1999;10(3):319–26.

Chen R, Tunstall-Pedoe H, Tavendale R. Environmental tobacco smoke and lung function in employees who never smoked: the Scottish MONICA study. *Occupational and Environmental Medicine* 2001;58(9):563–8.

Coultas DB. Health effects of passive smoking: 8. Passive smoking and risk of adult asthma and COPD: an update. *Thorax* 1998;53(5):381–7.

Coultas DB, Mapel D, Gagnon R, Lydick E. The health impact of undiagnosed airflow obstruction in a national sample of United States adults. *American Journal of Respiratory and Critical Care Medicine* 2001;164(3):372–7.

Cummings KM, Zaki A, Markello S. Variation in sensitivity to environmental tobacco smoke among adult non-smokers. *International Journal of Epidemiology* 1991;20(1):121–5.

Dahms TE, Bolin JF, Slavin RG. Passive smoking: effects on bronchial asthma. *Chest* 1981;80(5): 530–4.

Dales RE, Kerr PE, Schweitzer I, Ressor K, Gougeon L, Dickinson G. Asthma management preceding an emergency department visit. *Archives of Internal Medicine* 1992;152(10):2041–4.

Danuser B, Weber A, Hartmann AL, Krueger H. Effects of a bronchoprovocation challenge test with cigarette sidestream smoke on sensitive and healthy adults. *Chest* 1993;103(2):353–8.

Dayal HH, Khuder S, Sharrar R, Trieff N. Passive smoking in obstructive respiratory disease in an industrialized urban population. *Environmental Research* 1994;65(2):161–71.

Dennis RJ, Maldonado D, Norman S, Baena E, Martinez G. Woodsmoke exposure and risk for obstructive airways disease among women. *Chest* 1996;109(1):115–9.

Escolar JD, Martinez MN, Rodriguez FJ, Gonzalo C, Escolar MA, Roche PA. Emphysema as a result of involuntary exposure to tobacco smoke: morphometrical study of the rat. *Experimental Lung Research* 1995;21(2):255–73.

Fletcher C, Peto R, Tinker C, Speizer FE. *The Natural History of Chronic Bronchitis and Emphysema: An Eight-Year Study of Early Chronic Obstructive Lung Disease in Working Men in London.* New York: Oxford University Press, 1976.

Flodin U, Jonsson P, Ziegler J, Axelson O. An epidemiologic study of bronchial asthma and smoking. *Epidemiology* 1995;6(5):503–5.

Floreani AA, Rennard SI. The role of cigarette smoke in the pathogenesis of asthma and as a trigger for acute symptoms. *Current Opinion in Pulmonary Medicine* 1999;5(1):38–46.

Forastiere F, Mallone S, Lo Presti E, Baldacci S, Pistelli F, Simoni M, Scalera A, Pedreschi M, Pistelli R, Corbo G, et al. Characteristics of nonsmoking women exposed to spouses who smoke: epidemiologic study on environment and health in women from four Italian areas. *Environmental Health Perspectives* 2000;108(12):1171–7.

Greer JR, Abbey DE, Burchette RJ. Asthma related to occupational and ambient air pollutants in nonsmokers. *Journal of Occupational Medicine* 1993; 35(9):909–15.

Hirayama T. Non-smoking wives of heavy smokers have a higher risk of lung cancer: a study from Japan. *British Medical Journal* 1981;282(6259):183–5.

Hu FB, Persky V, Flay BR, Richardson J. An epidemiological study of asthma prevalence and related factors among young adults. *Journal of Asthma* 1997; 34(1):67–76.

Jaakkola MS, Jaakkola JJ, Becklake MR, Ernst P. Passive smoking and evolution of lung function in young adults: an 8-year longitudinal study. *Journal of Clinical Epidemiology* 1995;48(3):317–27.

Jaakkola MS, Jaakkola JJ, Becklake MR, Ernst P. Effect of passive smoking on the development of respiratory symptoms in young adults: an 8-year longitudinal study. *Journal of Clinical Epidemiology* 1996;49(5):581–6.

Jindal SK, Gupta D, Singh A. Indices of morbidity and control of asthma in adult patients exposed to environmental tobacco smoke. *Chest* 1994;106(3):746–9.

Jindal SK, Jha LK, Gupta D. Bronchial hyperresponsiveness of women with asthma exposed to environmental tobacco smoke. *Indian Journal of Chest Diseases & Allied Sciences* 1999;41(2):75–82.

Joad JP, Bric JM, Pinkerton KE. Sidestream smoke effects on lung morphology and C-fibers in young guinea pigs. *Toxicology and Applied Pharmacology* 1995;131(2):289–96.

Jones JG, Minty BD, Lawler P, Hulands G, Crawley JC, Veall N. Increased alveolar epithelial permeability in cigarette smokers. *Lancet* 1980;12(1):66–8.

Kalandidi A, Trichopoulos D, Hatzakis A, Tzannes S, Saracci R. Passive smoking and chronic obstructive lung disease [letter]. *Lancet* 1987;330(8571):1325–6.

Kanner RE, Connett JE, Altose MD, Buist AS, Lee WW, Tashkin DP, Wise RA. Gender difference in airway hyperresponsiveness in smokers with mild COPD: the Lung Health Study. *American Journal of Respiratory and Critical Care Medicine* 1994;150(4):956–61.

Kerstjens HA, Rijcken B, Schouten JP, Postma DS. Decline of FEV_1 by age and smoking status: facts, figures, and fallacies. *Thorax* 1997;52(9):820–7.

Knight A, Breslin AB. Passive cigarette smoking and patients with asthma. *Medical Journal of Australia* 1985;142(3):194–5.

Lam TH, Liu J, Hedley AJ, Wong CM, Ong SG. Passive smoking and respiratory symptoms in never-smoking women in Hong Kong. In: Slama K, editor. *Tobacco and Health.* New York: Plenum Press, 1995:547–9.

Lee LY, Gerhardstein DC, Wang AL, Burki NK. Nicotine is responsible for airway irritation evoked by cigarette smoke inhalation in men. *Journal of Applied Physiology* 1993;75(5):1955–61.

Lee PN, Chamberlain J, Alderson MR. Relationship of passive smoking to risk of lung cancer and other smoking-associated diseases. *British Journal of Cancer* 1986;54(1):97–105.

Leuenberger P, Schwartz J, Ackermann-Liebrich U, Blaser K, Bolognini G, Bongard JP, Brandli O, Braun P, Bron C, Brutsche M, et al. Passive smoking exposure in adults and chronic respiratory symptoms (SAPALDIA Study). *American Journal of Respiratory and Critical Care Medicine* 1994;150(5 Pt 1):1222–8.

Magnussen H, Jorres R, Oldigs M. Effect of one hour of passive cigarette smoking on lung function and airway responsiveness in adults and children with asthma. *The Clinical Investigator* 1992;70(3–4): 368–71.

Mannino DM, Siegel M, Rose D, Nkuchia J, Etzel R. Environmental tobacco smoke exposure in the home and worksite and health effect in adults: results from the 1991 National Health Interview Survey. *Tobacco Control* 1997;6(4):296–305.

Menon P, Rando RJ, Stankus RP, Salvaggio JE, Lehrer SB. Passive cigarette smoke-challenge studies: increase in bronchial hyperreactivity. *Journal of Allergy and Clinical Immunology* 1992;89(2):560–6.

Menzies D, Bourbeau J. Building-related illnesses. *New England Journal of Medicine* 1997;337(21):1524–31.

Moschandreas DJ, Relwani SM. Perception of environmental tobacco smoke odors: an olfactory and visual response. *Atmospheric Environment* 1992; 26B(3):263–9.

National Cancer Institute. *Health Effects of Exposure to Environmental Tobacco Smoke: The Report of the California Environmental Protection Agency.* Smoking and Tobacco Control Monograph No. 10. Bethesda (MD): U.S. Department of Health and Human Services, National Institutes of Health, National Cancer Institute, 1999. NIH Publication No. 99-4645.

National Heart, Lung, and Blood Institute. *Guidelines for the Diagnosis and Management of Asthma: Expert Panel Report 2*. Bethesda (MD): National Institutes of Health, National Heart, Lung, and Blood Institute, 1997. NIH Publication No. (NIH) 97-4051.

National Research Council. *Environmental Tobacco Smoke: Measuring Exposures and Assessing Health Effects*. Washington: National Academy Press, 1986.

Ng TP, Tan WC. Epidemiology of allergic rhinitis and its associated risk factors in Singapore. *International Journal of Epidemiology* 1994;23(3):553–8.

Norback D, Edling C. Environmental, occupational, and personal factors related to the prevalence of sick building syndrome in the general population. *British Journal of Industrial Medicine* 1991;48(7): 451–62.

Nowak D, Jörres R, Martinez-Müller L, Grimminger F, Seeger W, Koops F, Magnussen H. Effect of 3 hours of passive smoke exposure in the evening on inflammatory markers in bronchoalveolar and nasal lavage fluid in subjects with mild asthma. *International Archives of Occupational and Environmental Health* 1997a;70(2):85–93.

Nowak D, Jörres R, Schmidt A, Magnussen H. Effect of 3 hours' passive smoke exposure in the evening on airway tone and responsiveness until next morning. *International Archives of Occupational and Environmental Health* 1997b;69(2):125–33.

Oryszczyn M-P, Annesi-Maesano I, Charpin D, Paty E, Maccario J, Kauffmann F. Relationships of active and passive smoking to total IgE in adults of the Epidemiological Study of the Genetics and Environment of Asthma, Bronchial Hyperresponsiveness, and Atopy (EGEA). *American Journal of Respiratory and Critical Care Medicine* 2000;161(4):1241–6.

Ostro BD, Lipsett MJ, Mann JK, Wiener MB, Selner J. Indoor air pollution and asthma: results from a panel study. *American Journal of Respiratory and Critical Care Medicine* 1994;149(6):1400–6.

Paoletti P, Carrozzi L, Viegi G, Modena P, Ballerin L, Di Pede F, Grado L, Baldacci S, Pedreschi M, Vellutini M. Distribution of bronchial responsiveness in a general population: effect of sex, age, smoking, and level of pulmonary function. *American Journal of Respiratory and Critical Care Medicine* 1995;151(6):1770–7.

Piitulainen E, Tornling G, Eriksson S. Environmental correlates of impaired lung function in non-smokers with severe α_1-antitrypsin deficiency (PiZZ). *Thorax* 1998;53(11):939–43.

Pope CA III, Xu X. Passive cigarette smoke, coal heating, and respiratory symptoms of nonsmoking women in China. *Environmental Health Perspectives* 1993;101(4):314–6.

Rijcken B, Schouten JP, Xu X, Rosner B, Weiss ST. Airway hyperresponsiveness to histamine associated with accelerated decline in FEV_1. *American Journal of Respiratory and Critical Care Medicine* 1995;151(5):1377–82.

Robbins AS, Abbey DE, Lebowitz MD. Passive smoking and chronic respiratory disease symptoms in non-smoking adults. *International Journal of Epidemiology* 1993;22(5):809–17.

Saetta M, Turato G, Maestrelli P, Mapp CE, Fabbri LM. Cellular and structural bases of chronic obstructive pulmonary disease. *American Journal of Respiratory and Critical Care Medicine* 2001;163(6):1304–9.

Samet JM. Definitions and methodology in COPD research. In: Hensley MJ, Saunders NA, editors. *Clinical Epidemiology of Chronic Obstructive Pulmonary Disease*. New York: Marcel Dekker, 1989:1–22.

Samet JM. Adverse effects of smoke exposure on the upper airway. *Tobacco Control* 2004;13(Suppl 1): i57–i60.

Samet JM, Cain WS, Leaderer BP. Environmental tobacco smoke. In: Samet JM, Spengler JD, editors. *Indoor Air Pollution: A Health Perspective*. Baltimore: The Johns Hopkins University Press, 1991:152–60.

Samet JM, Lange P. Longitudinal studies of active and passive smoking. *American Journal of Respiratory and Critical Care Medicine* 1996;154(6 Pt 2):S257–S265.

Sandler DP, Comstock GW, Helsing KJ, Shore DL. Deaths from all causes in non-smokers who lived with smokers. *American Journal of Public Health* 1989;79(2):163–7.

Schwartz J, Zeger S. Passive smoking, air pollution, and acute respiratory symptoms in a diary study of student nurses. *The American Review of Respiratory Disease* 1990;141(1):62–7.

Seymour BW, Pinkerton KE, Friebertshauser KE, Coffman RL, Gershwin LJ. Second-hand smoke is an adjuvant for T helper-2 responses in a murine model of allergy. *The Journal of Immunology* 1997; 159(12):6169–75.

Shephard RJ, Collins R, Silverman F. "Passive" exposure of asthmatic subjects to cigarette smoke. *Environmental Research* 1979;20(2):392–402.

Sippel JM, Pedula KL, Vollmer WM, Buist AS, Osborne ML. Associations of smoking with hospital-based care and quality of life in patients with obstructive airway disease. *Chest* 1999;115(3):691–6.

Stankus RP, Menon PK, Rando RJ, Glindmeyer H, Salvaggio JE, Lehrer SB. Cigarette smoke-sensitive asthma: challenge studies. *Journal of Allergy and Clinical Immunology* 1988;82(3 Pt 1):331–8.

Tarlo SM, Broder I, Corey P, Chan-Yeung M, Ferguson A, Becker A, Warren P, Simons FE, Sherlock C, Okada M, et al. A case-control study of the role of cold symptoms and other historical triggering factors in asthma exacerbations. *Canadian Respiratory Journal* 2000;7(1):42–8.

Thun MJ, Day-Lally C, Myers DG, Calle EE, Flanders WD, Zhu B-P, Namboodiri MM, Heath CW Jr. Trends in tobacco smoking and mortality from cigarette use in Cancer Prevention Studies I (1959 through 1965) and II (1982 through 1988). In: Shopland DR, Burns DM, Garfinkel L, Samet JM, editors. *Changes in Cigarette-Related Disease Risks and Their Implication for Prevention and Control*. Smoking and Tobacco Control Monograph No. 8. Bethesda (MD): U.S. Department of Health and Human Services, Public Health Service, National Institutes of Health, National Cancer Institute, 1997a:305–82. NIH Publication No. 97-4213.

Thun MJ, Myers DG, Day-Lally C, Namboodiri MM, Calle EE, Flanders WD, Adams SL, Heath CW Jr. Age and the exposure-response relationships between cigarette smoking and premature death in Cancer Prevention Study II. In: Shopland DR, Burns DM, Garfinkel L, Samet JM, editors. *Changes in Cigarette-Related Disease Risks and Their Implication for Prevention and Control*. Smoking and Tobacco Control Monograph No. 8. Bethesda (MD): U.S. Department of Health and Human Services, Public Health Service, National Institutes of Health, National Cancer Institute, 1997b:383–413. NIH Publication No. 97-4213.

Thurlbeck WM. Emphysema then and now. *Canadian Respiratory Journal* 1994;1(1):21–39.

Tracey M, Villar A, Dow L, Coggon D, Lampe FC, Holgate ST. The influence of increased bronchial responsiveness, atopy, and serum IgE on decline in FEV1: a longitudinal study in the elderly. *American Journal of Respiratory and Critical Care Medicine* 1995;151(3):656–62.

Trédaniel J, Boffetta P, Saracci R, Hirsch A. Exposure to environmental tobacco smoke and adult nonneoplastic respiratory diseases. *European Respiratory Journal* 1994;7(10):173–85.

Trinder PM, Croft PR, Lewis M. Social class, smoking and the severity of respiratory symptoms in the general population. *Journal of Epidemiology and Community Health* 2000;54(5):340–3.

U.S. Department of Health and Human Services. *The Health Consequences of Involuntary Smoking. A Report of the Surgeon General*. Rockville (MD): U.S. Department of Health and Human Services, Public Health Service, Centers for Disease Control, Center for Health Promotion and Education, Office on Smoking and Health, 1986. DHHS Publication No. (CDC) 87-8398.

U.S. Department of Health and Human Services. *The Health Consequences of Smoking: A Report of the Surgeon General*. Atlanta: U.S. Department of Health and Human Services, Centers for Disease Control and Prevention, National Center for Chronic Disease Prevention and Health Promotion, Office on Smoking and Health, 2004.

U.S. Environmental Protection Agency. *Respiratory Health Effects of Passive Smoking: Lung Cancer and Other Disorders*. Washington: U.S. Environmental Protection Agency, Office of Research and Development, Office of Air and Radiation, 1992. Publication No. EPA/600/6-90/006F.

Venables KM, Chan-Yeung M. Occupational asthma. *Lancet* 1997;349(9063):1465–9.

Weiss ST, Utell MJ, Samet JM. Environmental tobacco smoke exposure and asthma in adults. *Environmental Health Perspectives* 1999;107(Suppl 6):891–5.

White JR, Froeb HF, Kulik JA. Respiratory illness in nonsmokers chronically exposed to tobacco smoke in the work place. *Chest* 1991;100(1):39–43.

Whittemore AS, Perlin SA, DiCiccio Y. Chronic obstructive pulmonary disease in lifelong nonsmokers: results from NHANES. *American Journal of Public Health* 1995;85(5):702–6.

Wiedemann HP, Mahler DA, Loke J, Virgulto JA, Snyder P, Matthay RA. Acute effects of passive smoking on lung function and airway reactivity in asthmatic subjects. *Chest* 1986;89(2):180–5.

Willes SR, Fitzgerald TK, Bascom R. Nasal inhalation challenge studies with sidestream tobacco smoke. *Archives of Environmental Health* 1992;47(3):223–30.

Willes SR, Fitzgerald TK, Permutt T, Proud D, Haley NJ, Bascom R. Acute respiratory response to prolonged, moderate levels of sidestream tobacco smoke. *Journal of Toxicology and Environmental Health, Part A* 1998;53(3):193–209.

Winneke G, Neuf M. Separating the impact of exposure and personality in annoyance response to environmental stressors, particularly odors. *Environment International* 1996;22(1):73–81.

Wright JL. Small airways disease: its role in chronic airflow obstruction. *Seminars in Respiratory Medicine* 1992;13(2):72–84.

Yates DH, Breen H, Thomas PS. Passive smoke inhalation decreases exhaled nitric oxide in normal subjects. *American Journal of Respiratory and Critical Care Medicine* 2001;164(6):1043–6.

Yates DH, Havill K, Thompson MM, Rittano AB, Chu J, Glanville AR. Sidestream smoke inhalation decreases respiratory clearance of ^{99m}Tc-DTPA acutely. *Australian and New Zealand Journal of Medicine* 1996;26(4):513–8.

Yunginger JW, Reed CE, O'Connell EJ, Melton LJ III, O'Fallon WM, Silverstein MD. A community-based study of the epidemiology of asthma: incidence rates, 1964–1983. *American Review of Respiratory Disease* 1992;146(4):888–94.

Zhang J, Qian Z, Kong L, Zhou L, Yan L, Chapman RS. Effects of air pollution on respiratory health of adults in three Chinese cities. *Archives of Environmental Health* 1999;54(6):373–81.

Chapter 10
Control of Secondhand Smoke Exposure

Introduction

This chapter examines measures to control exposure to secondhand smoke in public places, workplaces, and homes, including legislation, education, and approaches based on building designs and operations. The discussion reviews progress toward smokefree indoor spaces in the United States during the past three decades, including approaches that have been employed to reduce exposure, in the context of extensive scientific evidence on health effects and control measures. Table 10.1 provides a chronology of some landmark or exemplary efforts at all levels of government to limit exposure to secondhand smoke.

Historical Perspective

Over the past three decades, substantial progress has been made to control secondhand smoke exposure. The number of public and workplace policies restricting or not allowing smoking has increased; concomitantly, the prevalence of reported exposure to secondhand smoke in public places and workplaces has progressively declined, and the levels of the biomarker cotinine have fallen among U.S. nonsmokers. Cotinine levels dropped sharply during the 1990s, particularly among adults (Centers for Disease Control and Prevention [CDC] 2003). This trend stems from voluntary actions by employers and businesses, declining smoking prevalence, changing patterns of smoking in homes, and increasingly comprehensive and stringent government regulations at the local, state, and national levels (U.S. Department of Health and Human Services [USDHHS] 2000c). The findings and conclusions of previous Surgeon General's reports and other governmental scientific reports have played a critical role in supporting efforts to reduce secondhand smoke exposure, especially policy initiatives. These findings have been frequently cited by persons implementing policy changes.

The first Surgeon General's report to systematically review existing evidence on the health effects of secondhand smoke was the 1972 report, *The Health Consequences of Smoking* (U.S. Department of Health, Education, and Welfare [USDHEW] 1972). This report concluded that an atmosphere contaminated with tobacco smoke could cause discomfort in many persons, and levels of carbon monoxide (CO) measured in experiments in rooms filled with cigarette smoke could, on occasion, be harmful, particularly for individuals with preexisting diseases such as chronic obstructive pulmonary disease and coronary heart disease (CHD) (USDHEW 1972). Thus, the 1972 report raised the possibility that secondhand smoke could be detrimental to the health of some segments of the population. However, this report did not prompt widespread policy changes.

The 1986 report of the Surgeon General, *The Health Consequences of Involuntary Smoking* (USDHHS 1986), has had a great impact on tobacco control policy. It was the first report to focus exclusively on secondhand smoke and remains a milestone in the history of translating scientific evidence on secondhand smoke into policy initiatives. The report reached the following three major conclusions:

1. Involuntary smoking is a cause of disease, including lung cancer, in healthy nonsmokers.

2. The children of parents who smoke, compared with the children of nonsmoking parents, have an increased frequency of respiratory infections, increased respiratory symptoms, and slightly smaller rates of increase in lung function as the lung matures.

3. Simple separation of smokers and nonsmokers within the same air space may reduce, but does not eliminate, exposure of nonsmokers to environmental tobacco smoke (p. vii).

Although the 1986 Surgeon General's report had no direct regulatory consequences at the federal level,

Table 10.1   Summary of milestones in establishing clean indoor air policies in the United States

Year	Event
1971	The Surgeon General proposes a federal smoking ban in public places.
1972	The first report of the Surgeon General to identify secondhand smoke as a health risk is released.
1973	Arizona becomes the first state to restrict smoking in several public places.
	The Civil Aeronautics Board requires no-smoking sections on all commercial airline flights.
1974	Connecticut passes the first state law to apply smoking restrictions in restaurants.
1975	Minnesota passes a statewide law restricting smoking in public places.
1977	Berkeley, California becomes the first community to limit smoking in restaurants and other public places.
1983	San Francisco passes a law to place private workplaces under smoking restrictions.
1986	A report of the Surgeon General focuses entirely on the health consequences of involuntary smoking, proclaiming secondhand smoke a cause of lung cancer in healthy nonsmokers.
	The National Academy of Sciences issues a report on the health consequences of involuntary smoking.
	Americans for Nonsmokers' Rights becomes a national group; it had originally formed as California GASP (Group Against Smoking Pollution).
1987	The U.S. Department of Health and Human Services establishes a smoke-free environment in all of its buildings, affecting 120,000 employees nationwide.
	Minnesota passes a law requiring all hospitals in the state to prohibit smoking by 1990.
	A Gallup Poll finds, for the first time, that a majority (55 percent) of all U.S. adults favor a complete ban on smoking in all public places.
1988	A congressionally mandated smoking ban takes effect on all domestic airline flights of two hours or less.
	New York City's ordinance for clean indoor air takes effect; the ordinance bans or severely limits smoking in various public places and affects 7 million people.
	California implements a statewide ban on smoking aboard all commercial intrastate airplanes, trains, and buses.
1990	A congressionally mandated smoking ban takes effect on all domestic airline flights of six hours or less.
	The U.S. Environmental Protection Agency (EPA) issues a risk assessment draft on secondhand smoke.
1991	The National Institute for Occupational Safety and Health issues a bulletin recommending that secondhand smoke be reduced to the lowest feasible concentration in the workplace.
1992	Hospitals applying for accreditation to the Joint Commission on Accreditation of Healthcare Organizations are required to develop a policy prohibiting smoking by patients, visitors, employees, volunteers, and medical staff.
	The U.S. EPA releases its report classifying secondhand smoke as a Group A (known to be harmful to humans) carcinogen, placing secondhand smoke in the same category as asbestos, benzene, and radon.

Table 10.1   Continued

Year	Event
1993	Los Angeles passes a ban on smoking in all restaurants.
	The U.S. Postal Service eliminates smoking in all facilities.
	Congress enacts a smoke-free policy for Special Supplemental Food Program for Women, Infants, and Children (WIC) clinics.
	A working group of 16 state attorneys general releases recommendations for establishing smoke-free policies in fast-food restaurants.
	Vermont bans smoking in all public buildings and in many private buildings open to the public.
1994	The U.S. Department of Defense prohibits smoking in all indoor military facilities.
	The Occupational Safety and Health Administration proposes a rule that would ban smoking in most U.S. workplaces.
	San Francisco passes a ban on smoking in all restaurants and workplaces.
	The *Pro-Children Act* requires persons who provide federally funded children's services to prohibit smoking in those facilities.
	Utah enacts a law restricting smoking in most workplaces.
1995	New York City passes a comprehensive ordinance effectively banning smoking in most workplaces.
	Maryland enacts a smoke-free policy for all workplaces except hotels, bars, some restaurants, and private clubs.
	California passes comprehensive legislation that prohibits smoking in most enclosed workplaces.
	Vermont's smoking ban is extended to include restaurants, bars, hotels, and motels, except for those establishments holding a cabaret license.
1996	The U.S. Department of Transportation reports that about 80 percent of nonstop scheduled U.S. airline flights between the United States and foreign points will be smoke-free by June 1, 1996.
1997	President Clinton signs an executive order establishing a smoke-free environment for federal employees and all members of the public visiting federally owned facilities.
	The California EPA issues a report determining that secondhand smoke is a toxic air contaminant.
	Settlement is reached in the class action lawsuit brought by flight attendants exposed to secondhand smoke.
1998	The U.S. Senate ends smoking in the Senate's public spaces.
	California law takes effect banning smoking in bars that do not have a separately ventilated smoking area.
	The Minnesota tobacco document depository is created as a result of the tobacco industry settlement with the State of Minnesota and BlueCross BlueShield of Minnesota. U.S. tobacco companies are required to maintain a public depository to house more than 32 million pages of previously secret internal tobacco industry documents.

Table 10.1   Continued

Year	Event
2000	The New Jersey Supreme Court strikes down a local clean indoor air ordinance adopted by the city of Princeton on the grounds that state law preempts local smoking restrictions. A congressionally mandated smoking ban takes effect on all international flights departing from or arriving in the United States.
2002	New York City holds its first hearing on an indoor smoking ban that would include all bars and restaurants. The amended *Clean Indoor Air Act* enacted by the state of New York (Public Health Law, Article 13-E), which took effect July 24, 2003, prohibits smoking in virtually all workplaces, including restaurants and bars. The Michigan Supreme Court refuses to hear an appeal of lower court rulings striking down a local clean indoor air ordinance enacted by the city of Marquette, on the grounds that state law preempts local communities from adopting smoking restrictions in restaurants and bars that are more stringent than the state standard. Delaware enacts a comprehensive smoke-free law, and repeals a preemption provision precluding communities from adopting local smoking restrictions that are more stringent than state law. Florida voters approve a ballot measure that amends the state constitution to require most workplaces and public places, with some exceptions such as bars, to be smoke-free.
2003	Dozens of U.S. airports, including airline clubs, passenger terminals, and nonpublic work areas, are designated as smoke-free. Connecticut and New York enact comprehensive smoke-free laws. Maine enacts a law requiring bars, pool halls, and bingo venues to be smoke-free. State supreme courts in Iowa and New Hampshire strike down local smoke-free ordinances, ruling that they are preempted by state law.
2004	Massachusetts and Rhode Island enact comprehensive smoke-free laws. The International Agency for Research on Cancer issues a new monograph identifying secondhand smoke as "carcinogenic to humans."

Table 10.1   Continued

Year	Event
2005	The Centers for Disease Control and Prevention issues the *Third National Report on Human Exposure to Environmental Chemicals,* which documents that cotinine levels decreased 68 percent for children, 69 percent for adolescents, and 75 percent for adults from the early 1990s to 2002.
	Illinois becomes the second state, after Delaware, to completely repeal a state preemption provision precluding local smoking restrictions that are more stringent than the state standard. Illinois also became the first state to repeal a provision of this kind as a stand-alone action; Delaware had done so in conjunction with the enactment of a comprehensive statewide smoke-free law.
	Washington state passes Initiative Measure 901 (Clean Indoor Air Act).
	Montana enacts legislation that makes most workplaces and restaurants smoke-free.
	North Dakota enacts legislation that makes most workplaces smoke-free.
	Georgia enacts a law that makes some workplaces and public places, including some restaurants, smoke-free. The Georgia law allows communities to continue to enact more comprehensive local smoke-free ordinances.
	Vermont, which already has a law in place making restaurants smoke-free, enacts a provision making bars smoke-free as well.
	Maine, which has already made restaurants and bars smoke-free, strengthens its smoking restrictions in workplaces.
	A comprehensive Rhode Island law enacted in 2004 that makes workplaces, restaurants, and bars smoke-free took effect, and was further strengthened through the removal of two temporary exemptions.
2006	The District of Columbia enacts legislation requiring most workplaces and public places to be smoke-free. Bars and bar areas in restaurants are required to be smoke-free as of January 1, 2007.
	Colorado and New Jersey enact legislation requiring most workplaces and public places, including restaurants and bars, to be smoke-free. Both laws exempt casino floor areas.
	Utah, which already had a law in place mandating smoke-free restaurants, enacts legislation requiring most workplaces and bars to also be smoke-free.
	Arkansas enacts legislation requiring many workplaces and public places to be smoke-free; restaurants and bars that deny entry to persons under 21 years of age are exempt.
	Arkansas enacts a separate law making it illegal to smoke in a vehicle when a child is present who is younger than six years of age or who weighs less than 60 pounds.
	Puerto Rico enacts legislation requiring most workplaces and public places, including restaurants, bars, and casinos, to be smoke-free. The law also makes it illegal to smoke in a private vehicle with a child in a child's seat.

the report provided an important impetus to a trend that was already under way in California and, to a lesser extent, in other states toward local ordinances that restrict smoking in enclosed public places and workplaces. In fact, the three conclusions noted above (particularly the third one) were cited in the "Findings and Intent" section of many of these ordinances (Rigotti and Pashos 1991; National Cancer Institute [NCI] 2000b; American Lung Association [ALA] 2005; American Nonsmokers' Rights Foundation [ANR] 2005d). The 1986 Surgeon General's report also provided an impetus to the adoption of voluntary (or private) smoking restrictions by businesses (USDHHS 1986). The year 1986 also saw the publication of a report by the National Research Council (NRC 1986b) of the National Academy of Sciences on the health effects of secondhand smoke, which also concluded that secondhand smoke exposure is a cause of lung cancer in nonsmokers.

A second milestone in establishing a scientific foundation for efforts to reduce secondhand smoke exposure was the publication of the 1992 U.S. Environmental Protection Agency (EPA) report, *Respiratory Health Effects of Passive Smoking: Lung Cancer and Other Disorders* (USEPA 1992). The report concluded that secondhand smoke is a Group A carcinogen (i.e., a carcinogen that has been shown to cause cancer in humans). Specifically, the report found that secondhand smoke is a human lung carcinogen estimated to be responsible for approximately 3,000 lung cancer deaths of U.S. nonsmokers annually. The report also concluded that secondhand smoke exposure is causally associated with a number of health conditions in children, including lower respiratory tract infections, an increased prevalence of fluid in the middle ear, and additional episodes and an increased severity of symptoms in children with asthma.

Although the EPA report had no direct regulatory effect, the report provided additional scientific evidence and authoritative conclusions supporting the need for the adoption of smoking restrictions by governmental bodies and private businesses. It was widely cited by local advocates and policymakers, particularly the conclusion that secondhand smoke is a Group A carcinogen. The report helped to accelerate the trend to enact local clean indoor air ordinances and, in particular, local ordinances that went beyond restricting smoking to designated areas to eliminating smoking altogether in certain settings. Anticipating the report's potential impact, cigarette manufacturers made a concerted effort to block or delay its publication (Bero and Glantz 1993; Muggli et al. 2004) and filed a lawsuit challenging its conclusions once it

was published (*Flue-Cured Tobacco Cooperative Stabilization Corp. v. United States Environmental Protection Agency* [M.D.N.C. June 22, 1993], *cited in* 8.2 TPLR 3.97 [1993]). A 1998 U.S. District Court ruling vacated the report with regard to lung cancer based on procedural and scientific concerns (*Flue-Cured Tobacco Cooperative Stabilization Corp. v. United States Environmental Protection Agency*, 4 F. Supp. 2d 435 [M.D.N.C. 1998]). However, this court ruling was voided in 2002 when the U.S. Court of Appeals found that the report was not subject to judicial review, and the legal action was subsequently dismissed (*Flue-Cured Tobacco Cooperative Stabilization Corp. v. The United States Environmental Protection Agency*, No. 98-2407 [4th Cir., December 11, 2002], *cited in* 17.7 TPLR 2.472 [2003]).

A third milestone in assessing the evidence on secondhand smoke was the 1997 publication of the California Environmental Protection Agency (Cal/EPA) report, *Health Effects of Exposure to Environmental Tobacco Smoke* (Cal/EPA 1997), which was also disseminated in 1999 as a NCI monograph (NCI 1999). This was the first major report to conclude definitively that secondhand smoke exposure is a cause of heart disease in nonsmokers. The report also quantified the health burden that secondhand smoke imposes by providing ranges of estimates for the annual morbidity and mortality among U.S. nonsmokers from various health conditions attributable to secondhand smoke exposure. The estimates of deaths attributed to secondhand smoke in this report were widely cited in local policy debates. In addition, the finding that secondhand smoke exposure was a cause of heart disease was particularly significant because the potential impact on heart disease morbidity and mortality rates was greater than the impact as a cause of lung cancer. This conclusion was also a source of concern among persons already diagnosed with heart disease and persons with a family history of other risk factors for heart disease. A new, yet large, constituency thus became concerned about the risks from secondhand smoke exposure.

The 2001 report of the Surgeon General on women and smoking concluded that epidemiologic and other data support a causal relationship between secondhand tobacco smoke exposure from their spouse and CHD mortality among women who were nonsmokers. In addition, a 2002 CDC report estimated that secondhand smoke exposure causes more than 35,000 deaths annually of U.S. nonsmokers, which was the lower endpoint of the estimate in the Cal/EPA report (Cal/EPA 1997; USDHHS 2001; CDC 2002). A 2004 commentary published in the *British Medical Journal* reviewed recent evidence on the acute cardiovascular effects of even brief secondhand smoke exposures and suggested that clinicians should advise patients who already have or are at special risk for heart disease to avoid indoor environments where there are likely to be smokers (Pechacek and Babb 2004).

International reports reached similar conclusions on the causation of disease and other adverse health effects from exposure to secondhand smoke (National Health and Medical Research Council 1997; Scientific Committee on Tobacco and Health 1998; World Health Organization [WHO] 1999). By 2000, there was little debate within the scientific community as to whether secondhand smoke causes diseases and other adverse health effects in children and adults. Two reports, the 2000 National Toxicology Program's *9th Report on Carcinogens* (USDHHS 2000b) and the 2004 International Agency for Research on Cancer (IARC) Monograph, *Evaluation of Carcinogenic Risks to Humans: Tobacco Smoke and Involuntary Smoking* (IARC 2004), further buttressed the case that secondhand smoke exposure poses serious health risks. Both reports concluded that secondhand smoke is a human carcinogen and a cause of lung cancer in humans. Although estimates differ on the magnitude of the excess risk, researchers continue to study the potential role of secondhand smoke as a cause of other diseases.

A growing number of local communities and, more recently, states have adopted increasingly comprehensive clean indoor air laws. This momentum drew on the strong body of scientific evidence and related conclusions; the efforts of public health officials at the local, state, and national levels who stepped forward as champions of this issue; and the nongovernmental organizations and grassroots advocates who built the case for "nonsmokers' rights." Numerous employers have also implemented voluntary smoke-free workplace policies.

The tobacco industry has attempted to counter this movement toward widespread control of exposure to secondhand smoke. The industry recognized as early as 1978 that the secondhand smoke issue posed a serious threat to its interests. In 1978, the Roper Organization surveyed the public for the Tobacco Institute and characterized the increasing public concern about the health risks posed by secondhand smoke as "the most dangerous development to the viability of the tobacco industry that has yet occurred" (Roper 1978, p. 4). The report also noted the concern that "What the smoker does to himself may be his business, but what the smoker does to the non-smoker is quite a different matter" (p. 4) and predicted that, as the belief that secondhand smoke exposure could harm nonsmokers

became more widespread, public support for smoking restrictions would continue to grow (Roper 1978). In 1998, the Minnesota Tobacco Document Depository was created as a result of the tobacco industry settlement with the state of Minnesota and BlueCross BlueShield of Minnesota. U.S. tobacco companies were required to maintain and provide public access to more than 32 million pages of previously secret internal documents. A review of these documents revealed that the tobacco industry feared that governmental regulations on smoking in public places would affect profits (Muggli et al. 2001). This same report and many others based on the documents showed that the industry attempted to influence worldwide public opinion on the health effects of secondhand smoke by producing its own scientific research. Other tobacco industry documents also indicate that cigarette manufacturers feared that increasingly stringent smoking restrictions in workplaces would prompt some smokers to quit or reduce their smoking (Hirschhorn and Bialous 2001; Fichtenberg and Glantz 2002; Drope et al. 2004).

The tobacco industry documents suggest that this concern has been a major underlying motivation for efforts by cigarette manufacturers to prevent or reverse the adoption of any restrictions on smoking. These efforts have included casting doubts on scientific findings regarding the health effects of secondhand smoke and characterizing smoking restrictions as unnecessary and as infringements on the rights of smokers. The tobacco industry has maintained that hospitality businesses would suffer economically from the restrictions themselves, which are also characterized as burdensome and difficult to implement. At the same time, the tobacco industry has presented "common courtesy," separate nonsmoking and smoking sections, and, more recently, ventilation approaches as sufficient and less intrusive alternatives to smoke-free policies (Davis et al. 1990; Barnes and Bero 1996; Hirschhorn and Bialous 2001; Drope et al. 2004). When local clean indoor air ordinances have been adopted, cigarette manufacturers have sought to reverse them by working with organizations such as state and local restaurant associations and other hospitality business interests to organize petition drives and place the ordinances on the ballot (Traynor et al. 1993; NCI 2000b; Ritch and Begay 2001; Tsoukalas and Glantz 2003). Other tobacco industry efforts include filing lawsuits challenging the ordinances on a variety of grounds, organizing media campaigns attacking the ordinances, undermining implementation of local and state smoke-free laws, and securing passage of state laws that preempt local smoking restrictions that exceed the state standard (Kluger 1996; Siegel et al. 1997; Dearlove et al. 2002; Nixon et al. 2004; NCI 2005). Cigarette manufacturers also collaborated with other organizations to defeat or weaken statewide clean indoor air legislation (Kluger 1996; Magzamen and Glantz 2001). At one time, cigarette firms also tried to discourage private employers from adopting voluntary smoke-free workplace policies, but those efforts seem to have ended (Landman 2000).

Smoking Restrictions in Public Places and Workplaces

Although some states and cities had already passed measures to reduce secondhand smoke exposure, the momentum to regulate smoking in public places increased in 1986 when reports by the Surgeon General (USDHHS 1986) and the NRC (1986b) concluded that secondhand smoke is a cause of lung cancer in nonsmokers. These reports became an impetus to increasingly common and restrictive government and private business policies limiting smoking in public places (Rigotti and Pashos 1991; NCI 2000a; ALA 2005; ANR 2005d). The designation of secondhand smoke as a Group A carcinogen by the EPA stimulated even further restrictions on smoking in public places and workplaces (USEPA 1992; Brownson et al. 1995).

Federal Government Smoking Restrictions

In the United States, the most progress in adopting comprehensive laws making public places and workplaces smoke-free has occurred at the local level and, more recently, at the state level. Progress has been far more rapid at the local level, particularly in the early years of the campaign for smoke-free environments. Federal initiatives in this area have been relatively limited. Federal smoking restrictions adopted to date are limited to a few settings, most notably airplanes, facilities providing federally funded services to children, and federally owned facilities, including military installations (see "Federal Laws and Regulations" later in this chapter). Although these policies affect a large number of people and carry symbolic importance, the policies cover only a small portion of the public places and workplaces where people are exposed to secondhand smoke.

Local Ordinances

The strongest, most comprehensive smoke-free laws have typically originated at the local level (NCI 2000b; USDHHS 2000c). Local smoke-free policy

efforts have generally met with greater success than federal or—until recently—state initiatives (NCI 2000b). More than 110 local ordinances with 100 percent smoke-free provisions had been adopted in the United States before the first state law with such a provision (for restaurants) was enacted in Vermont in 1993. One reason for this is that local governmental bodies tend to be relatively responsive to public sentiment, which increasingly favors comprehensive smoke-free legislation. Local smoke-free policy initiatives also typically engage communities in an intensive process of public education and debate. This process raises public awareness regarding the health risks that secondhand smoke exposure poses to nonsmokers, increases public support for policy measures that provide protections from these risks, and changes public attitudes and norms regarding the social acceptability of smoking. These changes, in turn, lay the groundwork for successfully enacting and implementing the proposed policy, which reinforces and accelerates these changes in the norm (NCI 2000b). Several states, some with and some without previous experience with local smoke-free laws, have attempted in recent years to follow a similar process at the state level and have successfully enacted and implemented statewide smoke-free laws, some of which are quite comprehensive (CDC 2005b). However, local smoke-free air laws continue to play an important role in allowing comprehensive protections to be put in place in communities in states that are not prepared to enact comprehensive smoke-free legislation on a statewide basis (Jacobson and Wasserman 1997; NCI 2000b).

Until recently, state clean indoor air laws lagged behind their local counterparts in terms of strength and breadth of settings covered. Despite this progress at the state level, comprehensive clean indoor air laws at the local level continue to be more numerous, more widespread, and more successful.

The modern era of local ordinances for clean indoor air began in the early 1980s, following the enactment of clean indoor air laws in cities and in several states (Table 10.1) (NCI 2000b). In 1977, Berkeley, California became the first community to limit smoking in restaurants and in other public places. After the release of the 1986 Surgeon General's report on the health consequences of secondhand smoke, the rates at which local smoking restrictions were adopted accelerated (Figure 10.1). By 1988, nearly 400 local clean indoor air ordinances had been enacted throughout the United States (Pertschuk and Shopland 1989). Since 1989, this trend has become even more pronounced (Rigotti and Pashos 1991; USDHHS 2000c),

Figure 10.1   Number of municipalities with local laws covering smoking in workplaces, restaurants, and enclosed public places, generally, 1978–2006

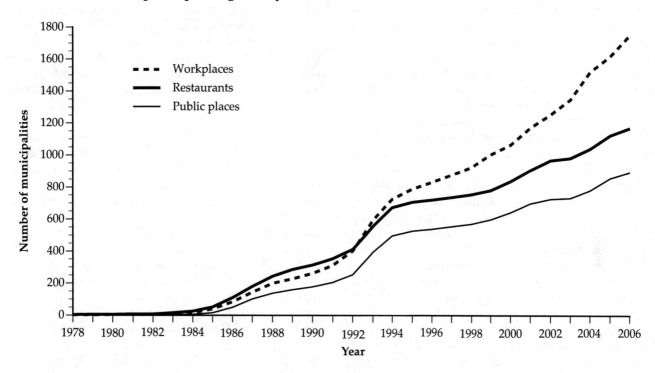

Source: American Nonsmokers' Rights Foundation, unpublished data, March 31, 2006.

and, as noted earlier, the publication of the 1992 EPA report provided an additional impetus.

A key factor in the widespread adoption of clean indoor air ordinances in U.S. communities during the past 20 years has been the emergence of a grassroots nonsmokers' rights movement (Kluger 1996; Glantz and Balbach 2000; NCI 2000b). Originating in California and gradually spreading nationwide, this movement initially consisted of community activists who were concerned about having to breathe secondhand smoke in restaurants and other public places and workplaces (Kluger 1996; NCI 2000b). Over time, the movement drew on the growing scientific evidence that was becoming available showing that secondhand smoke is not just an annoyance but a health hazard. In addition, the nonsmokers' rights activists increasingly joined forces with public health practitioners who were becoming aware of this fact. These practitioners were also beginning to realize that approaches that focused on fostering changes in social environments and norms were likely to have a greater impact in reducing tobacco use than strategies that focused on changing individual behavior. The

movement mobilized increasing numbers of nonsmokers who insisted that measures be taken to protect them (Kluger 1996; NCI 2000b). These efforts were spearheaded by organizations such as ANR, the three voluntaries—American Cancer Society (ACS), American Heart Association, and ALA—and loosely organized grassroots groups such as the Group Against Smoking Pollution (GASP). The groups behind this movement realized that the best chance of success lay at the local level after efforts at the state level had yielded disappointing results. Public health practitioners and advocates closely observed the experience in California, where efforts to adopt statewide clean indoor air protections were defeated in the California Legislature, and two statewide ballot initiatives (Propositions 5 and 10) were defeated in 1978 and 1980. Cigarette manufacturers had heavily financed opposition campaigns against all of those efforts (Kluger 1996; Glantz and Balbach 2000).

A model approach then emerged, first in California and subsequently in other states (Glantz 1987). The state tobacco control movement organized local coalitions of public health practitioners and advocates who engaged in an intensive process of public education and community mobilization. Most of these efforts were in place before launching a public campaign supporting a particular ordinance. The local coalitions assessed attitudes of the public and policymakers and often initiated a campaign when public support for the proposed ordinance was evident. On the other hand, ordinances were also introduced with less readiness to push tobacco control, as a process for change and as an educational approach. The ordinance itself was drafted to conform to the level of public readiness, with provisions only as strong as the public was willing to support. Similarly, the local coalitions did not bring an ordinance before a local governmental body until there was clear support from a majority of the policymakers. The vigorous debate that typically occurred after an ordinance was officially introduced provided substantial opportunities for health advocates to generate unpaid media coverage, further contributing to public education and public support. Public education and awareness contributed to changes in social norms regarding the acceptability of smoking in public places and workplaces—changes that were then solidified by the implementation of the ordinance. In the words of Stanton Glantz, one of the founders of ANR, "Ordinances only work to the extent that they sanctify a change in public attitudes" (Glantz 1998, p. 31).

In some states, once several communities had adopted ordinances, a number of other communities followed fairly quickly. The ordinances spread as residents and policymakers elsewhere in the state learned from the experiences of others that these measures were popular and workable and that the problems the opponents predicted—most notably economic hardship and enforcement difficulties—did not occur. In addition, as more communities in a state adopted ordinances, it became easier for one community to find and use a successful experience with an ordinance in a similar community as a model or example.

This model, first applied in California, was later applied to varying extents and with varying degrees of success in a number of other states, including Massachusetts, New Mexico, New York, Oregon, Texas, West Virginia, and Wisconsin. Ultimately, the majority of states where local smoke-free ordinances were not precluded by preemptive provisions in state law saw at least some communities enact such ordinances (NCI 2000b; Siegel 2002; Rogers 2003; ANR 2005d).

The first national organization to focus on the need for a local clean indoor air policy was ANR, which is still the recognized leader in the field. ANR has supported local efforts in a number of ways:

providing technical assistance, training, and strategic guidance to local coalitions; keeping them informed of the latest policy trends and opposition tactics; linking a coalition with local coalitions in other parts of the country that were encountering similar experiences; developing "best practices" guidelines (ANR 2002); and disseminating model ordinances. ANR maintains a database of local ordinances and their provisions in order to track progress in eliminating unintended loopholes and addressing legal issues (<http://no-smoke.org>).

In recent years, local progress in enacting clean indoor air policies has been furthered in some states by support from state tobacco control programs and other state organizations to develop and maintain a network of local coalitions through technical assistance and training on evidence-based tobacco control approaches, and through funding and a dedicated staff. California, Massachusetts, and Oregon were among the first states to achieve this level of organization, and other states followed suit (Siegel 2002). The American Stop Smoking Intervention Study for Cancer Prevention (ASSIST) was a major federal tobacco control initiative carried out during the 1990s, under the auspices of the NCI and the ACS (NCI 2005; see also <http://dccps.nci.nih.gov/tcrb/monographs/16/index.html>). Seventeen states received funding to conduct population-based policy interventions in four areas, including smoke-free air. State tobacco control programs in the ASSIST states were encouraged to support local and regional smoke-free policy efforts that included developing and maintaining community coalitions and providing technical assistance and dedicated staff. As a result of this focus, several ASSIST states made significant gains, such as enacting strong local smoke-free ordinances. Examples include Colorado, Maine, Minnesota, New Jersey, New Mexico, New York, and West Virginia (ANR 2005a). The experiences of these ASSIST states during this initiative also laid the groundwork for other subsequent smoke-free policy successes at local and state levels, once these states had transitioned to funding through CDC's National Tobacco Control Program. Robert Wood Johnson Foundation's SmokeLess States program also made a significant contribution to local progress in this area by highlighting a local clean indoor air policy as one of its priorities, by encouraging the state coalitions it funded to work with state tobacco control programs and other state organizations to support local clean indoor air policy efforts, and by providing these coalitions with sophisticated guidance (AMA 1998). In addition, studies in Massachusetts found that state funding of local boards of health was correlated with the adoption of local tobacco control ordinances, including local clean indoor air ordinances (Bartosch and Pope 2002; Skeer et al. 2004).

As a result of these local clean indoor air policy efforts, hundreds of U.S. communities have adopted some type of local smoking restriction. ANR reported that as of April 17, 2006, a total of 2,216 U.S. municipalities had some sort of smoking restriction in place, including 352 municipalities with smoke-free workplace ordinances, 292 municipalities with smoke-free restaurant ordinances, and 215 municipalities with smoke-free bar ordinances. In addition, 135 municipalities have adopted ordinances requiring all three settings to be smoke-free (ANR 2006a). These numbers mean that in the United States at that time, 29.0 percent of the people were covered by a local or state smoke-free workplace law, 40.3 percent were covered by a local or state smoke-free restaurant law, 31.3 percent were covered by a local or state smoke-free bar law, and 16.9 percent were covered by a comprehensive local or state law that made workplaces, restaurants, and bars smoke-free (ANR 2006b). Local jurisdictions that have recently enacted relatively comprehensive smoke-free legislation include several major metropolitan areas: Austin, Boston, Chicago, Columbus, Dallas, Indianapolis, Lincoln, and New York city. In the case of the first two cities, the municipal legislation was followed by a comprehensive statewide law (ANR 2006c).

As of March 2006, 896 local ordinances restrict or ban smoking in public places other than restaurants and workplaces (Figure 10.1). These ordinances specifically designate which agencies are responsible for enforcement: 27 percent of the ordinances cite health departments, 23 percent cite boards of health, 18 percent cite city or county administrators, 24 percent cite law enforcement, and 21 percent cite other agencies; 17 percent do not specify an enforcement agency or mechanism (ANR unpublished data, March 31, 2006). Because some municipalities have designated more than one enforcement agency, the percentages are not expected to add up to 100 percent. The implementation and enforcement of this legislation are just as important as its passage in achieving the policy goals (Nordstrom and DeStefano 1995; Weber et al. 2003).

The tobacco industry was quick to recognize the progress that advocates were making in advancing smoking restrictions at the local level. As early as 1986, Raymond Pritchard, Chairman of the Board of Brown and Williamson Tobacco Company, acknowledged that "our record in defeating state smoking restrictions has been reasonably good. Unfortunately, our record with respect to local measures—that is, in cities

and counties across the country—has been somewhat less encouraging....We must somehow do a better job than we have in the past in getting our side of the story told to City Councils and County Commissions. Over time we can lose the battle over smoking restrictions as decisively in bits and pieces—at the local level—as with state or federal measures" (Pritchard 1986, pp. 86, 88). As noted above, the tobacco industry has responded to local clean indoor air policy efforts by working with hospitality and gaming interests and other organizations to prevent local ordinances from being adopted and to attempt to reverse them once they have been enacted (Kluger 1996; Dearlove et al. 2002; Mandel and Glantz 2004; Nixon et al. 2004). One major approach that the industry has employed to accomplish both goals is supporting state laws that preempt local smoking restrictions that are stronger than the state standard (Siegel et al. 1997; Henson et al. 2002). During the mid-1990s, the tobacco industry made the passage of state preemption laws one of its major political objectives and experienced significant success in this area (Siegel et al. 1997; CDC 1999). Once in place, these laws have proved difficult to repeal, although there has been more success in this regard in recent years. To date, two states—Delaware and Illinois—have completely repealed a state preemption provision precluding local smoking restrictions (CDC 2005a). Delaware did so in 2002 in conjunction with enacting a comprehensive statewide smoke-free law, while Illinois did so in 2005 as a stand-alone action. In addition, several other states, including Louisiana, Nevada, North Carolina, and Tennessee, rescinded such preemptive provisions for certain settings. As of December 31, 2004, a total of 19 states had a preemptive provision in place for at least one of three settings—government worksites, private-sector worksites, and restaurants—up from 17 states at the end of 1998 (CDC 2005a). A *Healthy People 2010* objective calls for no states to have preemptive tobacco control laws in place by 2010 (USDHHS 2000a). Selected recent legislative and legal developments in this area are listed in Table 10.1.

In general, advocacy and public health organizations have resisted efforts to seek a statewide clean indoor air law until a state has had a critical mass of local ordinances in place for some time. This position is based on the concern that, in the absence of experience with implementing such ordinances and the grassroots support they generate, the final state legislation adopted is likely to be weak and, in many cases, to preempt stronger local ordinances. Moreover, even in cases where state smoke-free laws are not preemptive, they may lead to a decrease in the enactment of local smoke-free ordinances, perhaps because local policymakers perceive that the issue of secondhand smoke protection has been adequately addressed at the state level (Jacobson and Wasserman 1997). This concern has been borne out by experience in a number of states. The opposition to what were perceived as premature state clean indoor air laws was also based on the concern that even if a state that lacked pre-existing local ordinances succeeded in enacting a strong, nonpreemptive state law, the public would not be prepared to accept it because of the absence of the intensive public education, debate, and changes in norms that typically occur before the adoption of local ordinances, making it difficult to implement the law (Jacobson and Wasserman 1999; NCI 2000b; USDHHS 2000b).

Recent progress in enacting statewide smoke-free laws suggests that these concerns, while remaining valid in many cases, may not apply in certain situations (CDC 2005a,b). Several states (e.g., Connecticut, Delaware, Florida, and Rhode Island) that had little or no prior experience with local smoke-free ordinances have recently been able to enact relatively comprehensive statewide smoke-free laws (although in most cases these laws have retained preemption provisions where these provisions were already in place). Other states (e.g., Maine, Massachusetts, and New York) that have recently enacted relatively comprehensive statewide smoke-free laws had had previous experience with local ordinances. With time, the relative success experienced by these two categories of states in implementing their laws will provide insights into the issues described above. The experiences of these states will also shed light on a related question: whether states where local clean indoor air ordinances are preempted can achieve superior public health protections by first seeking to reverse the preemptive provision and pursue local smoke-free ordinances, or by skipping this step and proceeding directly to the pursuit of a comprehensive statewide smoke-free law (CDC 2005a,b).

State Laws and Regulations

Healthy People 2010 objective 27-13 calls for all states to adopt laws making enclosed workplaces and public places smoke-free (USDHHS 2000a). The first substantive modern state laws restricting smoking in public places were enacted in Arizona, Connecticut, and Minnesota in 1973–1975 (Table 10.1). Over the years, many other states enacted smoking restrictions (Kluger 1996; CDC 2005b). However, few of these restrictions were strong or comprehensive in

coverage. As recently as 2001, only a single state—California—had a statewide law in place making most enclosed workplaces and public places, including restaurants and bars, smoke-free (CDC 2005b). In 2002, Delaware became the second state to enact a comprehensive state law of this kind; this law also rescinded a preemption provision that had prevented communities from adopting local ordinances that were more stringent than the state standard. Since 2002, there has been rapid progress in this area, with a number of other states enacting and implementing similarly comprehensive smoke-free laws.

As of December 31, 2005, 49 states and the District of Columbia have mandated smoke-free indoor air to some degree or in some public places. These restrictions vary widely, from limited restrictions on public transportation to comprehensive restrictions in other public places and in worksites (Figure 10.2) (CDC, Office on Smoking and Health [OSH], State Tobacco Activities Tracking and Evaluation System, unpublished data; <http://www.cdc.gov/tobacco/statesystem>).

In addition (also as of December 31, 2005), 44 states and the District of Columbia have restricted smoking in government worksites: 22 states limit smoking to designated areas, 6 states require either no smoking or designated smoking areas with separate ventilation, and 16 states prohibit smoking entirely. Of the 31 states that restrict smoking in private worksites, 16 limit smoking to designated areas, 11 require a complete ban, and 4 require separate ventilation for smoking areas. Of the 34 states that regulate smoking in restaurants, only 11 states completely prohibit smoking (Delaware, Florida, Idaho, Maine, Massachusetts, Montana, New York, North Dakota, Rhode Island, Utah, and Washington). California and Connecticut require either a complete ban or separate ventilation for smoking areas (CDC, OSH, State Tobacco Activities Evaluation System, unpublished data; <http://www.cdc.gov/tobacco/statesystem>). As of April 2006, 11 states plus the District of Columbia have enacted comprehensive smoke-free laws throughout their jurisdictions that, when the laws take full effect as implemented in practice, will require almost all enclosed workplaces and public places, including restaurants and bars, to be smoke-free: California, Colorado, Connecticut, Delaware, Maine, Massachusetts, New Jersey, New York, Rhode Island, Utah, and Washington. The Colorado and New Jersey laws exempt casino floor areas. Together, these locales account for approximately 31 percent of the U.S. population. This estimate does not include the population covered by comprehensive local smoke-free laws in states

Figure 10.2 Cumulative number of state laws and amendments enacted for clean indoor air, 1963–2005

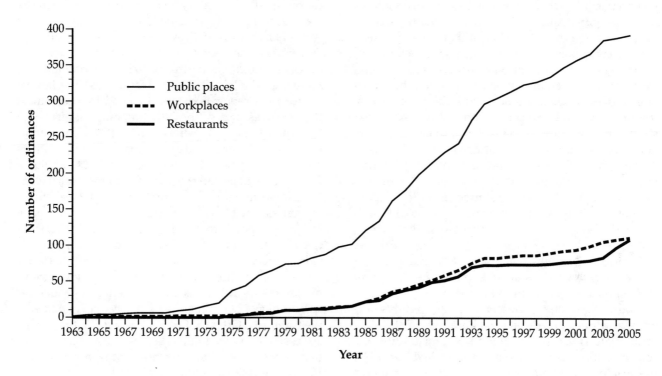

Source: U.S. Department of Health and Human Services, National Institutes of Health, National Cancer Institute, State Cancer Legislative Database, unpublished data, June 30, 2005.

that have not implemented comparable statewide legislation.

Of the numerous factors that appear to have contributed to this progress, perhaps the most important has been the adoption of comprehensive local clean indoor air ordinances in hundreds of communities across the United States, including high-profile cities such as New York City and Boston. These localities have demonstrated that the ordinances are popular, can be implemented with little difficulty, are met with high levels of compliance, and do not have a negative economic impact on restaurants and bars (New York City Department of Finance 2004) (see "Trends in Public Support for Smoking Restrictions," "Compliance with Workplace Smoking Policies," and "Economic Impact of Smoking Restrictions on the Hospitality Industry," later in this chapter). The trend toward these ordinances has also led some state restaurant associations and other hospitality interests to conclude that smoke-free laws were inevitable and it was preferable that these laws be implemented at the state level, where they would apply to all

communities. As a result, state restaurant associations in several states have shifted from opposing state clean indoor air legislation to taking a neutral or even a supportive position (Lindsay 2003; von Ziel-bauer 2003). The same concern that these laws should apply across the board has also led restaurant associations and proprietors in some states to advocate for state laws that applied to all types of hospitality businesses, including not only restaurants but also bars and gaming venues. More recently, the experiences of other states and even other countries (such as Ireland) in implementing comprehensive smoke-free laws should help to allay concerns, discredit opponents' claims, foster the sense of a natural and inevitable progression toward making workplaces and public places smoke-free, and convince state policymakers to emulate these examples.

Another major contributing factor to the adoption of comprehensive state laws has been the growing tendency to view smoke-free policies in hospitality businesses in the context of worker protection and workplace safety (beginning with the California state law), rather than as measures designed primarily to protect patrons. When framed in this context, a majority of the public and policymakers in many jurisdictions has come to the conclusion that restaurant and bar workers should be afforded the same health protections as employees in other occupations. Finally, the mounting scientific evidence regarding the health effects of secondhand smoke has clearly played a role in convincing the public and policymakers that strong steps needed to be taken to protect nonsmokers, including nonsmoking employees, from harm.

Even earlier, Maryland and Washington had implemented statewide workplace smoking restrictions through regulations, as opposed to legislation. In 1994, the Maryland Occupational Safety and Health Advisory Board proposed a regulation that would prohibit smoking in most workplaces in the state, including restaurants and bars (*Maryland Register* 1994). Despite strong statewide public support from both nonsmokers and smokers for these restrictions, the tobacco industry aggressively challenged this proposal and questioned the legal authority of the state to regulate smoking through an administrative rule rather than by statute (Shopland et al. 1995). In 1995, the original regulation was modified by legislative action to permit some exceptions for the hospitality industry, and the rules then went into effect. Also in 1994, the Washington State Department of Labor and Industries enacted an extensive indoor workplace smoking ban. Unlike the Maryland regulation, the Washington regulation applied only to office workplaces and did not cover hospitality workplaces such as restaurants and bars. A 1985 Washington state law restricting smoking in public places had specified exemptions for hospitality workplaces, and a temporary injunction aimed at removing the exemptions was dismissed by the state court. The ban went into effect without litigation (LeMier 1999). Health advocates in Washington have recently utilized several different approaches to attempt to extend the state's workplace smoking ban to cover hospitality settings, including the most recent effort to place a comprehensive measure that passed on the November 2005 ballot that makes almost all public places and workplaces in the state smoke-free. In 1990, the governor of North Dakota issued an executive order requiring state buildings under his jurisdiction to be smoke-free (George A. Sinner, memorandum, April 25, 1990).

California is currently considering regulating secondhand smoke as a toxic air contaminant. The process began in 2001 when Cal/EPA initiated an evaluation of the extent of Californians' secondhand smoke exposure and of the health effects associated with this exposure. In September 2005, Cal/EPA's Air Resources Board (ARB) released a report, *Proposed Identification of Environmental Tobacco Smoke as a Toxic Air Contaminant* (Cal/EPA 2005). This report updates and expands on a previous report on the health effects of secondhand smoke that Cal/EPA had published in 1997 (Cal/EPA 1997). NCI recognized the importance of the report and saw the need to disseminate it broadly as part of the NCI Smoking and Tobacco Control Monograph Series (NCI 1999). The report included revisions made in response to suggestions received during a public comment period following a 2003 release of a draft version of the report, as well as a section containing these comments and the agency's responses. The final report also incorporated revisions made in response to recommendations received from the California Scientific Review Panel on Toxic Air Contaminants, which had reviewed the document. The panel has approved the report and has recommended that ARB list secondhand smoke as a toxic air contaminant. The panel has also recommended that the California Office of Environmental Health Hazard Assessment list secondhand smoke as a toxic air contaminant that may disproportionately impact children. In January 2006, following a public hearing, the ARB formally designated secondhand smoke as a toxic air contaminant. This means that secondhand smoke will be listed as such a contaminant in the California Code of Regulations, and that the ARB is required by law to assess whether there is a need to further regulate outdoor secondhand smoke exposure among California residents.

Federal Laws and Regulations

As already noted, federal actions in this area have been comparatively few and relatively narrow in scope. Initial efforts at the federal level to control secondhand smoke exposure were largely directed at commercial airline flights. The flight attendants took an early and important role in advocating for smoke-free aircraft (Holm and Davis 2004). Their efforts began as early as 1966 and continued for decades, until smoke-free air travel was finally achieved in 2000.

In 1969, Ralph Nader petitioned the Federal Aviation Administration (FAA) to completely ban smoking on all passenger flights. Nader argued that smoking not only annoyed nonsmokers but also posed a significant danger to the health and safety of everyone on the airplane. Attorney John Banzhaf III then called for the FAA to separate smokers from nonsmokers on all domestic flights. The FAA rejected both requests. However, Surgeon General Jesse Steinfeld's 1971 public announcement about the harmfulness of indoor smoking and his call for a national nonsmokers' bill of rights (Steinfeld 1983) was received positively by the American public, possibly, in part, because most of the U.S. population did not smoke. Legislation was introduced in the U.S. Congress in 1971 (Holm and Davis 2004) to restrict smoking aboard all commercial aircraft, but the measure died in committee. However, that same year United Airlines voluntarily began to offer smoking and nonsmoking seating, and within a year most major U.S. carriers had followed suit, although not all airlines offered this option and open smoking was still the norm on many commercial flights. Furthermore, because these policies were voluntary, they were subject to change.

Using the conclusions of the 1972 Surgeon General's report (USDHEW 1972), Nader petitioned the Civil Aeronautics Board (CAB) to ban smoking aboard commercial aircraft on health grounds. The CAB at that time controlled most aspects of commercial aviation and was considered more consumer-oriented than the FAA. However, a December 1971 study examined the health effects of smoking aboard military and civilian transport aircraft and found, counter to data collected subsequently, no "persuasive evidence that exposure to tobacco smoke, in concentrations likely to occur in aircraft (assuming normal ventilation rates), is injurious to the health of nonsmokers" (Kluger 1996, p. 373). Despite low levels of measured pollutants, the study found that more than 60 percent of all nonsmoking passengers and 38 percent of smokers indicated they were annoyed by tobacco smoke from other passengers during a flight. The study was conducted jointly by several agencies within the U.S. DHEW, the U.S. Department of Transportation, and the FAA.

Citing a lack of supporting health data, the CAB rejected a complete ban on smoking and instead issued a rule based on passenger "comfort" that required all airlines to provide nonsmoking seating sections, effective July 1, 1973 (CAB 1972). This was the first federal regulation of secondhand smoke. The CAB ruling, however, only required that airlines set aside a limited number of nonsmoking seats. At the time of its implementation, only the last few rows of seats were reserved for this purpose and were available on a first-come, first-served basis. Once these seats were filled, remaining passengers were seated in the smoking section. The CAB later revised this rule to require more flexible seating arrangements, so that any passengers who requested it would be guaranteed a nonsmoking seat if they arrived at the gate at least 10 minutes before departure. With this change, the airlines could no longer assign a fixed number of seats for

smoking and nonsmoking passengers, and the smoking section aboard most flights became progressively smaller as more and more passengers requested nonsmoking seats.

In 1983, the CAB issued new regulations that banned smoking on flights of two hours or less, but revised that decision almost immediately. However, pressure for the ban increased as the evidence mounted on adverse health consequences from exposure to secondhand smoke. In 1986, NRC appointed a committee to examine issues of air quality in airplanes, and their report recommended a ban on smoking on all commercial flights within the United States (NRC 1986a). Congress passed legislation in 1987 (*Appropriations for the Fiscal Year 1988, and for Other Purposes* [Prohibition Against Smoking] 1987) prohibiting smoking on all regularly scheduled flights of two hours or less, which became effective in 1988. In 1990, federal law mandated that all domestic flights of six hours or less be smoke-free. In 2000, all flights to and from the United States were required to be smoke-free (Holm and Davis 2004).

The efforts of grassroots advocates and advocacy groups, including individual flight attendants, the flight attendants' union, ANR, and several local chapters of GASP, were instrumental in achieving this outcome. These groups effectively conveyed the perspective of flight attendants who were expected to accept exposure to a hazardous substance for long periods of time in a confined environment as part of their job description. This effort put a human face on the mounting scientific evidence that secondhand smoke exposure was harmful to nonsmokers and framed the issue as one of worker safety (Holm and Davis 2004). Another important factor contributing to the outcome of this effort was the mounting evidence that was emerging from a series of scientific studies showing that flight attendants were exposed to high levels of secondhand smoke and that neither ventilation nor separate smoking and nonsmoking sections were effectively reducing this exposure (Repace 2004a). For example, a 1988 study sponsored by NCI that used personal air nicotine monitors and measurement of cotinine in urine to assess nonsmoking flight attendants' exposure found that the secondhand smoke levels present on the aircraft produced measurable levels of cotinine in the urine of passengers and flight attendants, and that flight attendants assigned to work in nonsmoking sections were not protected from secondhand smoke exposure (Mattson et al. 1989).

In 1994, the Occupational Safety and Health Administration (OSHA) proposed regulations that would either prohibit smoking or limit it to separately ventilated areas in all U.S. workplaces (*Federal Register* 1994b), but ultimately withdrew the proposed rule in December 2001 (*Federal Register* 2001). The tobacco industry had orchestrated a concerted and intensive campaign to block it (Bryan-Jones and Bero 2003). In withdrawing the rule, OSHA suggested that the issue of secondhand smoke was being adequately addressed at the local and state levels, noting that "in the years since the proposal was issued, a great many state and local governments and private employers have taken action to curtail smoking in public areas and in workplaces" (*Federal Register* 2001, p. 64946). Public health groups acquiesced in the decision to withdraw the rule because they were concerned that the rule might turn out to contain weak smoking restrictions and to preempt stronger state and local action (Girion 2001).

However, the federal government has instituted increasingly broad and stringent regulations on smoking in its own facilities, culminating in a 1997 executive order making most federally owned buildings under the jurisdiction of the Executive Branch smoke-free. In addition, the *Pro-Children Act of 1994*, which was reauthorized under the *No Child Left Behind Act of 2001*, prohibits smoking in facilities that routinely provide federally funded services to children (see "Smoking Restrictions in Other Settings" later in this chapter). In November 2004, U.S. DHHS announced that it would move toward prohibiting tobacco use on the outdoor grounds of its facilities in 2005 (USDHHS 2004). In 2004, the Federal Bureau of Prisons implemented a nearly across-the-board smoke-free policy in 105 federal prisons (U.S. Department of Justice [USDOJ] 2004).

Smoking Restrictions in the Military

One arena in which the federal government has made significant progress in restricting indoor smoking is in the armed services. The U.S. military has imposed progressively more stringent smoking restrictions in its facilities. In 1994, the U.S. Department of Defense (DOD) issued an Instruction making all workplace settings under its control smoke-free (USDOD 1994). However, this Instruction exempted recreational and living facilities. The 1997 Executive Order issued by President Clinton, which made all indoor federally owned facilities smoke-free, extended the military policy to all indoor facilities except living quarters. A policy letter issued by Defense Secretary William Cohen in December 1999 gave morale, welfare, and recreational facilities such as bars, bowling alleys, and golf course clubhouses on military bases and installations a three-year grace period to become

smoke-free or to restrict smoking to separately ventilated smoking areas (Cole 2003). The deadline expired in December 2002, and most of these facilities have reportedly complied. Indoor military facilities where smoking continued to be permitted included barracks and housing. As of 2001, all guest rooms and common areas in Air Force lodging facilities were required to be smoke-free. As of March 2005, guest rooms at Army lodging facilities were also required to implement smoke-free policies. The Navy designated new and renovated lodging facilities as smoke-free, but existing guest smoking rooms will retain that designation until they undergo renovation (Tyler 2005).

In addition to protecting military personnel from secondhand smoke exposure, these smoking restrictions are intended to encourage cessation among military personnel who smoke and to discourage recruits from initiating smoking. Smoking prevalence among military personnel is higher than among the general population. DOD reported that 33.8 percent of military personnel (35.3 percent of men and 26.3 percent of women) smoked in 2002 (USDOD 2004). According to the 2002 National Health Interview Survey (NHIS), the corresponding figure for the general U.S. adult population was 22.5 percent (CDC 2004a). A DOD survey found that approximately 27 percent of U.S. Air Force personnel aged 17 through 64 years were smokers in 2002 (CDC 2004a). The same survey found that 35.6 percent of Army personnel, 36.0 percent of Navy personnel, and 38.7 percent of Marine personnel were smokers in 2002 (CDC 2004a). CDC estimated that current smoking cost the Air Force approximately $107.2 million that year, including $20 million for medical care expenditures and $87 million for lost workdays. DOD also estimated that current smoking among all beneficiaries of the U.S. military health care system costs an estimated $930 million in 1995, including $584 million for health care expenditures and $346 million in lost productivity (CDC 2000).

The military has set ambitious goals for reducing smoking to improve health and well-being among military personnel. Benefits include enhanced military readiness and reduced smoking-related health care costs. To achieve these goals, all four services now prohibit recruits from using tobacco products during basic training (Giordono 2002), the discounts on tobacco products in military commissaries have been reduced since 1996 (USDOD 1996), and all military personnel can choose from a range of smoking cessation services (see the sections on "Hospitals and Health Care Facilities" and "Nursing Homes" later in this chapter).

Private Sector Workplace Smoking Restrictions

In some cases, private employers have been required to implement workplace smoking restrictions in response to state or local laws or regulations. In other cases, employers have chosen to implement voluntary workplace smoking restrictions to protect their employees' health; increase productivity; reduce health care costs, other insurance costs, and maintenance and cleaning costs; or lessen legal liability for employee health conditions. A *Healthy People 2010* objective calls for all workplaces to adopt smoke-free workplace policies (USDHHS 2000a).

National data sets can be used to ascertain the level of workplace smoking restrictions among private firms in the United States. A survey conducted by the Bureau of National Affairs (1991) estimated that 85 percent of large workplaces had policies restricting smoking. The percentage of smoke-free workplaces increased substantially from 2 percent in 1986 to 7 percent in 1987 and to 34 percent in 1991. Similarly, data from the 1992 National Survey of Worksite Health Promotion Activities indicated that 87 percent of workplaces with 50 or more employees regulated smoking in some manner, and 34 percent prohibited it altogether (USDHHS 1993). In 1999, 79 percent of worksites with 50 or more employees had a policy that banned or limited smoking (USDHHS 1999).

There are fewer studies on the prevalence of smoking policies in small workplaces, where the majority of Americans work (U.S. Department of Commerce [USDOC] 2006). Smaller workplaces have been less likely than larger workplaces to implement smoking policies (CDC 1987b; USDHHS 1989). According to a comprehensive examination of workplace smoking policies in 1992–1993 from NCI's Tobacco Use Supplement to the U.S. Census Bureau Current Population Survey (CPS) (n = 100,561) (USDOC 1995), most indoor workers surveyed (81.6 percent) reported that an official policy governed smoking at their workplaces; nearly half reported that the policy could be classified as smoke-free—smoking was not permitted either in workplace areas or in common public use areas (Gerlach et al. 1997). This proportion varied by gender, age, ethnicity, and occupation. Respondents in blue-collar and service occupations, for example, were significantly less likely to report a smoke-free workplace policy. Although data were not specifically categorized by workplace size, the range of occupations suggests that the survey included a substantial proportion of persons who worked in smaller workplace environments. However, the data

suggest that there is substantial room for improvement among all workplace sizes in terms of smoke-free policy coverage.

A study drawing on data from the 1999 CPS Tobacco Use Supplement found that 69.3 percent of all U.S. indoor workers reported that they were covered by a workplace policy that made all public or common areas and work areas smoke-free, up from 46.5 percent in 1993 and 63.7 percent in 1996 (Shopland et al. 2004). A greater proportion of women (73.8 percent) than men (64.2 percent) reported working under such a policy. Substantial disparities in coverage by a smoke-free workplace policy were evident between white-collar workers (76.3 percent coverage) and blue-collar (52.2 percent coverage) and service workers (57.5 percent coverage), although these disparities have narrowed over time.

As part of the national Community Intervention Trial for Smoking Cessation (COMMIT), worksites in 22 communities were surveyed in 1989 and 1993 (Glasgow et al. 1992, 1996). In 1993, of the original sample, 66 percent of the worksites had developed written smoking policies, 76 percent had either smoke-free policies (no smoking anywhere indoors) or restrictive smoking policies (smoking allowed in only one or two areas), and 43 percent had smoking bans. These data reflect an increase of approximately 20 percentage points in the number of worksites with bans and a decrease of 7 percentage points in the number with restrictions during the five-year observation period (Glasgow et al. 1996).

A notable recent trend in this area is the tendency of some large private employers to adopt voluntary smoke-free or, in some cases, tobacco-free workplace campus policies that extend smoking and tobacco use policies to outdoor grounds. The policies are typically not primarily intended to reduce employees' secondhand smoke exposure, but to motivate and help employees who smoke or use other tobacco products to quit in the interests of promoting a healthy workforce and reducing employers' health care costs (Romero 2004). To this end, the policies are also typically coupled with an employer provision of expanded employee cessation services. Such policies have recently been adopted by a number of large companies. In particular, the policy adopted by Lowe's Home Improvement Company (Center for Health Improvement 2004) generated extensive publicity, perhaps in part because its corporate headquarters are located in a tobacco-growing state. These policies appear to be most likely adopted by organizations with a health-related mission (especially hospitals), as well as schools, colleges, and universities.

In November 2004, U.S. DHHS Secretary Tommy Thompson announced that U.S. DHHS would implement a tobacco-free campus policy in its facilities beginning in 2005 (USDHHS 2004). Other U.S. organizations have also adopted smoke-free or tobacco-free campus policies, including manufacturing companies and restaurant chains (<http://www.no-smoke.org/goingsmokefree.php?id=452>).

Attitudes and Beliefs About Secondhand Smoke

A number of nationally representative studies that assessed public attitudes toward smoking in public places have been published since the 1960s. The 1989 report of the Surgeon General considered studies from the previous three decades (USDHHS 1989). The most recent studies are the NCI's Tobacco Use Supplement to the CPS (USDOC 1985, 2004) and the NHIS (National Center for Health Statistics [NCHS] 2004). CPS is a monthly survey of about 50,000 households. Questions on smoking were included in September 1992, January 1993, and May 1993 (Gerlach et al. 1997), and the questions were repeated during the same months in 1995–1996, 1998–1999, and 2001–2002 (Shopland et al. 2001; CDC, NCHS, NHIS, public use data tapes, 2001–2002). In the text that follows, the dates of surveys are referred to as 1993, 1996, 1999, and 2002, respectively. The NHIS is a multipurpose health survey conducted by CDC. Because the CPS and NHIS represent the most recent data available using nationally representative samples, this Surgeon General's report includes extensive analyses of these data.

Trends in Beliefs About Health Risks of Secondhand Smoke

Surveys conducted in recent years consistently show that substantial majorities of the U.S. public believe that secondhand smoke exposure is a health hazard for nonsmokers. In both 1992 and 2000, NHIS asked respondents if they agreed with the statement that secondhand smoke is harmful. In both years, more than 80 percent of respondents agreed (Table 10.2). Individuals with more years of education were more likely to believe that secondhand smoke is harmful. According to data from the 2001 annual Social Climate Survey of Tobacco Control, 95 percent of the adults agreed that parental secondhand smoke was harmful to children, and 96 percent considered tobacco company claims that secondhand smoke is not harmful to be untruthful (McMillen et al. 2003).

The Gallup Organization surveyed U.S. adults in 2002–2004. A summary of the results reported that 54 percent considered secondhand smoke very harmful to adults, 32 percent considered secondhand smoke somewhat harmful, 9 percent believed that secondhand smoke was not too harmful, and 4 percent felt that it was not at all harmful (Blizzard 2004). Women were more likely than men to believe that secondhand smoke was very harmful (63 percent versus 44 percent, respectively). Groups aged 18 to 29 years were the most likely to believe that secondhand smoke was very harmful (61 percent), compared with 55 percent for respondents aged 30 to 49 years, 48 percent for respondents aged 50 to 64 years, and 53 percent for respondents aged 65 or more years.

Yañez (2002) cited results from a 2002 national survey commissioned by the Robert Wood Johnson Foundation, which found that Hispanic/Latino (63 percent) and African American (66 percent) voters were more likely than White voters (53 percent) to believe that secondhand smoke is a serious health hazard.

Trends in Public Support for Smoking Restrictions

The CPS data were examined to assess changes in public support for smoking restrictions in six specific indoor settings: hospitals, worksites, malls, restaurants, bars/cocktail lounges, and sports arenas (Gower et al. 2000; Hartman et al. 2002). Data from these settings are cited throughout this section. For each survey, respondents were queried, "In (setting)

Table 10.2   Percentage of respondents aged 18 years or older who believe that secondhand smoke is harmful, by selected characteristics, United States, 1992 and 2000

Characteristic	1992 (%)	2000 (%)
Geographic region		
Midwest	86.8	83.7
Northeast	87.0	85.3
South	84.9	81.6
West	86.6	84.6
Age (years)		
18–24	92.4	86.6
18–24 (smokers only)	83.2	76.8
25–44	88.4	85.2
25–44 (smokers only)	75.4	70.3
45–64	84.2	81.9
45–64 (smokers only)	65.6	59.4
≥65	78.5	78.4
≥65 (smokers only)	48.6	43.2
Smoking status		
Smokers	71.4	66.8
Nonsmokers	91.6	88.5
Gender		
Men	84.0	80.2
Women	88.2	86.4
Education (number of years)		
≤8	72.9	76.2
9–11	77.1	74.3
12	84.9	79.7
13–15	88.6	84.9
≥16	92.0	90.8
Income		
Below poverty	83.0	79.1
At or above poverty	87.7	84.8

Sources: Centers for Disease Control and Prevention, National Center for Health Statistics, National Health Interview Survey, public use data tapes, 1992, 2000.

do you think that smoking should be: (1) allowed in all areas; (2) allowed in some areas; or (3) not allowed at all?" (USDOC 1995, pp. 9–22).

Nationally, the proportion of people who think indoor public places should be smoke-free increased between 1993 and 2002 for most settings. By 2002,

there was a significant level of support among the public for banning smoking in a number of public settings, including indoor work areas, hospitals, indoor sports arenas, and malls; about 58 percent of respondents favored total smoking bans in restaurants (Table 10.3), and 34 percent favored bans in bars (Table 10.4). Factors associated with restrictions in each of the six indoor areas are presented below. Across most of the specific settings, unless exceptions are noted, women were more supportive of smoking bans than men, white-collar workers were more supportive than blue-collar workers, and older respondents were more supportive than younger respondents.

According to the Gallup survey of U.S. adults in 2004, 58 percent favored a statewide smoking ban that would make it illegal to smoke in all workplaces, restaurants, and bars; 40 percent opposed such a restrictive measure (Mason 2004). Nonsmokers were substantially more likely than smokers to favor the policy in question; 66 percent of the respondents who reported smoking in the past week opposed the policy.

Some evidence suggests that Hispanics and African Americans are more likely than non-Hispanic Whites to support smoking restrictions in certain settings. In the analysis by Yañez of the 2002 national survey commissioned by the Robert Wood Johnson Foundation, Hispanic and African American voters were more likely than White voters to believe that secondhand smoke poses serious health risks to restaurant waitstaff and office workers; that restaurant workers have no choice about being exposed to secondhand smoke and deserve the same protections as other workers; and that nonsmokers have the right to breathe clean air where they shop, work, and eat (Yañez 2002). The survey also found that Hispanic and African American voters were more likely than White voters to support laws prohibiting smoking in indoor workplaces, public buildings, and restaurants.

Using CPS data for 1993, 1996, and 1999, Gilpin and colleagues (2004) compared attitudes toward secondhand smoke between residents of California and the rest of the United States. California has had a large and comprehensive tobacco control program since 1988 that emphasized changing social norms around tobacco use. A 1995 law mandated smoke-free workplaces including restaurants; in 1998, smoking was prohibited in bars, clubs, and gaming rooms. In 1993, 58.5 percent of Californians agreed that smoking should be eliminated in at least four of six

Table 10.3   **Percentage of respondents aged 18 years or older who support smoke-free restaurants, by selected characteristics, United States, 1992–2002**

Characteristic	1992–1993 (%)	1998–1999 (%)	2001–2002 (%)
Overall	45.09	51.93	57.57
Geographic region			
Midwest	40.66	45.34	49.94
Northeast	45.15	51.63	58.77
South	43.52	48.31	52.90
West	52.57	64.88	71.61
Age (years)			
18–24	39.58	45.53	51.10
25–44	44.19	51.62	57.01
45–64	46.25	53.01	58.49
≥65	49.93	55.65	61.98
Smoking status			
Smokers	16.39	22.38	26.60
Nonsmokers	54.37	60.28	65.38
Gender			
Men	43.61	48.94	54.40
Women	46.36	54.64	60.49
Education			
Less than high school	45.33	51.95	57.68
High school diploma	39.91	46.27	52.14
Some college	44.91	51.70	56.70
Bachelor's/postgraduate	53.72	59.54	65.03
Income			
Below poverty	41.98	50.61	55.51
Borderline	44.69	50.38	54.67
Above poverty	45.53	52.08	57.79
Occupational status			
White collar	47.76	54.19	59.79
Blue collar	37.98	44.08	49.12
Farm	44.11	52.26	54.64
Service	39.50	47.98	53.38
Race/ethnicity			
Non-Hispanic White	43.40	49.40	55.11
Non-Hispanic Black	45.79	51.33	56.87
Hispanic	59.06	66.85	70.93
Non-Hispanic American Indian	41.51	47.11	55.79
Non-Hispanic Asian	55.34	64.82	69.33

Sources: U.S. Department of Commerce, Census Bureau, National Cancer Institute Sponsored Tobacco Use Supplement to the Current Population Survey, public use data tapes, 1992–1993, 1998–1999, 2001–2002.

Table 10.4 Percentage of respondents aged 18 years or older who support smoke-free bars, by selected characteristics, United States, 1992–2002

Characteristic	1992–1993 (%)	1998–1999 (%)	2001–2002 (%)
Overall	24.19	29.78	34.03
Geographic region			
Midwest	21.19	23.29	26.14
Northeast	25.23	31.24	35.63
South	25.29	29.12	32.32
West	24.75	36.33	43.31
Age (years)			
18–24	15.87	21.26	25.43
25–44	21.03	26.48	30.73
45–64	26.99	32.62	36.34
≥65	34.56	40.34	44.84
Smoking status			
Smokers	5.19	8.36	9.81
Nonsmokers	30.34	35.92	40.19
Gender			
Men	22.10	27.05	31.09
Women	25.96	32.30	36.77
Education			
Less than high school	28.99	35.54	38.79
High school diploma	21.63	26.75	30.92
Some college	21.55	27.51	31.07
Bachelor's/postgraduate	27.30	32.41	36.93
Income			
Below poverty	23.97	31.59	35.42
Borderline	26.34	32.18	34.83
Above poverty	23.86	28.79	32.90
Occupational status			
White collar	23.24	28.16	32.54
Blue collar	18.71	23.61	27.11
Farm	23.31	32.10	31.04
Service	20.23	27.17	30.87
Race/ethnicity			
Non-Hispanic White	22.97	27.28	31.17
Non-Hispanic Black	26.08	32.11	36.36
Hispanic	31.63	41.44	46.13
Non-Hispanic American Indian	20.95	25.52	31.45
Non-Hispanic Asian	30.58	40.76	45.19

Sources: U.S. Department of Commerce, Census Bureau, National Cancer Institute Sponsored Tobacco Use Supplement to the Current Population Survey, public use data tapes, 1992–1993, 1998–1999, 2001–2002.

venues they were queried about (restaurants, hospitals, work areas, bars, indoor sports venues, and indoor shopping malls) versus 46.5 percent of U.S. residents. By 1999, 75.8 percent of California residents were in agreement for at least four of the venues, but only 57.3 percent of other U.S. respondents showed similar support. Moreover, differences in support among demographic groups and by race and ethnicity were less pronounced in California by 1999 than in the rest of the United States. In 1999, Californians with a high school education or less (73.9 percent) showed more support for smoke-free policies compared with college graduates (65.9 percent) in all other states. The use of mass media by the California Tobacco Control Program to educate the public on the dangers of secondhand smoke included special efforts to reach racial and ethnic groups and appears to have reached all education levels (Gilpin et al. 2004). This and other studies and surveys have suggested that the presence of smoking restrictions itself contributes to public support for such restrictions, perhaps by contributing to changes in social norms. Once such restrictions have been implemented, this support appears to grow with the passage of time (Borland et al. 1990; Tang et al. 2003; RTI International 2004). This phenomenon appears to be especially pronounced among smokers. For example, an evaluation of the New York state tobacco control program found that the proportion of adults who supported the state's smoke-free law had increased from 64 percent in 2003 (before the law took effect) to 79 percent in 2005. Support among smokers nearly doubled, from 25 percent in 2003 to 46 percent in 2005. Support among nonsmokers increased from 74 to 84 percent during this same period (New York State Department of Health 2005).

Hospitals

Across all indoor settings, support for smoking bans was highest for hospitals. In fact, most hospitals in the United States have had smoking bans since 1992, when the Joint Commission on Accreditation of Healthcare Organizations (JCAHO) required accredited hospitals to be smoke-free (JCAHO 1992). By 2001, more than 83 percent of respondents to the CPS survey favored smoking bans in hospitals (Hartman et al. 2004). Individuals living in the West were most likely to support hospital smoking bans, and people in the South and Midwest were least likely. Support increased with increasing levels of education

of the respondent (USDOC, U.S. Census Bureau, NCI Tobacco Use Supplement to the CPS, public use data tape, 2002).

Restaurants

Public support for smoke-free restaurants increased from 45 percent in 1993 to 58 percent in 2002 (Table 10.3). Support for smoke-free restaurants was highest in California (which had banned smoking in restaurants and bars in 1998) and Utah, while tobacco-producing states (Kentucky, North Carolina, Tennessee, and West Virginia) reported the lowest levels of support (USDOC, U.S. Census Bureau, NCI Tobacco Use Supplement to the CPS, public use data tapes, 2001–2002). In general, support was higher in the Northeast and West than in the South and Midwest. In 2002, significantly more nonsmokers than smokers supported smoke-free restaurants (65 percent versus 27 percent, respectively). Support for smoke-free restaurants increased with higher income and education levels and higher occupational status.

Bars

Support for smoke-free bars also increased from 1993 to 2002, but remained lower than support for smoke-free policies in other settings (Table 10.4). In 1999, only California and a handful of U.S. communities outside California had implemented smoking bans in bars. In most locations, respondents would probably not have experienced this type of smoking restriction. Among states, support for smoking bans in bars in 2002 was highest in California; even before the 1998 statewide ban there had been ordinances banning smoking in bars in a number of California communities. In California, 54 percent of residents favored a total ban; among regions, support was highest among respondents from the West and Northeast. Overall, support for a ban on smoking in bars was four times higher among nonsmokers than among smokers (CDC 2005b). Studies also examined support for restricting but not eliminating smoking in bars (Table 10.5).

As of April 17, 2006, 10 states (California, Connecticut, Delaware, Maine, Massachusetts, New Jersey, New York, Rhode Island, Vermont, and Washington) have enacted and implemented state laws making bars smoke-free (ANR 2006a). In addition, as of April 17, 2006, 215 municipalities had ordinances in place requiring bars to be smoke-free (ANR 2006a).

Table 10.5 Percentage of respondents aged 18 years or older who believe smoking should be allowed in some areas of bars, by selected characteristics, United States, 1992–2002

Characteristic	1992–1993 (%)	1998–1999 (%)	2001–2002 (%)
Overall	44.18	42.65	40.64
Geographic region			
Midwest	44.37	44.57	42.55
Northeast	48.58	45.14	43.48
South	41.64	42.16	40.33
West	43.76	39.24	36.83
Age (years)			
18–24	46.20	43.19	42.34
25–44	46.53	44.77	42.19
45–64	42.54	41.83	39.89
≥65	38.82	37.94	35.44
Smoking status			
Smokers	41.84	40.45	40.00
Nonsmokers	44.94	43.28	40.80
Gender			
Men	42.16	41.67	40.28
Women	45.88	43.54	40.97
Education			
Less than high school	37.28	35.72	36.72
High school diploma	42.73	41.62	39.11
Some college	46.34	43.45	41.81
Bachelor's/postgraduate	50.11	47.65	44.52
Income			
Below poverty	38.75	37.53	36.68
Borderline	39.74	37.69	37.30
Above poverty	45.38	43.96	41.77
Occupational status			
White collar	48.48	46.15	43.78
Blue collar	40.51	40.60	38.90
Farm	39.52	38.13	39.58
Service	43.80	41.55	40.26
Race/ethnicity			
Non-Hispanic White	44.61	43.33	41.45
Non-Hispanic Black	44.99	44.60	42.09
Hispanic	39.32	35.91	35.10
Non-Hispanic American Indian	37.11	39.34	36.77
Non-Hispanic Asian	46.88	41.79	40.22

Sources: U.S. Department of Commerce, Census Bureau, National Cancer Institute Sponsored Tobacco Use Supplement to the Current Population Survey, public use data tapes, 1992–1993, 1998–1999, 2001–2002.

Other data collected after local and state bans were in place have suggested increased levels of support for these restrictions after their implementation. For example, in a poll conducted by the Field Research Corporation in 1998, when California's law prohibiting smoking in bars first went into effect, only 24 percent of smokers and 59 percent of all bar patrons supported the ban. However, a poll conducted in 2000 found that the level of support among smokers had almost doubled to 44 percent and support among all patrons had increased to 73 percent (California Department of Health Services 2000). This poll also found that 72 percent of bar patrons were concerned about the effects of secondhand smoke on their health and that 75 percent felt that it was important to have a smoke-free environment inside bars (Tang et al. 2003). Researchers found that approval among bar patrons of the California smoke-free bar law had increased from 60 percent three months after the law took effect in 1998 to 73 percent in 2000 (Tang et al. 2003). Compliance with the law has also increased over time (Weber et al. 2003). Approval for the law also increased among bar owners, managers, and employees. A study based on a telephone survey of randomly selected respondents reported that 50.9 percent of 650 bar owners, managers, and staff surveyed in 2002 stated that they preferred to work in a smoke-free environment, up from 17.3 percent of 651 surveyed in 1998 (p <0.001) (Tang et al. 2004). The study also found that 45.5 percent of respondents surveyed stated that they were concerned about the effects of secondhand smoke on their health, up from 21.6 percent in 1998 (p <0.001). Tang and colleagues (2004) concluded that a positive and significant attitudinal change occurred among California's bar owners, managers, and bartenders regarding the law.

Sports Arenas

Support for total smoking bans in indoor sports arenas also increased from 1993 to 2002; support was highest in the West and Northeast (Table 10.6).

Support for a total ban on smoking in sports arenas was second only to support for smoke-free hospital policies among indoor public places. Blacks had lower levels of support than did Whites or Hispanics. Overall, individuals with a higher socioeconomic status (SES) were more likely to support smoke-free indoor sports arenas.

Malls

The percentage of individuals supporting a total ban on smoking in malls increased substantially from 1993 to 2002 (Table 10.7). Support was highest in the West and Northeast, while respondents from the South and Midwest expressed lower levels of support. Smokers were significantly less likely than nonsmokers to support smoke-free malls (59 percent versus 81 percent, respectively), although it is notable that by 2002, an overall 59 percent of smokers supported smoke-free malls; the youngest (18 through 24 years) and oldest (≥65 years) age groups had similar levels of support and were more supportive than the two intermediate age groups. Hispanics and Asians were the most supportive, while African Americans, American Indians, and Whites had lower (but still high) levels of support. Support generally increased with increasing levels of education. Similar levels of support were seen across income levels.

Indoor Work Areas

Support for policies prohibiting smoking in indoor work areas also increased from 1993 to 2002. By 2002, nearly 75 percent of the respondents supported having smoke-free workplaces. The lowest levels of support were in the tobacco-producing states. Support was similar across age groups and increased with increasing levels of education. A large increase in support was seen between those with a high school diploma or some college education and those with a college degree or higher educational attainment (Table 10.8).

Table 10.6 Percentage of respondents aged 18 years or older who support smoke-free sports arenas, by selected characteristics, United States, 1992–2002

Characteristic	1992–1993 (%)	1998–1999 (%)	2001–2002 (%)
Overall	66.98	71.67	77.21
Geographic region			
Midwest	66.11	69.81	75.72
Northeast	67.12	72.52	79.09
South	64.43	67.83	72.91
West	71.96	79.01	83.92
Age (years)			
18–24	64.01	69.80	75.56
25–44	65.37	70.04	75.46
45–64	68.55	73.14	77.42
≥65	71.04	74.70	80.06
Smoking status			
Smokers	48.71	53.41	59.68
Nonsmokers	72.88	76.82	81.64
Gender			
Men	63.44	67.84	73.56
Women	69.97	75.17	80.60
Education			
Less than high school	64.75	69.60	77.37
High school diploma	64.71	68.42	73.79
Some college	67.07	72.03	76.83
Bachelor's/postgraduate	72.63	76.86	81.68
Income			
Below poverty	64.02	70.03	75.56
Borderline	65.73	69.71	74.25
Above poverty	67.53	72.17	77.72
Occupational status			
White collar	68.97	73.67	79.15
Blue collar	60.01	64.69	70.01
Farm	67.11	70.95	75.10
Service	64.47	70.57	76.50
Race/ethnicity			
Non-Hispanic White	66.48	70.83	76.67
Non-Hispanic Black	65.38	68.96	74.30
Hispanic	73.47	78.30	81.99
Non-Hispanic American Indian	68.12	69.64	75.75
Non-Hispanic Asian	73.84	79.96	84.29

Sources: U.S. Department of Commerce, Census Bureau, National Cancer Institute Sponsored Tobacco Use Supplement to the Current Population Survey, public use data tapes, 1992–1993, 1998–1999, 2001–2002.

Table 10.7   Percentage of respondents aged 18 years or older who support smoke-free malls, by selected characteristics, United States, 1992–2002

Characteristic	1992–1993 (%)	1998–1999 (%)	2001–2002 (%)
Overall	54.62	69.40	76.40
Geographic region			
Midwest	51.00	64.87	73.33
Northeast	56.46	71.55	78.15
South	51.52	65.60	72.31
West	61.92	78.37	84.48
Age (years)			
18–24	49.90	71.12	78.57
25–44	52.19	68.67	75.86
45–64	55.95	68.81	74.53
≥65	62.54	71.02	77.10
Smoking status			
Smokers	31.77	50.24	59.22
Nonsmokers	61.99	74.83	80.74
Gender			
Men	51.55	66.01	73.29
Women	57.21	72.49	79.28
Education			
Less than high school	57.54	68.86	77.35
High school diploma	51.64	65.82	72.63
Some college	53.02	69.63	76.19
Bachelor's/postgraduate	58.87	74.19	80.43
Income			
Below poverty	54.94	68.63	75.52
Borderline	56.27	68.03	73.85
Above poverty	54.42	69.72	76.82
Occupational status			
White collar	54.67	71.68	78.67
Blue collar	48.53	63.24	70.41
Farm	54.30	68.42	74.32
Service	51.76	68.50	76.10
Race/ethnicity			
Non-Hispanic White	53.05	67.97	75.38
Non-Hispanic Black	55.08	67.55	74.05
Hispanic	67.86	79.28	83.59
Non-Hispanic American Indian	51.35	66.01	74.73
Non-Hispanic Asian	63.84	78.15	83.59

Sources: U.S. Department of Commerce, Census Bureau, National Cancer Institute Sponsored Tobacco Use Supplement to the Current Population Survey, public use data tapes, 1992–1993, 1998–1999, 2001–2002.

Table 10.8   Percentage of respondents aged 18 years or older who support smoke-free indoor workplaces, by selected characteristics, United States, 1992–2002

Characteristic	1992–1993 (%)	1998–1999 (%)	2001–2002 (%)
Overall	58.06	68.17	74.48
Geographic region			
Midwest	52.72	61.85	68.39
Northeast	57.07	69.00	75.42
South	56.49	65.77	72.17
West	67.59	77.89	83.45
Age (years)			
18–24	55.02	67.27	72.78
25–44	56.68	68.46	75.25
45–64	58.79	67.75	73.64
≥65	62.92	68.77	74.60
Smoking status			
Smokers	30.60	43.82	51.11
Nonsmokers	66.92	75.05	80.37
Gender			
Men	53.48	63.37	70.14
Women	61.93	72.54	78.49
Education			
Less than high school	54.68	63.41	71.69
High school diploma	52.61	62.34	68.65
Some college	59.44	69.46	75.24
Bachelor's/postgraduate	68.46	77.52	83.13
Income			
Below poverty	52.73	63.83	70.14
Borderline	55.80	63.79	68.93
Above poverty	58.96	69.12	75.40
Occupational status			
White collar	63.60	74.59	80.75
Blue collar	46.46	56.98	63.78
Farm	52.56	63.92	67.95
Service	53.05	65.21	71.87
Race/ethnicity			
Non-Hispanic White	56.40	66.22	72.81
Non-Hispanic Black	57.97	67.81	73.70
Hispanic	71.99	78.81	83.18
Non-Hispanic American Indian	51.26	62.09	70.65
Non-Hispanic Asian	73.48	81.06	85.74

Sources: U.S. Department of Commerce, Census Bureau, National Cancer Institute Sponsored Tobacco Use Supplement to the Current Population Survey, public use data tapes, 1992–1993, 1998–1999, 2001–2002.

Policy Approaches

During the past 30 years, policies to restrict smoking in public places and in workplaces have been implemented with increasing success. Over time, the number, strength, and coverage of these policies have steadily increased. Although not subject to regulation, exposure in the home (the main source of exposure for most children at present) has also been the focus of intervention research designed, to the extent possible, to help smoking parents protect their children from secondhand smoke exposure and to help smokers protect nonsmoking spouses and other adult nonsmokers who live with them.

Smoke-Free Workplace Policies

Workplace smoking restrictions are implemented by employers for a variety of reasons, including responding to a local or state law or regulation; promoting a healthier workforce; protecting employees and patrons from secondhand smoke exposure; reducing health, life, disability, and fire insurance costs; and many others (CDC, Wellness Councils of America, ACS 1996; Task Force on Community Preventive Services 2005). These restrictions may apply to work areas, public or common areas (e.g., lobbies, cafeterias, or restrooms), or to all locations (Gerlach et al. 1997) and can take a variety of forms. For example, they may

- prohibit smoking or use of all tobacco products (including smokeless tobacco) on the entire workplace campus, including both indoor areas and outdoors areas such as parking lots;

- prohibit smoking or use of all tobacco products in indoor areas and restrict smoking outdoors to certain designated areas;

- prohibit smoking or use of all tobacco products in indoor areas and in specified outdoor areas;

- prohibit smoking or use of all tobacco products in indoor areas and outdoors within a designated distance from building entrances, exits, windows, and air ducts;

- prohibit smoking in indoor areas only;

- restrict smoking indoors to designated areas that are separately enclosed and ventilated; and

- restrict smoking indoors to designated areas that are not required to be separately enclosed and ventilated (CDC, ACS, Wellness Councils of America 1996).

Only policies that (at a minimum) require indoor facilities to be completely smoke-free provide effective protection from secondhand smoke exposure (USDHHS 2000c; Task Force on Community Preventive Services 2005). Such policies are also more effective in prompting employees who smoke to quit or to reduce their cigarette consumption (Fichtenberg and Glantz 2002; Bauer et al. 2005).

Smoking Restrictions in Private Workplaces

Data from NCI's Tobacco Use Supplement to the CPS for 1993, 1996, 1999, and 2002 (U.S. DOC, U.S. Census Bureau, NCI Sponsored Tobacco Use Supplement to the CPS, public use data tapes, 1993, 1996, 1999, 2002; Shopland et al. 2001; Hartman et al. 2002) track trends in worker protection from secondhand smoke exposure based on the percentage of indoor workers reporting that they work under a smoke-free workplace policy—defined as an official employer policy that prohibits smoking in both public or common areas and work areas. Nationally, coverage of workers by smoke-free policies increased substantially from 1993 to 2002. According to CPS data, 71 percent of all indoor workers were covered by a smoke-free policy in 2002, compared with 64 percent in 1996 and 47 percent in 1993. According to NHIS data from 2000 (USDHHS, CDC, NCHS, NHIS, public use data tape, 2000), 87 percent of respondents reported an employer workplace policy restricting smoking in some fashion, compared with only 44 percent in 1992. By 2000, 92 percent of workers who reported an employer workplace policy to restrict smoking described the policy as a smoking ban in all work areas. Between 1993 and 2002, the proportion of U.S. indoor workers reporting a smoke-free workplace policy increased more than 50 percent. Between 1999 and 2002, however, the rate of increase slowed, most likely reflecting the overall high levels of workplace smoking bans already achieved.

As already noted, a study drawing on 1999 CPS Tobacco Use Supplement data found that 69.3 percent of all U.S. workers reported a workplace policy that made all public or common areas and work areas smoke-free (Shopland et al. 2004). A greater proportion of women (73.8 percent) than men (64.2 percent) reported working under such a policy. Substantial disparities in smoke-free workplace policy coverage were evident between white-collar workers on the one hand and blue-collar and service workers on the other hand, with 76.3 percent, 52.2 percent, and 57.5 percent of these occupational groups, respectively, reporting that they were covered by a policy of this type, although the data reported indicate that these disparities have narrowed somewhat over time.

Variations by State

The CPS data showed significant variations among states in the proportion of indoor workers who reported coverage by a smoke-free workplace policy (Table 10.9) (Shopland et al. 2002). In 2002, this proportion ranged from a high of 85 percent among workers in Utah to 51 percent in Nevada. In 1993, less than 50 percent of indoor workers in 33 states reported working in smoke-free workplaces. In 1996, only two states—Arkansas and Nevada—still reported coverage rates of under 50 percent. In 2002, there were no states below this mark. At the other end of the spectrum, in 1993 only three states—Idaho, Utah, and Washington—documented that at least 60 percent of all indoor workers reported smoke-free policies. In 1996, 32 states plus the District of Columbia had achieved this level of coverage, and in 2002 the number had increased to 48 states plus the District of Columbia (Table 10.9). States with a significant tobacco growing or manufacturing presence, such as Georgia, Kentucky, North Carolina, South Carolina, and Virginia, have also experienced significant progress in the level of worker protection. The states that experienced the greatest proportional increases in smoke-free workplace policy coverage between 1993 and 1999 were North Carolina (>98 percent), Kentucky (>95 percent), and Arkansas (>92 percent), although this proportionally high gain reflects these states having levels of worker protection significantly below the rest of the nation in 1993 (Shopland et al. 2001).

Variations by Geographic Region

Some studies have also shown regional differences in workplace smoking policies. According to the CPS data, workers in the Midwest and the South had the lowest rates of smoke-free indoor workplace policies, whereas workers in the Northeast and the West had the highest rates (Figure 10.3 and Table 10.10). Between 1993 and 2002, however, indoor workers in the West reported the smallest relative increase in smoke-free workplace policies compared with workers in other regions. Nationwide, most of the observed gains occurred between 1993 and 1996 (Table 10.10).

Variations by Gender

Using CPS data, Sweeney and colleagues (2000) found that the prevalence of smoke-free indoor workplace policies also varied considerably by gender, with women significantly more likely than men to report working under a smoke-free workplace policy regardless of geographic region (Figure 10.4). This pattern occurred across all assessment periods.

Variations by Occupational Status

White-collar indoor workers reported significantly higher rates of smoke-free workplace policies compared with blue-collar or service workers (Figure 10.5). By 2002, more than 77 percent of white-collar workers in the United States reported working under a smoke-free policy, compared with just over 50 percent of blue-collar workers. Among all workers, however, Shopland and colleagues (2002) noted that there was a significant decline in the rate of increase in smoke-free policy coverage between 1996 and 1999 compared with 1993 and 1996. This decline could reflect reaching a ceiling effect at high levels of overall coverage (Shopland et al. 2002).

In 1999, only 43 percent of food service workers reported working in a smoke-free environment, of whom waiters and waitresses had the least protection (12.9 percent) of all job classifications among food service workers. One out of five workers in the occupational category of food service workers is a teenager, and more than half are female; wages paid to these full-time workers are among the lowest of any occupational group (Shopland et al. 2004). A study of serum cotinine concentration by occupation found

Table 10.9   Percentage of indoor workers aged 18 years or older who reported smoke-free workplace smoking policies by state, United States, 1992–2002

State	1992–1993 (%)	1995–1996 (%)	1998–1999 (%)	2001–2002 (%)
Alabama	38.98	55.46	64.50	66.80
Alaska	58.71	69.53	73.61	77.00
Arizona	57.30	64.96	68.67	72.19
Arkansas	33.27	48.77	63.79	64.56
California	58.77	75.84	77.57	80.09
Colorado	53.87	71.51	73.07	69.35
Connecticut	48.82	67.48	74.00	73.95
Delaware	50.30	65.51	71.33	72.54
District of Columbia	52.76	74.78	74.55	76.12
Florida	53.83	66.39	69.70	65.72
Georgia	48.28	57.10	67.00	63.51
Hawaii	47.06	60.71	72.39	62.20
Idaho	60.35	70.48	71.55	71.83
Illinois	40.24	60.91	67.91	69.55
Indiana	35.83	52.43	58.75	61.14
Iowa	44.92	61.78	70.32	70.72
Kansas	49.68	63.03	74.23	72.51
Kentucky	29.34	50.56	57.21	59.24
Louisiana	39.91	56.51	64.64	64.60
Maine	55.25	73.36	75.71	81.83
Maryland	53.30	82.58	81.99	77.81
Massachusetts	48.74	71.13	77.32	81.49
Michigan	39.70	53.54	61.54	65.67
Minnesota	54.82	68.49	74.30	75.05
Mississippi	40.72	53.84	62.34	66.93
Missouri	40.32	58.78	65.92	66.10
Montana	43.77	58.15	68.74	71.05
Nebraska	44.88	63.39	68.22	70.92
Nevada	33.84	40.14	48.65	50.94
New Hampshire	53.03	73.14	74.34	76.89
New Jersey	46.37	67.90	73.06	75.25
New Mexico	55.28	65.58	68.32	71.02
New York	42.91	64.96	72.91	77.06
North Carolina	30.90	55.34	61.23	67.87
North Dakota	47.69	61.22	67.27	72.63
Ohio	37.60	56.85	63.98	66.41
Oklahoma	41.62	58.26	67.93	70.96
Oregon	59.98	66.96	66.98	74.47
Pennsylvania	41.72	59.90	69.16	72.43
Rhode Island	45.69	69.75	72.12	77.00
South Carolina	38.57	59.16	63.88	65.97
South Dakota	43.61	62.36	60.99	65.45
Tennessee	36.23	53.96	63.62	66.21
Texas	51.35	65.02	66.49	68.19
Utah	65.54	83.70	84.56	84.86
Vermont	58.65	78.24	77.74	78.46
Virginia	43.83	62.92	71.08	72.39
Washington	67.93	72.67	74.74	71.94
West Virginia	38.11	59.63	64.17	69.84
Wisconsin	44.69	62.25	64.74	69.26
Wyoming	48.37	61.33	66.12	67.57

Sources: U.S. Department of Commerce, Census Bureau, National Cancer Institute Sponsored Tobacco Use Supplement to the Current Population Survey, public use data tapes, 1992–1993, 1995–1996, 1998–1999, 2001–2002.

Figure 10.3   Percentage of indoor workers aged 18 years or older who reported smoke-free workplace policies, by region, United States, 1992–2002

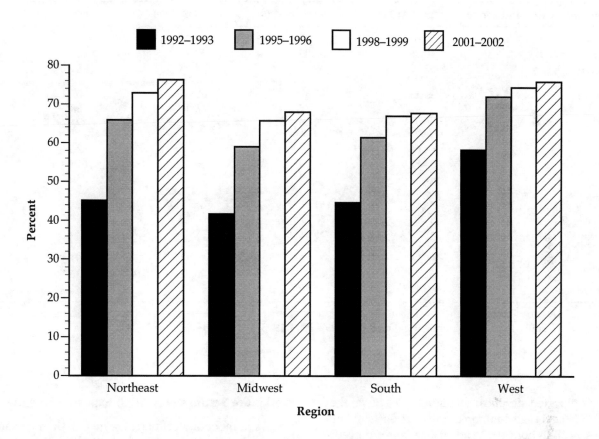

Sources: U.S. Department of Commerce, Census Bureau, National Cancer Institute Sponsored Tobacco Use Supplement to the Current Population Survey, public use data tapes, 1992–1993, 1995–1996, 1998–1999, 2001–2002.

that nonsmoking waiters and waitresses had the highest cotinine levels of any occupational group (Wortley et al. 2002).

Variations by Age

In the 1993 CPS data, younger workers, particularly males, were the least protected of all age groups; this trend persisted across survey years through 2002. Generally, smoke-free policy coverage for indoor workers increased with an increase in age except in the oldest age group (Table 10.11) (Shopland et al. 2002). The NHIS data (USDHHS, CDC, NCHS, NHIS, public use data tapes, 1992, 2000) showed a similar pattern.

Variations by Race and Ethnicity

Few differences were noted with respect to race and ethnicity among indoor workers (Figure 10.6). Hispanic workers who responded to the CPS reported slightly lower rates of coverage compared with Whites or Blacks in both 1996 and 1999, whereas the 1993 rates of all three groups were similar (Shopland et al. 2002). NHIS data yielded similar results (USDHHS, CDC, NCHS, NHIS, public use data tapes, 1992, 2000).

Variations by Smoking Status

In the 1993, 1996, 1999, and 2002 CPS data, indoor workers classified as lifetime nonsmokers and former

Table 10.10 Percentage of indoor workers aged 18 years or older who reported smoke-free workplace policies, by geographic region and gender, United States, 1992–2002

Geographic region and gender	1992–1993 (%)	1995–1996 (%)	1998–1999 (%)	2001–2002 (%)
Overall	46.65	63.85	69.34	71.15
Men	40.46	58.05	63.95	66.41
Women	51.70	69.02	74.08	75.21
Northeast	45.13	65.87	72.85	76.22
Men	38.45	60.75	68.46	72.19
Women	50.95	70.48	76.72	79.62
Midwest	41.69	58.99	65.70	67.94
Men	34.82	51.20	58.31	61.48
Women	47.37	65.99	72.23	73.54
South	44.64	61.43	66.96	67.64
Men	38.53	55.47	61.13	62.14
Women	49.13	66.41	71.82	72.11
West	58.28	72.00	74.35	75.86
Men	52.75	67.69	70.72	73.24
Women	63.16	76.20	77.81	78.28

Sources: U.S. Department of Commerce, Census Bureau, National Cancer Institute Sponsored Tobacco Use Supplement to the Current Population Survey, public use data tapes, 1992–1993, 1995–1996, 1998–1999, 2001–2002.

smokers reported significantly higher rates of smoke-free policy coverage compared with current smokers (Table 10.12). In both 1992 and 2000, a larger percentage of nonsmokers than smokers reported employer policies that restricted smoking in work areas, but this question was only asked of individuals who had reported the existence of an employer smoking policy (USDHHS, CDC, NCHS, NHIS, public use data tapes, 1992, 2000).

Variations by Educational Attainment

Using the CPS data across all years (Shopland et al. 2002), smoke-free worksite coverage was strongly associated with the worker's level of education (Figure 10.7). In 2002, about 57 percent of indoor workers with less than a high school education reported a smoke-free worksite, compared with 71 percent with some college education, and 81 percent with 16 or more years of education. The same trends were observed in the NHIS data (USDHHS, CDC, NCHS, NHIS, public use data tape, 2000), although the reported levels of smoke-free worksite policy coverage were higher for each educational category in the 2000 NHIS data (except those with less than a high school diploma) compared with the 1999 CPS data.

Workplace Settings with High Exposure Potential

A number of workplaces related to the entertainment and hospitality industries, including restaurants, bars, and casinos, continue to present the potential for high levels of worker exposure to secondhand smoke. This potential for higher exposure reflects the frequent exemption of these settings from state and local clean indoor air laws and the generally higher levels of smoking, primarily by patrons, in such locations.

Restaurant and bar workers are far less likely than other workers to be protected by smoke-free workplace policies, more likely than other workers to have these policies violated where they do exist, and more likely to be exposed to high levels of secondhand smoke on the job. Data from the CPS Tobacco Use Supplement document that workers in the food preparation and services occupation were less likely than employees in any other occupational category to report a workplace policy in place that designated both work areas and public or common areas as smoke-free (Shopland et al. 2004). As of 1999, only 42.9 percent of food preparation and service workers surveyed reported such a policy compared with 69.3 percent of U.S. indoor workers overall. For the more specific food service job categories of waiters/

Figure 10.4 **Percentage of indoor workers aged 18 years or older who reported smoke-free workplace policies, by gender, United States, 1992–2002**

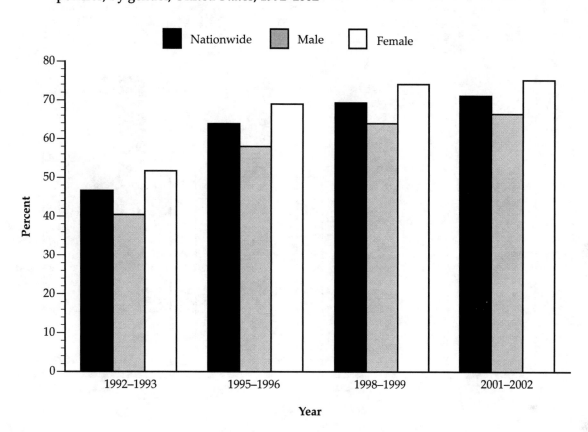

Sources: U.S. Department of Commerce, Census Bureau, National Cancer Institute Sponsored Tobacco Use Supplement to the Current Population Survey, public use data tapes, 1992–1993, 1995–1996, 1998–1999, 2001–2002.

waitresses and bartenders, the proportions of employees reporting such a policy were even lower: 27.7 percent and 12.9 percent, respectively. Moreover, while only 3.8 percent of all U.S. workers who worked under a smoke-free workplace policy reported that someone had smoked in their work area during the two weeks preceding the interview, the corresponding figure for food service workers was 6.4 percent (compared with 3.7 percent for nonfood service workers), and the figures for waiters/waitresses and bartenders were 12.9 percent and 32.2 percent, respectively (although in the latter two cases the confidence intervals [CIs] are quite wide).

Wortley and colleagues (2002) analyzed the objective indicator of cotinine levels among nonsmoking adult workers surveyed in the 1988–1994 Third National Health and Nutrition Examination Survey (NHANES III) who reported no home exposure to

cigarette smoke; their findings are consistent with these results. The study found that waiters/waitresses had the highest geometric mean serum cotinine level and the highest proportion of workers with a cotinine level above the accepted cutoff point used to indicate secondhand smoke exposure compared with any of the occupational categories examined. The study also reported higher cotinine levels among blue collar and service occupations and lower cotinine levels among white collar occupations. Occupations with higher worker cotinine levels tended to be those in which other studies have reported that smaller proportions of workers were protected by smoke-free workplace policies (Wortley et al. 2002).

In a review of studies with reported mean concentrations of several relevant airborne substances, such as CO, nicotine, and respirable suspended particulates, Siegel (1993) found that the levels of

Figure 10.5   Percentage of indoor workers aged 18 years or older who reported smoke-free workplace policies, by occupational status, United States, 1992–2002

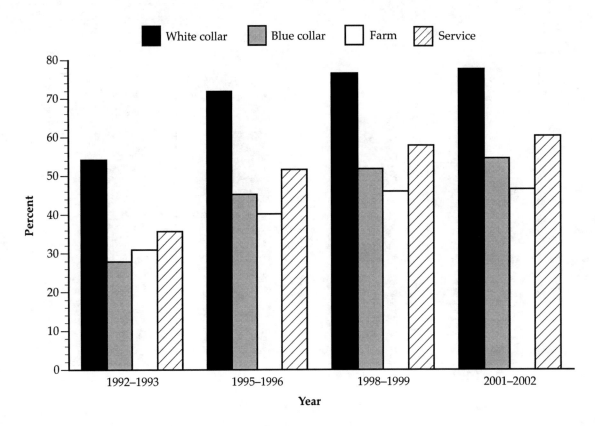

Sources: U.S. Department of Commerce, Census Bureau, National Cancer Institute Sponsored Tobacco Use Supplement to the Current Population Survey, public use data tapes, 1992–1993, 1995–1996, 1998–1999, 2001–2002.

secondhand smoke in restaurants were 1.6 to 2.0 times higher than in offices and 1.5 times higher than in homes with at least one smoker. Levels in bars were 3.9 to 6.1 times higher than in typical office settings and 4.4 to 4.5 times higher than in homes with at least one smoker. Siegel (1993) also reviewed epidemiologic studies that provided lung cancer risk estimates for food service workers. He concluded that compared with the general population, these workers have an estimated 50 percent greater risk of developing lung cancer, in part attributable to secondhand smoke exposure on the job.

Workers in casinos that allow smoking comprise another group at high risk for exposure to secondhand smoke (Davis 1998). A 1995 study of casino workers documented the presence of nicotine in the air inhaled by the workers and an increase

in serum cotinine levels across the work shift (Trout et al. 1998). The mean cotinine level in these workers was higher than for participants in NHANES III (1988–1991) who reported secondhand smoke exposure at work. A recent study found that patrons who had spent four hours in a casino where smoking was allowed experienced statistically significant increases in 4-(methylnitrosamino)-1-(3-pyridyl)-1-butanol, a tobacco-specific lung carcinogen (Anderson et al. 2003). The study concluded that exposure of a nonsmoker to secondhand smoke in a casino results in the uptake of this carcinogen. This finding has implications for casino employees who are likely to spend significantly more time than patrons in these environments. The authors noted that "on the basis of our results and other studies, one would expect that carcinogen levels in nonsmoking casino

Table 10.11   Percentage of indoor workers aged 18 years or older who reported smoke-free workplace policies, by age and gender, United States, 1992–2002

Characteristic (years)	1992–1993 (%)	1995–1996 (%)	1998–1999 (%)	2001–2002 (%)
Age				
18–24	39.65	55.54	60.34	63.19
25–44	47.40	64.17	69.16	70.93
45–64	48.82	67.35	73.82	74.91
≥65	46.51	63.49	69.77	72.85
Men				
18–24	33.29	50.12	54.92	58.52
25–44	40.83	58.29	63.74	66.05
45–64	43.35	61.61	68.66	70.31
≥65	41.94	58.02	62.86	68.26
Women				
18–24	44.64	60.43	64.86	66.89
25–44	52.89	69.57	74.17	75.34
45–64	53.15	72.18	78.09	78.65
≥65	49.77	67.97	75.63	76.46

Sources: U.S. Department of Commerce, Census Bureau, National Cancer Institute Sponsored Tobacco Use Supplement to the Current Population Survey, public use data tapes, 1992–1993, 1995–1996, 1998–1999, 2001–2002.

employees would increase as a result of ETS [environmental tobacco smoke] exposure at their worksite" (Anderson et al. 2003, p. 1545).

Siegel and Skeer (2003) identified additional specialized workplace settings that appear to have high potential for worker secondhand smoke exposure. The authors reviewed existing data on secondhand smoke exposure in bars, bowling alleys, billiard halls, betting establishments, and bingo parlors, measured by ambient nicotine air concentrations. Nicotine concentrations in these venues were 2.4 to 18.5 times higher than concentrations in offices or residences and 1.5 to 11.7 times higher than concentrations in restaurants. The authors concluded that these exposure levels may subject workers in those venues to (working) lifetime excess lung cancer mortality risks that substantially exceed the typical de manifestis risk level that triggers regulatory action (Siegel and Skeer 2003).

Data from the CPS Tobacco Use Supplement suggest that certain population groups are more likely to work in food preparation and service jobs and in other occupations where they are less likely than other workers to be covered by smoke-free workplace policies. These groups include teens and young adults (Gerlach et al. 1997), persons of low SES (Shopland et al. 2004), and Hispanics (Shopland et al. 2004).

Compliance with Workplace Smoking Policies

In the past, most studies focused on assessing whether workplace smoking policies were in place and describing the provisions of those policies. Less emphasis had been placed on assessing compliance with the policies. To ascertain worksite compliance with smoking policies, the 1996 and 1999 CPS asked all employees who reported working under an official policy that prohibited smoking in work areas and in public or common areas whether anyone had smoked in their work area at any time during the two-week period before their interview (USDOC 2004). In both 1996 and 1999, Shopland and colleagues (2001) noted very low rates of infractions overall (Table 10.13) and few differences by geographic region. In 1999, 3.8 percent of all U.S. workers covered by a smoke-free workplace policy reported that someone had smoked in their work area during the two weeks preceding the interview (Shopland et al. 2004). As noted earlier, this figure was substantially higher for food preparation and service workers (6.4 percent) compared with nonfood service workers (3.7 percent). The figures for waiters/waitresses and bartenders were 12.9 percent and 32.2 percent, respectively.

Figure 10.6   Percentage of indoor workers aged 18 years or older who reported smoke-free workplace policies, by race and ethnicity, United States, 1992–2002

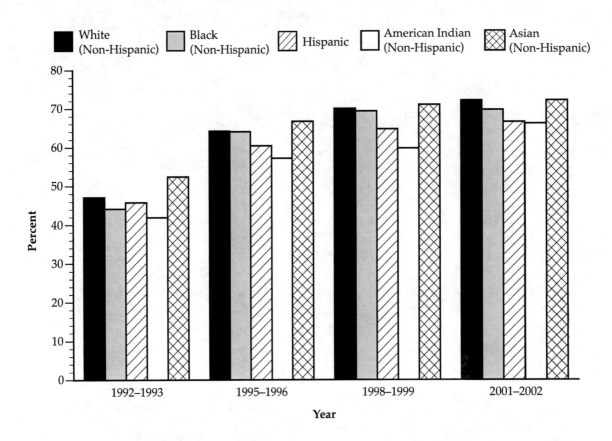

Sources: U.S. Department of Commerce, Census Bureau, National Cancer Institute Sponsored Tobacco Use Supplement to the Current Population Survey, public use data tapes, 1992–1993, 1995–1996, 1998–1999, 2001–2002.

Table 10.12   Percentage of indoor workers aged 18 years or older who reported smoke-free workplace policies, by smoking status, United States, 1992–2002

Smoking status	1992–1993 (%)	1995–1996 (%)	1998–1999 (%)	2001–2002 (%)
Smokers	36.9	53.7	59.2	61.2
Nonsmokers*	49.9	67.0	72.3	73.9

*Includes lifetime nonsmokers and former smokers.
Sources: U.S. Department of Commerce, Census Bureau, National Cancer Institute Sponsored Tobacco Use Supplement to the Current Population Survey, public use data tapes, 1992–1993, 1995–1996, 1998–1999, 2001–2002.

Figure 10.7   Percentage of indoor workers aged 18 years or older who reported smoke-free workplace policies, by level of education, United States, 1992–2002

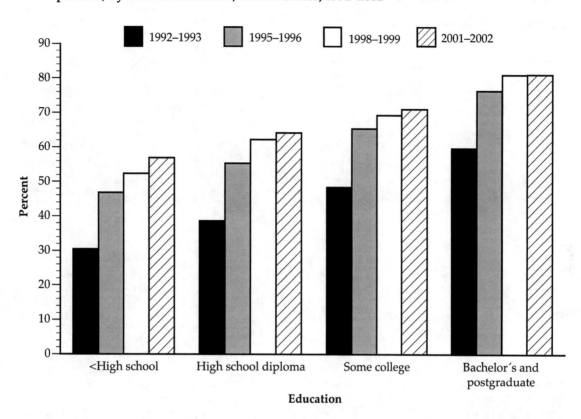

Sources: U.S. Department of Commerce, Census Bureau, National Cancer Institute Sponsored Tobacco Use Supplement to the Current Population Survey, public use data tapes, 1992–1993, 1995–1996, 1998–1999, 2001–2002.

Hyland and colleagues (1999b) assessed compliance in New York restaurants with an earlier, less stringent clean indoor air law that took effect in 1995. The study relied on three data sources: a population-based telephone survey of restaurant owners and managers, independent restaurant inspections conducted by the New York City Health Department, and complaint records maintained by the department. On the basis of the first two measures, the authors estimated that between 65 and 80 percent of restaurants were in full compliance with the law. The study found that 89 percent of restaurant proprietors reported that their indoor dining area was smoke-free and that inspections detected evidence of smoking in only 2 percent of the restaurants. Moreover, more than 80 percent of the restaurant proprietors reported that they were able to comply with the law with little or moderate effort, and 75 percent reported that they did not need to spend any money to achieve compliance.

The complaint records showed a decline over the longer term. The authors concluded that restaurants were able to comply with the law with relative ease and at little expense (Hyland et al. 1999b).

Weber and colleagues (2003) looked at long-term compliance trends under California's 1998 smoke-free bars law; some studies have suggested that rates of noncompliance with smoke-free policies may be especially high in this setting (Shopland et al. 2004). Weber and colleagues (2003) examined the results of a population-based annual inspection survey of free-standing bars and of bars within restaurants in Los Angeles County. The study found that the major problem at the outset of implementation was patron smoking in freestanding bars; only 45.7 percent of freestanding bars were in compliance in 1998. Patron smoking in bars within restaurants (92.2 percent compliance) and employee smoking in freestanding bars (86.2 percent compliance) and in bars within

Table 10.13 Percentage of indoor workers aged 18 years or older who reported compliance with workplace smoking bans, by geographic region and occupational status, United States, 1995–2002

Geographic region and occupational status	1995–1996 (%)	1998–1999 (%)	2001–2002 (%)
Northeast			
White collar	95.13	96.34	96.97
Blue collar	89.31	91.55	94.44
Farm*	86.51	79.98	90.93
Service	93.24	93.07	93.74
Midwest			
White collar	95.73	96.85	97.42
Blue collar	93.37	93.85	93.75
Farm*	95.41	97.51	83.88
Service	93.07	93.63	94.28
South			
White collar	95.71	97.04	97.76
Blue collar	92.36	94.85	95.10
Farm*	96.41	96.90	91.31
Service	92.16	95.30	95.60
West			
White collar	96.71	97.38	97.55
Blue collar	94.12	94.36	94.63
Farm*	100.00	95.78	96.74
Service	93.76	93.84	95.36

Note: Compliance with workplace smoking bans is defined as no one has smoked during the past two weeks in the area in which the respondent works.
*Data were statistically unreliable.
Sources: U.S. Department of Commerce, Census Bureau, National Cancer Institute Sponsored Tobacco Use Supplement to the Current Population Survey, public use data tapes, 1995–1996, 1998–1999, 2001–2002.

restaurants (96.5 percent compliance) were much less of a problem at baseline. By 2002, compliance (measured by the absence of patron smoking) had increased significantly in both freestanding bars (to 75.8 percent) and bars attached to restaurants (to 98.5 percent). Compliance (measured by the absence of employee smoking) had also increased by 2002 in both settings to 94.7 percent and 99.2 percent, respectively, although these increases were not significant. The authors concluded that the California law mandating smoke-free bars had effectively reduced patron and employee smoking in freestanding and attached bars in Los Angeles County and that laws of this type can be successfully implemented (Weber et al. 2003). Another study of the California smoke-free bar law found that the self-reported compliance of bar patrons who were current smokers increased from 75 percent three months after it took effect in 1998 to 86 percent in 2000 (Tang et al. 2003). The level of

compliance that bar patrons who were surveyed reported observing among other bar patrons increased from 71 to 80 percent (Tang et al. 2003).

An official report documenting compliance with a New York City smoke-free workplace law that took effect in 2003 concluded that compliance was high among restaurants and bars (New York City Department of Finance 2004). The New York City Health Department inspected 22,000 establishments and found that 97 percent were in compliance with the law. Compliance was measured by the absence of observed smoking by patrons or employees, the absence of ashtrays, and the presence of properly posted "No Smoking" signs. Similarly, an observational study found that within one month after the New York state smoke-free law took effect, the proportion of smoke-free restaurants, bars, and bowling facilities statewide increased from 31 to 93 percent (New York State Department of Health 2004).

Taken together, the Los Angeles and New York findings suggest that high rates of compliance with smoke-free workplace laws can be achieved even in bars, one of the settings where a higher level of resistance to such laws would be expected.

Evidence suggests that public education and public debate before the adoption of a smoke-free law, as well as during the period leading up to its implementation, can play an important role in paving the way for successful implementation of the law and achieving high compliance rates, especially in hospitality venues. To be effective, a smoke-free law should designate an appropriate and willing enforcement agency and establish a public complaint mechanism and make the complaints received through this mechanism be the driving force for enforcement (Jacobson and Wasserman 1997; California Department of Health Services 1998, 2001a; NCI 2000b; Emerson 2001; Kiser and Boschert 2001). In addition, the law should hold business proprietors, instead of or in addition to individual patrons, responsible for violations and should treat these violations as civil, as opposed to criminal, matters. Experience suggests that laws are likely to be easier to enforce if they are drafted simply and if they contain consistent provisions that apply to all similar settings and to all persons at all times with few, if any, exemptions and ambiguities. Local clean indoor air laws also may be easier to implement because of higher levels of public awareness and cooperation from local enforcement agencies (Jacobson and Wasserman 1997). Evidence indicates that with careful drafting, proper preparation, and the passage of time, clean indoor air laws—especially at the local level—can become largely self-enforcing.

Effect of Workplace Smoking Restrictions

Air Quality

A number of studies have assessed the impact of smoke-free air laws on air quality in restaurants, bars, and other hospitality venues, determined by levels of various markers, most commonly of particulate matter. These studies have consistently found that air quality has improved markedly following the implementation of clean indoor air laws. Repace (2004b) found that levels of respirable particles and particulate polycyclic aromatic hydrocarbons fell sharply in hospitality venues following the implementation of a statewide comprehensive clean indoor air law in Delaware. Similarly, a 2004 study (CDC 2004c) documented similar findings: particulate matter levels fell substantially in hospitality venues in New York state

after a comprehensive state law took effect; levels fell in every venue where smoking had been occurring at baseline.

Secondhand Smoke Exposure

The 2000 Surgeon General's report concluded that "smoking bans are the most effective method for reducing ETS exposure," and that "Optimal protection of nonsmokers and smokers requires a smoke-free environment" (USDHHS 2000c, p. 261). The 2005 *Guide to Community Preventive Services* concluded that "smoking bans and restrictions were effective in decreasing the amount of ETS by approximately 72%" and that "bans and restrictions were also effective in reducing exposure to ETS by approximately 60%" (Task Force on Community Preventive Services 2005, p. 48). The guide went on to say that it "recommends smoking bans and restrictions on the basis of strong evidence of effectiveness in decreasing both the amount of, and exposure to, environmental tobacco smoke" (p. 50).

Studies evaluating objective markers of secondhand smoke exposure among nonsmokers have confirmed self-reported data that suggest that smoke-free air policies in workplaces lead to reduced exposure. Marcus and colleagues (1992) published findings from a pilot study (n = 106) and from a larger study (n = 881) that examined the relationship between a workplace smoking policy, self-reported secondhand smoke exposure, and salivary cotinine concentrations in nonsmoking workers. In both studies, more restrictive workplace smoking policies were associated with a lower proportion of nonsmoking volunteers with detectable salivary cotinine levels. A recent study in New York City reported similar findings: cotinine levels decreased by 85 percent among nonsmoking restaurant and bar employees following the implementation of a statewide comprehensive clean indoor air law (New York City Department of Finance 2004).

A study that assessed air nicotine concentrations before and after implementation of a workplace smoking policy demonstrated a 98 percent reduction in nicotine concentrations following policy implementation (Vaughan and Hammond 1990). Hammond and colleagues (1995) collected 359 air nicotine samples at workstations of nonsmokers across 25 workplaces and found strong associations between workplace policies and nicotine concentrations. For example, the median nicotine concentration in open offices that allowed smoking was 8.6 micrograms per cubic meter ($\mu g/m^3$), compared with 1.3 $\mu g/m^3$ in workplaces that restricted smoking, and 0.3 $\mu g/m^3$ in sites that banned smoking.

A recent study from Massachusetts assessed data from a random-digit telephone dialing survey and found that adults living in towns with stronger restaurant and bar smoking regulations were more likely to report no exposure to secondhand smoke in restaurants and bars (Albers et al. 2004b). Another recent study, also from Massachusetts, documented similar findings: youth living in towns with stronger restaurant smoking restrictions were also more likely to report no exposure to secondhand smoke in restaurants (Siegel et al. 2004).

Farrelly and colleagues (2005) assessed second-hand smoke exposure levels among employees in restaurants, bars, and bowling facilities in New York state before and after implementation of a comprehensive state smoke-free law. Secondhand smoke exposure was assessed both by self-reported information collected through a telephone survey and by saliva cotinine levels. A total of 24 nonsmoking workers were included in the study. The study found that the proportion of workers reporting exposure to second-hand smoke at work fell by 85 percent from baseline to one year after the law took effect, from 91 percent (95 percent CI, 67–98) to 14 percent (95 percent CI, 4–37). Self-reported hours of secondhand smoke exposure at work during the past four days fell by 98 percent from 12.1 hours (95 percent CI, 8.0–16.3) to 0.2 hours (95 percent CI, -0.1–0.5 hours) (p <0.01). Average cotinine levels fell from 3.6 nanograms per milliliter (ng/mL) (95 percent CI, 2.6–4.7 ng/mL) to 0.8 ng/mL (95 percent CI , 0.4–1.2) over this same period. The proportion of workers reporting sensory irritation symptoms (including eye, nose, or throat irritation) in the past four weeks fell from 88 percent (95 percent CI, 66–96) to 38 percent (95 percent CI, 20–59) (p <0.01). In contrast, the proportion of workers reporting respiratory symptoms (including wheezing/whistling in the chest, shortness of breath, coughing in the morning, coughing during the day or at night, or bringing up phlegm) did not decrease significantly. Farrelly and colleagues (2005) concluded that the New York state smoke-free law has had its intended effect of protecting hospitality workers from secondhand smoke exposure.

Skeer and colleagues (2005) assessed self-reported workplace secondhand smoke exposure among a cross-sectional sample of 3,650 adults in Massachusetts who were employed outside the home. The data source was a larger longitudinal random digit-dialed telephone survey. Eighty-one percent of respondents reported working under a complete smoke-free workplace policy, 16 percent reported working under a policy that restricted smoking to designated areas, and 3 percent reported no workplace smoking restrictions. The study found that, overall, 27 percent of respondents reported being exposed to secondhand smoke in the workplace during the preceding week. Self-reported exposure was inversely related to the comprehensiveness of workplace smoking policies: 19.6 percent of workers reporting working under a smoke-free workplace policy reported exposure, compared with 49.9 percent of those covered by a workplace policy limiting smoking to designated areas and 75.1 percent reporting no workplace smoking policy or one that allowed smoking in most areas. Compared with employees who worked under a complete smoke-free workplace policy, employees whose workplace had no smoking restrictions in place had 10.27 times the odds of being exposed to secondhand smoke at work and 6.34 times the duration of exposure; employees who worked under a workplace smoking policy that limited smoking to designated areas had 2.9 times the odds of being exposed to secondhand smoke at work and 1.74 times the duration of exposure. Skeer and colleagues (2005) concluded that smoke-free workplace policies substantially reduce both the likelihood and the duration of workers' on-the-job secondhand smoke exposure. This appears to be one of the first studies to examine the relationship between workplace smoking policies and duration of workplace secondhand smoke exposure.

Studies thus demonstrate a strong relationship between the level of policy restriction and second-hand smoke exposure using three different measures of exposure: cotinine levels, air measurements, and self-reports.

Health Outcomes

Several studies have gone beyond assessing the impact of workplace smoking restrictions on second-hand smoke exposure and have examined their impact on actual health outcomes. These studies have found that smoke-free workplace laws appear to yield health benefits soon after implementation.

Eisner and colleagues (1998) examined the impact of the California smoke-free bars law on the respiratory health of bartenders. The investigators assessed respiratory symptoms and pulmonary function in 53 bartenders from a random sample of bars in San Francisco, California, before and eight weeks after the law took effect. Self-reported exposure to secondhand smoke at work declined from a median of 28 hours per week at baseline to 2 hours per week after the ban. Of the bartenders (74 percent) who reported respiratory symptoms such as cough or wheeze at baseline, 59 percent reported no symptoms at follow-up. There was a statistically significant improvement in pulmonary function using measurements of mean forced vital capacity and forced expiratory volume in one second following the ban. This finding suggests that the long-term exposure to secondhand smoke experienced by bartenders does have an adverse health effect, and smoking bans can effectively protect the health of these workers (Eisner et al. 1998).

Fichtenberg and Glantz (2000) assessed the impact of California's statewide tobacco control program, implemented in 1989, on heart disease mortality from 1980 to 1997, when heart disease mortality rates were steadily declining. The authors found a significant decrease in mortality after 1989 and estimated that there were 58,900 fewer deaths from heart disease between 1989 and 1997 because of the program (Fichtenberg and Glantz 2001). This benefit of the program might reflect reduction not only of active smoking but of involuntary smoking.

Sargent and colleagues (2004) reported that a comprehensive clean indoor air law in Helena, Montana, appeared to be associated with a significant reduction in the number of monthly hospital heart attack admissions during the six months that it was in effect (16 fewer admissions, 95 percent CI, -31.7 to -0.3). A commentary on the study reviewed recent literature on the acute cardiovascular effects of brief secondhand smoke exposures and noted that, although the study had important limitations and needed to be replicated, its findings were broadly plausible and suggest that comprehensive smoke-free measures might potentially produce quick and substantial reductions in heart disease morbidity and mortality (Pechacek and Babb 2004).

Smoking Behavior

Workplace smoking restrictions have the potential to change employees' smoking patterns by reducing opportunities to smoke, by altering workplace norms, and, in some cases, by providing more access to employer-provided cessation services. A series of studies described below examined the impact of smoking restrictions on the number of cigarettes smoked and on smoking rates among employees who are current smokers. Studies have found an association between workplace smoking policies, particularly more restrictive policies, and decreases in the number of cigarettes smoked per day, increases in attempts to stop smoking, and increases in smoking cessation rates.

An analysis of data from a five-year COMMIT follow-up of 8,271 employed adult smokers examined changes in the number of cigarettes smoked per day relative to workplace smoking policies. These self-reported surveys were conducted in 1988 and 1993 (Glasgow et al. 1997). Using multiple linear regression techniques, the investigators found a statistically significant reduction in the number of cigarettes smoked per day over the five-year period in workplaces where smoking was restricted to designated areas compared with workplaces without smoking restrictions. There was an even greater reduction in daily cigarette use among workers whose workplaces completely prohibited smoking; those employees were 25 percent more likely to make a cessation attempt and 25 percent more likely to successfully quit compared with workers in workplaces without smoking bans.

A similar analysis of the California Tobacco Survey data found that current daily smokers who worked in workplaces with some smoking restrictions were more likely to reduce the number of cigarettes they smoked per day compared with smokers who worked in workplaces with no smoking restrictions (odds ratio [OR] = 1.38 [95 percent CI, 0.95–2.00]) (Moskowitz et al. 2000). A greater effect was noted for daily smokers whose workplaces banned smoking (OR = 1.52 [95 percent CI, 1.14–1.71]). The study controlled for gender, age, race, ethnicity, education level, family income, and the number of cigarettes smoked per day one year before the survey (Moskowitz et al. 2000). Using 1993 and 1996 CPS data, Burns and colleagues (2000) collected data from indoor workers who were 25 through 64 years of age and who had smoked daily one year before their interviews in both surveys. Comparing smokers who worked in smoke-free workplaces with smokers who worked in workplaces with less stringent or no restrictions, the investigators found a statistically significant (p <0.001) shift toward smoking fewer cigarettes per day among workers in smoke-free workplaces. However, the authors were unable to directly attribute these reductions to workplace smoking restrictions because the CPS did not ask for the number of cigarettes smoked per day one year before the interview (Burns et al. 2000). Working in a smoke-free environment was also associated with a greater likelihood of being a former smoker or quitting for at least three months. A recent review of studies examining the impact of smoke-free workplaces on smoking behavior concluded, using a pooled estimate of the reviewed studies, that totally smoke-free workplaces were associated with a reduction in smoking prevalence of 3.8 percent and with a reduction in daily smoking among continuing smokers of 3.1 cigarettes per day (Fichtenberg and Glantz 2002). Extrapolating these findings to the U.S. workforce, Fichtenberg and Glantz (2002) estimated that if all U.S. workplaces became smoke-free, the per capita U.S. cigarette consumption would drop by 4.5 percent.

A cohort study drawing on telephone survey data collected as part of COMMIT found that employees in workplaces that changed to or maintained smoke-free workplace policies between 1993 and 2001 were 1.9 times more likely (OR = 1.92 [95 percent CI, 1.11–3.32]) than employees whose workplaces allowed smoking everywhere to have quit smoking by 2001 (Bauer et al. 2005). Continuing smokers reported consuming 2.57 fewer cigarettes daily on average. Employees working under smoke-free workplace policies in both 1993 and 2001 were 2.3 times more likely (OR = 2.29 [95 percent CI, 1.08–4.45]) than employees whose workplace allowed smoking everywhere to have quit by 2001, with continuing smokers reporting consuming 3.85 fewer cigarettes daily on average. Workplace policies that restricted smoking to designated areas did not have a significant effect on cessation. Worksite smoking policies were not related to the number of quit attempts reported. The proportion of respondents who reported working under a smoke-free workplace policy increased from 27 percent in 1993 to 76 percent in 2001. Bauer and colleagues (2005) concluded that smoke-free worksite policies help employees reduce their cigarette consumption and quit smoking.

A recent NCI monograph summarized the evidence on the impact of smoke-free workplace policies on the smoking behavior of employees:

> [Smoke-free workplace policies] ... have two effects on smokers as they are implemented. They increase the rate at which smokers attempt to quit, and they reduce the number of cigarettes smoked per day. Once restrictions on smoking in the workplace have been successfully implemented, they continue to have the effect of reducing the number of cigarettes smoked per day, and they increase the success rate of smokers who are attempting to quit. There may also be a small effect of increasing the frequency with which smokers attempt to quit (NCI 2000a, p. 118).

Additional benefits of these interventions (smoking bans and restrictions) include reductions in daily consumption of cigarettes among workers exposed to bans or restrictions and increases in tobacco use cessation by smokers exposed to workplace smoking bans (Task Force on Community Preventive Services 2005).

Recent evidence suggests that comprehensive smoke-free laws may have an effect on smoking behavior that extends beyond employees of the affected workplaces. Recent findings from New York City and Delaware indicate that, when implemented in conjunction with other evidence-based tobacco control activities, including cigarette excise tax increases, such laws may contribute to substantial and quick reductions in adult smoking prevalence among the general population (State of Delaware 2004; Frieden et al. 2005). In both cases, adult smoking prevalence fell by 11 percent in one year, with even sharper decreases in the smoking prevalence among young adults.

Based on a review of the applicable evidence, the *Guide to Community Preventive Services* concluded that "additional benefits of these interventions [smoking bans and restrictions] include reductions in daily consumption of cigarettes among workers exposed to bans or restrictions and increases in tobacco use cessation by smokers exposed to workplace smoking bans" (Task Force on Community Preventive Services 2005, pp. 50–51). The publication also concluded that smoking bans and restrictions ... helped to reduce cigarette consumption and to increase the number of people who quit smoking" (Task Force on Community Preventive Services 2005, p. 49).

Some studies have also found that smoke-free laws contribute to decreases in smoking among youth. For example, a national study found that adolescents who work in smoke-free workplaces are significantly less likely to be smokers than adolescents who work in workplaces with no smoking restrictions or with restrictions less than a smoking ban in a full work area (Farkas et al. 2000). A Massachusetts study found that youth living in towns with smoke-free restaurant laws were less than 50 percent as likely to progress to established smoking behaviors compared with youth living in towns with weak smoking restrictions in restaurants (Siegel et al. 2005). The *Guide to Community Preventive Services* found that "smoke-free policies also challenge the perception of smoking as a normal adult behavior. By changing this perception, these policies can change the attitudes and behaviors of adolescents, resulting in a reduction in tobacco use initiation" (Task Force on Community Preventive Services 2005, p. 48).

As noted earlier, numerous tobacco industry documents suggest that cigarette manufacturers have also recognized that workplace smoking restrictions, especially smoke-free policies, prompt some smokers to quit and lead continuing smokers to reduce their smoking. For example, one document states that "smoking bans are the biggest challenge we have ever faced. Quit rate goes from 5% to 21% when smokers work in non-smoking environments" (<http://legacy.library.ucsf.edu/tid/nyg12a00>). Another document states that "total prohibition of smoking in the workplace strongly affects industry volume. Smokers facing these restrictions consume 11%–15% less than average and quit at a rate that is 84% higher than average" (John Heironimus, memo to Louis Suwarna, January 22, 1992; <http://legacy.library.ucsf.edu/tid/rvv24e00>). The document goes on to note that "milder workplace restrictions, such as smoking only in designated areas, have much less impact on quitting rates and very little effect on consumption." The document concludes that "clearly, it is most important for PM [Philip Morris] to continue to support accommodation for smokers in the workplace." Finally, a third document states that "financial impact of smoking bans will be tremendous. Three to five fewer cigarettes per day per smoker will reduce annual manufacturer profits a billion dollars plus per year" (<http://legacy.library.ucsf.edu/tid/ijo42e00>). In fact, industry documents suggest that the concern that workplace smoking restrictions will cause smokers to quit or reduce their tobacco use is a major motivation for the industry's repeated efforts to prevent or reverse the adoption of such restrictions.

Social Norms

In addition to protecting nonsmokers from secondhand smoke and helping smokers to quit or reduce their cigarette use, it is also likely that smoking restrictions contribute to changes in public norms regarding the social acceptability of smoking, although relatively few studies have examined this issue. A study that relied on a random-digit telephone dialing survey in Massachusetts, which had a comprehensive program in place, examined the relationship between the strength of local restaurant smoking regulations and the perceived social acceptability of smoking in restaurants, bars, and in general among adults and youth (Albers et al. 2004a). The study also assessed the relationship between the strength of these regulations and perceptions of adult smoking prevalence and found that in towns with strong regulations, adults (but not youth) were more likely to consider smoking in restaurants and bars as unacceptable. In addition, adults and youth living in towns with strong regulations were generally more likely to think that most adults in their town perceived smoking in restaurants as unacceptable compared with their counterparts in

towns with less stringent or no regulations. Youth who lived in towns with strong regulations were also more likely to perceive that most adults in their town disapproved of smoking in general (i.e., not just in restaurants).

Finally, in towns with strong regulations, youth, but not adults, were more likely to perceive a lower prevalence of adult smoking. The 2005 *Guide to Community Preventive Services* states that "smoke-free policies also challenge the perception of smoking as a normal adult behavior. By changing this perception, these policies can change the attitudes and behaviors of adolescents, resulting in a reduction in tobacco use initiation" (Task Force on Community Preventive Services 2005, p. 48).

A number of studies have suggested that smoke-free laws, which depend for their successful implementation on prior changes in social norms, contribute to further changes in these norms over time once they are in place (NCI 2000b; Tang et al. 2003; Gilpin et al. 2004). One implication is that the presence of smoke-free policies leads to further public support for such policies (Borland et al. 1990; Tang et al. 2003; Gilpin et al. 2004; RTI International 2004).

Economic Impact of Smoking Restrictions on the Hospitality Industry

The economic impact of smoke-free regulations on restaurants and bars has been the subject of intense debate, often at local or state levels as bans have been considered. Owners of establishments who view regulations as negatively affecting sales or other aspects of how they conduct their business are reluctant to support such measures or may oppose them. The tobacco industry has consistently claimed that such measures lead to an approximate 30 percent or greater decline in sales (Traynor et al. 1993; Glantz and Charlesworth 1999; Dearlove et al. 2002). However, the industry claims are countered by many studies published during the last decade in the peer-reviewed scientific literature that assessed various objective economic impacts of these regulations on bars and restaurants. A number of these studies are described below. Regardless of the outcome measured, the studies found no evidence of negative economic impacts.

Studies that assessed the economic impact of clean indoor air laws have generally focused on restaurants and bars. Objective indicators of an economic impact on these establishments include sales tax receipts and revenues, employment, and the number of restaurant and bar licenses issued by state health departments and state liquor authorities. Although most of the studies have looked at sales tax data, employment and license data have the advantage of being available more quickly. Some studies have also included surveys that assessed self-reported intentions and behaviors of the customers of these food and beverage establishments. Economic impact studies have assessed the effects of both local and state clean indoor air laws.

Two of the first studies on the economic impact of clean indoor air laws on restaurants and bars were carried out by Glantz and Smith (1994, 1997). Both studies used sales tax data to assess the impact of local ordinances in California and Colorado. The first study found no effect on the fraction of total retail sales that went to restaurants or on the ratio of restaurant sales in communities with ordinances compared with restaurant sales in control communities without such ordinances that were also matched for population, income, smoking prevalence, and geographic location. The communities varied in population size from a few thousand to more than 300,000, and the length of time that the ordinances were in effect ranged from a few months to more than 10 years (Glantz and Smith 1994).

In a follow-up study that included additional analyses of sales data from the 15 cities included in the original study, Glantz and Smith (1997) again examined restaurant sales as a fraction of total retail sales before and after implementation of the ordinances. The investigators compared the ratio of restaurant sales in communities that had enacted ordinances with restaurant sales in communities without ordinances and found that local smoke-free restaurant ordinances did not have a significant effect on restaurant sales. This study also included data from seven communities in California (five cities and two counties) that had enacted ordinances requiring smoke-free bars that were matched with communities without such ordinances. The study examined sales from specific eating and drinking establishments with licenses to serve all types of liquor as a fraction of all retail sales and as a fraction of all sales by eating and drinking establishments. The authors detected no significant effect on bar sales as a fraction of total retail sales, on the ratio between bar sales in cities with and without ordinances, or on the ratio of sales from eating and drinking establishments that were licensed to serve all types of liquor compared with all sales from eating and drinking establishments (Glantz and Smith 1997). The length of time that smoke-free ordinances in bars had been in effect ranged from 25 to 65 months.

Other studies have reached similar findings. One study analyzed restaurant sales after a local ban on smoking had taken effect in a small suburb of Austin, Texas, and found, contrary to prior claims, no indication of reduced restaurant sales (CDC 1995). Other analyses of sales tax receipts have also found that over time, such ordinances had no effect on the fraction of total retail sales for eating and drinking establishments. A more recent study examined whether a smoking ban in El Paso, Texas, affected restaurant and bar revenues (CDC 2004b). In January 2002, the city implemented an ordinance banning smoking in all public places and workplaces, including restaurants and bars. The study, which examined sales tax and mixed-beverage tax data from 12 years before and 1 year after the ordinance was implemented, found that there were no statistically significant changes in restaurant and bar revenues after the ordinance was implemented.

Using taxable sales data from eating and drinking establishments in New York City, Hyland and colleagues (1999a) observed a 2.1 percent increase in sales following implementation of a citywide smoking ban in restaurants compared with sales two years before the law took effect. At the same time, taxable sales in eating and drinking establishments in the rest of the state declined by 3.8 percent. Using a nonrandomized pretest/posttest design and controlling for seasonal effects, Bartosch and Pope (1999) examined the impact of smoke-free restaurant ordinances in 35 cities and towns in Massachusetts between January 1992 and December 1995. The authors used aggregate meal tax data collected by the Massachusetts Department of Revenue before and after the ordinances took effect. The number of restaurants per community varied considerably, from less than 10 to more than 150. Cities and towns without a smoke-free restaurant policy served as comparison communities. The study documented that the enactment of a local smoke-free restaurant ordinance was not followed by a statistically significant changes in the taxable meals revenue that the town collected (Bartosch and Pope 1999).

An in-depth analysis of California tax revenue data from 1990 to 2002 found that the 1995 statewide smoke-free restaurant law was associated with an increase in restaurant revenues. The analysis also found that the 1998 statewide smoke-free bar law was associated with an increase in bar revenues (Cowling and Bond 2005).

Finally, a study of the California smoke-free bar law found that the proportion of bar patrons who reported that they were just as likely or more likely to visit bars that had become smoke-free increased from 86 percent three months after the law took effect in 1998 to 91 percent in 2000 (Tang et al. 2003).

A recent report from New York City assessed all four economic indicators (sales tax receipts, revenues, employment, and the number of licenses issued) and found no negative impact on restaurants and bars from city and state clean indoor air laws (New York City Department of Finance 2004). This study specifically examined various time periods before and after the laws took effect and reported increases in all four economic measures. Restaurant and bar business tax receipts had increased by 8.7 percent; employment in restaurants and bars had increased by about 2,800 seasonally adjusted jobs, amounting to an absolute gain of about 10,600 jobs; and there was a net gain of 234 active liquor licenses for restaurants and bars out of a total of 9,747 such licenses. In addition, a majority of respondents to a Zagat survey and a Zogby poll reported that the smoking restrictions would not have any effect on their patronage of restaurants and bars (New York City Department of Finance 2004). Moreover, the number of respondents who would patronize these establishments more frequently as a result of these restrictions exceeded the number of respondents who said their patronage would decrease. An evaluation of the New York state tobacco control program reached similar findings regarding the economic impact of New York's statewide smoke-free law. The report found that this law had no impact on sales in full-service restaurants and bars (New York State Department of Health 2005).

Studies have also assessed the economic impact of smoke-free restaurant laws on tourism. Glantz and Charlesworth (1999) examined hotel revenues and tourism rates in six cities before and after passage of 100 percent smoke-free restaurant ordinances and compared these revenues and rates with those of U.S. hotels overall. The results indicated that smoke-free restaurant ordinances do not adversely affect tourism revenues and may, in fact, increase tourism (Glantz 2000). More recently, Dai and colleagues (2004) used a variety of measures to assess the impact of a state clean indoor air law in Florida on gross sales and employment levels in the leisure and hospitality industry throughout the state and, more specifically, on restaurants, hotels, and tourism (Dai et al. 2004). The study found increases in the fraction of retail sales from restaurants, lunchrooms, and catering services and increases in the fraction of employment in drinking and eating places and the fraction of employment in the leisure and hospitality industry as a whole following implementation of the law. There were no significant changes in the fraction of retail sales from taverns, night clubs, bars, liquor stores, and recreational admissions or in the fraction of employment in

the hospitality industry after the law took effect. The authors concluded that they were not able to detect a significant negative effect of the state law on sales and employment in the leisure and hospitality industry. The study analyzed sales data from restaurants, lunchrooms, and catering services separately from sales data for taverns, night clubs, and bars, thus addressing a concern that analyzing sales data from eating and drinking places combined could potentially blur differential impacts on these sectors. Interestingly, the study found that the fraction of retail sales for restaurants, lunchrooms, and catering services (which were covered by the law) increased following implementation of the law, but the corresponding fraction did not increase for taverns, night clubs, and bars (which were not covered by the law). These findings suggest that there was no shift in patronage from hospitality venues that were required to be smoke-free to hospitality venues where smoking was still allowed.

Few studies have examined the impact of smoking restrictions on gaming venues (such as casinos), which may be due in part to the fact that, until recently, few gaming venues in the United States have been included in governmental smoking restrictions; some venues have implemented significant voluntary smoking policies of their own. A linear regression analysis of the economic impact of a comprehensive state smoke-free law on casinos in Delaware that drew on revenue data from the Delaware Video Lottery found that the law had no significant effect either on total revenues ($p = 0.126$) or the average revenue per video lottery terminal ($p = 0.314$) (Mandel et al. 2005). The study controlled for economic activity and seasonal effects. In another study, researchers analyzed financial information reported to the State Lottery Commission. Local ordinances in Massachusetts that made charitable bingo venues smoke-free did not appear to negatively affect the profits from those venues (Glantz and Wilson-Loots 2003).

Discrepancies between economic impact studies of clean indoor air laws conducted either by the tobacco industry or by non-industry–supported scientists can be traced in part to variations in the types of data analyzed. Studies commissioned by or for the tobacco industry to assess the economic impact of smoke-free restaurant and bar regulations have generally relied on proprietor predictions or estimates of changes in sales, rather than on actual sales or revenue data. Such estimates are subject to significant reporting bias and are viewed with skepticism because they do not constitute empirical data. Scollo and colleagues (2003) investigated the possible causes of these discrepancies by examining the quality of studies on economic effects of smoke-free policies. Studies showing a negative economic impact that was attributed to clean indoor air laws were 4 times more likely to have used a subjective outcome measure and 20 times more likely not to have been subject to peer review than studies that found no adverse economic impact. All of the studies that found a negative economic impact were supported by the tobacco industry (Scollo et al. 2003). No peer-reviewed study using objective indicators such as sales tax revenues and employment levels found an adverse economic impact of smoke-free laws on restaurants and bars.

In assessing the economic impact of smoke-free policies and laws, their beneficial effect in reducing health care costs must also be weighed. One study using a simulation model projected that implementation of smoke-free policies in all U.S. workplaces would result in 1.3 million smokers quitting, 950 million fewer cigarette packs being smoked, 1,540 myocardial infarctions and 360 strokes being averted, and $49 million in direct medical cost savings being realized, all within the first year (Ong and Glantz 2004). The number of acute health events averted and the costs saved would increase over time. The model took into account both the impact of smokers quitting and the impact of the elimination of workplace secondhand smoke exposure among nonsmoking employees, with reduced secondhand smoke exposure accounting for 59 percent of the averted myocardial infarctions and 50 percent of the cost savings from averted myocardial infarctions during the first year (Ong and Glantz 2004).

The 2005 *Guide to Community Preventive Services* concluded that "we found no adverse impacts on business or tourism as a result of these policies" (Task Force on Community Preventive Services 2005, p. 49). Recently, some business organizations have come to the conclusion that smoke-free policies and laws can actually have a positive economic impact, as reflected not only in increased productivity and savings in employee health care costs, other insurance costs, and cleaning and maintenance costs, but also in the image and business climate of a community. For example, the Chamber of Commerce in Louisville, Kentucky, recently came out in support of a proposed municipal smoke-free ordinance. The president of the Chamber explained that "We believe that this piece of legislation ... has reasonable controls and is responsible in terms of really making a difference in the community and ultimately helping us reach our vision of becoming an economic hot spot" (Gerth 2005). "We would generally be in favor of less regulation," said Carmen Hickerson, a spokeswoman. "But quality-of-life issues

are decisions that factor in to economic development. Those things have as much, or more, weight than traditional economic development tools, such as tax breaks" (Vereckey 2005).

Household Smoking Rules

Home smoking restrictions are private household rules that are adopted voluntarily by household members. They can include comprehensive rules that make homes smokefree in all areas at all times and less comprehensive rules that restrict smoking to certain places or times (e.g., allowing smoking only in specific rooms, designating certain rooms as smoke-free, allowing smoking only when no children are present, etc.) (Pyle et al. 2005). The only approach that effectively protects nonsmokers from secondhand smoke exposure is a rule making the home completely smoke-free (Levy et al. 2004).

Smoke-free home rules and other home smoking restrictions may be implemented for a variety of reasons, including

- to protect children in the household from secondhand smoke exposure;

- to protect pregnant women in the household from secondhand smoke exposure;

- to protect nonsmoking spouses or other nonsmoking adult household members from secondhand smoke exposure;

- to protect children or adults who have health conditions that are exacerbated by secondhand smoke exposure or who are at risk for health conditions that can be triggered by secondhand smoke (e.g., a child with asthma, an adult with or at special risk for heart disease);

- to help smokers in the household cut down their cigarette consumption;

- to help smokers quit;

- to help smokers who have quit maintain abstinence;

- to set a positive example for children and youth in the household, to prevent them from becoming smokers themselves;

- aesthetic, hygienic, economic, and safety considerations, including eliminating the odor of secondhand smoke, eliminating cigarette burns, and eliminating the risk of fires caused by discarded cigarettes; and

- simply because no one in the household smokes anymore (Ferrence et al. 2005).

Prevalence and Correlates

Reducing secondhand smoke exposure in the home is important because the home is a major source of exposure for children and for those nonsmoking adults who are not exposed elsewhere. Reducing exposure in this setting is challenging, however, because there are no clearly established interventions that effectively reduce exposure at home. In addition, because smoke-free home rules are adopted voluntarily, rather than imposed by government bodies or employers, the prevalence of these rules is an important indicator of changes in norms regarding the social acceptability of smoking. In the text that follows, the definition of "children" varies across the studies cited.

In the past decade, substantial increases have occurred in the number of U.S. households with private rules to limit secondhand smoke exposure within the home. Even smokers are increasingly adopting such rules. One of the best data sources available on children's secondhand smoke exposure in the home is the National Health Interview Survey (NHIS). This information can be derived from NHIS data by correlating data on smoking in the home with data on households with children. NHIS data shows that the proportion of children aged 6 years and younger who are regularly exposed to secondhand smoke in their homes fell from 27 percent in 1994 to 20 percent in 1998. A recent study by Soliman and colleagues (2004) examined data from the NHIS and found that the prevalence of secondhand smoke exposure in homes with children fell from 35.6 percent in 1992 to 25.1 percent in 2000. The prevalence of adult smoking fell by a smaller amount during this same period, from 26.5 to 23.3 percent, indicating that a portion of the reduced exposure can be explained by the increase in home smoking rules. Home exposures declined across all racial, ethnic, educational, and income groups that were analyzed. Farkas and colleagues (2000) analyzed data from adolescents aged 15 through 17 years from the 1993 and 1996 CPS. Of those respondents, 48 percent lived in smoke-free households in 1993 and 55 percent lived in smoke-free homes by 1996.

The CPS data show that the percentage of smoke-free homes increased by 40 percent between 1993 and 2002, from 43 to 66 percent (Table 10.14). Households with a smoker in the home had lower rates of smoke-free home rules than did households without a smoker; however, the prevalence of smoke-free rules in homes with smokers increased by 110 percent between 1993 and 1999. In a 1997 survey in Oregon, Pizacani and colleagues (2003) found similar differences in the prevalence of smoke-free home rules between nonsmoking households (85 percent) and households with one or more smokers (38 percent). These trends of smoke-free home rules were observed in all four regions of the country in the CPS data. Individuals living in the West reported higher rates of smoke-free homes, but the largest increases between 1993 and 2002 were in the South and the Midwest. Similarly, there were wide variations among states in the percentage of individuals reporting household smoking bans. Utah reported the highest rate (83 percent), followed by California (78 percent), Arizona (76 percent), and Idaho (74 percent) (Tables 10.14 and 10.15).

The presence of a child younger than 13 years of age was associated with only a slight increase in the rate of smoke-free homes compared with homes where there were no children under 13 years of age (Table 10.15). However, a survey of 598 adult smokers living in an inner-city neighborhood in Kansas City (Missouri) found that after adjusting for age, race, gender, and education, a rule banning smoking or restricting it to designated locations in the home was significantly more likely in households with a child (OR = 2.63 [95 percent CI, 1.70–4.08]) or a nonsmoking adult partner (OR = 2.07 [95 percent CI, 1.19–3.61]) (Okah et al. 2002).

Households with lower incomes reported lower rates of smoke-free home rules compared with higher income households. The amount smoked was higher in lower income homes, whether or not a smoker resided in the home (Okah et al. 2002).

EPA conducted a national telephone survey in 2003 on children's secondhand smoke exposure and childhood asthma among a random digit-dialed sample of U.S. households, involving 14,685 interviews (USEPA 2005). The survey yielded the following results:

- Approximately 11 percent of children aged six years and under were reported to be exposed to secondhand smoke on a regular basis (four or more days per week) in their home.

- Secondhand smoke exposure is significantly higher in households at and below the poverty level.

- Parents account for the vast majority of exposure in homes (almost 90 percent of the exposure), followed by grandparents and other relatives living in the home.

Table 10.14 Prevalence of smoke-free households, by state, United States, 1992–2002

State	1992–1993 (%)	1998–1999 (%)	2001–2002 (%)
Overall	43.16	60.23	66.03
Alabama	38.94	59.13	62.11
Alaska	50.93	60.87	69.35
Arizona	54.38	71.60	75.93
Arkansas	33.21	53.02	57.05
California	59.07	72.71	77.51
Colorado	48.27	65.16	70.28
Connecticut	44.70	60.05	70.50
Delaware	40.13	55.36	64.31
District of Columbia	41.36	56.60	67.46
Florida	50.20	65.95	71.75
Georgia	41.75	61.88	69.06
Hawaii	51.46	64.99	68.26
Idaho	50.56	70.34	74.13
Illinois	38.56	54.56	60.27
Indiana	33.85	47.85	57.30
Iowa	36.05	52.92	61.65
Kansas	39.87	59.33	64.22
Kentucky	25.69	38.87	49.96
Louisiana	37.30	58.24	65.50
Maine	39.40	54.38	62.95
Maryland	42.99	64.32	67.71
Massachusetts	40.25	60.09	70.51
Michigan	35.35	51.19	58.01
Minnesota	39.70	61.52	66.25
Mississippi	41.15	54.93	61.97
Missouri	34.47	53.74	56.62
Montana	43.09	60.97	67.06
Nebraska	39.93	59.54	63.78
Nevada	45.52	63.66	68.65
New Hampshire	38.37	56.54	66.98
New Jersey	45.54	61.33	68.26
New Mexico	45.55	62.67	71.66
New York	41.59	58.25	63.44
North Carolina	34.32	52.95	57.07
North Dakota	41.16	56.38	62.79
Ohio	35.10	51.44	56.41
Oklahoma	39.23	54.06	60.86
Oregon	49.99	68.04	73.54
Pennsylvania	39.93	56.34	60.24
Rhode Island	38.87	60.40	65.52
South Carolina	40.20	58.62	67.56
South Dakota	36.80	57.13	61.08
Tennessee	34.09	51.96	56.10
Texas	46.32	65.29	71.09
Utah	69.58	81.13	83.13
Vermont	39.05	59.65	64.62
Virginia	39.27	58.35	64.49
Washington	54.25	68.92	71.26
West Virginia	27.78	42.75	50.16
Wisconsin	36.66	55.39	61.76
Wyoming	38.57	57.96	60.83

Sources: U.S. Department of Commerce, Census Bureau, National Cancer Institute Sponsored Tobacco Use Supplement to the Current Population Survey, public use data tapes, 1992–1993, 1998–1999, 2001–2002.

Table 10.15   Prevalence of smoke-free households, by geographic region, socioeconomic status, and household smoking status, United States, 1992–2002

Geographic region, socioeconomic status, and household smoking status	1992–1993 (%)	1998–1999 (%)	2001–2002 (%)	% change from 1992 to 2002
Overall	43.16	60.23	66.03	52.99
Geographic region				
Northeast	41.61	58.57	64.89	55.95
Midwest	36.55	53.63	59.51	62.82
South	41.07	59.13	65.19	58.73
West	55.80	70.59	75.20	34.77
Socioeconomic status				
Low	36.95	53.00	57.78	56.37
High	44.74	61.86	67.49	50.85
Smoking status				
No smokers in the home	56.80	73.65	78.88	38.87
Smokers in the home	9.56	20.05	25.58	167.57
Child aged <13 years	45.71	66.49	72.81	59.29
Smoker in the home and child <13 years	12.78	28.62	36.48	185.45
No smoker in the home and child <13 years	62.66	80.50	85.21	35.99

Sources: U.S. Department of Commerce, Census Bureau, National Cancer Institute Sponsored Tobacco Use Supplement to the Current Population Survey, public use data tapes, 1992–1993, 1998–1999, 2001–2002.

- The presence of a child with asthma in the home was not associated with reduced exposure, even in homes with younger children. Children with asthma were just as likely to be exposed to secondhand smoke as children in general.

- The contribution of visitors to the regular exposure of children to secondhand smoke was negligible. In households with children aged 6 years or younger, only 0.3 percent of children were exposed to secondhand smoke by visitors alone. Similarly, only 0.5 percent of children under 18 were exposed solely by visitors.

The prevalence of smoke-free household rules has been studied in California, which has undertaken a campaign to promote smoke-free homes as part of its comprehensive statewide tobacco control program (Gilpin et al. 2001). The 1999 California Tobacco Survey found that 73.2 percent of California homes had a smoke-free rule in place. This finding represented an increase of 30 percent from 1993. In addition, nearly half (47.2 percent) of the smokers lived in a smoke-free home—an increase of 135 percent from 1993. An additional 21.8 percent of smokers lived in homes

with some smoking restrictions. Consistent with these increases, the percentage of children and adolescents protected from secondhand smoke exposure at home increased by 15 percent during that same time period to 88.6 percent (Gilpin et al. 2001).

Gilpin and colleagues (1999) used data from the 1996 California Tobacco Survey (n = 8,904) to evaluate factors associated with the adoption of smoke-free home rules. The data showed that male smokers were more likely than female smokers to report smoke-free homes, and household smoking bans were less likely with the increased age of current smokers in the household. Hispanic and Asian smokers were more likely to report smoke-free homes (58 percent and 43 percent, respectively) than were non-Hispanic Whites (32 percent); African Americans were the least likely to report smoke-free homes (23 percent). Living in a household with a child or with nonsmoking adults predicted a smoke-free household. After adjusting for demographics, the investigators noted that smokers were nearly six times more likely to report living in a smoke-free home if they lived with a nonsmoking adult and child compared with smokers who lived in homes without children or adult nonsmokers (59 percent versus 15 percent, respectively).

Effect of Household Smoking Rules on Secondhand Smoke Exposure

During the past two decades, several data sources have consistently shown that a large proportion of children in the United States were regularly exposed to secondhand smoke. For example, 1988 NHIS data revealed that 42.4 percent of children aged five years and younger lived with at least one smoker (Overpeck and Moss 1991). Data from the 1991 NHIS indicated that 31.2 percent of children aged 10 years and younger were exposed daily to secondhand smoke in their homes (Mannino et al. 1996). An important finding was that children from lower income families were significantly more likely to be exposed to secondhand smoke than were children from higher income families. For example, 41 percent of children from lower income families were exposed daily compared with only 21 percent of children from higher income families. CDC's 2005 *Third National Report on Human Exposure to Environmental Chemicals,* drawing on data from NHANES, reported that median cotinine levels measured during 1999–2002 have fallen by 68 percent among children, by 69 percent among adolescents, and by 75 percent among adults when compared with median levels from 1988–1991. However, the data also show that children's cotinine levels are twice as high as those of adults (CDC 2005d).

In an intervention study of low-income households with at least one child under three years of age, the median household nicotine concentration was 3.3 $\mu g/m^3$ (Emmons et al. 2001). A recent study that measured cotinine levels in infants and nicotine levels in household dust, in the air, and on household surfaces found that smoke-free home rules may substantially reduce, but may not completely eliminate, household contamination from secondhand smoke, including secondhand smoke exposure of infants (Matt et al. 2004). The study found that infants living with smokers in homes with smoke-free rules had lower cotinine levels compared with infants from homes with smokers without such rules, but cotinine levels were higher compared with infants from homes without smokers. The same was true of nicotine levels in household dust, in air, and on household surfaces. One possible explanation for this finding is that even with smoke-free home rules, secondhand smoke may enter the house in the air, on dust, or on the smoker's breath or clothing. And there is always the possibility that some smokers may not be consistently complying with the rules or may be overstating the rules. Exposure does not appear to be lower in homes with children who are at particular risk from secondhand

smoke, such as children with asthma. Kane and colleagues (1999) conducted home visits of 828 households in a lower income section of Buffalo (New York) to identify 167 persons of all ages with asthma and 161 persons without asthma. Self-reported household secondhand smoke exposure levels were similar in both groups—half of the households reported exposure.

Interventions to Reduce Home-Based Secondhand Smoke Exposure of Children

Because secondhand smoke exposure poses serious health risks to children and because the home is the major source of exposure for children, a number of public health practitioners, tobacco control programs, and other organizations at the local, state, and national levels have carried out activities intended to reduce children's secondhand smoke exposure in the home. As the lead federal government agency in this area, EPA has played an especially significant role at the national level. EPA has collaborated with the health care community, state and local tobacco control programs, and other organizations to marshal efforts to institutionalize smoke-free home rules (USDHHS 2003). The American Legacy Foundation also launched a media initiative in 2005 to promote smoke-free homes and vehicles (American Legacy Foundation 2005).

However, few interventions to reduce children's secondhand smoke exposure have been systematically evaluated. The *Guide to Community Preventive Services* found insufficient evidence for the effectiveness of community educational initiatives designed to reduce secondhand smoke exposure in the home (Task Force on Community Preventive Services 2005). In a systematic review, the *Guide* was able to identify only three relevant studies and only one study that met its criteria.

Table 10.16 summarizes a number of relevant studies. The early studies did not show a significant effect on objective exposure measures, although some showed reductions of self-reported exposure.

Two trials in the United States found substantial reductions in secondhand smoke exposure among healthy children as a result of an intervention (Table 10.16) (Hovell et al. 2000a; Emmons et al. 2001). In a randomized controlled trial of 291 smoking parents of young children, Emmons and colleagues (2001) used a motivational intervention to reduce household secondhand smoke exposure. Participants were low-income families, recruited through primary care settings, with children younger than three years of age.

Participants were randomly assigned to either the motivational intervention group or a self-help comparison group; follow-up assessments were conducted at three months and six months. The motivational intervention consisted of one 30- to 45-minute motivational interview session at the participant's home with a trained health educator and four follow-up telephone counseling calls. The intervention included feedback to participants regarding baseline levels of airborne nicotine and CO in their homes. Families in the self-help group were mailed a copy of a smoking cessation manual, a secondhand smoke reduction tip sheet, and a resource guide. Household nicotine levels were measured by a passive diffusion monitor. The six-month nicotine levels were significantly lower in motivational intervention households than in the self-help households. Repeated measures of analysis of variance across baseline, three-month, and six-month time points showed a significant time-by-treatment interaction—indicating that patterns over time differ by treatment group—whereby nicotine levels for the motivational intervention group decreased significantly, and nicotine levels for the self-help group increased but were not significantly different from baseline.

Hovell and colleagues (2000a) evaluated a seven-session, three-month counseling intervention with a randomized trial design involving 108 mothers who had a child under four years of age. Reported exposure of children declined from 27.3 cigarettes per week at baseline to 4.5 cigarettes per week at 3 months and to 3.7 cigarettes per week at 12 months in the counseled group. The investigators also observed reductions in exposure among the controls, but the reductions among the intervention participants were significantly greater. At the 12-month follow-up comparison between the intervention group and the controls, the level of self-reported exposure in the intervention group was 41.2 percent of the exposure of the controls from maternal smoking and 46 percent of the exposure of the controls from all sources combined (Hovell et al. 2000a). Urinary cotinine concentrations among children decreased by 4 percent in the intervention group but increased by 85 percent in the control group.

Other studies have evaluated family interventions designed to reduce secondhand smoke exposure among children with asthma. Hovell and colleagues (2002) demonstrated a significant impact on self-reported exposure among a general population of families with children who have asthma and an impact on self-reported exposure and cotinine levels among Hispanic families (Table 10.16).

Gehrman and Hovell (2003) reviewed 19 studies of interventions to reduce secondhand smoke exposure among children in the home setting that were published between 1987 and 2002. The interventions fell into two categories: (1) physician-based interventions, which consisted of information and recommendations delivered orally by a physician or nurse during a regularly scheduled appointment (e.g., a well-baby or immunization visit) in a pediatrician's office or other health care facility, and (2) home-based interventions, which consisted of counseling delivered by a nurse or a trained research assistant during a home visit. The main outcome of interest was children's secondhand smoke exposure, with parental smoking cessation as a secondary outcome of interest in some studies. Children's exposure was primarily measured through parental self-report, with some studies also measuring children's urinary cotinine levels. Of the 19 studies, 11 reported significant reductions in secondhand smoke exposure. However, only one of the eight studies that monitored children's cotinine levels reported significant differences in cotinine levels between treatment and control groups. Effect sizes (measured as Cohen's d) ranged from -0.14 to 1.04, with a mean effect size of 0.34. The review suggests that interventions in this area can achieve at least small to moderate effects.

Gehrman and Hovell (2003) concluded that home-based interventions, which tended to be more intensive in terms of frequency and duration of contact, generally appeared to be more effective than physician-based interventions, which tended to be less intensive. Seven of the eight exclusively home-based interventions assessed yielded significant effects, compared with 4 of the 10 physician-based interventions. The review also found that interventions that were explicitly based on behavior change theory (e.g., behavior modification theory, social learning/cognitive theory) appeared to be more likely to be effective, with eight of the nine interventions that fell into this category registering significant secondhand smoke reductions.

Gehrman and Hovell (2003) suggest that optimal interventions should combine physician- and home-based approaches, combine immediate steps to reduce children's secondhand smoke exposure with cessation support for parents who want to quit, be based on behavior change theory (especially in terms of providing participants with concrete skills and strategies to help them achieve the desired outcomes), foster participants' self-efficacy and provide them with ongoing reinforcement for positive behavior changes, and be sustained over time. The study also suggests

Table 10.16   Studies assessing the effectiveness of interventions to reduce home-based secondhand smoke exposure of children

Study	Target population	Assessment of secondhand smoke exposure	Response rates Follow-up rates
Woodward et al. 1987	New mothers who smoked (n = 184)	Maternal reports and infant urinary cotinine	>95% 85%
Chilmonczyk et al. 1992	Mothers of pediatric patients (n = 103)	Maternal reports and urinary cotinine	NR* 55%
Greenberg et al. 1994	New mothers, smokers, and nonsmokers (n = 933)	Maternal reports and infant urinary cotinine	47% 71%
Hovell et al. 1994	Families of children with asthma aged 6–17 years, recruited from asthma clinics (n = 91)	Child's self-monitoring and environmental monitoring (air nicotine levels)	NR NR
McIntosh et al. 1994	Families of children with asthma aged 6 months to 17 years, recruited from asthma clinics (n = 72)	Maternal self-reports of indoor smoking; child's urinary cotinine level	NR 67%
Groner et al. 2000	Mothers of children <12 years of age (n = 479)	Knowledge of effects of secondhand smoke on children; maternal smoking status; location of maternal smoking	48% NR
Hovell et al. 2000a	Mothers of children <4 years of age (n = 108)	Children's urinary cotinine levels; maternal reports; nicotine monitors	92% 94%
Emmons et al. 2001	Smoking parents of children <3 years of age (n = 291)	Household nicotine, participant carbon monoxide level	81.2% at 3 months 85.1% at 6 months

Intervention conditions	Findings
• Intervention: self-help materials (Bringing Up Baby Smoke-Free); 1 telephone counseling follow-up call • Minimal contact control: baseline and 3-month assessment • Follow-up only: 3-month assessment	• No differences in infants' secondhand smoke exposure (parent-reported levels) • No differences in infant cotinine levels • No differences in maternal smoking status
• Intervention: feedback from pediatricians regarding infant levels of urinary cotinine; tips for reducing secondhand smoke exposure • Control: assessment only	• No difference in infant cotinine level
• Intervention: 4 home visits from a study nurse during 6 months; self-help materials • Control: assessments only at 3 weeks of age, 7 and 12 months of age	• For nonsmoking mothers: difference of 0.5 cigarettes in the number of parent-reported cigarettes that the infant was exposed to • For smoking mothers: decrease of 5.9 cigarettes in infant exposure; no differences in infant cotinine levels or maternal cessation
• Intervention: behavioral counseling sessions with parent and child; self-monitoring (feedback about child's pulmonary function and symptoms) • Monitoring only control: self-monitoring of exposures • Usual treatment control: baseline and follow-up assessments at 2, 6, 9, and 12 months	• Significantly greater self-reported exposure reduction in intervention group (70%) versus monitoring control (42%) and usual care (34%) groups • No differences in air nicotine levels
• Usual care: secondhand smoke reduction education and advice to quit smoking indoors • Intervention: usual care plus written feedback about child's cotinine level	• No difference in indoor smoking or child's cotinine level
• Intervention 1: brief cessation counseling focusing on child secondhand smoke exposure plus self-help manual, reminder cards, and telephone calls • Intervention 2: brief counseling session focused on smoking's effects on maternal health; self-help materials, reminder cards, and telephone calls • Control: no cessation advice	• No impact on quit rate • Significant difference in change of smoking location and knowledge of secondhand smoke effects
• Intervention: telephone and in-person sessions totaling 7 hours to decrease exposure; signs and rewards provided • Control: nutritional counseling; brief cessation advice; brief advice not to expose kids to secondhand smoke	• Significant differences between groups by the time of reported childhood exposures to secondhand smoke from maternal reports and for total exposures to secondhand smoke • Significant differences between groups by time in cotinine levels
• Intervention: motivation interview and 4 follow-up calls • Control: self-help mailed printed materials	• 6 months: significant effects • Significant time-by-treatment interactions

Table 10.16   Continued

Study	Target population	Assessment of secondhand smoke exposure	Response rates Follow-up rates
Wilson et al. 2001	Secondhand smoke-exposed Medicaid-eligible children aged 3–12 years, treated for asthma at a hospital (n = 87)	Urinary cotinine/creatinine ratio; number of acute asthma visits; hospitalizations; smoking restrictions in the home; amount smoked; reported exposures of children; asthma control	59% provided 12 months of cotinine data
Hovell et al. 2002	Hispanic children with asthma (n = 204)	Reported secondhand smoke exposure; child urinary cotinine; parent saliva cotinine; air nicotine monitor	98% of intervention group completed all sessions

*NR = Data were not reported.

that future studies should explore approaches to increasing the effectiveness of physician-based interventions, for example, equipping mothers with skills to deal with spouses or other household members who are contributing to children's secondhand smoke exposure. In addition, studies should examine efficacy of other interventions, including group interventions (as opposed to one-on-one interventions), the use of motivational interviewing, exploring the link between reducing children's secondhand smoke exposure and increasing parental cessation, and interventions directed at children (as opposed to interventions directed at parents). The authors also emphasize the importance of evaluating interventions; they note, for example, that while "home-based interventions may be particularly promising, …future research should be done in a systematic, replicable manner so that investigators can make more direct comparisons" (Gehrman and Hovell 2003, p. 297). Finally, in addition to refining interventions directed at individual behavior change, efforts should be continued to increase public awareness and smoking restrictions.

Hovell and colleagues (2000b) examined the effectiveness of available approaches to reducing secondhand smoke exposure among children. The study identified three trials reporting that repeated counseling reduced quantitative measures of secondhand smoke exposure in asthmatic children and one controlled trial reporting that repeated physician counseling directed toward reducing secondhand smoke exposure increased parental cessation. Controlled trials of clinicians' one-time counseling

yielded null results. The study concluded that one-time clinical interventions appeared marginally effective or ineffective. Repeated minimal interventions, while not consistently yielding changes in secondhand smoke exposure, appeared to hold more promise. However, the study calls for further evaluations of this approach, specifically large-scale controlled trials.

Hovell and colleagues (2000b) also note that even the interventions that appeared to reduce secondhand smoke exposure rarely eliminated it completely and suggest that these interventions may need to be sustained over long periods of time. The study points to a need for further research on approaches that combine counseling to reduce children's secondhand smoke exposure with subsequent counseling to help parents quit smoking. Such counseling might include interventions to address situations where the mother, who typically is the patient receiving the counseling, is not the only smoker in the household or is not a smoker at all. Other interventions might be directed at children instead of parents. Still others might address the social disparities implicit in the increased prevalence of smoking and secondhand smoke exposure among low-SES populations and some racial/ethnic groups.

Hovell and colleagues (2000b) also examined a number of other strategies for reducing children's secondhand smoke exposure, including regulatory, policy, legal, and media approaches. The study concludes by noting the importance of pursuing interventions in this area within the context of a comprehensive approach to tobacco control.

Intervention conditions	Findings
• Intervention: behavioral counseling; review of cotinine results • Control: usual medical care	• Significant differences in acute asthma medical visits and hospitalizations • Nonsignificant differences in cotinine/creatinine ratios and home smoking policies
• Intervention: 1.5 hours of asthma management education; 7 sessions to reduce secondhand smoke exposure • Control: asthma management education	• Significant differences in reported exposures • Significant reductions in 4-month cotinine levels, but not in 13-month cotinine levels

In addition to the role of the health care sector in establishing smoke-free policies and changing norms related to smoking in health care settings, the role that pediatricians can play in reducing exposure of children to secondhand smoke has drawn increasing attention. The American Academy of Pediatrics has recommended that secondhand smoke exposure of children should be discussed as part of pediatric care, and providers should follow the Agency for Healthcare Research and Quality (formerly the Agency for Health Care Policy and Research) guidelines for working with parents to quit or reduce their smoking (Etzel and Balk 1999). The American Academy of Pediatrics has identified secondhand smoke exposure as a priority area and is collaborating with EPA and others to reduce childhood exposures.

Effect on Smoking Behavior

National data have confirmed findings from California that relate household smoking rules and workplace smoking policies to smoking status. Farkas and colleagues (1999) analyzed 1993 CPS data and found that, compared with smokers living under no household smoking restrictions, smokers living under a total household smoking ban were almost four times more likely to report an attempt to quit smoking during the previous 12 months compared with smokers with no household smoking restrictions (OR = 3.86 [95 percent CI, 3.57–4.18]). Smokers who lived in a home with a partial smoking ban were almost twice as likely to report an attempt to quit during the previous 12 months (OR = 1.83 [95 percent

CI, 1.72–1.92]). The investigators also noted a weaker relationship between workplace smoking bans compared with workplaces with no restrictions or restrictions less than a ban on smoking in work areas, and reporting an attempt to quit (OR = 1.14 [95 percent CI, 1.05–1.24]). Among smokers who attempted to quit in the previous year, smokers who lived under a household smoking ban had an OR of 1.65 (95 percent CI, 1.43–1.91) of abstaining for at least six months compared with smokers with no household smoking restrictions, while smokers who lived under a partial household smoking ban had an OR of 1.20 (95 percent CI, 1.05–1.38). Smokers with a workplace smoking ban who tried to quit had an OR of 1.21 (95 percent CI, 1.00–1.45) for abstaining for at least six months compared with smokers working under no workplace restrictions or some form of restriction less than a work area ban (Farkas et al. 1999).

In a recent prospective study of a population-based cohort of smokers identified from a previous telephone survey, Pizacani and colleagues (2004) found that smokers living under a full household smoking ban at baseline were twice as likely as smokers living with no ban or with a partial ban to attempt to quit and to abstain for at least one day over follow-up of about two years. The study also found that among smokers who were preparing to quit at baseline, a full ban was associated with a lower relapse rate and with more than four times the odds of abstaining for seven or more days at follow-up. These associations were not found among smokers in the precontemplation/contemplation stage of quitting. The authors concluded that full household smoking bans may facilitate cessation among smokers who are preparing to quit by increasing cessation attempts and may prolong the time to relapse among these smokers (Pizacani et al. 2004).

Important relationships have also been found between household and workplace smoking restrictions and smoking trends among adolescents. After adjusting for demographics, school enrollment, and having other smokers in the home, adolescents from smoke-free households were 26 percent less likely to be smokers than adolescents who lived in homes without smoking restrictions. Adolescents who worked indoors in smoke-free workplaces were 32 percent less likely to be smokers than adolescents whose indoor workplaces had a partial work area ban. Smoke-free home rules also increased the chances of quitting among adolescent smokers; respondents were 1.80 times more likely to be former smokers if they lived in smoke-free homes (Farkas et al. 2000). The findings of the surveys need to be interpreted with consideration of the difficulty in inferring causal directions from cross-sectional data. The cohort study of Pizacani and colleagues (2004) would not be subject to this potential limitation.

Smoking Restrictions in Institutional Settings

Institutional settings provide a particularly challenging venue for secondhand smoke control, because the rights of both those who live and those who work in the setting must be considered. Bans have been implemented in hospitals and other health care facilities over the last two decades. Prisons and nursing homes are two additional settings where restrictive smoking policies have been considered and enacted.

Hospitals and Health Care Facilities

Beginning in the 1980s, individual hospitals were made smoke-free. The experiences of two major medical institutions, the Johns Hopkins Hospital and the Mayo Medical Center, are well-documented (Hurt et al. 1989; Stillman et al. 1990) and demonstrate the importance of a comprehensive approach and provide a model for other institutions. In the early 1990s, smoking was systematically restricted in the inpatient health care setting as a result of two policy initiatives, one by the U.S. Department of Veterans Affairs (VA) and the other by JCAHO. In January 1991, VA, the nation's largest health care provider, announced that all 172 of its acute care hospitals would be smoke-free; at the time of implementation, the policy affected 4.5 million patients in the United States (Joseph and O'Neil 1992). The VA policy prohibited smoking by patients, visitors, and employees in acute care facilities but not in the 146 long-term and chronic care facilities. The VA policy also ended the distribution of free tobacco products, increased the price of cigarettes sold in VA facilities to market rates, and eventually halted the sale of cigarettes in these facilities altogether. However, Congress passed the *Veterans Health Care Act of 1992*, which required VA hospitals to establish "suitable" indoor or outdoor smoking areas with "appropriate" heating and air conditioning. This legislation, which was largely seen as reversing progress from the 1991 VA policy (Joseph 1994), required smoking facilities to be built or upgraded, but provided no additional funding. Current VA policy has moved beyond the use of indoor smoking areas and mandates that each VA health care facility establish and maintain a smoking area in a detached building that is accessible, heated, air-conditioned, and meets JCAHO and OSHA requirements for ventilation (USVA 2003). Only long-term care or mental health programs can have indoor smoking areas, which must be separately ventilated. Smoking is allowed on the grounds of all VA facilities as long as it does not interfere with safety and public access. Smoking has been similarly restricted or banned in other federal institutions that have a health care component, including the U.S. Army (Hagey 1989) and the Indian Health Service (CDC 1987a).

Perhaps the most influential smoking policy in the health care sector is the JCAHO accrediting standard that was issued in January 1991. This standard required hospitals to develop and implement policies prohibiting smoking in hospital buildings by patients, visitors, staff, employees, and volunteers no later than the end of 1993 (JCAHO 1992). This policy covers the 5,000 hospitals and 560 psychiatric institutions that are accredited by JCAHO, which include 85 percent of all acute care hospitals in the United States. Exceptions are allowed for patients receiving physician prescriptions, primarily for nicotine replacement therapies to assist with smoking cessation, that are based on medical criteria defined by the medical staff at each institution. This standard is just one of a number of standards considered by JCAHO in accrediting hospitals; a hospital may not be fully compliant with the standard and still receive accreditation (Longo et al. 1998).

After implementing the hospital-wide no-smoking policy at Johns Hopkins, a study was conducted to determine patient compliance by assessing whether inpatients refrained from smoking or went outside to smoke (Stillman et al. 1995). Using a prospective design from 1990 to 1992, 504 patients were interviewed when they were admitted to the hospital about their knowledge of, attitude toward, and adherence to the no-smoking policy. The researchers found that 77 percent of smokers had abstained from smoking while hospitalized; 88 percent of the patients complied with the policy. The study demonstrated that hospital policies that impose abstinence provide an opportunity to promote smoking cessation.

To evaluate compliance with smoke-free standards in health care facilities, Joseph and colleagues (1995) surveyed 1,278 hospitals accredited by JCAHO. The investigators assessed compliance 16 months after the implementation of the smoke-free standard and found that 65 percent of hospitals were in compliance; 55 percent of the smoke-free hospitals with smoke-free policies in place had provided outdoor shelters for smokers, 16 percent of the smoke-free hospitals regularly granted exceptions for indoor smoking, and 29 percent of the smoke-free hospitals never granted exceptions. Overall, patient complaints about smoke-free hospital policies were uncommon. Predictors of hospital compliance included administrative support for the policy and inpatient smoking cessation services. Predictors of hospital noncompliance included greater numbers of beds allocated for psychiatric treatment, greater numbers of beds allocated for substance abuse treatment, and the presence of an active task force to address smoking policy. The authors suggest that the last finding reflects that, while a task force may be needed to write the hospital smoking policy and formulate an implementation plan, it should not be needed once the policy has been implemented. In addition, experiences with local clean indoor air ordinances suggest that the formation of a task force may sometimes be employed as a delaying tactic and may indicate that policymakers are resistant to the proposed policy. The authors of the survey noted that "fear of the effect of restrictive smoking policies on psychiatric and substance abuse treatment populations is prevalent" (Joseph et al. 1995, p. 494). Furthermore, although the no-smoking standard did not apply to psychiatric and substance abuse treatment services, 43 percent of hospitals with psychiatric services had smoke-free psychiatric wards, and 35 percent of hospitals with inpatient substance abuse treatment programs had smoke-free substance abuse units (Joseph et al. 1995).

Two years following implementation of the JCAHO regulation, Longo and colleagues (1998) used annual survey data from the American Hospital Association and data from accreditation site visits by JCAHO to evaluate compliance with smoking bans among all U.S. hospitals except offshore military hospitals. For 1992–1993, they found that 96 percent of U.S. hospitals were in compliance with the JCAHO smoking ban. In fact, hospitals have the only industry-wide smoking ban in the United States (Brownson et al. 2002).

Another study drawing on data from a postal survey of administrators from a stratified random sample of 1,055 hospitals conducted in 1994 found that 55.2 percent of the hospitals surveyed met the standard, 41.4 percent exceeded the standard, and 3.4 percent were not in compliance with the standard (Longo et al. 1998). Of the hospitals that were found to meet or exceed the JCAHO standard, 53.7 percent had implemented their smoke-free policies before the standard was announced. Provisions of hospital policies that exceeded the JCAHO standard included provisions that prohibited smoking outdoors on hospital grounds or that allowed no exceptions for patients. Factors associated with exceeding the JCAHO standard included location in a non-tobacco-growing state, location in a metropolitan statistical area, having fewer than 100 beds, having unionized employees, being a children's hospital, and not having a psychiatric or substance abuse unit.

Most respondents rated their hospital's policy as very (60.3 percent) or moderately (36.6 percent) successful, with 3.3 percent rating the policy as only slightly successful or not at all successful (Longo et al. 1998). Hospitals that reported involving employees in planning or otherwise preparing for implementation (for example, by having employees serve on planning committees) were more likely to report having successful policies. The factors most frequently cited as prompting hospitals to implement smoke-free policies were the JCAHO standard (61.3 percent of respondents rated this factor as a very important influence), concern for employees' health (59.9 percent of respondents rated this as a very important influence), and public image (43.1 percent of respondents rated this as a very important influence). The factors most frequently cited as posing barriers to the successful implementation of smoke-free policies included negative employee morale (22.6 percent of respondents rated this as a moderate barrier and 2.4 percent as a severe barrier) and lack of acceptance of the policy by patients (22.2 percent of respondents rated this as a moderate barrier and 4.9 percent as a severe barrier) and visitors (20.3 percent of respondents rated this as a moderate barrier and 3.9 percent as a severe barrier). Longo and colleagues (1998) concluded that the presence of a pre-existing social norm in hospitals favoring smoke-free policies and the external catalyst provided by the JCAHO standard combined to make it possible for most U.S. hospitals to successfully implement smoke-free policies that met or exceeded the JCAHO standard.

Several other studies of smoke-free policy implementation in psychiatric and substance abuse treatment settings suggest that smoking bans can be implemented in these settings with a minimal impact on client recruitment and retention (Sterling et al. 1994), physical assaults, security calls, and discharges against medical advice (Haller et al. 1996; Velasco et al. 1996). In 2002, el-Guebaly and colleagues (2002) reported findings of a systematic review on smoking bans in mental health and addiction settings and identified 22 relevant studies on the impact of partial or total smoking bans. The bans did not lead to adverse consequences for therapy, nor was noncompliance an issue. An assessment of a no-smoking policy at the Ochner Clinic reported very high levels of support from both patients and employees both before and after implementation (Hudzinski and Frohlich 1990).

A study examined how smoke-free hospital policies affect employee smoking behavior (Longo et al. 1996). The study compared progression to cessation among 1,469 current and former smokers working under smoke-free hospitals to 920 current and former smokers employed in other workplaces that were not covered by smoke-free workplace policies over a five-year period following implementation of the smoke-free policies in hospitals, adjusting for socioeconomic, demographic, and smoking intensity variables. The study found that the quit ratios for these groups were 0.506 and 0.377, respectively. Longo and colleagues (1996) concluded that smoke-free hospital policies appear to help hospital employees quit smoking.

In recent years, a number of hospitals have expanded their smoking policies to prohibit smoking on their outdoor grounds, as well as in their enclosed facilities. These campus-wide policies often also prohibit the use of other tobacco products besides cigarettes. Hospitals often present such policies not only as a way to protect patients and staff from secondhand smoke exposure (for example, at hospital entrances) but also as projecting a positive, healthy image; sending a consistent message; and encouraging and supporting tobacco use cessation among both patients and staff.

Prisons

In 2002, U.S. prisons and jails housed more than 2 million persons (Harrison and Karberg 2003), and there were nearly 800,000 full-time, sworn law enforcement officers in the United States; many of these officers worked in prison settings. Estimates of smoking prevalence among U.S. prisoners are between 60 and 80 percent (Carpenter et al. 2001). In addition, the level of ventilation in correctional facilities may be inadequate relative to the number of prisoners because of overcrowded conditions (Hoge et al. 1994). Thus, in correctional facilities where smoking is allowed indoors, nonsmoking prisoners and staff are likely to be exposed to high levels of secondhand smoke. At the national level, both the American Correctional Association and the National Commission on Correctional Health Care have offered recommendations for smoking policies, but smoking regulations within correctional facilities have been implemented primarily at the local or state level.

A 1993 survey of the 50 state departments of corrections found that no prison system entirely banned smoking. By 1996, 7 state prison systems had banned smoking and 44 had placed limits on where inmates and staff could smoke; 70 percent of the facility representatives reported that the smoking policy at their institution had changed in the previous four years (Patrick and Marsh 2001). A national survey conducted in 1997–1998 of more than 900 correctional facilities found that 45 percent of these facilities still permitted smoking by either inmates or staff (Falkin et al. 1998). A 2003 survey of medical directors at state prisons, jails, and juvenile detention facilities found that 77 of the 100 respondents reported having a tobacco-free policy in place (National Network on Tobacco Prevention and Poverty 2004). However, only 16 of these correctional facilities applied these policies to staff as well as inmates. Nearly two-thirds of the facilities with tobacco-free policies reported adopting the policies because they were mandated to do so by federal case law, state law, or local ordinance. Many of the policies had not been updated for years. The facilities with tobacco-free policies estimated compliance rates of 81 percent for staff and 71 percent for inmates. Although 63 percent of all respondents reported assessing inmate tobacco use upon intake, more than 80 percent of the respondents reported that they provided no cessation programming in their facilities. In 2004, California adopted a law making all California prisons smoke-free (California State Assembly 2004). The legislation was presented primarily as a way to reduce the cost of state-funded inmate health care.

Also in 2004, the state of Washington implemented a similar measure (Sullivan 2004; Turner 2004). A 2004 article in the *Seattle Times*, citing the Washington State Department of Corrections as a source, reported that 21 states now ban smoking within their prisons (Sullivan 2004).

As of October 2005, 38 of 50 state correctional departments had enacted full or partial smoke-free protection policies (ANR 2005c). In 2004, the Federal Bureau of Prisons implemented an almost complete smoke-free policy in 105 federal prisons housing 180,000 inmates; smoking is still permitted in faculty housing, towers, and vehicles inhabited by one person (USDOJ 2004).

A recent survey of correctional employees in Vermont revealed relatively low levels of support for complete indoor and outdoor bans on inmate smoking, but significantly greater support for policies that ban indoor smoking and provide restricted outdoor smoking areas (Carpenter et al. 2001). These types of smoking restrictions decreased secondhand smoke levels in two Vermont prisons (Hammond and Emmons 2005). In July 1992, the Vermont Department of Corrections banned smoking in its six correctional facilities. This ban, however, was modified in December 1992 to allow for smoking outdoors. To assess the effect of the indoor smoking ban on secondhand smoke levels, airborne nicotine levels were measured at two of these facilities before the ban and four and nine months after its implementation. Before the ban, the average concentrations of nicotine were high, ranging from 1.3 to 24.6 $\mu g/m^3$ in living areas and from 0.4 to 3.4 $\mu g/m^3$ in central facilities, including the dining room, visiting room, and learning center. The smoking ban significantly reduced nicotine concentrations in the living areas to averages of 1.2 to 2.2 $\mu g/m^3$, although the trends in the central facilities were less clear (Hammond and Emmons 2005).

A 1993 Supreme Court ruling that has been cited in a number of subsequent court decisions refused to dismiss a Nevada inmate's claim that exposure to secondhand smoke resulting from being housed in a cell with a smoker violated the Eighth Amendment of the Constitution, which bars "cruel and unusual punishment" (*Helling v. McKinney* 113 S.Ct. 2475, 509 U.S. 25). The court stated that, if sustained, the allegation that prison officials had "with deliberate indifference, exposed him to ETS levels that pose an unreasonable risk to his future health" (p. 25) (even in the absence of immediate medical symptoms) might constitute a violation of that standard.

Nursing Homes

Evidence on the extent of smoking and secondhand smoke exposure in nursing homes is very limited. Smoking is particularly problematic in this setting because of concerns about exposing medically ill nonsmokers to secondhand smoke and about fire safety. Kochersberger and Clipp (1996) surveyed 106 administrators of VA nursing home care units. All of the respondents reported that their facilities permitted smoking. Adler and colleagues (1997) surveyed 114 nursing home social workers selected at random from a statewide association of social workers. Slightly less than half (45 percent) of the facilities where these individuals worked were smoke-free. Most of the social workers (60 percent) who worked at facilities that permitted smoking did not want the policy to change. In contrast, more than 75 percent of social workers at smoke-free facilities supported the policy.

Despite the challenges, there is a slow but increasing movement toward laws and policies that restrict or ban smoking in health care and assisted living facilities, including nursing homes. In 2004, JCAHO issued revised accreditation standards for long-term care facilities that included a new standard regulating smoking (JCAHO 2004). The standard (EC.1.30) states that long-term care facilities should restrict resident smoking, if allowed at all, to designated locations that are separate from care, treatment, or service areas. For example, Rhode Island enacted a law that went into effect in July 2001 banning smoking entirely in health care and assisted living facilities or confining smoking to areas that are separately enclosed and separately ventilated from those used by the general public (*An Act Relating to Health and Safety—Smoking in Public Places* 2001). In fact, facilities that permitted smoking experienced greater conflicts over smoking between residents and staff.

Public support for smoking bans in nursing homes has grown in recent years. A 2001 public opinion survey conducted in California by the Field Research Corporation found that 88.7 percent of respondents felt that nursing homes and other long-term care facilities should be smoke-free (California Department of Health Services 2001b).

One obstacle to enacting smoking restrictions in nursing homes is the hesitance of some policymakers to impose such restrictions in a residential setting (i.e., places of residence). Nursing homes are workplaces and homes to nonsmokers, some of whom might be especially susceptible to health effects associated with secondhand smoke exposure because of their advanced age. One study found traces of a tobacco-specific lung carcinogen in the urine of employees of a long-term care hospital; the employees were required as part of their jobs to spend time in a patient smoking lounge that was not separately ventilated (Parsons et al. 1998). In addition, fires caused by smoking pose a special hazard in nursing homes and other long-term care facilities (U.S. Fire Administration 2001).

Smoking Restrictions in Other Settings

Day Care

Day care settings present a potentially important source of secondhand smoke exposure for young children. In 1995, 75 percent of children (14.4 million) younger than five years of age were in some form of regular child care arrangement (Smith 1995). A national survey conducted in 1990 of 2,003 directors of licensed day care centers found that 99 percent of these facilities were in compliance with their state laws on smoking: 55 percent of the centers were smoke-free indoors and outdoors, 26 percent were smoke-free indoors only, and 18 percent allowed restricted indoor smoking. The best predictors of more stringent employee smoking policies were locations in the West or South, smaller size, and independent ownership (Nelson et al. 1993). This survey also found that of the 40 states that regulated employee smoking in day care facilities, only 3 states banned indoor smoking (Nelson et al. 1993). In a 2004 analysis by the ALA of state laws restricting smoking, researchers identified 44 states that regulated smoking in day care centers, of which 31 prohibited smoking, 5 allowed smoking only in enclosed and separately ventilated areas, and 8 had some other type of restriction (ALA 2004). These results only apply to licensed facilities and not necessarily to family day care or more informal arrangements, which may be less restrictive. A large proportion of children are in nonfederally funded settings; 50 percent of children in day care are cared for by a relative in an informal setting. The smoking rules in these settings have not been studied.

In 1994, the U.S. Congress passed the *Pro-Children Act of 1994*, which prohibits smoking in Head Start facilities and in kindergarten, elementary, and secondary schools that receive federal funding from the U.S. Department of Education, the U.S. Department of Agriculture, or the U.S. DHHS, with the exception of funding from Medicare or Medicaid. This legislation also applies to facilities that receive federal

funding to provide children with routine health care, day care, or early childhood development services. This measure was reauthorized under the *No Child Left Behind Act of 2001*. No nationally representative survey of day care facilities has been conducted since the enactment of the *Pro-Children Act of 1994*.

Schools

During the past decade, schools have increasingly adopted smoke-free policies to minimize prosmoking social norms, to reduce smoking initiation rates, and to protect children from secondhand smoke exposure in the school setting.

At the federal level, the *Pro-Children Act of 1994* prohibits smoking in facilities where federally funded educational, health, library, day care, or child development services are provided to children aged younger than 18 years (*Federal Register* 1994a). The *Pro-Children Act of 1994* was reauthorized under the *No Child Left Behind Act of 2001*.

Expanding upon the *Pro-Children Act of 1994*, the CDC Guidelines for School Health Programs to Prevent Tobacco Use and Addiction recommend a tobacco-free school policy that prohibits students, staff, and visitors from using tobacco products in school buildings, on school grounds, in school vehicles, and at school-sponsored events (including events held on and off school property) (CDC 1994). According to the guidelines, this policy should be in effect at all times, even when schools are out of session. The tobacco-free environment established by this policy protects children from secondhand smoke in school buildings and other areas that they frequent as part of their daily school experience and in particular eliminates exposure of children with asthma to secondhand smoke (CDC 2005c). These policies also reduce children's opportunities to use tobacco products and to witness others doing so, thus reinforcing the messages that children receive in school about the importance of healthy, tobacco-free lifestyles. Finally, tobacco-free school policies create young people who are prepared to—and in fact expect to—matriculate to smoke-free workplaces and communities (CDC 1994).

According to CDC's School Health Policies and Programs Study (SHPPS) 2000, 44.6 percent of schools reported tobacco-free school policies consistent with CDC recommendations, up from 36 percent in SHPPS 1994 (*Journal of School Health* 2001). The study also found that 45.5 percent of districts and 13 states reported such policies. Since 2000, the numbers of schools, districts, and states with tobacco-free school policies have continued to increase. Oregon is the most recent state to adopt such a policy. A *Healthy People 2010* objective calls for establishing comprehensive tobacco-free policies in all junior high schools, middle schools, and senior high schools (USDHHS 2000a). While substantial progress has been made on this objective, the target is not likely to be met by 2010 unless activity increases.

Colleges

To date, legislation has focused on smoking policies in elementary and secondary schools. No federal legislation has targeted smoking policies at colleges, although there appears to be increasing attention to this issue at the college level. In 1996, ALA surveyed colleges and universities featured in the 1996 edition of the *Princeton Review Student Access Guide to the Best 309 Colleges* (Meltzer et al. 1995). Seventy-three percent of the colleges surveyed permitted smoking, including 62 percent of those calling themselves "smoke-free." Across all colleges, 62.4 percent allowed smoking in individual dorm rooms. A 1999 survey of 393 student health center directors from four-year colleges found that 85 percent of the respondents considered student smoking on their campuses to be either a problem or a major problem (Wechsler et al. 2001a). Restrictions on smoking were common; 81 percent of the colleges prohibited smoking in all public areas, but only 26 percent prohibited smoking in all indoor areas, including student residence halls and private offices. The most restrictive policies were found among private-sector institutions, religious-affiliated institutions, and those in the West. Although 55.7 percent of the health centers offered smoking cessation programs for students, the colleges reported little student demand. But the smoking cessation programs were not uniformly strong. Only 31 percent of the schools with cessation programs offered individualized counseling; 25 percent offered comprehensive programs with counseling, screening, and assessments by a physician or health professional; and 19 percent offered pharmacologic aids for smoking cessation. The impact of college smoking policies was studied by Wechsler and colleagues (2001b) using a survey administered at 128 colleges. Students who entered college as non-smokers were about 40 percent less likely to be smoking at the time of the survey if they were living in smoke-free dorms. Wechsler and colleagues (2001b) also noted that current smokers who lived in smoke-free housing had lower cigarette consumption than those who lived in unrestricted housing.

In a study by Halperin and Rigotti (2003) that included interviews with key informants at the largest public university in each of the 50 states, 98 percent of the universities reported a smoking ban inside public buildings, 50 percent reported a ban outside building entrances, 54 percent reported a ban in student housing, and 30 percent reported a complete ban encompassing all three of these settings. In 2000, the American College Health Association recommended smoking bans in and around all campus buildings, including all campus housing and public areas (Fisher 2002). The impact of these recommendations has not yet been evaluated. In recent years, many colleges have expanded their smoking restrictions to include some outdoor areas, including, in some cases, making their entire campuses smoke-free.

Interstate Public Transportation

As noted earlier in this chapter (see "Historical Perspective"), the United States has prohibited smoking on all domestic airline flights of six hours or less since 1990. In addition, numerous airports in the United States have enacted smoke-free policies in the past several years. In 2002, researchers surveyed administrators about airport smoking policies at U.S. commercial service airports with more than 10,000 passenger boardings per year (CDC 2004d). Of the airports surveyed, 61.9 percent reported smoke-free policies in effect (defined as policies prohibiting smoking inside the airport by anyone, anywhere, and at any time). Larger airports, which account for the majority of passenger boardings, were less likely than smaller airports to have implemented such a policy. Smoke-free policies were reported by 41.9 percent of large-hub airports, 52.9 percent of medium-hub airports, 58.0 percent of small-hub airports, and 81.0 percent of no-hub airports. (The FAA assigns hub size designations based on the percentage of total U.S. passenger boardings that an airport accounted for during the previous calendar year.) These percentages of smoke-free policies, and in particular the figures for large-hub airports, have probably increased with the state clean indoor air laws that have been enacted since this survey was conducted. These laws typically apply to airports, and several of the states that have adopted comprehensive or relatively comprehensive laws are homes to major airports. ANR recently compiled a list of smoking policies at the nation's 10 busiest airports based on passenger traffic as of August 2001 (Baskas 2004). Five of these airports are entirely smoke-free indoors. The remaining five allow smoking in separate areas, but those smoking areas are not separately ventilated in most cases.

In 1971, the Interstate Commerce Commission (ICC) issued the first smoking regulations for interstate buses. The ICC mandated the creation of separate smoking sections in the rear of the buses. The ICC then ruled that as of January 6, 1972, the smoking area could not exceed 20 percent of the seats, but this order was not implemented. In 1976, the ICC amended the law to expand the smoking allotment to 30 percent. In 1990, the ICC banned smoking on interstate buses (*Federal Register* 1991).

Similar to buses, the initial 1971 ICC regulations for trains required that smoking on trains traveling on interstate routes be confined to designated areas (*U.S. Rail Passenger Service Act of 1970*). In 1976, ICC prohibited smoking in railroad food service cars and required separate coach cars for smoking and non-smoking passengers. In 1987, congressional legislation that threatened to withhold federal funds influenced the decision of the State of New York Metropolitan Transportation Authority (MTA) to ban smoking on the MTA Long Island Railroad (USDHHS 1989). In 1994, Amtrak banned smoking on all short and medium distance train travel.

Hotels

Recently, a number of hotels have implemented voluntary smoke-free policies that apply to common areas such as lobbies and to all guest rooms. Many other hotels have increased the proportion of their guest rooms that are designated nonsmoking. According to a *USA Today* article from November 2003, a PricewaterhouseCoopers study conducted in 2003 found that 84 percent of hotel rooms in eight major markets were designated nonsmoking, an increase from the 80 percent reported in 1998 (Yancey 2003). According to the American Hotel & Lodging Association, a trade organization in Washington, D.C., 65 percent of the rooms in nearly 8,000 properties surveyed in 2001 were designated nonsmoking—an increase from the 61.1 percent reported in 1998 (Yancey 2003).

Interviews with hotel executives suggest that these moves are in response to public demand, although important benefits include reduced cleaning costs and benefits to employees (Hospitality Net 2001). Some hotel proprietors report that even smokers are increasingly requesting smoke-free rooms (Yancey 2003). On the other hand, some proprietors also report that requests for smoking rooms increase in the short run when smoke-free laws are implemented, perhaps because smokers are no longer allowed to smoke in many other settings (Yancey 2003).

Multiunit Housing

As evidence regarding the health effects of secondhand smoke has accumulated, there has been growing concern about the impact of secondhand smoke exposure in multiunit housing settings. These settings include commercially owned apartments, condominiums, and public housing facilities, such as housing authorities and subsidized housing. Together with the workplace, the home is a major source of secondhand smoke exposure, especially for non-smokers who live with a smoker (Klepeis 1999; Cal/EPA 2005). Secondhand smoke from one unit in a multiunit housing complex can seep into an adjoining unit through shared air spaces or shared ventilation systems.

The main approach for addressing this issue has been education of landlords and property managers with the goal of having them implement voluntary no-smoking policies. In some cases, tenants have also taken legal action to achieve this outcome (Sweda 2004). These policies may apply to common spaces within the housing complex (such as lobbies, corridors, stairwells, elevators, laundry rooms, community rooms, and recreational areas), housing units rented to new tenants, or housing units rented to both new and existing tenants.

Until recently, landlords and property managers have been reluctant to restrict smoking in multiunit housing because of concerns about the legality of doing so and because of the perception that regulating tenants' smoking may constitute an intrusion on their privacy. However, tenants who live in multiunit housing have certain legal obligations and rights. These obligations and rights in many cases make it possible for landlords and property managers to restrict or eliminate smoking in apartments and for nonsmoking tenants to obtain relief from secondhand smoke seepage from adjoining units. In addition to protecting tenants from secondhand smoke exposure and avoiding legal action by nonsmokers who experience secondhand smoke seepage from neighboring units, landlords and property managers are in some cases motivated by additional factors, such as reductions in maintenance, cleaning costs, burns, fire danger, and property insurance premiums. Several organizations are providing information and technical assistance to landlords to encourage them to implement smoking restrictions in apartments and condominiums and are working with landlords to publicize smoke-free rentals through Web site listings (e.g., <http://www.smokefreeapartments.org>; <http://www.tcsg.org/sfelp/apartment.htm>; <http://www.mismokefreeapartment.org>).

A recent review of legal rulings in this area found that landlords, condominium associations, and other multiunit property holders may prohibit smoking for new, and in many cases existing, occupants (Schoenmarklin 2004). Courts do not recognize a legal right to smoke in such dwellings, whether the dwelling is publicly or privately owned. In addition, residents of multiunit dwellings have access to common law remedies for stopping secondhand smoke infiltration, including local safety and health codes. If a resident of a multiunit dwelling can demonstrate that secondhand smoke exposure limits a major life activity, the federal *Fair Housing Act of 1992* can be used to end the secondhand smoke incursion. Landlords and building owners can prohibit smoking in apartments and condominiums, protecting them from lawsuits related to secondhand smoke infiltration (Schoenmarklin 2004).

Similarly, a review of potential legal remedies for tenants affected by secondhand smoke seepage concluded that state regulations, such as sanitary codes, provide general language for protecting the health of residents in multiunit buildings (Kline 2000). Tenants can also use traditional claims of nuisance, warranties of habitability, and the right of quiet enjoyment.

The general health protection language of state regulations, along with evidence of the harmful effects of exposure to secondhand smoke, gives state agencies authority to regulate secondhand smoke infiltration between apartments in multiunit dwellings. In states where regulations do not exist, other legal remedies may be available, many premised on the existence of a harm to the nonsmoking resident (Kline 2000). In addition, residents who can prove that they have a disability, including multiple chemical sensitivity disorder or environmental illness, which is affected by exposure to secondhand smoke, have recourse under the *Fair Housing Act of 1992* (Schoenmarklin 2004).

In 2005, a housing court jury in Boston, Massachusetts, ruled that a couple could be evicted from a rented apartment based on other tenants' complaints that the secondhand smoke they generated was seeping into adjoining apartments (Ranalli and Saltzman 2005). The jury found that the couple's heavy smoking violated a clause that prohibited "any nuisance; any offensive noise, odor or fumes; or any hazard to health." They made this ruling even though the landlord had not included a specific nonsmoking clause in the lease.

Some government bodies have considered or enacted policies that restrict smoking in public housing. For example, a housing authority in Springfield, Illinois, adopted a policy phasing out smoking in common areas of public housing complexes (Bolinski

2003). Another housing authority in Auburn, Maine, adopted a policy that bans smoking in all units except those currently occupied by smokers, with these units gradually coming under the smoke-free policy as current tenants are replaced (Healthy Androscoggin 2004). The policy also prohibits smoking in housing authority buildings and within 25 feet of buildings, including common areas. Finally, a city council in Thousand Oaks, California, considered prohibiting smoking in its publicly subsidized apartments, including many or all residential units (Keating 2003; Lee 2003).

Other government bodies have gone further and taken steps to regulate smoking in private multiunit housing settings. For example, several cities in Alameda County, California, have local ordinances in place requiring that common areas in multiunit housing be smoke-free (Chen 2005). A Utah law stipulates that residential unit rental and purchase agreements may prohibit generation of tobacco smoke (Utah Condominium Ownership Act 2005). Finally, in 2003, legislation was introduced in the California legislature that would have regulated smoking in apartments and condominiums (LePage 2003b; Vogel 2003). Specifically, the legislation would have made indoor and outdoor common areas in these settings smoke-free, would have allowed landlords and homeowner associations to penalize residents whose secondhand smoke repeatedly seeps into neighbors' units, would have allowed tenants to bring legal actions against neighbors, and would have required all apartment and condominium units to be smoke-free by January 1, 2006, unless designated by their owners as smoking units. The sponsor ultimately withdrew the legislation, citing concerns that had been raised about it (LePage 2003a).

Outdoor Settings

In California, a state law banning tobacco use on all playgrounds and in "tot lot" sandbox areas took effect on January 1, 2002 (Hill 2002). The city of Los Angeles had already implemented a similar municipal law prohibiting smoking in all 375 city parks and recreation centers. Several other cities in California have also enacted smoke-free park measures (County of Los Angeles Department of Health Services 2001). These recent policy initiatives in California reflect a growing movement toward banning smoking in outdoor public places. The ANR reported that as of January 2005, a total of 577 jurisdictions had passed ordinances covering outdoor areas, including restrictions on smoking in outdoor areas near an enclosed building where smoking is prohibited and in sports or entertainment venues, as well as in places where the public congregates, such as parks, beaches, and plazas (ANR 2005b). These policies are presented as measures not only to protect children, youth, and nonsmoking adults from secondhand smoke, but also to set a healthy example for youth, reduce litter, and prevent infants from ingesting discarded cigarettes.

A recent trend in this area has been the adoption of local policies banning smoking on public beaches. A number of California communities have adopted such policies, as have some communities in other states (Evans 2003; Fuchs 2004). In 2004, the California legislature considered, but ultimately rejected, legislation that would have prohibited smoking at all California state beaches (Fuchs 2004). In addition to protecting nonsmokers from secondhand smoke, these measures are typically intended to remove a leading source of beach litter.

Finally, as noted above, many hospitals and schools, as well as a number of colleges and other workplaces, have implemented campus-wide policies that prohibit smoking on outdoor grounds in addition to indoor facilities in recent years. In addition to protecting nonsmokers from secondhand smoke, these policies are also intended to project a positive institutional image, convey a consistent pro-health message, undercut the perception that smoking is socially acceptable, discourage tobacco use initiation among students, and encourage and support tobacco use cessation among students, patients, and employees.

Legal Approaches

Nonsmokers have used the U.S. legal system to gain protection from the harm caused by secondhand smoke. The first successful case occurred in 1976 (*Shimp v. New Jersey Bell Telephone Co.*, 368 A.2d 408, 145 N.J. Super. 516 [1976]) where a New Jersey Superior Court ruled in favor of a nonsmoking office worker who sought relief from exposure to secondhand smoke in her worksite (USDHHS 2000c). Sweda (2004) reviewed 420 cases of exposure to secondhand smoke between 1976 and 2003. Cases were categorized by type: negligence, workers' compensation and disability benefits, discrimination based on disabilities, smoke seepage in a multiunit building, child custody disputes, prisoners' rights, assault and battery, and cases against tobacco companies. Sweda (2004) concluded that successful cases are instrumental in convincing businesses and others to adopt smoke-free policies. For example, in *Staron et al. v. McDonald's Corp.*, 51 F.3d 353 (2d Cir. 1995), plaintiffs sued

McDonald's based on the *Americans with Disabilities Act of 1990* (ADA 1990), which prohibits discrimination based on disabilities. The plaintiffs claimed that McDonald's restaurants were public accommodations that became inaccessible to customers with adverse reactions to tobacco smoke. A year after the suit was filed, McDonald's announced that all of its corporately owned restaurants would become smoke-free (Hilts 1994). This action paved the way for similar policies in other fast-food outlets. In 1995, the court ruled that a ban on smoking would be a reasonable modification.

Parmet and colleagues (1996) outlined the remedies available to persons with respiratory, cardiovascular, or other health conditions that are exacerbated by secondhand smoke exposure and that might qualify as disabilities under the terms of the ADA and the role that their physicians could play in helping them pursue these remedies. The commentary explained that such persons might be able to seek redress under the workplace and public accommodation discrimination provisions if policies allowing smoking in effect denied them the ability to work in or patronize these settings. The commentary draws a parallel between a restaurant allowing smoking and failing to provide a wheelchair ramp—both can in practice deny access to persons with specific disabilities and can thus be seen as constituting discrimination under the ADA. The commentary notes that physicians can play an important role by documenting that patients have serious health conditions that restrict their major life activities (e.g., breathing) and that are exacerbated by secondhand smoke. For example, physicians can provide patients with a letter to this effect that they can use in pursuing remedies with employers and managers of places of public accommodation. The commentary further suggests that, by educating such decision-makers and the general public that secondhand smoke is a serious health hazard, physicians can help resolve these situations through voluntary compliance and, ultimately, prevent them from occurring in the first place (Parmet et al. 1996).

In another novel approach, seven nonsmoking flight attendants sued the six major cigarette companies for illnesses resulting from exposure to tobacco smoke. *Broin v. Philip Morris Cos.*, No. 92-1405 (Fla., Dade Cty. Mar. 15, 1994), *cited in* 9.1 TPLR 2.1 (1994), was tried as a class action lawsuit on behalf of all flight attendants exposed to secondhand smoke and was settled in 1997. The settlement established and funded the Flight Attendants Medical Research Institute and provided a precedent that enabled individual flight attendants to sue tobacco companies for damages.

Although Sweda (2004) found a limited number of successful secondhand smoke cases, he observed, "the judicial branch has begun to recognize the need to protect the public—especially some of the most vulnerable members of our society—from the serious threat to their health that is exposure to SHS [secondhand smoke]" (p. i61).

Technical Approaches

Although policy approaches appear to be effective at reducing exposure, there are also technical strategies that have been used. This section reviews these strategies and evidence for their effectiveness.

Controlling Secondhand Smoke Exposure Indoors

Overview

Chapter 3 of this report (Assessment of Exposure to Secondhand Smoke) explained the foundation for engineering and policy options intended to reduce, restrict, or eliminate secondhand smoke exposure indoors. This chapter revisits the basic concepts of ventilation and air cleaning to provide an understanding of the various strategies proposed in building codes, ventilation designs, building operating procedures, and other practices to reduce or attempt to eliminate exposure of nonsmokers to tobacco smoke within a built environment. The discussion covers the evidence on the efficacy and effectiveness of these strategies. The literature review covers the relevant peer-reviewed evidence, but does not attempt to systematically capture the substantial non–peer-review or "gray" literature. This section first provides a simplified (time-averaged, steady-state form) mass balance equation for predicting indoor concentrations of a contaminant. This equation provides a foundation for considering the potential effectiveness of control strategies (Klepeis 1999; Ott 1999).

Mass Balance–Steady-State Equation

The mass balance model describes how the concentration of an indoor contaminant varies with the strength of the pollution source and the factors acting to reduce its concentration. Equation A expresses the physical factors governing concentrations of indoor airborne contaminants, including secondhand smoke:

$$\text{Equation A} \qquad C_{in} = \frac{PaC_{out} + Q_s/V}{a + k}$$

This form of the equation is simplified by the assumption that the air of the indoor environment is well mixed and that steady-state conditions exist. It is possible to computationally consider the temporal variation of each parameter in Equation A, as well as the multiple compartments within a space or building. With an expansion to multiple compartments (i.e., rooms or spaces), Equation A would include terms for describing air transfer between adjacent rooms or between areas (e.g., from a smoking section of a restaurant, club, or airplane to a nonsmoking area).

In Equation A, the indoor concentration (C_{in}) is in mass per unit volume and C_{out} is the outdoor concentration in the same units. For secondhand smoke, this term might be specified as μg per m³ for particles and for some gaseous species, and as ng/m³ for metals and other constituents of secondhand smoke that are present in small quantities. P is the unitless penetration coefficient. In the context of a building with a mechanical air handling unit (AHU), P would represent the fraction of a constituent in the incoming supply air that passes through filters and other system components such as cooling coils and ducts that would remove some of the constituents from the flowing air. For homes without air conditioning, P is the fraction of an airborne contaminant in the outdoor air that comes indoors through windows, doors, and cracks or down chimneys, driven by pressure differences across the exterior boundary of the structure. Penetration can be very high (approaching 100 percent) for particles of certain sizes, particularly small particles, and for inert (nonreactive) gases.

Penetration might, on the other hand, actually be zero if, for example, air-cleaning devices completely capture the contaminant.

The air exchange rate (a) describes the effective rate at which indoor air is replaced by outdoor air. The air exchange rate is expressed as inverse time, indicating the fraction of indoor volume that is exchanged in an hour. Most buildings do not have a "once through system" or complete mixing, where only air coming from the outdoors is used to replace all indoor air. Typically, an air exchange rate of one per hour might only be 65 percent effective in flushing out the indoor air. As discussed in Chapter 3 (see "Building Designs and Operations"), heating, ventilating, and air conditioning (HVAC) systems in buildings (and in airplanes) usually mix a portion of the outside air with a portion of the previously circulated indoor air to create the supply air that conditions indoor spaces. So the term PaC_{out} can be decomposed to include both components of the supply air: the ventilation component derived from outdoor air and the return (recirculated) air component.

The Q_s term represents the mass flux generation rate (mass/time) for internal sources of contaminants. For cigarettes, this term reflects the rate at which particles or specific gases are released and is thus an index of the strength of smoking as a source of indoor pollution. Data are available on emission rates of cigarettes (IARC 2000). Dividing Q_s by the volume (V) of a room, house, atrium, or other space yields a concentration flux term with units similar to the other terms in the numerator. In the context of secondhand smoke generation, smoking is a time-varying event. Detailed computational fluid dynamic models can estimate time-resolved concentrations associated with the smoking of a single cigarette. Steady-state models average source generation rates over hours to days. Estimating the volume term can be as straightforward as the simple calculation of the physical dimensions of a building, house, or room. In this case, volume refers to the space where air is "well mixed." Thus, there is an important distinction between estimated concentrations from a lit cigarette in still air versus the concentrations in a restaurant or a nightclub with substantial air movement and smokers dispersed throughout.

Equation A also shows that the flux terms in the numerator are divided by the air exchange rate (a) and a decay or removal rate (k). This k term represents the loss rate per unit of time through chemical or physical means, such as deposition on surfaces, air cleaning, or change of state or condition. For example, vapors might decay by condensing or adsorbing onto particles or through chemical transformations. The number of particles in particular size ranges might change because of agglomeration. Rates of loss of particles from the air reflect primarily diffusion to surfaces, sedimentation, coagulation, and evaporation. Vapors and gases do not settle out of the air, but they diffuse to surfaces, with possible re-emission, and can react with gaseous and particulate constituents of the air as well. The rate of loss to surfaces is enhanced by turbulence in the air, such as mixing by fans. The temperature of the surface also affects loss rates. By a mechanism called thermophoresis, particles and gases can be preferentially driven from warm surfaces such as radiators and light fixtures to cold surfaces. In addition, experiments reveal that concentrations of particle-bound polycyclic aromatic hydrocarbons decay twice as fast as respirable particle concentrations (Repace 2004b).

Policies for Controlling Secondhand Smoke

Although Equation A is a simple expression of a mass balance equation, it indicates all of the options for mitigating concentrations of secondhand smoke in indoor air. These options include source control, ventilation, and filtration. Among indoor air pollutants, secondhand smoke is unique in the possibility for full control. By eliminating sources indoors and preventing outdoor tobacco smoke from entering by distancing it from air intakes, the numerator of the equation becomes zero, and there is no secondhand smoke.

Equation B is derived from Equation A by considering tobacco smoke constituents only and by assuming that outdoor air contains no secondhand smoke components (i.e., $C_{out} = 0$). With these assumptions, Equation B implies that control options relate to increasing air exchange rates for ventilation or enhancing removal rates with air cleaning devices.

$$\text{Equation B} \qquad C_{in} = \frac{Q_s/V}{a + k} = \frac{Q_s}{V(a+k)}$$

Additional strategies include physically modifying the volume or area where smoking is allowed. Smokers might be separated from nonsmokers with controlled airflow that directs secondhand smoke to exhaust fans independently and separately exhausted from the HVAC system. This strategy is often used in restaurants or hotels that designate smoking and nonsmoking rooms or floors. Smoking lounges can be effective theoretically if the room is physically separated by walls and doors from surrounding spaces, internal pressure is negative to surrounding areas, and air from the room is not mixed back into the supply air for the building.

Field studies provide some indication of the potential for various strategies implied by the mass balance equation to affect secondhand smoke concentrations. Liu and colleagues (2001) assessed the effectiveness of control measures for secondhand smoke in a study of 118 smoking areas in 111 county and city buildings. The data were collected in California from 1991 to 1994, before the current statewide indoor smoking ban, but the findings are relevant to current building scenarios. Inspection of the smoking areas showed a range of operational and design problems, including the incomplete separation of smoking and nonsmoking areas, a failure to vent the smoking area to the outside, and the recirculation of secondhand smoke-contaminated air. Only 7 percent of the areas had the requisite features for the most complete control: exhausting smoke-contaminated air outside, no recirculation from the smoking area, and full walls from floor to ceiling. Measurement data showed that this control strategy could reduce concentrations in surrounding nonsmoking areas.

In some situations where smoking can be intense, such as gaming establishments, a combination of strategies and technological enhancements may be needed to reduce secondhand smoke concentrations in the absence of a smoking ban. Supplemental air cleaners recirculate room air that has passed through filters or electrostatic air cleaners. Some establishments use devices to generate charged ions that attach to smoke particles to increase their removal rates by electrostatic attraction to any surface in the room. A combination of turbulent mixing, as with fans, and an added electric charge may significantly increase particle removal. In yet another approach, appliance manufacturers claim that adding ozone (O_3) to the indoor air will accelerate oxidative reactions of some secondhand smoke constituents and decrease odor and secondhand smoke concentrations.

These mass balance considerations imply a range of policy options related to source control and ventilation, including elimination of the source term (Q_s), leading to no secondhand smoke indoors, and increasing the effectiveness of air exchange (a) to achieve targeted concentration values (C_{in}). These options have been widely debated; the advocacy and public health communities argue that smoking bans are necessary, and the tobacco industry has proposed that secondhand smoke concentrations can be controlled at acceptable levels through strategies of mutual accommodation between smokers and non-smokers, ventilation, and air cleaning (Bialous and Glantz 2002). The tobacco industry has attempted to assure that ventilation will be maintained as a strategy for achieving acceptable indoor air quality, even with smoking allowed.

The principles of public health protection underlying this discussion need to be considered. There is universal acceptance of the concept that outdoor air is a "public good," and for this reason, outdoor air quality is monitored in the United States to meet public health goals under the federal *Clean Air Act of 1990* (USEPA 2004). It is the obligation of government to protect the users (the general public) and maintain the quality of that public good (outdoor air), so users will not be harmed by contaminants released into the air by those who would pollute it. Indoor spaces are private as well as public. Consequently, the principles that have been applied to outdoor air may not apply directly to all indoor air, particularly in private places. In public places, where indoor air can be more readily construed as a public good, segregating smokers and banning smoking have become enforced approaches that are well accepted, and bans have become mandatory in many environments, including hospitals, schools, and childcare facilities.

In a limited way, the government has assumed an obligation to ensure that "workplace" air is free of specific airborne contaminants that can cause harm to the worker, as discussed earlier in this chapter. OSHA has standard-setting and enforcement responsibilities that are applied to the workplace. The FAA also has rule-making responsibilities affecting air quality for flight crews. In 1994, OSHA published a "Notice of Proposed Rulemaking on Indoor Air Quality" (*Federal Register* 1994b). The proposed rules included the requirement that employers either establish a designated smoking area with ventilation control or ban smoking. These rules would have eliminated secondhand smoke exposure to nonsmokers in the workplace by prohibiting work-related activities in the designated smoking area. Although lengthy hearings were held, these draft rules were never promulgated and have now been withdrawn (*Federal Register* 2001).

The WHO European Center established guiding principles for indoor air rights in its report *The Right to Healthy Indoor Air*, which provided a basis for excluding known hazardous substances from indoor air (Møhave and Krzyzanowski 2000, 2003). As discussed earlier in this chapter (see "Local Ordinances" and "State Laws and Regulations"), an increasing number of municipalities and states in the United

States, including California and New York City, have now completely banned smoking in workplaces and in public indoor environments. Yet the tobacco industry and some in the hospitality and gaming industries argue that with improved ventilation technologies, both smokers and nonsmokers can be accommodated (<http://www.philipmorrisusa.com/en/policies_practices/smoking_restrictions.asp>). Repace (2000a) counters that even with the optimistic assumption of a 90 percent reduction in secondhand smoke in bars and casinos by using the most advanced ventilation technologies, cancer and heart disease risks from secondhand smoke would not be reduced below the EPA limits for hazardous air pollutants in outdoor air. Although Repace's risk model is well documented, no regulatory entity or federal agency has relied upon Section 112 of the *Clean Air Act of 1990* as a framework for establishing indoor air quality goals for secondhand smoke at some de minimis risk level, and the tobacco industry places the emphasis on accommodation without specifying indoor air levels of secondhand smoke that would be acceptable (<http://www.philipmorrisusa.com/en/policies_practices/smoking_restrictions.asp>).

The American Society of Heating, Refrigerating and Air-Conditioning Engineers (ASHRAE) is the professional organization for the ventilation industries, and its membership includes thousands of practicing ventilation engineers in the United States. The ASHRAE Standing Standards Project Committee provides guidance on indoor space ventilation for achieving acceptable indoor air quality (American National Standards Institute/ASHRAE Standard 62-2001, *Ventilation for Acceptable Indoor Air Quality*) (ASHRAE 2001). The ASHRAE Standard 62-2001 provides the basis for municipal building codes and design specifications for HVAC equipment. The first version of Standard 62 was approved in 1973 with revisions in 1981 and 1989, and a process of revision is constantly ongoing (Bialous and Glantz 2002).

The 1989 revision of Standard 62 had implications for controlling secondhand smoke concentrations; the standard proposed that "acceptable indoor air quality," as defined by ASHRAE, could be achieved in the presence of "moderate" amounts of smoking by meeting ventilation requirements (ASHRAE 1989; Bialous and Glantz 2002). Bialous and Glantz (2002) provide a detailed account of Standard 62 and the involvement of the tobacco industry in deliberations around the standard. ASHRAE accepts the engagement of all affected parties in its activities.

Standard 62-2001 is the most recent version and is undergoing a process of continuous revision. It is important to point out that with the 1999 and 2001 revisions, there is no longer a footnote to the table providing ventilation recommendations that allow a moderate amount of smoking. The ASHRAE Board has acknowledged that allowing smoking indoors is incompatible with the stated goal of the standard, which is to "minimize the potential for adverse health effects" (Persily 2002, p. 329).

In 2005, ASHRAE published a position document on secondhand smoke that had the purpose of providing information on secondhand smoke to its members and of considering the implications of this information for building design and operation (ASHRAE 2005). The document, approved by ASHRAE's Board of Directors, recognized the consensus view that secondhand smoke exposure poses a risk to health. Among the conclusions were the following:

> There is a consensus amongst medical cognizant authorities that secondhand smoke is a health risk, causing lung cancer and heart disease in adults, and causing adverse effects on the respiratory health of children, including exacerbating asthma and increasing risk for lower respiratory infection. At present, the only means of eliminating health risks associated with indoor exposure is to ban all smoking activity. Although complete separation and isolation of smoking rooms can control secondhand smoke exposure in non-smoking spaces in the same building, adverse health effects for the occupants of the smoking room cannot be controlled by ventilation. No other engineering approaches, including current and advanced dilution ventilation, "air curtains" or air cleaning technologies, have been demonstrated or should be relied upon to control health risks from secondhand smoke exposure in spaces where smoking occurs, though some approaches may reduce that exposure and address odor and some forms of irritation. An increasing number of local and national governments, as well as many private building owners, are adopting and implementing bans on indoor smoking. At a minimum, ASHRAE members must abide by local regulations and building codes and stay aware of changes in areas where they practice, and should educate and inform their clients

of the substantial limitations and the available benefits of engineering controls. Because of ASHRAE's mission to act for the benefit of the public, it encourages elimination of smoking in the indoor environment as the optimal way to minimize secondhand smoke exposure (ASHRAE 2005).

Because indoor exposure to secondhand smoke in the United States continues, and because in many countries outside the United States there are limited or no restrictions on smoking, it is useful to review the various strategies to lessen the impact of smoking indoors and assess their efficacy. These approaches incorporate segregation of smokers from nonsmokers and include controlled and enhanced ventilation and air cleaning.

Technological Strategies for Controlling Secondhand Smoke

Some state and local ordinances require designated nonsmoking and smoking areas in public access facilities such as restaurants. Typically, these ordinances provide little guidance on how to achieve this separation or how effective it has to be in controlling concentrations in the nonsmoking areas. Also, studies have not addressed all of the factors that are potentially relevant to this determination (e.g., smoking rates, dilution measures, containment measurements, and biomarkers of exposure) across the broad spectrum of possible designs. Therefore, only general guidance is available based on engineering principles, and there is a limited literature.

In integrated spaces—spaces with no walls that accommodate multiple occupants or uses such as restaurants, casinos, and similar venues—pressure-driven airflow is the only method capable of directing secondhand smoke away from nonsmokers. With separate rooms and physical barriers, air supply and exhaust routes can be designed to more effectively isolate impacts. However, employees may not have the same options as patrons to avoid exposure, particularly if their work activities require them to enter designated smoking areas.

A second general strategy involves controlled ventilation. Possible methods include ashtrays to capture cigarette emissions, hoods placed over gaming tables or bars to remove secondhand smoke from the area proximate to smokers, and displacement ventilation. Displacement ventilation can orient air supply and air exhaust in a configuration that directs secondhand smoke away from nonsmoking patrons

and employees such as bartenders. Thus, displacement ventilation can be considered a design option for the separation strategy. Design criteria include a low-velocity air supply near the floor with the exhaust at the ceiling. Turbulence has to be reduced to limit the general mixing of secondhand smoke before it is exhausted. The location and balance of supply and exhaust air are as critical as the interior design is because barriers and heat sources such as lights and appliances can affect airflow. The movement of people stirs the air and actually causes bulk transport of air from smoking to nonsmoking areas, which reduces the effectiveness of separation strategies.

With efficient heat recovery devices for the exhaust air, it is becoming less costly to increase outdoor air supply rates. Because most office buildings have conventional HVAC systems that force conditioned supply air to mix with room air to achieve comfort conditions, the strategy to accommodate nonsmoking employees or visitors would simply be based on dilution. However, if complemented with improved filtration of the return air, it is possible to achieve greater reductions of some secondhand smoke constituents beyond what dilution alone can accomplish (ASHRAE 1999).

The concept is straightforward: process a portion of the air locally and remove secondhand smoke constituents with commonly used devices mounted on ceilings. The devices use the principle of electrostatic precipitation to remove particles or a series of filters to remove particles and odors. New devices have become available recently and include ultraviolet-activated photo catalytic systems that oxidize vapor phase organic compounds. With the addition of filters to this configuration, these devices could also remove particles. However, widespread application of these systems to effectively control secondhand smoke exposure in buildings has not yet been demonstrated.

Table 10.17 presents six technologies used in air cleaning systems (Daniels 2002). The devices that are effective for particles as well as for the vapor phase organic constituents of secondhand smoke might be more efficacious for controlling secondhand smoke. The effectiveness of these devices will be determined by the product of the volume of air processed and the removal efficiency of various constituents in comparison with the dilution rate achieved by the overall ventilation of the air delivered to the conditioned space. If the decay rate by supplemental air cleaning is comparable to or exceeds the dilution rate by air exchange, then a cleaning system may measurably reduce concentrations of secondhand smoke. If smokers are

Table 10.17 Comparison of air-cleaning systems

Characteristic	Technology					
	Electrostatic precipitation	Solid media filtration	Gas-phase filtration	Ozone (O_3) generation	Catalytic oxidation	Bipolar air ionization
Function	Electronic	Physical	Physico-chemical	Electronic	Physico-chemical	Electronic
Principle	High-voltage wire and plate	Flat, pleated, or high efficiency particulate air media	Sorption and reaction	Sparking discharge	Solid catalysts with or without ultraviolet	Dielectric barrier discharge
Process	Charging of particulate matter	Collection on porous media	Sorption and reaction	O_3 generation	Catalytic oxidation	Positive and negative ion generation
Active species	Charged particles	High surface area	Sorption and reaction sites	O_3	Reactive oxygen species	Reactive oxygen and charged species
By-products	O_3 if not cleaned regularly	Spent filters; contaminants	Spent media with contaminants	Significant O_3, atmospheric reactants	Exhausted or fouled catalysts, some VOCs*	Some O_3
VOCs	Sorption of VOCs on PM$^†_x$	NA‡	Adsorption/absorption	Chemical oxidation	Chemical oxidation	Chemical oxidation
PM$_x$	Collection on plates	Impact, settling, and diffusion	Collection on media	NA	NA	Agglomeration

*VOCs = Volatile organic compounds.
†PM = Particulate matter.
‡NA = Not applicable.
Source: Adapted from Daniels 2002.

clustered within a space and supplemental air cleaners can be appropriately placed to effectively capture secondhand smoke near the source, then the overall efficiency of an air-cleaning strategy can be further enhanced.

Effectiveness

Field and laboratory investigations have evaluated the secondhand smoke control strategies discussed above. Three extensive literature searches were conducted to identify articles related to the control of tobacco smoke in nonresidential settings. The searches included PubMed, Medline, Kompass, JICST-Eplus, BIOSIS Previews, Vizon SciTec, Dissertation Abstracts, Inside Conferences, ELSEVIER BIOBASE, PASCAL, National Institute for Occupational Safety and Health

(NIOSH), ABI/INFORM, BioBusiness, Wilson Business Abstracts, ToxFile, EMBASE Excerpta Medica Database, and Current Contents Search.

The search was restricted to published articles, abstracts, conference abstracts, proceedings, and dissertations relevant to the following key words: environmental tobacco smoke OR ETS AND (control OR controlling OR controls) AND (separation OR filtration OR removal OR local source capture OR isolation OR elimination OR reducing exposure OR controlled exposure OR mechanical OR ventilation OR HVAC OR air condition). The third search included all listings appearing through August 29, 2003.

The searches yielded 50, 55, and 83 abstracts, respectively, which were then reviewed and categorized. Full articles were obtained for those deemed relevant to the evaluation of smoking controls in non-residential settings based on bans, separation, and mechanical systems. Further culling retained only articles that reported environmental measurements of particles, nicotine, or other indicators of second-hand smoke concentrations and the few studies that conducted laboratory evaluations of equipment and smoking chambers (rooms). The studies reported here have evaluated strategies that fall into one of three categories: bans, separation with existing conventional HVAC systems, or separation with designed control systems (e.g., ventilation or air cleaning).

There are many studies of concentrations of secondhand smoke in office buildings, hospitals, restaurants, bars (which are called public houses [pubs] in the United Kingdom), airplanes, and homes, among other locations (Chapter 4, Prevalence of Exposure to Secondhand Smoke). Comparisons of these studies are complicated by the different methodologies and environmental measurements used to characterize various components of secondhand smoke and the differences in sampling protocols (Chapter 3, Assessment of Exposure to Secondhand Smoke). Nicotine has been most widely used as an indicator of secondhand smoke, but other components of tobacco smoke have been used as well, including the particle mass, particle number density, and light scattering. Oldaker and colleagues (1990) made short-term measurements (one hour) of nicotine, respirable suspended particles (RSP), and ultraviolet-absorbing particulate matter (UVPM) in more than 125 offices and four cities. Turner and colleagues (1992) documented secondhand smoke markers for office areas with samples from nearly 500 locations. Hedge and colleagues (1993) measured various secondhand smoke constituents in 27 office buildings classified by ventilation systems. Baek and colleagues (1997) reported on nicotine and volatile organic compound levels in 12 office buildings in Korea; 4 of these buildings had recently instituted nonsmoking policies. Jenkins and colleagues (2001) examined the day-to-day variability of secondhand smoke components in a single large office building that permitted unrestricted smoking. In addition to repeated measurements at 29 locations in the building, there were personal samples collected from 24 nonsmoking participants. Sterling and colleagues (1996) studied personal and fixed locations of exposures in two U.S. office buildings that did not restrict smoking. A number of studies during the past 10 years assessed nicotine and respirable particle levels in workplaces,

homes, and penal institutions (Hammond 2002; Hammond and Emmons 2005). Many of these studies were designed to assess the effectiveness of smoking bans and smoking restrictions such as separate designated areas or a designated smoking area either alone or in combination with mechanical systems.

The following sections summarize the articles that were reviewed and then categorized according to the information they provided on smoking bans, designated nonsmoking areas, and separate rooms with or without dedicated air handling systems. This discussion also includes studies that purported to demonstrate that with general building ventilation alone, the impact of secondhand smoke is not substantial.

Banning Smoking

Building on the earlier work of Becker and colleagues (1989) and Stillman and colleagues (1990), many studies have demonstrated the effectiveness of using markers to monitor for secondhand smoke, as well as the effectiveness of complete smoking bans to reduce the number of cigarettes smoked. Becker and colleagues (1989) measured and averaged seven-day nicotine concentrations one month before and six months after a smoking ban was instituted at Johns Hopkins Children's Center. Substantial and significant decreases of nicotine were noted in some areas, such as elevator lobby lounges, where levels dropped from 13 to 0.45 $\mu g/m^3$. However, levels of nicotine changed little in restrooms (7.33 versus 6.68 $\mu g/m^3$) and in outpatient clinics (0.28 versus 0.36 $\mu g/m^3$) where levels were already low.

Stillman and colleagues (1990) pursued a similar strategy to evaluate the effectiveness of a campaign to eliminate smoking from all areas of Johns Hopkins University medical institutions. The investigators monitored seven-day nicotine concentrations with passive samplers placed in randomly selected locations eight months before and again one month before the campaign. Median nicotine concentrations ($\mu g/m^3$) dropped significantly in cafeterias (7.06 versus 0.22 $\mu g/m^3$), waiting areas (3.88 versus 0.28 $\mu g/m^3$), offices (2.05 versus 0.12 $\mu g/m^3$), staff lounges (2.43 versus 0.12 $\mu g/m^3$), and corridors (2.28 versus 0.20 $\mu g/m^3$). Similar to the observations of Becker and colleagues (1989), restroom levels did not show a significant decline (17.71 versus 10.0 $\mu g/m^3$). Ott and colleagues (1996) also reported evidence that smoking bans can effectively reduce or eliminate secondhand smoke exposure in taverns.

As a result of California's smoking policies in public places, these investigators documented a 77 percent reduction in respirable particulate concentrations. Miesner and colleagues (1989) found concentrations of particulate matter less than 2.5 micrometers in diameter ($PM_{2.5}$) of less than 30 $\mu g/m^3$ in offices without smoking and 30 to 140 $\mu g/m^3$ in restaurants and bars that permitted smoking. Brauer and Mannetje (1998) similarly showed that $PM_{2.5}$ in restaurants that prohibited smoking averaged 38 $\mu g/m^3$ (7–65 $\mu g/m^3$ range), while unrestricted smoking in restaurants raised the mean to 190 $\mu g/m^3$ (47–253 $\mu g/m^3$ range). Cadmium (Cd) concentrations also showed a consistent decrease in restaurants with smoking bans (0.65–1.7 $\mu g/m^3$) compared with restaurants that permitted smoking (2.2–10 $\mu g/m^3$ for smoking).

Heloma and colleagues (2001) reported on an evaluation of workplace nicotine exposure from secondhand smoke and the effect of national smoke-free workplace legislation in Finland. In March 1995, the *Tobacco Control Act* was reformed to move from voluntary compliance to prohibition of smoking on all premises for both workers and customers in workplaces. The authors pointed out that employers could comply by either imposing a total smoking ban or establishing designated smoking areas. Two rounds of surveys and measurements were conducted: one before the stricter law went into effect and one shortly afterward. The investigators surveyed 12 medium and large workplaces from both industrial and service sectors. Approximately 1,000 employees participated in each survey. Reported exposure to secondhand smoke, as well as the amount of smoking, decreased significantly between the two surveys. Median nicotine levels, which were 1.2 $\mu g/m^3$ in industrial workplaces, 1.5 $\mu g/m^3$ in the service sector, and 0.4 $\mu g/m^3$ in offices, all showed substantial decreases for the year following the enactment of stricter antismoking rules: 0.05 $\mu g/m^3$, 0.2 $\mu g/m^3$, and 0.1 $\mu g/m^3$, respectively.

The study conducted by Heloma and colleagues (2001) represents the most substantial evaluation of smoking restrictions in the workplace. Although nicotine levels were reduced significantly in all three sectors that were surveyed, the investigators still detected measurable levels in the follow-up survey. The authors did not distinguish between workplaces that banned smoking entirely and those that provided a designated smoking area. Unfortunately, distributional information on nicotine concentrations was not provided. The smallest reduction in nicotine was for office settings (75 percent), followed by the service sector (87 percent). The data do not indicate whether persistent exposure resulted from noncompliance, drifting smoke, or recirculated air from the designated smoking area.

In Japan, more than half of all adult men smoke, and the typical office environment is a large open (non-partitioned) area (Mochizuki-Kobayashi et al. 2004). Thus, the exposure of nonsmoking workers to secondhand smoke in the Japanese workplace is extensive. In 1996, the Japanese government required employers to establish workplace smoking policies and procedures. Mizoue and colleagues (2000) from the University of Occupational and Environmental Health in Japan collaborated with Finnish and Swedish researchers to assess the effectiveness of various strategies to comply with the law. Approximately three-fourths of all nonsmokers reported some workplace exposure; 50 percent reported exposure to secondhand smoke of more than four hours per day. Unfortunately, markers for secondhand smoke were not collected in this survey of 3,224 municipal employees from a city in northern Kyushu, Japan. This survey was conducted six months after the national policy was implemented. Banning smoking reduced secondhand smoke exposure of nonsmokers, yet 25 percent still reported some workplace exposure, and 15.6 percent said the exposure occurred for four or more hours per day. The authors concluded that any policy less restrictive than eliminating (isolating) smoking from the work area was insufficient. This finding encouraged the government to pursue stricter rules in Japan's workplaces.

These studies clearly demonstrate that secondhand smoke exposure can be eliminated with a smoking ban, as predicted by the mass balance equation. However, the findings also indicate the need for full compliance with such bans because incomplete compliance will lead to continued exposure.

Separation Strategies

Carrington and colleagues (2003) conducted a study of secondhand smoke exposure in 60 randomly selected bars in Greater Manchester, United Kingdom. Separating smokers from nonsmokers reduced the concentrations of various secondhand smoke markers such as RSP, UVPM, and nicotine by about 50 percent in comparisons of smoking and nonsmoking sections (Table 10.18). However, the levels of secondhand smoke in the smoking and nonsmoking sections were unaffected by the various ventilation systems in place, which included electrostatic precipitators and extractor fans. The investigators also noted substantial variations in secondhand smoke

Table 10.18 Untransformed secondhand smoke marker concentrations (µg/m³) for smoking and nonsmoking areas in United Kingdom public houses

Secondhand smoke markers (location)	N	Minimum	Maximum	Median	Percentiles 75	Percentiles 25
RSPM* (smoking)	138	14.6	356.3	98.3	153.1	50.0
RSPM (nonsmoking)	23	20.8	164.6	68.8	108.3	41.7
UVPM† (smoking)	137	0.5	269.7	58.5	108.3	25.7
UVPM (nonsmoking)	22	5.7	132.1	32.9	69.2	15.5
FPM‡ (smoking)	137	<0.1	298.3	73.2	127.0	28.4
FPM (nonsmoking)	22	8.5	152.3	37.7	74.9	18.6
SolPM§ (smoking)	137	1.6	514.4	63.8	148.6	21.7
SolPM (nonsmoking)	22	6.8	158.9	29.7	76.6	12.8
Nicotine (smoking)	134	0.5	516.9	63.0	132.8	23.5
Nicotine (nonsmoking)	23	0.5	77.8	21.1	42.7	10.6

Note: N is the total number of sample locations for 60 pubs.
*RSPM = Respirable suspended particulate matter.
†UVPM = Ultraviolet light-absorbing particulate matter.
‡FPM = Fluorescent particulate matter.
§SolPM = Solanesol particulate matter.
Source: Adapted from Carrington et al. 2003.

concentrations across the bars in the study, but only provided an overall statistical analysis. The authors concluded that the Public Places Charter, which was initiated by the hospitality industry and the government of the United Kingdom to increase the number of nonsmoking facilities and provide better ventilation, was having only limited success in abating secondhand smoke exposure. The investigators suggested that better ventilation designs, which the bars in the study did not have, might significantly reduce secondhand smoke exposure (Carrington et al. 2003).

There were attempts to control secondhand smoke exposure in a university cafeteria by implementing both strategies: separating smokers from nonsmokers and increasing the ventilation (Hammond 2002). Nicotine levels in the smoking section averaged 31 µg/m³; in the nonsmoking section within 25 feet of the smoking section, concentrations were one-tenth of those levels; and nonsmoking sections that were farther away averaged levels of 0.7 µg/m³.

Results from tests conducted over a four-day period documented higher levels in some measurements than in the reported average values. This finding indicated that secondhand smoke had intruded into the nonsmoking areas.

In a study of 75 restaurants in 26 cities, Hammond (2002) reported a mean nicotine level of 3.7 µg/m³ and a 1,000-fold range in concentrations. Similar to the United Kingdom bar study, separating smokers reduced exposure to secondhand smoke, but there was no evidence that an increase in ventilation had any effect. The data suggest that in spatially separated strategies where half or more of the seating area was nonsmoking, secondhand smoke levels in the nonsmoking sections were reduced, but levels remained high (Hammond 2002).

Lockhart Risk Management Ltd. (1995) attempted to characterize smoking density in studies of pubs in Vancouver, British Columbia (Canada); Repace (2000b) reported the results. In 10 pubs where smokers were separated from nonsmokers, the Lockhart studies measured nicotine levels in both areas, counted the number of lit cigarettes, and from these numbers derived a density of active smokers per 100 cubic meters. Figure 10.8 shows a slight difference in nicotine levels between smoking and nonsmoking sections when the density of active smokers is taken into account. Nonetheless, the results demonstrated that some bars had either well-mixed air or poorly controlled airflow—nicotine levels in nonsmoking sections were only slightly reduced from those in the smoking sections.

Brauer and Mannetje (1998) also studied secondhand smoke exposure in restaurants and bars in Vancouver, British Columbia (Canada). The investigators collected six-hour integrated samples of PM less than 10 micrometers in diameter (PM_{10}) and $PM_{2.5}$ for mass concentrations and then extracted and analyzed the samples for Cd as a marker for cigarette smoke. Of the 20 restaurants sampled, 5 were classified as nonsmoking, 11 as restricted smoking with measurements from the nonsmoking area, and 4 as unrestricted smoking. The authors found that the three types of establishments differed in their mean PM_{10}, $PM_{2.5}$, and Cd concentrations, but did have some overlapping values from other possible sources. Nevertheless, the investigators noted a clear distinction among restaurant groups in the Cd levels. The mean and standard deviation for Cd in $\mu g/m^3$ were 0.97 (0.44) for nonsmoking restaurants, 1.3 (1.3) for restricted places, and 6.5 (3.4) for unrestricted places. The authors concluded that partial smoking restrictions substantially reduce but do not eliminate secondhand smoke exposure of nonsmokers, and nonsmokers and smokers alike might experience substantial particulate exposures from cooking emissions.

Separating smokers from nonsmokers does not alter the source strength in the mass balance model, but only moves nonsmokers away from the smoking area. Studies show that levels are lower on average in nonsmoking compared with smoking sections, but secondhand smoke is readily found in nonsmoking sections.

Designated Smoking Areas

Several researchers have investigated the use of designated smoking areas to control secondhand smoke (Vaughan and Hammond 1990; Pierce et al. 1996; Hammond 2002), and Wagner and colleagues (2002) have evaluated air leakage from a simulated smoking room. Vaughan and Hammond (1990) collected nicotine measurements in a modern office building before and after smoking was restricted to a snack

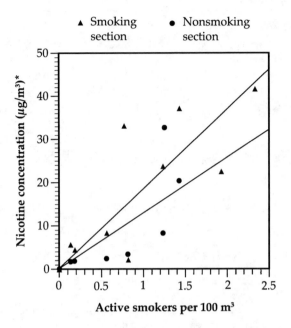

Figure 10.8   Nicotine levels measured in 10 Vancouver, British Columbia, pubs for the Heart and Stroke Foundation of British Columbia and Yukon, 1995

*$\mu g/m^3$ = Micrograms per cubic meter.
Source: Lockhart Risk Management Ltd. 1995. Reprinted with permission from Robert W. Lockhart.

bar on one floor. Measurements were made in areas and floors that were adjacent to and that shared the same AHU as the designated smoking area. Measurements were also collected from other locations (floors) in this building. Nicotine levels indicated that the policy successfully reduced exposure to secondhand smoke by 90 to 95 percent. However, a "spillover" effect into areas adjacent to the designated smoking area was apparent from nicotine levels that were four times higher than those in areas not sharing the same AHU with the smoking area. Smokers using the designated area were themselves subject to levels that were 1,800 times higher than the typical office nicotine levels before the new smoking policy took effect.

Hoping to achieve a better understanding of the effects that various design and operating parameters have on performance, Wagner and colleagues (2002) built a physical model of a smoking lounge at the Lawrence Berkeley National Laboratory. They found it essential to maintain the smoking room at a negative pressure with respect to adjacent areas to ensure that the tobacco smoke did not move out of the room into the surrounding air. To achieve this negative pressure, they established a separate exhaust for the room that exceeded supply and leakage. They also reported that the "pumping" action of a hinge-mounted door caused secondhand smoke to spill into adjacent areas. A sliding door is thus preferable to a standard swing-type door to reduce secondhand smoke leakage.

The spillage of secondhand smoke from a designated smoking lounge was evident in the study of an office building floor reported by Yamato and colleagues (1996). The smoking room (4 m × 4 m) at one end of a floor (45.5 m × 34 m) was equipped with three air cleaners with an effective air cleaning rate of once per minute. The ceiling exhaust provided two air changes per hour (ACH). Smoking was substantial, and average 24-hour suspended particulate concentrations in the smoking room during each of the two consecutive days studied ranged from 520 to 1,310 $\mu g/m^3$. Particle concentrations in the nonsmoking office area 25 m farther down the corridor were 30 and 50 $\mu g/m^3$ for each of the two days studied. However, the corridor, the hall leading to the stairs, and the kitchen located near the smoking room experienced concentrations three to seven times higher than in the nonsmoking office area. This case study indicated that with just four persons simultaneously smoking, air cleaners (even at one air change per minute) and exhaust ventilation were insufficient to maintain particle concentrations below the Japanese standard of 150 $\mu g/m^3$ for office buildings.

Pierce and colleagues (1996) conducted a set of experiments in an office suite of 3,100 square feet in a three-story building that totaled 45,000 ft^2. The building had a single roof-mounted AHU that supplied conditioned ducted air to ceiling diffusers and a ceiling plenum return (unducted). Ceiling-mounted fan coil units provided additional conditioning to the six exterior offices in the test suite. The conference room was 8 percent of the suite area (14 ft × 20 ft) and was the designated smoking lounge. Four air-cleaning devices were tested for effectiveness in reducing RSP, nicotine, CO, and other markers. The investigators made eight-hour measurements inside and outside the lounge as fixed and personal samples. Cigarettes were counted, and the entrance door to the lounge was kept closed except for entering and exiting. They studied six sets of conditions and reported that a baseline without smoking and one with smoking, but without auxiliary air cleaners operating, clearly demonstrated the impact of smoking. For example, nicotine levels went from below the level of detection to about

50 $\mu g/m^3$ inside the lounge, and RSP ranged up to 500 $\mu g/m^3$ for the smoking situation. The first device tested, Device 1, was a recirculating air cleaner (1,050 cubic feet [ft^3] per minute) with a 95 percent high efficiency particulate air (HEPA) filter and a bed of carbon, permanganate, and zeolite media. The authors did not report the volume of the lounge or the ventilation rate of the base building AHU. With the assumption that the room was 14 ft by 20 ft by 8 ft, Device 1 was capable of cleaning the entire volume of the lounge every two minutes, or 30 effective ACH. Even at this substantial volume flow, the concentration of nicotine, the secondhand smoke marker, only dropped to about one-half of the smoking/no device baseline, and the RSP levels were one-third to one-fifth of the smoking baseline levels. The CO levels were not affected, and the other secondhand smoke markers showed a 90 percent reduction.

Device 2 had a prefilter of unspecified efficiency and drew air at an unspecified rate past an O_3 generator. However, Pierce and colleagues (1996) did not report the generation rate or room O_3 concentrations. Apparently, this device did not lower any of the secondhand smoke markers.

Device 3 had an electrostatic prefilter, a V-bag filter that contained numerous V-shaped pockets to increase its surface area of unspecified efficiency, followed by a charcoal bed. The device was ceiling mounted and moved 650 ft^3 per minute. This system was capable of processing the room air every three to four minutes (if a very high removal efficiency could be achieved, the device would be equivalent to 15 to 20 ACH). Nicotine levels were slightly less than one-half of the baseline smoking condition. Particles and the other secondhand smoke markers did not appear to be reduced to any notable extent below the baseline smoking case. Nicotine levels in the lounge were 22.5 $\mu g/m^3$ and 19.8 $\mu g/m^3$ compared with 48 $\mu g/m^3$ and 54.2 $\mu g/m^3$ at baseline; RSP levels in the lounge were 380 $\mu g/m^3$ and 380 $\mu g/m^3$ compared with 155 $\mu g/m^3$ and 500 $\mu g/m^3$ at baseline (Pierce et al. 1996).

Device 4 drew in air at 750 ft^3 per minute past an electrostatic prefilter and a highly efficient (reported to be 99.999 percent) HEPA filter. It also had a carbon-adsorbing bed. Nicotine levels were again about one-half of the baseline smoking condition. The RSP and other secondhand smoke markers were reduced by 80 percent. This device, as with the others, did not reduce CO levels (Pierce et al. 1996).

The fixed location and personal monitoring collected outside the lounge provided some evidence that secondhand smoke might have spilled from the lounge and was then recirculated by the ceiling-mounted fan coil units or was present in the supply air from the AHU operating in the building. The investigators did not describe the smoking policy for the building nor did they adequately describe the ventilation system, but the nicotine measurements were informative. Because RSP comes from many sources, small differences in air concentrations cannot readily be interpreted. However, the UVPM and the fluorescent particulate matter analyses are more specific to secondhand smoke compared with RSP analyses (Nelson et al. 1992). The baseline case for these two markers without smoking indicated that secondhand smoke from other smokers in the building was not a concern. Measurements during the runs with the different air cleaning devices provided evidence of some incidental secondhand smoke exposure. Given the laboratory findings of Wagner and colleagues (2002), some spillage of secondhand smoke occurs with conventional swing doors if strict negative pressures are not maintained.

Pierce and colleagues (1996) generalized beyond the evidence documented in their study when they concluded that "auxiliary air cleaning devices operating concurrently with dilution ventilation can be effective in reducing the levels of nicotine and RSP in a designated smoking area" (Pierce et al. 1996, p. 57). Their study does not apply to all devices nor would it apply to all designated smoking areas within a building. These limited studies show that designated smoking areas also do not prevent exposure of persons outside of these areas to secondhand smoke. The strategy may require complicated engineering and a careful assessment of relevant building characteristics. Designated smoking areas may also adversely affect the health of smokers by exposing them to highly concentrated levels of secondhand smoke and would also subject any staff who enter to high concentrations (Siegel et al. 1995).

Smoking Bans Versus Unrestricted Smoking

Prohibiting smoking effectively reduces and can eliminate exposure to secondhand smoke in the workplace (Hammond et al. 1995). Using nicotine as a marker for cigarette smoking, Hammond and colleagues (1995) demonstrated that secondhand smoke could be reduced in offices and shops more effectively with a complete ban compared with partially restricted and unrestricted smoking policies. Figure 10.9 displays the frequency distribution for nicotine levels measured at the desks of nonsmokers under the three different conditions. The median nicotine

concentrations dropped from 8.6 to 1.3 $\mu g/m^3$ when smoking was restricted and to 0.3 $\mu g/m^3$ when smoking was prohibited. Similar shifts in the distribution of nicotine concentrations were seen in measurements from nonoffice workplace settings (Figure 10.10).

Jenkins and colleagues (2001) documented personal exposure measurements in a large, four-story office building with prevalent and unrestricted smoking. The air exchange rate was between 0.6 and 0.7 ACH. Of the 300 employees, 16 percent smoked regularly at work. Samples were analyzed for several secondhand smoke markers including nicotine. The nicotine levels in the nonsmoking offices and cubicles, as well as in the common areas, were in the range that Hammond and colleagues (1995) had measured in workplaces that restricted smoking. The article by Jenkins and colleagues (2001) pointed out that the secondhand smoke levels were lower than the levels OSHA had recorded in buildings with unrestricted smoking. A more appropriate analysis would include normalizing the results by occupant density, smoking prevalence, and effective ventilation rate. The building studied had a low occupancy density

Figure 10.9   Cumulative frequency distributions of weekly average nicotine concentrations at the desks of nonsmoking workers in open offices

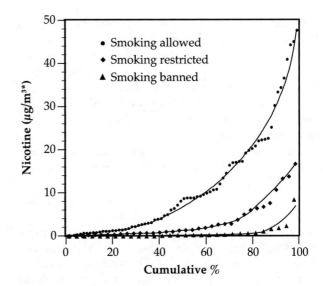

*$\mu g/m^3$ = Micrograms per cubic meter.
Source: Hammond et al. 1995.

Figure 10.10 Cumulative frequency distributions of weekly average nicotine concentrations in nonsmokers' work areas in shops and other nonoffice settings

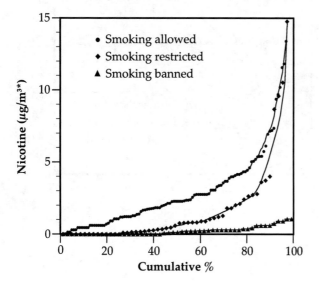

*$\mu g/m^3$ = Micrograms per cubic meter.
Source: Hammond et al. 1995.

of four persons per 1,000 ft²; six to eight persons per 1,000 ft² is more typical for office buildings. The building that Jenkins and colleagues (2001) studied was well ventilated with carbon dioxide levels of only 125 to 175 parts per million above outdoor values. The effect of dilution can also be seen when comparing these results with those of Hammond and colleagues (1995). Forty percent of the nicotine values that Hammond and colleagues (1995) had documented in a building with unrestricted smoking exceeded the upper values that Jenkins and colleagues (2001) obtained in cubicles and offices with smokers.

Sterling and colleagues (1996) also studied secondhand smoke exposure in two office buildings with unrestricted smoking. The authors collected eight-hour personal and fixed location samples of respirable particle mass and other markers for secondhand smoke. Secondhand smoke markers and respirable particulates provided similar results whether measured in fixed locations or by direct personal (non-smoker) assessments in one building, but less so in the second building. The lack of correspondence found in the second building was pronounced for particle phase measures but not for vapor phase components.

This finding suggests that nicotine and 3-ethenyl-pyridine vapor phase markers measured in fixed locations within a building might represent a personal exposure to secondhand smoke. Building 1 was a two-floor sealed office building (approximately 20,000 ft²) without operable windows and with 29.1 percent ventilation air; the HVAC was delivering an average of 18 ft³ per minute per person with an assumed 60 percent ventilation effectiveness. Rates were somewhat higher at the fixed-site locations. Building 2 was also a sealed building without operable windows; it was three times the size of Building 1 and contained two AHUs. Assuming an 80 percent mixing efficiency for the ventilation air, AHU 1 served 231 people and supplied outside ventilation air between 21.0 and 35.6 ft³ per minute per person. AHU 2 provided ventilation for 147 people who occupied the upper floor. AHU 1 ventilation air rates were between 20 and 36 ft³ per minute per person. AHU 2 had a somewhat lower range—between 11 and 32 ft³ per minute per person. This study documented the ventilation component, but not the actual amount or prevalence of smoking during the two days of monitoring. The occupancy density of Building 2 was less than typical, and both buildings had ventilation rates that exceeded ASHRAE standards in place at that time for office buildings. Therefore, the authors overstated their findings when they claimed, "the results demonstrate that with ventilation in accordance with current ASHRAE standards, dilution can be an effective means of controlling ETS-related constituents to low concentrations" (Sterling et al. 1996, p. 112).

Indoor particle concentrations for $PM_{2.5}$ were measured in the comprehensive EPA study of 100 office buildings in the United States (Womble et al. 1995, 1996). Smoking was permitted in 29 of these buildings. Although there are no apparent differences in the outdoor particle concentrations ($PM_{2.5}$) measured at air intakes, the $PM_{2.5}$ concentrations inside buildings that did not permit smoking appear to be higher than inside buildings where smoking was permitted, particularly during the summer (Figure 10.11). When the investigators compared the ventilation rates for smoking and nonsmoking buildings, the buildings where smoking was permitted had similar ventilation rates for the buildings studied in the winter but higher ventilation rates for the buildings studied in summer (Figure 10.12). Most buildings exceed the minimum ventilation rates recommended in the most recent ASHRAE standard. Of the buildings with smokers, the median ventilation rates were about twice the recommended ASHRAE standard (ASHRAE 1989).

Figure 10.11 Cumulative distribution of indoor PM$_{2.5}$* concentrations in 100 United States office buildings by smoking policy

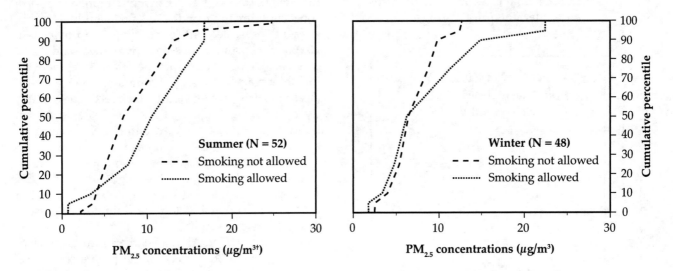

*PM$_{2.5}$ = Particulate matter less than 2.5 micrometers in diameter.
†µg/m^3 = Micrograms per cubic meter.
Source: Brightman 2005.

Figure 10.12 Cumulative distribution of ventilation rates in 100 United States office buildings by smoking policy

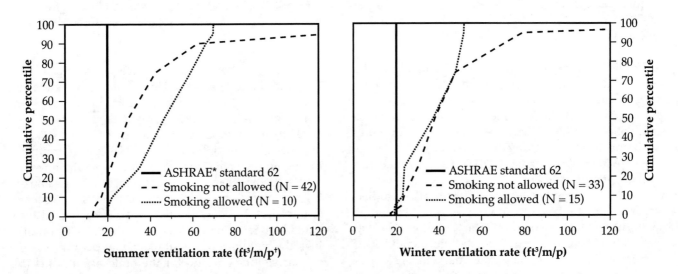

*ASHRAE = American Society of Heating, Refrigerating and Air-Conditioning Engineers.
†ft^3/m/p = Cubic feet per meter per person.
Source: Brightman 2005.

The PM$_{2.5}$ data from the EPA Building Assessment, Survey and Evaluation Study underscore the importance of including details on ventilation conditions, smoking rates, and occupant density, among other parameters, in drawing conclusions about the efficacy of dilution or even of partial restrictions to mitigate the impacts of secondhand smoke exposure (Womble et al. 1995, 1996).

Conclusions

1. Workplace smoking restrictions are effective in reducing secondhand smoke exposure.

2. Workplace smoking restrictions lead to less smoking among covered workers.

3. Establishing smoke-free workplaces is the only effective way to ensure that secondhand smoke exposure does not occur in the workplace.

4. The majority of workers in the United States are now covered by smoke-free policies.

5. The extent to which workplaces are covered by smoke-free policies varies among worker groups, across states, and by sociodemographic factors. Workplaces related to the entertainment and hospitality industries have notably high potential for secondhand smoke exposure.

6. Evidence from peer-reviewed studies shows that smoke-free policies and regulations do not have an adverse economic impact on the hospitality industry.

7. Evidence suggests that exposure to secondhand smoke varies by ethnicity and gender.

8. In the United States, the home is now becoming the predominant location for exposure of children and adults to secondhand smoke.

9. Total bans on indoor smoking in hospitals, restaurants, bars, and offices substantially reduce secondhand smoke exposure, up to several orders of magnitude with incomplete compliance, and with full compliance, exposures are eliminated.

10. Exposures of nonsmokers to secondhand smoke cannot be controlled by air cleaning or mechanical air exchange.

Overall Implications

Total bans on indoor smoking in hospitals, restaurants, bars, and offices will substantially reduce secondhand smoke exposure, up to several orders of magnitude with incomplete compliance, and, with full compliance, exposures will be eliminated. Absent a ban, attempts to control secondhand smoke exposure of nonsmoking occupants or patrons have mixed results. Uncontrolled air currents, mixed return air and ventilation air, and the lack of complete physical barriers lead to persistence of some secondhand smoke exposure with partial restriction strategies. The few studies that claim unrestricted smoking in offices meets ASHRAE standards do not provide convincing evidence that exposures of nonsmokers to secondhand smoke were adequately reduced (ASHRAE 1999). Specially designed smoking areas inside a building can effectively isolate secondhand smoke, but effectiveness depends on engineering design and on high volume exhaust separated from the main AHU to maintain a negative pressure within the physically isolated area. Mechanical air cleaning has not been sufficiently effective to permit exhaust air, transported or leaked air from a designated smoking area, or air from a physically separated smoking room or lounge to be remixed with ventilation air.

Ventilation rates substantially higher than the minimums recommended by ASHRAE (1999) might dilute some secondhand smoke constituents in some indoor settings to levels indistinguishable (statistically) from levels in buildings that restrict smoking. Perhaps, under such circumstances, indoor air quality might be perceived as acceptable at the 80 percent threshold criterion set by ASHRAE for persons voluntarily electing to be indoors in the presence of active smokers. However, this threshold criterion does not adequately account for possible health effects associated with exposure to secondhand smoke constituents even at low levels. Absent being able to specify acceptable levels of airborne contaminants and risks associated with secondhand smoke, concentration-based guidelines for secondhand smoke cannot be developed. Thus, exposure to secondhand smoke components cannot be controlled sufficiently through dilution ventilation or by typical air cleaning strategies if the goal is to achieve no risk or a negligible risk. The only effective controls that eliminate exposures of nonsmokers are the complete physical isolation of smoking areas with separate air exhausts or a total smoking ban within the structure. This conclusion echoes prior conclusions of federal agencies (USDHHS 1986; USEPA 1992; NIOSH 1991).

Despite wider adoption of smoking restrictions, exposures to secondhand smoke persist. Among adults, data from the 1991 NHIS Health Promotion and Disease Prevention Supplement indicate that 20.2 percent of lifetime nonsmokers and 23.1 percent of former smokers reported any exposure to secondhand smoke at home or at work (Mannino et al. 1997). Self-reported data from NHANES III (1988–1991) suggest that 37 percent of lifetime nonsmokers were exposed to secondhand smoke, and men (46 percent) were more likely than women (32 percent) to experience exposure (Steenland et al. 1998). Most nonsmokers were exposed in the workplace (20 percent) compared with those exposed at home (11 percent) or at both work and home (6 percent). However, Pirkle and colleagues (1996) used high-performance liquid chromatography atomspheric-pressure chemical ionization tandem mass spectrometry to analyze serum cotinine levels and found that 87 percent of nonsmokers had detectable levels. These investigators also noted that children, non-Hispanic Blacks, and males had higher levels than the rest of the populations that were studied (Pirkle et al. 1996).

Some evidence suggests that exposure among certain ethnic and gender groups may be higher. For example, Pletsch (1994) examined self-reported secondhand smoke exposure data from 4,256 Hispanic females aged 12 through 49 years who participated in the Hispanic Health and Nutrition Examination Survey (NCHS 1985). Pletsch (1994) found that 62 percent of Mexican American women, 59 percent of Puerto Rican women, and 52 percent of Cuban American women were regularly exposed to secondhand smoke at home, and 35 percent of Mexican American women, 28 percent of Puerto Rican women, and 49 percent of Cuban American women were regularly exposed at work.

According to NHIS data, most of the U.S. working population (76.5 percent) does not smoke (NCHS, public use data tape, 2002). In 2002, there were an estimated 100.3 million nonsmoking workers in the United States. In a study that compared exposure levels with OSHA's significant risk standards, more than 95 percent of the office workers exposed to secondhand smoke in the United States exceeded OSHA's significant risk level for heart disease mortality, and 60 percent exceeded the significant risk level for lung cancer mortality (Repace et al. 1998). Repace and colleagues (1998) estimated excesses of 4,000 heart disease deaths and 400 lung cancer deaths were attributable to workplace exposure.

On the basis of this review, it is clear that banning smoking from the workplace is the only effective way to ensure that exposures are not occurring. Despite reductions in workplace smoking, significant worker safety issues remain that only smoking bans can address. The home remains the most serious venue for secondhand smoke exposure.

References

Adler G, Greeman M, Rickers S, Kuskowski M. Smoking in nursing homes: conflicts and challenges. *Social Work in Health Care* 1997;25(4):67–81.

Albers AB, Siegel M, Cheng DM, Biener L, Rigotti NA. Relation between local restaurant smoking regulations and attitudes towards the prevalence and social acceptability of smoking: a study of youths and adults who eat out predominantly at restaurants in their town. *Tobacco Control* 2004a;13(4): 347–55.

Albers AB, Siegel M, Cheng DM, Rigotti NA, Biener L. Effects of restaurant and bar smoking regulations on exposure to environmental tobacco smoke among Massachusetts adults. *American Journal of Public Health* 2004b;94(11):1959–64.

American Legacy Foundation. More than 13 million American children regularly breathing secondhand smoke in their homes, cars: American legacy Foundation and the Ad Council launch first campaign to call attention to and educate public about dangers of secondhand smoke [press release]. Washington: American Legacy Foundation, January 11, 2005.

American Lung Association. *State Legislated Actions on Tobacco Issues*. 16th Edition, 2004. Washington: American Lung Association, 2005.

American Medical Association. *SmokeLess States National Tobacco Prevention and Control Program: Five Years of Making a Difference*. Chicago: American Medical Association, 1998.

American Nonsmokers' Rights Foundation. *Local 100% Smokefree Laws in All Workplaces, Restaurants, and Bars: Effective by Year*. Berkeley (CA): American Nonsmokers' Rights Foundation, 2005a.

American Nonsmokers' Rights Foundation. *Municipalities with Ordinances Covering Outdoor Air*. Berkeley (CA): American Nonsmokers' Rights Foundation, January 2005b.

American Nonsmokers' Rights Foundation. *100% Smokefree Correctional Facilities*. Berkeley (CA): American Nonsmokers' Rights Foundation, 2005c; <http://www.no-smoke.org/pdf/100smokefree prisons.pdf>; accessed: October 24, 2005.

American Nonsmokers' Rights Foundation. *Overview List–How Many Smokefree Laws?* Berkeley (CA): American Nonsmokers' Rights Foundation, 2005d.

Americans for Nonsmokers' Rights. Overview List— How Many Smokefree Laws?, April 17, 2006; <http://www.no-smoke.org/pdf/mediaordlist. pdf>; accessed: May 15, 2006a.

Americans for Nonsmokers' Rights. Percent of U.S. State Populations Coverd by Local or State 100% Smokefree Air Laws, April 17, 2006; <http:// www.no-smoke.org/pdf/percentstatepops.pdf>; accessed: May 15, 2006b.

Americans for Nonsmokers' Rights. States and Municipalities with Local 100% Smokefree Laws in Workplaces, Restaurants, or Bars, April 17, 2006 <http://www.no-smoke.org/pdf/100ordlist.pdf>; accessed: May 15, 2006c.

American Society of Heating, Refrigerating and Air-Conditioning Engineers. *ASHRAE Standard 62-1989: Ventilation for Acceptable Indoor Air Quality*. Atlanta: American Society of Heating, Refrigerating and Air-Conditioning Engineers, 1989.

American Society of Heating, Refrigerating and Air-Conditioning Engineers. *ANSI/ASHRAE Standard 62-1999: Ventilation for Acceptable Indoor Air Quality*. Atlanta: American Society of Heating, Refrigerating and Air-Conditioning Engineers, 1999.

American Society of Heating, Refrigerating and Air-Conditioning Engineers. *ASHRAE Standard 62-2001: Ventilation for Acceptable Indoor Air Quality*. Atlanta: American Society of Heating, Refrigerating and Air-Conditioning Engineers, 2001.

American Society of Heating, Refrigerating and Air-Conditioning Engineers. *Environmental Tobacco Smoke: Position Document*. Atlanta: American Society of Heating, Refrigerating and Air-Conditioning Engineers, 2005.

Americans for Nonsmokers' Rights, American Cancer Society, American Heart Association, American Lung Association, Campaign for Tobacco-Free Kids, SmokeLess States. *Fundamentals of Clean Indoor Air Policy* 2002. http://www.no-smoke.org/ goingsmokefree.php?dp=d13/p141.

Americans with Disabilities Act of 1990, Public Law 101-336, 104 Stat. 327.

An Act Relating to Health and Safety—Smoking in Public Places (January 2001), Chapter 69 of the *Public Laws of the State of Rhode Island and Providence Plantations*, Volume I:334–5; Rhode Island (Rhode Island House Bill 5883; <http://www.rilin.state.ri.us/ billtext/billtext01/housetext01/h5883.htm>; accessed: February 3, 2006).

Anderson KE, Kliris J, Murphy L, Carmella SG, Han S, Link C, Bliss RL, Puumala S, Murphy SE, Hecht SS. Metabolites of a tobacco-specific lung carcinogen in nonsmoking casino patrons. *Cancer Epidemiology, Biomarkers & Prevention* 2003;12(12):1544–6.

Appropriations for the Fiscal Year 1988, and for Other Purposes (Prohibition Against Smoking on Scheduled Flights and Tampering with Smoke Alarms), Public Law 100-202, *U.S. Statutes at Large* 101(1987):1329–82, I328(a).

Baek SO, Kim Y-S, Perry R. Indoor air quality in homes, offices and restaurants in Korean urban areas—indoor/outdoor relationships. *Atmospheric Environment* 1997;31(4):529–44.

Barnes DE, Bero LA. Industry-funded research and conflict of interest: an analysis of research sponsored by the tobacco industry through the Center for Indoor Air Research. *Journal of Health Politics, Policy and Law* 1996;21(3):515–42.

Bartosch WJ, Pope GC. The economic effect of smoke-free restaurant policies on restaurant business in Massachusetts. *Journal of Public Health Management and Practice* 1999;5(1):53–62.

Bartosch WJ, Pope GC. Local enactment of tobacco control policies in Massachusetts. *American Journal of Public Health* 2002;92(6):941–3.

Baskas H. Finding a smoking (or smoke-free) area at the airport, 2004; <http://www.usatoday.com/travel/columnist/baskas/2004-06-01-baskas_x.htm>; accessed: February 3, 2006.

Bauer JE, Hyland A, Li Q, Steger C, Cummings M. A longitudinal assessment of the impact of smoke-free worksite policies on tobacco use. *American Journal of Public Health* 2005;95(6):1024–9.

Becker DM, Conner HF, Waranch R, Stillman F, Pennington L, Lees PS, Oski F. The impact of a total ban on smoking in the Johns Hopkins Children's Center. *Journal of the American Medical Association* 1989;262(6):799–802.

Bero LA, Glantz SA. Tobacco industry response to a risk assessment of environmental tobacco smoke. *Tobacco Control* 1993;2(2):103–13.

Bialous SA, Glantz SA. ASHRAE Standard 62: tobacco industry's influence over national ventilation standards. *Tobacco Control* 2002;11(4):315–28.

Blizzard R. Second-hand smoke: harmful or hyperbole? Princeton (NJ): The Gallup Organization, 2004.

Bolinski J. High-rises to ban smoking. *The State Journal-Register* April 25, 2003;City/State Sect:19.

Borland R, Owen N, Hill D, Chapman S. Changes in acceptance of workplace smoking bans following their implementation: a prospective study. *Preventive Medicine* 1990;19(3):314–22.

Brauer M, Mannetje A. Restaurant smoking restrictions and environmental tobacco smoke exposure. *American Journal of Public Health* 1998;88(12):1834–6.

Brightman H. Health, comfort, and productivity in United States office buildings [dissertation]. Boston: Harvard School of Public Health, 2005.

Broin v. Philip Morris Cos., No. 92-1405 (Fla., Dade Cty. Mar. 15, 1994), *cited in* 9.1 TPLR 2.1 (1994).

Brownson RC, Davis JR, Jackson-Thompson J, Wilkerson JC. Environmental tobacco smoke awareness and exposure: impact of a statewide clean indoor air law and the report of the US Environmental Protection Agency. *Tobacco Control* 1995;4(2):132–8.

Brownson RC, Hopkins DP, Wakefield MA. Effects of smoking restrictions in the workplace. *Annual Review of Public Health* 2002;23:333–48.

Bryan-Jones K, Bero LA. Tobacco industry efforts to defeat the Occupational Safety and Health Administration indoor air quality rule. *American Journal of Public Health* 2003;93(4):585–92.

Bureau of National Affairs, Inc. *Smoking in the Workplace: 1991—SHRM-BNA Survey No. 55.* Bulletin to Management. Washington: Bureau of National Affairs, Inc., 1991.

Burns DM, Shanks TG, Major JM, Gower KB, Shopland DR. Restrictions on smoking in the workplace. In: *Population Based Smoking Cessation: Proceedings of a Conference on What Works to Influence Cessation in the General Population.* Smoking and Tobacco Control Monograph No. 12. Bethesda (MD): U.S. Department of Health and Human Services, Public Health Service, National Institutes of Health, National Cancer Institute, December 2000:99–128.

California Department of Health Services. *A Model for Change: the California Experience in Tobacco Control.* Sacramento (CA): California Department of Health Services, Tobacco Control Section, 1998.

California Department of Health Services. Support for smoke-free bars grows stronger in California [press release]. Sacramento (CA): California Department of Health Services, October 16, 2000.

California Department of Health Services. *Eliminating Smoking in Bars, Taverns and Gaming Clubs: The California Smoke-Free Workplace Act.* Sacramento (CA): California Department of Health Services, Tobacco Control Section, 2001a.

California Department of Health Services. Governor Davis announces a decrease in the smoking rate and support for more smoke-free environments [press release]. Sacramento (CA): California Department of Health Services, April 25, 2001b.

California Environmental Protection Agency. *Health Effects of Exposure to Environmental Tobacco Smoke.* Sacramento (CA): California Environmental Protection Agency, Office of Environmental Health Hazard Assessment, Reproductive and Cancer Hazard Assessment Section and Air Toxicology and Epidemiology Section, 1997.

California Environmental Protection Agency. *Proposed Identification of Environmental Tobacco Smoke as a Toxic Air Contaminant. Part B: Health Effects.* Sacramento (CA): California Environmental Protection Agency, Office of Environmental Health Hazard Assessment, 2005.

California State Assembly. Senate passes prison smoking ban [press release]. Sacramento (CA): California State Assembly, August 24, 2004.

Carpenter MJ, Hughes JR, Solomon LJ, Powell TA. Smoking in correctional facilities: a survey of employees. *Tobacco Control* 2001;10(1):38–42.

Carrington J, Watson AFR, Gee IL. The effects of smoking status and ventilation on environmental tobacco smoke concentrations in public areas of UK pubs and bars. *Atmospheric Environment* 2003;37(23):3255–66.

Center for Health Improvement. *Health Policy Guide: Smoke-Free Workplace.* Sacramento (CA): Center for Health Improvement, 2004 (<http://www.health.policycoach.org/doc.asp?id=3144>; accessed: May 16, 2004).

Centers for Disease Control and Prevention. Progress in chronic disease prevention: Indian Health Service facilities become smoke-free. *Morbidity and Mortality Weekly Report* 1987a;36(22):348–50.

Centers for Disease Control and Prevention. Progress in chronic disease prevention: Survey of worksite smoking policies—New York City. *Morbidity and Mortality Weekly Report* 1987b;36(12):177–9.

Centers for Disease Control and Prevention. Guidelines for school health programs to prevent tobacco use and addiction. *Morbidity and Mortality Weekly Report* 1994;43(RR-2):1–18.

Centers for Disease Control and Prevention. Assessment of the impact of a 100% smoke-free ordinance on restaurant sales—West Lake Hills, Texas, 1992–1994. *Morbidity and Mortality Weekly Report* 1995;44(19):370–2.

Centers for Disease Control and Prevention. Preemptive state tobacco-control laws—United States, 1982–1998. *Morbidity and Mortality Weekly Report* 1999;47(51&52):1112–4.

Centers for Disease Control and Prevention. Costs of smoking among active duty U.S. Air Force personnel—United States, 1997. *Morbidity and Mortality Weekly Report* 2000;49(20):441–5.

Centers for Disease Control and Prevention. Annual smoking-attributable mortality, years of potential life lost, and economic costs—United States, 1995–1999. *Morbidity and Mortality Weekly Report* 2002;51(14):300–3.

Centers for Disease Control and Prevention. *Second National Report on Human Exposure to Environmental Chemicals. Results.* Atlanta: U.S. Department of Health and Human Services, Centers for Disease Control and Prevention, National Center for Environmental Health, Division of Laboratory Sciences, 2003. NCEH Publication No. 02-0716.

Centers for Disease Control and Prevention. Cigarette smoking among adults — United States, 2002. *Morbidity and Mortality Weekly Report* 2004a;53(20):427–31.

Centers for Disease Control and Prevention. Impact of a smoking ban on restaurant and bar revenues—El Paso, Texas, 2002. *Morbidity and Mortality Weekly Report* 2004b;53(7):150–2.

Centers for Disease Control and Prevention. Indoor air quality in hospitality venues before and after implementation of a clear indoor air law—Western New York, 2003. *Morbidity and Mortality Weekly Report* 2004c;53(44):1038–41.

Centers for Disease Control and Prevention. Survey of airport smoking policies—United States, 2002. *Morbidity and Mortality Weekly Report* 2004d;53(50):1175–8.

Centers for Disease Control and Prevention. Preemptive state smoke-free indoor air laws—United States, 1999–2004. *Morbidity and Mortality Weekly Report* 2005a;54(10):250–3.

Centers for Disease Control and Prevention. State smoking restrictions for private-sector worksites, restaurants, and bars—United States, 1998 and 2004. *Morbidity and Mortality Weekly Report* 2005b;54(26):649–53.

Centers for Disease Control and Prevention. *Strategies for Addressing Asthma Within a Coordinated School Health Program, With Updated Resources.* Atlanta: Centers for Disease Control and Prevention, National Center for Chronic Disease Prevention and Health Promotion, 2005c.

Centers for Disease Control and Prevention. *Third National Report on Human Exposure to Environmental Chemicals.* Atlanta: U.S. Department of Health and Human Services, Centers for Disease Control and Prevention, National Center for Environmental Health, Division of Laboratory Sciences, 2005d. NCEH Publication No. 05-0570.

Centers for Disease Control and Prevention, Wellness Councils of America, American Cancer Society. *Making Your Workplace Smokefree: A Decision Maker's Guide*. Atlanta: U.S. Department of Health and Human Services, Centers for Disease Control and Prevention, 1996.

Chen S. *State of Tobacco Control in Alameda County 2004*. Emeryville (CA): American Lung Association of the East Bay, 2005.

Chilmonczyk BA, Palomaki GE, Knight GJ, Williams J, Haddow JE. An unsuccessful cotinine-assisted intervention strategy to reduce environmental tobacco smoke exposure during infancy. *American Journal of Diseases of Children* 1992;146(3):357–60.

Civil Aeronautics Board. Economic Regulations Docket No. 21708. Part 252 - Segregation of passengers who desire to be seated in specifically designated "smoking" areas aboard commercial aircraft operated by certificated air carriers, 1972; <http://legacy.library.ucsf.edu/tid/qfs90c00>; accessed: August 14, 2004.

Cole W. Smoking ban redefines military culture. *Honolulu Advertiser*, January 5, 2003.

County of Los Angeles Department of Health Services. Smoke-free zones in Los Angeles parks [press release], 2001. <http://www.no-smoking.org/august01/08-10-01-4.html>; accessed: August 14, 2004.

Cowling DW, Bond P. Smoke-free laws and bar revenues in California—the last call. *Health Economics* 2005;14(12):1273–81.

Dai C, Denslow D, Hyland A, Lotfinia B. *The Economic Impact of Florida's Smoke-Free Workplace Law*. Gainesville (FL): University of Florida, 2004.

Daniels SL. Control of volatile organic compounds and particulate matter in indoor environments of airports by bipolar air ionization. Paper presented at the Federal Aviation Administration Technology Transfer Conference; May 5–8, 2002; Atlantic City, New Jersey.

Davis RM. Exposure to environmental tobacco smoke: identifying and protecting those at risk [editorial]. *Journal of the American Medical Association* 1998; 280(22):1947–8.

Davis RM, Boyd G, Schoenborn CA. 'Common courtesy' and the elimination of passive smoking: results of the 1987 National Health Interview Survey. *Journal of the American Medical Association* 1990;263:2208–10. [See also erratum in *Journal of the American Medical Association* 1990;263(22):3025.]

Dearlove JV, Bialous SA, Glantz SA. Tobacco industry manipulation of the hospitality industry to maintain smoking in public places. *Tobacco Control* 2002;11(2):94–104.

Drope J, Bialous SA, Glantz SA. Tobacco industry efforts to present ventilation as an alternative to smoke-free environments in North America. *Tobacco Control* 2004;13(Suppl I):i41–i47.

Eisner MD, Smith AK, Blanc PD. Bartenders' respiratory health after establishment of smoke-free bars and taverns. *Journal of the American Medical Association* 1998;280(22):1909–14.

el-Guebaly N, Cathcart J, Currie S, Brown D, Gloster S. Public health and therapeutic aspects of smoking bans in mental health and addiction settings. *Psychiatric Services* 2002;53(12):1617–22.

Emerson E. *California Lessons in Clean Indoor Air: A Compilation of Campaign Stories, Implementation Tools, and Compliance Strategies*. Sacramento (CA): California Department of Health Services, Tobacco Control Section, 2001.

Emmons KM, Hammond SK, Fava JL, Velicer WF, Evans JL, Monroe AD. A randomized trial to reduce passive smoke exposure in low-income households with young children. *Pediatrics* 2001;108(1):18–24.

Etzel RA, Balk SJ, editors. *Handbook of Pediatric Environmental Health*. Elk Grove Village (IL): American Academy of Pediatrics, 1999.

Evans D. Solana Beach bans smoking on beaches. *San Diego Union-Tribune* October 8, 2003;ZONE Sect: NC-1.

Fair Housing Act of 1992.

Falkin GP, Strauss S, Lankenau S. Cigarette smoking policies in American jails. *American Jails* 1998; 12(3):9–14.

Farkas AJ, Gilpin EA, Distefan JM, Pierce JP. The effects of household and workplace smoking restrictions on quitting behaviors. *Tobacco Control* 1999;8(3):261–5.

Farkas AJ, Gilpin EA, White MM, Pierce JP. Association between household and workplace smoking restrictions and adolescent smoking. *Journal of the American Medical Association* 2000;284(6):717–22.

Farrelly MC, Nonnemaker JM, Chou R, Hyland A, Peterson KK, Bauer UE. Changes in hospitality workers' exposure to secondhand smoke following the implementation of New York's smoke-free law. *Tobacco Control* 2005;14(4):236–41.

Federal Register. Interstate Commerce Commission. Prohibition against smoking on interstate passenger-carrying motor vehicles (49 CFR Part 374), 56 *Fed. Reg.* 1745 (1991).

Federal Register. U.S. Department of Health and Human Services. Implementation of Pro-Children Act of 1994; notice to prohibit smoking in certain facilities, 59 *Fed. Reg.* 67713 (1994a).

Federal Register. U.S. Department of Labor, Occupational Safety and Health Administration. Indoor air quality (29 CFR Parts 1910, 1915, 1926 and 1928), 59 *Fed. Reg.* 15968 (1994b).

Federal Register. U.S. Department of Labor, Occupational Safety and Health Administration. Indoor air quality: withdrawal of proposal (29 CFR Parts 1910, 1915, 1926 and 1928), 66 *Fed. Reg.* 64946 (2001).

Ferrence R, Timmerman T, Ashley MJ, Northrup D, Brewster J, Cohen J, Leis A, Lovato C, Poland B, Pope M, et al. *Second Hand Smoke in Ontario Homes: Findings from a National Study.* Special Reports Series. Toronto: Ontario Tobacco Research Unit, 2005.

Fichtenberg CM, Glantz SA. Association of the California Tobacco Control Program with declines in cigarette consumption and mortality from heart disease. *New England Journal of Medicine* 2000;343(24):1772–7.

Fichtenberg C, Glantz SA. Controlling tobacco use [letter]. *New England Journal of Medicine* 2001;344(23):1797–9.

Fichtenberg CM, Glantz SA. Effect of smoke-free workplaces on smoking behaviour: systematic review. *British Medical Journal* 2002;325(7357):188.

Fisher L. Back to school: smoking policies in US college residence halls (fall 2002). *Cancer Causes and Control* 2002;13(8):787–9.

Flue-Cured Tobacco Cooperative Stabilization Corp. v. United States Environmental Protection Agency (M.D.N.C. June 22, 1993), *cited in* 8.2 TPLR 3.97 (1993).

Flue-Cured Tobacco Cooperative Stabilization Corp. v. United States Environmental Protection Agency, 4 F. Supp. 2d 435 (M.D.N.C. 1998).

Flue-Cured Tobacco Cooperative Stabilization Corp. v. The United States Environmental Protection Agency, No. 98-2407 (4th Cir., December 11, 2002), *cited in* 17.7 TPLR 2.472 (2003) (Overturning lower court's decision invalidating EPA's findings that secondhand smoke is a "known human carcinogen").

Frieden TR, Mostashari F, Kerker BD, Miller N, Hajat A, Frankel M. Adult tobacco use levels after intensive tobacco control measures: New York City, 2002–2003. *American Journal of Public Health* 2005;95(6):1016–23.

Fuchs B. Solana Beach smoking ban used as guide by coast cities. *San Diego Union-Tribune* September 12, 2004;NEWS Sect:A-1.

Gehrman CA, Hovell MF. Protecting children from environmental tobacco smoke (ETS) exposure: a critical review. *Nicotine and Tobacco Research* 2003;5(3):289–301.

Gerlach KK, Shopland DR, Hartman AM, Gibson JT, Pechacek TF. Workplace smoking policies in the United States: results from a national survey of more than 100,000 workers. *Tobacco Control* 1997;6(3):199–206.

Gerth J. Chamber to back smoke ban: business group's stance is new. *Louisville Courier-Journal* June 4, 2005;Sect News:1B.

Gilpin EA, Emery SL, Farkas AJ, Distefan JM, White MM, Pierce JP. *The California Tobacco Control Program: A Decade of Progress, Results from the California Tobacco Surveys, 1990–1999.* La Jolla (CA): University of California at San Diego, 2001.

Gilpin EA, Lee L, Pierce JP. Changes in population attitudes about where smoking should not be allowed: California versus the rest of the USA. *Tobacco Control* 2004;13(1):38–44.

Gilpin EA, White MM, Farkas AJ, Pierce JP. Home smoking restrictions: which smokers have them and how they are associated with smoking behavior. *Nicotine & Tobacco Research* 1999;1(2):153–62.

Giordono J. Navy smokers nervously eye tougher policies in civilian world. *Stars and Stripes,* December 31, 2002.

Girion L. OSHA drops plan for smoke-free workplace safety: Public health advocates say they urged the agency to drop the proposal for fear it would be watered down. *Los Angeles Times* December 19, 2001;Business Section:3.

Glantz SA. Achieving a smokefree society [editorial]. *Circulation* 1987;76(4):746–52.

Glantz SA. Big tobacco's worst nightmare. *Scientific American* 1998;279(1):30–1.

Glantz SA. Effect of smokefree bar law on bar revenues in California. *Tobacco Control* 2000;9(1):111–2.

Glantz SA, Balbach ED. *The Tobacco War: Inside the California Battles.* Berkeley (CA): University of California Press, 2000.

Glantz SA, Charlesworth A. Tourism and hotel revenues before and after passage of smoke-free restaurant ordinances. *Journal of the American Medical Association* 1999;281(20):1911–8.

Glantz SA, Smith L. The effect of ordinances requiring smoke-free restaurants on restaurant sales. *American Journal of Public Health* 1994;84(7):1081–5.

Glantz SA, Smith L. The effect of ordinances requiring smoke-free restaurants and bars on revenues: a follow-up. *American Journal of Public Health* 1997; 87(10):1687–93.

Glantz SA, Wilson-Loots R. No association of smoke-free ordinances with profits from bingo and charitable games in Massachusetts. *Tobacco Control* 2003;12(4):411–3.

Glasgow RE, Cummings KM, Hyland A. Relationship of worksite smoking policy to changes in employee tobacco use: findings from COMMIT. Community Intervention Trial for Smoking Cessation. *Tobacco Control* 1997;6(Suppl 2):S44–S48.

Glasgow RE, Sorensen G, Corbett K. Worksite smoking control activities: prevalence and related worksite characteristics from the COMMIT: Study, 1990. *Preventive Medicine* 1992;21(6):688–700.

Glasgow RE, Sorensen G, Giffen C, Shipley RH, Corbett K, Lynn W. Promoting worksite smoking control policies and actions: the Community Intervention Trial for Smoking Cessation (COMMIT) experience. *Preventive Medicine* 1996;25(2):186–94.

Gower KB, Burns DM, Shanks TG, Vaughn JW, Anderson CM, Shopland DR, Hartman AM. Section III: workplace smoking restrictions, rules about smoking in the home, and attitudes toward smoking restrictions in public places. In: Shopland DR, Hobart R, Burns DM, Amacher RH, editors. *State and Local Legislative Action to Reduce Tobacco Use.* Smoking and Tobacco Control Monograph No. 11. Bethesda (MD): U.S. Department of Health and Human Services, National Institutes of Health, National Cancer Institute, 2000:187–340. NIH Publication No. 00-4804.

Greenberg RA, Strecher VJ, Bauman KE, Boat BW, Fowler MG, Keyes LL, Denny FW, Chapman RS, Stedman HC, LaVange LM. Evaluation of a home-based intervention program to reduce infant passive smoking and lower respiratory illness. *Journal of Behavioral Medicine* 1994;17(3):273–90.

Groner JA, Ahijevych K, Grossman LK, Rich LN. The impact of a brief intervention on maternal smoking behavior. *Pediatrics* 2000;105(1 Pt 3):267–71.

Hagey A. Implementation of a smoking policy in the United States Army. *New York State Journal of Medicine* 1989;89(1):42–4.

Haller E, McNiel DE, Binder RL. Impact of a smoking ban on a locked psychiatric unit. *Journal of Clinical Psychiatry* 1996;57(8):329–32.

Halperin AC, Rigotti NA. US public universities' compliance with recommended tobacco-control policies. *Journal of American College Health* 2003;51(5):181–8.

Hammond SK. The efficacy of strategies to reduce environmental tobacco smoke concentrations in homes, workplaces, restaurants, and corrections facilities. In: Levin H, editor. *Indoor Air 2000.* Proceedings of the 9th International Conference on Indoor Air Quality and Climate; June 30–July 5, 2002; Monterey (CA). Vol. 2. Santa Cruz (CA): Indoor Air, 2002:115–20.

Hammond SK, Emmons KM. Inmate exposure to secondhand smoke in correctional facilities and the impact of smoking restrictions. *Journal of Exposure Analysis and Environmental Epidemiology* 2005; 15(3):205–11.

Hammond SK, Sorensen G, Youngstrom R, Ockene JK. Occupational exposure to environmental tobacco smoke. *Journal of the American Medical Association* 1995;274(12):956–60.

Harrison PM, Karberg JC. Prison and jail inmates at midyear, 2002. *Bureau of Justice Statistics Bulletin*, April 2003; <http://www.ojp.usdoj.gov/bjs/abstract/pjim02.htm>; accessed: October 4, 2004.

Hartman A, Willis G, Lawrence D, Gibson JT. The 2001–2002 tobacco use supplement to the Current Population Survey (TUS-CPS): representative survey findings. Bethesda (MD): U.S. Department of Health and Human Services, National Institutes of Health, National Cancer Institute, December 2004; <http://riskfactor.cancer.gov/studies/tus-cps/results/data0102/cps_results0102.pdf>; accessed: February 3, 2006.

Hartman A, Willis G, Lawrence D, Marcus S, Gibson JT. The 1998–1999 NCI tobacco use supplement to the Current Population Survey (TUS-CPS): representative survey findings. Bethesda (MD): U.S. Department of Health and Human Services, National Institutes of Health, National Cancer Institute, May 2002; <http://riskfactor.cancer.gov/studies/tus-cps/results/data9899/cps_results.pdf>; accessed: June 14, 2004.

Healthy Androscoggin. Auburn housing authority third in nation to go smoke-free [press release]. Auburn (ME): Healthy Androscoggin, September 20, 2004.

Hedge A, Erickson WA, Rubin G. Effects of restrictive smoking policies on indoor air quality and sick building syndrome: a study of 27 air-conditioned offices. *Proceedings of Indoor Air '93.* The Sixth International Conference on Indoor Air Quality and Climate; July 4–8, 1993; Vol. 1. Helsinki, 1993:517–22.

Helling v. McKinney, 113 S.Ct. 2475, 509 U.S. 25 (1993).

Heloma A, Jaakkola MS, Kahkonen E, Reijula K. The short-term impact of national smoke-free workplace legislation on passive smoking and tobacco use. *American Journal of Public Health* 2001;91(9):1416–8.

Henson R, Medina L, St. Clair S, Blanke D, Downs L, Jordan J. Clean indoor air: where, why, and how. *Journal of Law, Medicine, & Ethics* 2002;30 (3 Suppl):75–82.

Hill J. No-smoking zone growing: the statewide playground ban adds a 25-foot buffer. *Sacramento Bee* December 31, 2002;MAIN NEWS Sect:A3.

Hilts PJ. McDonald's bans smoking at all company-owned restaurants. *New York Times* February 24, 1994;Sect A:16(col 1).

Hirschhorn N, Bialous SA. Second hand smoke and risk assessment: what was in it for the tobacco industry? *Tobacco Control* 2001;10(4):375–82.

Hoge CW, Reichler MR, Dominguez EA, Bremer JC, Mastro TD, Hendricks KA, Musher DM, Elliott JA, Facklam RR, Breiman RF. An epidemic of pneumococcal disease in an overcrowded, inadequately ventilated jail. *New England Journal of Medicine* 1994;331(10):643–8.

Holm AL, Davis RM. Clearing the airways: advocacy and regulation for smoke-free airlines. *Tobacco Control* 2004;13(Suppl I):i30–i36.

Hospitality Net. San Diego Hotelier Joins Nascent Smoke-free Movement, September 4, 2001; <http://www.hospitalitynet.org/news/4009034.print>; accessed: February 25, 2005.

Hovell MF, Meltzer SB, Wahlgren DR, Matt GE, Hofstetter CR, Jones JA, Meltzer EO, Bernert JT, Pirkle JL. Asthma management and environmental tobacco smoke exposure reduction in Latino children: a controlled trial. *Pediatrics* 2002;110(5): 946–56.

Hovell MF, Meltzer SB, Zakarian JM, Wahlgren DR, Emerson JA, Hofstetter CR, Leaderer BP, Meltzer EO, Zeiger RS, O'Connor RD. Reduction of environmental tobacco smoke exposure among asthmatic children: a controlled trial. *Chest* 1994;106(2):440–6. [See also erratum in *Chest* 1995;107(5):1480.]

Hovell MF, Zakarian JM, Matt GE, Hofstetter CR, Bernert JT, Pirkle J. Effects of counselling mothers on their children's exposure to environmental tobacco smoke: randomised controlled trial. *British Medical Journal* 2000a;321(7257):337–42.

Hovell MF, Zakarian JM, Wahlgren DR, Matt GE. Reducing children's exposure to environmental tobacco smoke: the empirical evidence and directions for future research. *Tobacco Control* 2000b;9(Suppl II):ii40–ii47.

Hudzinski LG, Frohlich ED. One-year longitudinal study of a no-smoking policy in a medical institution. *Chest* 1990;97(5):1198–202.

Hurt RD, Berge KG, Offord KP, Leonard DA, Gerlach DK, Renquist CL, O'Hara MR. The making of a smoke-free medical center. *Journal of the American Medical Association* 1989;261(1):95–7.

Hyland A, Cummings KM, Nauenberg E. Analysis of taxable sales receipts: was New York City's Smoke-Free Air Act bad for business? *Journal of Public Health Management and Practice* 1999a;5(1):14–21.

Hyland A, Cummings KM, Wilson MP. Compliance with the New York City Smoke-Free Air Act. *Journal of Public Health Management and Practice* 1999b;5(1):43–52.

International Agency for Research on Cancer. *IARC Monographs on the Evaluation of Carcinogenic Risks to Humans: Some Industrial Chemicals*. Vol. 77. Lyon (France): International Agency for Research on Cancer, 2000.

International Agency for Research on Cancer. *IARC Monographs on the Evaluation of Carcinogenic Risks to Humans: Tobacco Smoke and Involuntary Smoking*. Vol. 83. Lyon (France): International Agency for Research on Cancer, 2004.

Jacobson PD, Wasserman J. *Tobacco Control Laws: Implementation and Enforcement*. Washington: RAND 1997.

Jacobson PD, Wasserman J. The implementation and enforcement of tobacco control laws: policy implications for activists and the industry. *Journal of Health Politics, Policy and Law* 1999;24(3):567–98.

Jenkins RA, Maskarinec MP, Counts RW, Caton JE, Tomkins BA, Ilgner RH. Environmental tobacco smoke in an unrestricted smoking workplace: area and personal exposure monitoring. *Journal of Exposure Analysis and Environmental Epidemiology* 2001;11(5):369–80.

Joint Commission on Accreditation of Healthcare Organizations. *Accreditation Manual for Hospitals. Volume 1: Standards*. Oakbrook Terrace (IL): Joint Commission on Accreditation of Healthcare Organizations, 1992.

Joint Commission on Accreditation of Healthcare Organizations. *Comprehensive Accreditation Manual for Long Term Care* (CAMLTC). Oakbrook Terrace (IL): Joint Commission on Accreditation of Healthcare Organizations, 2004.

Joseph AM. Is Congress blowing smoke at the VA? *Journal of the American Medical Association* 1994;272(15):1215–6.

Joseph AM, Knapp JM, Nichol KL, Pirie PL. Determinants of compliance with a national smoke-free hospital standard. *Journal of the American Medical Association* 1995;274(6):491–4.

Joseph AM, O'Neil PJ. The Department of Veterans Affairs smoke-free policy. *Journal of the American Medical Association* 1992;267(1):87–90.

Journal of School Health. School Health Policies and Programs Study (SHPPS) 2000: a summary report. *Journal of School Health* 2001;71(7):251–350.

Kane MP, Jaen CR, Tumiel LM, Bearman GM, O'Shea RM. Unlimited opportunities for environmental interventions with inner-city asthmatics. *Journal of Asthma* 1999;36(4):371–9.

Keating J. Lawyers OK no-smoking apartments in T.O. *Ventura County Star* June 16, 2003;News Sect:B1.

Kiser D, Boschert T. Eliminating smoking in bars, restaurants, and gaming clubs in California: BREATH, the California Smoke-Free Bar Program. *Journal of Public Health Policy* 2001;22(1):81–7.

Klepeis NE. Validity of the uniform mixing assumption: determining human exposure to environmental tobacco smoke. *Environmental Health Perspectives* 1999;107(Suppl 2):357–64.

Klepeis NE. An introduction to the indirect exposure assessment approach: modeling human exposure using microenvironmental measurements and the recent National Human Activity Pattern Survey. *Environmental Health Perspectives* 1999:107 (Suppl 2):365–74.

Kline RL. Smoke knows no boundaries: legal strategies for environmental tobacco smoke incursions into the home within multi-unit residential dwellings. *Tobacco Control* 2000;9(2):201–5.

Kluger R. *Ashes to Ashes: America's Hundred-Year Cigarette War, the Public Health, and the Unabashed Triumph of Philip Morris*. New York: Alfred A. Knopf, 1996.

Kochersberger G, Clipp EC. Resident smoking in long-term care facilities—policies and ethics. *Public Health Reports* 1996;111(1):66–70.

Landman A. Push or be punished: tobacco industry documents reveal aggression against businesses that discourage tobacco use. *Tobacco Control* 2000;9(3):339–46.

Lee G. Council to mull smoking ban; measure would target public housing units. *Los Angeles Daily News* June 14, 2003;News Sect:N4.

LeMier M. *Tobacco and Health in Washington State*. Olympia (WA): Washington State Department of Health, Office of Community Wellness & Prevention, Tobacco Prevention & Control Program, 1999.

LePage A. Bill to ban smoking in apartments put on hold. *Ventura County Star* May 16, 2003a;News Sect: A6.

LePage A. Driving home perils of smoking: a bill would restrict lighting up in condos and apartments. *Sacramento Bee* March 2, 2003b;Main News Sect:A1.

Levy DT, Romano E, Mumford EA. Recent trends in home and work smoking bans. *Tobacco Control* 2004;13(3):258–63.

Lindsay J. Push for smoking bans gains steam around Bay State. *Associated Press* March 9, 2003;Business News Sect;State and Regional.

Liu KS, Alevantis LE, Offerman FJ. A survey of environmental tobacco smoke controls in California office buildings. *Indoor Air* 2001;11(1):26–34.

Lockhart Risk Management Ltd. *Indoor Air Quality Survey of Restaurants, Pubs and Casinos*. Vancouver (British Columbia): Lockhart Risk Management Ltd., 1995. File 477-I1.

Longo DR, Brownson RC, Johnson JC, Hewett JE, Kruse RL, Novotny TE, Logan RA. Hospital smoking bans and employee smoking behavior: results of a national survey. *Journal of the American Medical Association* 1996;275(16):1252–7.

Longo DR, Feldman MM, Kruse RL, Brownson RC, Petroski GF, Hewett JE. Implementing smoking bans in American hospitals: results of a national survey. *Tobacco Control* 1998;7(1):47–55.

Magzamen S, Glantz SA. The new battleground: California's experience with smoke-free bars. *American Journal of Public Health* 2001;91(2):245–52.

Mandel LL, Alamar BC, Glantz SA. Smoke-free law did not affect revenue from gaming in Delaware. *Tobacco Control* 2005;14(1):10–2.

Mandel LL, Glantz SA. Hedging their bets: tobacco and gambling industries work against smoke-free policies. *Tobacco Control* 2004;13(3):268–76.

Mannino DM, Siegel M, Husten C, Rose D, Etzel R. Environmental tobacco smoke exposure and health effects in children: results from the 1991 National Health Interview Survey. *Tobacco Control* 1996;5(1):13–8.

Mannino DM, Siegel M, Rose, D, Nkuchia J, Etzel R. Environmental tobacco smoke exposure in the home and worksite and health effects in adults: results from the 1991 National Health Interview Survey. *Tobacco Control* 1997;6(4):296–305.

Marcus BH, Emmons KM, Abrams DB, Marshall RJ, Kane M, Novotny TE, Etzel RA. Restrictive workplace smoking policies: impact on nonsmokers' tobacco exposure. *Journal of Public Health Policy* 1992;13(1):42–51.

Maryland Register. Title 09. Department of Licensing and Regulation. Prohibition on smoking in an enclosed workplace. *Maryland Register* 1994;21(15):1304.

Mason H. Support for smoking bans smoldering in Britain, Canada. Princeton (NJ): The Gallup Organization, 2004.

Matt GE, Quintana PJE, Hovell MF, Bernert JT, Song S, Novianti N, Juarez T, Floro J, Gehrman C, Garcia M, et al. Households contaminated by environmental tobacco smoke: sources of infant exposures. *Tobacco Control* 2004;13(1):29–37.

Mattson ME, Boyd G, Byar D, Brown C, Callahan JF, Corle D, Cullen JW, Greenblatt J, Haley NJ, Hammond K, et al. Passive smoking on commercial air flights. *Journal of the American Medical Association* 1989;261(6):867–72.

McIntosh NA, Clark NM, Howatt WF. Reducing tobacco smoke in the environment of the child with asthma: a cotinine-assisted, minimal-contact intervention. *Journal of Asthma* 1994;31(6):453–62.

McMillen RC, Winickoff JP, Klein JD, Weitzman M. US adult attitudes and practices regarding smoking restrictions and child exposure to environmental tobacco smoke: changes in the social climate from 2000–2001. *Pediatrics* 2003;112(1):e55–e60.

Meltzer T, Custard ET, Katzman J, Knower Z. *Princeton Review Student Access Guide: The Best 309 Colleges.* 1996 ed. New York: Random House, 1995.

Miesner EA, Rudnick SN, Hu FC, Spengler JD, Preller L, Ozkaynak H, Nelson W. Particulate and nicotine sampling in public facilities and offices. *Journal of the Air Pollution Control Association* 1989;39(12):1577–82.

Mizoue T, Reijula K, Yamato H, Andderson K. Environmental tobacco smoke and control program in Japanese municipal workplaces. In: Seppen O, Seri J, editors. *Healthy Buildings 2000.* Proceedings of the Sixth International Conference on Healthy Buildings; August 6–10, 2000; Espoo, Finland. Vol. 2. Espoo, Finland: International Society of Indoor Air Quality and Climate, 2000;101–6.

Mochizuki-Kobayashi Y, Samet JM, Yamaguchi N, editors. *Tobacco Free Japan: Recommendations for Tobacco Control Policy.* A co-publication of Tobacco Free Japan and the Institute for Global Tobacco Control, Johns Hopkins Bloomberg School of Public Health. Tokyo: Tobacco Free Japan, 2004.

Møhave L, Krzyzanowski M. The right to healthy indoor air. *Indoor Air* 2000;10(4):211.

Møhave L, Krzyzanowski M. The right to healthy indoor air: status by 2002. *Indoor Air* 2003;13 (Suppl 6):50–3.

Moskowitz JM, Lin Z, Hudes ES. The impact of workplace smoking ordinances in California on smoking cessation. *American Journal of Public Health* 2000;90(5):757–61.

Muggli ME, Forster JL, Hurt RD, Repace JL. The smoke you don't see: uncovering tobacco industry strategies aimed against environmental tobacco smoke policies. *American Journal of Public Health* 2001;91(9):1419–23.

Muggli ME, Hurt RD, Repace J. The tobacco industry's political efforts to derail the EPA report on ETS. *American Journal of Preventive Medicine* 2004;26(2):167–77.

National Cancer Institute. *Health Effects of Exposure to Environmental Tobacco Smoke: The Report of the California Environmental Protection Agency.* Smoking and Tobacco Monograph No. 10. Bethesda (MD): U.S. Department of Health and Human Services, National Institutes of Health, National Cancer Institute, 1999. NIH Publication No. 99-4645.

National Cancer Institute. *Population Based Smoking Cessation: Proceedings of a Conference on What Works to Influence Cessation in the General Population.* Smoking and Tobacco Control Monograph No. 12. Bethesda (MD): U.S. Department of Health and Human Services, National Institutes of Health, National Cancer Institute, 2000a. NIH Publication No. 00-4892.

National Cancer Institute. *State and Local Legislative Action to Reduce Tobacco Use.* Smoking and Tobacco Control Monograph No. 11. Bethesda (MD): U.S. Department of Health and Human Services, National Institutes of Health, National Cancer Institute, 2000b. NIH Publication No. 00-4804.

National Cancer Institute. *ASSIST: Shaping the Future of Tobacco Prevention and Control.* Tobacco Control Monograph No. 16. Bethesda (MD): U.S. Department of Health and Human Services, National Institutes of Health, National Cancer Institute, 2005. NIH Publication No. 05-5645.

National Center for Health Statistics. Plan and operation of the Hispanic Health and Nutrition Examination Survey, 1982–84. *Vital and Health Statistics.* Series 1, No. 19. Hyattsville (MD): U.S. Department of Health and Human Services, Public Health Service, National Center for Health Statistics, 1985. DHHS Publication No. (PHS) 85-1321.

National Center for Health Statistics. Health Measures in the New 1997 Redesigned National Health Interview Survey (NHIS), April 8, 2004 (updated); <http://www.cdc.gov/nchs/about/major/nhis/hisdesgn.htm>; accessed: June 1, 2004.

National Health and Medical Research Council. *The Health Effects of Passive Smoking*. A scientific information paper. Canberra (Commonwealth of Australia): Canberra ACT, 1997.

National Institute for Occupational Safety and Health. *Environmental Tobacco Smoke in the Workplace: Lung Cancer and Other Health Effects*. Current Intelligence Bulletin 54. Cincinnati: U.S. Department of Health and Human Services, Public Health Service, Centers for Disease Control, National Institute for Occupational Safety and Health, Division of Standards Development and Technology Transfer, Division of Surveillance, Hazard Evaluations, and Field Studies, 1991. DHHS (NIOSH) Publication No. 91-108.

National Network on Tobacco Prevention and Poverty. *Tobacco Policy, Cessation, and Education in Correctional Facilities*. West Sacramento (CA): National Network on Tobacco Prevention and Poverty, 2004.

National Research Council. *Environmental Tobacco Smoke: Measuring Exposures and Assessing Health Effects*. Washington: National Academy Press, 1986a.

National Research Council. *The Airliner Cabin Environment: Air Quality and Safety*. Washington: National Academy Press, 1986b.

Nelson DE, Sacks JJ, Addiss DG. Smoking policies of licensed child day-care centers in the United States. *Pediatrics* 1993;91(2):460–3.

Nelson PR, Heavner DL, Collie BB, Maiolo KC, Ogden MW. Effect of ventilation and sampling time on environmental tobacco smoke component ratios. *Environmental Science & Technology* 1992;26(10):1909–15.

New York City Department of Finance. The State of Smoke-Free New York City: A One-Year Review. New York: New York City Department of Finance, New York City Department of Health and Mental Hygiene, New York City Department of Small Business Services, New York City Economic Development Corporation, March 2004; <http://www.nyc.gov/html/doh/downloads/pdf/smoke/sfaa-2004report.pdf>; accessed: February 3, 2006.

New York State Department of Health. *First Annual Independent Evaluation of New York's Tobacco Control Program*, Albany (NY): 2004. <http://www.health.state.ny.us/nysdoh/tobacco/reports/docs/nytcp_eval_report_final_11-19-04.pdf>.

New York State Department of Health. *Second Annual Independent Evaluation of New York's Tobacco Control Program*, Albany (NY): 2005. <http://www.health.state.ny.us/prevention/tobacco_control/docs/2005-09_independent_evalutation.pdf>.

Nixon ML, Mahmoud L, Glantz SA. Tobacco industry litigation to deter local public health ordinances: the industry usually loses in court. *Tobacco Control* 2004;13(1):65–73.

No Child Left Behind Act of 1994, Public Law 107-110, 115 Stat. 1425.

No Child Left Behind Act of 2001, Public Law 107-110, 115 Stat. 1425.

Nordstrom DL, DeStefano F. Evaluation of Wisconsin legislation on smoking in restaurants. *Tobacco Control* 1995;4(2):125–8.

Okah FA, Choi WS, Okuyemi KS, Ahluwalia JS. Effect of children on home smoking restriction by inner-city smokers. *Pediatrics* 2002;109(2):244–9.

Oldaker GB III, Perfetti PF, Conrad FC Jr, Conner JM, McBride RL. Results from surveys of environmental tobacco smoke in offices and restaurants. In: Kasuga H, editor. *Indoor Air Quality*. New York: Springer-Verlag, 1990:99–104.

Ong MK, Glantz SA. Cardiovascular health and economic effects of smoke-free workplaces. *American Journal of Medicine* 2004;117(1):32–8.

Ott WR. Mathematical models for predicting indoor air quality from smoking activity. *Environmental Health Perspectives* 1999;107(Suppl 2):375–81.

Ott WR, Switzer P, Robinson J. Particle concentrations inside a tavern before and after prohibition of smoking: evaluating the performance of an indoor air quality model. *Journal of the Air & Waste Management Association* 1996;46(12):1120–34.

Overpeck MD, Moss AJ. Children's exposure to environmental cigarette smoke before and after birth: health of our nation's children, United States, 1988. *Advance Data* 1991;202:1–11.

Parmet WE, Daynard RA, Gottlieb MA. The physician's role in helping smoke-sensitive patients to use the Americans With Disabilities Act to secure smoke-free workplaces and public spaces. *Journal of the American Medical Association* 1996;276(11):909–13.

Parsons WD, Carmella SG, Akerkar S, Bonilla LE, Hecht SS. A metabolite of the tobacco-specific lung carcinogen 4-(methylnitrosamino)-1-(3-pyridyl)-1-butanone in the urine of hospital workers exposed to environmental tobacco smoke. *Cancer Epidemiology, Biomarkers & Prevention* 1998;7(3):257–60.

Patrick S, Marsh R. Current tobacco policies in U.S. adult male prisons. *Social Sciences Journal* 2001; 38(1):27–37.

Pechacek TF, Babb S. Commentary: How acute and reversible are the cardiovascular risks of secondhand smoke. *British Medical Journal* 2004;328(7446): 980–3.

Persily A. The revision of Standard 62: what a difference a decade makes. In: Levin H, editor. *Indoor Air 2002*. Proceedings: 9th International Conference on Indoor Air Quality and Climate; June 30–July 5, 2002. Santa Cruz (CA): Indoor Air 2002, 2002:328–33.

Pertschuk M, Shopland DR, editors. *Major Local Smoking Ordinances in the United States: A Detailed Matrix of the Provisions of Workplace, Restaurant, and Public Places Smoking Ordinances*. Bethesda (MD): U.S. Department of Health and Human Services, Public Health Service, National Institutes of Health, and Americans for Nonsmokers' Rights, 1989. NIH Publication No. 90-479.

Pierce WM, Janczewski JN, Roethlisberger B, Pelton M, Kunstel K. Effectiveness of auxiliary air cleaners in reducing ETS components in offices. *ASHRAE Journal* 1996;38:51–7.

Pirkle JL, Flegal KM, Bernert JT, Brody DJ, Etzel RA, Maurer KR. Exposure of the US population to environmental tobacco smoke: the Third National Health and Nutrition Examination Survey, 1988 to 1991. *Journal of the American Medical Association* 1996;275(16):1233–40.

Pizacani BA, Martin DP, Stark MJ, Koepsell TD, Thompson B, Diehr P. Household smoking bans: which households have them and do they work? *Preventive Medicine* 2003;36(1):99–107.

Pizacani BA, Martin DP, Stark MJ, Koepsell TD, Thompson B, Diehr P. A prospective study of household smoking bans and subsequent cessation related behaviour: the role of stage of change. *Tobacco Control* 2004;13(1):23–8.

Pletsch PK. Environmental tobacco smoke exposure among Hispanic women of reproductive age. *Public Health Nursing* 1994;11(4):229–35.

Pritchard R. Tobacco industry speaks with one voice, once again. Candy Journal July 17–August 6, 1986. American Tobacco. Bates No. 950685111. http://legacy.library.ucsf.edu/tid/beb85f00.

Pro-Children Act of 1994, Public Law 103-227, Title XX, 1041–1044, Chapter 68, Subchapter X, Part B, 1041, 108 Stat. 271.

Pyle SA, Haddock CK, Hymowitz N, Schwab J, Meshberg S. Family rules about exposure to environmental tobacco smoke. *Families, Systems and Health* 2005;23(1):3–16.

Ranalli R, Saltzman J. Jury finds heavy smoking to be grounds for eviction: verdict is said to be one of first in nation. *Boston Globe* June 16, 2005.

Repace J. Banning outdoor smoking is scientifically justifiable. *Tobacco Control* 2000a;9(1):98.

Repace J. *Can Ventilation Control Secondhand Smoke in the Hospitality Industry?* Bowie (MD): Repace Associates, 2000b.

Repace J. Flying the smoky skies: secondhand smoke exposure of flight attendants. *Tobacco Control* 2004a; 13(Suppl I):i8–i19.

Repace J. Respirable particles and carcinogens in the air of Delaware hospitality venues before and after a smoking ban. *Journal of Occupational and Environmental Medicine* 2004b;46(9):887–905.

Repace JL, Jinot J, Bayard S, Emmons K, Hammond SK. Air nicotine and saliva cotinine as indicators of workplace passive smoking exposure and risk. *Risk Analysis* 1998;18(1):71–83.

Rigotti NA, Pashos CL. No-smoking laws in the United States: an analysis of state and city actions to limit smoking in public places and workplaces. *Journal of the American Medical Association* 1991;266(22): 3162–7.

Ritch WA, Begay ME. Strange bedfellows: the history of collaboration between the Massachusetts Restaurant Association and the tobacco industry. *American Journal of Public Health* 2001;91(4):598–603.

Rogers EM. *Diffusion of Innovations*. 5th ed. New York: Free Press, 2003.

Romero CL. No ifs, ands or butts; valley firms go zero tolerance on smoking. *The Arizona Republic* March 11, 2004;Business Sect:1D.

Roper Organization. *A Study of Public Attitudes Toward Cigarette Smoking and the Tobacco Industry in 1978, Volume I*. Roper Organization, Inc. 1978. American Tobacco. Bates No. 966071061/1341. <http://legacy.library.ucsf.edu/tid/jdc70a00.

RTI International. *First Annual Independent Evaluation of New York's Tobacco Control Program*. Research Triangle Park (NC): RTI International, 2004.

Sargent RP, Shepard RM, Glantz SA. Reduced incidence of admissions for myocardial infarction associated with public smoking ban: before and after study. *British Medical Journal* 2004;328(7446): 977–80.

Schoenmarklin S. *Infiltration of Secondhand Smoke into Condominiums, Apartments and Other Multi-Unit Dwellings*. St. Paul (MN): Tobacco Control Legal Consortium, 2004.

Scientific Committee on Tobacco and Health. Report of the Scientific Committee on Tobacco and Health. London: Scientific Committee on Tobacco and Health, March 20, 1998; <http://www.archive.official-documents.co.uk/document/doh/tobacco/report/htm>; accessed: February 3, 2006.

Scollo M, Lal A, Hyland A, Glantz S. Review of the quality of studies on the economic effects of smoke-free policies on the hospitality industry. *Tobacco Control* 2003;12(1):13–20.

Shimp v. New Jersey Bell Telephone Co., 368 A.2d 408, 145 N.J. Super. 516 (1976).

Shopland DR, Anderson CM, Burns DM, Gerlach KK. Disparities in smoke-free workplace policies among food service workers. *Journal of Occupational and Environmental Medicine* 2004;46(4):347–56.

Shopland DR, Gerlach KK, Burns DM, Hartman AM, Gibson JT. State-specific trends in smoke-free workplace policy coverage: the Current Population Survey Tobacco Use Supplement, 1993 to 1999. *Journal of Occupational and Environmental Medicine* 2001;43(8):680–6.

Shopland DR, Hartman AM, Gibson JT, Anderson CM. Environmental tobacco smoke in the workplace: Trends in the protection of U.S. workers. In: *Work, Smoking, and Health: a NIOSH Scientific Workshop*. Atlanta: U.S. Department of Health and Human Services, Centers for Disease Control and Prevention, National Institute for Occupational Safety and Health, 2002:52–62. NIOSH Publication No. 2002-148.

Shopland DR, Hartman AM, Repace JL, Lynn WR. Smoking behavior, workplace policies, and public opinion regarding smoking restrictions in Maryland. *Maryland Medical Journal* 1995;44(2):99–104.

Siegel M. Involuntary smoking in the restaurant workplace: a review of employee exposure and health effects. *Journal of the American Medical Association* 1993;270(4):490–3.

Siegel M. The effectiveness of state-level tobacco control interventions: a review of program implementation and behavioral outcomes. *Annual Review of Public Health* 2002;23:45–71.

Siegel M, Albers AB, Cheng DM, Biener L, Rigotti NA. Effect of local restaurant smoking regulations on environmental tobacco smoke exposure among youths. *American Journal of Public Health* 2004;94(2):321–5.

Siegel M, Albers AB, Cheng DM, Biener L, Rigotti NA. Effect of local restaurant smoking regulations on progression to established smoking among youths. *Tobacco Control* 2005;14(5):300–6.

Siegel M, Carol J, Jordan J, Hobart R, Schoenmarklin S, DuMelle F, Fisher P. Preemption in tobacco control: review of an emerging public health problem. *Journal of the American Medical Association* 1997;278(10):858–63.

Siegel M, Husten C, Merritt RK, Giovino GA, Eriksen MP. Effects of separately ventilated smoking lounges on the health of smokers: is this an appropriate public health policy? *Tobacco Control* 1995;4(1):22–9.

Siegel M, Skeer M. Exposure to secondhand smoke and excess lung cancer mortality risk among workers in the "5 B's": bars, bowling alleys, billiard halls, betting establishments, and bingo parlours. *Tobacco Control* 2003;12(3):333–8.

Skeer M, Chang DM, Rigotti NA, Siegel M. Secondhand smoke exposure in the workplace. *American Journal of Preventive Medicine* 2005;28(4):331–7.

Skeer M, George S, Hamilton WL, Cheng DM, Siegel M. Town-level characteristics and smoking policy adoption in Massachusetts: are local restaurant smoking regulations fostering disparities in health protection? *American Journal of Public Health* 2004;94(2):286–92.

Smith K. *Who's Minding the Kids? Child Care Arrangements*. Current Population Reports, P70-70. Washington: U.S. Department of Commerce, Economics and Statistics Administration, U.S. Census Bureau, Fall 1995.

Soliman S, Pollack HA, Warner KE. Decrease in the prevalence of environmental tobacco smoke exposure in the home during the 1990s in families with children. *American Journal of Public Health* 2004; 94(2):314–20.

Staron v. McDonald's Corp., 51 F.3d 353 (2d Cir. 1995).

State of Delaware. Delaware's smoking rate decreased by 11 percent in 2003 [press release]. Dover (DE): State of Delaware, Office of the Governor, July 2, 2004.

Steenland K, Sieber K, Etzel RA, Pechacek T, Maurer K. Exposure to environmental tobacco smoke and risk factors for heart disease among never smokers in the Third National Health and Nutrition Examination Survey. *American Journal of Epidemiology* 1998;147(10):932–9.

Steinfeld JL. Women and children last? Attitudes toward cigarette smoking and nonsmokers' rights, 1971. *New York State Journal of Medicine* 1983; 83(13):1257–8.

Sterling EM, Collett CW, Ross JA. Assessment of non-smokers' exposure to environmental tobacco smoke using personal-exposure and fixed-location monitoring. *Indoor and Built Environment* 1996;5:112–25.

Sterling RC, Gottheil E, Weinstein SP, Kurtz JW, Menduke H. The effect of a no-smoking policy on recruitment and retention in outpatient cocaine treatment. *Journal of Addictive Diseases* 1994;13(4):161–8.

Stillman FA, Becker DM, Swank RT, Hantula D, Moses H, Glantz S, Waranch HR. Ending smoking at the Johns Hopkins Medical Institutions: an evaluation of smoking prevalence and indoor air pollution. *Journal of the American Medical Association* 1990;264(12):1565–9.

Stillman FA, Warshow M, Aguinaga S. Patient compliance with a hospital no-smoking policy. *Tobacco Control* 1995;4(2):145–9.

Sullivan J. Smoking to be banned in state prisons July 1. *Seattle Times* March 20, 2004;News Sect:A1.

Sweda EL Jr. Lawsuits and secondhand smoke. *Tobacco Control* 2004;13(Suppl I):i61–i66.

Sweeney CT, Shopland DR, Hartman AM, Gibson JT, Anderson CM, Gower KB, Burns DM. Sex differences in workplace smoking policies: results from the current population survey. *Journal of the American Medical Women's Association* 2000;55(5):311–5.

Tang H, Cowling DW, Lloyd JC, Rogers T, Koumjian KL, Stevens CM, Bal DG. Changes of attitudes and patronage behaviors in response to a smoke-free bar law. *American Journal of Public Health* 2003;93(4):611–7.

Tang H, Cowling DW, Stevens CM, Lloyd JC. Change of knowledge, attitudes, beliefs, and preference of bar owner and staff in response to a smoke-free law. *Tobacco Control* 2004;13(1):87–9.

Task Force on Community Preventive Services. *The Guide to Community Preventive Services: What Works to Promote Health?* New York: Oxford University Press, 2005.

Traynor MP, Begay ME, Glantz SA. New tobacco industry strategy to prevent local tobacco control. *Journal of the American Medical Association* 1993;270(4):479–86.

Trout D, Decker J, Mueller C, Berneryt JT, Pirkle J. Exposure of casino employees to environmental tobacco smoke. *Journal of Occupational and Environmental Medicine* 1998;40(3):270–6.

Tsoukalas T, Glantz SA. The Duluth Clean Indoor Air Ordinance: problems and success in fighting the tobacco industry at the local level in the 21st century. *American Journal of Public Health* 2003;93(8):1214–21.

Turner J. State prison smoking ban starts Monday; state prison inmates can no longer buy tobacco and will not be allowed to use it after Monday. *News Tribune* October 28, 2004;South Sound Sect:A1.

Turner S, Cyr L, Gross AJ. The measurement of environmental tobacco smoke in 585 office environments. *Environment International* 1992;18(1):19–28.

Tyler G. Navy Lodge facilities going smoke-free, but progress is slow. *Stars and Stripes* January 18, 2005.

U.S. Department of Commerce. *The Current Population Survey: Design and Methodology*. Technical Paper No. 40. Washington: U.S. Department of Commerce, U.S. Census Bureau, July 1985.

U.S. Department of Commerce. *Current Population Survey, September 1995: Tobacco Use Supplement*. Technical documentation CPS-95. Washington: U.S. Department of Commerce, Economics and Statistics Administration, U.S. Census Bureau, 1995.

U.S. Department of Commerce. *Statistical Abstract of the United Status: 2004–2005*. 124th ed. Washington: U.S. Department of Commerce, Economics and Statistics Administration, U.S. Census Bureau, 2004.

U.S. Department of Commerce. Current Population Survey;<http://www.bls.census.gov/cps/cpsmain.htm>; accessed: February 3, 2006.

U.S. Department of Defense. *Instruction Number 1010,15*. Washington: U.S. Department of Defense, March 7, 1994.

U.S. Department of Defense. *Sale of Tobacco Products in Military Commissaries* [press release]. Washington: U.S. Department of Defense, August 23, 1996.

U.S. Department of Defense. *2002 Survey of Health Related Behaviors* [press release]. Washington: U.S. Department of Defense, March 8, 2004.

U.S. Department of Health and Human Services. *The Health Consequences of Involuntary Smoking: A Report of the Surgeon General*. Rockville (MD): U.S. Department of Health and Human Services, Public Health Service, Centers for Disease Control, Center for Health Promotion and Education, Office on Smoking and Health, 1986. DHHS Publication No. (CDC) 87-8398.

U.S. Department of Health and Human Services. *Reducing the Health Consequences of Smoking: 25 Years of Progress. A Report of the Surgeon General*. Rockville (MD): U.S. Department of Health and Human Services, Public Health Service, Centers for Disease Control, National Center for Chronic Disease Prevention and Health Promotion, Office on Smoking and Health, 1989. DHHS Publication No. (CDC) 89-8411.

U.S. Department of Health and Human Services. *1992 National Survey of Worksite Health Promotion Activities: Summary.* Washington: U.S. Department of Health and Human Services, Public Health Service, 1993.

U.S. Department of Health and Human Services. *1999 National Worksite Health Promotion Survey: Report of Survey Findings.* Northbrook (IL): Association for Worksite Health Promotion, 1999.

U.S. Department of Health and Human Services. *Healthy People 2010: Understanding and Improving Health.* Washington: U.S. Government Printing Office, 2000a.

U.S. Department of Health and Human Services. *9th Report on Carcinogens.* Research Triangle Park (NC): U.S. Department of Health and Human Services, Public Health Service, National Toxicology Program, 2000b.

U.S. Department of Health and Human Services. *Reducing Tobacco Use. A Report of the Surgeon General.* Atlanta: U.S. Department of Health and Human Services, Centers for Disease Control and Prevention, National Center for Chronic Disease Prevention and Health Promotion, Office on Smoking and Health, 2000c:198. (p. 198, updated for this publication by the Centers for Disease Control and Prevention, 2004).

U.S. Department of Health and Human Services. *Women and Smoking. A Report of the Surgeon General.* Rockville (MD): U.S. Department of Health and Human Services, Public Health Service, Office of the Surgeon General, 2001.

U.S. Department of Health and Human Services. Progress Review: Tobacco Use, May 14, 2003; <http://www.healthypeople.gov/Data/2010prog/focus27/default.htm>; accessed: May 15, 2006.

U.S. Department of Health and Human Services. HHS Secretary Tommy G. Thompson announces new initiatives to help Americans quit smoking [press release]. Washington: U.S. Department of Health and Human Services, November 10, 2004.

U.S. Department of Health, Education, and Welfare. *The Health Consequences of Smoking. A Report of the Surgeon General: 1972.* Washington: U.S. Department of Health, Education, and Welfare, Public Health Service, Health Services and Mental Health Administration, 1972. DHEW Publication No. (HSM) 72-7516.

U.S. Department of Justice, Federal Bureau of Prisons. Smoking/No Smoking Areas [program statement], U.S. Department of Justice, Federal Bureau of Prisons, March 22, 2004; <http://www.bop.gov/policy/progstat/1640_004.pdf>; accessed: February 6, 2006.

U.S. Department of Veterans Affairs. *Smoking policies for patients in VA healthcare facilities.* VHA Directive 98-006. Washington: Veterans Health Administration, July 1, 2003.

U.S. Environmental Protection Agency. *Respiratory Health Effects of Passive Smoking: Lung Cancer and Other Disorders.* Washington: Environmental Protection Agency, Office of Research and Development, Office of Air and Radiation, 1992. Publication No. EPA/600/006F.

U.S. Environmental Protection Agency. *1990 Clean Air Act,* SEC. 112, Hazardous Air Pollutants, 2004; <http://www.epa.gov/oar/caa/caa112.txt>; accessed: August 17, 2004.

U.S. Environmental Protection Agency. National Survey on Environmental Management of Asthma and Children's Exposure to Environmental Tobacco Smoke [fact sheet]; <http://www.epa.gov/smokefree/pdfs/survey_fact_sheet.pdf>; accessed: October 13, 2005.

U.S. Fire Administration. Older adults and fire. *Topical Fire Research Series* 2001;1(5).

U.S. Rail Passenger Service Act of 1970, Public Law 91-518, CFR 1124.1.

Utah Condominium Ownership Act (March 2, 2005), Chapter 8 of the *Utah Code Annotated,* Sec. 57-8-16.

Vaughan WM, Hammond SK. Impact of "designated smoking area" policy on nicotine vapor and particle concentrations in a modern office building. *Journal of the Air & Waste Management Association* 1990;40(7):1012–7.

Velasco J, Eells TD, Anderson R, Head M, Ryabik B, Mount R, Lippmann S. A two-year follow-up on the effects of a smoking ban in an inpatient psychiatric service. *Psychiatric Services* 1996;47(8):869–71.

Vereckey B. Louisville prepared to vote on smoking ban. *The Associated Press* August 6, 2005;Sect State and Regional.

Veterans Health Care Act of 1992, Public Law 102-585, *U.S. Statutes at Large* 106(1992):4943.

Vogel N. Smoking at home targeted: apartment and condo residents could face restrictions if a lawmaker's bill to control secondhand smoke is approved. *Los Angeles Times,* March 2, 2003.

von Zielbauer P. Connecticut House passes ban on workplace smoking. *The New York Times* May 8, 2003; Sect B:col 5.

Wagner J, Sullivan DP, Faulkner D, Gundel LA, Fisk WJ, Alevantis LE, Waldman JM. Measurements and modeling of environmental tobacco smoke leakage from a simulated smoking room. Abstract in: Proceedings of Indoor Air Quality 2002; <http://www.indoorair2002.org/assets/Indoor_Air_2002_Abstracts.pdf>; accessed: February 3, 2006.

Weber MD, Bagwell DAS, Fielding JE, Glantz SA. Long term compliance with California's Smoke-Free Workplace Law among bars and restaurants in Los Angeles County. *Tobacco Control* 2003;12(3):269–73.

Wechsler H, Kelley K, Seibring M, Kuo M, Rigotti NA. College smoking policies and smoking cessation programs: results of a survey of college health center directors. *Journal of American College Health* 2001a;49(5):205–11.

Wechsler H, Lee JE, Rigotti NA. Cigarette use by college students in smoke-free housing: results of a national study. *American Journal of Preventive Medicine* 2001b;20(3):202–7.

Wilson SR, Yamada EG, Sudhakar R, Roberto L, Mannino D, Mejia C, Huss N. A controlled trial of an environmental tobacco smoke reduction intervention in low-income children with asthma. *Chest* 2001;120(5):1709–22.

Womble SE, Girman JR, Ronca EL, Axelrad R, Brightman HS, McCarthy JF. Developing baseline information on buildings and indoor air quality (BASE '94): Part I–study design, building selection, and building descriptions. In: Maroni M, editor. *Healthy Buildings '95*. Proceedings of the Fourth International Conference on Healthy Buildings; September 11–14, 1995; Milan, Italy. Vol. 3, Espoo, Finland: International Society of Indoor Air Quality and Climate, 1995:1305–10.

Womble SE, Ronca EL, Girman JR, Brightman HS. Developing baseline information on buildings and indoor air quality (BASE '95). In: *IAQ '96, Paths to Better Building Environments/Health Symptoms in Building Occupants*. Atlanta: American Society of Heating, Refrigerating and Air Conditioning Engineers, 1996;109–17.

Woodward A, Owen N, Grgurinovich N, Griffith F, Linke H. Trial of an intervention to reduce passive smoking in infancy. *Pediatric Pulmonology* 1987;3(3):173–8.

World Health Organization. *International Consultation on Environmental Tobacco Smoke (ETS) and Child Health: Consultation Report.* Geneva: World Health Organization, Division of Noncommunicable Diseases, Tobacco Free Initiative, 1999. Report No. WHO/NCD/TFI/99.10.

Wortley PM, Caraballo RS, Pederson LL, Pechacek TF. Exposure to secondhand smoke in the workplace: serum cotinine by occupation. *Journal of Occupational and Environmental Medicine* 2002;44(6):503–9.

Yamato H, Hori H, Morimoto Y, Tanaka I. Environmental tobacco smoke and policies for its control. *Industrial Health* 1996;34(3):237–44.

Yancey KB. U.S. hotels respond to guests' no-smoke signals. *USA Today*, November 28, 2003; Sect D:01.

Yañez E. Clean Indoor Air and Communities of Color: Challenges and Opportunities. Washington: The Praxis Project, 2002; <http://www.thepraxisproject.org/tools/CIA_and_CoC.pdf>; accessed: March 7, 2005.

A Vision for the Future

This country has experienced a substantial reduction of involuntary exposure to secondhand tobacco smoke in recent decades. Significant reductions in the rate of smoking among adults began even earlier. Consequently, about 80 percent of adults are now nonsmokers, and many adults and children can live their daily lives without being exposed to secondhand smoke. Nevertheless, involuntary exposure to secondhand smoke remains a serious public health hazard.

This report documents the mounting and now substantial evidence characterizing the health risks caused by exposure to secondhand smoke. Multiple major reviews of the evidence have concluded that secondhand smoke is a known human carcinogen, and that exposure to secondhand smoke causes adverse effects, particularly on the cardiovascular system and the respiratory tract and on the health of those exposed, children as well as adults. Unfortunately, reductions in exposure have been slower among young children than among adults during the last decade, as expanding workplace restrictions now protect the majority of adults while homes remain the most important source of exposure for children.

Clearly, the social norms regarding secondhand smoke have changed dramatically, leading to widespread support over the past 30 years for a society free of involuntary exposures to tobacco smoke. In the first half of the twentieth century smoking was permitted in almost all public places, including elevators and all types of public transportation. At the time of the 1964 Surgeon General's report on smoking and health (U.S. Department of Health, Education, and Welfare [USDHEW] 1964), many physicians were still smokers, and the tables in U.S. Public Health Service (PHS) meeting rooms had PHS ashtrays on them. A thick, smoky haze was an accepted part of presentations at large meetings, even at medical conferences and in the hospital environment.

As the adverse health consequences of active smoking became more widely documented in the 1960s, many people began to question whether exposure of nonsmokers to secondhand smoke also posed a serious health risk. This topic was first addressed in this series of reports by Surgeon General Jesse Steinfeld in the 1972 report to Congress (USDHEW 1972). During the 1970s, policy changes to provide smoke-free environments received more widespread consideration. As the public policy debate grew and expanded in the 1980s, the scientific evidence on the risk of adverse effects from exposure to secondhand smoke was presented in a comprehensive context for the first time by Surgeon General C. Everett Koop in the 1986 report, *The Health Consequences of Involuntary Smoking* (U.S. Department of Health and Human Services [USDHHS] 1986).

The ever-increasing momentum for smoke-free indoor environments has been driven by scientific evidence on the health risks of involuntary exposure to secondhand smoke. This new Surgeon General's report is based on a far larger body of evidence than was available in 1986. The evidence reviewed in these 665 pages confirms the findings of the 1986 report and adds new causal conclusions. The growing body of data increases support for the conclusion that exposure to secondhand smoke causes lung cancer in lifetime nonsmokers. In addition to epidemiologic data, this report presents converging evidence that the mechanisms by which secondhand smoke causes lung cancer are similar to those that cause lung cancer in active smokers. In the context of the risks from active smoking, the lung cancer risk that secondhand smoke exposure poses to nonsmokers is consistent with an extension to involuntary smokers of the dose-response relationship for active smokers.

Cardiovascular effects of even short exposures to secondhand smoke are readily measurable, and the risks for cardiovascular disease from involuntary smoking appear to be about 50 percent less than the risks for active smokers. Although the risks from secondhand smoke exposures are larger than anticipated, research on the mechanisms by which tobacco smoke exposure affects the cardiovascular system supports the plausibility of the findings of epidemiologic studies (the 1986 report did not address cardiovascular disease). This 2006 report also reviews the evidence on the multiple mechanisms by which secondhand smoke injures the respiratory tract and causes sudden infant death syndrome.

Since 1986, the attitude of the public toward and the social norms around secondhand smoke exposure have changed dramatically to reflect a growing viewpoint that the involuntary exposure of nonsmokers to secondhand smoke is unacceptable. As a result, increasingly strict public policies to control involuntary exposure to secondhand smoke have been put in place. The need for restrictions on smoking in enclosed public places is now widely accepted in the United States. A growing number of communities, counties, and states are requiring smoke-free environments for nearly all enclosed public places, including all private worksites, restaurants, bars, and casinos.

As knowledge about the health risks of secondhand smoke exposure grows, investigators continue to identify additional scientific questions.

- Because active smoking is firmly established as a causal factor of cancer for a large number of sites, and because many scientists assert that there may be no threshold for carcinogenesis from tobacco smoke exposure, researchers hypothesize that people who are exposed to secondhand smoke are likely to be at some risk for the same types of cancers that have been established as smoking-related among active smokers.

- The potential risks for stroke and subclinical vascular disease from secondhand smoke exposure require additional research.

- There is a need for additional research on the etiologic relationship between secondhand smoke exposure and several respiratory health outcomes in adults, including respiratory symptoms, declines in lung function, and adult-onset asthma.

- There is also a need for research to further evaluate the adverse reproductive outcomes and childhood respiratory effects from both prenatal and postnatal exposure to secondhand smoke.

- Further research and improved methodologies are also needed to advance an understanding of the potential effects on cognitive, behavioral, and physical development that might be related to early exposures to secondhand smoke.

As these and other research questions are addressed, the scientific literature documenting the adverse health effects of exposure to secondhand smoke will expand. Over the past 40 years since the release of the landmark 1964 report of the Surgeon General's Advisory Committee on Smoking and Health (USDHEW 1964), researchers have compiled an ever-growing list of adverse health effects caused by exposure to tobacco smoke, with evidence that active smoking causes damage to virtually every organ of the body (USDHHS 2004). Similarly, since the 1986 report (USDHHS 1986), the number of adverse health effects caused by exposure to secondhand smoke has also expanded. Following the format of the electronic database released with the 2004 report, the research findings supporting the conclusions in this report will be accessible in a database that can be found at http://www.cdc.gov/tobacco. With an this expanding base of scientific knowledge, the list of adverse health effects caused by exposure to secondhand smoke will likely increase.

Biomarker data from the 2005 *Third National Report on Human Exposure to Environmental Chemicals* document great progress since the 1986 report in reducing the involuntary exposure of nonsmokers to secondhand smoke (CDC 2005). Between the late 1980s and 2002, the median cotinine level (a metabolite of nicotine) among nonsmokers declined by more than 70 percent. Nevertheless, many challenges remain to maintain the momentum toward universal smoke-free environments. First, there is a need to continue and even improve the surveillance of sources and levels of exposure to secondhand smoke. The data from the 2005 exposure report show that median cotinine levels among children are more than twice those of nonsmoking adults, and non-Hispanic Blacks have levels more than twice those of Mexican Americans and non-Hispanic Whites (CDC 2005). The multiple factors related to these disparities in median cotinine levels among nonsmokers need to be identified and addressed. Second, the data from the 2005 exposure report suggest that the scientific community should sustain the current momentum to reduce exposures of nonsmokers to secondhand smoke (CDC 2005). Research reviewed in this report indicates that policies creating completely smoke-free environments are the most economical and efficient approaches to providing this protection. Additionally, neither central heating, ventilating, and air conditioning systems nor separately ventilated rooms control exposures to secondhand smoke. Unfortunately, data from the 2005 exposure report also emphasized that young children remain an exposed population (CDC 2005). However, more evidence is needed on the most effective strategies to promote voluntary changes in smoking norms and practices in homes and private automobiles. Finally, data on the health consequences of secondhand smoke exposures emphasize the importance of the role of health care professionals in this issue. They must assume a greater, more active involvement in reducing exposures, particularly for susceptible groups.

The Health Consequences of Involuntary Exposure to Tobacco Smoke

The findings and recommendations of this report can be extended to other countries and are supportive of international efforts to address the health effects of smoking and secondhand smoke exposure. There is an international consensus that exposure to secondhand smoke poses significant public health risks. The Framework Convention on Tobacco Control recognizes that protecting nonsmokers from involuntary exposures to secondhand smoke in public places should be an integral part of comprehensive national tobacco control policies and programs. Recent changes in national policies in countries such as Italy and Ireland reflect this growing international awareness of the need for additional protection of nonsmokers from involuntary exposures to secondhand smoke.

When this series of reports began in 1964, the majority of men and a substantial proportion of women were smokers, and most nonsmokers inevitably must have been involuntary smokers. With the release of the 1986 report, Surgeon General Koop noted that "the right of smokers to smoke ends where their behavior affects the health and well-being of others" (USDHHS 1986, p. xii). As understanding increases regarding health consequences from even brief exposures to secondhand smoke, it becomes even clearer that the health of nonsmokers overall, and particularly the health of children, individuals with existing heart and lung problems, and other vulnerable populations, requires a higher priority and greater protection.

Together, this report and the 2004 report of the Surgeon General, *The Health Consequences of Smoking* (USDHHS 2004), document the extraordinary threat to the nation's health from active and involuntary smoking. The recent reductions in exposures of nonsmokers to secondhand smoke represent significant progress, but involuntary exposures persist in many settings and environments. More evidence is needed to understand why this progress has not been equally shared across all populations and in all parts of this nation. Some states (California, Connecticut, Delaware, Maine, Massachusetts, New York, Rhode Island, and Washington) have met the *Healthy People 2010* objectives (USDHHS 2000) that protect against involuntary exposures to secondhand smoke through recommended policies, regulations, and laws, while many other parts of this nation have not (USDHHS 2000). Evidence presented in this report suggests that these disparities in levels of protection can be reduced or eliminated. Sustained progress toward a society free of involuntary exposures to secondhand smoke should remain a national public health priority.

A Vision for the Future   669

References

Centers for Disease Control and Prevention. *Third National Report on Human Exposure to Environmental Chemicals*. Atlanta: U.S. Department of Health and Human Services, Centers for Disease Control and Prevention, National Center for Environmental Health, 2005. NCEH Publication No. 05-0570.

U.S. Department of Health and Human Services. *The Health Consequences of Involuntary Smoking. A Report of the Surgeon General*. Rockville (MD): U.S. Department of Health and Human Services, Public Health Service, Centers for Disease Control, Center for Health Promotion and Education, Office on Smoking and Health, 1986. DHHS Publication No. (CDC) 87-8398.

U.S. Department of Health and Human Services. *Healthy People 2010: Understanding and Improving Health*. Washington: U.S. Government Printing Office, 2000.

U.S. Department of Health and Human Services. *The Health Consequences of Smoking: A Report of the Surgeon General*. Atlanta: U.S. Department of Health and Human Services, Centers for Disease Control and Prevention, National Center for Chronic Disease Prevention and Health Promotion, Office on Smoking and Health, 2004.

U.S. Department of Health, Education, and Welfare. *Smoking and Health: Report of the Advisory Committee to the Surgeon General of the Public Health Service*. Washington: U.S. Department of Health, Education, and Welfare, Public Health Service, Center for Disease Control, 1964. PHS Publication No. 1103.

U.S. Department of Health, Education, and Welfare. *The Health Consequences of Smoking: A Report of the Surgeon General: 1972*. Washington: U.S. Department of Health, Education, and Welfare, Public Health Service, Health Services and Mental Health Administration, 1972. DHEW Publication No. (HSM) 72-7516.

Appendix

Publication lags, even short ones, prevent an up to-the-minute inclusion of all recently published articles and data. Therefore, by the time the public reads this report, there may be additional published studies or data. To provide published information as current as possible, this Appendix lists more recent studies that represent major additions to the literature.

Chapter 2
Toxicology of Secondhand Smoke

Bradley TP, Golden AL. Tobacco and carcinogens in the workplace. *Clinics in Occupational and Environmental Medicine* 2006:5(1):117–37.

Hecht SS. Carcinogenicity studies of inhaled cigarette smoke in laboratory animals: old and new. *Carcinogenesis* 2005;26(9):1488–92.

Hecht SS, Carmella SG, Le K-A, Murphy SE, Boettcher AJ, Le C, Koopmeiners J, An L, Hennrikus DJ. 4-(Methylnitrosamino)-1-(3-pyridyl)-1-butanol and its glucuronides in the urine of infants exposed to environmental tobacco smoke. *Cancer Epidemiology, Biomarkers & Prevention* 2006;15(5):988–92.

Houston TK, Person SD, Pletcher MJ, Liu K, Iribarren C, Kiefe CI. Active and passive smoking and development of glucose intolerance among young adults in a prospective cohort: CARDIA study. *British Medical Journal* 2006; doi:10.1136/bmj.38779.584028.55.

Husgafvel-Pursiainen K. Genotoxicity of environmental tobacco smoke: a review. *Mutation Research* 2004;567(2–3):427–45.

Neff RA, Simmens SJ, Evans C, Mendelowitz D. Prenatal nicotine exposure alters central cardiorespiratory responses to hypoxia in rats: implications for sudden infant death syndrome. *Journal of Neuroscience* 2004;24(42):9261–8.

Slikker W Jr, Xu ZA, Levin ED, Slotkin TA. Mode of action: disruption of brain cell replication, second messenger, and neurotransmitter systems during development leading to congnitive dysfunction—developmental neurotoxicity of nicotine. *Critical Reviews in Toxicology* 2005;35(8–9):703–11.

van der Vaart H, Postma DS, Timens W, Hylkema MN, Willemse BWM, Boezen HM, Vonk JM, de Reus DM, Kauffman HF, ten Hacken NHT. Acute effects of cigarette smoking on inflammation in healthy intermittent smokers. *Respiratory Research* 2005;6(1):22.

Wang Y, Zhang Z, Lubet R, You M. Tobacco smoke-induced lung tumorigenesis in mutant A/J mice with alterations in K-ras, p53, or Ink4a/Arf. *Oncogene* 2005;24(18):3042–9.

Chapter 3
Assessment of Exposure to Secondhand Smoke

Centers for Disease Control and Prevention. Indoor air quality in hospitality venues before and after implementation of a clean indoor air law—Western New York, 2003. *Morbidity and Mortality Weekly Report* 2004;53(44):1038–41.

Murphy SE, Link CA, Jensen J, Le C, Puumala SS, Hecht SS, Carmella SG, Losey L, Hatsukami DK. A comparison of urinary biomarkers of tobacco and carcinogen exposure in smokers. *Cancer Epidemiology, Biomarkers & Prevention* 2004;13(10):1617–23.

Repace J, Al-Delaimy WK, Bernert JT. Correlating atmospheric and biological markers in studies of secondhand tobacco smoke exposure and dose in children and adults. *Journal of Occupational and Environmental Medicine* 2006;48(2):181–94.

Chapter 4
Prevalence of Exposure to Secondhand Smoke

Blackburn CM, Bonas S, Spencer NJ, Coe CJ, Dolan A, Moy R. Parental smoking and passive smoking in infants: fathers matter too. *Health Education Research* 2005;20(2):185–94.

Panagiotakos DB, Pitsavos C, Chrysohoou C, Skoumas J, Masoura C, Toutouzas P, Stefanadis C. Effect of exposure to secondhand smoke on markers of inflammation: the ATTICA study. *American Journal of Medicine* 2004;116(3):145–50.

Chapter 5
Reproductive and Developmental Effects from Exposure to Secondhand Smoke

---

Kharrazi M, DeLorenze GN, Kaufman FL, Eskenazi B, Bernert JT Jr, Graham S, Pearl M, Pirkle J. Environmental tobacco smoke and pregnancy outcome. *Epidemiology* 2004;15(6):660–70.

McMartin KI, Platt MS, Hackman R, Klein J, Smialek JE, Vigorito R, Koren G. Lung tissue concentrations of nicotine in sudden infant death syndrome (SIDS). *Journal of Pediatrics* 2002;140(2):205–9.

Slotkin TA. Cholinergic systems in brain development and disruption by neurotoxicants: nicotine, environmental tobacco smoke, organophosphates. *Toxicology and Applied Pharmacology* 2004;198(2):132–51.

Wisborg K, Kesmodel U, Henriksen TB, Olsen SF, Secher NJ. Exposure to tobacco smoke in utero and the risk of stillbirth and death in the first year of life. *American Journal of Epidemiology* 2001;154(4):322–7.

Chapter 6
Respiratory Effects in Children from Exposure to Secondhand Smoke

---

Alati R, Al Mamun A, O'Callaghan M, Najman JM, Williams GM. In utero and postnatal maternal smoking and asthma in adolescence. *Epidemiology* 2006;17(2):138–44.

DiFranza JR, Aligne CA. Weitzman M. Prenatal and postnatal environmental tobacco smoke exposure and children's health. *Pediatrics* 2004;113 (4 Suppl):1007–15.

Gilliland FD, Berhane K, Li Y-F, Rappaport EB, Peters JM. Effects of early onset asthma and *in utero* exposure to maternal smoking on childhood lung function. *American Journal of Respiratory and Critical Care Medicine* 2003;167(6):917–24.

Gilliland FD, Li Y-F, Dubeau L, Berhane K, Avol E, McConnell R, Gauderman WJ, Peters JM. Effects of glutathione S-transferase M1, maternal smoking during pregnancy, and environmental tobacco smoke on asthma and wheezing in children. *American Journal of Respiratory and Critical Care Medicine* 2002;166(4):457–63.

Gilliland FD, Li Y-F, Peters JM. Effects of maternal smoking during pregnancy and environmental tobacco smoke on asthma and wheezing in children. *American Journal of Respiratory and Critical Care Medicine* 2001;163(2):429–36.

Gilmour MI, Jaakkola MS, London SJ, Nel AE, Rogers CA. How exposure to environmental tobacco smoke, outdoor air pollutants, and increased pollen burdens influences the incidence of asthma. *Environmental Health Perspectives* 2006;114(4): 627–33.

Jaakkola JJK, Nafstad P, Magnus P. Environmental tobacco smoke, parental atopy, and childhood asthma. *Environmental Health Perspectives* 2001;109(6):579–82.

Jaakkola MS, Piipari R, Jaakkola N, Jaakkola JJK. Environmental tobacco smoke and adult-onset asthma: a population-based incident case-control study. *American Journal of Public Health* 2003;93(12): 2055–60.

Lannerö E, Wickman M, Pershagen G, Nordvall L. Maternal smoking during pregnancy increases the risk of recurrent wheezing during the first years of life (BAMSE). *Respiratory Research* 2006;7(1):3.

Mannino DM, Moorman JE, Kingsley B, Rose D, Repace J. Health effects related to environmental tobacco smoke exposure in children in the United States: data from the Third National Health and Nutrition Examination Survey. *Archives of Pediatrics and Adolescent Medicine* 2001;155(1):36–41.

Moshammer H, Hoek G, Luttmann-Gibson H, Neuberger MA, Antova T, Gehring U, Hruba F, Pattenden S, Rudnai P, Slachtova H, et al. Parental smoking and lung function in children: an international study. *American Journal of Respiratory and Critical Care Medicine* 2006; doi:10.1164/rccm.200510-1552OC.

Zlotkowska R, Zejda JE. Fetal and postnatal exposure to tobacco smoke and respiratory health in children. *European Journal of Epidemiology* 2005;20(8):719–27.

Chapter 7
Cancer Among Adults from Exposure to Secondhand Smoke

Anderson KE, Carmella SG, Ye M, Bliss RL, Le C, Murphy L, Hecht SS. Metabolites of a tobacco-specific lung carcinogen in nonsmoking women exposed to environmental tobacco smoke. *Journal of the National Cancer Institute* 2001;93(5):378–81.

Brennan P, Buffler PA, Reynolds P, Wu AH, Wichmann HE, Agudo A, Pershagen G, Jöckel K-H, Benhamou S, Greenberg RS, et al. Secondhand smoke exposure in adulthood and risk of lung cancer among never smokers: a pooled analysis of two large studies. *International Journal of Cancer* 2004;109(1):125–31.

Brownson RC, Figgs LW, Caisley LE. Epidemiology of environmental tobacco smoke exposure. *Oncogene* 2002;21(48):7341–8.

deAndrade M, Ebbert JO, Wampfler JA, Miller DL, Marks RS, Croghan GA, Jatoi A, Finke EE, Sellers TA, Yang P. Environmental tobacco exposure in women with lung cancer. *Lung Cancer* 2004;43(2):127–34.

Enstrom JE, Kabat GC. Environmental tobacco smoke and tobacco related mortality in a prospective study of Californians, 1960–98. *British Medical Journal* 2003;326(7398):1057.

Kreuzer M, Gerken M, Kreienbrock L, Wellmann J, Wichmann HE. Lung cancer in lifetime nonsmoking men—results of a case-control study in Germany. *British Journal of Cancer* 2001;84(1):134–40.

Vineis P, Airoldi L, Veglia F, Olgiati L, Pastorelli R, Autrup H, Dunning A, Garte S, Gormally E, Hainaut P, et al. Environmental tobacco smoke and risk of respiratory cancer and chronic obstructive pulmonary disease in former smokers and never smokers in the EPIC prospective study. *British Medical Journal* 2005;330(7486):277.

Chapter 8
Cardiovascular Diseases from Exposure to Secondhand Smoke

Hill S, Blakely T, Kawachi I, Woodward A. Mortality among never smokers living with smokers: two cohort studies, 1981–4 and 1996–9. *British Medical Journal* 2004;328(7446);988–9.

Iribarren C, Darbinian J, Klatsky AL, Friedman GD. Cohort study of exposure to environmental tobacco smoke and risk of first ischemic stroke and transient ischemic attack. *Neuroepidemiology* 2004;23(1–2):38–44.

Kamholz SL. Pulmonary and cardiovascular consequences of smoking. *Clinics in Occupational and Environmental Medicine* 2006;5(1):157–71.

Kaur S, Cohen A, Dolor R, Coffman CJ, Bastian BA. The impact of environmental tobacco smoke on women's risk of dying from heart disease: a meta-analysis. *Journal of Women's Health* 2004;13(8):888–97.

Kiechl S, Werner P, Egger G, Oberhollenzer F, Mayr M, Xu Q, Poewe W, Willeit J. Active and passive smoking, chronic infections, and the risk of carotid atherosclerosis: prospective results from the Bruneck Study. *Stroke* 2002;33(9):2170–6.

McGhee SM, Ho SY, Schooling M, Ho LM, Thomas GN, Hedley AJ, Mak KH, Peto R, Lam TH. Mortality associated with passive smoking in Hong Kong. *British Medical Journal* 2005;330(7486):287–8.

Qureshi AI, Suri MF, Kirmani JF, Divani AA. Cigarette smoking among spouses: another risk factor for stroke in women. *Stroke* 2005;36(9):e74–e76.

Whincup PH, Gilg JA, Emberson JR, Jarvis MJ, Feyerabend C, Bryant A, Walker M, Cook DG. Passive smoking and risk of coronary heart disease and stroke: prospective study with cotinine measurement. *British Medical Journal* 2004;329(7459):200–5.

Zhang X, Shu XO, Yang G, Li HL, Xiang YB, Gao Y-T, Li Q, Zheng W. Association of passive smoking by husbands with prevalence of stroke among Chinese women nonsmokers. *American Journal of Epidemiology* 2005;161(3):213–8.

Chapter 9
Respiratory Effects in Adults from Exposure to Secondhand Smoke

Dhala A, Pinsker K, Prezant DJ. Respiratory health consequences of environmental tobacco smoke. *Clinics in Occupational and Environmental Medicine* 2006;5(1):139–56.

Eisner MD. Environmental tobacco smoke exposure and pulmonary function among adults in NHANES III: impact on the general population and adults with current asthma. *Environmental Health Perspectives* 2002;110(8):765–70.

Eisner MD, Klein J, Hammond SK, Koren G, Lactao G, Iribarren C. Directly measured second hand smoke exposure and asthma health outcomes. *Thorax* 2005;60(10):814–21.

Gilmour MI, Jaakkola MS, London SJ, Nel AE, Rogers CA. How exposure to environmental tobacco smoke, outdoor air pollutants, and increased pollen burdens influences the incidence of asthma. *Environmental Health Perspectives* 2006;114(4):627–33.

Jaakkola MS, Piipari R, Jaakkola N, Jaakkola JJK. Environmental tobacco smoke and adult-onset asthma: a population-based incident case-control study. *American Journal of Public Health* 2003;93(12): 2055–60.

Maziak W, Ward KD, Rastam S, Mzayek F, Eissenberg T. Extent of exposure to environmental tobacco smoke (ETS) and its dose-response relation to respiratory health among adults. *Respiratory Research* 2005;6(1):13.

Skorge TD, Eagan TML, Eide GE, Gulsvik A, Bakke PS. The adult incidence of asthma and respiratory symptoms by passive smoking *in utero* or in childhood. *American Journal of Respiratory and Critical Care Medicine* 2005;172(1):61–6.

Svanes C, Omenaas E, Jarvis D, Chinn S, Gulsvik A, Burney P. Parental smoking in childhood and adult obstructive lung disease: results from the European Community Respiratory Health Survey. *Thorax* 2004;59(4):295–302.

Upton MN, Smith GD, McConnachie A, Hart CL, Watt GC. Maternal and personal cigarette smoke synergize to increase airflow limitation in adults. *American Journal of Respiratory and Critical Care Medicine* 2004;169(4):479–87.

Chapter 10
Control of Secondhand Smoke Exposure

Anderson PA, Buller DB, Voeks JH, Borland R, Helme D, Bettinghaus EP, Young WF. Predictors of support for environmental tobacco smoke bans in state government. *American Journal of Preventive Medicine* 2006;30(4):292–9.

Centers for Disease Control and Prevention. Indoor air quality in hospitality venues before and after implementation of a clean indoor air law—Western New York, 2003. *Morbidity and Mortality Weekly Report* 2004;53(44):1038–41.

Centers for Disease Control and Prevention. Survey of airport smoking policies—United States, 2002. *Morbidity and Mortality Weekly Report* 2004;53(50): 1175–8.

Javitz HA, Zbikowski SM, Swan GE, Jack LM. Financial burden of tobacco use: an employer's perspective. *Clinics in Occupational and Environmental Medicine* 2006;5(1):9–29.

Johnsson T, Tuomi T, Riuttala H, Hyvärinen M, Rothberg M, Reijula K. Environmental tobacco smoke in Finnish restaurants and bars before and after smoking restrictions were introduced. *Annals of Occupational Hygiene* 2006; doi:10.1093/annhyg/me1011.

McMillen RC, Gresham K, Valentine N, Chambers C, Frese W, Cosby AG. The National Social Climate of Tobacco Control, 2000–2005, 2006; <http://www.ssrc.msstate.edu/socialclimate/reports/2005_National_Report.pdf >; accessed: May 10, 2006.

Siegel M, Barbeau EM, Osinubi OY. The impact of tobacco use and secondhand smoke on hospitality workers. *Clinics in Occupational and Environmental Medicine* 2006;5(1):31–42.

Winickoff JP, McMillen RC, Carroll BC, Klein JD, Rigotti NA, Tanski SE, Weitzman M. Addressing parental smoking in pediatrics and family practice: a national survey of parents. *Pediatrics* 2003;112(5):114–651.

List of Abbreviations

AB	aminobiphenyl
AC	adenylyl cyclase
ACH	air changes per hour
ACS	American Cancer Society
ADA	Americans with Disabilities Act of 1990
AHA	American Heart Association
AHU	air handling unit
ALA	American Lung Association
ALL	acute lymphocytic leukemia
ALSPAC	Avon Longitudinal Study of Pregnancy and Childhood
AMA	American Medical Association
ANR	American Nonsmokers' Rights
AOD	airway obstructive disease
AOM	acute otitis media
AOR	adjusted odds ratio
ARB	Air Resources Board
ARIC	Atherosclerosis Risk in Communities
ASHRAE	American Society of Heating, Refrigerating and Air-Conditioning Engineers
ASSIST	American Stop Smoking Intervention Study for Cancer Prevention
ATP	adenosine triphosphate
BALF	bronchoalveolar lavage fluid
B[a]P	benzo[a]pyrene
BAS	building automation system
BHR	bronchial hyperreactivity
BL	bronchiolitis
BMI	body mass index
BR	bronchitis
BRFSS	Behavioral Risk Factor Surveillance System
BSID	Bayley Scales of Infant Development
Ca	calcium
CAB	Civil Aeronautics Board
Cal/EPA	California Environmental Protection Agency
CAT	California Achievement Test
C/Co	concentration of contaminant
Cd	cadmium
CDC	Centers for Disease Control and Prevention
CFD	computational fluid dynamics

CHD	coronary heart disease
CI	confidence interval
CIN	cervical intraepithelial neoplasia
cm	centimeter
cm^3	cubic centimeter
CNS	central nervous system
CO	carbon monoxide
CO_2	carbon dioxide
COMMIT	Community Intervention Trial for Smoking Cessation
COPD	chronic obstructive pulmonary disease
CPS	Current Population Survey
CPS-I	Cancer Prevention Study I
CPS-II	Cancer Prevention Study II
CT	computed tomography
df	degrees of freedom
EC	European Communities
EEFR	end-expiratory flow rate
EIA	enzyme-linked immunoassay
ELISA	Enzyme-Linked ImmunoSorbent Assay
ENT	ear, nose, and throat
ENU	ethylnitrosourea
EP	ethenyl pyridine
EPA	Environmental Protection Agency
ETS	environmental tobacco smoke
FAA	Federal Aviation Administration
FEF	forced expiratory flow
FEFR	forced expiratory flow rate
FEV_1	forced expiratory volume in one second
fmol	femtomole
FPM	fluorescing particulate matter
FRC	functional residual capacity
ft^2	square feet
ft^3	cubic feet
FVC	forced vital capacity
g	gram
GASP	Group Against Smoking Pollution
GC–MS	gas chromatography–mass spectrometry
GLC	gas-liquid chromatography
Gluc	glucuronide

GM-CSF	granulocyte-macrophage colony-stimulating factor	**mg**	milligram
GSTM1	glutathione *S*-transferase form M1	**MI**	myocardial infarction
Hb	hemoglobin	**mL**	milliliter
HCFA	Health Care Financing Administration	**MMEF**	mean mid-expiratory flow
HDL	high-density lipoprotein	**MRC**	Medical Research Council
HEPA	high-efficiency particulate air	**MRI**	magnetic resonance imaging
hMG	human menopausal gonadotropin	**MSCA**	McCarthy Scales of Children's Abilities
1-HOP	1-hydroxypyrene	**MTA**	Metropolitan Transportation Authority
HPB	4-hydroxy-1-(3-pyridyl)-1-butanone	μ	micron
HPLC	high-performance liquid chromatography	μg	microgram
HVAC	heating, ventilating, and air-conditioning	μL	microliter
IARC	International Agency for Research on Cancer	μm	micrometer
IBD	inflammatory bowel disease	μmol	micromole
ICC	Interstate Commerce Commission	**nAChR**	nicotinic acetylcholine receptor
ICD	*International Classification of Diseases*	*NAT*	*N-acetyltransferase*
IFN-γ	interferon gamma	**NCHS**	National Center for Health Statistics
IgE	immunoglobulin E	**NCI**	National Cancer Institute
IgG1	immunoglobulin G1	**ng**	nanogram
IHD	ischemic heart disease	**NHANES**	National Health and Nutrition Examination Survey
IL	interleukin	**NHAPS**	National Human Activity Pattern Survey
IMT	intimal medial thickness	**NHIS**	National Health Interview Survey
ISAAC	International Study of Asthma and Allergy in Childhood	**NHMRC**	National Health and Medical Research Council
IU	International Units	**NHS**	Nurses Health Study
IUGR	intrauterine growth retardation	**NIH**	National Institutes of Health
JCAHO	Joint Commission on Accreditation of Healthcare Organizations	**NIOSH**	National Institute for Occupational Safety and Health
JPHC	Japan Public Health Center	**NMFS**	National Mortality Followback Survey
L	liter	**NNAL**	4-(methylnitrosamino)-1-(3-pyridyl)-1-butanol
LBW	low birth weight	**NNAL-Gluc**	glucuronide conjugate of NNAL
LC	liquid chromatography	**NNK**	4-(methylnitrosamino)-1-(3-pyridyl)-1-butanone
LD	less than detectable		
LDL	low-density lipoprotein	**NNN**	*N'*-nitrosonornicotine
LPS	lipopolysaccharide	**NO**	nitric oxide
LRI	lower respiratory illness	**NOS**	nitric oxide synthase
L/S	lectin/sphyngomyelin	**NPC**	nasopharyngeal carcinoma
m^2	square meter	**NPD**	nitrogen-phosphorus specific detector
m^3	cubic meter	**NR**	data were not reported
MAPK	mitogen-activated protein kinase	**NRC**	National Research Council
MDI	Mental Development Index	**NS**	not significant
MEE	middle ear effusion	**NTS**	nucleus tractus solitarius
MEFR	mid-expiratory flow rate	O_3	ozone
MeSH	Medical Subject Headings	**8-OH-dG**	8-hydroxydeoxyguanosine

OM	otitis media		**SGA**	small for gestational age
OME	otitis media with effusion		**sGaw**	specific airway conductance
OPPS	Ottawa Prenatal Prospective Study		**sGaw$_{EE}$**	specific airway conductance at end expiration
OR	odds ratio		**SHEEP**	Stockholm Heart Epidemiology Program
OSH	Office on Smoking and Health		**SHPPS**	School Health Policies and Programs Study
OSHA	Occupational Safety and Health Administration		**SIDRIA**	Italian Studies on Respiratory Disorders in Childhood and the Environment
OVA	ovalbumen		**SIDS**	sudden infant death syndrome
PAF-AH	platelet-activating factor acetylhydrolase		**s/kPa**	kilopascal
PAH	polycyclic aromatic hydrocarbon		**SO$_2$**	sulfur dioxide
PEF	peak expiratory flow		**SolPM**	solanesol particulate matter
PFT	pulmonary function test		**SPT**	skin-prick test
pg	picogram		**^{99m}Tc-DTPA**	technetium^{99m} labeled diethylenetriamine penta-acetate
PIF	peak inspiratory flow		**TEA**	thermal energy analyzer
PK-C	protein kinase C		**Th**	T-helper
PM	particulate matter		**TIA**	transient ischemic attack
PMA	phorbol 12-myristate 13-acetate		**TNF**	tumor necrosis factor
pmol	picomole		**T$_{PTEF}$:T$_E$**	the ratio of time to peak tidal expiratory flow to expiratory time
PMN	polymorphonuclear leukocyte		**TSNA**	tobacco-specific nitrosamine
PN	pneumonia		**tt-MA**	*trans,trans*-muconic acid
POR	prevalence odds ratio		**URI**	upper respiratory illness
ppb	parts per billion		**USDHEW**	U.S. Department of Health, Education, and Welfare
ppm	parts per million		**USDHHS**	U.S. Department of Health and Human Services
PPVT	Peabody Picture Vocabulary Test		**USDOC**	U.S. Department of Commerce
RAST	Radioallergosorbent Test		**USDOD**	U.S. Department of Defense
RAVEN	Raven Colored Progressive Matrices Test		**USDOJ**	U.S. Department of Justice
RDD	random-digit telephone dialing		**USVA**	U.S. Department of Veteran Affairs
RIA	radioimmunoassay		**UV**	ultraviolet
ROM	recurrent otitis media		**UVPM**	ultraviolet-absorbing particulate matter
RPM	respirable particulate matter		**Vmax$_{FRC}$**	maximal forced expiratory flow at functional residual capacity
RR	relative risk		**VOCs**	volatile organic compounds
RSP	respirable suspended particles		**WHO**	World Health Organization
RSV	respiratory syncytial virus		**WISC**	Weschler Intelligence Scale for Children
SCAN	central auditory processing task			
SCI	silent cerebral infarction			
SD	standard deviation			
SEER	Surveillance, Epidemiology, and End Results			
SES	socioeconomic status			

List of Tables and Figures

Chapter 7
Cancer Among Adults from Exposure to Secondhand Smoke

Index

Note: t following a number refers to a Table; f following a number refers to a Figure.

O